P9-CLA-845

Health Information
Management of a Strategic Resource

CONTENTS

EDITION 5

Health Information

Management of a Strategic Resource

Mervat Abdelhak, PhD, RHIA, FAHIMA
Managing Editor
Department Chair and Associate Professor
Health Information Management
School of Health and Rehabilitation Sciences
University of Pittsburgh
Pittsburgh, Pennsylvania

Mary Alice Hanken, PhD, RHIA, CHPS
Editor
Senior Lecturer
Health Informatics and Health Information Management Programs
  (Master's and Baccalaureate)
School of Public Health
University of Washington
Seattle, Washington

Quality Manager
Sound Mental Health
Seattle, Washington

ELSEVIER
SAUNDERS

3251 Riverport Lane
St. Louis, Missouri 63043

HEALTH INFORMATION: MANAGEMENT OF A
STRATEGIC RESOURCE, FIFTH EDITION

ISBN: 978-0-323-26348-1

Copyright © 2016, 2012, 2007, 2001, 1996 by Saunders, an imprint of Elsevier Inc.

All rights reserved. No part of this publication may be reproduced or transmitted in any form or by any means, electronic or mechanical, including photocopying, recording, or any information storage and retrieval system, without permission in writing from the publisher. Details on how to seek permission, further information about the Publisher's permissions policies and our arrangements with organizations such as the Copyright Clearance Center and the Copyright Licensing Agency, can be found at our website: www.elsevier.com/permissions.

This book and the individual contributions contained in it are protected under copyright by the Publisher (other than as may be noted herein).

Notices

Knowledge and best practice in this field are constantly changing. As new research and experience broaden our understanding, changes in research methods, professional practices, or medical treatment may become necessary.

Practitioners and researchers must always rely on their own experience and knowledge in evaluating and using any information, methods, compounds, or experiments described herein. In using such information or methods they should be mindful of their own safety and the safety of others, including parties for whom they have a professional responsibility.

With respect to any drug or pharmaceutical products identified, readers are advised to check the most current information provided (i) on procedures featured or (ii) by the manufacturer of each product to be administered, to verify the recommended dose or formula, the method and duration of administration, and contraindications. It is the responsibility of practitioners, relying on their own experience and knowledge of their patients, to make diagnoses, to determine dosages and the best treatment for each individual patient, and to take all appropriate safety precautions.

To the fullest extent of the law, neither the Publisher nor the authors, contributors, or editors, assume any liability for any injury and/or damage to persons or property as a matter of products liability, negligence or otherwise, or from any use or operation of any methods, products, instructions, or ideas contained in the material herein.

Library of Congress Cataloging-in-Publication Data
Health information (Abdelhak)
   Health information : management of a strategic resource / Mervat Abdelhak, managing editor ; Mary Alice Hanken, editor. – 5th edition.
      p. ; cm.
   Includes bibliographical references and index.
   ISBN 978-0-323-26348-1 (pbk. : alk. paper)
   I. Abdelhak, Mervat, editor.   II. Hanken, Mary Alice, editor.   III. Title.
   [DNLM: 1. Health Information Management–organization & administration.   2. Electronic Health Records–organization & administration. W 26.5]
   R858
   610.285–dc23
                                                                          2014034671

Senior Content Strategist: Linda Woodard
Senior Content Development Specialist: Diane Chatman
Publishing Services Manager: Hemamalini Rajendrababu
Project Manager: Kamatchi Madhavan
Design Direction: Renee Duenow

  Working together
to grow libraries in
developing countries

www.elsevier.com • www.bookaid.org

Printed in China
Last digit is the print number: 9   8   7   6   5   4   3   2   1

This edition of *Health Information: Management of a Strategic Resource*
is dedicated to Kathy Hanken.

Kathy died suddenly and unexpectedly on February 1, 2014, of an undiagnosed inflammation of
her heart muscle. She was our beloved daughter. Always a major part of the lives of our family members,
she was the frequent social spark for family events, the consulting chef for holiday and special
gatherings and always willing to pitch in and help. Kathy loved to travel and traveled with us and
with friends. She visited Africa twice with Jim, her Dad. Kathy attended several AHIMA annual
meetings. She also helped select restaurants when we attended AHIMA and editorial meetings
for the multiple editions of this book.

At the time of her death she had just opened a new restaurant at the University of Washington
called Local Point. She was the Executive Chef and General Manager. Several years ago after
working in fine dining restaurants in the Seattle area Kathy joined a team of fine dining chefs at
the University of Washington. Their mission was to change the dining experience of students at the
University. This mission-driven activity fit her well. She enjoyed working with students and
typically employed about 70-75 students a year in the restaurants she managed at the University.
We often shared stories about working with students and being a manager/leader. Kathy received
several awards for her work at the University and was an elected member of the professional
staff council. One of her hobbies was jewelry making. Many of her friends and family members
have gifts of her jewelry.

Kathy was a good daughter, sister, aunt and friend. We all have many fond memories. We miss her.

CONTRIBUTORS

Mervat Abdelhak, PhD, RHIA, FAHIMA
Managing Editor
Department Chair and Associate Professor
Health Information Management
School of Health and Rehabilitation Sciences
University of Pittsburgh
Pittsburgh, Pennsylvania

Meryl Bloomrosen, MBA, MBI, RHIA, FAHIMA
Consultant
Silver Spring, Maryland
Chapter 3: Health Information Infrastructure and Systems

Melanie S. Brodnik, PhD, RHIA
Associate Professor, Emeritus
Health Information Management & Systems
School of Allied Medical Professions
The Ohio State University
Columbus, Ohio
*Chapter 2: The Health Informatics and Information Management
  Profession*

Bonnie Cassidy, MPA, RHIA, FAHIMA, HHIMSS
Senior Director of HIM Innovation
Nuance Communications, Inc.
Burlington, Massachusetts
*Chapter 9: Health Information Systems: Collaboration, Analysis,
  Design, Implementation, Operation*

Kay Clements, MA, RHIA, CCS, CPC
Director and Associate Professor
Health Information Management Program
Department of Health Services Administration
School of Health Professions
University of Alabama at Birmingham
Birmingham, Alabama
Chapter 13: Data Analytics: Reporting, Interpretation, and Use

Mary Alice Hanken, PhD, RHIA, CHPS
Editor
Senior Lecturer
Health Informatics and Health Information Management
Department of Health Services
School of Public Health
University of Washington
Quality Improvement Manager, Sound Mental Health
Seattle, Washington
Chapter 5: Data Access and Retention
*Chapter 9: Health Information Systems: Collaboration, Analysis,
  Design, Implementation, Operation*
Chapter 14: Public Health Informatics

Anita Hazelwood, MLS, RHIA, FAHIMA
Professor and Program Director
Health Information Management
University of Louisiana at Lafayette
Lafayette, Louisiana
Chapter 17: Operational Management

Susan Helbig, MA, RHIA
Editor Ancillaries
Lecturer
Health Informatics and Health Information Management
Department of Health Services
School of Public Health
University of Washington
Seattle, Washington
Chapter 6: Electronic Health Record Systems
Chapter 16: Human Resource Management

Shannon Houser, PhD, MPH, RHIA
Associate Professor
Health Information Management Program
Department of Health Services Administration
School of Health Professions
University of Alabama at Birmingham
Birmingham, Alabama
Chapter 13: Data Analytics: Reporting, Interpretation and Use

Bryant Thomas Karras, MD
Public Health Informatics Officer
Washington State Department of Health
Public Health Laboratories
Shoreline, Washington
Chapter 14: Public Health Informatics

Jill Callahan Klaver, JD, RHIA
Medical Staff Quality Specialist
Crittenton Hospital Medical Center
Royal Oak, Michigan
Chapter 15: Privacy and Health Law

Amy Yarbrough Landry, PhD, MBA
Assistant Professor
Department of Health Services Administraton
School of Health Professions
University of Alabama at Birmingham
Birmingham, Alabama
Chapter 1: Health Care Systems

Gretchen F. Murphy, MEd, RHIA, FAHIMA
Director, Master's Program
Health Informatics & Health Information Management
Department of Health Services
School of Public Health
University of Washington
Seattle, Washington
Chapter 6: Electronic Health Record Systems

Bryon Pickard, MBA, RHIA
Director of Operations
Vanderbilt Medical Group Business Office
Vanderbilt University Medical Center
Nashville, Tennessee
Chapter 18: Revenue Cycle and Financial Management

Midge Noel Ray, PhD, RN, CCS
Associate Professor
Health Information Management
Department of Health Services Administration
School of Health Professions
University of Alabama at Birmingham
Birmingham, Alabama
Chapter 1: Health Care Systems

Melissa Saul, MS
Clinical Data Scientist
Adjunct Assistant Professor, HIM
Department of Biomedical Informatics
University of Pittsburgh
Pittsburgh, Pennsylvania
Chapter 8: Technology, Applications and Security

Donna J. Slovensky, PhD, RHIA, FAHIMA
Professor and Associate Dean for Academic & Student
   Affairs
School of Health Professions
University of Alabama at Birmingham
Birmingham, Alabama
Chapter 12: Performance Management and Patient Safety

Patrice L. Spath, MA, RHIT
Healthcare Quality Specialist
Brown-Spath & Associates
Forest Grove, Oregon
Chapter 12: Performance Management and Patient Safety

Marsha Steele, MEd, RHIA
Senior Lecturer
Health Informatics & Health Information Management
Department of Health Services
School of Public Health
University of Washington
Seattle, Washington
*Chapter 7: Classification Systems, Clinical Vocabularies and
   Terminology*

Mary Spivey Teslow, MLIS, RHIA
Assistant Professor
Health Information Administration Program
Western Carolina University
Cullowhee, North Carolina
Chapter 4: Health Data Concepts and Information Governance

Carol A. Venable, MPH, RHIA, FAHIMA
Retired - Professor and Department Head
Health Information Management
The University of Louisiana at Lafayette
Lafayette, Louisiana
Chapter 17: Operational Management

Valerie J.M. Watzlaf, PhD, RHIA, FAHIMA
Associate Professor
Department of Health Information Management
School of Health and Rehabilitation Sciences
University of Pittsburgh
Pittsburgh, Pennsylvania
Chapter 10: Statistics and Data Presentation
Chapter 11: Research and Epidemiology

PREFACE

INTENDED AUDIENCE

Health Information: Management of a Strategic Resource, 5th edition, and a set of integrated tools and online resources, have been developed for health information management (HIM) and health informatics (HI) students and practitioners who are interested in today's reliable systems and tomorrow's future direction to guide and influence practice, education, and research in HIM/HI. The purpose of this book is to develop and support health information professionals who are crucial to the success and efficacy of the health care system. The expertise HIM professionals bring to the exciting challenges of an integrated, technologically upgraded, secure set of systems is in great demand today. *Health Information: Management of a Strategic Resource* assists practitioners and students alike to realize the broader perspective of the scope and domains of HIM practice and to understand the expanded boundaries and roles that exist today and the opportunities that lie within our reach to influence professional advancement and tomorrow's practice. We also hope that this book will aid HIM professionals in viewing their profession with confidence, pride, and excitement.

Health Information: Management of a Strategic Resource serves as a valuable tool to others who are changing the health care system from a paper to an electronic environment. Finally, the book may realize its greatest value in expanding the expectations and understanding of health professionals—administrators, information systems professionals, researchers, policy developers, and others—about the role(s) of HIM professionals and the contributions they make to the quality of health care.

In today's fast-changing health care system, HIM professionals must lead the effort in changing to and improving electronic health record systems; expand their scope and domains of practice; use data, information, and technology in a new way; and assess their performance. HIM professionals must update their knowledge constantly and approach their expanded roles and functions with a new mind-set. In this book, our impressive list of contributors use fresh insight to present today's most reliable and workable systems. Provided is a new approach in addressing the fundamental and important issues within the HIM field.

CONCEPTUAL FRAMEWORK

The editors have designed the text based on a conceptual framework with an agreed-on set of assumptions instead of presenting a series of chapters with isolated information on tasks, tools, and functions. The following are the underlying assumptions on which chapter outlines were developed and contributors were selected:

1. Health information is indeed a strategic resource crucial to the health of individual patients and the population, as well as to the success of the health care institution or enterprise.
2. Health care must be patient centered.
3. Health care consumers are becoming more engaged and responsible for their own health.
4. Changing from a paper to an electronic health record is a given.
5. Health information professionals are leaders in the transformation to and improvement of electronic health record systems, aiding in the design, management, and use of health care data and health information systems.
6. Health care data are to be viewed as a continuum beginning with patient-specific data (clinical data), moving to aggregate data (such as performance data, utilization review, and risk management data), to knowledge-based data (used in planning and decision support), and then to comparative, community-wide data (population health data used in policy development) external to the enterprise or institution.
7. The quality of data and the data-to-information transformation are paramount to the efficacy of any information system; thus emphasis is on the use of information that has value in decision making, evaluation, planning, marketing, and policy development.
8. Data standards and terminologies are important for the functioning of electronic health information systems and the exchange of data between a variety of data users.
9. The integration and assimilation of technology in the health information professional's daily functions is a reality.
10. The transition to and constant fine-tuning of the electronic health record systems is an excellent opportunity, and the success of these systems depends on the scope and domain of practice of health information management professionals.
11. The quality of health care depends on a functioning information infrastructure with quality health care data.
12. Payment systems will change, but payers will still need to know what they are paying for, and systematic ways of describing individual's health status, preventive health, emerging problems, diagnoses and treatment are needed.

13. Health care providers and public health providers will need data as they work together to meet the goals and objectives of a healthier population at the community level, state level, and national level.

ORGANIZATION OF THE TEXT

Health Information: Management of a Strategic Resource is composed of 18 chapters by more than 20 contributors. Each chapter includes a chapter outline, key words, defined abbreviations, and objectives. Throughout the text, you will note Self-Assessment and Did You Know? boxes, as well as reference to the Evolve Resources. An exclusive website (Evolve) for our readers, is included to guide readers to additional information. The glossary provides a comprehensive listing of all the key words.

Chapter 1 (Health Care Systems) provides an overview of the health care system including topics on e-health, evidence-based medicine, and consumer centric health care. Chapter 2 (The Health Informatics and Information Management Profession), is a review of the HIM/HI professions with a focus on HIM and HI and their development, structure, goals, and roles.

Chapter 3 (Health Information Infrastructure and Systems), presents the private and public initiatives. Chapter 4 (Health Data Concepts and Information Governance) presents a variety of data elements required or collected, maintained, and used in the health care industry. The chapter also addresses the users of data and information systems and the role of HIM professionals in data collection, organization, and use. Chapter 5 (Data Access and Retention) addresses considerations related to the access, storage and retention of records in paper and electronic formats. Chapter 6 (Electronic Health Record Systems) addresses the fundamentals of an electronic health record (EHR), the transition process from a paper medical record to the electronic health record, and the ongoing development of EHR systems. The definition of a legal medical record is also presented. Chapter 7 (Classification Systems, Clinical Vocabularies, and Terminology) addresses clinical terminologies, vocabularies, and data standards.

Chapter 8 (Technology, Applications, and Security) covers various information technologies and their use in health care. Data quality and security and the role of HIM in these areas are a focus of this chapter. Chapter 9 (Health Information Systems: Collaboration, Analysis, Design, Implementation, Operation) addresses the analysis, design, implementation, and evaluation of health information systems with discussion of the tools and aids used in these phases.

Chapter 10 (Statistics and Data Presentation) provides the foundation for understanding health statistics and its use and for organizing and displaying results. Chapter 11 (Research and Epidemiology) helps the reader in designing research studies and understanding epidemiology with applications specific to health information management. Chapter 12 (Performance Management and Patient Safety) describes the various methods for assessing and improving the quality of care and services rendered in today's health care systems, while emphasizing the crucial role of health information management professionals in that area. Chapter 13 (Data Analytics: Reporting, Interpretation, and Use) provides a pragmatic view of how data are used in health care, from registries to reimbursement to research and clinical outcomes. Chapter 14 (Public Health Informatics) addresses the use of data to assess and improve health from a population perspective. Chapter 15 (Privacy and Health Law) addresses the legal issues pertinent to the practice of health information management and today's health care system.

Chapter 16 (Human Resource Management) explores the societal, legislative, organizational, functional, and personal objectives and activities of human resource management. Performance evaluation, employment law, multicultural workforce, and career planning are some of the topics addressed. Chapter 17 (Operational Management) addresses standards and methods of improvement including systems analysis, ergonomics, and design process. Reengineering and project management methods and activities are also addressed. Chapter 18 (Revenue Cycle and Financial Management) addresses financial planning and financial accounting methods, while emphasizing the role of the HIM professional in revenue management.

CROSSWALK TO THE AHIMA COUNCIL FOR EXCELLENCE IN EDUCATION COMPETENCY MAPS

Health Information, 5th edition, aligns with the 2014 HIM competencies identified by the AHIMA Council for Excellence in Education. The crosswalk below lists the domains and which chapters cover that information. Chapters are listed in order based on relevance to the domain. (For more information on the HIM competency maps, visit http://www.ahimafoundation.org/education/curricula.aspx.)

Domain	Abdelhak Chapter
Domain I. Data Content, Structure & Standards (Information Governance)	4, 5, 7, 13, 2, 6, 11, 14, 3
Domain II. Information Protection: Access, Disclosure, Archival, Privacy & Security	15, 5, 6, 8, 3
Domain III. Informatics, Analytics and Data Use	13, 10, 11, 12, 8, 9, 2, 14, 3
Domain IV. Revenue Management	18, 7, 1, 12, 17
Domain V. Compliance	15, 12, 1, 4, 16, 18, 17
Domain VI. Leadership	1, 15, 16, 18, 9, 15, 2, 9, 17

Domain I. Data Content, Structure & Standards (Information Governance)
Definition: Academic content related to diagnostic and procedural classification and terminologies; health record documentation requirements; characteristics of the healthcare system; data accuracy and integrity; data integration and interoperability; respond to customer data needs; data management policies and procedures; information standards.

Domain II. Information Protection: Access, Disclosure, Archival, Privacy & Security
Definition: Understand healthcare law (theory of all healthcare law to exclude application of law covered in Domain V); develop privacy, security, and confidentiality policies, procedures and infrastructure; educate staff on health information protection methods; risk assessment; access and disclosure management.

Domain III. Informatics, Analytics and Data Use
Definition: Creation and use of Business health intelligence; select, implement, use and manage technology solutions; system and data architecture; interface considerations; information management planning; data modelling; system testing; technology benefit realization; analytics and decision support; data visualization techniques; trend analysis; administrative reports; descriptive, inferential and advanced statistical protocols and analysis; IRB; research; patient-centered health information technologies; health information exchange; data quality.

Domain IV. Revenue Management
Definition: Healthcare reimbursement; revenue cycle; chargemaster; DOES NOT INCLUDE COMPLIANCE regulations and activities related to revenue management (coding compliance initiatives, fraud and abuse, etc.) AS THESE ARE COVERED IN DOMAIN V.

Domain V. Compliance
Definition: COMPLIANCE activities and methods for all health information topics. For example, how to comply with HIPAA, Stark Laws, Fraud and Abuse, etc.; coding auditing; severity of illness; data analytics; fraud surveillance; clinical documentation improvement.

Domain VI. Leadership
Definition: Leadership models, theories, and skills; critical thinking; change management; workflow analysis, design, tools and techniques; human resource management; training and development theory and process; strategic planning; financial management; ethics and project management.

ONLINE RESOURCES FOR STUDENTS, INSTRUCTORS, AND PRACTITIONERS

- **Evolve Resources:** The companion Evolve website provides course management tools that instructors can use to reinforce and expand on the concepts they deliver in class. Instructors can use the Evolve site to publish their class syllabus, outline, and lecture notes; to set up "virtual office hours" and e-mail communication; to share important dates and information through the online class calendar; to access the **TEACH Instructor Resources** which accompany the text; and to encourage student participation through chat rooms and discussion boards. For students, there are links to websites with related material and all the material contained in the **Study Guide**.
- The **Study Guide:** This online, interactive resource contains integrated tools available to students, educators, and practitioners, including pretest and chapter review questions and assignments, such as case studies, group exercises, field experience activities, and critical thinking questions.

- The **TEACH Instructor Resources:** This resource on the Evolve site includes answers to the study guide assignments and self-assessment questions; a PowerPoint "image library" of figures and tables from the textbook; lesson plans; lecture outlines; and a test bank with more than 1000 questions and answers in electronic form to assist in test construction, scoring, and the generation of grades and test statistics.

We would like to thank the contributors for their willingness to take part in this endeavor and share their expertise. Their insights, suggestions, and questions have greatly strengthened the book and Evolve (online resources), bringing our vision to life.

We shall be grateful to readers who have suggestions for additions or revisions or who are interested in sharing their experiences in using the book and the Evolve resources with us. We hope that *Health Information: Management of a Strategic Resource*, fifth edition, will be a valuable resource addressing the challenges that touch all of us.

Mervat Abdelhak, Managing Editor
Mary Alice Hanken, Editor

CONTENTS

SECTION IV
Data Management and Use

10 STATISTICS AND DATA PRESENTATION, 381

SECTION V
Management

Health Information
Management of a Strategic Resource

HEALTH CARE SYSTEMS

Midge Noel Ray • Amy Y. Landry

ⓔ Student Study Guide activities for this chapter are available on the Evolve Learning Resources site for this textbook. Please visit http://evolve.elsevier.com/Abdelhak.

CHAPTER CONTENTS

OBJECTIVES

After reading this chapter, the reader will be able to do the following:
✓ Define key words.
✓ Describe the evolution of the U.S. health care system, beginning with health care in the nineteenth century through Healthy People 2020.
✓ Identify and describe the regulators of health care, including government and nongovernment entities.
✓ Outline the role of the federal, state, and local governments in the provision of health care.
✓ Identify legislation that affects or regulates health care in the United States.
✓ Distinguish between the various health care organizations (HCOs) responsible for providing health care.
✓ Describe the classification of acute health care facilities, including bed size, ownership and control, population served, and services offered.
✓ Describe the organizational structures of the hospital as discussed within this chapter.
✓ Describe the role and responsibilities of the governing body and administrative heads employed in the HCOs.
✓ Outline the organizational structure of the professional staff, including the membership, clinical privileges, services, committees, and bylaws.
✓ Identify and define the scope of the ancillary and support services and departments in health care facilities.
✓ Describe categories of the health workforce, and address education, licensing, certification requirements, and areas of expertise.
✓ State current mechanisms of health care financing.
✓ Describe specific information technologies and how they affect the health care systems.

KEY WORDS

Accountable care organizations
Accreditation
Acute care
Advance directive
Alternative medicine
Ambulatory care
Ancillary services
Assisted living facility
Bed size (bed count)
Behavioral health
Benefit period
Beneficiaries
Capitation
Case management
Catchment area
Certification
Claim
Client
Clinical privileges

Coinsurance
Complementary and alternative medicine
Complementary medicine
Conditions of participation
Continuum of care
Contracted amount
Copayment
Critical access hospital
Deductible
Deemed status
Direct pay
Durable medical equipment
E-health
Electronic health record
Electronic medical record
Emergency department
Encounter
Episode of care

Evidence-based medicine
Ex officio
Fee-for-service
Fiscal intermediary
Gatekeeper
Governing body
Health care services
Health insurance exchange
Home health care
Horizontal integration
Hospice
Hospital
Hospital ambulatory care
Hospital formulary
Hospital inpatient
Hospital patient
Indigent
Indirect pay
Inpatient

Insurance
Integrated delivery system
Licensure
Life care centers
Long-term care
Managed care
Meaningful use
Medicaid
Medically indigent
Medicare
Morbidity
Mortality
Nursing care
Nursing facility
Observation unit
Osteopathic medicine
Out-of-pocket
Outpatient
Outsourcing

Palliative care
Participating providers
Patient
Patient assessment
Patient-centered care
Patient-centered medical home
Payer
Personal health record
Point of service
Practice Act

Preexisting condition
Preferred provider organization
Premium
Primary care
Proprietary
Prospective payment system
Provider
Rehabilitation
Reimbursement formula
Resident

Respite care
Retrospective payment system
Satellite clinic
Secondary care
Self-pay
Skilled nursing facility
Sliding-scale fee
Solo practice
Swing beds
Tertiary care

The Joint Commission
Third-party payer
Trauma center
Triage
TRICARE
Usual, customary, and reasonable
   charges
Utilization review
Vertical integration

ABBREVIATIONS

ACEN Accreditation Commission for Education in Nursing
ACF Administration for Children and Families
ACO Accountable Care Organizations
ACS American College of Surgeons
AHA American Hospital Association
AHIMA American Health Information Management Association
AHRQ Agency for Healthcare Research and Quality
AIDS acquired immunodeficiency syndrome
AMA American Medical Association
ANA American Nurses Association
ANSI American National Standards Institute
AOA American Osteopathic Association
AoA Administration on Aging
BCBS Blue Cross and Blue Shield
CAAHEP Commission on Accreditation of Allied Health Education Programs
CAH critical access hospital
CAHIIM Commission on Accreditation for Health Informatics and Information Management Education
CAM complementary and alternative medicine
CARF Commission on Accreditation of Rehabilitation Facilities
CDC Centers for Disease Control and Prevention
CDSS clinical decision support system
CEO chief executive officer
CFO chief financial officer
CHAMPUS Civilian Health and Medical Program for the Uniformed Services
CHAP community health accreditation program
CHC community health center
CIO chief information officer
CMS Centers for Medicare and Medicaid Services
CNA certified nursing assistant
CNO chief nursing officer
COBRA Consolidated Omnibus Budget Reconciliation Act
COCA Commission on Osteopathic College Accreditation
COO chief operating officer
COP (Medicare) Conditions of Participation
CRNA certified registered nurse anesthetist
DHHS Department of Health and Human Services
DME durable medical equipment
DO doctor of osteopathy
DRG diagnosis-related group
DSS decision support systems
ED emergency department
EHR electronic health record
EMR electronic medical record
EMTALA Emergency Medical Treatment and Active Labor Act
ESRD end-stage renal disease
FDA Food and Drug Administration
FI fiscal intermediary

FLEX Federation Licensing Examination
GDP gross domestic product
HCFA Health Care Financing Administration (now CMS)
HCO health care organization
HEW Health, Education, and Welfare
HFAP Healthcare Facilities Accreditation Program
HIM health information management
HIPAA Health Insurance Portability and Accountability Act
HL7 Health Level 7
HMO health maintenance organization
HRSA Health Resources and Services Administration
IDS integrated delivery system
IHS Indian Health Service
IOM Institute of Medicine
IPA independent practice association
JCAH The Joint Commission on Accreditation of Hospitals
LPN licensed practical nurse
LTC long-term care
MCAT Medical College Admission Test
MCO managed care organization
MD medical doctor
MMA Medicare Modernization Act
NBME National Board of Medical Examiners
NCCAM National Center for Complementary and Alternative Medicine
NCQA National Committee for Quality Assurance
NHII National Health Information Infrastructure
NHIN National Health Information Network
NIH National Institutes of Health
NP nurse practitioner
OIG Office of Inspector General
OSHA Occupational Safety and Health Administration
PA physician assistant
PCMH patient-centered medical home
PHR personal health record
PHS public health service
POS point of service
PPACA Patient Protection and Affordable Care Act
PPO preferred provider organization
PPS prospective payment system
QIO quality improvement organization
RN registered nurse
SCHIP State Children's Health Insurance Program
SNF skilled nursing facility
SSA Social Security Administration
TEFRA Tax Equity and Fiscal Responsibility Act
TJC The Joint Commission
VA Veterans Administration
VISN Veterans Integrated Service Networks
WEDI Workgroup on Electronic Data Interchange

Health information management (HIM) is a vital component of the health care delivery system. Therefore it is crucial for health information professionals to understand the structure of that system. This chapter introduces the reader to the health care system, including what the system is like and how it functions, and identifies its components. Topics include the history, influencing factors, payers, regulatory agencies, structure, operation, and workforce of health care systems in the United States.

EVOLUTION OF HEALTH CARE SYSTEMS IN THE UNITED STATES

From its inception hundreds of years ago to the present, the health care system has been continually evolving. In the United States, virtually every person is in some way a patient or a consumer of health care at some point. Most people are born either in a hospital or outside the hospital with the assistance of a health care professional. Other people come in contact with the health care system in a variety of ways, including physical examination, immunizations, employee physicals, school vision and hearing screens, emergency care, and public health service (PHS) announcements.

Before proceeding, see Box 1-1 for key definitions.

Health Care in the Nineteenth Century

The nineteenth century saw the development and organization of professional education and health-related associations.

BOX 1-1   Key Definitions

Care—*Care* is the management of, responsibility for, or attention to the safety and well-being of another person or other persons.[2]

Client—A *client* is a person who receives professional services; a patient in the behavioral health setting, adult day care, or home health care may be referred to as a client.

Health—*Health* is best defined by the World Health Organization as a state of complete physical, mental, and social well-being and not merely the absence of disease or infirmity.[1]

Health care services—*Health care services* are the processes that contribute to the health and well-being of the person. Services may be provided in a variety of health care settings, such as the hospital, ambulatory, or home setting, and include nursing, medical, surgical, or other health-related services.[2]

Inpatient—*Inpatient* refers to a patient who is receiving health care services and is provided room, board, and continuous nursing service in a unit or area of the hospital.[2]

Outpatient—An *outpatient* is a patient who is receiving health care services at a hospital without being hospitalized, institutionalized, or admitted as an inpatient.

Patient—A *patient* is an individual, including one who is deceased, who is receiving or using or who has received health care services.[2]

Payer—A *payer* is an organization or individual who provides the money to pay for health care services.

Provider—A *provider* is any entity that provides health care services to patients, including health care organizations (hospitals, clinics) and health care professionals.

Resident—A *resident* is a patient who resides in a long-term care facility.

The first school in the United States dedicated to training physicians was founded in 1765 in Philadelphia. Before this time, the only training an American physician received was by way of apprenticeship with an older physician. As the population in the United States grew and moved westward, the demand for more hospitals and physicians increased. To meet the growing need for more physicians, a large number of new medical schools were opened, most of which were profit oriented. By the end of the nineteenth century, there were no fewer than 400 medical schools in the United States, most of questionable quality.[1]

In 1847, a group of physicians formed the American Medical Association (AMA) for the primary purpose of establishing and supporting a code of ethics for physicians in their duties to their patients and the profession. The AMA initially examined the poor quality of medical education and the questionable ethics of practicing physicians. Today, membership in the AMA is open to any physician in good standing and includes local, city, and state medical societies. The AMA is dedicated to promoting the science and art of medicine, improving public health, making health care policy, and servicing the professional needs of its members.[2]

The American Hospital Association (AHA) was founded in 1898 for the purpose of promoting public welfare by providing better health care in hospitals. The AHA offers education for health care leadership and provides health care information on trends and issues. The AHA maintains data on hospital profiles and represents hospital interests in legal, legislative, and regulatory matters, all of which are directed at improving the nation's health care system.[3]

In the late nineteenth century, states became involved in health care when mental health reformers pushed for an innovation, that "insanity" be managed as a medical or mental disorder. State governments established mental institutions for the confinement of the mentally ill rather than housing them in the poorhouses and prisons. However, because of inadequate funding, mental institutions soon became overcrowded, and living conditions were deplorable.

In the mid-1800s, there was evidence of the earliest forms of managed care. Plantation owners in Hawaii; mining companies in Pennsylvania and Minnesota; and lumber companies in Washington, Wisconsin, and Michigan tried to attract and keep immigrant workers by offering medical care for their workers. The companies contracted with local physicians and hospitals for a set number of beds. Some of the companies even built medical clinics and hospitals. Physicians who agreed to contract with these companies were ostracized from the local medical societies and were even threatened with revocation of their medical licenses.[4]

Twentieth-Century Reforms

In the early 1900s, most hospitals were viewed as boardinghouses for the poor and sick; physicians did not take histories and perform physical examinations on admission and seldom did they document assessments or diagnoses. The private sector, however, showed little interest in serving the population as a whole; the assumption was that local government would pay for health care for the poor.[5]

Between the 1870s and 1920s, the number of U.S. hospitals increased from fewer than 200 to more than 6000. Private benevolence was responsible for establishing hundreds of new hospitals that were not interested in serving the poor. By 1910, there were as many hospitals per 1000 population as there are today, and, as is still true today, part of the population was not being served.

In 1910, Abraham Flexner conducted a study on the quality of medical education in the United States. The famous Flexner Report identified serious problems and inconsistencies that existed in medical education. As a result, many of the profit-oriented schools were closed, and those that remained open underwent significant curriculum revision. In addition, the AMA initiated an accreditation process that ranked schools according to their performance. The Flexner Report established a model for medical education that is still used in many medical schools today.

In 1913, the American College of Surgeons (ACS) was founded. One of its purposes was to develop a system of hospital standardization that would improve patient care and recognize hospitals that had the highest ideals. To establish the standards, the ACS began collecting data from health records. At this time, the ACS realized that health record documentation was inadequate. In 1917, the ACS founded the Hospital Standardization Program, which laid the groundwork for establishing standards of care. The first ACS report revealed that of the 692 hospitals surveyed, only 89 met minimum standards, and some of the most prestigious hospitals did not meet approval. After issuing this report, the ACS adopted the Minimum Standards, which identified the essential standards for proper care and treatment of hospital patients. The Minimum Standards included specifications that established an organized medical staff, required that certain diagnostic and therapeutic facilities be available, and that a health record be written for every patient. The standards specified, among other things, that the record be complete, accurate, and accessible.[5] In fact, the standards for health care in use today continue to encompass the documentation requirements identified in 1919 (Box 1-2).

Although hospital admissions increased dramatically from 1935 to the end of World War II in 1945, the unemployed, disabled, older adults, and others who could not pay were excluded. The economy was growing, and technologic advances continued in the medical field. The need for more hospitals and high-quality health care accessible to all Americans increased. In 1946, Senators Lister Hill and Harold H. Burton sponsored the Hospital Survey and Construction Act. This legislation, known as the Hill-Burton Act, provided funding for the construction of hospitals and other health care facilities on the basis of state need. For the next 25 years, as a result of this program, hospital construction and expansion flourished.

In the early 1950s, the ACS Hospital Standardization Program was overburdened by the huge increase in the numbers of hospitals, nonsurgical specialties, and the perception that medical care was becoming more sophisticated. As a result,

---

BOX 1-2 Medical Record Specifications Identified in the Minimum Standards by the American College of Surgeons, 1919

A complete case record should be developed, including the following:
- Patient identification data
- Complaint
- Personal and family history
- History of current illness
- Physical examination
- Special examinations (consultations, radiography, clinical laboratory)
- Provisional or working diagnosis
- Medical and surgical treatments
- Progress notes
- Gross and microscopic findings
- Final diagnosis
- Condition on discharge
- Follow-up
- Autopsy findings in the event of death

Adapted from American College of Surgeons: Minimum standards, 1919, *Bull Am Coll Surg* 8:4, 1924.

The Joint Commission on Accreditation of Hospitals (JCAH) was founded in 1952 and adopted the Hospital Standardization Program from the ACS.[5]

In the 1950s, Americans began to want more technology, accessible to all people at an affordable cost. As advances were made in the medical field, the demand for health care services and the cost to provide those services grew. The attitude became "more is better." In addition, medical advances extended life expectancy, resulting in an increase in the older adult population. With the growing older adult population came a growth in the incidence of chronic diseases. As hospital care became more expensive, those who were uninsured or underinsured—primarily the poor and older adults—could not access the health care system. Up to this point, the federal and state governments did little to control hospital costs. However, in 1965, Congress amended the Social Security Act of 1935, Public Law 89-97, establishing both Title XVIII, Health Insurance for the Aged (now called Medicare), and Title XIX, which extended the Kerr-Mills Medical Assistance Program (now called Medicaid). Medicare is a federally funded program that provides health insurance for older adults and certain other groups, and Medicaid supports the states in paying for health care for the indigent.[6] A person who is indigent is without the means for subsistence—poor or impoverished. At this time, the federal government became a significant player in the health care delivery system because it not only funded and operated the Medicare program but also assisted the states with the Medicaid program. These programs are discussed further in the section on financing health care later in this chapter. In response to the federal government's establishing and regulating the Medicare and Medicaid programs, states began writing more and, in some cases, their first regulatory codes.

In the 1960s, there was a proliferation of various health care facilities, including long-term care (LTC), psychiatric and substance abuse facilities, and programs for the developmentally disabled. The JCAH not only redefined the standards to be the optimal achievable, as opposed to minimum standards, but also began developing standards for the various types of health care facilities.[5] In 1987, the JCAH reflected its broader scope by changing its name to *The Joint Commission on Accreditation of Healthcare Organizations* (Box 1-3). It has been known as The Joint Commission (TJC) since early 2007.

Toward the turn of the century, there were not only concerns regarding the cost of health care and quality but also increased awareness of patient safety. In 1999, the Institute of Medicine (IOM) published *To Err Is Human*, which reported that between 44,000 and 98,000 deaths per year are attributable to medical errors at a cost of approximately $17 billion to $29 billion. Medical errors include adverse drug events, mismatched blood types, and surgery on the wrong patient or limb. With this report has come increasing attention to patient safety and bringing more information to the point of care with the use of technology.[7] In 2004, the World Health Organization began supporting dialogue among health leaders, consumers, and health ministers to discuss patient safety.

SELF-ASSESSMENT QUIZ

1. Of all the legislation, identify and describe the one that has contributed the most to construction of health care facilities.

BOX 1-3   Historical Landmarks Affecting Health Care Systems

1910: Flexner Report, published by Abraham Flexner, revealed serious problems that existed in medical education. The report served as an impetus to establishing the accreditation of medical schools by the American Medical Association (AMA).

1913: American College of Surgeons (ACS) was founded for the purposes of establishing standards of care and recognizing those hospitals that have high ideals.

1917: ACS established the Hospital Standardization Program, which began testing basic standards of care.

1919: ACS adopted the Minimum Standards, which identified factors that are essential to proper care and treatment of hospital patients.

1935: Social Security Act was passed, which provided grants for old-age assistance and benefits, unemployment compensation, and aid to dependent children, maternal and child welfare, and other groups. It also established Social Security.

1946: Hospital Survey and Construction Act (Hill-Burton Act) was passed, which provided funding for the construction of health care facilities and equipment on the basis of state need.

1952: Joint Commission on Accreditation of Hospitals (JCAH) was founded, which adopted the Hospital Standardization Program from the ACS; in the late 1980s, JCAH changed its name to *The Joint Commission on Accreditation of Healthcare Organizations.*

1953: Department of Health, Education, and Welfare (HEW) was formed for the purpose of addressing issues related to the health, education, and welfare of the people of the United States.

1961: The Community Health Services and Facilities Act provided grants for the establishment of voluntary health planning agencies at the local level; it resulted in community health centers to serve low-income areas.

1965: Title III of the Older Americans Act established funding for transportation and for chore, homemaker, and home health aides for older adults.

1965: Congress amended the Social Security Act of 1935 (PL 89-97), which established Title XVIII, Health Insurance for the Aged (Medicare), and Title XIX, Medical Assistance Program (Medicaid).

1970: The Occupational Safety and Health Act was passed, which mandated employers to provide a safe and healthy work environment and therefore resulted in the development of standards.

1977: The Committee on Allied Health Education and Accreditation was founded by the AMA for the purpose of accrediting allied health programs; it disbanded in 1994.

1980: HEW was reorganized into the Department of Health and Human Services (DHHS), a federal cabinet-level department responsible for health issues, including health care and costs, welfare of various populations, occupational safety, and income security plans.

1982: The Tax Equity and Fiscal Responsibility Act, PL97-248, established a mechanism for controlling the cost of the Medicare program; this act set a limit on reimbursement and required the development of the prospective payment system (later to be known as *diagnosis-related groups*).

1985: Consolidated Omnibus Budget Reconciliation Act established the Emergency Medical Treatment and Active Labor Act, which is known as the "Patient Antidumping Law." It established criteria for the transfer and discharge of Medicare and Medicaid patients between two acute-care hospitals.

1987: The Nursing Home Reform Act, effective in 1990, required nursing facilities (long-term care facilities) to employ sufficient nursing personnel, 24 hours per day, to provide care to each resident according to the care plan.

1989: The Omnibus Budget Reconciliation Act brought attention and support to the production and dissemination of scientific and policy-relevant information that improves quality, reduces cost, and enhances effectiveness of health care and established the Agency for Health Care Research and Quality.

1990: The Patient Self-Determination Act resulted from the *Cruzan v. Missouri* (1990) case in which the court upheld patient wishes at the end of life. The Act increased the public's awareness of state laws governing patient options and rights, as well as advance directives.

1991: DHHS commissioned the Workgroup on Electronic Data Interchange to identify ways to increase the number of claims processed electronically, which would reduce administrative costs.

1992: The Computer-Based Patient Record Institute was created for the purpose of developing strategy that supports the development and adoption of the computer-based patient record.

1996 (implemented in 1998): Health Insurance Portability and Accountability Act is directed at improving access, affordability, and adequacy of health insurance; established a fraud- and abuse-detection program for health plans. It includes provision for administrative simplification that addresses privacy and security of personal health information and uniform definitions for transactions and code sets.

2010: President Obama signed the Patient Protection and Affordable Care Act into law. This was the largest reform of health care since the creation of Medicare and Medicaid in 1965. It is primarily targeted at increasing access to care and improving quality of health care.

? DID YOU KNOW?

Health care fraud and abuse costs as much as $100 billion a year. Often the fraud involves health care personnel who have access to patient information and sell that information to organized crime groups. The crime groups then use the data to "steal" money from Medicare in false claims.

Health Care in the Twenty-First Century

The health care system in the United States has evolved into a complex system composed of multiple types of facilities, providers, payers, regulators, and consumers who are demanding more and better health care. There is a proliferation of sophisticated technology for both medical practice and information management. The technology available in financial, administrative, and clinical information systems affects the quality, cost, and efficiency of health care systems. The technological advances in medicine support prevention, early diagnosis, shorter hospital stays, patient safety, and increased outpatient services and home health care.

In 2011 U.S. health care spending totaled approximately $2.7 trillion and composed approximately 17.9% of the U.S. gross domestic product (GDP). The United States spent $8,608 per person on health care, yet millions of people were uninsured or could not access the system. Those without insurance either could not afford coverage or could not find an insurance company willing to sell them a policy at any price. Prior to the passage of the Patient Protection and Affordable Care Act (PPACA) in 2010, insurance companies could cancel contracts with patients who had expensive (catastrophic costs) health care needs, as is the case with chronic conditions such as cancer, kidney disease, and heart disease. Geographic access to health care providers has also been an issue for individuals living in areas where little or no health care is available and who lack transportation.[9]

Advances in technology and scientific developments have supported a healthier lifestyle and a longer life expectancy. For women, life expectancy increased from 48.3 years in 1900 to 81 years in 2010, and for men, from 46.3 years to 76.2 years.[10] This longer life expectancy has resulted in an aging population, and the United States is looking forward to tremendous growth in the need for home health and LTC.

Despite escalating costs and difficulty accessing health care, consumers continue to demand more and better care. The result is a health care system that is evolving into a more patient- or consumer-centric culture. Patient-centered care allows patients to have more control over their care and access to their health care information. Evidence of patient-centered care includes the following:

- Making cost and quality data on hospitals and providers available to the consumer, such as the "Quality Check" function on the website for TJC where consumers can check on the accreditation findings of HCOs.
- Supporting patients in setting up their own personal health records (PHRs) by making provider records accessible to patients through Internet portals and other methods.

- Protecting the patient's privacy and security of health information by legislation.
- Increasing communication between patient and provider by e-mail or voicemail.

The American Health Information Management Association (AHIMA) has defined a PHR in the following way:

> The personal health record (PHR) is an electronic, lifelong resource of health information needed by individuals to make health decisions. Individuals own and manage the information in the PHR, which comes from healthcare providers and the individual. The PHR is maintained in a secure and private environment, with the individual determining rights of access. The PHR does not replace the legal record of any provider.[11]

Increasing costs and limited access to health care for all citizens created tremendous pressure to reform the U.S. health care system. President Obama signed the PPACA into law in March of 2010, and one of its primary goals is to expand access to health insurance for all citizens through an individual mandate and Medicaid expansion. By March of 2014, all U.S. citizens were required to obtain some sort of health insurance coverage, or be penalized under the PPACA. The law also includes provisions focused on controlling costs, increasing prevention, and improving the overall quality of the health care system.[9]

This health reform law presents the most sweeping changes to the health care system in the United States since the enactment of Medicare and Medicaid in 1965. As this represents a significant reform, the law has many critics. The Supreme Court of the United States reviewed the constitutionality of the law in 2012. The Court ruled that although the majority of the law is fine as it stands, the Medicaid expansion requirement was coercive. Therefore states have the ability to opt out of this portion of the legislation. As of 2013, twenty-five states, including the District of Columbia, have opted to move forward with the Medicaid expansion, providing coverage to citizens up to 133% of the federal poverty level. However, 22 states are opting out of this expansion, and 4 states are still debating their participation.[12]

CRITICAL THINKING

Review the literature on health care reform and write a 500 to 600 word description of two or three sections of the plan. Include the basic concepts (what it is about, who is affected, and how), date of implementation, and projected effect.

Healthy People

Since the year 2000, the U.S. Department of Health and Human Services (DHHS) has established science-based objectives for the United States that promote health and the prevention of disease. In the initial report, Healthy People 2000, DHHS used national data systems to identify opportunities and formulate goals for health improvement. This process has been replicated during the past 3 decades, and it has been estimated that the United States has made progress toward achieving approximately 71% of the Healthy People target.

The most recent initiative is Healthy People 2020. The health goals established in Healthy People 2020 were generated based on input from experts in the areas of public health, prevention, and health services delivery. Additionally, input from the public also factored heavily into the generation of the new objectives. Healthy People 2020 includes four primary goals:

- Attain high-quality, longer lives free of preventable disease, disability, injury, and premature death.
- Achieve health equity, eliminate disparities, and improve the health of all groups.
- Create social and physical environments that promote good health for all.
- Promote quality of life, healthy development, and healthy behaviors across all life stages.

Additionally, Healthy People 2020 is encouraging the development of user friendly applications for those individuals who are working toward the new national health objectives at both the state and local levels.[13]

REGULATORY AGENCIES AND ORGANIZATIONS

External forces that regulate the health care industry include, but are not limited to, the DHHS, TJC, the American Osteopathic Association (AOA), the Community Health Accreditation Program (CHAP) of the National League for Nursing, the Commission on Accreditation of Rehabilitation Facilities (CARF), and the state departments of public health. The regulatory activities of health care facilities are primarily directed at quality, utilization, and cost of care, whereas the regulatory activities that affect educational programs and the health care workforce are directed at quality and supply of manpower.

Federal Government as Regulator

The federal government has been involved in the regulation of the health care systems since the early part of the century, primarily in the consumer's interest. In 1906, the Pure Food and Drug Act was passed because of the unsanitary conditions that prevailed in the food production industry, and in 1938 the Food, Drug, and Cosmetic Act was passed to regulate the food, drug, and cosmetic industry. This act mandated that manufacturers prove safety, specify composition and method of manufacture, and provide labeling and package inserts. Interestingly, it was not until 1962 that manufacturers were required to prove efficacy (i.e., how effective a product is).

Department of Health and Human Services

The principal agency of the federal government responsible for the numerous regulatory programs that affect the health industry is the DHHS, formerly the Department of Health, Education, and Welfare (HEW). HEW, created in 1953, underwent numerous reorganizations that led to the creation of the DHHS in 1980. The organization of the DHHS is complex and includes numerous administrations, divisions, offices, centers, and agencies; the highest ranking official is the secretary of the DHHS, who advises the president of the United States on issues regarding health, welfare, income security plans, and programs and projects of the DHHS. The DHHS has regional offices that work with the states and communities in carrying out various programs.

Organization of DHHS

The organizational structure of the DHHS encompasses various agencies, centers, and offices, some of which are discussed in the following section and identified in the DHHS organizational chart illustrated in Figure 1-1. The DHHS organizational structure was recently amended to include an Office of Health Reform, which was established to oversee the implementation of PPACA.

Office of Inspector General

The responsibility of conducting and monitoring audits, inspections, and investigations regarding programs or projects sponsored by the DHHS is delegated to the Office of Inspector General (OIG). For example, this office investigates cases of alleged fraud and abuse that occur in Medicare and Medicaid programs and recommends corrective action in such cases.

Administration for Children and Families

The Administration for Children and Families (ACF) is committed to the development of children, youth, and families and to supporting activities that improve and enrich these groups. This agency administers and funds state grants regarding such issues as adoption, runaway and homeless youth, prevention and treatment of child abuse, and child welfare services.

Administration on Aging

The Administration on Aging (AoA) was created in response to the Amendment to the Older American Act of 1965. It supports a range of programs that offer services and opportunities for older Americans. The AoA is an advocate for older persons; it works to increase awareness of the contribution that older Americans make and alerts the public regarding the needs of older people.

Agency for Healthcare Research and Quality

The Agency for Healthcare Research and Quality (AHRQ) was established by the Omnibus Budget Reconciliation Act of 1989, which placed greater emphasis on health services research. The primary focus is to produce and disseminate scientific and policy-relevant information that improves the quality, reduces the cost, and enhances the effectiveness of health care.

Agency for Toxic Substances and Disease Registry

The Agency for Toxic Substances and Disease Registry is committed to protecting both workers and the public from

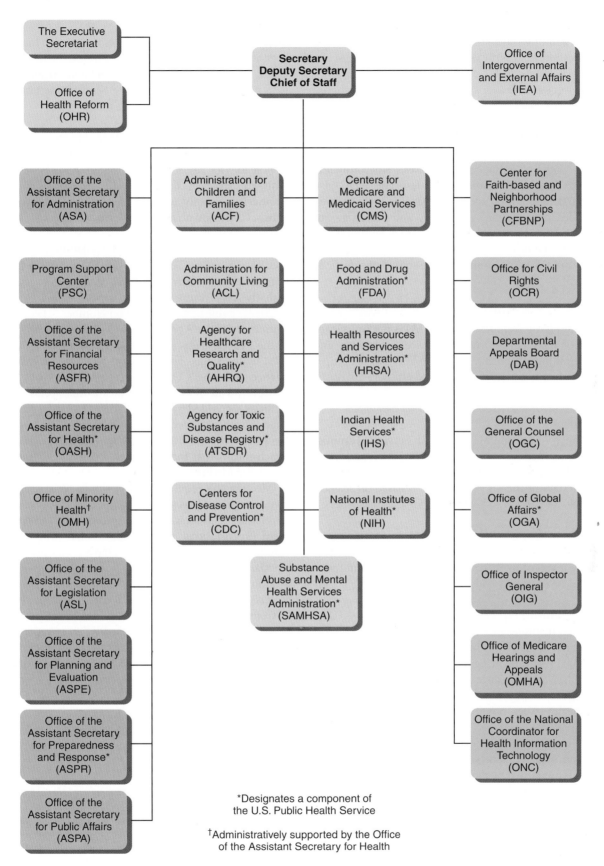

FIGURE 1-1 Organizational structure of the U.S. Department of Health and Human Services. (From U.S. Department of Health and Human Services: http://www.hhs.gov/about/orgchart. Accessed December 12, 2013.)

exposure to and the adverse effects of hazardous substances. The agency, among other functions, collects, analyzes, and disseminates information regarding mortality rates, disease, and hazardous substances; establishes registries for long-term follow-up; and develops programs for public response to health emergencies.

Centers for Disease Control and Prevention

The Centers for Disease Control and Prevention (CDC) is concerned with communicable diseases, environmental health, and foreign quarantine activities. The CDC also works with state and local agencies regarding these matters and provides consultation, education, and training. For example, the CDC has established recommendations (standards) called "Universal Precautions" that are guidelines for health care workers to minimize the spread of infectious substances.

Food and Drug Administration

The Food and Drug Administration (FDA) is responsible for the safety of foods, drugs, medical devices, cosmetics, and radiation-emitting equipment. Responsibilities include proper labeling, product information, safety, and efficacy.

Substance Abuse and Mental Health Services Administration

The Substance Abuse and Mental Health Services Administration is concerned with the effective prevention and treatment of addictive and mental disorders. The administration emphasizes state-of-the-art practice that is based on science, high quality, and access to health care for these disorders.

Health Resources and Services Administration

The Health Resources and Services Administration (HRSA) is primarily involved in the distribution of major grant funding to state governments and the private sector.

National Institutes of Health

The National Institutes of Health (NIH) is a major medical research center composed of numerous institutes and centers (e.g., National Institute on Aging, National Center for Nursing Research, National Cancer Institute). It is a major source of funding for health-related research (e.g., aging, cancer, women's health issues, obesity, nutrition).

Surgeon General

The surgeon general reports to the assistant secretary for health and is appointed by the president of the United States to serve a 4-year term. The primary role of the surgeon general is to provide leadership and management for the PHS Commissioned Corps and to serve as advisor on public health and scientific issues, including current and long-term health issues, emergency preparedness and response, protection and enhancement of the health of the nation, and provision of leadership on health initiatives such as prevention of spread of infectious diseases and tobacco cessation.

Indian Health Service

The Indian Health Service (IHS) is responsible for providing health care through a network of hospitals, health centers, health stations, school health centers and through contracts with private providers to eligible Native Americans.

Centers for Medicare and Medicaid Services

The Centers for Medicare and Medicaid Services (CMS), formerly Health Care Financing Administration (HCFA), is responsible for the Medicare program and the federal government's role in the Medicaid programs, with special emphasis on quality and utilization control. Through its programs, CMS is involved in the health care of older adults, the disabled, and the poor.

The CMS establishes rules and regulations that govern the Medicare program. To be eligible for Medicare and Medicaid reimbursement, providers must demonstrate compliance with the conditions of participation (COP), which were originally published in Regulation Number 5, Federal Health Insurance for the Aged. Revisions to the COP are published in the Federal Register. Compliance with the COP is regulated by the states. The review of HCOs to determine compliance with the COP is the responsibility of the states. However, Title XVIII, the Medicare Act, specifies that the facilities accredited by TJC and the AOA be deemed in compliance with the Medicare Conditions of Participation for Hospitals[5]; those accredited are said to have deemed status, which means that the accredited facility meets the requirements for Medicare COP.

Meeting the requirements of the COP is referred to as *being certified*. However, the term certification is also used to refer to the process by which government and nongovernment organizations evaluate educational programs, health care facilities, and individuals as having met predetermined standards. To ensure high-quality care, the CMS established a national network of Quality Improvement Organizations (QIOs) for each U.S. state and territory and for the District of Columbia. The QIOs work with health care providers and consumers to promote a high quality of care and to investigate complaints about care. The QIOs also work to protect the Medicare trust fund and ensure that payments are made for only medically necessary services.

> ### ✓ SELF-ASSESSMENT QUIZ
>
> 2. Medicare helps to pay health care costs for all of the following people EXCEPT:
>   a. Those age 65 and older
>   b. Indigent people of all ages
>   c. People with permanent kidney disease
>   d. People on disability for a minimum of 24 months

Social Security Administration

Before 1995, the Social Security Administration (SSA) was located within the organizational structure of the DHHS. However, in 1995 it became an independent agency.

The SSA manages the social security program for older adults, disabled and blind people, and for survivors (dependents). The social security program is financed by contributions from employees, employers, and self-employed people, which are placed in a fund. When earnings stop or are reduced because of retirement, death, or disability, the fund pays monthly cash amounts to supplement the loss of income.

Occupational Safety and Health Administration

In 1970, Congress passed the Occupational Safety and Health Act, which mandated that employers provide a safe and healthy work environment. The Occupational Safety and Health Administration (OSHA) is responsible for developing standards and regulations and conducting inspections and investigations to determine compliance, and it proposes corrective actions for noncompliance in matters related to occupational safety and health. Other agencies involved in establishing standards for occupational safety and health include government agencies, such as the CDC, and professional organizations, such as the ACS. The guidelines, recommendations, and standards are directed at protecting employees from occupational health hazards, such as minimizing the risk of contracting disease from asbestos in old buildings, contracting acquired immunodeficiency syndrome (AIDS) in health care facilities, and developing repetitive motion injuries such as carpal tunnel syndrome.

 SELF-ASSESSMENT QUIZ

3. What is the role of the surgeon general, and who appoints the surgeon general to serve?

The Role of States

State governments have regulatory involvement in the health care systems through state-owned and state-operated facilities, the funding of medical education and teaching hospitals, the certification of health care facilities according to the Medicare COP, maintenance of public health departments, and licensing of health care facilities and health occupations. Hospital ownership, medical education, certification, and licensing of health occupations are discussed in other sections; therefore only the states' roles in public health departments and in licensing health care facilities are addressed in this section.

State Health Departments

The organization of state health departments varies from state to state but is a joint venture between the state and the local communities. The health care provided is usually directed toward maternal and child health care, communicable diseases, and chronic diseases. The maternal and childcare services usually provide obstetric care, family planning, well-baby checkups, vaccinations, and other services. Health care for communicable diseases involves teaching the patient and community about transmission and prevention of certain diseases, diagnosing and treating communicable diseases such as measles and gonorrhea, and tracking the source of the communicable disease. Some of the chronic diseases that the public health department might manage are mental illness, substance abuse, hypertension, and diabetes. HIM professionals need to be knowledgeable about the organization of the state health department in the state where they reside or practice; information is usually available through the county health department.

State and local health departments have important roles in collecting information through vital statistics and communicable disease reporting, in ensuring safe drinking water and environment, and in bioterrorism.

Public health is a general term that refers to a wide array of activities directed at promoting the health of populations. Activities include efforts directed at prevention and early detection of disease and promotion of health in the general and in special populations. Many of the programs and activities are conducted by the states and funded by state and federal monies. The programs and activities include, among other activities, immunizations, behavior modification through education, health screenings and periodic examinations, and therapeutic interventions. For example, to reduce tobacco use, numerous state and federal initiatives are directed at educating the public about the risk of tobacco use, advice about how to quit, funding for counseling and advising patients on smoking cessation, and a hotline for consumers desiring to quit.

DID YOU KNOW?

Tobacco use is the leading cause of preventable morbidity and mortality in the United States. It causes numerous cancers including lung, mouth, bladder, and stomach cancers; heart disease, such as coronary artery disease and peripheral vascular disease; cerebrovascular attack; and emphysema and chronic obstructive pulmonary disease, and pneumonia.

Licensure of Health Care Facilities

Licensure gives legal approval for a facility to operate or for a person to practice within his or her profession (Table 1-1). Virtually every state requires that hospitals, nursing homes, and pharmacies be licensed to operate, although the requirements and standards for licensure may differ from state to state. State licensure is mandatory. Federal facilities such as those of the Department of Veterans Affairs do not require state licensure.

TABLE 1-1	Regulation of Health Care Providers	
	State Government	National Nongovernmental
Health care professionals	Licensure	Registration/certification
Health care facilities	Licensure	Accreditation

Although licensure requirements vary, health care facilities must meet certain basic criteria that are determined by state regulatory agencies. The standards address such concerns as adequacy of staffing, personnel employed to provide services, physical aspects of the facility (equipment, buildings), and services provided, including health records. Survey for licensure is typically performed annually, and the standards are usually considered to be minimally acceptable for operation. Some states also accept TJC accreditation as proof of meeting licensure requirements.

Legislation

Following is a brief discussion of selected legislation that has had a major effect on health care delivery in the United States.

The Consolidated Omnibus Budget Reconciliation Act (COBRA) of 1985 was written out of a concern for the management of indigent patients. COBRA established the Emergency Medical Treatment and Labor Act (EMTALA), which is known as the "Patient Antidumping Law." EMTALA established criteria for Medicare-certified facilities and physicians responsible for the transfer and discharge of patients. The law requires that every patient, regardless of ability to pay, who arrives at an emergency department (ED) with an emergency medical condition, including active labor, be provided a medical screening examination and stabilizing medical care. If the facility is unable to provide stabilizing treatment or if the patient requests, a transfer to an appropriate facility should be made.[14]

In 1989, the Omnibus Budget Reconciliation Act was passed, which emphasizes the production and dissemination of scientific and policy-relevant information that improves the quality, reduces the cost, and enhances the effectiveness of health care. This act promoted the development of outcome measures (criteria) for health care quality.

The Patient Self-Determination Act of 1990 was a result of the Supreme Court's ruling in *Cruzan v. Missouri* (1990) that upheld patient wishes, although the decision meant inevitable death for the patient. The act is intended to increase the public's awareness of the respective state laws governing patient options for health care, patient rights, and advance directives. An advance directive is a legal, written document that specifies patient preferences regarding future health care or specifies another person to make medical decisions in the event the patient has an incurable or irreversible condition and is unable to communicate his or her wishes; the patient must be competent at the time the document is prepared and signed. The advance directive guides the health care team in making decisions about life-sustaining treatment and organ donation and usually designates a person to assume authority for the patient. The statute requires providers to develop written policies and procedures on self-determination and to document in each health record regardless of whether an advance directive has been signed. The HIM or risk management department is responsible for ensuring that the proper documentation is in each health record. (See Chapter 14, Privacy and Health Law, for further information.)

Prior to PPACA, some individuals with complex medical conditions that were expensive to treat had difficulty maintaining insurance coverage. Payers would frequently drop high-cost individuals, making it almost impossible to secure insurance coverage. As an answer to this issue, Congress passed the Health Insurance Portability and Accountability Act (HIPAA) in 1996, which is a comprehensive law dealing with a variety of health care issues mainly directed at improving access, affordability, and adequacy of health insurance. One of the main provisions of HIPAA is to provide for the portability of group health insurance when a person changes employers. Before the enactment of HIPAA, employees often had to wait for coverage themselves or for one of their dependents because of preexisting conditions such as asthma or high blood pressure. HIPAA allowed for continuous coverage when a person changed from one group insurance plan to another. The act also established tax breaks for purchasers of LTC insurance and self-employed purchasers of health insurance and created a fraud and abuse program for health plans.

HIPAA includes many other provisions that affect the operation of HCOs. Some that have had the greatest effect on HIM can be found in the administrative simplification section. The privacy and security rules are included in this section. The privacy rule applies to protected health information in any format created or used by health care providers, health care plans, and health care clearinghouses. The HIPAA security rule is concerned with the protection of the electronic health information. The advent of HIPAA has brought about expanded roles and responsibilities for HIM professionals—that is, protecting privacy and maintaining the security of electronic health care transactions and records. The federal regulations standardize the privacy and security practices in the health care industry throughout the United States. Before HIPAA, laws differed among states.

The Health Information Technology for Economic and Clinical Health (HITECH) Act was signed into law in 2009. HITECH was part of the American Recovery and Reinvestment Act of 2009, and its purpose was to promote the meaningful use of health information technology. This act includes incentive payments to providers who adopt and use electronic health records (EHRs) beginning in 2011. Those physicians and health care providers opting not to adopt EHRs will be penalized after 2015. Adoption alone is not sufficient; providers must demonstrate the meaningful use of this technology.

Finally, the recent PPACA was signed into law in 2010. As discussed in the earlier portion of this chapter, PPACA was created primarily to expand access to health insurance coverage. Through PPACA, health insurance exchanges or electronic marketplaces will be created in each state to allow individuals to directly compare and purchase health insurance coverage. Currently, most individuals purchase insurance coverage through their employer. However, exchanges will offer an alternative mechanism for this transaction. In addition to increasing access to health insurance coverage through the individual mandate and Medicaid expansion, PPACA also has provisions for improving quality and a national prevention and wellness strategy.

Accreditation

The process by which a private nongovernmental organization or agency performs an external review and grants recognition to a program of study or institution that meets certain predetermined standards is called *accreditation.* The review process and the standards are devised and regulated by professional organizations such as TJC and the AOA. Although the process is voluntary, there are financial and legal incentives for HCOs to attain accreditation. Advantages of accreditation are numerous and include the following:

- Required for reimbursement for certain patient groups
- Validates the quality of health care institutions, programs, and services
- Provides a competitive edge over nonaccredited facilities

The HIM department plays a crucial role in accreditation because the review of health information data is a major part of the accreditation process. The HIM professionals should have access to and be familiar with the standards contained in the most current accreditation manual for the type of HCO in which they are employed.

The Joint Commission

TJC is a private, nonprofit organization that establishes guidelines and standards for the operation and management of health care facilities with emphasis on the health care functions crucial to patient care. The mission of TJC is "to continuously improve health care for the public, in collaboration with other stakeholders, by evaluating HCOs and inspiring them to excel in providing safe and effective care of the highest quality and value."[15]

The standards are based on HCOs being responsible for providing a high quality of health care to the people they serve while efficiently using resources. Currently, when an organization is found to be in substantial compliance with TJC standards, accreditation is awarded. TJC does on-site, unannounced, accreditation surveys between 18 and 39 months from the previous survey with an emphasis on the safety and quality of care, treatment, and services.[15]

TJC accredits numerous types of HCOs. Some examples of the HCOs for which standards are developed include hospitals, behavioral HCOs, LTC organizations, home care organizations, ambulatory care organizations, pathology and clinical laboratory services, office-based surgery practices, and managed care organizations (MCOs).[14] As mentioned earlier, TJC has information available on its website for consumers to check on the accreditation status of health care facilities.

American Osteopathic Association

Much like TJC, the AOA has a voluntary program that accredits osteopathic medical colleges and health care facilities. Its mission is to promote osteopathic medicine through education, research, and delivery of quality health care that is cost-effective. Osteopathic medicine is based on the theory that all body systems are interconnected, and therefore the focus of health care is directed at the whole person.[16] Because two thirds of the body is composed of muscle and bone, osteopathic medicine places a great deal of emphasis on the musculoskeletal system. The hospitals that are accredited are recognized by the DHHS as having "deemed status," and therefore are eligible to receive Medicare funds. The AOA's Healthcare Facilities Accreditation Program (HFAP) offers voluntary accreditation to a wide variety of HCOs, including hospitals, ambulatory care facilities, mental health facilities, and substance abuse facilities. Programs that are accredited meet or exceed the standards for educational quality that have been established by the AOA's Commission on Osteopathic College Accreditation (COCA).[17]

Commission on Accreditation of Rehabilitation Facilities

Founded in 1966, CARF is an independent accrediting agency for rehabilitation facilities. Rehabilitation is the processes of treatment and education that leads the disabled person to the achievement of maximum independence and function and a personal sense of well-being. The mission of CARF is to promote the quality, value, and optimal outcomes of services for people with disabilities. As a result of this mission, CARF sets and maintains standards directed at improving quality of care, conducting research, identifying competent organizations that provide rehabilitative services, and providing an organized forum in which people served, providers, and others can participate in quality improvement.[18]

Community Health Accreditation Program

The independent, nonprofit organization that accredits community-based HCOs, including home health and hospice agencies, is the CHAP. Unlike those of other accrediting bodies, CHAP standards are consumer oriented, with more emphasis on the patient perspective than on the clinical aspect of care. Like TJC, HCOs accredited by CHAP are deemed to have met the Medicare COP.[18]

National Committee for Quality Assurance

The National Committee for Quality Assurance (NCQA) is a private, nonprofit, organization that offers accreditation, certification, recognition, and performance measurement to various HCOs. Its mission is to improve the quality of health care. One component of the quality improvement plan is the Health Plan Employer Data and Information Set, which is a standardized set of performance measures designed to allow purchasers and consumers to compare the performance of managed-care plans.[19]

Regulatory Mechanisms of Health Occupations

Numerous agencies, organizations, and pieces of legislation regulate the education and practice of the various health occupations. The regulatory activities include state licensure of practitioners, accreditation of educational programs, certification of practitioners, and legislation that governs practice. A few of these activities are discussed here. Licensure, like that of HCOs, is required to practice the profession, whereas registration and certification are voluntary processes and are not required by law to practice that profession. Individual HCOs may require certification or registration as a condition of employment.

American Medical Association

The AMA, previously discussed, is a professional organization for physicians that is involved in the accreditation of medical schools, residency programs, and certain allied health programs.

American Osteopathic Association's Commission on Osteopathic College Accreditation

The COCA is the only accrediting organization for osteopathic medical education in the United States. Programs that are accredited meet or exceed the standards for educational quality that have been established by the AOA.[17]

Commission on Accreditation of Allied Health Education Programs

The Commission on Accreditation of Allied Health Education Programs (CAAHEP) accredits 25 health-science occupations and more than 2100 programs and is recognized as the largest accrediting organization in the field of health sciences. CAAHEP works with professional organizations in the accreditation process.[20] For example, CAAHEP works with the American Association of Respiratory Care in accrediting respiratory therapy educational programs.

Commission on Accreditation for Health Informatics and Information Management Education

The Commission on Accreditation for Health Informatics and Information Management Education (CAHIIM) is an independent, accrediting organization for degree-granting programs in health informatics and information management. CAHIIM accreditation means that an educational program has voluntarily undergone a rigorous review process and has been determined to meet or exceed the standards set by the sponsoring professional organization, the AHIMA in cooperation with the Commission.[21]

Accreditation Commission for Education in Nursing

The accrediting body for schools of nursing that offer diplomas or associate, bachelor's, master's, and doctoral degrees in nursing is the Accreditation Commission for Education in Nursing (ACEN). The ACEN establishes standards for the nursing curriculum, including programs for registered nurses (RNs) and licensed practical nurses (LPNs). The purpose of the ACEN is to support the interests of nurse educators, nurses, and the public by ensuring high-quality education through accreditation.[22]

State Licensure of Practitioners

In the licensing of practitioners, states have the right to control the entry into certain professions through licensure and the right to revoke the license. The license itself is a permit issued by the state that authorizes a person to practice in a specified area; without this permission, such practice is illegal.

Each state establishes its own licensing requirements and restricts certain activities to those who are licensed by that state. Licensure requirements involve completion of a program of study and examination by the state. Restrictions are specific for the license. For example, prescribing and dispensing medications were at one time restricted to licensed physicians. Today, however, many states have given prescriptive authority to nurse practitioners (NPs) and others. The health occupations that require licensure to practice include medicine, osteopathy, nursing, nursing home administration, dentistry, podiatry, and numerous others, depending on the state. Some professions, such as occupational therapy, are both licensed and certified.

The state law that defines the rights and scope of practice of each profession and the requirements to attain a license is often called the Practice Act. In the case of nursing, it is called the *Nursing Practice Act*. Because these laws and regulations define the scope of practice, they are often an area of contention between professions when the scopes overlap. The Practice Acts also define the conditions for endorsement (reciprocity) between states. Although endorsement varies from state to state, most states require a current and active license from another state, graduation from an approved educational program, and a minimum number of years of practice.

HEALTH CARE DELIVERY SYSTEMS

Continuum of Care

The continuum of care is the full range of health care services provided, moving from the least acute and least intensive to the most acute and most intensive, or vice versa. The level and type of care provided are determined by the needs of the patient. Table 1-2 identifies the components of the continuum of health care services.

Primary care is the care provided at the point of first contact (encounter) with the health care provider in an ambulatory care setting. Ideally, the care is continuous and comprehensive, and may involve episodes of care for a specific condition during a period of relatively continuous care. The provider coordinates and manages all aspects of the patient's health care, including the preventive care and use of consultants and community resources as appropriate. Primary care encompasses preventive care (comprehensive care) and acute care. Health care services directed at preventing disease or injury, minimizing the consequences of existing conditions, and promoting health are the major objectives of preventive care. Annual physical examinations,

TABLE 1-2   Continuum of Health Care Services

Health Care Service	Description	Examples of Setting
Preventive care	Care directed at preventing injury or condition. Examples: immunizations, genetic testing, use of safety belts	Physician office, public health departments, clinics
Primary care	Care provided at point of first contact; includes preventive care, acute care, early detection, and intervention	Physician office, public health departments, clinics
Specialist care	Care directed at specific body organ or system or specific disease	Specialists such as gastroenterologists, cardiologists, and psychiatrists
Long-term care	Medical and nonmedical care provided for chronic, debilitating conditions such as Alzheimer's disease, chronic obstructive pulmonary disease, quadriplegia	Home health care, long-term care facilities
Rehabilitative care	Care directed at restoring disabled person to maximum physical, mental, and vocational health; goal is independence and productivity	Inpatient and outpatient rehabilitation facilities, home health care, and rehabilitation departments of hospitals and long-term care
Respite care	Short-term care in which care is provided to patient for purpose of providing caregiver with time off and rest	Patient or family home; adult day care; long-term care facilities
End-of-life care	Hospice care provided to patients in last 6 months of life; includes the palliative and supportive	Patient or family home care, skilled nursing home care of terminally ill patients and their families

immunizations, family planning, vision and hearing screens, health education, and early detection of disease are examples of preventive medicine. Acute care, in contrast, implies the treatment of common illnesses and injuries, such as nausea, vomiting, and abrasions. Providers of primary care are family practitioners, internists, pediatricians, obstetricians, gynecologists, physician assistants (PAs), and NPs; the care is commonly provided in one of many ambulatory care settings. Primary care providers often serve as gatekeepers. When physicians serve a gatekeeping function, they regulate a patient's access to more specialized physicians, and ensure the patient only receives a higher level of care when medically appropriate. This function may be mandated by payers, as is often the case in a managed care environment. The focus of primary care is on prevention through regular physical examinations and other care services (education, immunization, family planning, emergency care). If a patient needs to see a specialist, the gatekeeper must make the referral and thereby controls the access to all other care.

The patient-centered medical home (PCMH) is a new model of primary care, which emphasizes care coordination and communication. The idea is that a patient will form a relationship with a primary care provider, and that provider will provide support and coordination for that individual's health care needs. The PCMH encourages five primary functions, including comprehensive care, patient-centered care, coordinated care, accessible services, and quality and safety.[23]

Secondary care, a term not as widely used as primary or tertiary care, implies care by a specialist, usually through referral from the primary care physician. Secondary care may be obtained in an outpatient setting, or it may be obtained in a community based hospital. Tertiary care is a term used for the care provided at facilities with advanced technologies and specialized intensive care units, such as teaching institutions and university medical centers. The providers are specialists who are widely recognized for their expertise in specific areas of medicine and include specialists such as endocrinologists, hematologists, oncologists, thoracic surgeons, and neurosurgeons.

Ambulatory Care

Ambulatory care is a comprehensive term for all types of health care provided in an outpatient setting; the patient travels to and from the facility on the same day and is not hospitalized, institutionalized, or admitted as an inpatient. For example, a resident of a nursing home may be transported to the outpatient department at the hospital for a mammogram (radiograph of the breast) and then returned to the nursing home later the same day. This person is a resident (inpatient) of the nursing home but an outpatient of the hospital.

There are two major types of ambulatory (or outpatient) care:

- Care provided in freestanding medical centers: Examples of freestanding medical centers include physicians' solo, partnership, or group practices; public health departments; community health centers (CHCs); and urgent care centers.
- Care provided in organized settings that function independently of the physicians providing the care: The settings for this type of ambulatory care include hospital-owned clinics, outpatient departments, ambulatory treatment units, EDs, ancillary services, and urgent care centers. Note that urgent care centers and others may be in either type of setting, depending on ownership of the facility. The physician may be an employee of the urgent care facility or may be the owner and provider.

Physician Practices

Physician practices have historically been private practices; however, with health care reform, physicians are collaborating, networking, and forming alliances with other providers, including managed-care programs and hospitals, all of which are described in the section on financing of health care. Additionally, many individual and groups of physicians are implementing a PCMH strategy. This emphasizes a relationship between a patient and a physician, in which the physician is responsible for coordinating patient care.

Private Practice

The term *private practice* usually refers to physicians or other health care providers who are established in an independent practice that is for profit. Although providers of health care include numerous professionals (dentists, podiatrists, chiropractors) who can by law practice independently, this discussion focuses on the physician as the provider. The primary mode by which physicians provide health care is within their private medical office (practice), although this is changing.

Some physicians are self-employed and legally the sole owners of their practices; these solo practices are on the decline. Most physicians in solo practices have an informal arrangement with other physicians to "take call" when they are not available. "Take call" refers to the practice of one physician managing care for another physician's patients, which allows the physician to take time away from work.

A partnership is a legal agreement between two or more physicians to share certain expenses and profits. The term *partnership* may apply to group practice (three or more physicians) if the group has entered a legal agreement to share certain assets and liabilities as determined by the agreement. The agreement specifies that the physicians are employees of the practice, with all monies generated and expenses from the practice to be pooled and redistributed to the physicians according to the agreement. The size, composition, organizational structure, and financial arrangements of the groups are highly varied. Some group practices may have arrangements that involve sharing certain central services and still maintaining the physicians' individual practices. For example, each physician has his or her own office but may purchase office equipment and supplies or contract with a medical transcription service as a group. This concept allows the physician to remain independent and be competitive in the marketplace.

The group practice may be composed of many physicians of the same specialty or may be a multispecialty group. An example of a same-specialty practice is a group of obstetricians and gynecologists or a group of ophthalmologists. The group shares office space, equipment, nursing and support staff, and patient call (providing care 24 hours a day). The multispecialty group offers services in at least two specialty areas. A women's center is a good example of a multispecialty group practice; the providers at a women's center may include pediatricians, obstetricians, gynecologists, infertility specialists, and gerontologists. Many of the larger groups have their own ancillary services, such as a clinical laboratory and radiology units.

Corporate Practice Model

Reimbursement and regulatory requirements are becoming increasingly complex for physicians. The burden of running one's own business, in addition to practicing high quality medicine, can be overwhelming. Many physicians are seeking employment in group practices owned by health systems, hospitals, MCOs, or other entities. This type of corporate medicine allows physicians to focus less on the business aspects of running a physician practice and more on patients and clinical quality. With the implementation of health reform and an emphasis on wellness, the trend of physician employment will increase in the next decade.

Community Health Centers

In 1961 the Community Health Services and Facilities Act provided grants for the establishment of voluntary health planning agencies at the local level. These demonstration projects were developed to serve low-income areas. CHCs were designed to provide comprehensive care in a catchment area that has limited or nonexistent health services for certain populations or special health needs. A catchment area is a defined geographic area that is served by a health care program, project, or facility such as a hospital or mental health center. Services provided are usually directed at population groups and range from immunizations, diagnostic testing, and screening to nutrition counseling and family planning.

Funding for CHCs comes from a variety of sources, including monies from private, state, and federal grants; federal funds from the PHS and the Bureau of Community Health Services of DHHS; and funds from local or state health departments. Care at the centers may be provided at no charge, or the cost may be based on the patient's ability to pay, which is referred to as a sliding scale fee.

Community-Based Care

The term *community-based care* refers to the delivery of services that go beyond an institutional setting and reach out into the community. These services may include adult day care centers, clinics at public schools, visits by medical staff to homeless shelters, house calls to the homebound and older adults, meal services provided to older adults in need (Meals on Wheels Association of America), and mobile vans to provide testing and screening. Community-based programs are financed by a combination of funding that includes Medicare, Medicaid, other federal and state moneys, private donations, and other sources. In 1965, Title III of the Older Americans Act established funding for transportation and for chore, homemaker, and home health aides for older adults, all of which are forms of community-based care.

Surgicenters and Urgent Care Centers

Free-standing surgical facilities in which surgical procedures can be safely performed on the day of admission or on an outpatient basis are called *surgicenters* or *ambulatory surgery centers*. Many hospitals offer outpatient surgery. Patients need to be well enough to withstand the surgery and go home afterward. Urgent care, medical walk-in, and convenience care centers are for patients who need routine care or who have minor but urgent health problems. The facilities are usually open at least 12 hours a day, 7 days a week, and do not require appointments. The patient population is composed of those who do not have an established relationship with a physician in the area, those who are not established with any physician, and those whose physician is not accessible at the time of need.

Hospital Ambulatory Care

Hospital ambulatory care is "hospital-directed" health care that is provided to patients who are not admitted as inpatients and for which the hospital is responsible, regardless of the location of the health care. Hospital ambulatory care services include satellite clinics, observation units, outpatient departments, ancillary services, and other specialty clinics.

Satellite Clinics

Hospitals may own and operate one or more ambulatory care facilities called satellite clinics that are not located on the campus of the main hospital. Satellite clinics are established in areas that are convenient to the patients, such as places of employment, or in areas that are closer to a specific patient population.

Observation Unit

The observation unit of the hospital is a unit, department, or beds for the observation of patients who need assessment, evaluation, or monitoring because of a significant degree of instability or disability that does not require admission to the hospital as an inpatient. For the Medicare patient, CMS suggests that the physician use 24 hours as a benchmark; that is, if the patient is expected to require hospital care for 24 or more hours or meets the inpatient criteria for hospital admission (or both), the physician should admit the patient as an inpatient as opposed to an observation patient. The observation period should not exceed 36 to 48 hours.

Outpatient Departments

In outpatient departments or clinics of a hospital, primary care, or specialized medical care is provided to patients who are not admitted. In addition to primary care, outpatient departments diagnose and treat conditions that are not emergent in nature and yet require intervention within a short period, such as earaches, nausea, vomiting, diarrhea, muscle sprains, dizziness, headaches, and conjunctivitis. The specialty clinics that many hospitals operate include preadmission testing, pediatrics, obstetrics, gynecology, orthopedics, and surgery; the larger tertiary hospitals may offer clinics for such specialties as low-birth-weight neonatal care, high-risk pregnancy, sports medicine, and cancer.

Outpatient surgery departments include units within the hospital as well as satellite surgery centers that perform surgery for which admission is not required.

Ancillary Services (Professional Service Departments)

Ancillary services provide diagnostic and therapeutic services at the request of a physician to both inpatients and outpatients; the departments include radiology (medical imaging), clinical laboratory, physical therapy, occupational therapy, respiratory therapy, cardiographics, pharmacy, and other services. Hospital ancillary departments may provide treatment for conditions such as cancer and heart disease. A patient may seek outpatient radiation therapy or chemotherapy.

For example, physicians who are not equipped or trained to perform certain diagnostic procedures such as colonoscopy refer the patient to the appropriate ancillary department for the procedure. Ancillary services differ from other areas of the hospital because the hospital is able to charge patients or third parties directly and therefore generate revenue for the hospital. They are under the direction of physicians.

Hospitals

There is no single definition of the word *hospital*, and the hospital of the present is undergoing tremendous change because of pressures to contain cost and support a continuum of care that is of high quality and accessible to all. The hospital description provided in this section characterizes the traditional, stand-alone hospital.

The AHA defines a hospital as a health care facility that has an organized medical and professional staff, inpatient beds available 24 hours a day, and the primary function of providing inpatient medical, nursing, and other health-related services for surgical and nonsurgical conditions and usually provides some outpatient services, especially emergency care.[3]

Hospitals may be classified in numerous ways, including the following:
- Ownership
- Number of beds
- Length of stay
- Clinical classification
- Patients
- Organization

Recently, the critical access hospital (CAH) has evolved to meet the needs of a population that does not have adequate acute care facilities. A hospital classified as a CAH receives reimbursement enhancements for meeting the needs of an underserved area. A CAH is certified by the state as being necessary to the residents in the community or no hospital or other CAH is within 35 miles of the CAH. The CAH provides acute inpatient care, has no more than 25 beds, and has an annual average length of stay of 96 hours.[3]

SELF-ASSESSMENT QUIZ

4. Why are some people without adequate access to health care?

Ownership

Hospitals are either government owned (federal, state, or local) or nongovernment owned. Government-owned hospitals are not for profit, whereas nongovernment-owned hospitals may be for profit or not for profit.

Government-Owned Hospitals

Federally owned hospitals receive funding and administrative direction from the branch of the government that owns them. The federal government finances health care services and facilities for active and retired military personnel, their dependents, veterans, merchant marines, Native Americans, Native Alaskans, and other groups. For some of these groups—for example, the merchant marines—the health care provided is contracted out, whereas other groups, such as the American Indians, have their own government-funded and operated health care facilities.

The Department of Veterans Affairs (VA) medical centers are federally owned health care facilities that provide health benefits to people who have served in the U.S. military. Eligibility for hospital care requires that the person have a service-related condition or disability or be unable to pay for health care. Currently the VA owns and operates 152 hospitals and more than 1400 sites that provide care including ambulatory care and community-based outpatient clinics, nursing homes, and rehabilitation treatment programs. The VA is organized into 21 Veterans Integrated Service Networks (VISNs) that oversee and manage the various VA health care facilities. The Department of Defense provides health care for active and retired military personnel and their dependents. The facilities owned and operated by the department include the Army, Navy, Air Force, and Marine Corps, all of which offer comprehensive health care either on military bases or in regional centers.[24]

Much like federally owned hospitals, state, county, and city hospitals are guided by the respective government, depending on the needs of the population served. State hospitals include facilities for mental illness, the developmentally disabled, chronic disease, and medical education. County, district, and city hospitals are usually established to meet the health care needs of their communities. These hospitals are governed by locally elected officials.

Nongovernment-Owned Hospitals

The two types of nongovernment-owned hospitals are as follows:
- For profit
- Not for profit

The for-profit hospitals, also called proprietary, private, or investor-owned hospitals, are governed by the individual, partnership, or corporation that owns them. Larger corporations may own numerous hospitals or hospital chains and offer stock that is publicly traded. These facilities are operated in a manner to benefit the owners and investors financially.

The not-for-profit (voluntary) hospitals include those that are owned by churches and religious orders (e.g., Catholic,

Protestant) and those that are owned by industries, unions, and fraternal organizations or just community hospitals. Not-for-profit hospitals are usually exempt from paying local, state, and federal taxes in exchange for providing benefits to the community such as indigent care. The faith-based hospitals may incorporate aspects of the religion in their philosophy about care and leadership of the hospital. For example, Catholic hospitals may prohibit sterilization procedures performed for the purpose of birth control.

Bed Size (Bed Count)

The total number of inpatient beds with which the facility is equipped for patient admissions is its bed size (bed count). A facility is licensed by the state for a specific number of beds.

Length of Stay

The average length of stay for a hospital determines whether the hospital is classified as a short-term (acute) care facility or LTC facility. If the average length of stay is less than 30 days, the hospital is classified as a short-term (or acute) care facility; if the average length of stay is 30 or more days, the hospital is classified as a LTC facility.

Clinical Classification

According to the AHA, there are four major types of hospitals[3]:
- General
- Special
- Rehabilitation and chronic disease
- Psychiatric

Note that some references and literature classify rehabilitation and chronic disease hospitals and psychiatric hospitals as specialty hospitals.

General Hospital

The general hospital provides patient services, both diagnostic and therapeutic, for various medical conditions. These services include the following[3]:
- Radiographic services
- Clinical laboratory services
- Operating room services

Specialty Hospital

The specialty hospital provides diagnostic and therapeutic services for patients with a specific medical condition. Many hospitals provide health care for specific groups of people, such as children (pediatric hospitals) or women (women's hospitals). In addition, specialty hospitals provide care for specific conditions or diseases, such as mental illness (psychiatric hospitals), cancer (cancer hospitals), or burns (burn hospitals).

Rehabilitation and Chronic Disease Hospital

The rehabilitation and chronic disease facility provides diagnostic and therapeutic services to patients who are disabled or handicapped and require restorative and adjustive services. Of vital importance in these facilities are the physical therapy, occupational therapy, speech therapy, and psychological and social work services that are provided.

Psychiatric Hospital

The primary purpose of the psychiatric hospital is to provide diagnostic and therapeutic services for patients with a mental illness or a psychiatric-related illness. The primary focus of the health care is to provide behavioral health services, which includes psychiatric, psychological, and social work services to the patient.

Hospital Patients

People who are receiving or using health care services for which the hospital is liable or held accountable are considered to be hospital patients. Hospital patients include inpatients, observation patients, ambulatory care patients, emergency patients, and newborn inpatients. To be considered a hospital inpatient, the patient generally stays overnight and is provided room, board, and nursing service in a unit or area of the hospital. All other types of hospital patients are discussed under the appropriate service areas.

Organization

The following discussion is typical of the traditional hospital setting for a general acute care facility. However, with health care reform, hospitals are undergoing quantum changes, including the formation of joint ventures and alliances and partnering with MCOs, physicians, and other HCOs. Hospitals operate under numerous organizational schemes; a few of these are described in this section.

Historically, most hospitals have been organized in a hierarchical form in which the individuals at the top have authority that passes downward through a chain of command (Figure 1-2). This vertical operation gives the governing body the ultimate authority, followed by the chief executive officer (CEO). The organization includes a governing body, administration, medical staff, department heads or directors, supervisors, and numerous subordinates down to the staff and line workers. Communication is fairly restricted to the vertical. Physicians do not fall within the chain of command unless they are employees of the hospital. Certain physician specialties are more likely to be employed by the hospitals. These include pathologists, hospitalists, and, in some cases, anesthesiologists and emergency medicine physicians.

The matrix organization is increasing in popularity because it is flexible and supports multidimensional organization. The matrix organization supports general managers who focus on managing people and processes as opposed to strategy and structure. As the health care system has grown to be very complex, it has become increasingly difficult for one person (i.e., the CEO) to manage the organization effectively, so the matrix organization will have talented leaders who are focused on certain processes. The matrix organization gives way to horizontal, informal communications that embrace individual capabilities. Employees have dual responsibilities and may have two or more supervisors, but they have a shared vision that supports the organization as a whole.

Another type of organizational scheme that is growing in popularity is service line management. With this model, the

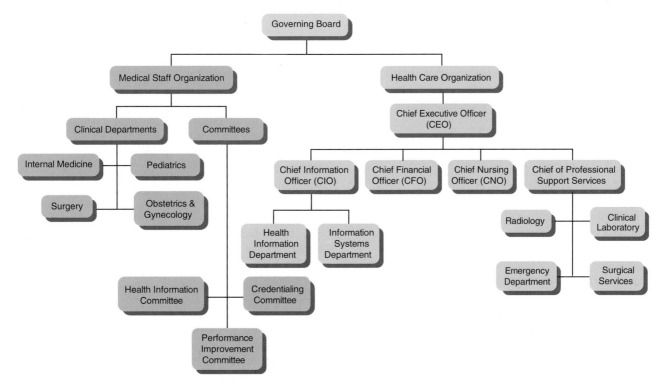

FIGURE 1-2 Health care facility organization chart. Health information management department may report to chief information officer, chief operating officer, or chief financial officer.

hospital may be organized around product line categories, such as obstetric, rehabilitation, and cardiology units, as opposed to departments, such as nursing, pharmacy, and respiratory therapy. Each service line will have dedicated support staff such as marketing, human resources, and so on.

Governance Structure

Although most hospitals today are forming alliances with other health care providers or are part of multihospital systems, this discussion of the organization is specific to the freestanding hospital. The organizational chart of a typical traditional hospital is shown in Figure 1-2.

The governing body or board, often called the *board of trustees, board of governors,* or *board of directors,* is a group of individuals who have the ultimate legal authority and responsibility for the operation of the hospital, including the quality and cost of care. The governing body of a voluntary (not-for-profit) hospital is usually composed of between 6 (for smaller hospitals) and 25 (for larger hospitals) board members who are not paid. Board members of for-profit hospitals typically receive financial compensation for participation. Board membership is usually made up of influential business and community leaders who have a vested interest in their community and perhaps a skill that would be of value to the board. For example, a business executive can provide support for the business aspect, and an attorney would have a better understanding of the legal issues. The medical staff has the right to be represented on the governing board. The CEO, medical staff, and other insiders may be members of the governing board but may or may not have voting privileges; the nonvoting members are often referred to as ex officio members.

According to TJC standards,[15] a hospital is required to do the following:
- Identify how it is governed and the key individuals involved.
- Establish policy and promote performance improvement.
- Provide for management and planning for the institution.
- Adopt bylaws addressing legal accountability and responsibilities to patients served.
- Provide for appropriate medical staff.
- Establish a criteria-based process for selecting a qualified and competent CEO.
- Provide for compliance with applicable laws and regulations.
- Provide for collaboration of leaders in developing, reviewing, and revising policies and procedures.
- Provide for conflict resolution.

The governing board functions according to bylaws established by the board, has regular meetings with documented minutes of the meetings, and has subcommittees that assist in the responsibilities of the governing board. The bylaws delineate the purposes of the organization, the composition and responsibilities of the board, meeting requirements, duties and responsibilities of officers and committees, selection of board members and officers, and revisions and amendments of the bylaws.

The governing board has standing committees and special committees. Standing committees may include the executive committee (conducts interim business), finance committee, medical staff, nominating committee, personnel, physician recruitment, and long-range planning. Special committees or task forces are created for specific projects or tasks and are disbanded on completion of the project or task.

The governing board has the ultimate responsibility for the quality of patient care and it depends on the HIM department to provide documentation to assist in and support decision making and long-range planning for the hospital. TJC has identified numerous information processes for which the governing body and organizational leaders are responsible, including obtaining, managing, and using information to improve patient care, governance, management, and support processes.[15] The governing body and administration depend on the HIM department not only to perform these processes in a timely, accurate manner, but also to ensure the accessibility, security, confidentiality, and integrity of the data in compliance with internal and external regulations.

Leadership

Leadership differs from hospital to hospital, depending on the hospital's size and organizational scheme. TJC states that the primary role of the leadership is planning, directing, coordinating, providing, and improving health care that responds to community and patient needs and improves health care outcomes. Leadership may be composed of a wide variety of organizational leaders or only a few, some of whom are briefly described here.

Chief Executive Officer

The CEO, also called *hospital administrator* or *president,* is recruited and selected by the governing board. This person is the principal administrative official of the hospital or other health care facility. At one time, the CEO was responsible for the day-to-day operation of the hospital. Today, however, the CEO's primary role involves creating hospital strategy, and ensuring that this strategy is implemented. Although the CEO is responsible for the hospital's operations, the direct oversight of daily operations is often relegated to a chief operating officer (COO).

The CEO serves as a liaison between the governing board and the medical staff. TJC standards stipulate that effective leadership of the hospital does the following[15]:
- Develops a strategic plan that supports the organization's mission, vision, and values.
- Communicates the mission, vision, and plan throughout the organization.
- Provides the framework to accomplish the goals that fulfill the vision.

At least annually, the plan for providing patient care should be reviewed to determine whether it meets identified patient needs and is consistent with the hospital mission; the plan should be revised as appropriate. The HIM department is involved in the preparation of much of the documentation, especially the following[25]:

- Clinical information
- Accreditation standards
- Risk management
- Utilization review
- Quality of patient care

Chief Operating Officer

The COO of a hospital is ultimately responsible for its day-to-day operations. A COO provides leadership, direction, and administration of operations in compliance with the mission and strategic plan of the organization. He or she oversees the operation of specific departments. For example, the COO may be responsible for coordinating hospital activities, such as ancillary or support services and other functional areas.

Chief Information Officer

The chief information officer (CIO) holds an executive position with primary responsibility for information resources management in the organization. He or she is involved in strategic planning, management, design, integration, and implementation of health information systems. Health information systems embrace the financial, administrative, and clinical information needs of the health care facility or organization. In hospitals, the usual departments that report to the CIO are information systems, telecommunications, HIM, and management engineering.

Chief Financial Officer

The financial operations of a health care institution are under the direction of the chief financial officer (CFO), who is sometimes called *director of finance* or *fiscal affairs director*. Although the title may vary, this person is often a director or hospital vice president who reports directly to the CEO or some other level in the administration. The CEO and the CFO also report to a finance committee within the governing body of the hospital. The finance committee is an advisory group within the board that is responsible for reviewing the hospital's financial position and making fiscally related decisions. According to TJC, the board and the CEO are responsible for the control and use of all financial resources.[15] The daily financial operation, however, is usually delegated to the CFO.

The financial department of a health care institution, under the direction of the CFO, is responsible for functions such as accounting, inventory control, payroll, accounts payable and receivable, cash management, billing, credit and collections, budgeting, cost accounting, fund accounting, and internal control. The functions within the finance arena involve the recording and reporting of financial information, the management of cash and other hospital assets, and planning and control. The CFO has overall responsibility for these areas and acts as an adviser to the CEO and the governing board on both daily operational issues and plans for the future.

Other Hospital Leadership

In addition to the leaders outlined in the previous discussion, hospitals may have a variety of leaders depending on the organization's size and scope. Chief nursing officers (CNOs) are clinical leaders that oversee the hospital's nursing staff. Some organizations have a chief quality officer who is responsible for ensuring good clinical quality of care. Additionally, other executives such as vice presidents, associate administrators, and so on, may exist to oversee particular areas of a hospital. Typically larger hospitals have larger leadership structures.

Medical Staff (Professional Staff Organization)

The medical staff is a formally organized staff of licensed physicians and other licensed providers as permitted by law (e.g., dentists, podiatrists, chiropractors) with the authority and responsibility to maintain proper standards of medical care. The medical staff is governed by its own bylaws, rules, and regulations, which must be approved by the hospital's governing board. TJC standards state that the primary responsibility of the medical staff is the quality of the professional services provided by the members with clinical privileges and the responsibility of being accountable to the governing body. **Clinical privileges** refer to the permission granted by the appropriate authority (governing board) to practitioners to provide well-defined patient care services in the granting institution on the basis of licensure, education, training, experience, competence, health status, and judgment. Each member of the medical staff has delineated clinical privileges that identify the specific patient care services the member may provide or perform independently in the hospital.[15]

The medical staff responsibilities include recommending to the governing board staff appointments and reappointments, credentialing (which is delineating clinical privileges), continuing medical education, and maintaining a high quality of patient care.

The organizational scheme of the medical staff includes officers, committees, and clinical services. TJC requires that there be an executive committee empowered to conduct medical staff business between staff meetings and be responsible to the governing body. In smaller hospitals, the medical staff as a whole serves as the executive committee. The executive committee is composed of members of the medical staff and an ex officio member from administration, usually the CEO or the CEO's designee.

The members of the medical staff are organized into areas of clinical services and departments that are usually representative of the medical specialties. Each service or department has an appointed director, department head, or chairperson. The services that are common to most hospitals are internal medicine, surgery, anesthesiology, pediatrics, obstetrics and gynecology, psychiatry, neurology, radiology and diagnostic imaging, and pathology. These are briefly defined in Table 1-3.

TABLE 1-3 Medical Specialties

Specialty	Description and Examples of Diagnoses and Procedures
Anesthesiology	Study and art of anesthesia administration, with and without loss of consciousness: epidural anesthesia, spinal anesthesia, inhalation of ether, analgesia maintenance
Cardiology	Study of cardiovascular system and treatment of its diseases: rheumatic heart disease, coronary artery disease, myocardial infarction, congestive heart failure
Cardiovascular surgery	Surgical specialty of the heart and blood vessels: coronary artery bypass graft, coronary arthrectomy, aneurysmectomy
Clinical informatics	Subspecialty that combines patient care and informatics knowledge that optimizes delivery of health care
Dermatology	Study and treatment of skin and diseases and conditions of skin: basal cell carcinoma, exfoliative dermatitis, pityriasis rosea, biopsies and excisions of lesions, cellulitis, acne vulgaris
Endocrinology	Study and treatment of the endocrine glands: diabetes mellitus (types I and II), thyroiditis, Addison's disease, adrenal virilism
Family medicine	Medical specialty that provides continuing, comprehensive health care for individuals and families; this is a specialty in breadth that integrates the biological, clinical, and behavioral sciences; scope encompasses all ages, both sexes, each organ system, and every disease entity
Gastroenterology	Study of digestive system and treatment of its disorders, including esophagus, stomach, intestines, liver, pancreas, and gallbladder, and ulcers, gastroenteritis, pylorospasm, gastritis, Crohn's disease
General surgery	Surgical specialty concerned with surgical treatment of diseases of the abdominal organs, skin, and breast: cholecystectomy, hernia repairs, appendectomies
Gynecology	Surgical specialty concerned with study of female reproductive and urinary systems and treatment of disorders: endometriosis, cystitis, herpes genitalia, mastitis, uterine prolapse, infertility
Hematology	Study and treatment of blood, blood-forming tissues, and blood disorders: anemias, leukemia, hemophilia, thrombocytopenic purpura, bone marrow biopsy
Hospitalist	Medical specialty in which primary focus is the general medical care of hospitalized patients: patient care, teaching, research, and leadership
Infectious disease	Study and treatment of diseases caused by pathogenic microorganisms, including contagious and noncontagious infections: AIDS, syphilis, tuberculosis, hepatitis, wound infections
Internal medicine	Study and treatment of disease of internal organs with nonsurgical therapy: hypertension, rheumatoid arthritis, meningitis
Interventional radiology	Subspecialty of radiology that involves performing invasive diagnostic and therapeutic procedures using imaging guidance on vascular structures and other body tissues; procedures include angiography, angioplasty, placement of drainage catheters, and radiofrequency ablation of tumors
Nephrology	Study and treatment of kidney and its diseases: acute and chronic kidney failure, polycystic kidney disease, nephrolithiasis, pyelonephritis, glomerulonephritis
Neurology	Study and treatment of nervous system and its diseases: cerebral palsy, brain abscess, cerebrovascular attack, Alzheimer's disease, Parkinson's disease
Neurosurgery	Surgical specialty involving study of nervous system and treatment of disorders: hydrocephalus, meningomyelocele, brain abscess, carpal tunnel syndrome
Obstetrics	Surgical specialty concerned with management of pregnancy, including prenatal, perinatal, and postnatal stages: normal pregnancy, placenta previa, eclampsia, ectopic pregnancy, gestational diabetes
Oncology	Study and treatment of cancer, including benign and malignant: melanoma, squamous cell carcinoma, multiple myeloma, Hodgkin's disease, leukemia
Ophthalmology	Surgical specialty concerned with study of eye and treatment of visual problems: cataracts, corneal transplant, diabetic retinopathy, visual acuity, optic nerve damage
Orthopedics	Surgical specialty dealing with musculoskeletal system, including prevention of disorders and restoration of function: arthritis, fractures, scoliosis, joint replacements, osteomyelitis
Otorhinolaryngology	Surgical specialty dealing with study and treatment of disorders of ears, nose, and throat: acute tracheitis, tonsillectomy and adenoidectomy, sinusitis, otitis media, deviated nasal septum
Pediatrics	Study and care of children, including normal growth and development: chickenpox, cystic fibrosis, pneumonia, immunizations, diarrhea, gastritis, mumps
Plastic and reconstructive surgery	Surgical specialty concerned with repair, restoration, and reconstruction of body structures: blepharoplasty, scar revision, liposuction, breast reduction and reconstruction, dermabrasion
Psychiatry	Study, diagnosis, and treatment of mental illness: anorexia nervosa, clinical depression, alcohol withdrawal syndrome, senile dementia
Pulmonary medicine	Study, diagnosis, and treatment of lung disorders: pneumonia, chronic obstructive pulmonary disease, asthma, cystic fibrosis, bronchiectasis, respiratory failure

TABLE 1-3	Medical Specialties—cont'd
Specialty	Description and Examples of Diagnoses and Procedures
Radiology	Use of radiant energy in study, diagnosis, and treatment of disease: computed tomography, radiography, echocardiography, magnetic resonance imaging, radiation therapy
Thoracic surgery	Surgical specialty dealing with study and treatment of thorax and its disorders: pneumonectomy, diaphragmatic hernia, lung abscess, thoracotomy, bronchial lavage
Urology	Surgical specialty concerned with study and treatment of male genitourinary system and female urinary system: vasectomy, nephrolithiasis, benign prostatic hyperplasia, transurethral resection of prostate

AIDS, Acquired immunodeficiency syndrome.

 CRITICAL THINKING

Create a table that briefly defines the following disorders and that identifies at least two specialties that would manage a patient with the disorder. The disorders are diabetes mellitus type I, Alzheimer's disease, glomerulonephritis, ulcerative colitis, gout, cholelithiasis, Meniere's disease, gestational diabetes, and prostatitis.

Essential Services

TJC identifies hospital services that must be provided on a regular basis and that are necessary for patient assessment and care. Patient assessment is the process of obtaining appropriate and necessary information about each individual seeking entry into a health care setting or service. The following services are essential to this function.[15]

Nursing Care

The nursing service is usually organized under the direction of a nurse executive (CNO, director, vice president), with nursing supervisors, department heads, charge nurses, and staff nurses. The nurse executive has the responsibility and authority to establish nursing standards, policies, and procedures that are in compliance with state law and professional standards.

Within an HCO, there are different levels of nursing, including staff nurse, nurse manager, clinical nurse specialist, and private duty nurse. The staff nurse provides direct patient care in a specific unit with assigned patients. For example, an RN or a LPN may be the staff nurse assigned to five patients in the well-baby nursery during the evening shift. The nurse manager may be a head nurse, nursing supervisor, or department head who is responsible for certain units or staff. This person makes patient assignments and staffing decisions and is responsible for the quality of care provided by the nursing staff. The clinical nurse specialist is considered an expert in a specialized area, such as neonatology or pain management. This person is an RN with advanced education or experience in the area of expertise. The clinical nurse specialist also works in research, education, administration, and consultation.[26] The private duty nurse is an RN or LPN who is employed by an external agency or individual to provide direct patient care to one patient for 8 to 12 hours for a certain period.

Some facilities may employ nursing assistants who, depending on the work environment, are known by many names, including certified nursing assistants (CNAs), patient care technicians, nurses aides, orderlies, and home health aides. The nursing assistants are eligible for certification that involves training and clinical experience obtained on the job. On completion and examination, they become CNAs. Nursing assistants work under the supervision of a nurse and they provide basic patient care, such as assisting the patient with bathing, dressing, and eating and obtaining vital signs.

Nursing care is based on a process that involves assessment, diagnosis, outcomes and planning, implementation, and evaluation of patient care, and the documentation in the health record must reflect this process. The HIM department often collaborates with the nursing service in collecting, analyzing, and disseminating data; in developing reports; and in addressing issues related to the health record. Issues of critical importance are the authenticity, completeness, timeliness, integrity, and security of both the paper and the EHR.

Diagnostic Radiology Services

The diagnostic radiology department (medical imaging department) functions in the diagnosing of diseases and conditions by using ionizing radiation (e.g., radiography, computed tomography, radioactive isotopes), ultrasonography, and magnetic resonance imaging. TJC requires health care facilities to provide diagnostic testing, including imaging, that is relevant both to determining the patient's health care needs and to the treatment of the patient.[15] An example of a diagnostic radiology procedure is mammography (breast radiography), which may be performed for the purpose of diagnosing breast cancers; an example of a therapeutic procedure is radiation therapy, which is performed for the purpose of treating malignant neoplasms (cancers).

The radiology department is headed by a radiologist (a physician), who may be called the chief or director of radiology. Under the direction of the radiologist is the technical staff, which includes physicians (radiation therapists, radiation physicists), radiology technologists, and radiation therapy technologists. Radiation therapy is often a separate department as well.

Nuclear Medicine

Nuclear medicine may be considered part of the radiology department, or it may be a separate department. It is distinguished from radiology, however, because the procedures involve the use of radioisotopes (radionuclides) for diagnosing and treating the patient. Unlike that in radiography, the image created in nuclear medicine gives information not only about the structure but also about the function of the organ or tissue under study. Examples of diagnostic procedures performed in nuclear medicine are nuclear scans of the thyroid, heart, and liver and radioimmunoassays, which are used to detect hormones and drugs in blood samples.

The staff in nuclear medicine, which is under the direction of a physician who specializes in nuclear medicine, includes nuclear medicine technicians or staff from the radiology department.

Dietary (Nutrition) Services

The dietetic service considers all nutritional aspects of the patient and patient care and provides high-quality nutrition to every patient. According to TJC, nutritional care must be provided in a timely and effective manner. Such care consists of nutritional assessment; nutritional therapy; diet preparation, distribution, or administration; nutritional education; and monitoring of the nutritional care of patients.[15]

Nutritional care is interdisciplinary and therefore involves not only dietetic services but also other members of the health care team, such as physicians and nurses. Dietetic services employ clinical dietitians, who are responsible for the therapeutic care of patients. Additional dietary staff is employed to assist with the preparation, serving, and delivery of food and the maintenance of dining services for the staff and visitors.

Pathology and Clinical Laboratory Services

This ancillary area assists in the prevention, diagnosis, and treatment of disease by examination and study of tissue specimens, blood and body secretions, and wound scrapings and drainage. The pathology and clinical laboratory department functions in serology, histology, cytology, bacteriology, hematology, blood bank, organ bank, biochemistry, and tissue preparation. These departments are commonly subunits of the pathology department.

Pathology and clinical laboratory services employ a variety of health professionals—medical laboratory technologist, medical laboratory technician, histotechnologist, and cytotechnologist—all of whom work under the direction of a pathologist.

Emergency Services

Emergency care service is a vital component of the acute care facility that provides care around the clock to patients who present with conditions that are urgent, life-threatening, or potentially disabling. The ED functional areas include a trauma area, examination rooms, psychiatric observation rooms, and observation beds. Coming through the ED is one of the primary ways patients are admitted into the hospital. A patient in the ED can be managed in one of the following ways: treated and discharged to home, treated and admitted for observation, treated and admitted to an inpatient unit, assessed and sent to surgery, stabilized and transferred to another facility, or, in the event of death, transferred to the morgue. Emergency services are primarily provided by physicians and RNs who specialize in emergency medicine.

In the ED, the patient has usually had the acute onset of a serious condition, such as a myocardial infarction (heart attack) or closed head injury, or has a complication of a chronic condition, such as ketoacidosis, which may occur with diabetes mellitus. When the patient arrives, the ED staff performs triage. The term *triage* is a French word originating from care on battlefields, where quick decisions had to be made regarding who could wait for care, who needed immediate care, and who was beyond benefiting from care. In the ED, triage is the process of sorting out for the purpose of early assessment to determine the urgency and priority for care and to determine the appropriate source of care. Triage promotes efficiency and effectiveness in the management of the diverse patient group arriving in the ED.[27]

In the United States, emergency patients are a diverse group because the need for care may range from relatively minor to serious, urgent, or life-threatening. People who do not have access to health care often use the ED for non-emergency problems. The inability to access health care may be due to numerous factors, such as an inability to pay, being either underinsured or uninsured, or not having a health care provider available in the area or at the time of need. In some areas, urgent care centers are not available, and patients use the ED for minor health problems.

In the United States, trauma is the leading cause of death in the 34 years or younger age group, and many of those deaths occur in EDs that are not recognized as trauma centers. To minimize the morbidity and mortality rate related to trauma, trauma centers were developed. Morbidity refers to the extent of illness, injury, or disability in a given population, and mortality means the death rate in a given population. A trauma center is an emergency care center that is specially staffed and equipped to handle trauma patients; most trauma centers are equipped with an air transport system. EDs are accredited by the ACS, and accredited EDs are verified to meet the criteria established by the *Resources for Optimal Care of the Injured Patient: 2006*. The designated level of care (Level I, II, or III) is crucial to the decision making of emergency personnel (paramedics, emergency medical technicians) in determining which facility is best suited to handle the health care needs of the transported patient. The assigned level of care is based on the center's hours of operation; availability of trauma surgeon, nurses, and other trained staff; and access to laboratory, radiology, surgery, anesthesia, equipment, and drugs. Emergency centers ranked as Level I offer the most comprehensive emergency care 24 hours a day, with at least one trauma surgeon or appropriate substitute on duty and access to various specialists. In addition to other criteria, the Level I trauma centers must admit at least 1200 trauma patients per year. Level II and Level III emergency services are also staffed 24 hours a day but have more lenient requirements for the availability of specialty physicians and nurses. EDs that are accredited to provide Level I or II care are recognized as trauma centers.[27]

Pharmaceutical Service

The pharmaceutical service is responsible for maintaining an adequate supply of medications, providing nursing units with floor stock, and preparing and dispensing medications with appropriate documentation. The pharmacist also prepares the intravenous fluids with any necessary additives and monitors adverse effects of drugs. Floor stock is an inventory of drugs that is maintained on each nursing unit; the stock varies in each unit, depending on the type of unit (e.g., cardiac intensive care vs. a pediatric unit). The pharmaceutical service will maintain a hospital formulary that provides information on drugs that are approved and maintained by the HCO. The hospital formulary contains information on drugs including, but not limited to, names, dosages and strengths, packaging, characteristics, and clinical usage.

The pharmaceutical service is under the direction of a state-licensed pharmacist, who is assisted by pharmaceutical technicians.

Physical Rehabilitation Services

The diagnosis and treatment of certain musculoskeletal and neuromuscular diseases and conditions are responsibilities of physical medicine and rehabilitation. This area covers physical therapy, occupational therapy, speech therapy, and audiology. Physical therapists are state licensed and trained to use light, heat, cold, water, ultrasound, electricity, and manual manipulation to improve or correct a musculoskeletal or neuromuscular problem. They often teach the patient exercises that will help to strengthen specific muscle groups or assist the patient to ambulate (walk) with an artificial limb. Occupational therapists work with the patient to minimize disability and teach the patient to compensate for the disability. For example, a patient who is permanently confined to a wheelchair and needs to resume housekeeping responsibilities may be taught how to shop for groceries or how to prepare a meal. Speech pathologists are concerned with human communication; they teach the patient how to compensate for difficulty with speech or the inability to speak. For example, a patient who stutters is taught speech exercises to help control or minimize the stuttering. Audiology is the science of hearing, and an audiologist would examine, evaluate, and prescribe therapy to patients with a hearing deficit.

Respiratory Care Services

Respiratory care services encompass diagnostic and therapeutic procedures for a wide variety of patients. The service is responsible for assisting with the provision of care for patients with various acute and chronic lung conditions. Responsibilities include administering oxygen, performing pulmonary function studies, administering inhalants such as bronchodilators, performing chest physiotherapy, obtaining and analyzing arterial blood gases, setting up and maintaining mechanical ventilators, and assisting in cardiopulmonary resuscitation. These therapists work under the direct order of a physician and provide respiratory care in all patient care areas of the hospital, as necessary.

Social Services

The department of social services is staffed by medical and psychiatric social workers who work with the patient and family members to help them understand the social, economic, and emotional factors related to therapy and recovery; identify and coordinate necessary community and medical care resources; and collaborate with and educate the hospital staff regarding social service concerns. Social workers are often responsible for discharge planning, thereby supporting the continuum of care.

Other Services

Information on additional hospital services, such as case management, pastoral care, ethics, patient representatives, patient escort, plant technology and safety management, and central supply, may be obtained by surveying area health care facilities.

Health Information Management

Although this book is devoted to HIM, a brief discussion is included to round out the functions of the hospital. The HIM department, or medical records department, is primarily responsible for the management of all paper and electronic patient information. It must develop and maintain an information system that is consistent with the mission of the health care facility and in compliance with regulatory and accrediting agencies. The department is responsible for the organization, maintenance, production, and dissemination of information, including privacy, data security, integrity, and access. Some of the functions of the department include clinical data management, transcription of medical and surgical notes, coding of diagnoses and surgical procedures, disclosing health information to authorized users, and retrieving and storing medical information. With the technological advances in information management, the increased demands for patient data, and the push for cost containment, efficiency, and accessibility of health care, the area of HIM is rapidly evolving and growing. As we move toward the EHR, new opportunities and challenges will evolve, and many of the roles and functions will change.

Subacute Care

Subacute care is a transitional level of care that may be necessary immediately after the initial phase of an acute illness. It is more commonly used with patients who have been hospitalized and are not yet ready for return to the LTC facility or to home care. The patient does require more advanced or specialized nursing care than is normally provided in the nursing facility or in home health programs. The location of subacute care may be a designated area of either the hospital or a nursing facility or may be provided by a home health agency.

Home Care (Home Health Care)

Home health care is the provision of medical and nonmedical care in the home or place of residence to promote, maintain, or restore health or to minimize the effect of disease or disability.[2] With the exception of hospice, the location of the health care services distinguishes home health from other types of care facilities and programs. Home care services mainly provide care for rehabilitation therapies and postacute care. Home health services are a medical adjunct to acute care, which extends the continuum of care from the inpatient to the home setting.

The patient population for home health care is dominated by older adults, although younger adults and children use the service. Home health care for the older adult population is viewed as achieving cost savings compared with longer hospital stays or LTC. It is also life enriching because it enables patients to remain in the comfort of their homes.

Home health has grown rapidly since 1965, when the Medicare program was established and allowed reimbursement for home care. The Medicare definition of home health care stipulates that the needed nursing care, physical therapy, or speech therapy must be skilled intermittent care provided under a physician's written direction and plan of care in the residence of the homebound client.[28] Simply put, Medicare requires that the home care provided be physician directed and that it involve regularly scheduled home visits. For example, a home care patient who is receiving oxygen therapy may be initially visited four times a week for one week by an RN. One of the goals of therapy is to have the patient or family assume responsibility for care, with visits by the RN being reduced to once or twice a week. However, if the patient is living alone and needs assistance with self-care, then a nurse's aide, in addition to the RN, may visit every other day to assist with personal care.

Long-Term Care Facilities

LTC is health care that is provided over a long period (30 or more days) to patients who have chronic diseases or disabilities. The facilities providing the LTC are considered to be nonacute care facilities. The type of care a patient can receive is highly variable and ranges from personal care and social, recreational, and dietary services to skilled nursing or rehabilitation care.[5] Patients admitted to LTC facilities are usually called *residents* because the patient resides in the facility. The term *nursing home* is a layperson's term for any and all LTC facilities; the appropriate term is skilled nursing facility (SNF).

Skilled nursing facilities are required by law to employ sufficient nursing personnel on a 24-hour basis to provide care to each resident according to the care plan.[5] Among other things, nursing facilities are required to provide skilled nursing care and related services for patients who require medical, nursing, or rehabilitative care. Examples of SNF care include wound care, intravenous injections, and physical or speech therapy. The need for custodial care (i.e., assistance with bathing, eating, and dressing) does not qualify the patient for Medicare coverage in a SNF. However, Medicare will cover these services along with the activities of daily living for patients requiring skilled nursing care or rehabilitative services.[28]

To be certified as a Medicare or Medicaid provider, a nursing facility must comply with the COP. An LTC facility is licensed by the state to provide a designated level of care, which may simply be personal care or room and board, or may require skilled nursing. A facility may be licensed to provide different levels of care; if so, the number of beds for each level of care is designated.

The patient population in LTC facilities is primarily older adults who are unable to live independently, but it also includes people of all ages who are convalescing, are being rehabilitated, or who have a chronic condition that requires long-term health care services (e.g., Alzheimer's disease, senile dementia).

There are several types of LTC facilities.

Assisted Living

An assisted living facility typically offers housing and board with a broad range of personal and supportive care services. Most residents of assisted living facilities privately pay for services, as they are often not covered by any insurer.

Domiciliary or Custodial (Residential)

Supervision, room, and board are provided for people who are unable to live independently. Most residents need assistance with activities of daily living (e.g., bathing, eating, dressing).

Independent Living Facility

An independent living facility is composed of apartments and condominiums that allow residents to live independently; assistance (e.g., dietary, health care, social services) is available as needed by residents.

Life Care Centers

Also called retirement communities, life care centers provide living accommodations and meals for a monthly fee. They offer a variety of services, including housekeeping, recreation, health care, laundry, and exercise programs.

Nursing Facility

Nursing facility is a comprehensive term for an LTC facility that provides nursing care and related services for residents who require medical, nursing, or rehabilitative care. A sufficient number of skilled nursing personnel must be employed on a 24-hour basis to provide care to residents according to the care plan.

Swing Beds

Hospital swing beds are designated beds that have the flexibility of serving as acute care or postacute long-term beds. Certain small, rural hospitals or CAHs that are Medicare certified are allowed to have swing beds for acute or SNF health care. Among other things, the patient using the swing bed for postacute care must have been an inpatient in an acute care facility for 3 consecutive days and on discharge is admitted to the swing bed hospital for posthospital extended care. The costs for the posthospital extended care are covered by

Medicare Part A. The concept of swing beds was established by the Social Security Act.

Hospice Care

The concept of hospice, meaning "given to hospitality," dates back to the medieval period, when weary travelers were provided a place for shelter and rest. Today, a hospice is a multidisciplinary health care program that is responsible for the palliative and supportive care of terminally ill patients and their families, with consideration for their physical, spiritual, social, and economic needs. Palliative care consists of health care services that relieve or alleviate patient symptoms and discomforts, such as pain and nausea; it is not curative. The primary goal of a hospice is to allow patients to die with dignity in their homes or a homelike environment. Most hospice patients have cancer, but many hospices accept other terminally ill patients, such as those with AIDS or end-stage kidney, heart, or lung disease.

The type of program that is suitable often depends on the patient's condition and the support available in the patient's home (Table 1-4). For the patient who remains in the home, most hospices require that a primary caregiver be identified who will assist with care; the primary caregiver may be a spouse, family member, friend, or live-in companion. Other hospice programs, such as skilled nursing facilities, may have units or beds for hospice patients who are unable to remain in their homes. Hospice patients may require hospitalization for acute symptom management (pain, vomiting, infection) or when the primary care person needs a respite or break.

Hospice programs are physician directed and multidisciplinary in that numerous caregivers are involved in providing care. Caregivers for hospice include nurses, social workers, nurse's aides, clergy, dietitians, and trained volunteers who run errands, mow grass, do housekeeping chores, cook, and perform other necessary jobs that allow the patient to remain in the home.

TABLE 1-4 Models of Hospice Care

Type	Description
Home health agency–based	Owned and operated by private, freestanding home health agencies; care provided in home
Hospital-based	Owned and operated by hospital: rooms or departments allotted for hospice care; care provided in facility or home
Independent community–based	Usually nonprofit; governed by community board, independent; care provided in home
Nursing facility–based	Owned and operated by a nursing facility; rooms or units allotted for hospice care; care provided in facility
Other models	Owned by religious orders, health maintenance organizations, combinations of the other models

Reimbursement for hospice care comes from Medicare, Medicaid, private pay, third-party payers, community funds, and other sources.

Respite Care

Respite care is a type of short-term care in which the focus is on giving caregivers time off yet continuing the care of the patient. This may involve someone spending the day with the patient in the home, admitting the patient to an adult or child day care, or providing temporary institutionalization. Respite care is often provided to caregivers of terminally ill patients or severely disabled children or adults.

> **? DID YOU KNOW?**
>
> Racial and ethnic minorities experience a different quality of care than other patients. In nursing homes, facilities with higher percentages of minorities report lower quality of care and lower financial performance.

Complementary and Alternative Medicine

Complementary and alternative medicine (CAM) refers to therapies (usually not included in Western medicine) that may or may not have been proven to be effective. Complementary medicine includes those practices that could be used along with conventional therapies. For example, aromatherapy might be used to relax a patient after a surgical procedure, whereas alternative medicine consists of those practices that would be used in lieu of conventional medicine. For example, patients may choose to use dietary supplements of soy protein to lower blood cholesterol as opposed to the cholesterol-lowering medications whose efficacies have been proven. The CAM therapies include herbal remedies, massage therapy, natural food diets, acupuncture, and biofeedback. The NIH established the National Center for Complementary and Alternative Medicine (NCCAM) to explore the science, train researchers, and disseminate authoritative information to the public and professionals regarding CAM.

> **✓ SELF-ASSESSMENT QUIZ**
>
>
> 5. Identify the five different terms that might be used to identify a patient, and state what health care facilities (or organizations) would use these terms.

E-Health

E-health is the use of emerging information and communication technology, especially the Internet, to improve or enable health and health care. The field of e-health includes a range of functions and capabilities such as specialized search engines focused on various kinds of health care; provider and payer websites, some of which give consumers access to their own information or the ability to communicate with the provider, make appointments, or renew prescriptions; support groups; web-based physician consultations;

self-care or monitoring systems; telemedicine; and disease management. As with other Internet-related sectors, the status of the e-health arena is extremely fluid and characterized by rapid developments in the commercial and noncommercial sectors.

Adult Day Care Services

An adult day care service is a health care program that provides supervision, medical and psychological care, and social activities for older adults (referred to as clients) who reside at home. These clients either cannot stay alone or prefer the social interaction during the day. Services provided may include intake assessment, health monitoring, occupational therapy, personal care, activities, transportation, and meals.[3]

Mobile Diagnostic Services

A growing trend is to transport health care services to the patient, especially in the area of diagnostic procedures and preventive services. Mammography and magnetic resonance imaging require expensive equipment that may not be available in small communities and rural areas. Mobile units from larger health care facilities are now transporting this advanced equipment and staff to these areas. Preventive services such as immunizations, blood pressure measurement, and cholesterol screening are easily provided from mobile units, which may even be staffed by volunteer health professionals.

Contract Services

The use of contract services, also called outsourcing, by HCOs is increasing. Contract services may include food, laundry, housekeeping, medical waste disposal, release of information services, transcription, coding, collections, and clinical services such as physical therapy, emergency care, and speech pathology. With the increase in the use of contract services, providers are expecting improved quality with cost containment.

CRITICAL THINKING

A 74-year-old woman is in the end stages of Alzheimer's disease and lives at home, where her 80-year-old husband provides care for her. He has caregivers who visit every day for 4 hours to assist with her care. She is confined to her bed and wheelchair, and no longer communicates verbally. She is not expected to live beyond the next 4 months. Identify at least four types of health care services and two specialists appropriate for this patient and the family. Explain each of your choices.

Health Care Delivery Systems

In recent years, integrated delivery systems (IDS), which involve various ownerships and linkages among hospitals, physicians, and insurers, have evolved. An IDS is a vertical integration of HCOs, defined as a network of HCOs that provide or arrange to provide a continuum of services to a population; the network assumes the clinical and fiscal responsibility for the outcomes and health status of the population. The IDS may include an acute care facility, a subacute care facility, an LTC facility, a pediatric hospital, a rehabilitation facility, a psychiatric hospital, and numerous physicians and may provide mobile diagnostic services. The IDS is formed for the purpose of (1) providing more cost-effective care than an array of HCOs, (2) contracting with providers who take responsibility for the quality of care and provide the care in a cost-effective manner, and (3) protecting the autonomy of participating providers. By participating in an IDS, providers have input into how the IDS is run and get more patient referrals.

Health reform under PPACA has facilitated the creation of accountable care organizations (ACOs). ACOs are groups of providers that collaborate with the goal of giving high quality, coordinated care to Medicare patients. The providers involved in ACOs may include physicians, hospitals, home health agencies, and other health care delivery organizations. The goal of ACOs is to coordinate care for a particular patient population to ensure that care is delivered efficiently and effectively. In addition to quality improvement, cost savings is another important goal of ACOs. Although most ACOs are in the early stages of development, generating an integrated model of health care for particular patient populations is quickly becoming the goal for most health care systems. This form of care coordination is likely to expand beyond the Medicare population.

Although the IDS is a vertical integration, a merging of HCOs offering services at the same point on the continuum of care is a horizontal integration. For example, an acute care hospital may join with another hospital that provides similar services but to a different population or at a different location.

HEALTH CARE PROFESSIONALS

The health care systems in the United States are labor intensive, using large numbers of highly skilled health care professionals and practitioners. There are more than 200 health occupations in the United States. The places of employment are just as varied, including hospitals, medical offices, insurance companies, nursing facilities, pharmacies, MCOs, schools, correctional facilities, and pharmaceutical and medical supply companies.

Wilson and Neuhauser[29] defined health care professionals as having the following attributes:

- Certification or licensure is required for membership in the profession.
- A national or regional professional association exists.
- A defined body of scientific knowledge and certain technical skills are required for practice.
- A code of ethics exists.
- Members of the profession practice with a degree of authority and have expertise for decision making in their area of competence.

Health Care Team

Almost all health care is provided by a multidisciplinary team of professionals. Being a member of the health care team requires that each person be responsible for his or her area of expertise with consideration for the contributions of other team members. The ultimate goal is comprehensive care for the patient as a whole. The health care team is composed of individuals who work either directly or indirectly to accomplish the goals of patient care. A physician directs the health care team by determining the plan of care, with team members complementing and supplementing each other's contributions. The makeup of the team depends on the patient's needs, the setting for health care, and the physician. For example, the health care team for a patient who is a resident in an LTC facility consists of a primary care physician (perhaps a gerontologist), nursing staff (RN, LPN), a dietitian, a physical therapist, a recreation therapist, a nursing assistant, and a pharmacist. A patient in this setting is not likely to need a nurse anesthetist or surgeon.

Terms such as *technologist, technician, therapist, paraprofessional, assistant,* and *aide* are often used to describe certain health care providers. *Technologist* and *therapist* imply education at or above the bachelor degree level; *technician* and *assistant* indicate education or training at or above the associate degree level; and *assistant* and *aide* refer to on-the-job training.

Most health care occupations can be classified into one of the following categories:

- Independent practitioner
- Dependent practitioner
- Supporting staff

The independent practitioner category includes those who by law may provide a range of services without the consent or approval of a third party. The dependent practitioner category includes those who by law may deliver a limited range of services (often specified by law) under the supervision or authorization of the independent practitioner. Some health occupations may move from one category to another, depending on state law; for example, NP and nurse midwife may be in either the dependent or the independent category on the basis of responsibilities and place of employment. The term *midlevel practitioner* refers to individuals, other than physicians, dentists, or podiatrists, who can dispense controlled substances within their professional practice. The midlevel practitioner is a dependent practitioner who may be a nurse midwife, nurse anesthetist, or PA, among others. The third category is the supporting staff, who function under the supervision or authorization of independent or dependent practitioners.[5] A fourth category that must be identified is the noncaregiving group, which includes all people who have no direct patient contact yet make significant contributions to the health care systems.

Physicians

The primary leader of the traditional health care team is most often the physician; some exceptions to this are the independent practices of NPs, podiatrists, chiropractors, optometrists, and nurse midwives. A physician is qualified by formal education and legal authority through licensure to practice medicine. Typically, physicians have practiced medicine by using clinical guidelines and policies that were primarily derived from expert opinion and clinical judgment. Today, there is a trend toward physicians using evidence-based medicine to make medical decisions, which means that the guidelines or medical decision making is supported by research.[2]

Types

There are two types of physicians: doctor of medicine (MD) and doctor of osteopathic medicine (DO). Both types of physicians are licensed by each state as medical practitioners who may diagnose, provide treatment, perform surgery, and prescribe medication. They both complete 4 years of medical education, a supervised internship or residency program, and state licensing examinations. The DO practices comprehensive medicine that uses manipulative therapy along with more traditional forms of therapy.

Medical Education and Training

The framework for medical education as we know it today dates back to 1910, when Abraham Flexner published a report that identified numerous serious deficiencies and inconsistencies in medical education. As a result of this report, most medical schools follow the Flexner model.

Today, admission to medical school requires 3 to 4 years of undergraduate work in the sciences and a competitive score on the Medical College Admission Test (MCAT). Medical school (undergraduate medical education) consists of medical science courses and clinical experience. The medical degree is awarded on completion of medical school. However, a person must still pass an examination to obtain a state license to practice medicine.

Licensure

The Federation Licensing Examination (FLEX) is a standardized licensure test developed by the Federation of State Medical Boards of the United States. The scores for successful completion vary from state to state.

An alternative to the FLEX is an examination developed by the National Board of Medical Examiners (NBME). The Board is dedicated to preparing and administering high-quality examinations for state licensure, collaborating with the state licensing boards in achieving goals of quality, supporting quality in medical education, and developing and evaluating testing methods, medical knowledge, and competence. The three-part NBME examination allows the student to be tested at intervals during training. After passing the NBME examination or FLEX and completing 1 year of residency, a medical physician may apply for state licensure, which authorizes him or her to practice medicine.

After graduation from medical school, the physician may complete a residency that consists of several years of training in a teaching hospital; during residency, the physician works under the supervision of licensed physicians. The residency program is considered to be graduate medical education. Depending on the chosen specialty, the residency may vary from 3 to 7 years. Because of the large numbers of physicians who require a residency program, a National Residency Matching Program was established to match applicants with hospital preferences, much like a clearinghouse for the residency program. The hospital residency programs are accredited by the Accreditation Council on Graduate Medical Education, which is composed of representatives from the public, residents, federal government, and professional organizations, including the AMA, AHA, and American Board of Medical Specialties.

Although there is an increasing demand for generalists (i.e., family practitioners, internists), many physicians seek certification in a specialty area. There are many specialties and subspecialties in the practice of medicine, such as neurology, hematology, oncology, cardiology, and pediatrics. Examples of surgical specialties and subspecialties are orthopedics, obstetrics, gynecology, and neurosurgery. To become board certified, the physician must meet certain requirements established by the Board of Certification, which is under the jurisdiction of the specialty. For example, to become board certified, surgeons must demonstrate additional training time and proven competence, and complete rigorous examination. In addition, physicians who are accepted for a fellowship at a specialty college are highly respected by the medical profession in their area of expertise.

Physician Assistant

The PA is a midlevel practitioner trained to assist the physician in various capacities, including evaluating, monitoring, and diagnosing patients. In addition, PAs may perform routine therapeutic procedures, counsel, and refer patients as necessary. Some states grant the PA prescriptive authority. Most PAs are employed in primary care and have proved to be cost-effective.

A surgeon assistant is a PA who has specialized in surgery. In addition to assisting the surgeon during operative procedures, the surgeon assistant performs other health care services including physical assessments and patient education.

Nursing

In the United States, nursing is the single largest health care profession; as of 2009, there were more than 2.5 million RNs employed in the United States.[30] They are employed in a wide variety of facilities, including hospitals, physician offices, patient homes, schools, camps, occupational and industrial settings, public health facilities, and private practice. Therefore it is important for the HIM professional to have a good understanding of the roles and responsibilities of the nurse in health care systems.

According to the American Nurses Association (ANA), the responsibilities of RNs include the following:

- Perform physical exams and health histories,
- Provide health promotion, counseling and education,
- Administer medications, wound care, and numerous other personalized interventions,
- Interpret patient information and make critical decisions about needed actions,
- Coordinate care, in collaboration with a wide array of health care professionals,
- Direct and supervise care delivered by other health care personnel, and
- Conduct research in support of improved practice and patient outcomes.[26]

Nursing practice includes but is not limited to clinical practice, administration, education, research, consultation, and management. Nursing care standards have been developed by professional organizations, such as the ANA; the standards address policies, procedures, and written mechanisms. Although nursing care is integrated and provided throughout various settings, nursing practice itself is regulated by the individual states as stipulated by the Nurse Practice Act of each state.

Nursing Care Models

Nursing care may be provided by various models, including primary nursing, patient-focused care, and team nursing. The term *primary* implies that one nurse is responsible for the management of care for each assigned patient. With primary nursing, the RN is responsible for the entire patient stay, 24 hours a day. The RN develops a written plan of care for each patient assignment. All other nurses who are providing care to this patient follow, update, and revise the plan of care as necessary.

Types and Education

The major types of nursing are registered nursing and licensed practical nursing (sometimes called *licensed vocational nursing*). Table 1-5 outlines the education and training of nurses and their various roles and responsibilities. To practice as an RN, one must graduate from a state-approved school of nursing and pass a state licensing examination.

Specialties

In addition to the various educational levels of nursing, many specialties and subspecialties are available, including the following:

- A certified nurse midwife is an RN who has completed advanced training in a program accredited by the American College of Nurse–Midwives and who is certified as a nurse midwife. The primary focus of health care is on well-woman gynecologic and low-risk obstetric care, including prenatal, labor and delivery, and postpartum care.[26]
- A certified registered nurse anesthetist (CRNA) is an RN with specialized training in the administration and control of anesthesia and in the evaluation and management of a patient's physiology during the preoperative, operative, and postoperative periods. Requirements for practice include completion of a master's degree in a nurse anesthetist program accredited by the American Association

TABLE 1-5   Education for Professional Nurses

Degree and Level Attained	Years of College	Examples of Roles and Responsibilities
Doctor of Science in Nursing (DNS) or Doctor of Philosophy (PhD)	3–5 years graduate work (postbaccalaureate) with clinical	Researcher, educator, administrator, clinician, director of nursing
Master of Science in Nursing (MSN)	5–6 academic years with clinical	Nurse practitioner, clinical nurse specialist, administrator, director of nursing, supervisor, nurse manager
Baccalaureate degree (BSN)	4 full years with clinical	Nursing supervisor, head nurse, charge nurse, nurse manager
Associate degree	2 years with clinical	Charge nurse, nurse manager, staff nurse
Diploma	27–36 months with clinical	Charge nurse, nurse manager, staff nurse
Licensed practical nurse (LPN) or licensed vocational nurse (LVN)	1 year with clinical	Staff nurse, nurse manager; works under the supervision of registered nurse, physician, or some other professional authorized by state law

of Nurse Anesthetists and successful completion of a national certification examination.[26]

- A NP is an RN who is prepared to provide primary and preventive health care services. NPs practice in all types of health care settings, such as clinics, hospitals, schools, and private practice. They usually specialize in a specific area, such as family practice, pediatrics, public health, geriatrics, or maternal–infant care. Certification for NPs is offered by professional organizations such as the National Board of Pediatric Nurse Practitioners.[30]

Allied Health Professionals

The federal government has defined an allied health professional (PL 102-408, the Health Professions Education Amendment of 1991) as a health professional other than an RN or a PA who (1) has received a certificate or an associate, bachelor's, master's, or doctoral degree or postdoctoral training in a science relating to health care and (2) shares in the responsibility for the delivery of health care services or related services, including the following:

- Identification, evaluation, and prevention of diseases and disorders
- Dietary and nutritional services
- Health promotion services
- Rehabilitation services
- Health systems management services
- Those meeting the federal government's definition, such as HIM professionals

Allied health professionals are involved in every facet of care, including diagnostic and therapeutic procedures, education, counseling, and evaluation and management of care, all of which are directed at assisting the physician with patient care. Many allied health professionals are employed in an ancillary department of the hospital. As health care delivery has advanced in sophisticated technology and specialization, the area of allied health has grown tremendously. There are hundreds of health care occupations in the United States, some of which are found in HIM, medical technology, respiratory therapy, occupational therapy, physical therapy, and nutritional therapy.

Although not true for HIM professionals, most allied health personnel function by order of physicians. In hospitals that are organized by departments, allied health professionals are employed in a specific department; in hospitals that are organized by function, allied health professionals may be cross-trained in several areas and employed in units that provide patient-focused care. Allied health professionals were also discussed in the section on the organization of hospitals.

SELF-ASSESSMENT QUESTION

6. List at least four types of health care professionals and describe their role, training, and requirements (credentials) for practice.
7. Search the literature for the three levels of trauma centers described in this chapter and distinguish among the levels.
8. Describe and distinguish between SNF, assisted living, and independent living for older adult patients.

FINANCING HEALTH CARE

Paying for health care services in the United States is a complex system that involves multiple payers and numerous mechanisms of payment. Payment methods may be direct pay or indirect pay. Payment by the patient to the provider is referred to as self-pay, out-of-pocket pay, or direct pay. Indirect pay involves payment by a third party to the provider on behalf of the patient. Indirect payers may be the government, insurance companies, managed-care programs, or self-insured companies.

Insurance is a purchased contract (policy) in which the purchaser (insured) is protected from loss by the insurer's agreeing to reimburse for such loss. When the patient contracts with a health insurance company to provide health care coverage, payments for health care are considered indirect; in coinsurance, the insured is partially liable for the debt. Many people are employed by companies that offer health care insurance at a group rate; the company may finance its own insurance company (self-insured companies) or contract with an insurance company to provide coverage. Some employers (purchasers) may pay for the insurance in its entirety, some share the cost of premiums, and others merely negotiate the group rate and the employee bears the entire cost.

Some health care providers are beginning to contract directly with employers to provide health care, eliminating the insurance carriers; this direct contracting reduces costs. Additionally, employers can negotiate costs with high-quality providers on behalf of their employees. Health insurance exchanges have been introduced under PPACA. Beginning in October of 2013, health insurance exchanges became available for the residents of each state. Some exchanges are administered by the states, and some states have opted to let the federal government run the exchanges. These exchanges are electronic marketplaces through which individuals can shop for health insurance. They provide information about different plans that can be directly compared. Additionally, various levels of benefits are defined through these exchanges. Health insurance exchanges were created to facilitate the uptake of health insurance as a result of the individual mandate that requires all citizens to have health insurance coverage. Individuals who are not eligible for a group insurance plan through their employers, or who opt to purchase insurance independent of their employment use these exchanges.

One of the largest nonprofit insurance companies in the United States is Blue Cross and Blue Shield of America (BCBS). BCBS is composed of Blue Cross, which is insurance that covers certain hospital services, and Blue Shield, which is insurance that covers certain physician services and other health care services. Like other insurance companies, BCBS negotiates numerous health care contracts with employers, professional organizations or associations, schools, and

individuals. The coverage, benefits, costs, deductibles, grace periods, and other policy specifications vary from group to group (Box 1-4).

Reimbursement

Reimbursement is critical to the livelihood of every health care facility and provider. In the United States, reimbursement for health care is a function of multiple payers, some of which are discussed in this section. The agreement between the third-party payers and the providers concerning what will be paid for and how much will be paid to the provider is called the reimbursement formula. These formulas are quite complicated and differ according to what was negotiated between the provider and the third-party payer. These are often referred to as the contracted amount.

Historically, payment for health care services has been by the retrospective payment system. With this payment method, charges for health care services are determined after the health care is provided. The actual amount paid may be based on fee-for-service or on the usual, customary, and reasonable charges. Fee-for-service is a reimbursement method in which the cost is based on the provider's charge for each service (e.g., charges for each x-ray test, laboratory test). Hospitals are paid on the basis of the number of days the patient needed care and the resources used during the course of treatment, such as medications, laboratory tests, and medical supplies. The usual, customary, and reasonable charges are based on the physician's usual charge for the service, the amount that physicians in the area usually charge for the same service, and whether the amount charged is reasonable

---

BOX 1-4   Terminology Common to Health Insurance Policies

Beneficiary—A *beneficiary* is one who is eligible to receive or is receiving benefits from an insurance policy or a managed-care program.

Benefit—A *benefit* is the amount of money paid for specific health care services or, in managed care, the health care services that will be provided or for which the provider will be paid.

Benefit period—The **benefit period** is the time frame in which the insurance benefits are covered; varies from policy to policy.

Claim—A **claim** is a request for payment by the insured or the provider for services covered.

Copayment—A *copayment* is a type of cost sharing in which the insured (subscriber) pays out-of-pocket a fixed amount for health care services.

Coverage—*Coverage* refers to the types of diseases, conditions, and diagnostic and therapeutic procedures for which the insurance policy will pay.

Deductible—The *deductible* is the amount of cost that the beneficiary must incur before the insurance will assume liability for the remaining cost.

Exclusion—An *exclusion* is a specific condition or hazard for which a health care policy will not grant benefit payments; often includes preexisting conditions and experimental therapy.

Fiscal intermediary—A *fiscal intermediary* is a contractor that manages the health care claims.

Insurance—*Insurance* is a purchased contract (policy) in which the purchaser (insured) is protected from loss by the insurer's agreeing to reimburse for such loss.

Out-of-pocket costs—*Out-of-pocket costs* are monies that the patient pays directly to the health care provider.

Payer—A *payer* is the party financially responsible for reimbursement of health care costs.

Policy—A *policy* is a written contract between insurance company and subscriber (insured) that specifies the coverage, benefits, exclusions, copayments, deductibles, benefit period, and so on.

Preexisting condition—A *preexisting condition* is a disease, injury, or condition identified as having occurred before a specific date.

Premium—A *premium* is a payment required to maintain policy coverage; usually paid periodically.

Reimbursement—*Reimbursement* is payment by a third party to a provider of health care.

Rider—A *rider* is a policy amendment that either increases or decreases benefits.

Subscriber—A *subscriber* is a person who elects to enroll or participate in managed care or purchase health care insurance.

Third-party payer—A *third-party payer* is the party (insurance company, state or federal government, other) responsible for paying the provider on behalf of the insured (subscriber, patient, member) for health care services rendered.

for the service provided. In low-income community or public health programs, the cost for care may be based on the patient's ability to pay, referred to as a sliding scale fee.

Another form of reimbursement, the capitation method, is common in managed-care programs. In the capitation method, a prepaid, fixed amount is paid to the provider for each person (per capita) served, regardless of how much or how often the patient receives health care services.[4]

Managed Care

The HIM professional needs to develop an understanding of managed care because it greatly affects the health care field and has unique information needs. Managed care is a generic term for a health care reimbursement system that is designed to minimize use of services and contain costs while ensuring the quality of care. The term *managed care* encompasses a continuum of practice arrangements, including health maintenance organizations (HMOs), preferred provider organizations (PPOs), and other alternative delivery systems. The characteristics of the various managed-care programs are highly varied; some are discussed here.

MCOs contract with employers, unions, individuals, and other purchasers to provide comprehensive health care to people who voluntarily enroll in the plan. On the basis of the arrangement, the MCO provides the health care services or arranges for services while controlling the cost and use of those services. With this in mind, one can see that some models integrate health insurance, delivery, and payment within one organization and exercise control over use. Providers who agree to participate in the managed-care plans may be salaried employees, paid fee-for-service or by capitation, or may negotiate a unique financial arrangement.

Health Maintenance Organizations

The oldest of the managed-care plans is the HMO, which integrates health care delivery with insurance for health care. The HMO was actually in existence before the concept of managed care. The health care services may be provided directly or by contract with other providers. The concept of prepaying a fixed amount per person (capitation) for health care services dates back to 1906, when a group of physicians offered health care services to a lumber company. The Western Clinic of Tacoma, Washington, offered the lumber company health care services for a fixed amount per capita. One of the largest and best known of the HMOs is Kaiser Permanente in California, a nonprofit HMO that is hospital based, employs full-time physicians, and provides comprehensive care.

The HMO models feature the following characteristics:
- Subscribers voluntarily enroll in the plan.
- Providers voluntarily agree to participate in the plan.
- An explicit contractual responsibility for providing health care services is assumed by the HMO.
- A prefixed periodic payment or capitation is made by the HMO to the provider regardless of how much or how often the patient uses the services.

- The financial risk is borne by the HMO and the provider.
- Patients receive no coverage when using providers outside of the HMO network or receive care from a provider without a referral from a primary care physician.

The three types of HMOs are the following:
- A staff model is an organization in which salaried physicians are employed by the HMO to provide care only for HMO subscribers; providers practice within the same facility. The HMO owns and operates ambulatory care facilities that include ancillary services and physician offices. Inpatient care is usually under contract with local health care facilities.
- In a group model an HMO contracts with group practices and hospitals to provide comprehensive health care services to subscribers. The groups of physicians are usually multispecialty.
- In a network type the HMO contracts with a variety of providers to provide health care to subscribers; a physician's patient population may include not only the HMO's patients but also other HMO and non-HMO patients.

The independent practice association (IPA) is a group of physicians organized into a health care provider organization that furnishes services to patients who have signed up for a prepayment plan in which the physician services are supplied by the IPA. The patient population of the physician participating in such an association includes both HMO and non-HMO patients.[4]

Preferred Provider Organizations

A PPO is a network of physicians or HCOs that enter into an agreement with payers or employers to provide health care services on a discounted fee schedule in return for increased patient volume. Patients are encouraged to use these providers by having a lower deductible, copayment, and coinsurance for services given by these providers. Patients are discouraged from using nonparticipating providers by paying higher nonnegotiated fees for their copays and deductibles. However, they still receive some coverage.

Case Management

Case management is an aspect of health care that refers to all activities, including assessment, treatment planning, referral, and follow-up, that ensure the provision of comprehensive and continuous services and the coordination of payment and reimbursement of care.[5] The individual responsible for coordinating all the care is designated the case manager (gatekeeper, primary care provider). This concept becomes crucial when the MCO is managing the care of patients with complex conditions such as cancer, AIDS, or chronic obstructive pulmonary disease. In these complex cases, the MCO (or providers) may employ case managers who coordinate and monitor the secondary and tertiary care that is needed. The case manager is an experienced health care professional who is knowledgeable about the clinical aspect of the patient's condition and the available resources.

Point-of-Service Plan

The point-of-service (POS) plan may be integrated in a number of managed-care plans, including the HMO. The POS plan merely requires the enrollee (patient) to select a provider at the time, and each time, care is provided. The managed-care plan may be a POS plan or may offer POS as an option. The selected provider may or may not be a participant in the MCO. If enrollees are required to select a provider at the time they are enrolled in the managed-care plan, it is called a *point-of-enrollment plan.*

Utilization Management

In an attempt to control the cost of health care, many payers require some form of utilization review. Utilization review is the process of evaluating the efficiency and appropriateness of health care services according to predetermined criteria.

Government's Role as Payer

The bulk of the government's spending on health care goes to the Medicare and Medicaid programs. In 1965, the federal government spent $5.5 billion on health and the cost in 2009 was expected to be about $2.5 trillion. As a result of the spiraling costs, the federal government is pressing for changes to contain health care costs. Because both Medicare and Medicaid are modeled after private insurance companies, much of the terminology is common to many insurance policies.

Medicare

Eligibility, Coverage, and Benefits

The Medicare program is designed to help pay health care costs for those aged 65 years and older and for other groups, including people with permanent kidney damage (referred to as end-stage renal disease [ESRD]) and those receiving disability benefits for a minimum of 24 months. The specific requirements for Medicare eligibility are published in the annual Medicare handbook available on the Medicare website. People who are enrolled in Medicare or Medicaid programs are called beneficiaries.[28]

The Medicare program consists of Parts A, B, C, and D, which cover different medical costs and are governed by different rules.

Hospital insurance, called Part A, helps to pay for inpatient hospital care, inpatient care in a nursing facility, home health care, and hospice care. Part A pays for the hospital costs that include a semiprivate room, meals, nursing service, medications, laboratory tests and radiology, intensive care, operating and recovery room, medical supplies, rehabilitation services, and preparatory services related to kidney transplantation. The physician's fees are not covered by Part A, although the beneficiary is hospitalized and receiving physician services.[28]

Medicare medical insurance, Part B, is a voluntary insurance program designed to supplement the cost of inpatient and outpatient care that is not covered under Part A. Part B coverage includes the physician's fee for services such as diagnostic tests, medical and surgical services, radiography, durable medical equipment (DME), ambulance service, home health, radiation therapy, and other outpatient services.[28] DME is equipment such as wheelchairs, oxygen equipment, walkers, and other devices prescribed by the physician for use in the home.

Medicare Part C, also known as *Medicare Advantage,* is available to beneficiaries who are enrolled in Medicare Parts A and B. Medicare Part C offers various managed-care plans, including HMO, POS, and PPO plans, among others, and private fee-for-service plans previously discussed. Depending on the type of plan selected, services may include preventive care and drug benefits and may have additional monthly premiums because of the extra benefits.[28]

The Medicare Prescription Drug, Improvement, and Modernization Act of 2003, commonly known as the *Medicare Modernization Act* (MMA), expanded Medicare coverage. The law provides for outpatient prescription drug coverage, expanded health plan options, and improved access to health care for rural Americans; it also covers preventive care services, such as flu shots and mammograms.

Medicare Part D, also known as the *Medicare Prescription Drug Plan,* is an insurance that covers the cost of prescription drugs. There are numerous plans, and the coverage and cost depend on the plan selected. Some plans have higher deductibles but may cover more expensive drugs. The beneficiary pays a monthly premium and a deductible and a part of the drug cost. Medicare prescription drug coverage is available through either Medicare Part C or Part D.[28]

✓ **SELF-ASSESSMENT QUESTION**

9. If a patient purchases a prescription drug at the local drug store, which Medicare program provides the prescription drug coverage?
   a. Part A
   b. Part B
   c. Part C
   d. Part D

Reimbursement Under Medicare

Hospitals, physicians, and other health care providers are reimbursed for services delivered to a Medicare beneficiary through a fiscal intermediary (FI). The intermediary is an organization that has contracted to manage the processing of claims and payments to the providers for Medicare Part A, according to federal regulations. The federal government assigns local insurance companies or BCBS plans to act as intermediaries and operate under contract to process Medicare claims. The fiscal intermediaries vary within states or regional areas. From 1966 to 1983, hospitals were paid by the retrospective payment system. Charges for inpatient services were submitted directly to the Medicare Part A FI and were paid on the basis of the reasonable cost of providing the care.

Financing of Medicare

The Medicare program is administered by the CMS of the DHHS. Financing of Part A is primarily by payroll tax, unless the beneficiary does not qualify for federal retirement benefits (Social Security); Part B is financed by federal appropriations with monthly premiums paid by the Medicare beneficiary.

The Medicare beneficiary is required to pay deductibles and copayments for health care services covered by Part A. In addition, the beneficiary pays monthly premiums, the deductible, and a percentage of the charges for Medicare Part B. A deductible is the cost that must be incurred by the patient beneficiary before the insurer assumes liability for the remaining charges. Copays and deductibles are also required for prescription drug coverage under Medicare Part D.[28]

In 1982, Congress passed the Tax Equity and Fiscal Responsibility Act (TEFRA), Public Law 97-248, which mandated the development of a mechanism for controlling the cost of the Medicare program and created the prospective payment system (PPS), a reimbursement method in which the amount of payment is determined in advance of services rendered. Rates are established annually by the CMS. Under this system, the reimbursement for hospital inpatient care of Medicare patients is determined by a classification scheme called diagnosis-related groups (DRG), and reimbursement for physician services is based on the resource-based relative value scale. If a particular inpatient case requires more than the average number of days in the hospital or consumes expensive hospital resources, the hospital may lose money on that patient. Conversely, patients who require fewer resources save the hospital money. Providers have to maintain quality and yet be careful not to order excessive tests or extend treatment beyond what is considered medically necessary by the CMS. Prospective reimbursement systems are used in all types of organizations along the continuum of care, including hospital ambulatory care, skilled nursing facilities, and home health care.

Medicaid

Originally called the *Medical Assistance Program,* Medicaid was established by Title XIX of the Social Security Act. Medicaid is a joint program between the state and the federal governments to provide health care to welfare recipients in the different states. Like other government programs, Medicaid has changed somewhat since its inception in 1965. This discussion is restricted to the program as it exists at the time of publication.

Eligibility for coverage is determined by the individual states but must provide for welfare recipients, poor children younger than 5 years, certain low-income pregnant women, and medically indigent people. The medically indigent are those whose incomes are above what would normally qualify for Medicaid but whose medical expenses are high enough to bring their adjusted income to the poverty level. A great deal of variability exists from state to state. Each state sets its own limits regarding income that is considered to be at poverty level. Although the states vary in coverage and eligibility, they must comply with the federal guidelines.

The federal government identifies certain essential services that Medicaid must provide. These include inpatient and outpatient hospital care, physician services, laboratory and radiology services, skilled nursing care for those older than 21 years, home health care, family planning services, and early and periodic screening, diagnosis, and treatment of individuals under age 21 years. Each state can choose to provide additional health care benefits, such as medical care services by licensed practitioners other than MDs, dental care, physical therapy, eyeglasses, and prescription drugs.

The federal government shares in the cost of the Medicaid program with each state. The percentage of cost sharing varies on the basis of the per capita (per person) income of the state. In addition, the states can set copayments and deductibles for the medically indigent and for the optional services for welfare recipients.

Medicaid Reimbursement

Each state sets its own terms for Medicaid reimbursement to hospitals and health care providers. In some areas of the country, Medicaid recipients are encouraged to join managed-care plans.

Because of the variation in coverage and the fact that there is still a population that does not qualify for Medicaid yet cannot afford or access health care, the program has been under scrutiny.

Under PPACA, an expansion plan for Medicaid was created in which each state would expand eligibility to 133% of the federal poverty level. However, the Supreme Court deemed this unconstitutional and coercive, so states can opt out of the expansion. Currently, 25 states are pursuing the expansion.

State Children's Health Insurance Program

The Balanced Budget Act of 1997 created the State Children's Health Insurance Program (SCHIP). This state-administered program offers health insurance for uninsured children up to age 19 years. It is designed to provide health insurance to families that may not be eligible for Medicaid because of their income. Each state establishes its own guidelines for enrollment, eligibility, and services. The basic services include hospitalizations, physician visits, immunizations, and ED visits.

TRICARE

The Department of Defense provides health care for active and retired military personnel and their dependents. Health care for active-duty and retired military personnel and their families and survivors is currently covered by TRICARE, formerly the Civilian Health and Medical Program for the Uniformed Services (CHAMPUS).

Workers' Compensation

Each state has workers' compensation insurance laws. This insurance pays for medical expenses and lost income, protection against lost occupational skills, and capacity and death benefits for survivors for workers who were injured or became ill as a result of work. Workers' compensation is funded by employer insurance programs. Most workers' compensation programs will pay lost wages and health care costs.

TECHNOLOGY IN HEALTH INFORMATION

Point-of-Care Clinical Information Systems

Point-of-care clinical information systems (POS information systems) allow caregivers to capture and input data where health care service is provided and may be at the time of patient care. A point-of-care system can collect data directly from monitoring devices such as those in intensive care units. Many systems for point-of-care documentation are moving to wireless systems, giving clinicians more flexibility; accurate, timely reporting; and patient-focused care.

Electronic Data Exchange

Electronic data exchange provides the ability to edit, submit, and pay health care claims by way of electronic transfer. In 1991, the Workgroup on Electronic Data Interchange (WEDI) was commissioned by the secretary of DHHS to reduce the cost of health care administration by increasing the number of claims processed electronically. Today the primary objective of WEDI is to improve health care quality by managing the electronic information exchange and management in an efficient and effective manner. Electronic data exchange requires a level of standardization in the way the data are formatted, making it easier for different computer systems to exchange data. The Transaction and Code Set Regulations of the section of the HIPAA Administrative Simplification Rules address the standardization of the transactions between providers and payers.

Decision Support Systems

A decision support system (DSS) is a computerized system that gathers information from various sources and uses analytical models to assist providers in clinical decision making regarding administrative, clinical, and cost issues. For example, a clinical decision support system (CDSS) called *Quick Medical Reference* provides information about signs, symptoms, diagnosis, and treatment of more than 700 diseases. Other clinical DSS software programs provide reminders or make recommendations on the basis of clinical guidelines.

Electronic Health Record

Transitioning from the paper medical record to the EHR continues to present numerous challenges that include privacy, data security, technology, policy, people, and processes. The most commonly used standards for developing electronic clinical and administrative data sets were established by the Health Level 7 (HL7) of the American National Standards Institute (ANSI). The standards are focused on the exchange, management, and integration of electronic health care information for HCOs.

Electronic patient records that are developed by individual health care providers and organizations are electronic medical records (EMRs) that are composed of whole files as opposed to individual data elements. There are hundreds of types of information systems that make up the EMR. The EMR is primarily used by a specific entity. The data from the EMR are the source of data for the EHR. The EHR represents the ability to easily share medical information by way of interfaces among stakeholders including patients, providers, payers and insurers, and government agencies. Wherever the patient seeks health care, the information should follow and be accessible. Among other things, data sharing by EHR is important in forming health care policy, public health reporting, aggregating data for research, billing, and managing patient accounts.

National Health Information Infrastructure

The challenges of medical errors, inconsistent quality, and escalating health care costs has prompted the need for a National Health Information Infrastructure or Network (NHII or NHIN) that encompasses an EHR system for all providers and the ability to communicate electronically so that a complete EHR is assembled at the point of care. The IOM has released numerous reports that call for the need to develop the NHII. The NHII will be a network of local health information structures that allow for the exchange of health information within the community, including clinician information systems, consumer health information, ancillary health systems, DSSs, educational components, and communication and networking systems that allow for integration of information across sites.[7] Although the project is to be developed and operated by the private sector, the DHHS has taken the lead in trying to move the initiative forward by convening stakeholder meetings and disseminating the vision.

National Call for EHRs

The IOM of the National Academy of Science is a nonprofit organization that serves as an advisor to the nation on issues related to improving health. The IOM has addressed issues such as the number of uninsured Americans, immunization safety, autism, health literacy, childhood obesity, privacy of personal health care data, and the disclosure to the public of cost and quality information about institutions and clinicians.[7]

A report from the General Accounting Office identified the following ways in which the EHR can improve health care delivery:

- Provides data that are more accessible, of better quality, versatile for display, and easier to retrieve—all of which support decision making.

- Enhances outcomes research by capturing clinical data from large databases.
- Improves hospitals' efficiency by reducing cost and enhancing staff productivity.

The integration of clinical data management into a common database allows the HCOs to develop strategies that support quality, control cost, and examine processes to improve efficiency. The integration further supports the collaboration and coordination of efforts by all health care professionals.

Clinical information systems are critical to address the changing health care environment needs for containing costs, improving quality, and providing accessible health care, all of which are vital components of health care reform.

FUTURE ISSUES

Until recently, the primary stakeholders in health care were the HCOs, providers, and payers. Today and more so in the future, the health care industry will have a greater awareness and recognition of the consumer as an important stake-holder. Consumers are more informed, participating in health care decision making and taking more responsibility for their health care. In addition, in an arena that is balancing the business of health care, technology, and social welfare goals, there continues to be concern for quality, cost, and access to care.

With the evolution of the EHR, there continues to be serious concerns about data security and confidentiality. HIM professionals will have numerous opportunities to affect the direction of health care by addressing issues of security and integrity of the EHR, practice standards, regulatory issues, and documentation that improves patient care quality, as well as by facilitating the development and use of the PHR. The continued growth in ambulatory care, LTC, and home health care has brought to the forefront the information needs in these areas. HIM professionals are and will continue to be of vital importance to the information needs of every component of health care systems but particularly with regard to the innovative programs that are emerging and the needs that the EHR movement has brought about.

CHAPTER REVIEW

1. Which of the following terms is based on the patients ability to pay for health care?
   a. indirect pay
   b. sliding scale fee
   c. catchment area
   d. out-of-pocket pay

2. A hospital that receives reimbursement for meeting the needs of an underserved area is a:
   a. tertiary care facility
   b. critical access hospital
   c. proprietary hospital
   d. managed care organization

3. The primary goal of accountable care organizations is to:
   a. ensure that care is delivered efficiently and effectively.
   b. control the overall cost of care that is delivered.
   c. promote more patient and family involvement in care.
   d. coordinate care across the continuum of care.

4. Which one of the following statements is NOT true about an HMO?
   a. providers voluntarily agree to participate in the plan.
   b. subscribers volunteer to participate.
   c. the HMO assumes responsibility for providing health care services.
   d. no financial risk is borne by the HMO and the provider.

5. People who receive Medicare benefits are called:
   a. subscribers
   b. patients
   c. residents
   d. beneficiaries

6. An aspect of health care that refers to all activities, including assessment, treatment planning, referral, and follow-up, that ensures the provision of comprehensive and continuous care is called:
   a. tertiary care
   b. continuum of care
   c. case management
   d. point of care

7. What do you call the reimbursement that is negotiated between a provider and third party payer?
   a. usual, customary, and reasonable charges
   b. contracted amount
   c. sliding scale fee
   d. retrospective payment system

8. If a patient purchases a prescription drug at the local drug store, which Medicare program provides the prescription drug coverage?
   a. Part A
   b. Part B
   c. Part C
   d. Part D

9. A report from the General Accounting Office identified health care delivery benefits of the electronic health record. These include all of the following EXCEPT:
   a. the data are more accessible, of better quality, and easier to retrieve.
   b. the system enhances outcomes research by capturing clinical data from large databases.
   c. the system reduces the incidence of fraud and abuse that occurs because of poor documentation.
   d. the hospitals' efficiency is improved by reducing costs and enhancing staff productivity.

10. Short-term care with a focus on giving caregivers time off is called:
    a. respite care
    b. hospice care
    c. palliative care
    d. domiciliary care

11. A reimbursement method in which the amount of payment to the health care facility is determined in advance of services rendered is called:
    a. retrospective payment system
    b. fee for service system
    c. prospective payment system
    d. capitation reimbursement system

12. Of the following, which health care professional is the single largest profession in the United States?
    a. physicians
    b. nurses
    c. dentists
    d. physical therapists

13. An older adult patient who is receiving care for her skin wounds and physical therapy is most likely to be in an independent living facility.
    a. true
    b. false

REFERENCES

1. Ackerknecht EH: Medicine of ancient civilization. In Ackerknecht EH, editor: *A short history of medicine*, 4 ed., Baltimore, 1982, Johns Hopkins Press, pp 21–26.
2. American Medical Association: http://www.ama-assn.org. Accessed June 6, 2014.
3. American Hospital Association: *About the AHA*, 2013: http://www.aha.org/about/index.shtml. Accessed June 6, 2014.
4. Knight W: What is managed care?. In *Managed care: what it is and how it works*, Gaithersburg, MD, 1998, Aspen Publishers, pp 19–43.
5. Roberts JS, Coale JG, Redman RR: A history of The Joint Commission on Accreditation of Hospitals, *JAMA* 258:936–940, 1987.
6. Sultz HA, Young KM: Financing health care. In *Health care USA—Understanding its organization and delivery*, 4 ed., Gaithersburg, MD, 2004, Aspen Publishers.
7. Institute of Medicine: *To err is human: building a safer health system*, 2000, National Academy Press. http://www.nap.edu/books/0309068371/html. Accessed June 6, 2014.
8. U.S. Department of Health and Human Services: *National health expenditures 2011 highlights*: http://www.cms.gov/Research-Statistics-Data-and-Systems/Statistics-Trends-and-Reports/NationalHealthExpendData/Downloads/highlights.pdf. Accessed June 6, 2014.
9. Summary of the Affordable Care Act, Kaiser Family Foundation: http://kaiserfamilyfoundation.files.wordpress.com/2011/04/8061-021.pdf. Accessed June 6, 2014.
10. *Health, United States, 2011*, Centers for Disease Control and Prevention http://www.cdc.gov/nchs/data/hus/hus12.pdf#018.
11. AHIMA: The Role of the Personal Health Record in the EHR, *J AHIMA* 76(7):64A-D, 2005.
12. Status of State Action on the Medicaid Expansion Decision, as of September 3, 2013, Kaiser Family Foundation, http://kff.org/health-reform/state-indicator/state-activity-around-expanding-medicaid-under-the-affordable-care-act/. Accessed June 6, 2014.
13. Introducing Healthy People 2020: http://www.healthypeople.gov/2020/about/default.aspx. Accessed June 6, 2012.
14. Centers for Medicare and Medicaid Services: Emergency Medical Treatment and Labor Act: http://www.cms.gov/EMTALA/01_Overview.asp#TopOfPage. Accessed June 6, 2014.
15. The Joint Commission, 2013: http://www.jointcommission.org. Accessed June 6, 2014.
16. American Osteopathic Association (updated 2013): http://www.osteopathic.org. Accessed June 6, 2014.
17. DO-Online. The Home for Osteopathic Medical Profession. Accreditation and program approval, 2009: www.osteopathic.org/inside-aoa/accreditation/Pages/default.asp.
18. CARF International. Quick facts about CARF (2013): http://www.carf.org/About/QuickFacts/. Accessed June 6, 2014.
19. National Committee for Quality Assurance: Quality measurement guidelines: http://www.ncqa.org/tabid/440/Default.aspx. Accessed June 6, 2014.
20. Commission on Accreditation of Allied Health Education Programs: What is CAAHEP?, 2009: www.caahep.org/content.aspx?ID-63.
21. Commission on Accreditation of Health Informatics and Information Management Education: http://www.cahiim.org. Accessed June 6, 2014.
22. Accreditation Commission for Education in Nursing: Mission, Purpose, Goals: http://acenursing.org/mission-purpose-goals. Accessed June 6, 2014.
23. Agency for Healthcare Research and Quality: Patient centered medical home resource center, 2013: http://pcmh.ahrq.gov/portal/server.pt/community/pcmh__home/1483/PCMH_Defining%20the%20PCMH_v2.
24. Veterans Administration Office of Human Resources and Administration: About VHA, 2013, http://www.va.gov/health/aboutVHA.asp.
25. Agency for Healthcare Research and Quality: Emergency severity index, version 4: http://www.ahrq.gov/research/esi/esi1.htm#chapter1. Accessed June 6, 2014.
26. American Nurses Association: What nurses do, 2013: http://www.nursingworld.org/EspeciallyForYou/What-is-Nursing/Tools-You-Need/RNsAPNs.html. Accessed June 6, 2014.
27. American College of Surgeons, Committee on Trauma: New verification site visit outcomes, 2009: http://www.facs.org/trauma/verifivisitoutcomes.html. Accessed June 6, 2014.
28. Centers for Medicare and Medicaid Services: Medicare program—general information, 2013: http://www.cms.hhs.gov/MedicareGenInfo.
29. Wilson FA, Neuhauser D: Health manpower. In *Health services in the United States*, 2 ed., Cambridge, MA, 1987, Ballinger, p 61.
30. ACHE Key Industry Facts, 2011. The American College of Healthcare Executives. www.ache.org/pubs/research/key_industry_2013.pdf.

CHAPTER 2

THE HEALTH INFORMATICS AND INFORMATION MANAGEMENT PROFESSION

Melanie S. Brodnik

ⓔ Student Study Guide activities for this chapter are available on the Evolve Learning Resources site for this textbook. Please visit http://evolve.elsevier.com/Abdelhak.

CHAPTER CONTENTS

OBJECTIVES

After reading this chapter, the reader will be able to do the following:
✓ Define the key words.
✓ Discuss the patient record as a source of health data and information.
✓ Trace the early evolution of patient records in health care.

✓ Describe key forces that have influenced the evolution of the patient record.
✓ Discuss how technology has influenced the demand for electronic health records and a national health information infrastructure (NHII).
✓ Trace the early evolution of the health information management profession.

✓ Describe the effect of information technology on the health information management profession and the issues the profession faces in an electronic health care environment.

✓ Discuss the requirements for initial and continuing certification within the health information management profession and the profession's commitment to lifelong learning.

✓ Describe the benefits of seeking and maintaining professional certification.

✓ Identify the governance and volunteer structure of the American Health Information Management Association and what membership has to offer the professional.

✓ Discuss the principles found within the American Health Information Management Association Code of Ethics and how they apply in today's health care environment.

KEY WORDS

Accreditation
Accredited record technician
AHIMA Foundation
American Recovery and
 Reinvestment Act
Certification
Certified coding associate
Certified coding specialist
Certified coding specialist—
 physician based
Certified health data analyst
Certified in healthcare privacy
Certified in healthcare privacy and
 security
Certified in healthcare security
Code of ethics
Commission on Accreditation for
 Health Informatics and
 Information Management
 Education

Commission on Certification for
 Health Informatics and
 Information Management
Communities of Practice
Computer-based Patient Record
 Institute
Conditions of participation
Credential
Data
E-health
Electronic health information
 management
Electronic health record
Electronic medical record
Fee-for-service
Fellow of the American Health
 Information Management
 Association
Foundation of Research and
 Education in Health Information

Management (now AHIMA
 Foundation)
Health informatics
Health information exchange
Health information technology
Health Information Technology for
 Economic and Clinical Health Act
HIM Profession Core Model
Health Insurance Portability and
 Accountability Act
Hybrid record
Information
The Joint Commission
Knowledge
Legal health record
Licensure
Longitudinal record
Medicaid
Medicare

National Health Information
 Infrastructure
Office of the National Coordinator for
 Health Information Technology
Patient record
President's Information Technology
 Advisory Committee
Profession
Prospective payment
Record
Regional health information
 organizations
Registered health information
 administrator
Registered health information
 technician
Registered record librarian
Registration
Secondary patient data

ABBREVIATIONS

AAMRL American Association of Medical Record Librarians
ACS American College of Surgeons
AHA American Hospital Association
AHIMA American Health Information Management Association
AMA American Medical Association
AMIA American Medical Informatics Association
AMRA American Medical Record Association
ARLNA Association of Record Librarians of North America
ARRA American Recovery and Reinvestment Act
ART Accredited record technician
BOD Board of Directors
CAHIIM Commission on Accreditation of Health Informatics and Information Management Education
CCA Certified coding associate
CCHIIM Commission on Certification for Health Informatics and Information Management
CCS Certified coding specialist
CCS-P Certified coding specialist–physician based
CDIP Clinical documentation improvement practitioner
CEE Council for Excellence in Education
CEU Continuing education unit
CHDA Certified health data analyst
CHP Certified in healthcare privacy
CHPS Certified in healthcare privacy and security
CHS Certified in healthcare security
CHTS Certified healthcare technology specialist
CoPs Communities of Practice
CPRI Computer-based Patient Record Institute
CSA Component state association

e-Health Electronic health
e-HIM Electronic health information management
EHR Electronic health record
EMR Electronic medical record
FAHIMA Fellow of the American Health Information Management Association
FORE Foundation of Research and Education (now AHIMA Foundation)
HI Health informatics
HIE Health information exchange
HIIM Health informatics and information management
HIM Health information management
HIPAA Health Insurance Portability and Accountability Act
HIT Health information technology
HITECH Health Information Technology for Economic and Clinical Health Act
HOD House of Delegates
ISP Independent study program
JCAH Joint Commission on the Accreditation of Hospitals
JCAHO Joint Commission on the Accreditation of Healthcare Organizations
LHR Legal health record
MD Medical doctor
NHII National Health Information Infrastructure
ONC Office of the National Coordinator for Health Information Technology
PHR Personal health record
PITAC President's Information Technology Advisory Committee
RHIA Registered health information administrator
RHIT Registered health information technician
RRL Registered record librarian

This chapter traces the evolution of the patient record and the health information management (HIM) profession in the United States to its current status. The primary professional association for HIM professionals in the United States is the American Health Information Management Association (AHIMA). Its mission and role in HIM education, program accreditation, credentialing of professionals, support of professional development opportunities, code of ethics, and key initiatives to move the profession forward are discussed. The history of the profession (that is, a discipline that has formalized itself through specialized educational training and a specific code of conduct) is intricately linked to the development of landmark changes in the health care system. The roles of HIM professionals are diverse, and the variety of opportunities has increased in ways the early founders of the profession could never have imagined. However, one main thread continues to bind the past to the future—the goal of supporting quality health care through quality information.

HEALTH INFORMATION MANAGEMENT—A PROFESSION IN TRANSITION

HIM has been defined as a profession that "is responsible for ensuring the availability, accuracy, and protection of the clinical information that is needed to deliver health care services and to make appropriate health care related decisions."[1] Whether the information is in paper or electronic form, the goal of HIM is to manage, provide, and protect quality information in support of quality health care. The HIM profession and health care industry in general are experiencing a fundamental change in the way health care data and information are collected, accessed, analyzed, and managed as a result of advances in information technology and government mandates. Paper-based patient records are rapidly being replaced by electronic health records (EHR) that purport to improve patient care, control health care costs, support patient safety and provide better public health surveillance. Federal legislation such as the Health Information Technology for Economic and Clinical Health Act (HITECH) as part of the American Recovery and Reinvestment Act (ARRA) of 2009 and the Health Insurance Portability and Accountability Act (HIPAA) have fostered the increased use of EHRs and health information technology (HIT) and the increased demand for a workforce competent in managing EHR systems and the data generated by such systems. HIT in this context refers to managing health information and the exchange of health information in a digital format.[2]

Since its inception in 1928, the HIM profession has served to improve patient care through better documentation practices while protecting the privacy and security of patient information. Throughout the years the profession has adapted its practices in support of the many changes occurring in health care delivery including the transition to EHRs and increased uses of HIT. The roles and functions of HIM professionals have similarly adapted and are now rapidly transitioning to include additional responsibilities in HIT, leadership, information governance, data stewardship, and health care analytics. HIM professionals work collaboratively with health care providers and others in the field of health informatics (HI) to establish a health care information infrastructure that supports quality health care while balancing the patient's right to privacy with legitimate uses of information for administrative, financial, clinical, research, and public health purposes. Health informatics in general refers to the science of how health information is captured, transmitted, and used in health using information technology and computer science.[2] As health care has come to rely on such technology and science, informatics has become an important component of practice within the HIM profession.

THE PATIENT RECORD—SOURCE OF HEALTH DATA AND INFORMATION

The patient record is a primary source of health data and information for the health care industry. The record can be paper based, electronic, or a combination of both, referred to as a hybrid record. Data refer to raw facts, characters, or symbols that, when organized and processed to produce meaning, result in information. Knowledge is derived from information after it is organized, analyzed, and synthesized by the user. A record is a body of known or recorded facts regarding someone or something. When an individual seeks care or treatment from a health care provider, a record of that care or treatment is generated. The data collected from and on the patient are stored in the patient record. The record may be called a *patient record, medical record, health record, clinical record, resident record, client record,* and so forth, depending on the nature and philosophy of the health care setting in which the record was generated. In addition, the record may be labeled as an EHR or electronic medical record (EMR) if HIT is used to generate the record. In any case, the patient record is created as a direct result of the health care delivered in that setting. It is the legal documentation of care provided to an individual by the medical or health care professionals who practice in the setting. The data, information, or record may have the term clinical preceding it to denote that the data, information, or record relates specifically to the care and treatment of a patient.

Health information in general includes a wide range of data that are used for multiple purposes. The data span birth to death and wellness to illness.[2] Data that commonly compose health information are found in Box 2-1. The data and information documented in the record and the record in total are used for the following purposes:

- Documenting health care services provided to an individual to support continuing communication and decision making among health care providers
- Establishing a record of health care services provided to an individual that can be used as evidence in legal proceedings
- Assessing the effectiveness and efficiency of the health care services provided

BOX 2-1	Types of Data Included in Health Information

Clinical data—captured during the process of diagnosis and treatment; support direct patient care; and are used for health care reimbursement, planning, and research purposes.

Epidemiologic databases—aggregate data about a population, reveal disease trends.

Demographic data—used to provide unique identification of individual, patient, health care provider.

Financial data—derived from care process, used individually for patient billing, reimbursement, and in aggregate for understanding clinical cost of health care, rules for reimbursement and organizations of financial well-being.

Research data—collected as part of care or gathered for specific research purposes or clinical trials.

Reference data—refer to literature, research outcomes, protocol, formulary, care plan, clinical alert or reminder, and so on that enhance clinical knowledge or operational decision making.

Coded data—data translated into a code using standard nomenclature or classification system that may be aggregated, analyzed, and compared for decision-making purposes.

Source: Health information management: Professional definitions from the AHIMA 1999 and 2000 Committees on Professional Development, 2001.

- Documenting health care services provided to support reimbursement claims that are submitted to payers
- Supplying data and information that supports strategic planning, administrative decision making, public health surveillance, research activities and public policy development related to health care, such as regulations, legislation, and accreditation standards

The use of data contained in the patient record has increased with the growing complexity of health care decision making and the increasing complexity of the health care delivery system. Whether patients receive treatment in a hospital, long-term care facility, ambulatory clinic, or physician office, patients are likely to encounter a variety of health care providers working collaboratively to provide the most effective treatment or care for these patients. This situation creates a heightened reliance by care providers on the patient record as a means of communication and as a source of data for decision making.

Documentation within the patient record is the basis for health care billing and reimbursement. Third-party payers such as insurance companies and the federal government through programs such as Medicare and Medicaid use the data documented in the record as proof of the care delivered to the patient. Without appropriate documentation to support the care given, the health care setting or provider will not be reimbursed for services rendered.

The data and information in the patient record are used to substantiate whether the patient received quality care or treatment in the most effective and efficient way possible. Because the cost of health care represents a large portion

of the United States' gross national product, efforts to control spiraling health care costs while providing quality health care place extra importance on the patient record.

Not only are the data and information within the patient record used to substantiate the care given for reimbursement and quality proposes, the record is also a legal document that confirms whether treatment was delivered in a manner appropriate for the given health problem. The record is used to show proof in a court of law of what transpired during the course of a patient's illness and treatment. As a legal document, the patient record is defined as a record that is "generated at or for a healthcare organization as its business record and is the record that would be released upon request."[3] It is the **legal health record** (LHR) of the organization.

The patient record is a valuable source of data for research such as comparative effectiveness research, program evaluation, education, public health studies, and population health management. Data from the record that are stored in government and private databases are often termed **secondary patient data** and are used in the aggregate for these purposes. Published data on acquired immunodeficiency syndrome, sexually transmitted diseases, diseases caused by certain infections, and outbreaks of illness such as severe acute respiratory syndrome or the H1N1 flu rely on careful documentation in the patient record or source document. Hospital mortality rates are published, as are performance reports on health care organizations. More and more health plans provide performance information to consumers, often referred to as "report cards," to help the consumers evaluate and select the health plan that is best suited to them.[4] Data and subsequent information generated from patient care are even more important as efforts focus on identifying the most effective way to deliver quality care for the least amount of expense.

✅ SELF-ASSESSMENT QUIZ

1. What is the difference between HIM, HIT, and HI?
2. Name at least two pieces of legislation that have fostered the implementation of EHRs.
3. Name and describe at least four types of data that commonly compose health information.
4. What does the term *legal health record* refer to?

EVOLUTION OF THE PATIENT RECORD

The importance that patient records play in today's health care environment is clear. How did patient records evolve as a primary source of health care data and information, and what forces influenced this evolution? In addition, what are the milestones in the history of this evolution that have brought us to today's need for EHR systems and an NHII?

Early History

The value of recording patient information has been recognized since prehistoric times. The methods used to record early attempts to treat disease were primitive and differ markedly from the electronic information systems now in use. Prehistoric cave paintings are thought to be the earliest accounts of treating the sick. The paintings depict skull trephination and amputation of fingers and other parts of the extremities. As civilizations developed, stone carvings were made in addition to drawings, and eventually pen and paper became the mode for recording words and thoughts.[5]

Methods for maintaining patient records were slow to develop, and the earliest institutions used some abbreviated form. Many hospitals appear to have used a ledger to record at least minimum information about a patient—for example, name, address, date of birth, and major health problem. The use of ledgers for record keeping was popular in other businesses as well. They were used by banks, hotels, and other commercial enterprises. Many pioneer record keepers, such as Thomas Jefferson, George Washington, and Benjamin Franklin, used ledger-style recordings, so it is not surprising that health care initially adopted a similar system of documentation.

Early U.S. hospitals such as the New York Hospital, established in 1771, did not begin recording patient clinical information until approximately 1790. Pennsylvania Hospital, established in Philadelphia in 1792 under the leadership of Benjamin Franklin, included entries of the patient's name, address, and ailment in bound ledger books, many of which were made in Franklin's handwriting. Charity Hospital in New Orleans similarly entered its first medical records in large ledgers. Because many of its earliest patients were seamen, the terminology used in the records often reflects a nautical influence. Massachusetts General Hospital, established in 1821, maintained patient records from its beginning. These records were sufficiently comprehensive to enable the cataloging of diseases and operations.[6] One Virginia hospital, established in 1911, maintained its early clinical records in leather-bound volumes that contained between 50 and 100 patient records per volume.

The ledger style of recording patient care was most popular in these early hospitals. As the record-keeping process became more detailed and interest in learning from treatment experience increased, the minimal ledger entry was no longer sufficient. Early record keepers in hospitals looked beyond ledgers to find ways of making patient records more accessible and useful by moving from ledgers to individual patient records. These records were organized into systems that allowed easier retrieval of a patient's record and the data within the document.

In the early hospitals, only a small circle of health care providers had access to the patient records. The records were brief and contained carefully handwritten entries. In time the information recorded in the patient record was organized into various types of reports such as patient history and physical examination, operative report, progress report, nursing notes, laboratory results, and other ancillary service reports. To help in the learning process of health care providers, some hospitals filed the records of similar diseases or treatments together. Others set up disease and treatment indexes, which enabled them to associate particular patient records with a specific index. When the typewriter was invented in 1874, early hospitals adopted this new form of "information technology" to process their health care data. They began typing the lengthy handwritten documents within the patient record such as operative reports and history and physical examinations. Over time, patient records came to contain scores of documents in a wide variety of formats accessed by a wide variety of legitimate users for multiple reasons. With an increased need to access patient data on a more real-time basis, the paper form of the record no longer meets the demands placed on it. The paper record can be in only one place at one time, and the data, once entered into the paper record, cannot be manipulated to show trends or relationships among data as may be uniquely required by an individual user of the record. Many forces have influenced the importance of patient records and the data therein, as well as the need to move the paper-based record to an electronic format.

Influential Forces

Accreditation

By the turn of the twentieth century, hospitals were viewed as boardinghouses for the poor and sick, and issues related to the shortcomings of medical education and the quality of documentation in patient records surfaced. To address these issues, voluntary organizations and state and federal governments began efforts to standardize and regulate the delivery of health care. The American Medical Association (AMA) and American Hospital Association (AHA) were already 50 years old by the turn of the century. However, the organization that was most aware of the need for quality patient records was the American College of Surgeons (ACS). The ACS brought to the forefront the realization that, to assess the quality of physician education and the resulting treatment provided to patients, those performing the assessment needed data, and the primary source of these data was the patient record.

To elevate the quality of surgery being performed in hospitals, the ACS established minimum standards that included specifications for the content of the patient's record and required that certain activities be documented within a predefined time frame. In 1918, the ACS began to survey hospitals to see whether the standards were being met and found that "only 89 of the 692 hospitals of 100 or more beds surveyed met the minimum standards."[7] The ACS provided leadership and funding for the accreditation activity and also helped form the professional organization now known as AHIMA, which is discussed later in this chapter.

The other voluntary organizations of the AMA, AHA, American College of Physicians, and the Canadian Hospital Association joined the ACS to support the early accreditation body. The Canadian Hospital Association eventually withdrew from the body and formed its own accreditation program in Canada. In 1952, the remaining voluntary member organizations formed the Joint Commission on the Accreditation of Hospitals (JCAH) to carry on with the hospital accreditation program. Over the years, the JCAH expanded its accreditation activity to incorporate all types of health care organizations, all of which must maintain patient records (sometimes called *resident, client,* or *medical records*). It changed its name to the Joint Commission on the Accreditation of Healthcare Organizations (JCAHO) to reflect the expansion of its accreditation activities and, in 2007, renamed itself again as The Joint Commission. Throughout the years, The Joint Commission has set expectations for quality patient care with the patient record as the primary source of data to substantiate this care. Standards related to the content of patient records and the processes for storing, retrieving, and protecting patient data and records have been identified and make up a chapter within the accreditation manuals devoted specifically to information management.[8]

Licensing of Health Care Facilities

Running parallel to the accreditation programs offered by the early voluntary organizations and later The Joint Commission, states began programs to license facilities. Although many of the state licensing codes focused heavily on the physical facility to ensure safe surroundings, they also included sections on the basic requirements for a patient record and patient record system. State licensing boards, or in some cases registration boards, required that health care facilities accredited by The Joint Commission must also meet the state licensing requirements to be authorized to provide health care services. As standards and regulations evolved, health care facilities were required to adhere to whichever standard or regulation was more stringent. In general, the voluntary Joint Commission accreditation review involves standards that are more stringent than state-mandated minimum requirements. However, at times the state licensing requirements are more defined than Joint Commission standards. For example, states may require a specific retention period for patient records, whereas the Joint Commission standard for record retention may simply require that the organization have a retention policy for patient records.

Paying for Health Care

In time, as the U.S. population grew and more hospitals were built to meet the need for health care services, various methods for funding the services emerged. Private health insurance appeared in the first half of the century, and federal programs for insuring selected segments of the population appeared in 1965. These third-party payer sources have contributed to the demand for health care data, as found in the patient record. Also, these third-party payers have heavily influenced methods for documenting in the patient record and fast and accurate retrieval of this documentation for reimbursement purposes.

Employers began to add benefits to workers' compensation packages in the form of health insurance as early as 1929. Major expansion of health insurance benefits and programs occurred in the 1950s and 1960s, followed by another major thrust for funding health care through managed-care plans. Over the years, insurance companies and managed-care organizations have increased the quantity and specificity of the documentation required from the patient record to support each claim for health care services that is submitted for payment. Likewise, state and federal governments have done the same through Medicare and Medicaid programs.[9]

In 1965, Congress added provisions to the Social Security Act that created the Medicare and Medicaid programs (see Chapter 1). This event resulted in the addition of regulations at the federal and state levels for patient records. Many of the basic Joint Commission standards were incorporated into the federal regulations known as the conditions of participation.[10] The conditions of participation spelled out for health care providers the regulations that they must follow to be reimbursed for the health care given to patients who use Medicare and Medicaid as their payment source. One regulation required that each admission of a patient to the hospital was subject to review and potential denial of payment if the admission was judged, after the fact, to be unnecessary. The federal government set up a monitoring system for Medicare patients that reviewed the appropriate use of hospital resources and the quality of patient care. Much of the review focused on the patient record as the primary source of information. The phrase "if it isn't documented, it wasn't done" became a mantra during this time in an attempt to communicate the increasing importance of proper documentation in the patient record under the Medicare review program.

The Medicare and Medicaid programs were essentially a fee-for-service style of reimbursement. If a service was provided that the programs had agreed to cover, a payment would be received at a discounted rate. The system encouraged more services to generate more payment. Spiraling health care costs over the next 15 years led Congress to search for ways to control these costs. One solution was to move from a fee-for-service style of reimbursement to a prospective payment method. The prospective payment method compared with the fee-for-service method of reimbursement is based on payment rates that are established in advance and that reflect an average of what a service should cost. Thus between 1980 and 2002, Congress moved to a prospective payment system method of reimbursing health care for seven health care services: ambulatory surgery centers (1980), inpatient acute care hospitals (1983), skilled nursing facilities (1998), home health agencies (2000), outpatient hospital services (2001), inpatient rehabilitation facilities (2002), and long-term care hospitals (2002).[9] The patient record became, and still is, the primary data source used to justify each claim submitted for the respective prospective payment systems. Thus the need to improve methods of collecting, processing, communicating, and managing data from patient records is paramount to meeting the demands for increased information and quality patient care.

Technology

Throughout the twentieth and into the twenty-first centuries, innovation and adoption of technology has increasingly been used as a tool to support diagnostic, therapeutic, monitoring, and educational activities associated with direct patient care. The results produced through the application of technology in patient care were reported in the primary patient record; however, the actual scan or image produced by the application was stored in another location. As information technology matured over the years and the demand for more information increased, new approaches to the patient record emerged. Data may become part of the record without forcing the data to appear on paper; that is, data from images, voice, and sound can be an integral part of a primary patient record that is electronic in format.

In the 1980s, a breakthrough in the processing of data and information occurred when personal computers and data communication technologies entered the marketplace and became more affordable. These technologies enabled hospitals and other health care providers to increase their reliance on HIT as a means of staying competitive in an increasingly information-intensive industry. The challenge was to move the paper-based patient record to an EHR format. In such a format, the patient record can be composed of electronic databases (or repositories of data) that contain the health care information generated on the patient while treated in a given health care facility. The data within the database can be accessed and arranged in multiple ways such as a longitudinal record from birth to death of a patient, an in-depth view of a single, current health problem of how one individual is being managed, or the records (data) of many individuals merged to provide information on the outcome of particular treatments across a population of patients.

In 1989 the Institute of Medicine addressed this challenge by undertaking a study to improve patient records through the use of information technology. The Institute of Medicine convened a committee of industry experts who reported in 1991 that health care professionals and organizations should be encouraged to adopt computer-based patient records as a standard for all records related to patient care. They defined the patient record of the future as one that "will reside in a system specifically designed to support users by providing accessibility to complete and accurate data, alerts, reminders, clinical support systems, links to medical knowledge and other aids."[11] If the patient record was computerized, it could allow multiple users to access data at the same time. Researchers could also access the data in aggregate form if they were looking for data on a certain type of treatment but did not need to identify an individual patient. One recommendation of the study was that the "public and private sectors join in establishing a Computer-based Patient Record Institute (CPRI) to promote and facilitate development, implementation, and dissemination of the [computer-based patient record]."[11] The institute was formed and functioned throughout the 1990s in support of computerizing patient records.

During the 1990s there was continuous growth of information and communication technologies, including the Internet, web-based applications, wireless communication, and telephony in regard to patient care and treatment. As a result, the concept of electronic health (e-health) emerged. E-health refers to the following:

> Health services and information delivered or enhanced through the Internet and related technologies. In a broader sense, the term characterizes not only a technical development, but also a state-of-mind, a way of thinking, an attitude, and a commitment for networked, global thinking, to improve health care locally, regionally, and worldwide by using information and communication technology.[12]

By the end of the 1990s, we saw a growing reliance on e-health in all phases and aspects of health care and life. The need for public health preparedness and disease surveillance systems to address terrorism and other public health concerns on a national and global basis emerged. There was a growing emphasis on bringing the consumer of health care into the picture as a way to improve care and control costs. The concept of consumers taking charge of their health care by keeping their own personal health record (PHR) and linking the caregiver and consumer through HIT was seen as important to the future of health care delivery.

Up to this time, providers were adopting applications to capture, process, and retrieve data electronically from all or parts of the patient record. As a result, patient records in some instances became a combination of paper, digitized information, and imaged documents. We began to see patient records and patient record systems in some organizations change from strictly paper-based documents to a hybrid record. A *hybrid record* refers to a record that includes both paper and electronic documents and uses both manual and electronic processes to store and retrieve the documents.[13]

By the early 2000s a complete EHR was still not the norm of practice for a variety of reasons, including a lack of data standards and interoperability, investment costs, acceptance of HIT by staff, and availability of staff to implement EHR systems. However, to address these barriers, the federal government and a number of public-private organizations began working on ways to speed up the adoption of EHRs as a means to improve the quality, safety, efficiency, and cost of health care.[14]

In January 2004 President George W. Bush highlighted the importance of information technology in health care in his State of the Union Address. He stated, "By computerizing health records, we can avoid dangerous medical mistakes, reduce costs, and improve care."[13] The following April, President Bush issued an executive order that called for widespread adoption of interoperable EHRs within 10 years and established the position of the National Coordinator for Health Information Technology.[15] Subsequently, in June 2004 the President's Information Technology Advisory Committee (PITAC) published a report that suggested to reduce health care costs, control medical and medication errors, reduce needless duplication of diagnostic tests, and monitor public health and bioterrorism concerns the government should enable ways to develop a twenty-first-century EHR system.[14]

The PITAC proposed a framework for a health care information infrastructure that would be composed of four elements: EHRs for all Americans; computer-assisted clinical decision support; computerized provider order entry; and secure, private, interoperable, e-health information exchange.[14] The PITAC report was followed by a progress report from the Office of the National Coordinator for Health Information Technology (ONC) which laid out strategic action to achieve a vision of consumer-centric and information-rich health care. To achieve this vision, the ONC supported numerous efforts to implement EHRs and regional health information organizations, now identified as health information exchanges (HIEs).[16] Since these documents were published, the federal government has taken an action-oriented role in facilitating the adoption of HIT and EHR systems, which will be discussed in more detail later in the book. In addition, a number of federal grants have been funded and legislation enacted in support of the ONC efforts.[17] The HITECH Act of 2009 called for the Centers for Medicare and Medicaid Services to establish an incentive payment program for health care providers who adopt and demonstrate meaningful use of certified EHR systems. In addition, leadership and support for EHR adoption and HIEs was granted to ONC through the HITECH Act.[18]

Today, when asked what constitutes a patient record, one has to look beyond a hard copy, paper-based document to a broader view of an EHR that fulfills several purposes as well as serving as the core for HIEs. As health care has become more complex, the patient record has evolved to address these complexities. It has emerged from prehistoric cave drawings to paper records to hybrid records and now to electronic records. In an electronic format, attention has been paid to health care data and information and how it translates to patient records that are generated and reside within a health care delivery organization or records that become part of HIE entities. In an electronic format, the patient record also enables the collection and use of secondary data for data analytics, business intelligence, health care policy analysis, and other major investigative purposes. Changes in electronically stored health care information and the patient record have given rise to the need for HIM professionals to assume a leadership role in information governance and stewardship as the health care industry transitions from paper-based patient records to EHR systems.

SELF-ASSESSMENT QUIZ

5. What professional organization was most aware of the need for quality patient records in the early part of the twentieth century and later established standards for the content of the records?
6. To be reimbursed for Medicare and Medicaid, an organization must comply with what federal regulations?
7. What is the difference between fee-for-service and prospective payment reimbursement methods?
8. The term *hybrid record* refers to what type of patient record?

EVOLUTION OF THE HEALTH INFORMATION MANAGEMENT PROFESSION

Early History

The early efforts by the medical profession to upgrade the education of physicians and to evaluate the quality of care provided to patients have a direct link to the beginning of the HIM profession in the United States. The HIM profession evolved from the need for accurate and complete records regarding the care and treatment of patients as one means to improve and standardize health care. The ACS's standardization program was the catalyst for organizing and educating a group of people who could assist hospitals in meeting the informational needs of accrediting bodies and medical educators. Hospital medical record departments were forming, and a knowledgeable workforce was needed to implement and manage methods of collecting, storing, and retrieving patient data and records. In 1928 Dr. Malcolm MacEachern, director of hospital activities at the ACS and an important leader in the hospital standardization movement, recognized that more was needed to bring about change in the quality of patient records.[7] He invited medical record workers from the United States and Canada to attend a meeting of the Clinical Congress of the ACS. The meeting program and exhibits were devoted to medical record documentation and standard-setting efforts of the ACS. The meeting resulted in the medical record workers organizing to form the Association of Record Librarians of North America (ARLNA). Grace Whiting Myers, Librarian Emeritus of Massachusetts General Hospital, was elected the first president of the association.[7] Establishment of the ARLNA was the first step toward professionalization of the discipline of HIM.

The first annual meeting of the ARLNA was held in Chicago the following year. Fifty-three charter members adopted the association's constitution and bylaws and identified ways to communicate and educate a medical record workforce. At the close of the meeting, the members decided to communicate through the publication of a quarterly journal, Bulletin of the Association of Record Librarians of North America. In addition, a committee was formed to develop a course of study for medical record librarians. This course of study laid the groundwork for the profession's development of education programs at the associate, baccalaureate, and master's degree levels.[19] Efforts of this committee are discussed in more detail in the section, "Formation of Education Programs."

Along with the development of standardized educational curriculum, the ARLNA determined that it needed to set standards for its members and formed a Board of Registration in 1933. The board developed rules and regulations for registering members as a registered record librarian (RRL). The rules and regulations set by the board in essence "certified" that the individual met certain criteria or standards that entitled him or her to bear the credential RRL.[20] Additional certifications have been added over the years and are discussed later in the chapter under the section "Professional Certification."

By 1939 the young association had revised its bylaws to allow for state associations to become affiliates of the national association. The Canadian members of the association eventually broke away and formed their own association in 1944.[21] The ARLNA subsequently changed its name to the American Association of Medical Record Librarians (AAMRL). It opened its first executive office in Chicago with the help of the AHA and moved to its own headquarters in 1946.[22] Throughout the next 30 years association activities focused on building a professional body of knowledge that supported academic program growth, program accreditation, professional certification, and continuing education. In 1970 the association changed its name to the American Medical Record Association (AMRA) and changed its name again in 1991 to the AHIMA.[22]

1990s

Each change in the association's name was to accommodate the expanding roles and responsibilities of its members that resulted from changes in the health care industry. The 1991 name change reflected the profession's look toward the future when paper-based patient records would be replaced with EHRs and HIM practice would move into an electronic age of information management. Throughout the 1990s the association expanded its role in shaping health care policy; advocating legal and regulatory changes while advancing confidentiality, privacy, and security concerns; and understanding the potential roles health information managers would assume in an e-health care environment and the education they would need to assume these roles.[23] In 1996 the association published Vision 2006, a strategic document that focused the association's efforts on multiple fronts including the identification of seven emerging roles for HIM professionals. Many additional roles have since been identified as the profession has expanded its responsibilities with increased reliance on HIT (Box 2-2).[23,24]

At the end of the 1990s, e-health had permeated the health care landscape and HIM professionals found that the skills

used to manage paper medical record systems could easily transfer to managing in an e-health environment.[25]

2000s Forward

As the profession entered the twenty-first century it was evident that HIM professionals would be key participants in the industry's move to EHRs and the use of data for business intelligence purposes. The AHIMA E-health Task Force reported in 2002 that:

> The knowledge and expertise of managing the handwritten medical records containing source patient data has evolved from independent management of paper medical records in settings across the continuum of care to scanning the paper documents for multiple user access, to entering data into automated systems that generate electronic patient data, to integrated delivery systems that electronically manage the patient across the continuum of care, to network integration and e-health information management.[25]

The Task Force also identified roles that HIM professionals were suited to perform as the profession transitioned to an electronic health information management (e-HIM) environment.[25] In 2003 the e-HIM Task Force reported on its visions of health information and e-HIM practice in 2010.[26] The e-HIM vision statement moved health information out of a paper environment into an electronic environment and defined HIM as the "body of knowledge and practice that ensures the availability of health information to facilitate real-time health care delivery and critical health-related decision making for multiple purposes across diverse organizations, settings, and disciplines."[26] The e-HIM Task Force identified roles and competencies that HIM professionals were likely to assume as HIM practice moved toward an electronic environment (Box 2-3).[26]

Two years later, in 2005, the Task Force reassessed the environment and noted progress toward the industry's increasing adoption of HIT, the federal role in facilitating this adoption, efforts toward establishing national and regional HIEs, and growing interest in PHR use. The 2010 vision statement for health information was revised as follows:

> The future state of health information is electronic, consumer-centered, comprehensive, longitudinal, accessible, credible, and secure. Ownership of health information is a shared responsibility between the consumer and provider.[27]

Recommendations from the e-HIM Task Force's initial report were used to guide AHIMA activities in the areas of workforce development, industry partnerships and collaborations, professional self-development, education reform, research, and grantsmanship. Addressing concern for workforce needs, AHIMA engaged in a major study that was completed in 2005.[28] The study confirmed that with conversion of paper-based medical record systems to EHR systems, traditional HIM department functions were experiencing, and will continue to experience, significant changes, whether in a hospital, long-term care, or other type of health care

---

BOX 2-2

Vision 2006 Emerging Roles of Health Information Management Professionals

- Information privacy and security officer
- Clinical data specialist
- Decision support analyst
- Patient information coordinator
- Data quality manager
- Clinical data repository manager
- Corporate health information management director

BOX 2-3   HIM Professional Roles and Competencies in an e-HIM Environment

HIM Professional Roles

Business process engineer
Clinical research protocol designer and manager
Clinical trials manager
Clinical vocabulary manager
Consumer advocate
Data analyst
Data facilitator
Data/information broker
Data/information presenter
Data sets, nomenclature, and classification standards developer
Data miner
Data navigator
Data quality and integrity manager
Data resource manager
Data security, privacy, confidentiality manager
Data translator
Information systems designer
Work and data flow analyst

Competencies in e-HIM

- Establishing and guiding national, local, and state health information policy development and implementation
- Establishing and implementing policies, practices, and procedures governing all aspects of HIM
- Establishing and implementing standards for privacy, security, and confidentiality of health information

- Establishing and implementing policies and standards for monitoring of data integrity, accuracy, validity, authenticity, and version control
- Developing health information format and content standards to ensure the collection of accurate, timely, and complete health information
- Facilitating communication of health information across organizational health care teams and among different entities
- Facilitating the concurrent use of health information for multiple purposes (such as for direct patient care, outcomes measurement and evaluation, wellness and prevention, research, public health and policy development)
- Managing compliance, regulatory, accreditation, licensure, and (re)certification programs and activities
- Analyzing and synthesizing qualitative and quantitative health information for various and diverse needs and audiences
- Developing, designing, and implementing clinical vocabularies
- Translating and interpreting health information for consumers and their caregivers
- Helping consumers to access and obtain diverse and often complex health information
- Informing and educating consumers about health information issues
- Providing the context to understand, analyze, and interpret health information
- Helping providers understand data flow and reporting requirements within the context of dynamic rules, regulations, and guidelines
- Leading business process redesign efforts

HIM, Health information management.
Source: A vision of the e-HIM future: A report from the AHIMA e-HIM Task Force: http://library.ahima.org/xpedio/groups/public/documents/ahima/bok1_020477.pdf. Accessed November 2, 2013.

provider organization or agency. The movement is toward a virtual department; thus each function within the department must be reengineered, and in some cases eliminated, as EHRs are implemented.

The study also confirmed that HIM professionals work not only in hospitals but in more than 40 types of job settings with more than 200 job titles.[28] HIM professionals work wherever health data are collected, organized, and analyzed, including accounting and consulting firms, insurance companies, and research centers. A little more than 50% of HIM professionals work in health care provider organizations and the remaining number work in nonprovider settings. An increasing number of HIM professionals are involved in software development, marketing, and implementation as members of the information system staff within health care organizations or within software vendor environments. Many are engaged in entrepreneurial business ventures that demonstrate their ability to blend business knowledge with the professional discipline. HIM professionals are in positions with responsibility for setting standards and policies governing how health care data are collected, maintained, and disseminated. They are advocates for, and trainers of, the users of health care information and are data quality experts and advisors on the appropriate uses and interpretation of health care data. As health data

terminology managers, HIM professionals work with standards for EHR implementation and coding systems that support reimbursement and revenue applications. HIM professionals may function as privacy and security officers who protect the access and release of health care data. Some HIM professionals are partners with HIT professionals and health care providers in the planning, design, and implementation of EHR systems and regional HIEs.[28]

With growing emphasis on the implementation of EHRs and HIEs in the later part of the 2000s, AHIMA, in collaboration with the American Medical Informatics Association (AMIA), hosted a workforce summit to identify the need for a health care workforce capable of "innovating, implementing, and using health communications and information technology."[29] As a follow-up to the summit, AHIMA and AMIA formed a Joint Workforce Task Force in 2007 to identify the core competencies expected of a health care workforce that uses EHRs on a daily basis.[30] The Task Force developed an "EHR Core Competencies Matrix Tool" that identified competencies all employees should possess to use computer technologies and electronic information effectively in today's health care workplace. The competencies were categorized into five domains as follows:

1. Health information literacy and skills (13 competencies)
2. HI skills using the EHR (12 competencies)

3. Privacy and confidentiality of health information (21 competencies)
4. Health information and data technical security (8 competencies)
5. Basic computer literacy skills (18 competencies)[28]

Running parallel to this activity was the federal government's understanding that to achieve an electronic health care infrastructure and the use of EHRs, a health care workforce would have to be educated in HIT. With the passage of the ARRA in 2009 came support through the ONC to fund an "Health IT Workforce Development Program."[31] The goal of the program was to train a workforce to help providers implement EHRs for the purpose of improving quality, safety, and cost-effective health care. The program included training modules delivered through more than 70 community colleges and nine university-based training programs. The program also provided funding for the development of competency certification examinations that, if successfully completed, enabled an individual to use the credential *HIT PRO*. In July 2013 the AHIMA assumed responsibility for administering the examinations, which are discussed later in the chapter. To date, some 9600 individuals have completed the examinations.

Based on previous workforce activities, increasing reliance on technology, and data analytics the AHIMA Board of Directors developed a HIM Profession Core Model to reflect potential roles, settings, and effect of the profession in the next decade.[32] The model consists of five functional components with a sixth under review that relate to a HIM professional's direct interaction with patient health information (Box 2-4). In addition, the model identifies four areas of practice identified as extenders that "support, advance, extend and contribute" to the functional components.[32] For each of the functional components job roles have been identified along with value statements that further support the functional component. Job roles have also been identified for the four extenders as well as specific job settings applicable to both functional components and extenders. The job settings have been grouped into nine categories that best reflect the diversity of HIM work environments.[32]

The Core Model provides a way for the HIM professional to look at current and future opportunities as the profession continues to evolve and expand its responsibilities. The need for HIM professionals as well as other disciplines versed in HIT continues to grow as emerging technologies require qualified individuals to help others access information to support clinical decision making, research, revenue cycle management, and personal health management. The AHIMA continues to "play a critical role in the growth and success of the HIM profession"[28] by engaging in major initiatives that support HIM practice, advancing the roles of HIM professionals through cutting-edge academic programs, offering certification opportunities and providing professional development resources such as practice guidelines.

SELF-ASSESSMENT QUIZ

9. Identify four major milestones the HIM profession accomplished in its early history between 1928 and 1991.
10. What is the 2010 AHIMA e-HIM Task Force's revised definition of *health information?*
11. AHIMA used the e-HIM Task Force report to guide its activities in what areas?
12. What are the five competency domains identified in the AHIMA/AMIA Joint Workforce Task Force expected of a health care workforce that uses EHRs on a daily basis?
13. What was the goal of the federal Health IT Workforce Development Program?
14. The HIM Profession Core Model consists of what five functional components?

Formation of Education Programs

Education has been a building block of the HIM profession since 1928 when at its annual meeting ARLNA members formed a committee to develop a curriculum for the education of medical record librarians. The curriculum was finalized in 1932 and used to establish academic programs for medical record librarians. The first academic programs for

BOX 2-4 HIM Profession Core Model Elements

Extensions	Functional Components	Job Settings
• Education	• Data/information analysis, transformation and decision support	• Health care provider organizations
• Policy	• Information dissemination and liaison	• Health care data organizations
• Research	• Health information resource management and innovation	• Health care payer organizations
• Standards	• Information governance and stewardship	• Health care supplier organizations
	• Quality and patient safety (under further development)	• Planning organizations, regulators, and industry support
		• Educational institutions
		• Research institutions
		• Third-party compliance organizations
		• Consumer organizations

HIM, Health information management.
American Health Information Management Association. A new view of HIM: introducing the core model, Review Draft. 2011: http://library.ahima.org/xpedio/groups/public/documents/ahima/bok1_049283.pdf. Accessed November 2, 2013.

medical record librarians were provisionally approved in 1934.[22] Early programs were in hospitals and required from 2 to 4 years of college, with some requiring graduation from an approved nursing school. As programs were established, it became apparent that uniform standards for all medical record programs were needed; thus the "Essentials of an Acceptable School for Medical Record Librarians" were developed by the ARLNA in 1943.[22] This document became the foundation for the association's program accreditation process, described later.

By 1952, 19 schools offered formal educational programs for medical record librarians.[22] Although these formal educational programs were established at a number of sites, the number of professionals graduating did not meet the needs of the hospitals. This led to the decision to train another level of personnel to aid the medical record librarian. In 1953, six schools for training medical record technicians were approved. These programs were 9 to 12 months in length and located in hospitals; no formal academic credit was granted. After completion of the technician program, the graduate was eligible to write a certification examination. On successful completion of the examination, the individual was granted the credential accredited record technician (ART).[33] During the 1960s and 1970s, education programs at both the medical record librarian and medical record technician levels transitioned to 2- and 4-year college or university settings. This transition occurred as the profession's body of knowledge grew, and expanded skills in the work setting were required of program graduates.

In addition to the formal education programs found in universities and colleges, the professional association developed a correspondence course in 1961 to train more support staff at the technician level. Hospital-based technician programs were not producing enough graduates at the time to meet the workforce needs. Over time, the course was revised, and additional college requirements were added to the program in an effort to make the educational preparation of its graduates relatively comparable to that of graduates of the 2-year associate degree program.[34] In 1991, when the professional association changed its name to the *AHIMA*, the college and university programs also changed their program names to HIM. The correspondence course followed suit and was renamed the Independent Study Program for the Health Information Technician (ISP for HITs). By 1998, it was determined that the ISP for HITs was no longer necessary because of the growth of community or technical college technician programs. The ISP was discontinued December 31, 2001.

As of this writing, there are 336 accredited programs in HIM. There are 57 baccalaureate degrees, 271 associate degrees, 5 master's degrees in HIM and 3 master's degrees in HI programs, with the number of programs at all degree levels continuing to expand. Many baccalaureate degree programs also offer a postbaccalaureate degree option for those individuals who already possess a baccalaureate or advanced degree but wish to pursue the HIM degree. The curriculum in HIM programs has evolved over time to accommodate the increased demands for a workforce well educated in the use of HIT, health care data, and information management.

Major changes in HIM curriculum occurred in the mid-1990s as a result of the previously mentioned e-Health, e-HIM, and Workforce Task Forces. Curriculum models were developed for associate, baccalaureate, and master's degree programs that reflected content and competencies required of HIM professionals in the 21st century.[35–37] Models were developed as part of ongoing discussions of the profession's future and need for graduate education as a natural progression in the evolution of the HIM profession. The content domains of the curriculum models were integrated into the accreditation standards for baccalaureate, associate, and master's degree programs in HIM and HI.[38–41] A decision to incorporate the broader field of HI into the master's curriculum model was made because it was thought that others involved in the use of computers to manage health care data and information would be interested in pursuing an advanced degree in the subject area.

To better delineate the three academic levels in 2004, the AHIMA Education Strategy Committee developed a framework for HIM education, which provided a general descriptor for graduates of each of the academic program levels.[42] The descriptors emphasize the roles of HIM graduates in both a paper and electronic work environment. A brief synopsis of the descriptors follows.

Associate Degree HIM—Possesses technical expertise in health data collection, analysis, monitoring, maintenance, and reporting activities in accordance with established data quality principles, legal and regulatory standards, and professional best practice guidelines. These functions encompass, among other areas, processing and using health data for billing, compliance, and surveillance purposes.

Baccalaureate Degree HIM—Possesses expertise to develop, implement, or manage individual, aggregate, and public health care data collection and reporting systems. These systems ensure quality, integrity, availability, and preservation of health care data in support of patient safety and privacy, confidentiality, and security of health information.

Master's Degree HIM—Engages in executive-level, enterprise-wide, administrative, research, or applied HI activities. Focus is on evolving strategic and operational relevance and robustness of clinical information resources in health care industry and public health sector. Performs research to advance body of knowledge and standards associated with the management of health information.[42]

Subsequently, the curriculum models and content domains for the baccalaureate and associate degree HIM programs were updated in 2005, and the graduate curriculum model was updated in 2006.[35–37] Each update supported revisions to program accreditation standards. With movement of the health care industry to more patient-centric and evidence-based medicine along with greater pressures to adopt HIT and EHRs, the Education Strategy Committee in 2006, assessed the environmental factors influencing HIM practice and proposed a new vision for HIM education to be achieved by 2016.[43] A key priority in Vision 2016 was movement of the profession toward graduate education at the master's level. In 2010 the Education Strategy Committee revisited *Vision 2016* and set in motion the establishment of the Council for Excellence in Education (CEE).[44] The CEE functions to determine academic strategy for the profession. It has taken *Vision 2016* and transitioned it to *Reality 2016* in an effort to ensure that the profession will continue to evolve and meet the demands of a changing health care environment. Part of *Reality 2016* is to once again update the entry-level competencies and content that comprises HIM curriculum for associate, baccalaureate, and master's degree programs. Revisions to the competencies and content are under way as the profession continues to adapt to the dramatic changes in the way the industry "creates, uses, manages and disperses health information."[44]

Accreditation of Educational Programs

Because of close ties to the AMA and ACS and their accreditation program for medical schools, the AHIMA (formally ARLNA) developed an accreditation program for medical record librarian programs in 1943. The term accreditation is defined as a voluntary, nongovernmental process that educational programs elect to participate in as a means to demonstrate to the public that a program meets or exceeds stated standards of educational quality. The program accreditation for medical record librarians began in 1943, as noted earlier, and in 1953, the 2-year medical record technician degree programs were added to the accreditation agenda. The Essentials of an Acceptable School for Medical Record Librarians became the Standards for Health Information Management Education (Baccalaureate Degree and Associate Degree Programs). These standards represent the minimum requirements an education program must follow to achieve program accreditation.

From 1943 to 2004, the association collaborated with the AMA's Council on Allied Health Education and Accreditation and later the Council on Accreditation of Allied Health Educational Programs to accredit the HIM associate and baccalaureate degree programs at colleges and universities in the United States and its territories. In 2004, AHIMA established its own accrediting body for education programs, the Commission on Accreditation for Health Informatics and Information Management Education (CAHIIM). Given the increased importance of HI in the delivery of health care, the need for a qualified workforce in HIT, and the use of informatics in the HIM body of practice, the accrediting organization chose to incorporate responsibility for accrediting HI programs into its charge. CAHIIM functions as an independent accrediting organization that serves the public interest by establishing and enforcing quality accreditation standards for HIM and HI educational programs.[45] The CAHIIM recognizes programs that meet standards and assesses student achievement as it strives to promote, evaluate, and improve the quality of undergraduate and graduate education in HIM and HI in the United States and internationally.

The CAHIIM previously offered an approval process for master's degree programs in HIM and applied HI, which it converted to a formal accreditation process in January 2010. One other approval program is offered by AHIMA, but it does not fall under the responsibility of CAHIIM. The AHIMA Approval Committee for Certificate Programs is responsible for the Coding Education Program Approval Process, which approves coding programs.

Professional Certification

The focus of accreditation is on demonstrating to the public that a program or organization meets or exceeds stated standards of quality. An individual can also demonstrate to the public that he or she meets or exceeds stated standards of competence by obtaining professional certification. Licensure, certification, or registration is used by government and nongovernment agencies as a means to protect the public from individuals who have not met the standards of practice prescribed by a given state or profession. Individuals who do meet these standards are given the right to use specific credentials denoting that they have demonstrated a level of competence in their domain of practice. Individuals who obtain credentials are required to maintain their credential over time by meeting continuing education requirements as delineated by the agency or organization that supports the credential.

Licensure occurs at the state level and is overseen by a state licensing board or agency. An individual must meet eligibility requirements required by the state before the individual is granted a license to practice. Demonstration of eligibility is usually through successful completion of an education program and passing of a licensing examination. Most health professionals that treat or touch patients in some way are required to be licensed by the state in which they practice. For example, occupational therapists, physical therapists, and respiratory therapists must complete certain educational requirements and take state licensing examinations before they are allowed to practice in a state. Demonstrated success of these two requirements enables these practitioners to use the credential *licensed* (L) in their occupational title, such as *licensed occupational therapist*. Some health care professionals, such as occupational therapists, possess both a license and a certification credential, *registered occupational therapist*.

How do certification and registration differ from licensure? Certification refers to "the process through which a nongovernmental agency or association grants recognition of competence to an individual who has met predetermined qualifications specified by that agency or association."[46] Registration entails entering on an official list an individual who has been certified as eligible by set qualifications of an organization or agency. In regard to HIM, professional certification began in 1933 when the AHIMA (formally ARLNA) formed a Board of Registration to set standards for its members. One standard set by this new certifying body was that an individual had to be 21 years of age and of good moral and ethical character.[20] No formal examination of the candidate was required at that time. The credential bestowed on the individual who met these early standards was RRL.

By 1952 an examination component was added to the eligibility requirements and remains in place today. Certification examinations are constructed from detailed job analysis studies of individuals working in the profession. The analyses are updated every 3 to 5 years by the examination body. The job analysis study verifies the tasks performed by practitioners, which is then used to develop test specifications and questions for a given certification examination. Over the years, the profession's certification process has expanded to reflect the education and responsibilities of HIM professionals practicing in a variety of roles.

The AHIMA's certifying body is the Commission on Certification for Health Informatics and Information Management (CCHIIM). Previously, the commission was known as the *Council of Certification*. In 2009 the name of the certifying body was expanded to include future certification opportunities for HI professionals in addition to HIM professionals. The CCHIIM is responsible for "establishing, implementing, and enforcing standards and procedures for certification and recertification of health informatics and information management (HIIM) professionals."[47] The CCHIIM offers nine certification examinations that, if successfully completed, lead to nine distinct credentials, each of which are discussed in turn:

- Registered health information administrator (RHIA)
- Registered health information technician (RHIT)
- Certified coding associate (CCA)
- Certified coding specialist (CCS)
- Certified coding specialist—physician based (CCS-P)
- Certified health data analyst (CHDA)
- Certified in healthcare privacy and security (CHPS)
- Clinical documentation improvement practitioner (CDIP)
- Certified healthcare technology specialist (CHTS)

Registered Health Information Administrator and Registered Health Information Technician

The RHIA and RHIT credentials (formally RRL and ART, respectively) focus on HIM at an entry level of practice. Both credentials require that an individual pass a certification examination and be a graduate of an HIM education program that meets at least one of the following criteria:

- Accredited by the CAHIIM
- Approved by a foreign association with which AHIMA has a reciprocity agreement

An individual wishing to take the RHIA examination must have successfully met the academic requirements of a CAHIIM-accredited HIM program at the baccalaureate degree level or have a certificate of completion from a CAHIIM-accredited HIM program, plus a baccalaureate degree from a regionally accredited college or university. An individual wishing to take the RHIT examination must have successfully met the academic requirements of a CAHIIM-accredited HIM program at the associate degree level. The RHIA functions in the managerial areas of health

services and information systems and the uses of health-related data for planning, delivering, and evaluating health care. The RHIT typically functions in the technical areas of health data collection, analysis, and monitoring and often specializes in coding diagnoses and procedures for reimbursement purposes.[47]

Certified Coding Associate, Certified Coding Specialist, Certified Coding Specialist— Physician Based

In 1992 AHIMA moved into specialty certification as it recognized the need to offer credentials in specific areas of practice related to medical diagnostic and procedural coding. Coders are technical specialists who are a part of the health information services team in a health care organization. Their primary function is to apply national and facility-specific guidelines in the assignment of diagnosis and procedure codes to clinical data based on their review of the documentation in the patient record. Accuracy in coding is extremely important for revenue, reimbursement, and research purposes, as discussed earlier in the section on the evolving patient record. To address the increasing need for coders who possessed the necessary competence to engage in quality coding, AHIMA implemented both entry-level and advanced coding credentials. Coding is also a knowledge and skill component in the entry-level credentialing examinations for RHITs and RHIAs.

Three coding certification options are available. They are the CCA, CCS, and CCS-P. The education eligibility requirements for these three credentials vary based on the credential type. The CCA, an entry-level coding credential, was implemented in 2002. A high school diploma from a U.S. high school or equivalent educational background is required. The recommended amount of experience for this credential is 6 months or completion of an AHIMA-approved coding certificate program or other formal training program.[47] The CCS credential was implemented in 1992 and in 1997, the CCS-P was established. The CCS examination focuses on inpatient coding systems, whereas the CCS-P examination focuses on ambulatory or outpatient care coding. There are five eligibility requirement options for these examinations. An individual need only meet one of the requirements. Both the CCS and CCS-P credentials are for the more experienced coder. It is suggested that an individual have at least 2 or more years of coding experience to be successful on these examinations or have their CCA and 1 year of experience.[47]

Certified Health Data Analyst

Movement to EHRs and increased use of health care data has called for individuals who can acquire, manage, analyze, interpret, and transform data into quality information. In 2009 AHIMA implemented the CHDA credential to offer individuals who possess these skills an avenue for recognition of expertise in health data analysis and mastery of this domain of practice. Eligibility requirements for this credential include (1) an associate degree and 5 years of experience,

(2) RHIT and 3 years of experience, or (3) a baccalaureate or master's degree with 1 year of health care data experience.[47]

Certified in Healthcare Privacy and Security

In 1996 HIPAA required that health care providers, payers, and plans appoint privacy and security officials to carry out mandatory duties as prescribed in the HIPAA regulations. The regulations asked for privacy officers who would be responsible for the development and implementation of privacy-related policies and procedures and security officials whose duties would be the management and supervision of security measures to protect personal patient information.[47] In 2002 the AHIMA first implemented and sponsored the certified in healthcare privacy (CHP) credential followed by the certified in healthcare security (CHS) credential. Subsequently, in 2007 the two credentials were combined to form the credential CHPS.

The CHPS credential validates an individual's expertise in the design, implementation, and administration of comprehensive privacy and security protection programs in all types of health care settings. Eligibility for the CHPS examination requires that an individual must have met at least one of the following criteria: (1) a baccalaureate degree and a minimum of 4 years of experience in health care privacy and security management; (2) an advanced graduate degree (e.g., juris doctor, medical doctor [MD], doctor of philosophy) and 2 years of experience in health care privacy and security management; (3) an RHIA with a minimum of 2 years of experience in health care privacy and security management; or (4) an RHIT with a minimum of 4 years of experience in health care privacy and security management, or an associate degree and 6 years of experience in health care privacy and security management.[47]

Clinical Documentation Improvement Practitioner

The CDIP is a relatively new credential established to address the need for individuals who specialize in knowledge of documentation requirements relevant to compliant coding and billing demands. The knowledge base of a CDIP includes supporting efforts to ensure quality health information and the integrity of the patient record.[47] Eligibility for this examination includes an RHIA, RHIT, CCS, CCS-P, registered nurse, MD, or doctor of osteopathy and 2 years of experience in clinical documentation improvement, or an associate degree or higher and 3 years of experience.

Certified Healthcare Technology Specialist

The CHTS examinations are an outcome of the 2009 ARRA Health IT Workforce Development Program. In 2013 the HIT-PRO examinations were converted to the AHIMA CHTS credentials. These examinations assess the competency of HIT professionals in the following roles:
- Clinical/practitioner consultant
- Practice workflow and information management redesign
- Implementation manager
- Implementation support specialist
- Technical/software support staff
- Trainer

There are no formal eligibility requirements for the examination, but one assumes that an individual has completed one of the workforce development programs, or has sufficient work experience to be successful on the examination.[47]

 SELF-ASSESSMENT QUIZ

15. What is the difference between the three academic program levels in HIM?
16. What is the responsibility of the CEE?
17. What is the name of the organization that accredits academic programs in HIM?
18. What is the difference between licensure, certification or registration?
19. What is the name of the certifying body that credentials HIM professionals?
20. What two CCHIIM credentials require that an individual be a graduate of an accredited HIM program to take the certification examination?

Importance of Professional Certification

The importance of certification should not be underestimated. Research indicates that individuals who are certified tend to promote quality work outcomes.[48] In 2005 AHIMA surveyed employers seeking their opinion on the value of industry credentials. Survey results revealed that employers think favorably of industry credentials. Credentialed employees help reduce exposure to fraud and abuse and improve the delivery of quality health care. Employers tend to hire individuals with a credential over those without one and prefer credentials when promoting employees. Credentialed employees tend to earn more than noncredentialed employees. Employers also reported that the credential tells them the individual has met certain education requirements, possesses a certain competency level as proven by examination, and must stay informed through continuing education requirements.[49] Thus the importance of obtaining certification and maintaining one's credentials cannot be overemphasized. A credential can be important to professional success and future opportunities in the marketplace.

Other HIM-Related Professional Organizations and Relevant Credentials

The function of managing health information and patient records especially since the advent of computer technology in medicine and HIT has given rise to a number of individuals and corresponding professional associations who also work with and manage health data, information, and patient records in some way. Many of these individuals and associations have collaborative working relationships with AHIMA and its members, such as the previously mentioned AMIA. Some of these associations offer credentialing opportunities to their members, whereas some organizations do not function as a professional association but as a certification entity offering specialty certification options. Some of the more common associations who complement AHIMA and the work of HIM professionals are included in Box 2-5.

BOX 2-5   Professional Associations

The following associations represent only a small sample of professional associations that represent individuals involved in some aspect of health information management and who work collaboratively or in partnership with the AHIMA and its members.

Association of Healthcare Documentation Integrity (AHDI; http://www.ahdionline.org)—formerly the American Association for Medical Transcription (AAMT), the AHDI represents the clinical documentation sector (profession of medical transcription), setting standards for education and practice in the field of health data capture and documentation. Membership is open to any individual or business involved in the field of health data capture and documentation. AHDI offers a certification option for medical transcriptionists.

American Medical Informatics Association (AMIA; http://www.amia.org/about-amia)—AMIA represents the biomedical and health informatics sector, with a focus on advancing use of health information and communications technology in clinical care and clinical research, personal health management, public health and population, and translational science with the objective of improving health. Its membership comprises interdisciplinary, diverse groups (physicians, nurses, health information managers, researchers, scientists, etc.) involved in organization, analysis, management, and use of information in health care.

Health Information and Management Systems Society (HIMSS; http://www.himss.org/about)—HIMSS focuses on global leadership in the use of health care information technology and management systems for the betterment of health care. Membership comprises an interdisciplinary, diverse group (chief information officers, systems engineers, computer and information systems professionals, physicians, nurses, health information managers, etc.) involved in initiatives to promote information and management systems to ensure quality patient care. HIMSS offers a certification option for health care information and management systems professionals—Certified Professional in Healthcare Information and Management Systems (CPHIMS).

National Cancer Registrars Association (NCRA; http://www.ncra-usa.org)—NCRA represents the cancer data management profession and serves to educate and credential cancer registry professionals whose purpose is to capture information that is used to manage cancer, and ultimately cures. Membership is open to anyone working in the cancer registry arena. NCRA offers a certification option for cancer registry professionals.

Depending on the job function of the HIM professional, an individual may belong to several of the mentioned organizations and hold several credentials. There are a number of other specialty credentials that HIM professionals may consider, depending on personal interests and career focus. Each credential has its own set of eligibility and, in some cases, continuing education requirements. A few of the more common credentials and their sponsoring organizations are listed in Box 2-6.

BOX 2-6   Health Information Management–Related Credentials and Certification Organizations

- **CPEHR**—Certified Professional in Electronic Health Records, offered by the Health IT Certification
- **CPHIE**—Certified Professional in Health Information Exchange, offered by the Health IT Certification
- **CPHIT**—Certified Professional in Health Information Technology, offered by the Health IT Certification
- **CPHIMS**—Certified Professional in Health Information Management Systems, offered by the Health Information and Management System Society
- **CPHQ**—Certified Professional Health Quality, offered by the Health Care Quality Board
- **CMT**—Certified Medical Transcriptionist, offered by Association of Healthcare Documentation Integrity
- **CHC**-Certified in Healthcare Compliance, offered by Compliance Certification Board
- **CPC**—Certified Coding Professional, offered by the American Academy of Professional Coders
- **CTR**—Certified Tumor Registrar, offered by the National Cancer Registrars Association
- **RCC**—Radiology Certified Coder, offered by the Radiology Coding Certification Board

Maintenance of Certification and Lifelong Learning

Once a person receives a credential through the AHIMA's certification process, that person is required to maintain the credential by engaging in continuing education activity. Early in the profession's history it was recognized that the astonishing rate of change in medical science and the delivery of health care would require continuing learning on the part of HIM professionals to stay current in the discipline. The AHIMA was an early proponent of lifelong learning, offering its first formal continuing education institute in 1939.[22] In 1973, AHIMA adopted a formal maintenance of certification program that required the acquisition of a certain number of continuing education units (CEUs) on the basis of the credential. Standards for maintaining certification were defined along with CEU-qualifying activities.

Maintenance of the certification program is continually updated to reflect changes in practice and the addition of new credentials to the program. A prescribed number of CEUs must be obtained within a 2-year reporting cycle. The number of CEUs an individual must acquire during this time frame depends on the type and number of AHIMA credentials held.[50] For example, if an RHIA also holds a CHDA credential, then the individual would be required to obtain 40 CEUs during the 2-year reporting cycle (30 CEUs for the RHIA and 10 CEUs for the additional credential of CHDA). Overall, 80% of all CEUs must be earned in the domain of HIIM. Basically, the HIIM domain encompasses the following content areas where CEUs may be obtained:

- Technology: existing and emerging technologies for the collection of clinical data, the transformation of clinical data to useful health information, and the communication and protection of information

- Management development: organizational management theory and practices and human resource management techniques to improve departmental adaptability, innovation, service quality, and operational efficiency
- Clinical data management: data analysis of quality and clinical resources appropriate to the clinical setting including database management, coding compliance using coding or payment systems to ensure cost-effectiveness of services rendered
- Performance improvement: quality processes to ensure quality data are generating consistent, timely quality information; to develop systems that are flexible and adaptable in a constantly changing health care environment
- External forces: regulatory requirements and appropriate compliance initiatives (policies, procedures, protocols, and technology) for hospitals and other entities, including required practices for accrediting bodies and federal and state rules and regulations
- Clinical foundations: understanding of human anatomy and physiology, the nature of disease processes, protocols of diagnosis and treatment of major diseases including drugs, laboratory and other tests; to apply to reading, coding, and abstracting of medical information to support quality care and associated databases
- Privacy and security: current health care regulations that promote protection of medical information and electronic transmission of health information; patient advocacy related to privacy rights[50]

Although individuals who hold an AHIMA credential are required to maintain their credentials through continuing education activities, there is overall support among AHIMA members for the concept of lifelong learning. Lifelong learning is the responsibility of every individual who wishes to enter and survive in a work environment that continually faces global, economic, and technologic changes. The AHIMA members' affirmation of lifelong learning is delineated in the 2004 resolution "Lifelong Learning: The Guiding Principles for Professional Development."[51] To support learning activities, AHIMA offers educational content from AHIMA events as well as numerous audio seminars, webinars, online learning programs, and publications.

Fellowship Program

In 1999 the AHIMA implemented a fellowship program that is open to any individual who is an active, honorary, or senior member of AHIMA. The program is designed to recognize AHIMA members who have made significant and sustained contributions to the profession over time. Contributions can be made in any one or all of the following areas: innovation and knowledge sharing, meritorious service, and excellence in practice or education. The fellowship program is designed to bring together senior HIM professionals as an organizational resource and to provide an incentive to members to contribute to the advancement of the profession.[52]

Eligibility for fellowship requires that an individual have a minimum of 10 years of full-time professional experience in

HIM or a related field, 10 years of continuous AHIMA membership, evidence of sustained and substantial professional achievement, and a minimum of a master's degree. The fellowship program also offers a candidacy provision for those individuals who do not meet the criteria but wish to work toward fellowship over time. The process for fellowship designation requires that an individual complete an application that is reviewed for approval by the AHIMA Fellowship Committee. On approval by this committee, fellow status is conferred, and the individual may use the credential Fellow of the American Health Information Management Association (FAHIMA). It is a lifetime recognition that is subject to continuing AHIMA membership and compliance with the AHIMA Code of Ethics.[52]

 SELF-ASSESSMENT QUIZ

21. What is the value of professional certification?
22. What are the content areas that a credentialed HIM professional must obtain continuing education credits in?
23. Why is lifelong learning important to the HIM professional?
24. What is the purpose of the AHIMA fellowship program?

AMERICAN HEALTH INFORMATION MANAGEMENT ASSOCIATION TODAY

The AHIMA has enjoyed a long history of accomplishments, many of which were discussed earlier in the chapter. It has organized and reorganized itself throughout its history to meet the needs of its members and the changing dynamics of the HIM profession. Today, the AHIMA is more than 85 years old. Its membership is more than 71,000, and it continues to grow at a rate of 5% per year. Members are classified as *active, student, new graduate,* or *emeritus;* thus its membership structure allows anyone interested in HIM to join the association[53] (Box 2-7).

The benefits of AHIMA membership are numerous. The AHIMA is a member-centered organization (Figure 2-1) that provides members with key resources to assist with all aspects of HIM practice. Most important, the AHIMA champions and represents the profession in advocacy matters and key professional alliances, which keeps the profession in the forefront of issues related to its members and their professional domain of practice. Its core values center on leadership, respect, quality, and integrity, which support the association's vision of "leading the advancement and ethical use of quality health information to promote health and wellness worldwide."[54]

The AHIMA is headquartered in Chicago and with a satellite office in Washington, DC. It is a federation made up of 52 component state associations (CSAs), including the District of Columbia and Puerto Rico. The CSAs are affiliated with AHIMA and agree to support and carry out certain member benefits and activities that support the overall goal of the national association. The work of the AHIMA is carried out through a volunteer and staff structure.

BOX 2-7 American Health Information Management Association (AHIMA) Membership Categories

- **Active**—any individual interested in the AHIMA purpose and willing to abide by the Code of Ethics. Active members in good standing are entitled to all membership privileges including the right to vote.
- **Student**—students formally enrolled in an AHIMA-accredited or AHIMA-approved program, including programs pending accreditation or approval, or AHIMA's Coding Basics, that do not already have an AHIMA credential are eligible to apply for student membership. Eligibility is verified with the program director. Special benefits for student members: AHIMA Mentor Program, Student Community of Practice, and Student Connection e-news.
- **New Graduate**—New Graduate membership is for AHIMA Student Members only. After graduation from an AHIMA-accredited HIT, HIA, approved coding, or master's program, AHIMA Student Members may join as a New Graduate Member at a reduced annual dues rate. This is limited to 1 year.
- **Emeritus**—in recognition of service to the profession, current AHIMA members aged 65 years and older are eligible for this membership type.

The volunteer structure of the association is responsible for setting the policies of the organization and for providing direction to a wide variety of essential AHIMA activities. The AHIMA governs itself through its national Board of Directors (BOD) and a House of Delegates (HOD).[55,56] The board is elected by the membership and comprises a president, president-elect, past president director, and nine directors.

The chief executive officer of the association is an ex officio member of the board and is hired by the BOD. The BOD manages the property, business, and affairs of the association, including overseeing its strategic direction and its intellectual and financial assets.

The HOD is the legislative body of the association and serves to advise the BOD in regard to the needs of the members, profession, and industry. For example, the HOD advises the BOD in the development and modification of the association's strategic direction and plans. The HOD is composed of members who are elected leaders from their respective CSAs. The number of delegates from each state varies depending on the number of active members in the state and will vary from one to a maximum of five delegates per any one state. Governance of the HOD consists of a House leadership group, envisioning collaborative and various ad hoc task forces that serve as a needed.[56] There is a strong collaborative working relationship between the BOD and the HOD because both groups work in tandem to move the profession forward strategically and provide industry leadership in matters related to HIM.

In addition to the BOD and HOD, the volunteer structure of the association consists of the CAHIIM and CCHIIM, whose functions were discussed earlier, as well as committees, practice councils, and task forces. Members on the CAHIIM and CCHIIM are elected through national balloting and appointments, and membership on the committees, practice councils, and task forces are by appointment or self-nomination. In 2013, there were 26 volunteer groups at the national level excluding the CAHIIM and CCHIIM. The number varies by year on the basis of the strategic direction

FIGURE 2-1 The American Health Information Management Association (AHIMA) is a member-centered organization, with support resources for its members. *CAHIIM,* Commission on Accreditation for Health Informatics and Information Management Education; *CCHIIM,* Commission on Certification for Health Informatics and Information Management.

and need of the association. Collectively, more than 1000 members serve the AHIMA and CSAs in a volunteer capacity. Volunteerism has been at the heart of the association's activities for more than 85 years and continues to serve as a driving force in moving the profession forward.

Working in tandem with the volunteer structure are more than 100 association employees. The AHIMA staff is responsible for carrying out the day-to-day operation of the association. The staff works collaboratively with the volunteer structure to support the association's vision, mission, and values. In addition, the staff works with the volunteer structure to carry out the strategic priorities set each year by the association leadership. Since the early 2000s these priorities have focused on HIT issues encompassing EHRs, HIEs, privacy and security, standards for data interchange, and systems interoperability. In addition, priorities have called for improvements in the way medical and surgical information is coded for reimbursement and research purposes. This entails using the newest edition of the *International Classification of Diseases*, tenth edition, and other classification and nomenclature systems.

To facilitate its strategic thinking process, each year AHIMA leadership, along with its industry partners and others engage in an environmental scanning to identify issues and trends that may affect the health care industry and HIM profession. Data collected in the scanning process are grouped into the following categories:

- Business and economic climate trends
- Demographic trends
- Legislation and regulation trends
- Technology and science trends
- Other key trends[57]

The information gleamed from environmental scanning enables the AHIMA BOD in tandem with the HOD to set strategic goals in support of the profession. In 2013 the following strategic goals were identified as a result of the industry's movement toward information governance and the use of information for business intelligence purposes:

- Informatics: Transform data into health intelligence.
- Information governance: Be recognized as the experts in health information governance.
- Innovation: Increase thought leadership and evidence-based HIM research.
- Leadership: Develop HIM leaders across all health care sectors.
- Public good: Empower consumers to optimize their health through their personal health information.[58]

Over the next 3 to 5 years, AHIMA, as an industry leader, will continue to offer guidance and support to its members and the health care industry in general as demands increase for HIT and the use of health information.

American Health Information Management Association Communications

Communication is fundamental to supporting an association's members. The AHIMA communicates with its members though a variety of methods including publications such as e-newsletters, practice briefs, electronic alerts, and professional journals—*Journal of the American Health Information Management Association*,[59] *Perspectives in Health Information Management*,[60] and *Educational Perspectives in Health Informatics and Information Management*.[61] The latter two journals, *Perspectives* and *Educational Perspectives* are online, peer-reviewed research journals that foster the profession's commitment to research and scholarship in practice and education. To facilitate professional development, networking, and sharing among association members with similar issues and concerns, AHIMA implemented a web-based communication capability called Communities of Practice (CoPs). The CoPs provided members with up-to-date news, latest trends in HIM, links to numerous resources, and the association's online library, the Book of Knowledge. It brought members with like interests together to solve problems, network, career build, and much more.[62] In 2013 the CoPs received a new look and orientation that now offers online discussion opportunities for both AHIMA members and nonmembers. The CoPs transitioned to "Engage Online Communities," which include public communities as well as AHIMA member–only communities.[63] The public communities focus on HIM domains of practice such as coding, classification, and reimbursement; HI; information governance; and standards to name a few.[63] To further networking, collaboration opportunities, and sharing of resources, AHIMA has established communication links through Facebook, LinkedIn, Twitter, and YouTube services.

AHIMA FOUNDATION: RESEARCH AND EDUCATION IN HEALTH INFORMATION MANAGEMENT

An important indicator of the profession's growth as a discipline is evident in the activities of the AHIMA Foundation (formally known as the Foundation of Research and Education in Health Information Management [FORE]). The foundation was originally founded in 1962 and functions as a separate, incorporated affiliate organization of AHIMA with its own Board of Directors appointed by AHIMA. The Foundation exists to support people, research, resources, and education in the HIM profession. Its role is to provide financial and intellectual resources that support innovation and advancement in HIM for the betterment of the profession, health care, and the public.[64] The foundation's focus is on building tomorrow's workforce (students and faculty), empowering today's workforce (HIM professional), and building a solid research and policy base in HIM. In support of building tomorrow's workforce the foundation appointed a Senior Director of Academic Affairs and facilitated establishment of a CEE, whose purpose is to determine academic strategy to help HIM educational programs meet the industry's demands for high quality graduates. The foundation's efforts to empower today's workforce includes offering professional development opportunities such as a *Thought*

Leaders lecture series and a career map tool that enables an individual to view potential professional roles based on degree levels.[64] The foundation actively supports evidence-based health information research and establishing strategic alliances to advance innovation in the profession. The foundation has funded projects that include benchmarking and best practices research, HIM workforce studies and curriculum, and faculty support. The foundation also offers scholarships, professional recognition awards, and more.

THE PROFESSIONAL CODE OF ETHICS

A code of ethics guides the practice of individuals who choose a given profession. It sets forth the values and principles defined by the profession as acceptable behavior within a practice setting. The HIM profession enacted its first set of ethical principles in 1957 and has revised the code five times over the years with the latest revision occurring in 2011. Revisions of the code over the years demonstrate the importance that AHIMA places on making sure the code is relevant to all members irrespective of credential, membership status, practice functions, or work settings. The code is kept up to date and in line with the changing practice patterns and responsibilities of the HIM professional. The most recent revision of the code addresses issues related to technology, health care, and association management.[65] The code consists of eleven ethical principles and related guidelines. The guidelines assist in interpreting the principle and further delineate behaviors and situations to help clarify a principle.[65] Principles of the code are fundamental to the role of a HIM professional in the work environment. HIM professionals are in positions of responsibility in which they must ensure that the processes followed keep the organization in compliance with its various licensing, accrediting, and legal obligations. In addition, they are in positions in which confidential information is entrusted to them. HIM professionals extend this trust by serving as advocates for the protection and monitoring of such information. The code also speaks to the profession's fundamental duty to engage in lifelong learning and activities that will guide future development of systems to meet the changing needs of the health care industry.[66]

LOOKING TO THE FUTURE

HIT is allowing the transfer and linkage of data well beyond the walls of a health care facility. This technology is supporting the conversion of patient records to EHRs and EHR systems. Such a conversion cannot be successful unless the data to be transferred, manipulated, and aggregated are well defined, valid, and reliable.

As more data become available in electronic form, more potential uses and users will emerge. The capabilities of technology must be tempered with expertise related to information governance to ensure appropriate uses of the data and legitimate users. The pioneering HIM professionals used the resources of the day to help create accurate records that documented patient care. Today's professionals have the same responsibilities but many more challenges, as the value and volume of health information increases and the growing number of users and uses of the information also increases. As HIM professional roles and responsibilities change to accommodate the demands of the health care industry and health care reform, it is important that the profession maintain leadership in the governance and management of patient data, information, and EHR systems. HIM professionals and the AHIMA will continue to play a key role in the future of health care and the complex, integrated information system needed to support the delivery of efficient, quality care in an expanding and transforming health care system.

CHAPTER REVIEW

1. Who is responsible for setting the policies of the organization and for providing direction to the variety of AHIMA activities?

2. What is the responsibility of the AHIMA BOD?

3. What role does the HOD play in AHIMA governance?

4. What is the purpose of environmental scanning?

5. What five goals did the AHIMA BOD and HOD include in the 3- to 5-year strategic plan?

6. What is the role of the AHIMA Foundation?

7. What is the purpose of a code of ethics?

REFERENCES

1. American Health Information Management Association: *Pocket Glossary of Health Information Management and Technology,* Chicago, 2010, American Health Information Management Association.
2. American Health Information Management Association: Health Information 101: http://www.ahima.org/careers/healthinfo?tabid=what. Accessed November 5, 2013.
3. e-HIM Work Group on Defining the Legal Health Record: The legal process and electronic health records, *J Am Health Inform Manage Assoc* 76:96A–96D, 2005.
4. National Healthcare Quality Report, Agency for Healthcare Research and Quality, 2012: http://www.ahrq.gov/research/findings/nhqrdr/nhqr12/index.html. Accessed October 15, 2013.

5. Bettman CC: *Pictorial history of medicine,* Springfield, IL, 1979, Charles C Thomas, p 16.
6. Huffman EK: *Health information management,* ed 10, Berwyn, IL, 1994, Physicians' Record, p 3.
7. American Medical Record Association: The years of growth and development, *Med Record News* 50(66), 1978.
8. Joint Commission Resources Manuals: http://www.jointcommission.org/standards_information/hap_requirements.aspx. Accessed October 15, 2013.
9. Casto AB, Layman E: *Principles of healthcare reimbursement,* Chicago, 2013, American Health Information Management Association.
10. Conditions of Coverage and Conditions of Participation, Center for Medicare and Medicaid Services: http://www.cms.gov/Regulations-and-Guidance/Legislation/CFCsAndCoPs/index.html?redirect=/CFCsAndCOPs. (Accessed October 15.).
11. Institute of Medicine: *The computer-based patient record: an essential technology for health care,* rev ed, Washington, DC, 1997, National Academy Press.
12. Eysenbach G: What is e-health? *J Med Internet Res* 3:e20, 2001.
13. American Health Information Management Association: *Complete medical record in a hybrid EHR environment, I: Managing the transition* (Practice Brief), Updated 2010, Chicago, American Health Information Management Association.
14. President's Information Technology Advisory Committee, National Coordination Office for Information Technology Research and Development: Revolutionizing health care through information technology, 2004: http://www.nitrd.gov/Pitac/reports/20040721_hit_report.pdf. Accessed October 15, 2013.
15. Bush GW: Executive Order 13335: *Incentives for the use of health information technology and establishing the position of the national health information technology coordinator,* April 27, 2004: http://edocket.access.gpo.gov/2004/pdf/04-10024.pdf. Accessed October 15, 2013.
16. Thompson TG, Brailer DJ: *The decade of health information technology: delivering consumer-centric and information-rich health care: framework for strategic action,* Washington, DC, 2004, Department of Health and Human Services, National Coordinator for Health Information Technology, 2004. http://www.providersedge.com/ehdocs/ehr_articles/the_decade_of_hit-delivering_customer-centric_and_info-rich_hc.pdf Accessed October 15, 2013.
17. Agency for Health Research and Quality: *Summary of AHRQ health information technology portfolio 2011 annual report and project summaries. Agency for Health Research and Quality,* Publication No 12-0053-EF, November 2012.
18. Office of the National Coordinator for Health Information Technology: *Update on the adoption of health information technology and related efforts to facilitate the electronic use and exchange of health information: A report to Congress,* January 2012. http://www.healthit.gov/sites/default/files/pdf/january-2012-update-on-hit-adoption-report-to-congress.pdf Accessed October 15, 2013.
19. Bulletin of the Association of Record Librarians of North America, 1(1) 1930.
20. Huffman EK: Requirements and advantages of registration for medical record librarians, *Bull Am Assoc Med Record Librarians North Am* 12(4):102, 1941.
21. Amendments to the Constitution and By-Laws, (Adopted at the Tenth Annual Convention), *Bull Assoc Record Librarians North Am* 10(1)1939, 14.
22. American Medical Record Association: The years of growth and development, *Med Record News* 49:84–90, 1978.
23. Kloss L: Vision 2006: 10 years of advancing professional success, lessons for the decade to come, *J Am Health Inform Manage Assoc* 77:28–34, 2006.
24. *Evolving careers,* Chicago, 1998, American Health Information Management Association.
25. E-health Task Force: Your job in the e-health era, *J Am Health Inform Manage Assoc* 73:32–35, 2002.
26. A vision of the e-HIM future: a report from the AHIMA e-HIM Task Force, 2003: http://library.ahima.org/xpedio/groups/public/documents/ahima/bok1_020477.pdf. Accessed September 5, 2013.
27. Bloomrosen M: e-HIM: from vision to reality, *J Am Health Inform Manage Assoc* 76:36–41, 2005. http://library.ahima.org/xpedio/groups/public/documents/ahima/bok1_028133.hcsp?dDocNamebok1_028133 Accessed October 15, 2013.
28. *Embracing the future: new times, new opportunities for health information managers, summary findings from the HIM Workforce Study, 2005:* Chicago, 2005, American Health Information Management Association Foundation. http://library.ahima.org/xpedio/groups/public/documents/ahima/bok1_027398.pdf Accessed October 15, 2013.
29. American Health Information Management Association: *Building the workforce for health information transformation, 2006:* http://www.amia.org/sites/amia.org/files/Workforce_2006.pdf Accessed June 12, 2014.
30. American Medical Informatics Association: Health information management and informatics core competencies for individuals working with electronic health records, *Joint Work Force Task Force* 2008, http://library.ahima.org/xpedio/groups/public/documents/ahima/bok1_040723.pdf Accessed October 15, 2013.
31. Health Resources and Services Administration: Health IT training opportunities and requirements: http://www.hrsa.gov/healthit/workforce/training.html. Accessed November 2, 2013.
32. American Health Information Management Association: A new view of HIM: introducing the core model, Review Draft. 2011. http://library.ahima.org/xpedio/groups/public/documents/ahima/bok1_049283.pdf. Accessed November 2, 2013.
33. Medical record technician, *J Am Assoc Medical Record Librarians* 24:208–209, 1953.
34. American Medical Record Association: The years of growth and development, *Med Record News* 50(1)1978, 83.
35. American Health Information Management Association: *Curriculum model associate degree education in health information management framework for HIM education, 2005:* http://library.ahima.org/xpedio/groups/public/documents/internal_accreditation/bok1_036799.pdf Accessed October 22, 2013.
36. American Health Information Management Association: *Curriculum model baccalaureate degree education in health information management framework for HIM education, 2005:* http://library.ahima.org/xpedio/groups/public/documents/internal_accreditation/bok1_036800.pdf Accessed October 22, 2013.
37. American Health Information Management Association: *Program approval manual for health information management applied health informatics graduate degree levels, 2006:* Chicago, 2006, American Health Information Management Association http://library.ahima.org/xpedio/groups/public/documents/internal_accreditation/bok1_036804.pdf Accessed November 6, 2013.
38. Commission on Accreditation for Health Informatics and Information Management: *Standards and interpretations for accreditation of master's degree programs in health informatics, 2010:* http://cahiim.org/Files-Standards/2012_HI_Masters_Stndrds_elec.pdf Accessed October 22, 2013.
39. Commission on Accreditation for Health Informatics and Information Management: *Standards and interpretations for accreditation of master's degree programs in health information management, 2008:* http://www.cahiim.org/Files-Standards/2012_HIM_Masters_Stndrds_elec.pdf Accessed November 5, 2013.
40. Commission on Accreditation for Health Informatics and Information Management: *Standards and interpretations for accreditation of baccalaureate degree programs in health information management, 2012:* http://cahiim.org/Files-Standards/2012_HIM_Bacc_Stndrds_elec.pdf Accessed October 22, 2013.
41. Commission on Accreditation for Health Informatics and Information Management: *Standards and interpretations for accreditation of associate degree programs in health information management, 2012:* http://cahiim.org/Files-Standards/2012_HIM_Assoc_Stndrds_elec.pdf Accessed October 22, 2013.
42. Russell L, Patena K: Preparing tomorrow's professionals: a new framework for HIM education, *J Am Health Inform Manage Assoc* 75:23–26, 2004.
43. American Health Information Management Association: *Vision 2016: a blueprint for quality education in health information management, September 24, 2007:* http://library.ahima.org/xpedio/groups/public/

documents/ahima/bok1_035517.pdf#xml=http://library.ahima.org/xpedio/idcplg?IdcService=GET_XML_HIGHLIGHT_INFO&QueryText=%28Vision+2016%3a+A+Blueprint+for+Quality+Education+in+Health+Information+Management%29%3Cand%3E%28xPublishSite%3Csubstring%3E%60BoK%60%29&SortField=xPubDate&SortOrder=Desc&dDocName=bok1_035517&HighlightType=PdfHighligh Accessed November 5, 2013.

44. Calhoun M, Rudman W, Watzlaf V: Vision 2016 to reality 2016: building a profession, *J Am Health Inform Manage Assoc* 83:19–23, 2013.

45. American Health Information Management Association, Commission on Accreditation of Health Informatics and Information Management Education: http://www.cahiim.org/index.html. Accessed November 5, 2013.

46. American Health Information Management Association: Certification: http://www.ahima.org/certification. Accessed November 5, 2013.

47. Commission on Certification for Health Informatics and Information Management (CCHIIM). Candidate guide: http://www.ahima.org/~/media/AHIMA/Files/Certification/Candidate_Guide.ashx. Accessed October 15, 2013.

48. Parker W, Smith G: *Certification as a predictor of quality performance. Presented at the National Organization for Competency Assurance, Annual Educational Conference,* 2004. Miami, FL.

49. American Health Information Management Association: *Employers value credentials in healthcare—an AHIMA survey, 2005:* http://library.ahima.org/xpedio/groups/public/documents/ahima/bok1_042081.pdf Accessed October 15, 2013.

50. Commission on Certification for Health Informatics and Information Management: Recertification guide maintenance of certification: http://www.ahima.org/~/media/AHIMA/Files/Certification/Recertification_Guide.ashx. Accessed October 15, 2013.

51. Lifelong Learning Resolution (Lifelong Learning Resolution [2004 convention wrap-up]), *J Am Health Inform Manage Assoc* 76(64), 2005.

52. American Health Information Management Association: Fellowship program: http://www.ahima.org/about/recognition?tabid=fellowship. Accessed October 15, 2013.

53. American Health Information Management Association: Membership: http://www.ahima.org/membership. Accessed October 15, 2013.

54. American Health Information Management Association: Mission vision and values: http://www.ahima.org/about/aboutahima?tabid=mission. Accessed November 5, 2013.

55. American Health Information Management Association: Board of directors: http://www.ahima.org/about/governance?tabid=board. Accessed November 5, 2013.

56. American Health Information Management Association: House of Delegates: http://www.ahima.org/about/governance?tabid=hod. Accessed December 8, 2014.

57. Desai A: Environmental scan illuminates the path ahead for HIM, *J Am Health Info Manage Assoc* 84:48–52, 2013.

58. American Health Information Management Association: 2014-2017 Drive the power of knowledge strategic plan: http://library.ahima.org/xpedio/groups/public/documents/ahima/bok1_050165.pdf. Accessed November 5, 2013.

59. American Health Information Management Association: http://journal.ahima.org. Accessed December 8, 2014.

60. American Health Information Management Association: Perspectives in Health Information Management: http://perspective.ahima.org. Accessed December 8, 2014.

61. American Health Information Management Association: Educational Perspectives in Health Information Management: http://eduperspectives.ahima.org/. Accessed October 15, 2013.

62. Lane L: Communities of practice: harnessing the power of knowledge, *J Am Health Inform Manage Assoc* 73:24–27, 2002.

63. AHIMA's engage communities connect him professionals: http://journal.ahima.org/2013/09/12/ahimas-engage-communities-connect-him-professionals/. Accessed November 5, 2013.

64. American Health Information Management Association: The AHIMA foundation: http://www.ahimafoundation.org. Accessed October 15, 2013.

65. American Health Information Management Association: *AHIMA code of ethics, 1957, 1977, 1988, and 1998: Revised and adopted by AHIMA House of Delegates, October 2, 2011:* http://library.ahima.org/xpedio/groups/public/documents/ahima/bok1_024277.hcsp?dDocName=bok1_024277 Accessed October 15, 2013.

66. Hart-O'Connor S: Ethics update: revisions strengthen AHIMA's code of ethics, *J Am Health Manage Assoc* 83:40–41, 2012.

CHAPTER

3

HEALTH INFORMATION INFRASTRUCTURE AND SYSTEMS

Meryl Bloomrosen

ⓔ Student Study Guide activities for this chapter are available on the Evolve Learning Resources site for this textbook. Please visit http://evolve.elsevier.com/Abdelhak.

CHAPTER CONTENTS

OBJECTIVES

After reading this chapter, the reader will be able to do the following:
✓ Define the key words.
✓ Identify public and private sector initiatives and organizations in health information technology and health information exchange.
✓ Illustrate and understand the role of health information management in designing, developing, and implementing electronic health information technology and exchange policies and processes across organizations and multiple stakeholders.

✓ Understand the complex political, technical, legal, logistical, privacy-security, and clinical work flow factors contributing to the discussions of health information technology and exchange among and across multiple data sources and users.
✓ Identify potential management issues facing health care and information management professionals resulting from the migration and implementation of health information technology and systems.
✓ Understand the role and importance of (administrative and clinical) data content and messaging standards in achieving the goals of transforming the health care system.

KEY WORDS

Health information technology
Electronic health record
Nationwide health information network

ABBREVIATIONS

AHIC   American Health Information Community
AHRQ   Agency for Healthcare Quality and Research
AHIP   America's Health Insurance Plan
ANSI   American National Standards Institute
AQA   Ambulatory Quality Alliance
ARRA   American Recovery and Reinvestment Act of 2009
CAH   critical access hospital
CAP   College of American Pathologists
CDS   clinical decision support
CEHRT   certified electronic health record technology
CHI   Consolidated Health Informatics
CLIA   Clinical Laboratory Improvement Amendments of 1988
CMS   Centers for Medicare and Medicaid Services
CPOE   computerized physician order entry
DHHS   Department of Health and Human Services
DICOM   Digital Imaging Communications in Medicine
DSS   decision support system
EHRs   electronic health records
EMR   electronic medical record
eRX   electronic prescribing
FACA   Federal Advisory Committee Act
FCC   Federal Communications Commission
FDA   Food and Drug Administration
FHA   Federal Health Architecture
HCCF   Healthcare Connect Fund
HIE   health information exchange
HIM   health information management
HIPAA   Health Insurance Portability and Accountability Act
HIT   health information technology
HITECH   Health Information Technology for Economic and Clinical Health
HL7   Health Level 7
HRSA   Health Resources and Services Administration
IHTSDO   International Health Terminology Standards Development Organisation

IEEE 1073   Institute of Electrical and Electronics Engineers 1073
IOM   Institute of Medicine
ISO   International Organization for Standardization
LHNCBC   Lister Hill National Center for Biomedical Communications
LOINC   Logical Observation Identifier Name Codes
MU   meaningful use
NCPCP   National Council on Prescription Drug Programs
NCVHS   National Committee for Vital and Health Statistics
NDF-RT   National Drug File–Reference Terminology
NHII   National Health Information Infrastructure
NIH   National Institutes of Health
NIST   National Institute for Standards and Technology
NLM   National Library of Medicine
NRC   National Resource Center
NwHIN   Nationwide Health Information Network
OCR   Office for Civil Rights
ONCHIT   Office of the National Coordinator for Health Information Technology
ORHP   Office of Rural Health Policy
PCORI   Patient-Centered Outcomes Research Institute
PHI   personal health information
PHR   personal health record
PPACA   Patient Protection and Affordable Care Act
PSO   patient safety organization
QIO   quality improvement organization
RHIOs   regional health information organizations
ROI   return on investments
S&I   standards and interoperability
SDE   state-designated entity
SDO   standards development organization
SNOMED-CT   Systematized Nomenclature of Medicine—Clinical Terms
USDA   U.S. Department of Agriculture

HEALTH INFORMATION TECHNOLOGY IN HEALTH CARE

Many aspects of the health care industry are highly siloed and fragmented, which has led to ongoing and untenable levels of administrative complexity and compromises to quality and efficiency of care. One of the top-ranking challenges faced by most providers and many other stakeholders is the accuracy, completeness, timeliness, and efficiency of access to patient information. Historically, patient data were most frequently recorded and stored in paper-based systems and shared across organizations every day through low-technology modes such as fax, mail, and courier, causing unnecessarily high labor and nonlabor expenses. Patients were potentially misdiagnosed and mistreated because of a lack of quality, timely, and easily accessible data at the point of care.*,†,1

The earliest activities devoted to health information technology (HIT) implementation focused first on the automation of administrative functions, such as patient registration and claims processing. Subsequently, attention moved to address clinical functions and to achieve improvements in patient safety and care delivery. Most recently, numerous activities[2-4] have addressed how to provide for the exchange of clinical and administrative information[5-7] within and across settings and sites of care,[8-10] and how to facilitate use of data across organizations using standardized electronic communications methods and approaches. Increasingly and more recently there are initiatives such as the Electronic Data Methods Forum (a program funded by the Agency for Healthcare Quality and Research [AHRQ]) to advance the national dialogue on the use of electronic clinical data for the conduct of comparative effectiveness research,

---

Health information technology is broadly defined as the use of information and communication technology in health care.

†Electronic health record (EHR) systems are defined by the Institute of Medicine's letter report on the key capabilities of an electronic health record system. It was envisioned that ultimately EHR systems will include the ability to collect

longitudinal data for and about a person in an electronic format; to provide immediate electronic access to person and population level information by authorized users; to provide knowledge and decision-support tools that enhance the safety, quality, and efficiency of health care; and to support efficient processes for health care delivery.

quality improvement, and clinical decision support (CDS) by facilitating exchange and collaboration between the various other federally funded projects.[11] Another prominent activity is the move toward patient centeredness. For example, the Patient-Centered Outcomes Research Institute (PCORI) is authorized by Congress to conduct research to provide information about the best available evidence to help patients and their health care providers make more informed decisions. PCORI's research is intended to give patients a better understanding of the prevention, treatment, and care options available, and the science that supports those options.[12]

Previous efforts to address the national need for appropriate exchange of health data have largely operated independent of each other. Today, numerous initiatives are under way to coordinate and integrate activities and to leverage lessons learned from one activity to another.[13] For example, during the 2000s we have seen the implementation of nationwide efforts toward administrative simplification under the Health Insurance Portability and Accountability Act (HIPAA) of 1996, the related rise in electronic claims processing, and the Medicare and Medicaid electronic health record (EHR) incentive programs. The Health Information Technology for Economic and Clinical Health (HITECH) Act[14] seeks to improve American health care delivery and patient care through an unprecedented investment in HIT. Title IV, Division B, of the HITECH Act establishes incentive payments under the Medicare and Medicaid programs for eligible professionals and EHs that meaningfully use certified EHR technology (CEHRT). The Centers for Medicare and Medicaid Services (CMS) is charged with managing the Medicare and Medicaid EHR incentive programs.[15]

The Medicare and Medicaid EHR incentive programs provide incentive payments to eligible professionals, eligible hospitals and critical access hospitals (CAHs) to adopt, implement, upgrade, or demonstrate meaningful use (MU) of CEHRT.[16] Issued by CMS, MU rules define the minimum requirements that providers must meet through their use of CEHRT to qualify for the payments for various (incremental) stages of MU. The EHR incentive program asks providers to use the capabilities of their EHRs to achieve benchmarks that can lead to improved patient care. Standards and certification criteria for EHRs are issued by the Office of the National Coordinator for Health Information Technology (ONCHIT), and identify the standards and certification criteria for the certification of EHR technology, so eligible professionals and hospitals may be assured that the systems they adopt are capable of performing the required functions.[17]

In March 2010, President Obama signed the Patient Protection and Affordable Care Act (PPACA).[18] The law puts in place comprehensive health insurance reforms that will roll out over 4 years and beyond. On June 22, 2010, President Obama announced new interim final regulations, the Patient's Bill of Rights, that include a set of protections that apply to health coverage starting on or after September 23, 2010, 6 months after the enactment of the PPACA.[19] The Departments of Health and Human Services, Labor, and Treasury collaborated on the Patient's Bill of Rights, which will help children (and eventually all Americans) with preexisting conditions gain coverage and keep it, protect all Americans' choice of doctors, and end lifetime limits on the care consumers may receive. These new protections created an important foundation of patients' rights in the private health insurance market that puts Americans in charge of their own health.[20]

It has long been recognized that providers need data to treat their patients and to choose among treatment options, approaches, and modalities: payers require data to verify eligibility for treatment and to determine medical necessity for care, researchers need data for various comparative outcomes measurement projects, and regulators and policy makers require data to make prudent and cost-effective decisions that will ensure the public health and well-being of our country's citizens. The national policy agenda for HIT, health information exchange (HIE), and EHRs as implemented in the public and private sectors has been developing rapidly and is seen as a top priority.[21] These policy discussions have concluded that health data and information should be universally digitized and appropriately available. Improving patient safety and increasing the quality and efficiency of health care are primary motivating factors in most public and private sector efforts. Increasingly, multiple and previously diverse activities are being coordinated and leveraged together so that ideally we can all achieve the economic and social benefits that are optimistically promised.

This peak in activity seemed to be propelled with the President's 2004 State of the Union Address, followed by the creation of the Department of Health and Human Services (DHHS) ONCHIT and the release of the Strategic Framework, the federal funding of HIT projects by several agencies of the DHHS, and the numerous bills introduced in Congress that address various aspects of HIT and HIE. The concept of a national health information infrastructure envisions providing electronic information necessary for decision making at the time it is needed, in the place where it is needed, and to the people who need it. It will connect physicians, hospitals, health care purchasers and payers, researchers, public health professionals, and consumers. It is envisioned as a comprehensive, knowledge-based network of interoperable systems of clinical, public, and personal health information (PHI).[22] Early attention to the importance of improving access to health information led to increasing efforts for the creation of a National Health Information Infrastructure (NHII) network, an endeavor working toward a vision of an effective, efficient, high-quality health care system that harnesses the power of shared data to improve the health of all Americans. Subsequently, the concept of the NHII was defined by DHHS as an Internet-based architecture that links disparate health care information systems together to allow patients, physicians, hospitals, community health centers, and public health agencies across the country to share clinical information securely.[23] Over the years, the concepts of and approaches to achieving the NHII network have evolved into the development of the Nationwide Health Information Network (NwHIN)—a set of standards, services, and policies that enable the secure exchange of health information over the

Internet. The NwHIN is *not* a physical network that runs on servers at the DHHS, nor is it a network that stores patient records.[24]

SELF-ASSESSMENT QUIZ

1. True or False? Meaningful Use rules define the minimum requirements that providers must meet through their use of CERHT to qualify for the payments for various stages of meaningful use.
   a. True
   b. False
2. The NwHIN is the following:
   a. A set of standards, services, and policies that enable the secure exchange of health information online
   b. A physical network that runs on servers at the U.S. DHHS
   c. A network that stores patient records

BACKGROUND

For decades, the need for an improved HIT infrastructure has been a recurring theme in Institute of Medicine (IOM) reports, recommendations by the National Committee on Vital and Health Statistics (NCVHS), and innumerable testimonies before congressional committees.

In the IOM's report, "Crossing the Quality Chasm,"[25] the members of the institute, among other things, recommended the following:

> *Recommendation 19: Congress, the executive branch, leaders of health care organizations, public and private sector purchasers, and health informatics associations and vendors should make a renewed national commitment to building an information infrastructure to support health care delivery, consumer health, quality measurement and improvement, public accountability, clinical and health services research, and clinical education. This commitment should lead to the elimination of most handwritten clinical data by the end of the decade.*

In particular, HIT was identified as a critical environmental force that would significantly improve health care quality. Numerous activities in both the public and private sectors were quickly expanded.[26,27] Some of the more notable recent events are described here.

The DHHS AHRQ has been interested in the subject of EHRs for decades. The agency has identified gaps in knowledge relating to the use of HIT and provided recommendations on important thematic areas. The Agency continues to fund and support research on a number of topics, including the effect of HIT on important health-related outcomes; more research on HIT in diverse health care settings; the need to demonstrate the value of HIT in improving patient safety and quality of care, including direct and indirect and tangible and intangible benefits; the need to study incentives and disincentives to the adoption and use of HIT; the need for technical assistance to providers, organizations, and communities to implement HIT successfully in their environment; and the need to develop and disseminate evidence-based, executable knowledge content and decision-support tools to

support clinical decision making. AHRQ and several other federal agencies, such as the Office of Rural Health Policy (ORHP) and the Office for the Advancement of Telehealth at the Health Resources and Services Administration (HRSA) and the CMS continue to collaborate and to leverage their resources and expertise.[28] AHRQ continues to support development and use of HIT to address key issues; for example, "Health IT Enabled Quality Measurement" is an AHRQ report issued in 2013 as a result of research on the status of using HIT tools to collect and assess quality data. AHRQ continues to encourage the use of technology to collect, organize, and disseminate health information to improve care.[29] In early 2014, AHRQ identified additional funding opportunities for basic health IT research and to fill gaps in the field that will lead to improved design of health IT systems.[30]

The IOM released several reports such as "Crossing the Quality Chasm" that detail these needs, and various other organizations have focused industry attention on electronic health information and information technology.[31–36] Recent IOM reports have focused attention on the learning health system, availability of digital data, and HIT and patient safety.[37–39]

Many different components of the federal government touch on health care, and increasingly, federal leadership in HIT is more focused and coordinated. Although there is some integration of these efforts, until recently there has been neither a single voice for this effort nor a holistic set of goals for change. The position of National Coordinator was created in 2004, through an Executive Order, and legislatively mandated in the HITECH Act of 2009 (Figure 3-1).[40]

ONCHIT is the principal federal entity charged with coordination of nationwide efforts to implement and use the most advanced HIT and the electronic exchange of health information. The ONCHIT has been given the responsibility for coordinating HIT efforts throughout the federal government. ONCHIT authors regulations that set the standards and certification criteria EHRs must meet to assure health care professionals and hospitals that the systems they adopt are capable of performing certain functions. HHS has also issued rules and regulations to govern the MU of health IT. As part of the outreach effort, a variety of programs, projects, and policies that involve HIT were implemented throughout the HHS.[41] The DHHS Rural HIT Task Force, specifically the ONCHIT and the HRSA, worked with the U.S. Department of Agriculture (USDA) to ensure that rural health care providers can use USDA's Rural Development grants and loans to support the acquisition of health IT infrastructure. HHS and USDA signed a memorandum of understanding linking rural hospitals and clinicians to existing capital loan programs that enable them to purchase software and hardware needed to implement HIT. Two key USDA rural development programs that can help expand HIT infrastructure in rural America are the following:

- The Community Facilities Program provides direct and guaranteed loans as well as grants for community facilities projects in rural areas. This program may help offset the costs of EHR implementation for rural health care providers.

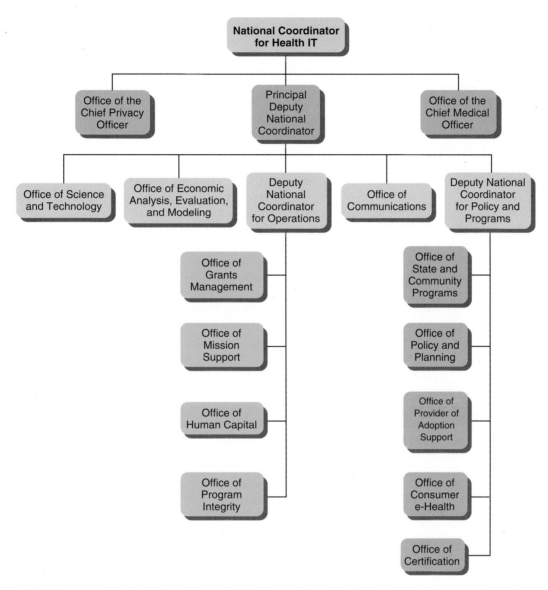

FIGURE 3-1 Organizational chart of the Office of the National Coordinator for Health Information Technology. *IT,* Information technology. HealthIT.gov: About ONC: http://www.healthit.gov/news room/about-onc. Accessed March 18, 2014.

- The Distance Learning and Telemedicine Grant Program may provide grants to help bring telemedicine services to rural communities.[42]

The American Recovery and Reinvestment Act (ARRA) of 2009 provided for the creation of an HIT policy committee and an HIT standards committee under the auspices of the Federal Advisory Committee Act (FACA).

The HIT policy committee makes recommendations to the national coordinator for HIT on a policy framework for the development and adoption of a nationwide health information infrastructure, including standards for the exchange of patient medical information. ARRA provides that the HIT policy committee shall at least make recommendations on the areas in which standards, implementation specifications, and certifications criteria are needed in eight specific areas.

The HIT standards committee is charged with making recommendations to the national coordinator for HIT on standards, implementation specifications, and certification criteria for the electronic exchange and use of health information. Initially, the HIT standards committee will focus on the policies developed by the HIT policy committee's initial eight areas. In developing, harmonizing, or recognizing standards and implementation specifications, the health IT standards committee will also provide for the testing of the same by the National Institute for Standards and Technology (NIST).[43]

FEDERAL INVOLVEMENT IN HEALTH INFORMATION TECHNOLOGY

The DHHS's involvement in HIT and health information standards has been long standing. The goal is to develop and implement a nationwide interoperable HIT infrastructure, improve the quality and efficiency of health care, and help consumers manage their care and safety. For many years the federal government supported research into clinical and applied informatics, health information management (HIM), and the use of computers in clinical practice with the objective to increase the use of computers in health care. Over the years, a number of initiatives have gained considerable momentum to establish messaging and data content standards. Table 3-1 provides an overview of these activities.[44]

DHHS agencies such as the AHRQ, the Food and Drug Administration (FDA), the HRSA, the CMS, the ONCHIT, and others have made adoption of technologies a priority (see Chapter 1, Figure 1-1).[45]

In a general sense, these efforts have the following purpose:

- Provide funding for HIT to improve the quality, safety, and efficiency of the nation's health care system.
- Have health care practitioners use information technology to assist in the delivery of patient care and to document that care.
- Establish standard ways to exchange data electronically for health care delivery, research, public health, and payment.

- Make investments to identify and speed the adoption of new technologies throughout the health care system.
- Foster the development of data standards.
- Advance the use of EHRs and accelerate secure sharing of health information among providers.

The DHHS has long played a leadership role in fostering the development of data standards. Previous efforts included the Consolidated Health Informatics (CHI) initiative and support for the NHII. Both activities have resulted in the adoption of interoperability for federal programs. The CHI initiative was one of the Office of Management and Budget's eGov initiatives to adopt health information interoperability standards, particularly health vocabulary and messaging standards, for implementation in federal government systems. Most of these standards were developed by nongovernmental standards development organizations (SDOs). Approximately 20 departments and agencies, including the DHHS, the Department of Defense, and the Department of Veterans Affairs, were active in the CHI governance process.

TABLE 3-1 Selected HIT/HIE Federal Initiatives

Consolidated Health Informatics Initiative	DHHS

The CHI is one of several projects launched as part of the president's e-Government initiative, which aims to improve government efficiency, effectiveness, and responsiveness to citizens while making it easier for citizens to obtain services and interact with the federal government. The CHI involved all federal agencies relating to health care, including the Department of Defense, Department of Veterans Affairs, the CMS, the Centers for Disease Control and Prevention, and the National Institutes for Health. This project will provide the basis for a simplified and unified system for sharing and revising medical information among government agencies and their private health care providers and insurers, ultimately leading to a single mechanism for making records accessible. As of October 1, 2006, the FHA program began operating under a new strategic framework. This framework does not contain a separate CHI initiative, and rather, involves FHA partners directly in the national standards harmonization process. Through this approach, federal government systems and processes will be fully aligned with the president's HIT goals and objectives of interoperability, improved quality of care, and increased efficiency.*

Health Alert Network	CDC

CDC's HAN is the CDC's primary method of sharing cleared information about urgent public health incidents with public information officers; federal, state, territorial, and local public health practitioners; clinicians; and public health laboratories. CDC's HAN collaborates with federal, state, territorial, and city and county partners to develop protocols and stakeholder relationships that will ensure a robust interoperable platform for the rapid distribution of public health information.†

National Committee on Vital and Health Statistics http://www.ncvhs.hhs.gov/fullcmte.htm

The NCVHS serves as the statutory [42 U.S.C. 242 k(k)] public advisory body to the Secretary of Health and Human Services in the area of health data and statistics. In that capacity, the Committee provides advice and assistance to the Department and serves as a forum for interaction with interested private sector groups on a variety of key health data issues.

The Committee is composed of 18 individuals from the private sector who have distinguished themselves in the fields of health statistics, electronic interchange of health care information, privacy and security of electronic information, population-based public health, purchasing or financing health care services, integrated computerized health information systems, health services research, consumer interests in health information, health data standards, epidemiology, and the provision of health services. Sixteen of the members are appointed by the Secretary of Health and Human Services for terms of 4 years each, with approximately four new members being appointed each year. Two additional members are selected by Congress.

National Electronic Disease Surveillance System	CDC

The NEDSS facilitates electronically transferring public health surveillance data from the health care system to public health departments. It is a conduit for exchanging information that supports NNDSS. Today, when states and territories voluntarily submit notifiable disease surveillance data electronically to CDC, they use data standards and electronic disease information systems and resources supported in part by NEDSS. This ensures that state data shared with CDC are submitted quickly, securely, and in an understandable form.‡

TABLE 3-1 Selected HIT/HIE Federal Initiatives—cont'd

National Vaccine Program Office	CDC

The NVPO is responsible for coordinating and ensuring collaboration among the many federal agencies involved in vaccine and immunization activities. NVPO provides leadership and coordination among federal agencies as they work together to carry out the goals of the National Vaccine Plan. The National Vaccine Plan provides a framework, including goals, objectives, and strategies, for pursuing the prevention of infectious diseases through immunizations. Additionally, NVPO staffs the NVAC, which was established to comply with Section 2105 of the Public Health Service Act (42 U.S. Code 300aa-5). Its purpose is to advise and make recommendations to the Assistant Secretary for Health in his or her capacity as the Director of National Vaccine Program on matters related to program responsibilities.[§]

Office of the National Coordinator for Health Information Technology and Standards Committees
http://www.healthit.gov/facas/

The ARRA of 2009 provided for the creation of an HIT Policy Committee and an HIT Standards Committee under the auspices of the FACA. The HIT Policy Committee makes recommendations to the National Coordinator for HIT on a policy framework for the development and adoption of a nationwide health information infrastructure, including standards for the exchange of patient medical information. The ARRA provides that the HIT Policy Committee shall at least make recommendations on the areas in which standards, implementation specifications, and certifications criteria are needed in eight specific areas. The HIT Standards Committee is charged with making recommendations to the National Coordinator for HIT on standards, implementation specifications, and certification criteria for the electronic exchange and use of health information. Initially, the HIT Standards Committee will focus on the policies developed by the HIT Policy Committee's initial eight areas. Within 90 days of the signing of ARRA, the HIT Standards Committee must develop a schedule for the assessment of policy recommendations developed by the HIT Policy Committee, to be updated annually. In developing, harmonizing, or recognizing standards and implementation specifications, the HIT Standards Committee will also provide for the testing of the same by the NIST.

ARRA, American Recovery and Reinvestment Act; *CDC,* Centers for Disease Control and Prevention; *CHI,* Consolidated Health Informatics; *CMS,* Centers for Medicare and Medicaid Services; *DHHS,* Department of Health and Human Services; *FACA,* Federal Advisory Committee Act; *FHA,* Federal Health Architecture; *HAN,* Health Alert Network; *HIE,* health information exchange; *HIT,* health information technology; *NCVHS,* National Committee on Vital and Health Statistics; *NEDSS,* National Electronic Disease Surveillance System; *NIST,* National Institute for Standards and Technology; *NNDSS,* National Notifiable Diseases Surveillance System; *NVAC,* National Vaccine Advisory Committee; *NVPO,* National Vaccine Program Office.
*eGov: Presidential initiatives: http://www.whitehouse.gov/sites/default/files/omb/assets/omb/egov/c-3-6-chi.html. Accessed June 26, 2014.
[†]Centers for Disease Control and Prevention: Health Alert Network (HAN): http://emergency.cdc.gov/han/. Accessed June 26, 2014.
[‡]Centers for Disease Control and Prevention: National Notifiable Diseases Surveillance System (NNDSS): http://wwwn.cdc.gov/nndss/script/nedss.aspx. Accessed June 26, 2014.
[§]U.S. Department of Health & Human Services: National Vaccine Program Office (NVPO): http://www.hhs.gov/nvpo/index.html. Accessed June 26, 2014.

? DID YOU KNOW?

The Standards and Interoperability (S&I) Framework within the ONCHIT was formed to orchestrate input from the public and private sectors to create harmonized HIT specifications for use throughout the United States.[46] The S&I Framework was established to enable health care stakeholders to drive higher interoperability and greater HIE to improve quality of care.[47] The S&I Framework is a collaborative community of participants from the public and private sectors who are focused on providing the tools, services, and guidance to facilitate the functional exchange of health information.[48]

CHI adopted uniform standards for electronic exchange of clinical information to be used across the federal health enterprise. On March 21, 2003, the DHHS and the Departments of Defense and Veterans Affairs announced the first set of uniform standards for the electronic exchange of clinical health information to be adopted across the federal government. The standards all federal agencies adopted include the following:

- Health Level 7 (HL7) messaging standards ensure that each federal agency can share information that will improve coordinated care for patients, such as entries of orders, scheduling appointments and tests, and better coordination of the admittance, discharge, and transfer of patients.
- National Council on Prescription Drug Programs (NCPDP) standards for ordering drugs from retail pharmacies standardize information between health care providers and the pharmacies. These standards were adopted under HIPAA (1996) and ensure that parts of the three federal departments that aren't covered by HIPAA will also use the same standards.
- Institute of Electrical and Electronics Engineers (IEEE) 1073 series of standards allow for health care providers to plug medical devices into information and computer systems that allow health care providers to monitor information from an intensive care unit or through telehealth services on Indian reservations and in other circumstances.
- Digital Imaging Communications in Medicine (DICOM) standards enable images and associated diagnostic information to be retrieved and transferred from various

manufacturers' devices and from medical staff work stations.

- Laboratory Logical Observation Identifier Name Codes (LOINCs) standardize the electronic exchange of clinical laboratory results.

In 2004 the DHHS and the Departments of Defense and Veterans Affairs announced the adoption of standards agreed to by the CHI initiative to allow for electronic exchange of clinical information across the federal government. The standards built on the existing set of standards adopted by the DHHS in 2003. The new standards agreed to by federal agencies were used as agencies develop and implement new information technology systems.

The specific new standards included the following:

- HL7 vocabulary standards for demographic information, units of measure, immunizations, and clinical encounters, and HL7's Clinical Document Architecture standard for text-based reports
- The College of American Pathologists (CAP) Systematized Nomenclature of Medicine—Clinical Terms (SNOMED-CT) for laboratory result contents, nonlaboratory interventions and procedures, anatomy, diagnosis and problems, and nursing

The DHHS has made this available for use in the United States at no charge to users. SNOMED-CT is owned, maintained, and distributed by the International Health Terminology Standards Development Organisation (IHTSDO). SNOMED-CT provides the core general terminology for the EHR and contains more than 300,000 active concepts with unique meanings and formal logic-based definitions organized into hierarchies. When implemented in software applications, SNOMED-CT can be used to represent clinically relevant information consistently, reliably, and comprehensively as an integral part of producing EHRs.[45]

- Laboratory LOINCs to standardize the electronic exchange of laboratory test orders and drug label section headers

LOINC is a universal code system for identifying laboratory and clinical observations. LOINC was initiated in 1994 by the Regenstrief Institute and developed by Regenstrief and the LOINC committee as a response to the demand for electronic movement of clinical data from laboratories that produce the data to hospitals, physicians' offices, and payers who use the data for clinical care and management purposes. LOINC's initial scope included laboratory and other clinical observations, and expanded to include radiology procedures in 2000. The current version of LOINC includes more than 72,000 terms, including laboratory tests, clinical measures like vital signs and anthropomorphic measures, clinical document titles, standardized survey instruments, and more. Under a contract awarded by the National Institute of Biomedical Imaging and Bioengineering, the developers of two advanced medical terminologies have begun work to harmonize and unify terms for radiology procedures.

DID YOU KNOW?

The International Organization for Standardization (ISO) is the world's largest developer of voluntary international standards. International standards give state-of-the-art specifications for products, services, and good practice, helping to make industry more efficient and effective.[49] An international standard is the result of an agreement between the member bodies of ISO. It may be used as such, or may be implemented through incorporation in national standards of different countries.[50] ISO is a network of national standards bodies. ISO members[51] are the foremost standards organizations in their countries and there is only one member per country.[52]

The American National Standards Institute (ANSI)[53] has coordinated the development of voluntary consensus standards in the United States since it was founded in 1918 and has represented the needs and views of U.S. stakeholders in standardization forums around the globe. ANSI is the U.S. member body to ISO.[54]

Creating standardized radiology procedure names will improve the quality, consistency, and interoperability of radiology test results in electronic medical record (EMR) systems and HIE.

In late 2013 the Radiological Society of North America, which owns and maintains the RadLex medical terminology for radiology, and the Regenstrief Institute, which owns and maintains the LOINC terminology standard for medical tests and measurements, were awarded a project by the National Institute of Biomedical Imaging and Bioengineering to produce a single unified source of names and codes for radiology procedures with a cooperative governance process.[55]

HIPAA transactions and code sets have been created for electronic exchange of health-related information to perform billing or administrative functions. These are the same standards now required under HIPAA for health plans, health care clearinghouses, and those health care providers who engage in certain electronic transactions.

A set of federal terminologies related to medications have been created, including the FDA's names and codes for ingredients, manufactured dosage forms, drug products, and medication packages; the National Library of Medicine's (NLM) RxNORM for describing clinical drugs; and the Veterans Administration's National Drug File–Reference Terminology (NDF-RT) for specific drug classifications.

The Human Gene Nomenclature is used to exchange information regarding the role of genes in biomedical research in the federal health sector, and the Environmental Protection Agency's Substance Registry System is used for nonmedicinal chemicals of importance to health care.

In 2003 DHHS asked the IOM and HL7 to design a functional model and standard for the EHR. DHHS also announced that the department has signed an agreement with the CAP to license the college's standardized medical vocabulary system and make it available without charge throughout the United States. The IOM issued its report, titled "Key Capabilities of an Electronic Health Record System," in 2003. In October 2003, the General Accounting Office released a report called, "Information Technology: Benefits Realized for Selected Health Care Functions."

? DID YOU KNOW?

As of October 1, 2006, the Federal Health Architecture (FHA) program operates under a strategic framework that does not contain a separate CHI initiative. Rather, it involves FHA partners directly in the national standards harmonization process. Through this approach, federal government systems and processes will be fully aligned with the President's HIT goals and objectives of interoperability, improved quality of care, and increased efficiency.

Historically, DHHS agencies such as the AHRQ, the National Institutes of Health (NIH), and the NLM have awarded financial contracts and grants to conduct research and to promote the use of HIT through the development of networks for sharing clinical data and projects for planning, implementing, and demonstrating the value of HIT. The goals of these research projects are to:

- Improve patient safety by reducing medical errors.
- Increase health information sharing among providers, laboratories, pharmacies, and patients.
- Help patients transition between health care settings.
- Reduce duplicative and unnecessary testing.
- Increase our knowledge and understanding of the clinical, safety, quality, financial, and organizational value and benefits of HIT.

✓ SELF-ASSESSMENT QUIZ

3. DHHS and the Departments of Defense and Veterans Affairs adopted the first set of uniform standards in 2003. When was the next set of standards adopted?
   a. 2004
   b. 2006
   c. 2012
4. DHHS agencies award contracts and grants to conduct research to meet which of the following goals:
   a. Improve patient safety by reducing medical errors.
   b. Help patients transition between health care settings.
   c. Reduce duplicative and unnecessary testing.
   d. All of the above.

In July 2004 DHHS released the "Framework for Strategic Action: The Decade of Health Information Technology: Delivering Consumer-Centric and Information-Rich Health Care." The goals of this 10-year plan were to transform the delivery of health care by building a new health information infrastructure, including EHRs, and a new network to link health records nationwide. The plan established three interrelated core strategies:

- Promoting EHR adoption by clinicians
- Supporting the creation of regional health care information organizations (RHIOs)
- Facilitating interoperability on a national scale

The ONCHIT issues its Federal HIT Strategic Plan annually, and recently issued a special report titled "Health Information Technology Patient Safety Action and Surveillance Plan." The Health IT Patient Safety Action and Surveillance Plan ("Safety Plan" or "Plan") addresses the role of HIT within DHHS's commitment to patient safety and builds on the recommendations made in the 2011 IOM report "Health IT and Patient Safety: Building Safer Systems for Better Care." The Plan has two related objectives:

- Use HIT to make care safer.
- Continuously improve the safety of health IT.[56]

ONCHIT and the AHRQ are supporting research and development of evidence-based tools and interventions designed for various stakeholder audiences, including HIT developers, implementers, clinical staff, and patient safety organizations (PSOs).[57,58]

The State Health Information Exchange Cooperative Agreement Program, authorized by Section 3013 of the Provincial Health Services Authority as amended by the ARRA, was designed to promote HIE across the health care system. The appropriate and secure electronic exchange of health information will improve care coordination, clinical outcomes, and the patient experience. Widespread adoption and MU of HIT is foundational to the development of a high-performance health care system.[59]

STATE HEALTH INFORMATION EXCHANGE COOPERATIVE AGREEMENT PROGRAM

In March 2010 ONCHIT completed the announcement of State HIE Cooperative Agreement Program awardees. In total, 56 states, eligible territories, and qualified state-designated entities (SDE) received awards. The State HIE Cooperative Agreement Program funds states' efforts to rapidly build capacity for exchanging health information across the health care system both within and across states. Awardees are responsible for increasing connectivity and enabling patient-centric information flow to improve the quality and efficiency of care. Key to this is the continual evolution and advancement of necessary governance, policies, technical services, business operations, and financing mechanisms for HIE over each state, territory, and SDE's 4-year performance period. This program is building on existing efforts to advance regional and state-level HIE while moving toward nationwide interoperability. On January 27, 2011, an additional $16 million was made available to states through ONCHIT's Challenge Grants program.[60]

The ONCHIT has supported expert research on various aspects of the HIE. This work will support ONCHIT's State HIE Cooperative Agreement Program grantees as they work to implement and sustain their work.[61]

The ONCHIT-funded Beacon Communities compiled and synthesized their lessons learned from building health IT infrastructure, driving population health improvement and testing innovative approaches during the 3-year program.

This information is now available in six learning guides offering proven strategies and actionable information that can be adapted by hospitals, health systems, individual practices, and health-focused community organizations to help them advance community-level health care transformation using health IT.[62]

In August 2013, the ONCHIT reported that between 2008 and 2012, information exchange among hospitals and other providers increased 41%, and 6 in 10 hospitals by 2012 could transfer and use health information with a provider outside the hospital or its own network.

AHRQ's HIT Portfolio (research initiative) on HIT is critical to the nation's strategy to bring health care into the twenty-first century by advancing the use of information technology. The AHRQ initiative included millions of dollars in grants and contracts to support and stimulate investment in HIT, especially in rural and underserved areas. Through these and other projects, AHRQ and its partners wanted to identify challenges to HIT adoption and use, solutions and best practices for making HIT work, and tools that will help hospitals and clinicians successfully incorporate new information technology. Over the years, the portfolio included grants to numerous health care stakeholders who are at various levels of HIT adoption and contracts to stakeholders such as states to launch HIE networks. AHRQ's Health IT Portfolio develops and disseminates evidence and evidence-based tools about the effect of HIT on health care quality. To accomplish this, the AHRQ Portfolio:

- Anticipates the future needs of the health care system and supports development of innovative HIT solutions.
- Identifies and fills current gaps in knowledge about HIT.
- Leverages the capability of HIT to improve the quality, safety, efficiency, and effectiveness of health care.[63]

The AHRQ National Resource Center (NRC) for Health Information Technology,[63] which was launched in September 2004, plays a pivotal role in achieving the goals of DHHS to modernize health care through the best and most effective use of information technology. The NRC encourages adoption of HIT by sharing the knowledge and findings that result from the real-world laboratory created in AHRQ's HIT initiative, as well as from other resources. The NRC supports the work of the HIT projects funded by AHRQ and other federal partners and will provide direct technical assistance and consulting services to individual projects during all phases of the work to develop and use HIT. Particular focus was placed on providing services to support challenges facing HIT implementation in rural settings.

? DID YOU KNOW?

Over the years, numerous reports have been developed and disseminated such as "Health Information Technology Leadership Panel: Final Report" published by DHHS. This report cites investment in information technology as an essential high priority for the American health care system and the U.S. economy.

In 2005 DHHS announced the formation of a national collaboration, the American Health Information Community (AHIC), to advance efforts to reach President Bush's call for most Americans to have EHRs within 10 years. The AHIC was created to help nationwide transition to EHRs—including common standards and interoperability—in a smooth, market-led way. The AHIC, formed under the auspices of the FACA, provided input and recommendations to the DHHS on how to make health records digital and interoperable and ensure that the privacy and security of those records are protected.[64] As of 2009, AHIC was called the *National eHealth Collaborative* and succeeded AHIC, which was a federal advisory committee established in 2005, and AHIC Successor, Inc., founded in 2008 to transition the original organization into a nonprofit public–private partnership to accelerates effective use of health IT to create a more patient- and family-centered health care system with better outcomes and greater value.[56,65]

CMS contracts with one organization in each state, as well as the District of Columbia, Puerto Rico, and the U.S. Virgin Islands to serve as that state or jurisdiction's quality improvement organization (QIO) contractor. QIOs are private, mostly not-for-profit organizations staffed by professionals, mostly doctors and other health care professionals, who are trained to review medical care and help beneficiaries with complaints about the quality of care and to implement improvements in the quality of care available throughout the spectrum of care.[66] Under the direction of CMS, the QIO program consists of a national network of QIOs, responsible for each U.S. state, territory, and the District of Columbia. QIOs work with consumers and physicians, hospitals, and other caregivers to refine care delivery systems to make sure patients get the right care at the right time, particularly patients from underserved populations. The program also safeguards the integrity of the Medicare Trust Fund by ensuring that payment is made only for medically necessary services and investigates beneficiary complaints about quality of care. By law, the mission of the QIO Program is to improve the effectiveness, efficiency, economy, and quality of services delivered to Medicare beneficiaries. The QIO program focuses on three aims: better patient care, better population health, and lower health care costs through improvement.[67]

ONCHIT is responsible for coordinating federal activities relating to HIT.

In February 2014 a final rule amended the Clinical Laboratory Improvement Amendments (CLIA) of 1988 regulations[68] to allow laboratories to give a patient, or a person designated by the patient as his or her personal representative, access to the patient's completed test reports on the patient's or representative's request. At the same time, the final rule eliminates the exception under the HIPAA privacy rule to an individual's right to access his or her protected health information when it is held by a CLIA-certified or CLIA-exempt laboratory. The final rule was issued jointly by three agencies within HHS: CMS, the Centers for Disease Control and Prevention, and the Office for Civil Rights, which is responsible for enforcing the HIPAA Privacy Rule.[69]

Over the years, DHHS has awarded many contracts to public–private groups to accelerate the adoption of HIT and the secure portability of health information across the United States. These groups have strategic partnerships to develop the building blocks necessary for achieving the U.S. government's goal of widespread adoption of interoperable EHRs.

The HIT partnerships were designed to do the following:
- Create and evaluate processes for harmonizing health information standards.
- Develop criteria to certify and evaluate HIT products.
- Develop solutions to address variations in business policies and state laws that affect privacy and security practices that may pose challenges to the secure communication of health information.

With support of the NIH, the Clinical and Translational Science Award (CTSA) program was launched in 2006 and has expanded to approximately 60 academic medical institutions across the country. The CTSA Consortium aims to improve human health by transforming the research and training environment to enhance the efficiency and quality of clinical and translational research. The CTSA program supports a national consortium of medical research institutions that are transforming the way biomedical research is conducted. Its goals are to accelerate the translation of laboratory discoveries into treatments for patients, to engage communities in clinical research efforts, and to train a new generation of clinical and translational researchers.[70]

The CTSA program has enabled innovative research teams to speed discovery and advance science aimed at improving our nation's health. Led by NIH's National Center for Advancing Translational Sciences, the CTSA program encourages collaborative teams of investigators to tackle complex health and research challenges and then find ways to turn these discoveries into practical solutions for patients. These teams are already making progress across a broad range of diseases and conditions, such as cancer, diabetes, neurologic disorders, and heart disease.[71]

The Lister Hill National Center for Biomedical Communications (LHNCBC), established by a joint resolution of the United States Congress in 1968, is an intramural research and development division of the NLM. Seeking to improve access to high-quality biomedical information for individuals around the world, the Lister Hill Center conducts and supports research and development in the dissemination of high-quality imagery, medical language processing, high-speed access to biomedical information, intelligent database systems development, multimedia visualization, knowledge management, data mining, and machine-assisted indexing. An important focus of the LHNCBC is the development of Next Generation EHRs to facilitate patient-centric care, clinical research, and public health, an area of emphasis in the NLM Long Range Plan 2006-2016.[72]

The NLM is the U.S. member of the IHTSDO and, as such, distributes SNOMED-CT at no cost in accordance with the member rights and responsibilities outlined in the IHTSDO's articles. The IHTSDO's uniform international license terms for SNOMED-CT will replace the U.S.-wide license terms NLM negotiated with the CAP in 2003, giving U.S. users broader rights to distribute derivative products internationally. The new license terms have been incorporated into the License for Use of the Unified Medical Language System (UMLS) Metathesaurus. SNOMED-CT is a comprehensive clinical terminology, originally created by the CAP and, as of April 2007, owned, maintained, and distributed by the IHTSDO, a not-for-profit association in Denmark. The CAP continues to support SNOMED-CT operations under contract to the IHTSDO and provides SNOMED-related products and services as a licensee of the terminology. SNOMED-CT is one of a suite of designated standards for use in U.S. federal government systems for the electronic exchange of clinical health information.[73] The ONCHIT and CMS have adopted SNOMED-CT as one of the key vocabularies for MU, EHR certification, and HIE. SNOMED-CT has been specified in the federal regulations published in September 2012,[74] in which it is recommended for documenting patient problems, encounter diagnosis, procedures, family health history, and smoking status.[75]

With the advances in the Internet and cloud computing, other federal agencies are involved with health- and HIT-related issues and public policies. These agencies include the Federal Communications Commission (FCC). FCC has several projects and initiatives to improve and enhance wireless communications and broadband connectivity nationwide

The FCC oversees the Rural Health Care Program, which is currently made up of four programs: the Healthcare Connect Fund (HCCF), the Telecommunications Program, the Internet Access Program, and the Rural Health Care Pilot Program.

In 2012 the FCC convened a summit with industry leaders to discuss opportunities to accelerate the adoption and use of mobile health care technologies. Since then, participants formed the "mHealth Task Force" to develop recommendations for industry and government action to harness the potential of mobile devices to improve health outcomes and lower costs of care.[76,77]

In December 2012 the FCC created the HCCF to expand access by health care providers to robust broadband networks. Building on lessons learned from 50 pilot projects testing how to most effectively use broadband to improve the quality and reduce costs of health care in rural areas, the HCCF reforms modernize the FCC's existing universal service Rural Health Care Program to expand the benefits of telemedicine nationwide.[78]

CONGRESS

Congress is also playing a significant leadership role—bipartisan support of the development, adoption, and use of HIT to improve health care has progressed over the years. Typically, multiple bills are introduced by both parties each legislative session that include significant components related to HIM, applied health informatics, HIT, and

HIE.[79] It is widely acknowledged that the ability to appropriately exchange health information confidentially and securely across health care systems, technologies, care settings, technology platforms, and communities is needed to achieve the nation's triple aim of transforming health care, improving clinical outcomes, and controlling costs.[80,81]

 SELF-ASSESSMENT QUIZ

5. Which program focuses on accelerating the translation of laboratory discoveries into actual patient treatments?
   a. NIH's National Center for Advancing Translational Sciences
   b. CTSA
   c. LHNCBC

ROLE OF THE PRIVATE SECTOR

The private sector has also demonstrated significant leadership with the emergence of several initiatives and programs designed to improve health care through information technology. Examples of such activities and organizations are shown in Table 3-2.

The private sector has also been very active in conferences and programs to provide seed funding and technical support to states, regions, and communities involved in HIE and Connecting for Health,[82] a public-private collaborative launched and funded by the Markle Foundation, with additional support from the Robert Wood Johnson Foundation, getting consensus among multiple stakeholders on a Roadmap for Electronic Connectivity, and several large employers

---

TABLE 3-2   Representative Private Sector Activities and Organizations

AcademyHealth: http://www.academyhealth.org/

AcademyHealth is a leading national organization serving the fields of health services and policy research and the professionals who produce and use this important work. Together with our members, we offer programs and services that support the development and use of rigorous, relevant, and timely evidence to increase the quality, accessibility, and value of health care, to reduce disparities, and to improve health. A trusted broker of information, AcademyHealth brings stakeholders together to address the current and future needs of an evolving health system, inform health policy, and translate evidence into action.

Ambulatory Care Quality Alliance: http://www.ambulatoryqualityalliance.org/

The AQA's vision is to be a major contributor to achieving the National Quality Strategy through a multi-stakeholder approach which embraces patient-centered team-based care.
The AQA has evolved since its inception in September 2004 when the American Academy of Family Physicians (AAFP), the American College of Physicians (ACP), America's Health Insurance Plans (AHIP), and the Agency for Healthcare Research and Quality (AHRQ) joined together to lead an effort for determining, under the most expedient time frame, how to most effectively and efficiently improve performance measurement, data aggregation, and reporting in the ambulatory care setting. Originally known as the *Ambulatory Care Quality Alliance,* the coalition is now known as the *AQA Alliance.* The AQA is a large voluntary multistakeholder collaborative of physicians and other clinicians, consumers, purchasers, health plans, and others who strive to meet its responsibilities in an effective, efficient, public, and transparent manner.

American Health Information Management Association: http://www.ahima.org/about/aboutahima

The American Health Information Management Association (AHIMA) is the premier association of health information management (HIM) professionals worldwide. Serving 52 affiliated component state associations and more than 71,000 members, it is recognized as the leading source of "HIM knowledge," a respected authority for rigorous professional education and training. Founded in 1928 to improve health record quality, AHIMA has played a leadership role in the effective management of health data and medical records needed to deliver quality health care to the public.

American Medical Informatics Association: www.amia.org

AMIA aims to lead the way in transforming health care through trusted science, education, and the practice of informatics. AMIA connects a broad community of professionals and students interested in informatics. AMIA is the bridge for knowledge and collaboration across a continuum, from basic and applied research to the consumer and public health arenas.

American Nursing Informatics Association: https://www.ania.org/about-us

ANIA is an organization originally founded in 1982 as the Capital Area Roundtable on Informatics in NursinG (CARING). CARING was developed and organized by nurses in 1982 as a nonprofit undertaking to provide a forum for the advancement of automated health care information systems. In 1992 the American Nursing Informatics Association was formed in Southern California to provide networking, education, and information resources that enrich and strengthen the roles of nurses in the field of informatics. In 2007 the organizations held their first joint annual conference and officially merged in 2010. After much thought and discussion, the Board of Directors proposed to change the official organization name to the "American Nursing Informatics Association" (ANIA) with a logo tagline of "where caring and technology meet."

Association of Medical Directors of Information Systems: http://www.amdis.org/

Founded in 1997, the Association of Medical Directors of Information Systems is the premier professional organization for physicians interested in and responsible for healthcare information technology. AMDIS Members are the thought leaders, decision makers, and opinion influencers dedicated to advancing the field of Applied Medical Informatics and thereby improving the practice of medicine.

TABLE 3-2 Representative Private Sector Activities and Organizations—cont'd

Bridges to Excellence: http://www.hci3.org/node/1/

Bridges to Excellence programs recognize and reward clinicians who deliver superior patient care. Their programs measure the quality of care delivered in provider practices. They emphasize managing patients with chronic conditions, who are most at risk of incurring potentially avoidable complications. Our Recognitions cover all major chronic conditions, plus office systems—and a real Medical Home measurement scheme to promote comprehensive care delivery and strong relationships between patients and their care teams.

Physicians, nurse practitioners, and physician assistants who meet our performance benchmarks can earn a range of incentives, sometimes including substantial cash payouts. Insurers and employers fund these payouts from the savings they achieve through lower health care costs and increased employee productivity.

California HealthCare Foundation: http://www.chcf.org/

CHCF is a nonprofit grantmaking philanthropy based in Oakland, California. Founded in 1996, the staff of about 50 people issues around $35 million in grants each year from an endowment of $700 million. CHCF does not participate in lobbying or fundraising.

College of Healthcare Information Management Executives: http://www.cio-chime.org/

The College of Healthcare Information Management Executives (CHIME) is the professional organization for chief information officers and other senior health care IT leaders. CHIME enables its members and business partners to collaborate, exchange ideas, develop professionally, and advocate the effective use of information management to improve the health and health care in the communities they serve.

Connecting for Health: http://www.markle.org/health/connecting-health

Connecting for Health was created as a public-private collaboration with goals to improve people's health and advance the quality of health care in the United States through innovations in information technology. We have tackled the challenges of creating a networked health information environment that has enabled secure and private information sharing.

eHealth Initiative: http://www.ehidc.org/

eHealth Initiative is a national organization that represents stakeholders in the health care industry and has a coalition of over 200 organizations. Members include clinicians; consumers; providers; health care purchasers; health plans; health IT suppliers; laboratories; pharmaceutical companies; medical device manufacturers; pharmacies; public health agencies; quality improvement organizations; academic groups; technology companies; telehealth groups; health care quality organizations; state, regional, and community-based health care organizations.

Healthcare Information and Management Systems Society: http://www.himss.org/AboutHIMSS/index.aspx?navItemNumber=17402

HIMSS is a global, cause-based, not-for-profit organization focused on better health through information technology (IT). HIMSS leads efforts to optimize health engagements and care outcomes using information technology. HIMSS is a part of HIMSS WorldWide, a cause-based, global enterprise producing health IT thought leadership, education, events, market research, and media services around the world. Founded in 1961, HIMSS WorldWide encompasses more than 52,000 individuals, of which more than two-thirds work in health care provider, governmental, and not-for-profit organizations across the globe, plus over 600 corporations and 250 not-for-profit partner organizations, that share this cause.

Leapfrog Group: http://www.leapfroggroup.org/

The Leapfrog Group is a voluntary program aimed at mobilizing employer purchasing power to alert America's health industry that big leaps in health care safety, quality, and customer value will be recognized and rewarded. Among other initiatives, Leapfrog works with its employer members to encourage transparency and easy access to health care information as well as rewards for hospitals that have a proven record of high quality care. The Leapfrog Hospital Survey is the gold standard for comparing hospitals' performance on the national standards of safety, quality, and efficiency that are most relevant to consumers and purchasers of care. Hospitals that participate in The Leapfrog Hospital Survey achieve hospital-wide improvements that translate into millions of lives and dollars saved. Leapfrog's purchaser members use Survey results to inform their employees and purchasing strategies. In 2009, 1206 hospitals across the country completed The Leapfrog Hospital Survey.

National Association of Health Data Organizations: http://www.cdc.gov/nceh/tracking/partners/nahdo.htm

The National Association of Health Data Organizations (NAHDO) is a national, not-for-profit membership organization dedicated to improving health care through the collection, analysis, dissemination, public availability, and use of health care data for policy and market uses.

National Committee for Quality Assurance: http://www.ncqa.org/

The National Committee for Quality Assurance is a private, 501(c)(3) not-for-profit organization dedicated to improving health care quality. Since its founding in 1990, NCQA has been a central figure in driving improvement throughout the health care system, helping to elevate the issue of health care quality to the top of the national agenda. NCQA has helped to build consensus around important health care quality issues by working with large employers, policymakers, doctors, patients, and health plans to decide what's important, how to measure it, and how to promote improvement. That consensus is invaluable—transforming our health care system requires the collected will and resources of all these constituencies and more.

Public Health Data Standards Consortium: http://www.phdsc.org/

The Public Health Data Standards Consortium (The Consortium) is a non-profit, membership-based organization of federal, state, and local health agencies; professional associations; academia; public and private sector organizations; international members; and individuals. Their goal is to empower the health care and public health communities with health information technology standards to improve individual and community health. In 1998, the founding members of this organization first recognized a need for an organized common voice from public health in the national health care standardization efforts. The Consortium became a not-for-profit organization in July 2003.

Continued

TABLE 3-2 Representative Private Sector Activities and Organizations—cont'd

Public Health Informatics Institute: http://www.phii.org/

The Public Health Informatics Institute is a program of the Task Force for Global Health, a 501(c)(3) non-profit organization. PHII is known for its expertise as a neutral convener of public health professionals and their stakeholders, transforming health practitioners' ability to apply information effectively in order to improve health outcomes worldwide.

Public Health Information Network http://www.cdc.gov/phin/

The Centers for Disease Control and Prevention's (CDC) Public Health Information Network (PHIN) is a national initiative to increase the capacity of public health agencies to electronically exchange data and information across organizations and jurisdictions (e.g., clinical care to public health, public health to public health, and public health to other federal agencies). To do so, PHIN promotes the use of standards and defines functional and technical requirements for public health information exchange.

The mission of PHIN is to establish and support shared policies, standards, practices, and services that facilitate efficient public health information access, exchange, use, and collaboration among public health agencies and with their clinical and other partners. The vision of PHIN is an integrated health care and public health system using information effectively to advance population health and well-being. Programmatic activities for the PHIN initiative including strategic planning, administration, management, and operations reside in the Division of Informatics Practice, Policy, and Coordination (DIPPC) in CDC's Public Health Surveillance and Informatics Program Office (proposed).

---

and health plans conducting "market experiments" involving incentives to practicing clinicians, hospitals, and other providers for improving quality using HIT (e.g., Bridges to Excellence).[83]

In spring 2013 a group of private sector organizations (Allscripts, athenahealth, Cerner, Greenway, and RelayHealth) announced the formation of the CommonWell Health Alliance. Envisioned to be a not-for-profit association, the Alliance is dedicated to the vision that a patient's data should be available to patients and providers regardless of where care occurs.[84]

COMPELLING REASONS TO IMPLEMENT HEALTH INFORMATION TECHNOLOGY

Several key reasons for accelerated implementation of HIT for administrative and clinical data capture, collection, and exchange have been identified and reported. It is important to note that, generally, these benefits were often documented to be unique to the specific setting and are not necessarily applicable to other settings. Nevertheless, providers have and continue to implement a wide range of clinical and administrative applications within their organizations, integrated delivery systems, office practices, and health plans. Several reports on research projects describe various and diverse methods to develop systems.[85-91]

In an effort to provide high-quality care in a more cost-effective manner, health care providers have implemented various systems. Frequently noted applications and information technology–enabled processes are depicted in Table 3-3.

Developers and implementers of HIT systems generally believe that HIT implementations offer benefits. Although the specific benefits may vary and often relate to the unique features and levels of system functionality, the literature overwhelmingly notes the benefits of HIT applications. Some have been well documented, such as improved quality of care, better patient access, improved patient satisfaction,

TABLE 3-3 Representative Applications and Information Technology–Enabled Processes

Administrative and Financial

- Accreditation and licensure reporting
- Appointment scheduling
- Bar coding
- Billing
- Claims submission, reconciliation, and adjudication
- Claims processing
- Clinical data registries, data collection, and reporting
- Communications
- Customer service
- E-mail (communications between providers and patients)
- Enrollment and eligibility verification
- Financial management
- HEDIS data collection
- Internet, Intranet, and web applications
- Internet access for patient and provider communications
- Meaningful use reporting
- Patient identity management
- Patient record linkage or matching
- Patient registration
- Prevention outreach
- Public health reporting (i.e., immunization, newborn screening, lead poisoning)
- Scanning documents
- Syndrome and disease surveillance

Clinical Care

- Automated clinical guidelines and protocols
- Case management
- Clinical alerts and reminders
- Clinical data warehousing and data mining
- CPOE
- CDSS
- Digital imaging, capture, and transmission
- Disease management
- Disease registries
- EHRs

TABLE 3-3	Representative Applications and Information Technology–Enabled Processes—cont'd

- Electronic monitoring systems
- eRX
- Fitness tracking
- Immunizations tracking
- Infectious disease management programs
- Imaging
- Medication history
- Order entry, management, and results reporting
- Patient reminders
- Personal health records
- Physician alerts
- Picture archiving and communications systems
- Results routing and reporting
- Speech recognition and transcription
- Telemedicine, telehealth, and teleradiology

CDSS, Clinical decision support system; *CPOE*, computerized physician order entry; *EHR*, electronic health record; *eRX*, electronic prescribing; *HEDIS*, Healthcare Effectiveness Data and Information Set.

and increased system efficiencies. Case studies and articles describe numerous examples of how HIT is being used in many initiatives, having been successfully implemented over many years. Generally, there is widespread agreement that HIT has had and will continue to have an enormously positive effect on health care practice and delivery, enhanced patient safety, and ultimately lower costs.[92,93]

Increasingly, research is demonstrating the great potential for HIT applications such as EHRs, e-prescribing, computerized physician order entry (CPOE), and CDS to improvements in nearly all areas related to improving population health. Rapid diffusion and adoption of evidence-based HIT innovation promises to revolutionize health in the United States by reducing medical errors, improving the quality of care delivered, controlling health care costs, empowering individuals to understand and address their health care needs, and supporting public health surveillance. The federal AHRQ identified five goals for the adoption of HIT[94]:

- Improve patient safety by reducing medical errors.
- Increase health information sharing between providers, laboratories, pharmacies, and patients.
- Help patients transition between health care settings.
- Reduce duplicative and unnecessary testing.
- Increase our knowledge and understanding of the clinical safety, quality, financial and organizational value, and benefits of HIT.

Beyond provider adoption of HIT, real population-level gains from these systems will occur when standardization allows for a basic level of interoperability and data sharing across systems, providers, communities, and regions. For example, the American Society for Testing and Materials, a standards development organization, has designed and adopted a health informatics standard titled "Specification for Continuity of Care (E2369-05)" in support of the AHRQ goal of helping patients transition between health care settings. The continuity of care document has specific data items that have been agreed on and are supported by many medical associations and societies as useful in transitioning patients between health care settings and providers. The standard uses extensible markup language to identify the data components.

Examples of potential identified benefits of using HIT are noted in Table 3-4.

The value of HIT and HIE may differ depending on the stakeholder and specific application(s) (Table 3-5).[95]

Examples of quantifiable benefits indicate that methods to measure benefits vary widely. Some report performing formal return-on-investment (ROI) or cost-benefit analyses before investing in HIT resources. Others describe measuring the financial outcomes in the sense of quantifiable improvements in operating expenses and new revenue for their health systems.[96–102]

Generally, measures of success vary widely and include formal and informal analyses of financial results. Some use an ROI method to assess the financial effects of service-related operating expenses compared with revenue gains from improved service delivery. In some instances, the measurable financial improvements attributed to or facilitated by an information system have included the ability to control or reduce operating expenses (such as those related to personnel, printing, or storage costs) or to expand the services offered by the health care organization. It is generally reported that successful HIT implementations require significant investments of time and therefore a system's financial return should also be measured over time; benefits are not immediate.[103–105]

Others measure benefits in more qualitative terms, such as attaining business objectives, maintaining operational viability, and retaining critical staff. For instance, one benefit to implementing patient access to personal health records (PHRs), patient–physician electronic messaging, and automated appointment scheduling is better communication, less hassle, and improved patient satisfaction. HIT also enhances continuity of patient care through better communication between and among practitioners, providers, and patients.

Other research has identified potential challenges and unintended consequences of HIT implementation and use.[106–109] For example, the IOM reviewed the available evidence and the experience from the field on how the use of HIT affects the safety of patient care and made recommendations on how public and private actors can maximize the safety of HIT-assisted health care services. The IOM's final report provided recommended options and opportunities for public and private interventions that may improve the safety of care that incorporates the use EHRs and other forms of HIT. The IOM Committee on Patient Safety and Health IT released its report on November 10, 2011.[110]

TABLE 3-4 Potential Benefits for Using Health Information Technology

Clinical Related	Administrative, Financial, and Organizational Related
Reduced medication and other medical errors	Increased staff productivity
Fewer and avoided adverse events	Reductions in staff time spent handling test results
Improved quality of care	Decrease in telephone calls requesting patient information
Ability to respond more quickly to patient needs	Decrease in mailing and faxing patient information
Enhanced customer/patient service	Streamlined administrative processes
Better communication between patients, caregivers, and clinicians	Improved data quality for research and clinical trials
More accurate, timely, and complete clinical care documentation	More accurate and complete clinical care documentation
Better communication across care delivery team	More timely public health reporting
Enhanced care coordination	Less redundant data entry
Integrating patient data with clinical decision support databases, pharmacy and laboratory data, and emergency systems	Significant job enhancement for nurses
	Better compliance with regulatory requirements
Developing networked CPOE	More accurate, legible, and timely clinical documentation
Helping identify and prevent adverse drug events	Increased access to timely data
Developing chronic disease treatment systems, including diabetes patient registries	Increased job satisfaction
	Improved work flow and work processes
Creating clinical DSSs	Enhanced communication across care team
Improve patient transitions between health care facilities and home	Better communication between patients, caregivers, and clinicians
Enable clinicians to assess patient information at the point of care	Better communication across care delivery team
More timely and comprehensive infection control processes	More timely, complete, and accurate capture of codes and charges
Increased time for hands-on patient care	Fewer rejected claims
Improved patient confidence in care	Improvements in electronic claims processing
Better information for clinical decisions and treatment options	Increased operating efficiencies
Reduced practice variation	Economies of scale
Improved patient satisfaction	Decreased costs associated with staffing and paper storage
Reduce medical errors and improve overall patient safety	Enhanced recruitment of qualified clinicians
Increase the identification and reporting of medical errors and adverse events	Fewer duplicative tests
	Decreased operating costs
Decrease in the number of actual errors and adverse events	Reduced storage and transcription costs
Decreased patient waiting times	Reduced per claim processing costs
Better patient compliance with treatment plans	Reduced supply costs
Streamlined disease and case management	More timely payment and reimbursement
	Reduction in duplicate tests and diagnostic procedures
	Fewer inpatient hospitalizations
	Fewer emergency department admissions
	Shorter hospital stays

CPOE, Computerized physician order entry; *DSS,* decision support system.

 SELF-ASSESSMENT QUIZ

6. AHRQ identified five goals for the adoption of HIT. Which is not one of those goals?
   a. Help patients transition between health care settings.
   b. Improve medication safety by rewriting the names and spelling of drugs.
   c. Reduce duplicative and unnecessary testing.
   d. None of the above.

OBSTACLES TO HEALTH INFORMATION TECHNOLOGY ADOPTION

Despite the promise of information technology, physicians and hospitals were not adopting clinical information systems at a very rapid rate. There were three primary reasons for this slow rate of adoption. First, although these systems had been shown to provide financial benefits, little, if any, of these benefits (including avoiding office visits, reduction in acute care, and improved compliance with medications) accrue to the small office providers who pay for the systems. Instead, the benefits were enjoyed by other organizations, including health plans and employers. Second, provider organizations that implemented new information technology systems often made difficult modifications to their existing clinical and administrative work flow and decision-making processes. Not surprisingly, clinicians who worked in these organizations were often reluctant to make such changes, particularly in the absence of any perceived benefits to the organization. Finally, there were—and still are—barriers to connecting these systems to allow for information sharing among disparate organizations through regional and national interoperability. These barriers include perceived legal limitations on such information sharing and the limited capacity of health care organizations to organize regionally.[111]

According to earlier studies by the RAND Corporation, the U.S. health care system could save lives and $162 billion annually with widespread use of HIT. The study examined

TABLE 3-5 Value by Stakeholder Perspective

Stakeholder Perspective	Overall Benefit
Providers and clinicians	Timely access to data for improved decision making Rapid access to data at point of care Reduced clerical and administrative costs More efficient and appropriate patient referrals and care management Increased safety in prescribing and monitoring medication compliance Timely alerts to contraindications Improved coordination of care Enhanced revenue through decrease in rejected claims
Payers	Improved customer service Improved disease and care management Improved information to support research, audit, and policy development Reduced administrative costs
Public health agencies	More comprehensive and timely data Enhanced clinician and provider participation Easier integration of data from disparate sources Earlier detection of potential disease outbreaks More timely detection of cases that suggest a local epidemic Enhanced outcomes analysis Better bioterrorism preparedness Enhanced and unified syndrome surveillance
Patients and consumers	Improved quality of care Better coordination of care Safer care Decreased costs of care Informed consumer choice Fewer redundant tests
Data providers (i.e., commercial laboratories, pharmacies, PBMS)	Enhanced public relations Decreased write-offs from unnecessary or duplicative tests Decreased EDI costs Increased data processing efficiencies Reduced administrative costs Increased patient compliance

EDI, Electronic data interchange; *PBMS,* Pharmacy Benefit Management System.

HIT's potential health and financial benefits. Cost savings stem from several sources, including CPOE, increased efficiency in hospitals and physician practices, reduced length of hospital stay and administrative costs, and optimized drug use.[112,113]

There were also several issues related to attaining implementation of HIT. Although there had been significant progress on articulating and working toward this vision, significant obstacles to HIT adoption existed. Several studies found financial benefits in the use and implementation of CPOE.[114] A survey of members of the American Academy of Family Physicians found that slightly less than one fourth of respondents use an EHR.[115] The report cites a number of barriers to more widespread adoption of this technology (including financial, leadership, and knowledge barriers). HIT implementation is complex and costly, requiring detailed knowledge of health care financing issues, clinical processes, patients' and providers' perspectives, and expectations, organizational management, technical applications, and important legal issues.

In another study RAND specifically looked at CPOE systems and found the following:

- Electronic prescribing (eRX) systems may greatly reduce medication errors, thereby maximizing patient safety and health.
- Menus that aid in selecting appropriate medication doses and other specific features are important for achieving these goals.
- Currently used electronic prescribing systems vary widely in their features and capabilities and may not produce the best results for patient safety and health, but it should be possible to implement approximately two thirds of the guidelines in the next 3 years.[116,117]

Another report compared health care with the use of information technology in other industries. It estimated potential savings and costs of widespread adoption of EMR systems, models important health and safety benefits, and concludes that effective EMR implementation and networking could eventually save more than $81 billion annually—by improving health care efficiency and safety—and that HIT-enabled prevention and management of chronic disease could eventually double those savings while increasing health and other social benefits. However, this is unlikely to be realized without related changes to the health care system.[118]

The NIST Health IT Usability initiative is focused on establishing a framework that defines and assesses HIT usability. The goal of the research efforts is to create a detailed specification of an objective, repeatable procedure for measuring and evaluating the usability of HIT systems. The initiative examines the human factors critical to designing usable EHRs and helps guide industry in usability engineering practices.[119] NIST has issued several reports, including the following:

- NISTIR 7769: Human Factors Guidance to Prevent Healthcare Disparities with the Adoption of EHRs
- NISTIR 7741: NIST Guide to the Processes Approach for Improving the Usability of Electronic Health Records
- NISTIR 7742: Customized Common Industry Format Template for Electronic Health Record Usability Testing
- NISTIR 7743: Usability in Health IT: Technical Strategy, Research, and Implementation
- NISTIR 7804: Technical Evaluation, Testing and Validation of the Usability of Electronic Health Records
- NISTIR 7865: A Human Factors Guide to Enhance EHR Usability of Critical User Interactions When Supporting Pediatric Patient Care
- NISTIR 7952: Toward a Shared Approach for Ensuring Patient Safety with Enhanced Workflow Design for Electronic Health Records—Summary of the Workshop

In addition, financial returns associated with HIT implementation were sometimes viewed as too diffuse to justify investment from individual health system actors. Because of these obstacles, in part, the health sector lagged behind almost every other field in the application of information technology. Where elements of such technology exist in health care settings today, too often they are still not interoperable, which greatly reduces their effectiveness.

Health care is delivered by various providers across multiple settings. Clinical information is complex and there were few incentives in place for information sharing across settings. Organizational and change management issues are also challenging in a clinical environment. Some of these challenges are listed in Table 3-6.

HEALTH INFORMATION NETWORKS

There is widespread recognition of the need for HIT and exchange/interoperability at the national level, and many local, state, and regional health information networks already exist or are in developmental stages. The creation of an NwHIN offered the opportunity to increase information exchange between the clinical care community and the clinical and biomedical research communities.[120] Studies have shown that clinical applications must interconnect if small and medium-size physician practices are to achieve the majority of the clinical decision benefit of an EHR. Such interconnectivity provides sufficient sources of data for patient information and it supports vital functionality, including advanced decision-support systems. To connect clinical applications, however, the health care industry must deploy a common technical framework based on open standards, built on the Internet

as a network of networks, and health care organizations must work together to share information.[97]

Numerous HIOs that facilitate HIE have emerged in many states throughout the country. Many states have one or more regional or community-based HIT projects or prototype HIEs that have received federal or private-sector funding. These efforts include the design, planning, development, implementation, and evaluation of the exchange and linkage of data among and across multiple stakeholders.[121] In addition to regional or state level organizations and entities, subnetwork organizations (SNOs) have been proposed by some as critical to the success of efforts to establish nationwide interoperability. Each region or subnetwork needs an entity to oversee its health information environment. Regional subnetworks have a public interest responsibility to address the needs of the entire population and all health information providers. Some subnetworks will be geographically based and others will be functional or organizational, crossing geographic boundaries. Some of these enterprise or private subnetworks (e.g., a large health system or research network) may not be subject to the same public interest governance and policy obligations.[122]

There is still no standard definition or single model at this time, but a framework for appropriate functions and organizational models is emerging.[123,124] Health care is delivered by various providers across multiple settings. Because patients receive care from multiple providers over an increasingly dispersed geographic area, the challenge in collecting, coordinating, and accessing relevant, meaningful, and timely data has been and continues to be challenging. Further, little is known about the benefits, challenges, and experiences associated with sharing or exchanging information at the community level between and among providers, institutions, and other organizations. However, the more widespread use of the Internet, and the continued refinement of communications and telecommunications technologies and the adoption of content and messaging standards, provides an additional opportunity to address the current fragmentation of clinical information among multiple providers and across sites of care.

There are an increasing number of efforts at HIE. Table 3-7 depicts a number of characteristics of these emerging and operational efforts.[121]

The eHealth Initiative has tracked the growth and progress of health care data exchange efforts across the United States. The 2013 survey covers nearly 200 respondents and demonstrates ongoing challenges related to sustainability, interoperability, and patient engagement.[125]

In 2004 AHRQ awarded contracts to develop statewide networks allowing major purchasers of health care, public and private payers, hospitals, ambulatory care facilities, home health care providers, and long-term care providers to use HIT to communicate and share information.

The Robert Wood Johnson Foundation seeks to improve the health and health care of all Americans. Project Health-Design was a groundbreaking national program of Robert Wood Johnson Foundation's Pioneer Portfolio, designed

TABLE 3-6 Potential Challenges

Technology costs	There are high costs for HIT software, hardware, upgrades, and maintenance. Systems and products are costly and practically unaffordable. Providers do not have ready access to the up-front operating capital required for HIT investment. Regardless of the application or the vendor, HIT requires significant up-front investment. Providers face competing priorities for limited resources. There are ongoing work flow and work processes regarding implementation and training.
Legacy systems	Systems that were implemented in the earlier decades were often installed as stand-alone systems and the costs to replace or to integrate these systems are significant, as are costs for continuing systems maintenance and upkeep. Many legacy and stand-alone systems exist. There are significant costs to integrate these different, isolated, and fragmented systems. HIT is expensive and it has been difficult to generate the significant capital needed for the initial and continuing HIT investments.
Implementation costs	HIT implementation requires significant resources in terms of capital, time, and staffing; level of access to this capital varies.
Developing and maintaining system interoperability	There are a wide range of available systems and applications, further complicating the ability to convey information from one system to another without costly custom interfaces. Health care is complex and no two providers or institutions are identical. A successful solution in one setting is not necessarily transferable to another. Vendors vary greatly in terms of their stability, the levels of their system capabilities and functionality, and their ability to successfully implement and support their proposed solutions. Systems are often not compatible or interoperable—they cannot talk to one another. Electronic connections must exist among all providers and institutions. Currently there is fragmented use of technology with minimal interoperability and the continued existence of many legacy systems. Providers cannot easily communicate with each other because systems cannot exchange information. Providers have merged into or formed larger delivery systems, often resulting in numerous disparate and sometimes duplicative systems. The EHR as envisioned by many implies total consolidation of all patient data from before birth to the present, accessible by those with a need to know, and available at all points of care. This will require full interoperability within and among all health care organizations. Additionally, vendor and technology neutrality is essential.
Ensuring authorized access to and privacy of personal health information	Can data be exchanged so that patient privacy is ensured? Maintaining confidential personal information is essential, especially with the implementation of increasingly advanced technology. Balancing federal privacy requirements with state-level regulations is challenging. Developing and implementing agreements to facilitate HIE but governing data access and protecting patient privacy are critical.
Developing and implementing standards	This lack of data content and transmittal and messaging standards prevents interoperability and sharing of data. Although standards development organizations such as ASTM and HL7 have developed content and messaging standards, their work has not been fully integrated. Standards are developed by voluntary private groups and ratified as national standards by the American National Standards Institute. The fact that a standard has been approved does not mean that it is adopted by the health care or health information vendor community. ASTM did initial work in standards related to privacy and confidentiality before HIPAA. These reference standards are still available for use as organizations and vendors continue to address continued concerns about privacy and confidentiality—balancing the needs for public access to information with the need for patient privacy and systems security.
Identifying the business case and value proposition	Providers that invest in and implement HIT absorb the full cost of system acquisition and implementation, but the benefits accrue to many others (insurers, benefit managers, employers, regulators). Those who stand to benefit the most from provider HIT implementation are typically not the ones who pay for it. Efforts are being made to create incentives for HIT adoption and to reduce the risk of technology investments.
Connecting providers and clinicians	Efforts are being made to help streamline quality and health status reporting and monitoring and to reduce redundant data collection and reporting. Motivating clinicians to adopt technologies (such as EHRs) remains difficult because of business and clinical process and work flow disruptions during initial implementation. Additionally, the upfront technology investments and costs are high and the financial benefits of HIT often accrue to others.

ASTM, American Society for Testing and Materials; *EHR,* electronic health record; *HIE,* health information exchange; *HIPAA,* Health Insurance Portability and Accountability Act; *HIT,* health information technology; *HL7,* Health Level 7.

to spark innovation in personal health technology. The program advances a vision of PHRs as springboards for action and improved health decision-making.[126] Project Health-Design's first nine teams embarked on a user-centered design process to create HIT tools that ranged from a mobile medication management system that alerts children with cystic fibrosis when to take various medicines to a personal digital assistant that tracks patient-sourced pain and activity data.[127] They offer open source access to many Project HealthDesign artifacts and work products, including publications, research instruments, development documentation, guides and other resources.[128]

In 2012 the Robert Wood Johnson Foundation awarded $359 million in grants in seven program areas:
- Childhood obesity
- Coverage
- Global health
- Human capital
- Pioneer
- Public health
- Quality/equality
- Vulnerable populations[86,127]

In this era of rapidly changing technologies and innovation and the effect of various environmental, political, and societal

TABLE 3-7   Selected Characteristics of Health Information Exchanges

Goals

- Reduce costs.
- Provide economies of scale.
- Offer extensive cost-recovering health-related services to providers, related agencies, and consumers.
- Support a fully integrated, longitudinal health record.
- Provide services to multiple stakeholders.
- Allow competitors to collaborate to share information.
- Provide technology-based information services to help maintain optimal health for all residents of community.
- Move administrative transactions between health care purchasers, payers, and providers.
- Improve the completeness and accuracy of health information.

Functionality

- Results retrieval
- Clinical messaging and document delivery
- Data entry
- Reporting
- Clinical decision support
- Public health:
  - ○ Case detection (electronic laboratory reporting)
  - ○ Cancer research (supported by National Cancer Institute)
  - ○ Showing outcome results
  - ○ Prompting physicians to screen
  - ○ Immunization registry
  - ○ Syndromic surveillance by emergency department chief complaint
- Secure exchange of confidential information
- Secure encryption of e-mail
- Digital signature of e-mail
- Digital signature for other documents
- Laboratory reporting

Data Exchanged

- Emergency department and outpatient visits
- Inpatient laboratory results
- Hospitalization discharge summaries
- Radiology reports
- Tumor registry data
- Anatomic pathology reports
- Immunizations
- Ambulatory notes
- Vital signs
- Visit reasons and diagnoses
- Medication profile
- Cardiac testing (echocardiograms, catheterizations, etc.)
- Radiology images
- Gastroenterology reports
- Problem lists and diagnoses
- Laboratory results
- Medications
- Allergies
- Immunizations
- Patient identification data
- Facility and practitioner identification data

Goals

- Promote the adoption of data standards and implement electronic data exchange.
- Encourage stakeholders to share the information needed to make good health care decisions, monitor patient populations, and support value-based purchasing.
- Improve inefficient information systems and provide for the open, secure exchange of information among trading partners.
- Protect the privacy and confidentiality of individuals while balancing the need to monitor health care performance and quality.

Functionality

- Laboratory reporting
- Birth reports
- Death reports from funeral homes
- Reportable events
- Disease registries
- Trauma registries
- Scheduling
- Local and national laboratory e-mail
- Billing data access for physician offices
- Local and national laboratory electronic access
- Identity correlation service—correlates multiple patient identities across disparate systems.
- Information locator service—identifies where clinical data reside on a correlated patient and accesses requested records for an authorized user
- Access control service—supports HIPAA compliance by enabling user-defined security rules, including role-based access and logging of all data access events
- Clinician and consumer portals—gives clinician end users the ability to perform customized patient searches and locate clinical results while using a browser-based user interface. The consumer/patient portal gives views of the same information and is managed by the patient's caregiver.

Data Exchanged

- Emergency department facility identification, emergency department practitioner type
- Emergency department payment data
- Emergency department arrival and first assessment data
- Chief complaint, triage acuity, mode of arrival, vitals signs
- Emergency department history and physical examination data
- Coded cause of injury ICD-10 codes
- Emergency department procedure and results data
- Emergency department disposition and diagnosis data
- Emergency department disposition, ICD-9 and ICD-10 coded diagnoses
- Laboratory results
- Radiology results (images, voices, file/dictation, reports)
- Pharmacy results (medication history)
- Administrative data (eligibility, referrals, authorizations)

HIPAA, Health Insurance Portability and Accountability Act; ICD, International Classification of Diseases.

factors on the delivery of health care, we need more than ever to understand the evolution of successful HIE and the potential of HIE to address these issues. Identifying the factors critical to success and the impediments to moving forward are essential to realizing the full potential of HIE. Regionally based collaborative efforts are seen as an increasing critical element to advance the broader adoption and use of HIT.

Today's proponents of HIE still have high hopes for improving care and cutting costs by sharing information among providers, payers, and purchasers.[129,130]

Communities need to assess their readiness for local and regional data sharing by conducting a rigorous review of the technical, clinical, and organizational capacity and capabilities and the level of community commitment and the availability of local leadership to spearhead the effort. Communities also need to address the various policy and regulatory changes, and security and privacy, medical malpractice, and practice transformation.[131]

ROLE OF HEALTH INFORMATION MANAGEMENT AND HEALTH INFORMATICS

HIT and HIE offer enormous opportunity for the U.S. health care system. It is becoming increasingly apparent that investments in HIT and HIE provide significant returns across a variety of metrics. HIT systems and applications provide increased delivery system efficiencies and cost savings, contribute to greater patient safety and better patient care, and achieve clinical and business process improvements. Patients and consumers benefit from the comprehensive adoption of HIT and the ability to share data within and across sites of care and among clinicians. Ultimately, other stakeholders such as employers, payers, policy makers, public health officials, and regulators will benefit from the ability to share and exchange data.[132-136]

The ability to exchange information quickly and accurately within and across delivery and research systems is paramount in health care delivery. But to realize the true potential, much more work must be undertaken. Over the past several years, health system leaders and the federal government have recognized the potential for electronic health information to transform the quality and efficiency of care delivery. There is growing adoption and use of EHRs, computerized order entry, and other technology-enabled automation components that compose an EHR system. There is a flurry of activity associated with development and implementation of community, state, and regional HIE.[136,137] Establishment of standards for content and message delivery and receipt are in various stages of agreement and execution. HIM professionals' contribution to determining how the meanings of clinical and administrative terms are defined and represented is essential.

HIM and applied health informatics skills can help address and resolve the HIM challenges likely to be encountered, including those related to the activities listed in Table 3-8.

TABLE 3-8 Health Informatics and Information Management Activities

- Adopting and implementing EHRs
- Analyzing clinical and administrative data
- Assessing and establishing organizational and community readiness
- Assessing work flow analysis and redesign
- Ensuring and facilitating patient identity management
- Ensuring clinician and provider adoption and use
- Ensuring compliance and regulation
- Ensuring data content and quality
- Complying with accreditation and licensing requirements
- Convening stakeholders for HIE efforts
- Defining organizational goals and program focus
- Defining the business and legal medical record
- Demonstrating value and benefit
- Determining data definitions and representation
- Determining user authentication verification processes and policies
- Developing agreements to facilitate HIE
- Developing and conducting user training and orientation
- Developing and testing features and functions
- Developing the vision for secured access to EHRs
- Developing the vision for secured access to personal health information
- Developing, implementing, and overseeing data access and sharing strategies, policies, and procedures
- Encouraging use and adoption of HIT and HIE
- Ensuring secure transactions
- Establishing confidentiality, privacy, and security policies and procedures
- Establishing consensus on data standards
- Establishing data and record ownership and control
- Facilitating collaboration among participating stakeholders
- Facilitating negotiation and data collection from data sources
- Implementing access and authentication policies and procedures
- Implementing data and transmission standards
- Implementing stakeholder and participant agreements
- Integrating consumer personal health record data and information
- Maintaining and managing the legal medical record
- Managing and overseeing access and authentication functions and activities
- Managing and overseeing data and information governance
- Participating in technology selection, implementation, and deployment
- Participating in various standards-setting organizations
- Participating in business process reengineering of clinical and administrative practices
- Planning for data and systems backup and contingencies
- Planning, designing, and developing health care information systems
- Promoting HIT and HIE as a priority
- Protecting the patient and public interests
- Revamping procedures, processes, and work flow
- Setting and establishing HIM practices, principles, policies, and procedures
- Training and educating providers and consumers
- Transitioning from legacy systems

EHR, Electronic health record; *HIE,* health information exchange; *HIM,* health information management; *HIT,* health information technology.

KEY CONCEPTS

Across the health care industry, stakeholders are committed to improved quality and efficiency of care and better patient safety. Many envision a twenty-first century health care system that is:

- Integrated and linked by information technology
- Consumer centered
- Using new drugs, technologies, and clinical procedures

This vision requires that health care be delivered efficiently and cost effectively. Key players in the industry are mobilizing around their collective and diverse interests in facilitating HIT and are supporting activities to further the adoption and deployment of HIT. We are seeing a rapid acceleration of continuing activities to help ensure the success of current efforts building on numerous efforts undertaken earlier.[138–144]

HIT has been identified as essential in transforming the U.S. health care system—making it safer and more efficient, and improving the quality of care for patients overall. HIT applications and systems such as EHRs, electronic prescribing (eRX), bedside bar coding, CPOE, and decision support systems (DSS) are widely seen as central to reducing errors and improving quality. Increasingly mobile health technologies and applications as well as telemedicine and telehealth capabilities are gaining attention.[145]

In their quest to improve the quality of patient care, many health care providers continue to take advantage of information and communications technology. Unfortunately, their ongoing difficulty in investing scarce resources into increasingly expensive HIT, as well as the current lack of standardization across HIT systems and challenges with usability,[146–152] has hampered the widespread adoption and implementation of these technologies.

The ability to capture, manage, and use electronic data and information is also essential to continuously improving excellence in health services research and public policy. A consensus has emerged that the nation's health and health care delivery system must replace its outdated and frequently error-plagued paper-based approach to HIM, and data and information governance. More recently, efforts are underway to plan, develop, and implement a national approach to collecting and sharing information among and across health care providers, payers, patients, and policy makers to achieve the national vision of improved health care for all citizens. The role of HIM and applied health informatics in these efforts is essential to their success.

Health care and public policy decisions rely on ready access to clear, concise, and up-to-date information—information that is increasingly complex and highly dynamic. Yet the health care industry continues to face challenging issues. The industry grapples with high and increasing levels of competition, ongoing and overlapping heavy legislative and regulatory burdens, and competing demands for better quality, lower costs, and increased access to services.

HIT solutions have long been and continue to be touted as the industry's solution to these problems. HIT has been around

for decades, but the industry is still a long way from full implementation. It is increasingly apparent that HIT will provide efficiencies, contribute to greater patient safety and better patient care, allow for increased delivery systems efficiencies, and achieve clinical and business process improvements. Ultimately, the industry will benefit greatly from the comprehensive automation of health care and related processes.

HIT can drive across-the-board positive changes and enhance value in care delivery. In particular, applications such as EHRs, eRX, and bedside bar coding have been identified and promoted as necessary to facilitate a safer and more efficient health care system. Ultimately, more widespread adoption of HIT will eliminate or reduce duplicative information gathering and will ensure delivery of health care based on timely, relevant, and complete information.

The U.S. health care industry is in the midst of a revolution that holds the promise of improved quality and efficiency, after years of halting progress, missteps, and a few striking but isolated successes in the application of HIT to the delivery of health care. Recently, national leaders in government and industry have recognized anew the critical importance of rapidly motivating, facilitating, and achieving the vision of a unified NHII based on locally implemented information technology.

Great challenges remain, however.[153–158] Among others, these ongoing and sometimes relentless challenges include ongoing development and implementation of standards for capturing and sharing data, dealing with privacy, security, and confidentiality concerns, achieving widespread adoption throughout the industry across diverse providers and settings, demonstrating a convincing case that HIT investments improve quality of care and represent sound business decisions, ensuring project sustainability, and developing and maintaining a trained workforce skilled in HIT, HIM, and health informatics.

These technologies are readily available for increasingly more widespread adoption by providers, including physicians, health plans, and hospitals. Evidence demonstrates the efficacy of these tools in addressing health status problems that result from process failures. However, HIT studies predict varying rates of EHR adoption in the future despite the current adoption incentives programs, such as MU.

HIT offers enormous potential, but it remains slowed by challenges and barriers. With regard to the opportunities presented by HIT, it is becoming increasingly apparent that HIT can provide savings, contribute to greater patient safety, enhance patient care, allow for increased delivery systems efficiencies, and achieve clinical and business process improvements. As such, HIT can drive across-the-board positive changes and enhance value in care delivery. In particular, applications such as EHRs, eRX, and bar coding have been identified and promoted as necessary to facilitate a safer and more efficient health care system. Patients and their caregivers will benefit from the comprehensive adoption of HIT and the ability to share data within and across sites of care and among providers. Ultimately, other stakeholders such as employers, payers, and regulators will benefit from the ability to share and exchange data.

CHAPTER REVIEW

1. Which committee makes recommendations to the national coordinator for health IT on standards, implementation specifications, and certification criteria for the electronic exchange and use of health information?
   a. HIT policy committee
   b. HIT standards committee
   c. ARRA

2. How many organizations does CMS contract with in each state to serve as that state's QIO contractor?
   a. one
   b. two
   c. four

3. The AHRQ research portfolio does the following:
   a. anticipates the future needs of the health care system and supports development of innovative HIT solutions.
   b. identifies and fills current gaps in knowledge about HIT.
   c. leverages the capability of HIT to improve the quality, safety, efficiency, and effectiveness of health care.
   d. all of the above.

4. The S&I framework within the ONCHIT:
   a. was formed to orchestrate input from the public and private sectors.
   b. helps create harmonized HIT specifications for use throughout the United States.
   c. enables health care stakeholders to drive higher interoperability and greater HIE to improve quality of care.
   d. all of the above.

5. The ANSI:
   a. coordinates the development of voluntary consensus standards in the United States.
   b. represents the needs and views of international but not U.S. stakeholders.
   c. ANSI is not the U.S. member body to ISO.

6. The PCORI conducts research to provide information about the best available evidence to help patients and their health care providers make more informed decisions and is:
   a. authorized by Congress
   b. an agency within the department of HHS
   c. part of the NIH

7. The EHR incentive programs provide incentive payments to eligible professionals, eligible hospitals, and CAHs:
   a. to adopt, implement, upgrade, or demonstrate meaningful use of CEHRT
   b. to donate technology to underserved and rural areas
   c. to participate in clinical trials

8. Which of the following entities is charged with managing the federal EHR incentive programs?
   a. CMS
   b. ONCHIT
   c. congress

9. Which of the following organizations is the principal federal entity charged with coordination of nationwide efforts to implement and use the most advanced HIT and the electronic exchange of health information?
   a. CMS
   b. AHRQ
   c. ONCHIT

10. The law that ended preexisting condition exclusions for children (health plans can no longer limit or deny benefits to children younger than 19 because of a preexisting condition) is:
    a. HIPAA
    b. HITECH
    c. PPACA

11. The CLIA of 1988:
    a. eliminated the exception under the HIPAA privacy rule to an individual's right to access his or her protected health information when it is held by a CLIA-certified or CLIA-exempt laboratory.
    b. created the exception under the HIPAA security rule to an individual's right to access his or her protected health information when it is held by a CLIA-certified or CLIA-exempt laboratory.
    c. determined that patients may not access their protected health information when it is held by a CLIA-certified or CLIA-exempt laboratory.

12. Project HealthDesign was a groundbreaking national program of Robert Wood Johnson Foundation's Pioneer Portfolio, designed to spark innovation in:
    a. personal health technology
    b. EHR
    c. robotics

REFERENCES

1. Institute of Medicine: Letter report on the key capabilities of an electronic health record system: http://www.iom.edu/Reports/2003/Key-Capabilities-of-an-Electronic-Health-Record-System.aspx. Accessed November 11, 2014.
2. Hripcsak G, Bloomrosen M, Flatelybrennan P, et al: Health data use, stewardship, and governance: ongoing gaps and challenges: a report from AMIA's 2012 Health Policy Meeting, J Am Med Inform Assoc 21(2):204–211, 2014.
3. Bloomrosen M, Detmer DE: Informatics, evidence-based care, and research: implications for national policy: a report of an American Medical Informatics Association health policy conference, J Am Med Inform Assoc 17(2):115–123, 2010.
4. Gupta D, et al: Evaluation of a deidentification (De-Id) software engine to share pathology reports and clinical documents for research, Am J Clin Pathol 121(2):176–186, 2004.
5. Bloomrosen M, Detmer D: Advancing the framework: use of health data—a report of a working conference of the American Medical Informatics Association, J Am Med Inform Assoc 15(6):715–722, 2008.
6. Safran C, Bloomrosen M, Hammond WE, et al: Expert Panel: Toward a national framework for the secondary use of health data: an American

Medical Informatics Association White Paper, *J Am Med Inform Assoc* 14 (1):1–9, 2006 Oct 31, Epub.

7. Sabharwal R, Holve E, Rein A, Segal C: *Approaches to using protected health information (PHI) for patient-centered outcomes research (PCOR): regulatory requirements, de-identification strategies, and policy*, AcademyHealth, March 2012, Electronic Data Methods Forum.

8. Wellner B, et al: Rapidly retargetable approaches to de-identification in medical records, *J Am Med Informatics Assoc* 14 (5):550–563, 2007.

9. Malin B, Kantarcioglu M, Cassa C: A survey of challenges and solutions for privacy in clinical genomics data mining. In *Privacy-aware knowledge discovery: novel applications and new techniques*, New York, 2011, CRC Press.

10. Hersh WR, Cimino J, Payne PRO, et al: Recommendations for the use of operational electronic health record data in comparative effectiveness research, *eGEMs* 1(1), 2013, Article 14.

11. Electronic Data Methods Forum: http://www.edm-forum.org/publicgrant/home/. Accessed June 22, 2014.

12. Patient-Centered Outcomes Research Institute: http://www.pcori.org/. Accessed June 22, 2014.

13. http://www.healthit.gov/sites/default/files/utility/final-federal-health-it-strategic-plan-0911.pdf. Accessed February 2006.

14. HealthIT.gov: Index for excerpts from the American Recovery and Reinvestment Act of 2009 (ARRA): http://www.healthit.gov/sites/default/files/hitech_act_excerpt_from_arra_with_index.pdf. Accessed June 22, 2014.

15. http://www.healthit.gov/policy-researchers-implementers/health-it-legislation.

16. Centers for Medicare and Medicaid Services: HER incentive programs: http://www.cms.gov/Regulations-and-Guidance/Legislation/EHRIncentivePrograms/index.html?redirect=/EHRIncentivePrograms/. Accessed June 22, 2014.

17. HealthIT.gov: Certification policy and programs: http://www.healthit.gov/policy-researchers-implementers/certification-and-ehr-incentives#standards-certification-criteria. Accessed June 22, 2014.

18. US Department of Health and Human Services: Key features of the Affordable Care Act: http://www.hhs.gov/healthcare/facts/timeline/index.html. Accessed June 22, 2014.

19. Centers for Medicare and Medicaid Services: The Center for Consumer Information and Insurance Oversight: http://www.cms.gov/CCIIO/Programs-and-Initiatives/Health-Insurance-Market-Reforms/Patients-Bill-of-Rights.html. Accessed June 22, 2014.

20. US Department of Health and Human Services: Key features of the Affordable Care Act by Year: http://www.hhs.gov/healthcare/facts/timeline/timeline-text.html. Accessed June 22, 2014.

21. Starr P: Smart technology, stunted policy: developing health information networks, *Health Aff* 16:91–105, 1997.

22. National Health Information Infrastructure: http://aspe.hhs.gov/sp/NHII/. Accessed August 14, 2006.

23. *State and regional experience in health information collection, sharing and reporting: a review of national and regional demonstration projects resources innovations and opportunities, Wisconsin Public Health and Health Policy Institute*, University of Wisconsin Medical School, Madison, 2005, Department of Population Health Sciences.

24. HealthIT.gov: Nationwide Health Information Network (NwHIN): http://www.healthit.gov/policy-researchers-implementers/nationwide-health-information-network-nwhin. Accessed June 22, 2014.

25. Committee on Quality of Health Care in America: *Institute of America: Crossing the quality chasm: a new health system for the 21st century*, Washington, DC, 2001, National Academies Press.

26. Office of the National Coordinator for Health Information Technology: Health IT strategic framework: Executive summary (July 2004): http://www.healthit.gov/sites/default/files/utility/final-federal-health-it-strategic-plan-0911.pdf. Accessed November 11, 2014.

27. *Summary of Nationwide Health Information Network (NHIN) Request for Information (RFI) responses June 2005*, Washington, DC, 2005, U.S. Department of Health and Human Services Office of the National Coordinator for Health Information Technology.

28. Agency for Healthcare Research and Quality: A summary of the proceedings: http://www.ahrq.gov/data/hitmeet.htm. Accessed August 14, 2006.

29. Agency for Healthcare Research and Quality: Health IT evaluation toolkit: http://healthit.ahrq.gov/health-it-tools-and-resources/health-it-evaluation-toolkit. Accessed June 23, 2014.

30. Agency for Healthcare Research and Quality: Health IT funding opportunities: http://healthit.ahrq.gov/funding-opportunities. June 24, 2014.

31. Corrigan JM, Greiner A, Erickson SM, editors: Institute of Medicine: Fostering rapid advances in health care: learning from system demonstrations. In: *Health care finance and delivery systems*, Washington, DC, 2002, Committee on Rapid Advance Demonstration Projects.

32. Institute of Medicine: *The future of the public's health in the 21st century*, Washington, DC, 2002, Committee on Assuring the Health of the Public in the 21st Century.

33. Institute of Medicine: *Who will keep the public healthy: educating public health professionals for the 21st century*, Washington, DC, 2002, Committee on Educating Public Health Professionals for the 21st Century.

34. Institute of Medicine: *Key capabilities of an electronic health record system*, Washington, DC, 2003, Committee on Data Standards for Patient Safety Institute of Medicine.

35. Aspden P, Corrigan JM, Wolcott J, et al, editors: Committee on Data Standards for Patient Safety: achieving a new standard of care, In Washington, DC, 2003, Institute of Medicine.

36. Adams K, Corrigan JM, editors: *Committee on Identifying Priority Areas for Quality Improvement: priority areas for national action: transforming healthcare quality*, Washington, DC, 2003, Institute of Medicine.

37. National Research Council: *Health IT and patient safety: building safer systems for better care*, Washington, DC, 2012, The National Academies Press.

38. National Research Council: *Digital data improvement priorities for continuous learning in health and health care: workshop summary*, Washington, DC, 2013, The National Academies Press.

39. National Research Council: Sharing clinical research data: workshop summary, Washington, DC, 2013, The National Academies Press.

40. HealthIT.gov: About ONC: http://www.healthit.gov/newsroom/about-onc. Accessed June 24, 2014.

41. HealthIT.gov: Policymaking, regulation, and strategy: http://www.healthit.gov/policy-researchers-implementers/policymaking-regulation-strategy. Accessed June 24, 2014.

42. HealthIT.gov: Rural healthcare initiative: http://www.healthit.gov/policy-researchers-implementers/rural-healthcare-initiative. Accessed June 24, 2014.

43. HealthIT.gov: Federal advisory committees (FACAs): http://www.healthit.gov/facas/?tid=125. Accessed June 24, 2014.

44. The White House Office of Management and Budget: http://www.whitehouse.gov/sites/default/files/omb/assets/egov_docs/FY10_UPI_CodingScheme.pdf. Accessed November 11, 2014.

45. US Department of Health and Human Services: HHS organizational chart: http://www.hhs.gov/about/orgchart/. Accessed June 24, 2014.

46. The Office of the National Coordinator for Health Information Technology: Standards and interoperability framework: http://www.healthit.gov/sites/default/files/pdf/fact-sheets/standards-and-interoperability-framework.pdf. Accessed June 24, 2014.

47. S&I Framework: http://www.siframework.org/. Accessed June 24, 2014.

48. S&I Framework: What is the S&I framework? http://www.siframework.org/whatis.html. Accessed June 24, 2014.

49. International Organization for Standardization: About ISO: http://www.iso.org/iso/home/about.htm. Accessed June 24, 2014.

50. International Organization for Standardization: http://www.iso.org/iso/home/standards and http://www.iso.org/iso/home.

51. International Organization for Standardization: *ISO membership manual*: http://www.iso.org/iso/iso_membership_manual_2013.pdf. Accessed June 24, 2014.

52. International Organization for Standardization: ISO members: http://www.iso.org/iso/home/about/iso_members.htm. Accessed June 24, 2014.

53. American National Standards Institute: About ANSI overview: http://www.ansi.org/about_ansi/overview/overview.aspx?menuid=1. Accessed June 24, 2014.

54. International Organization for Standardization: United States (ANSI): http://www.iso.org/iso/home/about/iso_members/iso_member_body.htm?member_id=2188. Accessed June 24, 2014.

55. Vreeman D: RSNA and Regenstrief Institute launch effort to unify radiology procedure naming, *LOINC Regenstrief:* http://loinc.org/news/rsna-and-regenstrief-institute-launch-effort-to-unify-radiology-procedure-naming.html/. Accessed June 24, 2014.

56. The Office of the National Coordinator for Health Information Technology: *Health information technology patient safety action and surveillance plan:* http://www.healthit.gov/sites/default/files/safety_plan_master.pdf. Accessed June 24, 2014.

57. HealthIT.gov: Health IT and patient safety tools and resources: http://www.healthit.gov/policy-researchers-implementers/health-it-and-patient-safety-tools-and-resources. Accessed June 24, 2014.

58. Agency for Healthcare Research and Quality: Patient safety organization (PSO) program: common formats: http://www.pso.ahrq.gov/formats/commonfmt.htm. Accessed June 24, 2014.

59. HealthIT.gov: State health information exchange: http://www.healthit.gov/policy-researchers-implementers/state-health-information-exchange. Accessed June 24, 2014.

60. HealthIT.gov: State health information exchange: http://www.healthit.gov/policy-researchers-implementers/state-health-information-exchange. Accessed June 24, 2014.

61. HealthIT.gov: Health information exchange research: http://www.healthit.gov/policy-researchers-implementers/health-information-exchange-research. Accessed June 24, 2014.

62. HealthIT.gov: Beacon community program: http://www.healthit.gov/policy-researchers-implementers/beacon-community-program. Accessed June 24, 2014.

63. Agency for Healthcare Research and Quality: http://healthit.ahrq.gov/. Accessed June 24, 2014.

64. US Department of Health and Human Services: http://www.healthit.gov/sites/default/files/oncfy09cj.pdf. Accessed January 2, 2007.

65. Healthcare Management and Information Systems Society: HIMSS Foundation: http://www.nationalehealth.org/about-national-ehealth-collaborative. Accessed June 24, 201.

66. Centers for Medicare and Medicaid Services: Quality improvement organizations: http://www.cms.gov/Medicare/Quality-Initiatives-Patient-Assessment-Instruments/QualityImprovementOrgs/index.html?redirect=/QualityImprovementOrgs/. Accessed June 24, 2014.

67. American Health Quality Association: http://www.ahqa.org/pub/189_817_5174.cfm. Accessed August 14, 2006.

68. Health Information Technology: Initial Set of Standards, Implementation Specification and Certification Criteria for Electronic Health Record Technology: Interim Final Rule, Federal Register 1/10/13 Part III DHHS, 45 CFR Part 170.

69. Centers for Medicare and Medicaid Services: Press release: HHS strengthens patients' right to access lab test reports: http://www.cms.gov/Newsroom/MediaReleaseDatabase/Press-releases/2014-Press-releases-items/2014-02-03.html. Accessed June 24, 2014.

70. Clinical and Translational Science Awards: About the CTSA consortium: https://www.ctsacentral.org/about-us/ctsa. Accessed June 24, 2014.

71. National Center for Translational Sciences: Clinical and translational science awards: http://www.ncats.nih.gov/files/ctsa-factsheet.pdf. Accessed June 24, 2014.

72. Lister Hill National Center for Biomedical Communications: About: http://lhncbc.nlm.nih.gov/about. Accessed June 24, 2014.

73. US National Library of Medicine: Unified medical language system (UMLS): SNOMED clinical terms (SNOMED CT): http://www.nlm.nih.gov/research/umls/Snomed/snomed_main.html. Accessed June 24, 2014.

74. Electronic Health Record Certification Criteria and the Office of National Coordinator Health Information Technology Certification Program, Regulatory Flexibility, Improvements and Enhanced Health Information Technology Exchange Final Rule *Federal Register* 79(176) 2014 Part IV DHHS 45 CFR Part 170.

75. The International Health Terminology Standards Development Organisation: *IHTSDO delivering SNOMED CT: the global clinical terminology:* http://ihtsdo.org/fileadmin/user_upload/Docs_01/Publications/SNOMED_CT/SnomedCt_MeaningfulUse_20130214.pdf. Accessed June 24, 2014.

76. Goldman J, Jarrin R, Trauner D: *mHealth Task Force: findings and recommendations:* http://www2.itif.org/2012-mhealth-taskforce-recommendations.pdf. Accessed June 24, 2014.

77. Federal Communications Commission: Fact sheet—mHealth task force recommendations: http://www.fcc.gov/document/fact-sheet-mhealth-task-force-recommendations. Accessed June 24, 2014.

78. Healthcare connect fund: http://transition.fcc.gov/Daily_Releases/Daily_Business/2013/db0225/DOC-319092A1.pdf. Accessed June 24, 2014.

79. Library of Congress: List of bills introduced in the 113th Congress: http://thomas.loc.gov/home/Browse.php. Accessed June 24, 2014.

80. Institute for Healthcare Improvement: The IHI triple aim: http://www.ihi.org/offerings/Initiatives/TripleAIM/Pages/default.aspx. Accessed June 24, 2014.

81. Berwick DM, Nolan TW, Whittington J: The triple aim: care, health, and cost, *Health Aff (Millwood)* 27(3):759–769, 2008. http://dx.doi.org/10.1377/hlthaff.27.3.759.

82. Markle: http://www.markle.org/health. Accessed June 24, 2014.

83. Markle: T6: Record locator service: technical background from the Massachusetts prototype community: http://www.markle.org/health/markle-common-framework/connecting-professionals/t6. Accessed June 24, 2014.

84. Forbes: http://www.forbes.com/fdc/welcome_mjx.shtml. CommonWell Health Alliance in Healthcare Technology News http://news.avancehealth.com/2013/03/commonwell-health-alliance.html. Accessed June 24, 2014.

85. National Committee on Vital and Health Statistics: *Information for health: a strategy for building the national health information infrastructure,* Washington, DC, 2001, National Committee on Vital and Health Statistics.

86. General Accounting Office: *Information technology: benefits realized for selected health care functions,* publication No. GAO-04-224, Washington, DC, 2003, General Accounting Office.

87. Agency for Healthcare Quality and Research: Case study finds computerized ICU information system care can significantly reduce time spent by nurses on documentation, October 10, 2003, press release.

88. Ball M, Garets DE, Handler T: *Leveraging IT to improve patient safety, Yearbook of Medical Informatics of the International Medical Informatics Association,* 2003, Heidelberg, Germany.

89. Bates DW, Gawande AA: Improving patient safety with information technology, *N Engl J Med* 348:2526–2534, 2003.

90. Vogel LH: Finding value from IT investments: exploring the elusive ROI in healthcare, *J Healthc Inf Manag* 17:20–28, 2003.

91. Newell L, Christensen D: Who's counting now? ROI for patient safety initiatives, *J Healthc Inf Manag* 17:29–35, 2003.

92. Hillestad R, Bigelow J, Bower A, et al: Can electronic medical record systems transform health care? Potential health benefits, savings and costs, *Health Aff* 24:1103–1117, 2005.

93. Cutler DM, Feldman NE, Horwitz JR: U.S. adoption of computerized physician order entry systems, *Health Aff* 24:1654–1663, 2005.

94. Agency for Healthcare Research and Quality: *Health IT to advance excellence in health care,* publication No. 05-M021, Rockville, MD, 2005, Agency for Healthcare Research and Quality. http://healthit.ahrq.gov, Accessed August 14, 2006.

95. Frisse M: Lessons learned from state and RHIOs: organizational, technical and financial aspects. Presented at the Third Annual Connecting Communities Learning Forum and Exhibition: http://www.ehidc.org/resource-center/publications/view_document/393-webinar-materials-connecting-communities-workgroup-advancing-behavioral-health-information-exchange and http://www.ehidc.org/hie-toolkit. Accessed November 11, 2014.

96. Health information technology, *Health Aff* 24(5):1148–1366, 2005.

97. Working Group on Financial, Organizational, and Legal Sustainability of Health Information Exchange: Financial, legal and organizational approaches to achieving electronic connectivity in healthcare, Connecting

for Health: http://www.markle.org/publications/1257-financial-legal-and-organizational-approaches-achieving-electronic-connectivity-he. Accessed September 1, 2006.

98. Lee J: Computerized physician order entry (CPOE) systems, Research Synthesis, AcademyHealth (2002): http://www.academyhealth.org/Training/content.cfm?ItemNumber=1690. Accessed November 11, 2014.

99. Coye MJ, Bernstein WS: Perspective: improving America's health care system by investing in information technology, *Health Aff* 22:56–58, 2003.

100. Bates DW, Leape LL, Cullen DJ, et al: Effect of computerized physician order entry and a team intervention on prevention of serious medication errors, *JAMA* 280:1311–1316, 1998.

101. Bates DW, Spell N, Cullen DJ, et al: The costs of adverse drug events in hospitalized patients, *JAMA* 277:307–311, 1997.

102. Classen DC, Pestotnik SL, Evans RS, et al: Adverse drug events in hospitalized patients: excess length of stay, extra costs, and attributable mortality, *JAMA* 277:301–306, 1997.

103. Leape LL, Bates DW, Cullen DJ: Systems analysis of adverse drug events, *JAMA* 274:34–43, 1995.

104. Leapfrog Group: *Computerized physician order entry (CPOE): fact sheet*, Washington, DC, 2000, http://www.leapfroggroup.org/media/file/FactSheet_CPOE2.pdf. Accessed August 11, 2002.

105. Hillestad R, Bigelow J, Bower A, et al: Can electronic medical record systems transform health care? Potential health benefits, savings, and costs, *Health Aff* 24:1103–1117, 2005.

106. Bloomrosen M, Starren J, Lorenzi NM, Ash JS, Patel VL, Shortliffe EH: Anticipating and addressing the unintended consequences of health IT and policy: a report from the AMIA 2009 Health Policy Meeting, *J Am Med Inform Assoc* 18(1):82–90, 2011.

107. Sittig DF, Singh H: A new sociotechnical model for studying health information technology in complex adaptive healthcare systems, *Qual Saf Health Care* 19(Suppl 3):i68–i74, 2010.

108. Harrison MI, Koppel R, Bar-Lev S: Unintended consequences of information technologies in health care—an interactive sociotechnical analysis, *J Am Med Inform Assoc* 14(5):542–549, 2007, Epub 2007 Jun 28.

109. Campbell EM, Sittig DF, Ash JS, Guappone KP, Dykstra RH: In reply to: e-Iatrogenesis: the most critical consequence of CPOE and other HIT, *J Am Med Inform Assoc*, 14:388, 2007 [Epub ahead of print.].

110. http://www.iom.edu/Reports/2011/Health-IT-and-Patient-Safety-Building-Safer-Systems-for-Better-Care.aspx.

111. Frisse ME: State and community-based efforts to foster interoperability, *Health Aff (Millwood)* 24:1190–1196, 2005.

112. Fonkych K, Taylor R: The state and pattern of health information technology adoption: http://www.rand.org/pubs/monographs/MG409/index.html. Accessed February 2006.

113. Girosi F, Meili R, Scoville R: Extrapolating evidence of health information technology savings and costs: http://www.rand.org/pubs/monographs/MG410/. Accessed February 2006.

114. Kaushal R, Jha AK, Franz C, et al: Return on investment for a computerized physician order entry system, *J Am Med Informatics Assoc* 13:261–266, 2006.

115. Center for Health Information Technology: http://healthit.ahrq.gov. Accessed November 11, 2014.

116. Bower AG: The diffusion and value of healthcare information technology: http://www.rand.org/pubs/monographs/MG272-1/. Accessed September 1, 2006.

117. Bell D, Marken RS, Meili R, et al: Electronic prescribing systems: making it safer to take your medicine? http://www.rand.org/pubs/research_briefs/RB9052/. Accessed September 1, 2006.

118. Hillestad R, Bigelow J, Bower A, et al: Can electronic medical record systems transform health care? Potential health benefits, savings and costs, *Health Aff* 24:1103–1117, 2005.

119. National Institute of Standards and Technology: Usability: http://www.nist.gov/healthcare/usability/. Accessed June 24, 2014.

120. *Accelerating research through the National Health Information Network,* Presented, Washington, DC, January 7, 2005, FasterCures and the Markle Foundation.

121. Frisse M, Marchibroda J, Welebob E: HIE takes shape in the states, *J AHIMA* 76:24–28, 2005, 30.

122. Connecting for Health: http://www.markle.org/health/connecting-health. Accessed November 11, 2014.

123. Qual-IT United Hospital Fund: www.uhfnyc.org. Accessed September 2, 2006.

124. Goldsmith J, Blumenthal D, Rishel W: Federal health information policy: a case of arrested development, *Health Aff* 22:44–55, 2003.

125. eHealth Initiative: What to expect from your HIE: http://www.ehidc.org/resource-center/white-papers-and-briefs/view_document/328-white-paper-what-to-expect-from-your-hie-data-exchange. Accessed June 24, 2014.

126. Project Health Design: http://www.projecthealthdesign.org/. Accessed June 24, 2014.

127. Project Health Design: About: http://www.projecthealthdesign.org/about. Accessed June 24, 2014.

128. Project Health Design: Artifacts: http://www.projecthealthdesign.org/artifacts. Accessed June 24, 2014.

129. Results from the research into the financial value of healthcare information exchange and interoperability HIMSS annual conference, presented February 23, 2004, Orlando, Florida.

130. Center for Information Technology Leadership: Healthcare information exchange and interoperability: www.himss.org. Accessed August 14, 2006.

131. MacDonald K, Metzger J: *Connecting communities: strategies for physician portals and regional data sharing—including results from a recent survey by the College of Healthcare Information Management Executives, 2004.* www.cio-chime.org, Accessed September 2, 2006.

132. Lorenzi NM: Strategies for creating successful local health information infrastructure initiatives, 2003 Contract No. 03EASPE00722: http://aspe.hhs.gov/sp/nhii/LHII-Lorenzi-12.16.03.pdf. Accessed January 2, 2007.

133. Beauchamp N, Eng TR: *Sustaining eHealth in challenging times Summary report at the Third Annual eHealth Developers Summit,* Tempe, AZ, November 6-8, 2002, eHealth Institute.

134. Community Health Information Networks: SunHealth Alliance and First Consulting Group, *Healthc Inf Manage* 2:15–20, 1995.

135. Rybowski L, Rubin R: *Building an infrastructure for community health information: lessons from the frontier,* Seattle, WA, 1998, Foundation for Health Care Quality.

136. Frisse M: State and community-based efforts to foster interoperability, *Health Aff* 24:1190–1196, 2005.

137. McDonald CJ, Overhage JM, Barnes M, et al: The Indiana network for patient care: a working local health information infrastructure. An example of a working infrastructure collaboration that links data from five health systems and hundreds of millions of entries, *Health Aff (Millwood)* 24:1214–1220, 2005.

138. Gottlieb LK, Stone EM, Stone D, et al: Regulatory and policy barriers to effective clinical data exchange: lessons learned from MedsInfo-ED. This pilot project can obtain the medication history for a majority of five million covered patients from only six data sources, *Health Aff (Millwood)* 24:1197–1204, 2005.

139. Agency for Healthcare Research and Quality: *Healthcare informatics standards activities of selected federal agencies (a compendium),* Rockville, MD, 1999, Agency for Healthcare Research and Quality.

140. Agency for Healthcare Research and Quality: *Summary report: current healthcare informatics standards activities of federal agencies,* Rockville, MD, 1999, Agency for Healthcare Research and Quality.

141. Agency for Healthcare Research and Quality: *Patient safety reporting systems and research in HHS: Fact sheet,* Rockville, MD, 2001, Agency for Healthcare Research and Quality.

142. Agency for Healthcare Research and Quality: *Bioterrorism preparedness and response: use of information technologies and decision support systems, Summary, Evidence Report/Technology Assessment,* publication No. Rockville, MD, 2002, Agency for Healthcare Research and Quality.

143. Agency for Healthcare Research and Quality: *Medical informatics for better and safer health care, Summary, Research in Action, 2002:* publication No. 02-0031, Rockville, MD, 2002, Agency for Healthcare Research and Quality. http://www.ahrq.gov/data/informatics/informatria.htm, Accessed August 14, 2006.

144. Agency for Healthcare Research and Quality: *Case study finds computerized ICU information system care can significantly reduce time spent by nurses on documentation,* press release, October 10, Rockville, MD, 2003, Agency for Healthcare Research and Quality.

145. mHealth and FDA Guidance, *Health Affairs,* http://www.healthaffairs.org/healthpolicybriefs/brief.php?brief_id = 104. Accessed June 24, 2014.

146. Middleton B, Bloomrosen M, Dente MA, et al: American Medical Informatics Association. Enhancing Patient Safety and Quality of Care by Improving the Usability of Electronic Health Record System: Recommendations from AMIA 20: e1-e8, 2013.

147. Patterson ES, Zhang J, Abbott P, et al: Enhancing electronic health record usability in pediatric patient care: a scenario-based approach, *Jt Comm J Qual Patient Saf* 39(3):129–135, 2013.

148. Landman AB, Redden L, Neri P, et al: Using a medical simulation center as an electronic health record usability laboratory, *J Am Med Inform Assoc* 21(3):558–563, 2014 Nov 18. http://dx.doi.org/10.1136/amiajnl-2013-002233.

149. Ant Ozok A, Wu H, Garrido M, Pronovost PJ, Gurses AP: *Usability and perceived usefulness of personal health records for preventive health care: a case study focusing on patients' and primary care providers' perspectives,* Appl Ergon, 45(4):1106–1115, 2013.

150. Kushniruk A, Kaipio J, Nieminen M, Nøhr C, Borycki E: Comparing approaches to measuring the adoption and usability of electronic health records: lessons learned from Canada, Denmark and Finland, *Stud Health Technol Inform* 192:367–371, 2013, PubMed PMID: 23920578.

151. Enhancing patient safety and quality of care by improving the usability of electronic health record systems: recommendations from AMIA, *J Am Med Inform Assoc* 20(e1):e2–e8, 2013.

152. Top 10 health technology hazards for 2014, *Health Devices,* https://www.ecri.org/Forms/Documents/2014_Top_10_Hazards_Executive_Brief.pdf. Accessed June 24, 2014.

153. Agency for Healthcare Research and Quality: *Expert panel meeting: health information technology,* Rockville, MD, 2003, Agency for Healthcare Research and Quality.

154. Jeffries J: New e-HIM initiative will reinvent HIM practice, support infrastructure, *J AHIMA* 74:70, 2003.

155. Bloomrosen M: e-HIM: From vision to reality, *J AHIMA* 76:36–41, 2005 [expanded online version].

156. Wing P, Langelier MH: The future of HIM: employer insights into the coming decade of rapid change, *J AHIMA* 75:28–32, 2004.

157. American Health Information Management Association and American Medical Informatics Association: Building the work force for health information transformation: http://www.amia.org/sites/amia.org/files/Workforce_2006.pdf. Accessed November 11, 2014.

158. Yasnoff WA, Humphreys BL, Overhage JM, et al: A consensus action agenda for achieving the national health information infrastructure, *J Am Med Inform Assoc* 11:332–338, 2004.

4 CHAPTER

HEALTH DATA CONCEPTS AND INFORMATION GOVERNANCE

Mary Teslow

ⓔ Student Study Guide activities for this chapter are available on the Evolve Learning Resources site for this textbook. Please visit http://evolve.elsevier.com/Abdelhak/.

CHAPTER CONTENTS

Health Record Flow and Processing
  Medical Transcription
Methods to Ensure Data Quality
  Record Content Review and Retrospective Completion
Data Quality Monitoring Methods and Solutions
  Quality Assessment and Improvement Study of Patient Record
    Documentation
      Quantitative Analysis
      Qualitative Analysis
      Legal Analysis
  Special Concerns of Alternative Care Settings
  Clinical Staff Activities Related to Data Quality
      Medical Record Committee
      Continuing Record Reviews
      Clinical Documentation Improvement
  Organization Structure That Encourages Data Quality
      The Joint Commission Information Management Standards
      Information Resources Management Committee
      Information Governance
  Characteristics of Data Quality
      Definitions
      Accessibility
      Accuracy
      Comprehensiveness
      Consistency
      Currency
      Data Definition
      Granularity
      Precision
      Relevance
      Timeliness
      Data Integrity
Data Needs Across the Health Care Continuum
  Minimum Data Sets
  Acute Care
      Data Needs
      Uniform Hospital Discharge Data Set
      Special Forms and Views
      Issues in Data Collection and Quality
  Ambulatory Care
      Data Needs
      Uniform Ambulatory Care Data Set

  Data Elements for Emergency Department
      Systems
      Special Forms and Views
      Issues in Data Collection and Quality
  Long-Term Care
      Data Needs
      MDS 3.0: Minimum Data Set for Long-Term Care Facility
        Resident Assessment Instrument
      Special Forms and Views
      Issues in Data Collection and Quality
  Long-Term Subacute Care
  Rehabilitation
      Inpatient Rehabilitation Facility
        Patient Assessment Instrument
      Issues in Data Collection and Quality
  Home Health Care
      Data Needs
      Outcome and Assessment Information Set
      Special Forms and Views
      Issues in Data Collection and Quality
  Continuity Assessment Record Evaluation
  Hospice
      Special Forms
      Issues in Data Collection and Quality
  Behavioral Health
      Data Needs
      Special Forms and Views
      Issues in Data Collection and Quality
  Personal Health Record
      Data Needs
      Special Forms and Views
      Issues in Data Collection and Quality
Patient-Centered Care
  Patient-Centered Medical Home
  Patient Portal
Electronic Health Record Initiatives
Summary and Management Issues
Chapter Review
Appendixes (Found on the Evolve site)
Appendix A: Sample Health Record Reports
References

OBJECTIVES

After reading this chapter, the reader will be able to do the following:

✓ Define key words.
✓ Define, compare, and contrast data and information.
✓ Describe the five unique roles of the health record.
✓ Discuss the importance of data in the care of the patient.
✓ Describe the major users of health care data and the importance of addressing the needs of each.
✓ Identify the steps in the management decision-making process, with particular attention to step 2, the collection of data.
✓ Evaluate and apply principles of forms and computer view design.
✓ Define the characteristics of data quality.

✓ Explain the importance of quality data and the mechanisms and controls used to ensure quality.
✓ Identify concerns related to data and the protection of patient confidentiality.
✓ Discuss the importance of consistency and comparability in data collection both within an institution and across the health care delivery system.
✓ Define information governance and its role in enterprise-wide data quality structures.
✓ Describe the concept and importance of a personal identification number.
✓ Identify the major information and data sets, their scope, and special features.
✓ Identify the values and uses of uniform data sets.

✓ Identify the basic forms and format of the paper-based health record.

✓ Compare and contrast the purposes and techniques related to record analysis, including quantitative, qualitative, and legal.

✓ Describe the purposes and techniques related to clinical record reviews.

✓ Compare and contrast the records for ambulatory care, acute care, long-term care and rehabilitation, home care, hospice, and behavioral health care.

✓ Describe the personal health record, its importance, formats, and relationship to the patient's health record.

✓ Describe the role of the health information manager in data collection and in determining the content of the clinical record.

KEY WORDS

Abbreviation list
Abstracting
Advocacy
Aggregate data
Attending physician
Authentication
Barcode
Barcode reader
Chart order
Conditions for coverage
Conditions of participation
Consultation
Continuing record review

Continuity assessment record evaluation
Continuum of care
Data
Database
Data set
Delinquent record
Demographic
Document
Documentation
Electronic data interchange
Encounter
Graphical user interface

Information
Information governance
Legal analysis
Legal health record
Licensed independent practitioner
Longitudinal patient record
Optical character recognition
Patient-centered medical home
Patient health record
Patient portal
Personal health record
Practitioner
Primary patient record

Promulgated
Provider
Public health
Qualitative analysis
Quantitative analysis
Secondary patient record
Stakeholders
Statistical analysis
Third-party payer
Unique identifier
View

ABBREVIATIONS

AAAHC   American Association of Ambulatory Health Care
ADLs   activities of daily living
AHDI   Association for Healthcare Documentation Integrity
AHIMA   American Health Information Management Association
AMA   against medical advice
ARNP   advanced registered nurse practitioners
ASC   ambulatory surgery center
ASTM   American Society for Testing and Materials
CAMH   *Comprehensive Accreditation Manual for Hospitals*
CARE   continuity assessment record evaluation
CARF   Commission on Accreditation of Rehabilitation Facilities
CDC   Centers for Disease Control and Prevention
CDI   clinical documentation improvement
CDS   clinical documentation specialists
CfC   conditions for coverage
CIO   chief information officer
CMS   Centers for Medicare and Medicaid Services
CoP   conditions of participation
CTO   chief technology officer
DEEDS   Data Elements for Emergency Department Systems
DHHS   Department of Health and Human Services
DIKW   Pyramid—data, information, knowledge, wisdom pyramid
DQM   data quality management
ECG   electrocardiogram
ED   emergency department
EDI   electronic data interchange
EHR   electronic health record
EMPI   enterprise master patient (person) index
GUI   graphical user interface
H&P   history and physical
HCO   health care organization
HEDIS   Healthcare Effectiveness Data and Information Set
HIE   health information exchange

HIM   health information management
HIMSS   Healthcare Information and Management Systems Society
HIPAA   Health Insurance Portability and Accountability Act
ICD   *International Classification of Diseases*
IG   information governance
IGRM   Information Governance Reference Model
IOM   Institute of Medicine
IRF-PAI   Inpatient Rehabilitation Facility Patient Assessment Instrument
LHR   legal health record
LIP   licensed independent practitioner
LTSC   long-term subacute care
MAR   medication administration record
MCO   managed-care organization
MDS   minimum data set
MPI   master patient (person) index
NCHS   National Center for Health Statistics
NCIPC   National Center for Injury Prevention and Control
NCR   no carbon required
NCQA   National Committee on Quality Assurance
NCVHS   National Committee on Vital and Health Statistics
NEDSS   National Electronic Disease Surveillance System
NMDS   Nursing Minimum Data Set
NMMDS   Nursing Management Minimum Data Set
NwHIN   Nationwide Health Information Network
OASIS   Outcome and Assessment Information Set
OCR   optical character recognition
PACS   picture archiving and communication system
PHI   personally identifiable health information
PHR   personal health record
POA   present on admission
POMR   problem-oriented medical record
QI   quality improvement

RHIO   regional health information organization
ROS   review of systems
SOAP   Subjective, Objective, Assessment, Plan
SSN   Social Security numbers

TJC   The Joint Commission
UACDS   Uniform Ambulatory Care Data Set
UHDDS   Uniform Hospital Discharge Data Set
UPIN   unique physician identification number

The United States health care delivery system continues to evolve in both size and complexity and is projected to reach almost 20% of the gross domestic product by 2020. The system is an elaborate and dynamic mosaic composed of consumers with diverse needs and an increasing array of providers in multiple types of facilities and locations, as well as an intricate management system monitored by payers, regulators, and accrediting bodies. Working together, their goal is to provide consumers with high-quality care that is accessible and cost-effective.

The patient record is the information centerpiece of the health care decision-making process, both for individual patient treatment and for its potential to collect or aggregate data (which does not identify any specific patients) for research and other purposes. In either electronic or paper form, it contains the essential data and information to answer the key questions related to the who, what, when, where, why, and how of patient care (Box 4-1).

HEALTH DATA USERS AND USES

Users and Uses of Health Data

Many users—both individuals and groups—rely on health data and demand quality in the data collected, analyzed, interpreted, and reported, including those described in this section. Figure 4-1 illustrates this environment and the numerous external forces that influence the patient's care and its documentation.

Patients

Patients use their health data to understand their health care and to become more active partners in maintaining or improving their health. Data can also be used in monitoring care when additional treatment is necessary. For example,

patients with diabetes or hypertension can make a difference by actively participating in controlling and monitoring their condition. Data are also used by patients to document the services received, to serve as proof of identity or disability, and to verify billed services. The American Health Information Management Association (AHIMA) has taken an advocacy position in promoting understanding of the personal health record (PHR) through its consumer education programs and a related website (http://www.myphr.com). The PHR is described later in this chapter.

Health Care Practitioners

Physicians, nurses, and other clinicians who are treating the patient use the record as a primary means of communication among themselves. Practitioners at the follow-up facility or agency to which the patient is transferred after discharge rely on the data for continuing care. In a residential facility, nursing staff review and evaluate the data to develop care plans outlining important nursing interventions. Health care practitioners in every setting use the clinical record as a resource.

Health Care Providers and Administrators

The term health care provider is broad based. It includes organizations that deliver health care services, such as hospitals, outpatient clinics, long-term care facilities, home care agencies, and hospices. Providers also can be individual practitioners or part of a multiprovider practice. The health record collects the data that document the provision of services. Providers use these data to evaluate care, monitor the use of resources, and receive payment for services rendered. Administrators analyze financial and patient case mix information for business planning, risk management, and marketing activities. Information is increasingly being viewed as an enterprise business asset, which has led to the development of information governance (IG) initiatives discussed later in this chapter.

Third-Party Payers

Data are the basis of claims processing to pay for the health care services provided. Third-party payers include private insurance companies, managed-care organizations (MCOs), and fiscal intermediaries who process claims for Medicare and Medicaid. Because the purpose of health data is to document the steps taken to prevent illness and promote wellness and the course of illness and treatment, the data become the basis for determining the appropriate payment to be made. Although capitated care may change the current billing systems, payers still want to know the services provided for the dollars spent. Even if transaction-based bills as we know them today disappear, data will be needed to document services provided. Billing data are currently the basis for reporting and managing costs of care. Payers for

BOX 4-1	Essential Health Data and Information Questions

Who?
Who are the patient, the provider, and the payer?
What?
What services were provided and at what cost?
When?
When were the services provided?
Where?
Where were the services provided?
Why?
Why were the services provided, or what was the justification for the services?
How?
How effective were the services, or what was the outcome?

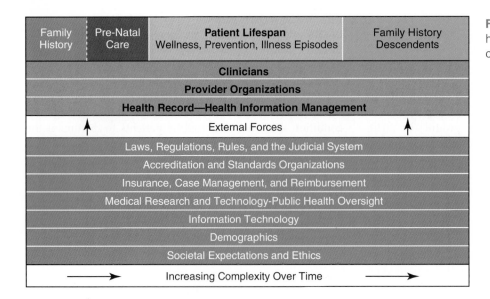

Family History	Pre-Natal Care	Patient Lifespan Wellness, Prevention, Illness Episodes	Family History Descendents
		Clinicians	
		Provider Organizations	
		Health Record—Health Information Management	
↑		External Forces	↑
		Laws, Regulations, Rules, and the Judicial System	
		Accreditation and Standards Organizations	
		Insurance, Case Management, and Reimbursement	
		Medical Research and Technology-Public Health Oversight	
		Information Technology	
		Demographics	
		Societal Expectations and Ethics	
→		Increasing Complexity Over Time	→

FIGURE 4-1 The influence of the health care environment on patient care and its documentation.

government insurance plans (i.e., Medicare and Medicaid) also actively monitor the appropriateness of the care and services given to a patient.

Utilization and Case Managers

Health care data include descriptions of care given and the justification for services. All organizational resources, including supplies, equipment, services, and providers, can be taken into consideration in a utilization review. Case management seeks to coordinate care so that the patient is cared for in the most clinically cost-effective manner. The emphasis is on disease management, especially for patients with chronic problems such as diabetes, hypertension, and asthma. Criteria are available for some facets of the case management process, such as admission, continued stay, and discharge from an inpatient facility and day-to-day management of specific chronic problems.

Quality of Care Committees

It is essential that the delivery of health care be monitored continuously—both concurrently and retrospectively. The basis for these reviews and the performance of quality assessment is the data recorded at the time care is given. Quality assessment and improvement committees use the information as a basis for analysis, study, and evaluation of the quality of care given to the patient. Studies by the Institute of Medicine (IOM) beginning in 1999 have dramatically increased the focus on patient safety and the use of data to improve care. The National Physician Data Bank uses secondary health care data to ensure that only qualified physicians practice medicine.

Accrediting, Licensing, and Certifying Agencies

Accrediting, licensing, and certifying agencies review patient records to provide public assurance that quality health care is being provided. The documented care and related data serve as evidence in assessing compliance with standards of care and in accrediting and licensing various health care organizations (HCOs).

Governmental Agencies and Public Health

Governmental agencies at the local, state, and federal levels use health care data to determine the appropriate use of governmental financial resources for health care facilities and educational and correctional institutions. Reviews are done on a continuing and retrospective basis. **Public health** is concerned with threats to the overall health of a community on the basis of population-based health data analysis in contrast to medical health care, which focuses on the treatment of the individual. Governments at all levels establish public health departments and programs that include surveillance and control of infectious disease, prevention such as vaccination programs, and promotion of healthy behaviors. At the national level, the Centers for Disease Control and Prevention (CDC) leads and coordinates these efforts.

Health Information Exchanges

Health information exchanges (HIEs), also called *regional health information organizations* (RHIOs), are collaborations to move clinical data across various health information systems within a geographic area. A variety of models are emerging, with a number of projects being developed at the state level. The goal of the partner organizations is to provide patient-centered care that improves quality, safety, efficiency, timeliness, and accessibility. HIEs and RHIOs use common, nonproprietary standards for content and exchange and are the building blocks of the U.S. Nationwide Health Information Network (NwHIN).

Employers

Health care data are used to evaluate and assess job-related conditions and injuries and to determine occupational hazards that may impede effective performance in the workplace. Workers' compensation is one state-based example. Employers also use the data to determine the extent of employee disabilities, to improve working conditions, and to manage employee benefit programs. The cost of health care benefits to both employers and employees has continued to rise. Health data are used to select health insurance companies, evaluate quality, and manage costs. Increasingly employers are offering incentives to employees to improve their health.

Attorneys and the Courts in the Judicial Process

Attorneys and the courts use the records as documentary evidence of a patient's course of treatment to protect the legal interests of the patient, health care providers, treating facility, and the public. Health care data are often the basis of evidence for the adjudication of both civil and criminal cases. The documentation may support the claims made by the individuals in a case, and it is often the only evidence available. In addition, data may aid in determining the need for admission of the mentally ill for treatment.

Planners and Policy Developers

State health departments use information related to vital statistics, disease incidence and prevalence, reports of child and elder abuse, and so on to provide aggregate data for public policy development and for intervention in individual situations as needed. The CDC coordinates these data nationally. Data are the basis for supporting the continuing need for services and the addition of new services by an HCO. Health care delivery is a dynamic process that requires the evaluation of current needs and future demands for the individual provider and the community in general.

Educators and Trainers

Within the health care setting, many individuals are learning the skills of quality health care service delivery. Data documentation assists these people in connecting the theory learned in the classroom to the practical aspects of care. Conferences and presentations about care already delivered are useful in training health care personnel. Data from the patient record are the basis for many continuing education programs and conferences that review treatment outcomes.

Researchers and Epidemiologists

Clinical research is a significant aspect of the improvement of care and assessment of the effectiveness of treatment and improved methods for future care. Researchers may also study the cost-effectiveness of patient care, review patient outcomes, and assess the use of technology. Epidemiologists help with early disease detection such as an outbreak of *Escherichia coli* infections. Health services research and policy studies provide information regarding the health care system.

Media Reporters

Radio, television, print, and web-based journalists report data that the public needs to know, such as health hazards, diseases that affect public health, and new developments in medical research. HCOs have been slow to engage social media mostly because of legal concerns. Early efforts have been limited to broadcast announcements of educational events and other community health news.

Decision Making

Used in every setting in which care is provided, the data in the patient record are the essential resource for clinical and administrative decisions. These data are often arranged and displayed to meet the various needs of diverse users.

Knowledge Hierarchy

Data are gathered consistent with the characteristics of data quality, arranged and displayed to add context and create useful information, given meaning leading to knowledge, and acted on with insight to make wise decisions. This progression is referred to as the *Knowledge Hierarchy* or the data, information, knowledge, wisdom (DIKW) pyramid, and is attributed to Ackoff.[1] Figure 4-2 includes the value added at each step and an example illustrating the use of birth certificate data, including weight, to reduce the number of

Step	Description	Value Added	Example: Low-Birth-Weight Babies
Wisdom	Knowledge + Insight + Action	Actionable intelligence: establish and reach measurable goals; wiser decisions	Public health programs and services established or revised, education campaigns
Knowledge	Information + Meaning	Connections: comparison, consequences, conversations	Comparisons to prenatal care, socioeconomic status, trends, benchmarking, etc.
Information	Data + Context	Interpretation: contextualized, categorized, calculated, condensed	Data analyzed and reported, e.g., mothers' age, race, residence
Data	Foundation for information	Observation: discrete, objective facts, figures, etc.	Individual birth certificates filed, including birth weight

FIGURE 4-2 Data, information, knowledge, wisdom pyramid and value added.

low-birth-weight babies. Definitions of the levels vary with more agreement at the levels of data and information.

Definitions

Data are a collection of elements on a given subject; the raw facts and figures expressed in text, numbers, symbols, and various media; and facts, ideas, or concepts that can be captured, communicated, and processed either manually or electronically. Elements are consistent with the characteristics of data quality. The subsequent levels depend on this foundation. The word *data* is plural and is used whenever more than one data element is described. *Datum* appropriately describes a single data element.

Information is data that have been processed into meaningful form—either manually or by computer—to make them valuable to the user. Data and information are not synonymous. Information adds context to a representation and tells the recipient something that was not known before. For example, graphing blood sugar levels over time reveals a trend not apparent from individual values. What is information for one person may not be information for another.

Knowledge is information that is further enhanced with meaning. Information is more clearly understood, such that it explains the how and the why about something. Knowledge bases are increasingly available as resources for both clinicians and administrative staff as part of information systems and electronic health records (EHRs).

Wisdom places knowledge in a framework to allow it to be applied in different situations in a measurable way to make wiser decisions and to establish and reach goals.

Decision-Making Process

Effective decision making proceeds through the following steps:
1. Problem identification
2. Data collection and analysis
3. Development of alternatives
4. Selection of the best alternative
5. Action
6. Follow-up and evaluation

Data collection is not an isolated function. It has a significant effect on both the efficiency and the effectiveness of the decision-making process. Well-defined and accurately collected data enhance the likelihood of an effective decision—but do not guarantee it.

Overseeing the use of patient data in planning, management, and research has long been the purview of health information managers. To be efficient, health information management (HIM) professionals must carefully consider the purposes for data collection and gather sufficient data items, but no more than required. Significant costs are associated with data collection, including staff time for entry, review, and management, and computer time and storage. Cost-effectiveness requires resistance to the "more-is-better" philosophy. The reason to collect data is to satisfy an identified need for the retention, retrieval, and use of data and to generate meaningful information and knowledge. After the essential data items are identified, it is generally agreed that

data should be captured only once and used by all portions of the system that require access to that particular data item. Health care documentation is often done in narrative form, which requires extraction of key pieces of data. Advances in EHRs permit the combination of discrete data fields with narrative content to add context. As we standardize health data and encourage use of discrete data, and as systems become more astute at automating the data extraction process, clinical data will be even more available.

The wide variety of uses for the data in the patient record provide the HIM manager with the challenge of collecting the necessary data to support and promote the efficiency and effectiveness on behalf of the patient, the provider, and the facility, as well as public health. Each of these constituencies benefits from the reliability and validity promoted by consistent definitions of data elements. Such definitions aid in facilitating data exchange and reducing misunderstandings. Standards are the foundation of a consistent data collection plan that supports the needs of individuals, organizations, and the health care delivery system at large.

✓ SELF-ASSESSMENT QUIZ

1. Which users require patient-identifiable data, and which do not?
2. Why are data standards key to meeting the needs of multiple stakeholders?
3. Are *data* and *information* synonyms? If not, why not?

OVERVIEW OF THE PATIENT RECORD

The Unique Roles of the Patient Health Record

A patient's health record plays five unique roles[2]:
1. It represents that patient's health history; that is, it is a record of the patient's health status and the health services provided over time.
2. It provides a method for clinical communication and care planning among the individual health care practitioners serving the patient.
3. It serves as the legal document describing the health care services provided.
4. It is a source of data for clinical, health services, and outcomes research.
5. It serves as a major resource for health care practitioner education.

Patient Health Record

The patient health record collects the data and information and generates reports—either on paper or electronically—on a single patient. It is the primary legal record documenting the health care services provided to a person in any aspect of the health care system. The term includes routine clinical records of care in any health-related setting, preventive care, lifestyle evaluation, research protocols, and various clinical databases. This repository of information is generated by health care practitioners as a direct result of interaction with the patient or with individuals who have personal knowledge of the patient (or with both). The record contains information about the patient and other individuals as they relate to the health of the patient. The term *patient health record* is generally synonymous with *medical record, health record, patient care record, primary patient record, client record,* and *resident record*. It should be noted that *health record* is a more comprehensive term that includes prevention and screening data whereas *medical record* more typically refers to encounters related to illness.

Primary Patient Record

The primary patient record is the record used by health care practitioners while providing patient care services to review patient data or document their own observations, actions, or instructions.

Secondary Patient Record

The secondary patient record is a subset derived from the primary record and contains selected data elements. Such secondary records or databases aid both clinicians and non-clinical individuals (that is, those not involved in direct patient care) in supporting, evaluating, and advancing patient care. *Patient care support* refers to administration, regulation, and payment functions. *Patient care evaluation* refers to quality assurance, utilization review, and medical or legal audits. *Patient care advancement* refers to research.

Legal Health Record

As mentioned earlier, the health record is the primary business record created by and for an HCO. As content and media have become more complex, the boundaries of the health record have become less clear and the concept of the legal health record (LHR) has emerged. To address these evolving issues, the AHIMA appointed a task force, subsequently publishing and updating a "Practice Brief on the Legal Health Record."[3] The resulting guidance is that the LHR is the portion of the record that will be disclosed, with appropriate authorization, to parties outside the organization. It is the responsibility of each organization to define its LHR.

Longitudinal Patient Record

The longitudinal patient record is a comprehensive patient record compiled and accessible over the individual's life span from birth to death. It is a valuable resource for clinical decision making that provides easy access to medical history, contains costs by reducing repeated diagnostic testing and treatments, and promotes patient safety through medical alerts and information on allergies, drug reactions, and drug-drug or drug-food interactions.

Paper-based records have been unable to achieve the advantages of longitudinal records because of their lack of standardization, difficulty in organizing, and limited access. One of the substantial advantages of moving to an EHR, or linkage of records, is the opportunity to create longitudinal patient records. The Veterans Administration has led the way in creating longitudinal electronic patient records to serve its patient population.

 DID YOU KNOW?

Benjamin Franklin began the first health records at Pennsylvania Hospital in 1752. He served as secretary and recorded the patient's name, address, disorder, and dates of admission and discharge. His ledgers can still be seen today.

DATA COLLECTION STANDARDS

The patient health record is currently a combination of discrete data elements and narrative in mixed media, including paper, electronic, voice, images, and waveforms. A variety of organizations and agencies in the public and private sectors are engaged in extensive efforts to standardize the record, including the development of data content and collection standards.

Governmental

Efforts to standardize health care data have existed since early efforts to record mortality and then morbidity data. Beginning in the 1990s, striking changes occurred in health and health care and in health data and information systems. Both the national environment for health information systems and the nature of the information systems have changed dramatically. The new electronic information environment is raising new privacy and security issues and magnifying the importance of ensuring that current policies are appropriate for new technologies.

One must keep in mind that although various agencies, committees, organizations, and individuals are working to develop new standards, others are currently collecting data at an accelerating rate. Multiple governmental, professional, and private groups are working toward a consensus on standards for both record content and electronic data transfer. It behooves all stakeholders to be aware of the goals, mandates, and activities of the others and to maintain effective communication within the health information community. The AHIMA works diligently representing its membership in these areas.

 DID YOU KNOW?

All of the government agencies are part of the Executive Branch of the federal government. They have quasilegislative and quasijudicial authority in their area of responsibility.

Department of Health and Human Services

Collection, analysis, and dissemination of health-related information are crucial aspects of the responsibilities of the Department of Health and Human Services (DHHS; http://www.hhs.gov). The DHHS also plays a national

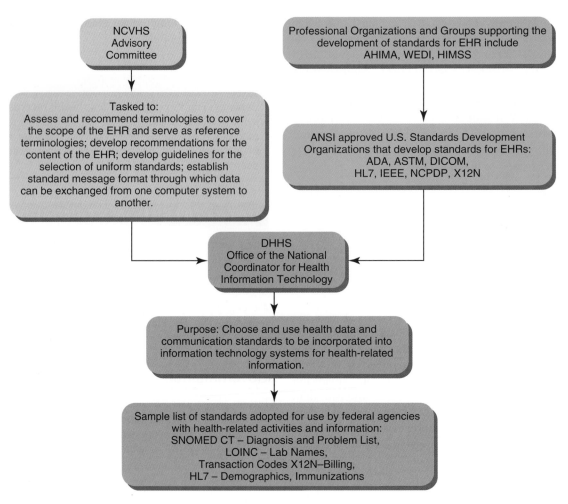

FIGURE 4-3 Federal and private sector activities that support the development and use of standards for electronic health record (EHR) systems. *ADA,* Americans with Disabilities Act; *AHIMA,* American Health Information Management Association; *ANSI,* American National Standards Institute; *ASTM,* American Society for Testing and Materials; *DHHS,* Department of Health and Human Services; *DICOM,* Digital Imaging and Communications in Medicine; *HIMSS,* Healthcare Information and Management Systems Society; *HL7,* Health Level 7; *IEEE,* Institute of Electrical and Electronics Engineers; *LOINC,* Logical Observation Identifier Name and Code; *NCPDP,* National Council of Prescription Drug Programs; *NCVHS,* National Committee on Vital and Health Statistics; *SNOMED-CT,* Systemized Nomenclature of Medicine—Clinical Terms; *WEDI,* Workgroup for Electronic Data Interchange; *X12N,* Data Interchange Standards Association ASC X12 Insurance Subcommittee.

leadership role in health data standards and health information privacy policy and is charged with the responsibility for implementation of the administrative simplification provisions of the Health Insurance Portability and Accountability Act of 1996 (HIPAA). In addition, the DHHS engages in cooperative efforts with standards organizations, professional organizations, state and local governments, other countries, and the international community to foster health data standards, comparability, and cross-national research. Figure 4-3 illustrates the scope of the federal government's involvement in health data standard activities.

Centers for Medicare and Medicaid Services
The Centers for Medicare and Medicaid Services (CMS) is the DHHS division responsible for developing and enforcing

regulations, including the conditions of participation (CoPs) and conditions for coverage (CfCs) that HCO s must meet to begin and continue participating in the Medicare and Medicaid programs (http://www.cms.gov). These minimum health and safety standards are the foundation for improving quality and protecting the health and safety of beneficiaries. CMS also ensures that the standards of accrediting organizations recognized by CMS (through a process called *deeming*) meet or exceed the Medicare standards set forth in the CoPs and CfCs.

❓ DID YOU KNOW?

The CoPs are published in the *Federal Register* and can be found online at https://www.federalregister.gov/

Health and Human Services Data Council

The DHHS Data Council coordinates all health and non-health data collection and analysis activities of the department, including an integrated health data collection strategy, coordination of health data standards, and health information and privacy policy issues, including the administrative simplification provisions of HIPAA (http://aspe.hhs.gov/datacncl).

National Committee on Vital and Health Statistics

The National Committee on Vital and Health Statistics (NCVHS) is the statutory public advisory body to the DHHS on health data, statistics, and national health information policy. This committee serves as a national forum for the collaboration of interested parties to accelerate the evolution of public and private health information systems toward more uniform, shared data standards within a framework protecting privacy and security. The NCVHS encourages the evolution of a shared, public-private national health information infrastructure that will promote the availability of valid, credible, timely, and comparable health data. With sensitivity to policy considerations and priorities, the NCVHS provides scientific and technical advice and guidance regarding the design and operation of health statistics and information systems and services and coordination of health data requirements. It also assists and advises the DHHS on HIPAA implementation and informs decision making about data policy by DHHS, states, local governments, and the private sector (http://www.ncvhs.hhs.gov).

National Center for Health Statistics

To clarify the names and acronyms, mention is made here of the National Center for Health Statistics (NCHS), which may easily be confused with the NCVHS. The NCHS is a part of the CDC of the DHHS, and it is the federal government's principal vital and health statistics agency. The NCHS provides a wide variety of data with which to monitor the nation's health. Although the data provided by the NCHS are used by policy makers in Congress and the administration, medical researchers, and others in the health community, the NCHS should not be mistaken for the NCVHS, which is a public policy advisory board (http://www.cdc.gov/nchs).

Overview of Information and Data Sets

The NCVHS has been the leading government agency in the area of standardization of health information, primarily through uniform data sets, since its initial charter in the 1950s. It addresses the need for uniform, comparable standards across geographic areas, populations, systems, institutions, and sites of care to maximize the effectiveness of health promotion and care and minimize the burden on those responsible for generating the data. To this end, the NCVHS has advised the DHHS on such matters as federal-state relationships, nomenclatures and classification systems, core data sets, and access and confidentiality issues.

TABLE 4-1 Federal Information and Data Sets

Acronym	Name	Purpose
CARE	Continuity Assessment Record Evaluation	An item set to standardize assessment of patients' medical, functional, cognitive, and social support status across acute and postacute settings
DEEDS	Data Elements for Emergency Department Systems	Uniform specifications for data entered into hospital emergency department records
MDS	Minimum Data Set for Long-Term Care	Comprehensive functional assessment of long-term care patients
OASIS	Outcome and Assessment Information Set	Core items of comprehensive assessment for adult home care patients; forms basis for measuring patient outcomes
UACDS	Uniform Ambulatory Care Data Set	Improve ability to compare data in ambulatory care settings
UHDDS	Uniform Hospital Discharge Data Set	Uniform collection of data on inpatients; used by federal and state agencies

The data sets promulgated by the NCVHS have become de facto standards in their areas for data collection by federal and state agencies and by public and private data-abstracting organizations. They have influenced both the CoPs and the claim forms on which Medicare and Medicaid data sets are based. Table 4-1 lists the existing federal data sets, which are discussed in detail later in this chapter. These data sets are intended to describe significant minimal data about patients, residents, or clients. It is important to remember, however, that, although these data are essential to the patient record and patient care, additional data are necessary for a comprehensive record that supports the delivery of that care.

Core Health Data Elements

The achievements of the NCVHS regarding minimum data sets (MDSs) have been significant. However, the ever-expanding sites of care, combined with the increasing use of electronic data, have made it imperative that all health data collection activities, when possible, use standardized data elements and definitions. Standardized data elements are also vitally important in the managed care field, in which there is a need to follow individuals through a continuum of care and at multiple sites. Performance monitoring and outcomes research are two additional areas that are currently hampered by the inability to link data sets from various sources because of varying data elements and definitions.

In 1996 the NCVHS completed a 2-year project to review the current state of health-related core data sets and to promote consensus by identifying areas of agreement on core health data elements and definitions. The goal has been to develop a set of data elements with agreed-on standardized definitions, not to specify a data set for mandated external reporting. The list of recommended data elements is by no means exhaustive and, unlike the result of earlier activities, is not a "data set" to be used in a specific setting.[4]

The 42 data elements are listed in Table 4-2. Consensus has been reached on definitions for the majority of these elements; for others, definitions must still be finalized; for a third group, additional study and testing are necessary. For the first 12 elements, with the exception of a unique identifier, information may not have to be collected at each encounter. Standard electronic formats are recommended to the extent that they have been developed. A column has been added to provide comparison with the American Society for Testing and Materials (ASTM) International Standard E1384-07, which is described in more detail in Chapter 6.

Centers for Disease Control and Prevention

The implementation of data sets and the core data elements have provided additional opportunities for research, reporting, and prevention. The CDC has developed the National Electronic Disease Surveillance System (NEDSS). NEDSS promotes the use of content and exchange standards to advance the development of efficient, integrated, and interoperable public health surveillance systems at the federal, state, and local levels. NEDSS-compatible systems can be used by state health departments for the surveillance and analysis of notifiable diseases. As with other data collection activities, it is important to balance the burden of collection and analysis with the value of the resulting information. Surveillance should provide the minimum necessary data fields to understand the current disease situation. NEDSS strives to meet this goal by streamlining case reporting for providers and their staff by standardizing forms, content, and so on. Improved data quality and consistency will decrease the burden on data analysts. This web-based strategy is intended to monitor and assess disease trends, guide prevention and intervention programs, inform public health policy and policy makers, identify issues necessary to public health research, provide information for community and program planning, and protect confidentiality while providing information to those who need to know. NEDSS is a major component of the Public Health Information Network, which is facilitated by the CDC (http://www.cdc.gov).

Nongovernmental

Accrediting Organizations

A wide variety of accrediting organizations set voluntary standards regarding health record data. Although it is

TABLE 4-2   Comparison of Core Health Data Elements

NCVHS*	ASTM E1384-07[†]
Personal/enrollment data	X
Personal/unique identifier (b)	X
Date of birth	X
Sex	X
Race and ethnicity	X
Residence	X
Marital status	X
Living/residential arrangement (a)	X
Self-reported health status (b)	X
Functional status (b)	X
Years of schooling	X
Patient's relationship to subscriber/person eligible for entitlement	X
Current or most recent occupation and industry (b)	X
Encounter Data	
1. Type of encounter (b)	X
2. Admission date (inpatient)	X
3. Discharge date (inpatient)	X
4. Date of encounter (outpatient and physician services)	X
5. Facility identification (a)	X
6. Type of facility/place of encounter (a)	X
7. Health care practitioner identification (outpatient) (a)	X
8. Provider location or address of encounter (outpatient)	X
9. Attending physician identification (inpatient) (a)	X
10. Operating clinician identification (a)	X
11. Health care practitioner specialty (a)	X
12. Principal diagnosis (inpatient)	Problem
13. Primary diagnosis (inpatient)	Problem
14. Other diagnoses (inpatient)	Problem
15. Qualifier for other diagnoses (inpatient)	Problem
16. Patient's stated reason for visit or chief complaint (outpatient) (a)	Problem
17. Diagnosis chiefly responsible for services provided (outpatient)	Problem
18. Other diagnoses (outpatient)	Problem
19. External cause of injury	Problem
20. Birth weight of neonate	X
21. Principal procedure (inpatient)	X
22. Other procedures (inpatient)	X
23. Dates of procedures (inpatient)	X
24. Procedures and services (outpatient)	
25. Medications prescribed	
26. Disposition of patient (inpatient) (a)	
27. Disposition (outpatient)	X

TABLE 4-2	Comparison of Core Health Data Elements—cont'd	
NCVHS		**ASTM E1384-07**
28. Patient's expected sources of payment (a)		X
29. Injury related to employment		X
30. Total billed charges (a)		X

*National Committee on Vital and Health Statistics (NCVHS) footnotes: as of August 1996. (a) Element for which substantial agreement has been reached but for which some amount of additional work is needed; (b) element which has been recognized as significant but for which considerable work remains to be undertaken. A lack of footnote indicates that these elements are ready for implementation.

†ASTM E1384-07 is described in more detail in Chapter 6.

voluntary, organizations choose to be accredited for several reasons. Accreditation may reduce reviews by the state and federal government (called *deeming*) and may facilitate payment for services and assure consumers and payers that a high quality of care is provided.

The Joint Commission

The Joint Commission (TJC) is by far the oldest and best known organizational accrediting body. It has developed accreditation standards across many settings in the health care continuum. Standards for each of the settings address information management and the record of care and treatment. Specifics are covered later in this chapter (http://www.jointcommission.org).

 DID YOU KNOW?

TJC began in 1953 as The Joint Commission on Accreditation of Hospitals. The name has evolved as accreditation has expanded to more types of HCOs. It is not a government agency.

National Committee on Quality Assurance

The National Committee on Quality Assurance (NCQA) is the source for information about the quality of the nation's managed care plans, which is used by consumers and employers in making health care choices. NCQA uses the Healthcare Effectiveness Data and Information Set (HEDIS) to measure performance (http://www.ncqa.org).

Other Accrediting Bodies

Various other specialty accrediting bodies exist, such as the American Osteopathic Association, the Commission on Accreditation of Rehabilitation Facilities (CARF), and the American Association of Ambulatory Health Care (AAAHC).

Standards-Setting Bodies

ASTM International

ASTM International is one of the largest voluntary standards development organizations in the world. It is a trusted source for technical standards related to the EHR, including information infrastructure and security, amendments to and use of signatures in documents, and code sets (http://www.astm.org).

Professional Organizations

The quality of health care data relies on the excellence of data collection at the time of service, the information system model design and implementation, data monitoring and evaluation, and the services provided by or under the direction of the HIM professional. In addition to continuing assessment of the quality of health data, continuous monitoring and evaluation of the quality of HIM services (based on practice standards) must be essential activities in all HCOs or non-HCOs that have these services.

Professional organizations take leadership positions and are advocates for best practices in their segment of the industry. They promote education and lifelong learning by providing resources, including publications, seminars, and online learning, as well as opportunities for certification. Membership in professional organizations provides access to resources and colleagues who support maintaining a high level of professional competence and ethical practice. Four important examples follow.

American Health Information Management Association

AHIMA is dedicated to the effective management of personal health information necessary to deliver quality health care to the public (http://www.ahima.org). Of particular importance are professional practice guidelines called *Practice Briefs*. They present best practices and are excellent for personal continuing education and evaluation of present organizational practices. The Engage online communities provide an opportunity to network with other AHIMA members. These communities provide valuable resources for specialty areas of practice.

DID YOU KNOW?

AHIMA was started in 1928 at the request of the American College of Surgeons to provide quality medical records for their Board Certification program. At the time it was called the *Association of Record Librarians of North America.*

Healthcare Information and Management Systems Society

Healthcare Information and Management Systems Society focuses on the optimal use of health care information technology and management systems for the betterment of human health (http://www.himss.org).

American Medical Informatics Association

The American Medical Informatics Association provides leadership in the development and implementation of information systems to improve patient care (http://www.amia.org).

Association for Healthcare Documentation Integrity

The Association for Healthcare Documentation Integrity (AHDI) is committed to the creation of quality health record reports from dictation produced by medical language specialists as well as the evolution of the medical transcription industry (http://www.ahdionline.org).

Researchers and Other Groups

A variety of informatics researchers and specialty groups are developing and testing data sets. An example is the work done at the University of Iowa on a Nursing Management Minimum Data Set (NMMDS), which is a research-based management data set that includes 17 across-settings elements. NMMDS is designed to meet the nurse executive's need for a specific nursing management data capture system that will produce accurate, reliable, and useful data for decision making. Additional projects explore the usefulness of large data repositories with three MDSs, including NMMDS, the Nursing Minimum Data Set (NMDS), and the Uniform Hospital Discharge Data Set (UHDDS), as well as the American Nurses Association Quality Indicators that support effectiveness research. It is reasonable to anticipate significant growth in this research.

 SELF-ASSESSMENT QUIZ

4. Identify three governmental and three nongovernmental bodies related to health care data.
5. What is the role of professional organizations in setting and supporting data standards?
6. Reflect back on the value of membership in your professional organization.

BASIC PRINCIPLES OF DATA COLLECTION

Documentation Responsibilities

Documentation in the health record refers to clinical information in various formats communicated among health care providers. It also serves as the official business record and supports compliance, reimbursement, and other functions. It is the responsibility of each HCO to identify who may provide care and then document that care in the patient record. The foundation for these decisions is state licensure laws, which specify the legal scope of practice for health care providers. State laws vary, and current laws must be consulted. For example, Washington State allows advanced registered nurse practitioners (ARNPs) to practice independently and prescribe medications. ARNPs are required to have a

physician resource identified in case they need assistance or consultation. Other clinicians, such as certified nurse mid-wives and physician assistants, have varying levels of independent practice, which may require supervision and a countersignature on documentation. Additional consideration should be given to reimbursement issues, including Medicare and Medicaid.

The organization's decisions are specified in policies and procedures and, if there is an organized medical staff, in the medical staff bylaws, rules, and regulations. TJC defines a licensed independent practitioner (LIP) as "any individual permitted by law and by the organization to provide care, treatment, and services without direction or supervision." The senior physician primarily responsible for the care and treatment of the patient, particularly during an acute care hospital admission is referred to as the attending physician. The process of credentialing, including the scope of privileges, is discussed in more detail in later chapters.

 DID YOU KNOW?

There are many medical specialties and subspecialties. You can find a list at The American Board of Medical Specialties at https://www.abms.org/who_we_help/physicians/specialties.aspx.

User Needs

Understanding standards, rules, and regulations is a solid foundation for developing a quality health record. However, before one can be confident that a fully functioning record has been designed, it is essential to consider the specialized needs of all the users of the record, including the organization as an entity and all internal and external users. Discussion takes place in committees, including those described in the TJC standards, and in other groups within the facility, as well as with department heads, and may include special interests from research to marketing. TJC requires that the organization define the components of a complete medical record. In addition, when both paper-based and electronic components are used, the content must be the same. Clinical record content is also described in federal regulations and in state laws and regulations.[5] Understanding the flow of data and information throughout the HCO and larger health system ensures that computer views (or screens) and paper forms are designed to facilitate the collection of data elements as care is provided. Training and practice in the design of computer views and paper forms and computer-based data capture techniques make the HIM professional a valuable management resource.

General Documentation Forms and Views

Although there are various data collection standards, accrediting and regulatory bodies and professional organizations do not require or recommend particular forms or views for documenting patient care. Although organizations are responsible for creating their own tools, it is not necessary to start from scratch. Books, journals, newsletters, and vendor catalogs offer examples. Local professional organizations and networking with colleagues can also lead to valuable suggestions on what has worked well and what has not.

To provide a starting point, forms commonly included in the paper health record are listed in Table 4-3 and described in the next section. (See Appendix A: Sample Health Record Reports on Evolve.) Any differences in application are discussed under the appropriate care setting. Acute care hospitals tend to be the most complex care setting and have the widest variety of forms. Views meet the same needs but through their smaller, more flexible logical structure. A more complete understanding of the role of each form or view will develop through the balance of this chapter, related topics in other chapters, and continuing professional education and experience.

Patient Identification

All forms and views must identify the patient, including all sides and segments of multipart paper forms and all screens of computer views. In most settings, a unique identifier number is assigned to link the patient to his or her record. This number is used to collect all patient data in the correct record or to be accessed by computer database query. The patient name and number are contained in a database called the master patient (person) index (MPI). It is the most essential tool for any health information department that numbers its records because it is the link between the patient's name and number. As more providers merge into health systems, MPIs are increasingly merged into an enterprise MPI (EMPI). The MPI/EMPI as it relates to access and retention of the clinical record and as one of the building blocks in an EHR system is discussed further in Chapter 7.

Administrative Forms

As the U.S. population becomes more diverse, consideration needs to be given to having some health record forms translated into the languages most common in the community. Administrative forms are most likely to require alternate versions.

Registration Record

Basic demographic, or patient identification data, and financial data are routinely collected for every patient in every care setting unless the patient or the patient's representative is unable to provide these data. The data are collected before care is rendered and include sufficient items to identify the patient positively, such as name, address, date of birth, next of kin, payment arrangements, and a patient identification number. Basic clinical data are also supplied on this form. In the outpatient setting, patients may be asked to complete some or all of this information.

TABLE 4-3 Overview of Common Health Record Forms and Views

Administrative Forms
- Registration record
- Consent to treatment
- Acknowledgment of HIPAA privacy notice
- Consent to release information
- Acknowledgment of patient's rights
- Advance directives
- Consent to special procedures
- Patient's legal status
- Property/valuables list
- Service agreement
- Transfer/referral form
- Birth certificate
- Death certificate

Clinical Forms
- Registration record
- Emergency record
- Problem list
- Medical history/review of systems
- Psychiatric/psychological history
- Physical examination
- Encounter record
- Interdisciplinary patient care plan
- Physician's orders
- Progress notes
- Consultation report
- Discharge/interval summary
- Discharge instructions to patient

Operative Forms
- Anesthesia report
- Recovery room report
- Operative report
- Pathology report

Obstetrical Data
- Antepartum record
- Labor and delivery record
- Postpartum record

Neonatal Data
- Birth history
- Neonatal identification
- Neonatal physical examination
- Neonatal progress notes

Nursing Forms
- Nursing notes
- Graphic sheet
- Medication sheet
- Special care units

Ancillary Forms
- Electrocardiograph
- Laboratory reports
- Radiology/imaging reports
- Radiation therapy
- Therapeutic services (e.g., PT, RT, OT)
- Case management/social services

HIPAA, Health Insurance Portability and Accountability Act; *OT*, occupational therapy; *PT*, physical therapy; *RT*, respiratory therapy.

The registration record is one of the most commonly computerized forms. It may also be called an identification sheet, face or summary sheet, or admission-discharge record.

Consent to Treatment

All care settings must receive a consent for treatment from the patient or guardian. Special legal considerations exist in emergency situations. The body of the form contains a statement indicating that the patient agrees to receive basic, routine services, diagnostic procedures, and medical care. An additional statement explains that treatment outcomes cannot be guaranteed.

Acknowledgment of HIPAA Privacy Notice

As part of the HIPAA privacy rule, covered entities are required to provide patients with a *Notice of Privacy Practices* and update this notice as needed. They are also required to make a good faith effort to obtain a written acknowledgment of receipt of the notice, except in emergency situations. This acknowledgment may be combined with other forms signed at registration or admission. If there are changes in privacy practices, an updated version of the notice should be posted in public locations of the facility, placed on the organization's website, and made available to individuals receiving services.

Consent to Release Information

The patient's signature authorizes the exchange of personally identifiable health information (PIHI) between the provider and other organizations. Most commonly, this specifies release of health information compiled during the episode of care to third-party payers. It may also permit the provider to request relevant health information from previous providers. In addition to written translation, verbal translation may also be necessary. It is generally understood that the provider has permission to release medical information for continuation of care. Confidentiality and legal considerations must be followed carefully in designing this form.

Acknowledgment of Patient Rights

This form lists the patient's rights while the patient is under care. A patient must be informed of his or her rights at the initiation of care, and there should be written evidence of this. One method of obtaining the evidence is to have the patient sign a copy and place it in the record as proof of the patient's being informed. If there are any changes in these rights, an updated copy should be signed and dated by the patient or guardian and added to the record.

Advance Directives

Advance directives give instructions regarding the patient's or guardian's wishes in special medical situations. The Patient Self-Determination Act, effective December 1991, requires that all patients older than 18 years be given written information about their rights under state laws so that they can make decisions concerning medical care, including their right to refuse or accept medical or surgical treatment. Also covered under the law is information regarding a patient's right to formulate advance directives, such as living wills and durable powers of attorney for health care. Although the law requires that patients be informed, it does not require that the advance directives be included in the chart. Patients are increasingly considering these options, discussing them with their family and personal advisers such as clergy and attorneys, and then executing the appropriate documents and including appropriate information in the record. Washington State, for example, provides a website where citizens can draft their advanced directive for both health care and mental health care.

Consent to Special Procedures

A special consent is required to authorize any nonroutine diagnostic or therapeutic procedure before it is performed on the patient. For special consents to be valid, the physician must explain the procedure in lay terms, the risks of having or refusing the procedure, available alternative procedures, and the likely outcome. Again, no guarantees are given. Signature by the patient or guardian confirms that the explanation has been given and understood and that the procedure has been agreed to. In addition to written translation, verbal translation may also be necessary. Both the CMS CoPs and TJC require that the medical staff bylaws, rules, and regulations address informed consent, including which procedures are covered. Consent must always be obtained, with the properly executed form on the chart before surgery. In emergencies, when consent is unavailable, the reason should be documented (e.g., "Patient unconscious").[5]

Property and Valuables List

An inventory of property and valuables brought by the patient should be created if the care involves an admission. Any items secured on the patient's behalf should be noted. Items such as visual aids, dentures, mobility devices, and prostheses are included, and the list is signed by the patient or a representative of the patient and a representative of the facility. Patients should be discouraged from retaining expensive, nonmedical items in their rooms.

Birth and Death Certificates

State laws require the filing of vital records, including birth and death certificates. The forms and procedures vary by state; frequently, copies are kept in the patient record.

Clinical Forms
Registration Record

In a hospital setting the registration record, discussed earlier, may also contain the attending physician's statement of diagnoses, intended procedures, and any allergies or sensitivities. In a clinic setting the registration record may contain a chief complaint and allergies as stated by the patient. The requirement for clinical data in the registration record has been increasing. For example, pay-for-performance initiatives require the reporting of diagnoses that are present on admission (POA) so that they may be differentiated from hospital errors. Additional benefits include any necessary third-party authorization for services can be obtained, appropriate unit or room assignment can be made, and nursing care can begin. Standard terminology should be used and abbreviations and symbols avoided. The acute care registration and admission-discharge paper record may also contain data on consultations and the disposition of the patient, including whether an autopsy was performed on a deceased patient. If the organization places the data into a database, then all "registration related" data could be present and used as appropriate.

History and Physical Examination

The medical history and physical (H&P) is a single report with the two segments as described in the following two sections. In acute care, TJC requires a report of a comprehensive H&P be completed and available within 24 hours, or sooner if surgery is to be performed. TJC permits an interval H&P examination when a patient is admitted within 30 days for the same condition.[5] In this circumstance, the H&P is updated as necessary. This key document is typically dictated and transcribed. A written note is provided in the chart while the report is being prepared.

Medical History and Review of Systems

The medical history, including a review of systems (ROS), forms the foundation for establishing a provisional diagnosis and developing a treatment plan. If the patient cannot reliably provide this important information, it should be obtained from the most knowledgeable available source. The source should be identified. In some settings the patient completes this form in advance of the visit. As with other forms or views, standardization is important. An outline of the sequence of data items may be printed on the form or represented as fields to be completed on one or more views. Computerization, with the options of alerts and alarms, makes it easier to ensure that all essential data items have been captured. Whichever technology is used, the tone should be impartial and reflect the patient's statements.

The components of the medical history consist of the chief complaint or a description of the symptoms that caused the patient to seek medical attention, the history of the current illness, medical history, family history, social history including health maintenance, and an ROS (Table 4-4). TJC also

---

TABLE 4-4　Medical History—Typical Segments and Content

Purpose: The medical history is a conversation to gather and document information from the patient. It is also important to establish a trusting and supportive relationship and to offer information and counseling. The scope and focus of the health history vary according to the clinical setting, the patient's agenda and problem, and the clinician's goals. Patients may complete a questionnaire prior to the visit which is a resource for the visit. The following is a classic representation, though the sequence may vary.

Segments	Complaints and Symptoms
Patient ID and Reliability	Patient is identified by age and gender. (Name is on the record.) The source of the history and the source's reliability are noted. The source of any referral is also noted so a response can be provided. Time of evaluation should be included, particularly in emergency situations.
CC: Chief complaint(s)	Concise and succinct description of why patient is seeking medical attention in his or her own words; complaints or goals
HPI: History of present illness	Builds on the CC and provides a detailed chronological account of development of patient's illness, from appearance of first symptom to present situation. Includes pertinent negatives and current medications. A helpful mnemonic is *PORCH:* prescription, over-the-counter, recreational, compliance, herbal.
PMH: Past medical history	Summary of childhood and adult illnesses and conditions, such as infectious diseases, number and gender of sexual partners, pregnancies, accidents, and hospitalizations Allergies and drug sensitivities or no known allergies, no known drug allergies Past surgical history: previous operations
FH: Family history	Age and health or cause of death of each immediate family member. Diseases among relatives in which heredity or contact might play a role, such as allergies, cancer, and infectious, psychiatric, metabolic, endocrine, cardiovascular, and renal diseases. May include a genetic hereditary diagram (genogram).
SH: Social and personal history	Daily routine, activities of daily living: dietary, sleep, and exercise patterns; use of caffeine, tobacco, alcohol, and other drugs and related substances, etc. Education and occupation, home environment and significant others, important experiences, leisure activities, religious affiliations and beliefs Health maintenance: immunizations, screening tests, safe sex, safety measures such as seat belts, bicycle helmets, smoke alarms, etc. Anticipatory guidance offered as appropriate.
ROS: Review of systems	Systematic inventory of each major body system designed to document presence or absence of common subjective symptoms that includes the following types of data:
General constitution	Usual weight, recent weight changes, fever, weakness, fatigue
Skin	Rashes, lumps, sores, itching, dryness, color change, moles, eruptions, dryness, cyanosis, jaundice; changes in skin, hair, and nails
Head	Headache (duration, severity, character, location), head injury, dizziness, lightheadedness (*HEENT* may be used for head, eyes, ears, nose, throat)

Continued

TABLE 4-4   Medical History—Typical Segments and Content—cont'd

Segments	Complaints and Symptoms
Eyes	Glasses or contact lenses, last eye examination, change in vision, glaucoma, cataracts, pain, redness, dry eyes, excessive tearing, double vision, blurred vision, spots, specks, flashing lights
Ears	Hearing, including use or nonuse of hearing aids, tinnitus, dizziness, pain, vertigo, earaches, infection, discharge
Nose	Head colds, epistaxis, discharges, obstruction, postnasal drip, sinus pain, itching, hay fever
Mouth and throat	Condition of teeth and gums, last dental examination, sores or soreness, redness, hoarseness, difficulty in swallowing, dentures, dry mouth
Neck	Lumps, "swollen glands," goiter, pain, or stiffness
Breasts	Lumps, pain or discomfort, nipple discharge, self-examination, last mammogram
Respiratory system	Chest pain, wheezing, cough, dyspnea, sputum (color and quantity), hemoptysis, asthma, bronchitis, emphysema, pneumonia, tuberculosis, pleurisy, last chest x-ray
Cardiovascular system	High blood pressure, chest pain, palpitations, rheumatic fever, heart murmur, orthopnea, dyspnea, paroxysmal nocturnal dyspnea, edema, tachycardia, vertigo, faintness, past electrocardiogram or other test results
Hematologic and lymphatic systems	Anemia, easy bruising or bleeding, past transfusions and any reactions
Gastrointestinal system	Appetite, thirst, indigestion, food intolerance, nausea, vomiting, anorexia, bulimia, hematemesis, change in bowel habits, frequency of bowel movements, rectal bleeding, black tarry stools, diarrhea, constipation, flatus, hemorrhoids, jaundice, liver or gallbladder trouble
Urinary system	Frequent urgency or painful urination, nocturia, hematuria, incontinence, urinary infection, kidney stones
Genitoreproductive system	*General:* birth control, sexually transmitted diseases, exposure to human immunodeficiency virus, sexual preference, interest, satisfaction *Male:* sores, discharge from penis, hernias, testicular pain or masses, erectile dysfunction, perineal numbness *Female:* age at menarche, regularity, frequency and duration of menstruation, dysmenorrhea, menorrhagia, bleeding between periods or after intercourse, tampon use, pregnancies, births, abortions, symptoms of menopause, last Papanicolaou smear
Peripheral vascular and extremities	Intermittent claudication, leg cramps, varicose veins, past clots, thrombophlebitis
Musculoskeletal system	Joint pain or stiffness, arthritis, gout, backache, muscle pain, cramps, swelling, redness, limitation in motor activity, previous traumas including fractures and other injuries
Endocrine system	Thyroid disease; heat and cold intolerance; excessive sweating, thirst, hunger, or urination
Neurologic system	Mood, attention, speech, memory loss, headaches, fainting, blackouts, seizures, paralysis, tingling, tremors
Psychiatric disorders	Nervousness, tension, mood including depression, memory, insomnia, headache, nightmares, personality disorders, anxiety disorders, mood disorders, suicidal ideation, obsessive-compulsive disorder, flashbacks

requires that a developmental age evaluation and educational needs assessment be included when the patient is a child or adolescent. All symptoms (positive data) should be documented, and the term *normal* (or negative data) should be discouraged except in summary statements.[5]

Physical Examination

The physical examination adds objective data to the subjective data provided by the patient in the history. Together, they provide the foundation from which the practitioner can establish a diagnosis and begin to develop a treatment plan. The examination should include all body systems (Table 4-5) and consider the patient's age, sex, and symptoms. Any existing diagnostic data or physical findings are also included. A definitive diagnosis may not be possible, in which event a provisional (tentative) diagnosis may be used. If several diagnoses potentially fit the patient's clinical presentation, this list of alternatives is called a differential diagnosis. In addition, a clinical impression and an intended course of action are required.

Interdisciplinary Patient Care Plan

Most care sites are required to have an interdisciplinary patient care plan. Exceptions are the physician's office or clinic and the acute care hospital, where the physician plan and other practitioners' plans are documented separately. The care plan is the foundation around which patient care is organized because it contains input from the unique perspective of each discipline involved. It includes an assessment, statement of goals, identification of specific activities or strategies to achieve those goals, and periodic assessment of goal attainment. The care plan is initiated when a patient is admitted or begins care, and it is periodically updated. The discipline responsible for implementing each part of the plan is identified. The plan is reviewed and revised as often as the organization, regulatory agencies, and accrediting bodies require, when goals are achieved, or as the circumstances of the patient change. Changes in the care plan can be easily summarized at discharge. Because of its central role in planning and providing care, the care plan is a valuable tool in evaluating both individual patient care and overall organizational patient care performance.

| TABLE 4-5 | Physical Examination—Typical Segments and Content |

Purpose: Guided by the subjective information obtained from the review of systems in the medical history, the clinician seeks and documents objective information through the physical examination. The following is a classic "head-to-toe" sequence, although there are variations. How complete various segments are will vary by setting and the patient's chief complaint.

Segments	Content
General constitutional	Apparent state of health, signs of distress, posture, weight, height, skin color, dress and personal hygiene, reactions to persons and things, facial expression, awareness, speech manner, orientation, mood
Vital signs	Temperature, pulse, respiration, blood pressure, pain
Skin	Color, vascularity, lesions, edema, moisture, temperature, texture, thickness, mobility and turgor, hands and nails
Head	Hair, scalp, skull, face (may appear as *HEENT*)
Eyes	Visual acuity and fields; position and alignment of the eyes, eyebrows, eyelids; tearing; conjunctivae; sclerae; corneas; irises; size, shape, equality, reaction to light and accommodation of pupils; extraocular movements, ophthalmoscopic examination
Ears	Auditory acuity, auricles, canals, tympanic membranes, discharge
Nose and sinuses	External nose, airways, mucosa, septum, sinus tenderness, discharge, bleeding, smell
Mouth and throat	Lips, oral mucosa, gums, teeth, tongue, palate, tonsils, pharynx, palate, uvula, postnasal drip, sores, lesions
Neck	Stiffness, thyroid, trachea, vessels, lymph nodes, salivary glands, jugular venous distention
Thorax and lungs	Anterior and posterior, shape, symmetry, retractions, percussion Breath sounds: adventitious sounds, fremitus, breath sounds, friction, spoken voice, whispered voice
Breasts, axillae	Symmetric, tenderness, dimpling, masses, scars, discharge from nipples, axillary nodes
Cardiovascular system	Location and quality of apical impulse, thrill, pulsation, rhythm, sounds, murmurs, friction rub, jugular venous pressure and pulse, carotid artery pulse
Abdomen	Contour, peristalsis, scars, rigidity, rebound, tenderness, spasm, masses, distention, fluid, hernia, bowel sounds and bruits, palpable organs
Genitourinary system	*Male:* scars, lesions, discharge, penis, scrotum, epididymis, varicocele, hydrocele, rectal examination *Female:* external genitalia, Skene's glands and Bartholin's glands, vagina, cervix, uterus, adnexa, rectal examination, Papanicolaou smear
Musculoskeletal system	Spine and extremities, deformities, swelling, redness, tenderness, range of motion, muscle tone, weakness
Lymphatics	Palpable cervical, axillary, inguinal nodes; location; size; consistency; mobility and tenderness
Blood vessels	Pulses, color, temperature, vessel walls, veins, varicose veins
Neurologic system	Cranial nerves, coordination, reflexes, biceps, triceps, patellar, Achilles, abdominal, Babinski, Romberg, gait, compare right and left, distal and proximal; sensory: pain, temperature, touch, position, vibration
Mental status	If not done during the examination: mood, thought processes and content, abnormal perceptions, insight and judgment, memory and attention, information and vocabulary, calculating abilities, abstract thinking, dementia screening
Diagnosis(es)	Impression: single diagnosis, provisional diagnosis, or differential diagnosis

HEENT, Head, ears, eyes, nose, and throat.

Physician or Practitioner's Orders

LIPs, as identified in the organization's policies and procedures and medical staff bylaws, rules, and regulations, communicate their plans for the patient by giving written or verbal orders or directions to the nursing staff and other practitioners. Orders are necessary for any type of treatment or diagnostic procedure such as medications, surgeries, and so on. Standing orders are a set of routine orders used for patients with a particular diagnosis or to prepare for or follow up a procedure. This type of order is discouraged, particularly with managed care, because the actions may not all be medically necessary for all patients. However, treatment guidelines and protocols that incorporate best practices for treating particular problems are being used. Orders based on these protocols provide a basic set of orders modified to address an individual patient's situation. Because they initiate actions, it is particularly important that all orders are dated and signed by the LIP giving the order. TJC requires that verbal orders or telephone orders for the exchange of critical test results be verified through a "read back" procedure. In addition, these orders must be authenticated within the time specified by state or federal law and regulations as well as the medical staff bylaws, rules, and regulations, if the organization has an organized medical staff.[5]

With the exception of office visits, orders are necessary for admission and discharge from facilities and for treatments such as radiation therapy. An admission order is written at the initiation of care, and a discharge order should be written for every patient when the physician determines that release is appropriate. Lack of a discharge order may indicate that the patient left against medical advice (AMA). If this situation occurs, the circumstances should be documented in the progress notes and discharge summary. Some variations on physician's orders can be encountered in special settings, such as residential or behavioral health. For example, in ambulatory behavioral health, a team may prepare a treatment plan that includes the services to be provided. The treatment plan then contains "orders" for treatment and may be signed by one or more of the clinicians involved in the client's treatment. Hospital orders are now typically managed through a computerized physician order entry system.

Progress Notes

Progress notes are interval statements that document the patient's illness or condition and response to treatment as specifically as possible. Which practitioners write progress notes varies with the health care setting. For example, physicians write the majority of progress notes in their offices, and these notes are the focal point when patients are admitted for care. Because nurses coordinate and provide most of the patient care in home health, their notes are most prominent. In mental health, progress notes feature the primary clinician's documentation of counseling. Progress notes may be integrated, with all providers writing sequentially on the same sheets, or they may be separated, with physicians, nurses, and other providers writing separately, perhaps on custom-designed forms or views. The computer views can be organized by date, type, author, or some other variable.

Regardless of where the progress notes are located, any practitioner who writes such notes is responsible for recording observations about the patient's progress and response to treatment from the perspective of his or her profession. For example, physician progress notes for admitted patients should include an admission note, subsequent notes, and a final note. The admission note provides an overview of the patient at admission and adds any relevant information that is not included in the H&P. The frequency of subsequent progress notes depends on the patient's condition and the site of care and its medical staff bylaws, rules, and regulations. Acute care notes are written daily, whereas long-term care notes may appropriately be written monthly. All treatments provided and the patient's responses to each are to be included, as are any complications the patient may have. When care of the patient is transferred from one physician to another, the physician releasing the patient should write a summary of the patient's course to that point. At the end of the admission, along with the discharge order, a final note is written stating the patient's general condition and instructions for the patient's activity, diet, medications, and any follow-up appointments. If the patient dies during the admission, the final notes describe the circumstances regarding the death, the findings, the cause of death, and whether an autopsy was planned.

Consultation Report

A **consultation** report contains an opinion about a patient's condition by a practitioner other than the attending physician. Opinions may be sought from pharmacists, dietitians, physical and occupational therapists, dentists, other physicians, and so on. The opinion is based on a review of the patient record, an examination of the patient, and a conference with the attending physician. Many organizations, particularly in acute care, combine the request section, where the attending physician states the reason for consultation, with a space for the response, where the consultant details his or her findings and recommendations. Each signs his or her respective section.

The CMS CoPs for hospitals require that the medical staff bylaws, rules, and regulations address the status of consultants. To be considered a consultant, a practitioner must be well qualified by training, experience, and competence to give an opinion in the specialty in which the advice is sought. It is the responsibility of the attending physician to request a consultation. The categories of patients for which consultations must be requested are as follows:
- Patients who are not good medical or surgical risks
- Patients whose diagnoses are obscure
- Patients whose physicians have doubts about the best therapeutic measures to be taken
- Patients who are involved in situations in which there is a question of criminal activity

In emergencies, exceptions may be made. The CoPs also state that routine procedures, such as radiologic studies, electrocardiograms (ECGs), tissue examinations, and proctoscopic and cystoscopic procedures, are not normally considered consultations.

Discharge and Interval Summary

The discharge and interval summary, or clinical résumé, concisely reviews the patient's course. It is typically associated with admissions, but it may be provided in other care settings. The summary begins with the reason for admission and includes chronological descriptions of significant findings from examinations and tests and procedures and therapies performed along with the patient's response. Details regarding discharge are also recorded, including the condition on discharge related to the condition on admission and follow-up instructions specifying medications, level of physical activity, diet, follow-up care, and patient teaching. Because the discharge summary is frequently referred to, standard terminology is essential, and abbreviations and ambiguous terms such as "improved" should be diligently avoided. All relevant diagnoses established by the time of discharge and all operative procedures performed should be recorded in standard terminology that indicates topography and etiology as necessary. When final diagnoses and procedures are listed on more than one form, attention must be paid to their agreement. In special cases, a final progress note may substitute for a discharge summary. Patients admitted for less than 48 hours with minor problems, uncomplicated deliveries, and normal neonates are examples. The discharge summary should be written or dictated immediately after discharge and authenticated.

Discharge Instructions to Patient

In addition to the instructions regarding patient after care included in the formal discharge summary, there is typically a separate form reviewed with the patient, family, or caregiver at the time of discharge. As with the formal discharge summary, it includes recommendations for diet and activity levels, medications, and referrals for follow-up care. For those patients who have undergone surgery or other procedures, specific directions may also be provided. Case Management and Social Services may be involved to coordinate items, such as durable medical equipment. These instructions are typically given by the patient's nurse. To promote a smooth transition to the next stage of care, the instructions should be as clear as possible. It is best practice that they be given both verbally and in writing in the language appropriate for the patient and/or caregiver. A copy of the instructions and any other relevant material are provided at discharge. In addition to the provider, the signature of the person receiving the instructions is included.

Operative Forms

Data from each operative event are collected by using a set of forms or views that are considered a unit. The consent for surgery and the pathology report are added to the forms described next.

Anesthesia Report

Procedures that require more than a local anesthetic also require an anesthesia report. Preoperative medication is recorded with time, concentration, and effect. The anesthetic agent is then documented, including the amount, route of administration, effect, and duration. The patient's condition throughout the procedure is described, including vital signs, blood loss, transfusions, and intravenous fluids given. The report should also describe any surgical manipulation that may affect anesthesia care, any complications during anesthesia, and any treatments unlikely to be documented elsewhere. The practitioner administering the anesthesia (either a nurse anesthetist or an anesthesiologist) records the data and signs the report.

Special anesthesia-specific notes are also required before and after surgery. The preanesthesia note, usually found in the progress notes, describes the planned procedure, the examination of the patient, and the choice of anesthetic. Also discussed are laboratory results, any drug history, any past or potential problems, and preanesthesia medications. The postanesthesia note may be in the progress notes, the recovery room record, or the anesthesia report. It documents the patient's condition, specifying the nature and extent of any complications. The postanesthesia note should be completed within 24 hours after surgery. Both notes are signed by the practitioner responsible for administering the anesthesia. TJC requires at least one postanesthesia visit that describes the presence or absence of anesthesia-related complications.[5] A visit is usually considered to occur apart from the operative or recovery area. Notes must specify time and date, with one visit occurring soon after surgery and another after the patient has completely recovered. The patient's condition may require additional visits. Although it is preferable that these notes be made by a physician or oral surgeon, any practitioner with pertinent comments regarding the patient's anesthesia care may add notes. If anesthesia personnel are unavailable to provide the documentation, the physician or dentist discharging the patient may complete the notes.

Recovery Room Record

The recovery room is designed to care for patients immediately after surgery or anesthesia. A separate form is typically used to record complete observation from the time the patient arrives in the recovery room until departure for the nursing unit or other destination. TJC requires that this form include the patient's condition and level of consciousness when entering and leaving the unit; vital signs; status reports of infusions, surgical dressings, tubes, catheters, or drains; and any treatment provided in the unit. The postanesthesia note may be documented on this form and, depending on its design, may be signed by a physician, nurse, or both.[5]

Operative Report

All patients who undergo surgery must have an operative report included in their records. The top portion provides identifying data, including the names of the surgeon and any assistants, and the date, duration, and name of the procedure. A postoperative diagnosis is required. A preoperative diagnosis, which should be entered in the progress notes before surgery, is also desirable for easy comparison. The body of the report contains a full description of the surgical approach, normal and abnormal findings, organs explored, procedures, implants, ligatures, sutures, and the number of packs, drains, and sponges used, and the condition of the patient at the conclusion of surgery. The report should be written or dictated immediately after surgery, included in the record as soon as possible, and signed by the surgeon. If this is not possible, continuity of care can still be maintained by writing a timely and detailed operative note in the record.

Pathology Report

A pathology report documents tissue examinations that may be microscopic in addition to being macroscopic (gross). The tissue may have been removed from the patient during a specialized procedure, such as a biopsy, or during surgery. It may have been expelled, such as in an abortion, or be the entire body, as when an autopsy is performed. Occasionally, objects such as coins are submitted as well. As in a consultation, the tissue or object is identified, a clinical diagnosis provided, and an opinion requested. The pathologist examines the specimen and, at a minimum, writes a report describing its gross diagnostic features. A policy decision needs to be made regarding which specimens require only a gross examination and diagnosis. This decision may vary, depending on how and where the pathologist practices, but involves the medical staff in acute care. When a microscopic examination is performed, it is the basis for the diagnosis. The pathologist dictates and signs the transcribed report, and the original is included in the patient's record.

Autopsy Report

When the report documents an autopsy, the pathologist summarizes the patient's illness and treatment, followed by a detailed report of gross findings and an anatomic diagnosis at autopsy. An autopsy is a lengthy procedure, and as many as 60 days may pass before reports are completed. A provisional autopsy diagnosis should be recorded in the patient's record within 3 days. Both reports are also signed by the pathologist.

Obstetrical Data

Another set of forms or views is collected for obstetrical care. Again, any appropriate consent for surgery or associated pathology report is added to the forms described next. The American College of Obstetricians and Gynecologists identifies the recommended content for these forms in its *Standards for Obstetric-Gynecologic Services.*

Antepartum Record

The antepartum or prenatal record begins in the office or clinic of the obstetrician or nurse midwife. Ideally started early in the pregnancy, the record includes a comprehensive H&P examination as described previously, with particular attention to menstrual history, reproductive history including live births and abortions, a risk assessment, and attendance at any childbirth classes. An example entry of a woman's reproductive history is "gravida 2, para 1, Ab 1," where gravida represents pregnancies; para, live births; and Ab, abortions, either spontaneous or elective. Beyond routine laboratory tests, the blood group and Rh factor, rubella status, cervical cytologic examination, and a syphilis screen should be checked. Women may choose to have their children at home, in a birthing center, or in a hospital. Whichever site is selected, a copy or abstract of current prenatal information should be available at the birthing site by at least the estimated thirty-sixth week of pregnancy. Arrangements should also be made for access to this information and to hospital care in case of an emergency in a birthing center or at home.

DID YOU KNOW?

Gravida is derived from the weight or gravity of the pregnant belly.

Labor and Delivery Record

This record tracks the patient from admission through delivery to the postpartum period. The antepartum record should be reviewed with attention to the special items already described. An evaluation is then made by the physician or nurse midwife, including an updated history or a complete history if there is no antepartum record, noting data on contractions, status of membranes, presence of significant bleeding, time and content of the patient's last intake of food or fluid, drug intake and allergies, choice of anesthesia, and plans to breast- or bottle-feed. The mother is monitored frequently, as is the child, with a fetal monitor. In the normal case, this is done by a nurse. At delivery, details regarding the mother are recorded, similar to those of a surgery. The neonate is also described, including his or her Apgar score

(an infant rating system at 1 and 5 minutes after birth), sex, weight, length, onset of respiration, abnormalities, and treatment to the eyes. Any fetal monitoring strips are identified and annotated with relevant data; they become part of the patient record. For multiple births, individual notations are made.

Postpartum Record

Postpartum data include information about the condition of the mother after delivery. The record may be a special form, or it may be included in the progress notes. In either case, attention is paid to assessing the lochia and condition of the breasts, fundus, and perineum as well as the usual postoperative status. Nursing staff continue this documentation as long as it is relevant.

Neonatal Data

As a live birth takes place, each new person is given his or her own record and record number included in the MPI/EMPI. A separate record is not created for fetal deaths. The neonatal record includes the regular H&P and progress notes, with the addition of special identification data. The record for healthy neonates is usually brief.

Neonatal Identification

While the neonate is still in the delivery room, two identical bands are prepared noting the mother's number and the neonate's sex and time of birth. One band is placed on the mother and the other is placed on the neonate. A band number and identification form about the mother and neonate are also prepared. Both bands and forms should be checked by two responsible practitioners before the neonate leaves the delivery room. Footprinting and fingerprinting, if performed, also require special forms. The nurse in charge of the delivery room is responsible for the identification process and signs the sheets along with any participating obstetrician.

Birth History

The birth history record may be shared with the mother's record, including pertinent history regarding pregnancy, any diseases, and delivery. The Apgar score, any prematurity or anomalies, and any problems that occur before transfer to the nursery are noted. Nurses or physicians sign the appropriate sections.

Neonatal Physical Examination

The neonatal physical examination repeats the birth data and concentrates on a detailed description of the neonate's appearance. The attending physician, typically a pediatrician, should examine the apparently healthy neonate as soon as possible and before discharge.

Neonate Progress Notes

The American Academy of Pediatrics recommends frequent recording of vital signs until the neonate is stable (usually within 12 hours after birth). TJC in particular requires that neonates who receive oxygen therapy should have the concentration recorded at intervals as written in the policies and procedures of the facility's nursery. If the infant should remain in the hospital for additional days, more notes are made. These notes and any other forms are added to the infant's record and signed by the LIP.[5]

Nursing Forms

Although nurses document on many forms within the record, the following forms are used exclusively by the nursing staff. Nurses typically perform an assessment that is used to develop a nursing care plan. Nurses should write their conclusions as nursing diagnoses. Nursing diagnoses are based on the patient's response to the alteration in health (medical condition), whereas a medical diagnosis is based on the physiologic or medical condition of the patient.

Nursing Notes

Nurses may write nurses' notes or contribute to integrated progress notes. Regardless of the form, these notes describe the patient and his or her condition in objective, behavioral terms. Quantitative data are encouraged. The documentation begins with an admission note, including notification of the attending physician of the admission. Subsequent notes are written as needed and include nursing interventions and the patient's response. The documentation ends with a discharge note. If the patient should die, a death note is written, including notification of the physician.

Graphic Sheet

A graphic sheet is used to plot the patient's vital signs (temperature, pulse and respiratory rates, and blood pressure). Additional information may be noted, including weight and intake and output of fluids and solids. The frequency of entries depends on the patient's condition. Paper forms usually provide space for six entries a day for several days, and additional sheets are added as needed. Nurses typically sign the form once and thereafter initial their entries. Computer views provide similar trending and authentication.

Medication Administration Record

The medication administration record (MAR) provides a detailed record of the medications administered. The date, time, name of drug, dose, and route of administration are included. If there is an adverse reaction or if it is not possible to administer a scheduled dose, this is also noted, and an explanation is given in the nurses' notes. The practitioner giving the dose initials the entry.

IOM reports first highlighted the cost and consequences of medication errors. Current best practices include medication reconciliation which compares all the medications a patient is taking, including over-the-counter drugs with medication orders. The goal is to reduce errors such as omissions, duplications, dose errors, or drug interactions. It should be done each time there is a transition in care involving new or rewritten medication orders. Transitions include changes in setting, level of care, service, or practitioner.

Special Care Units

Special units such as the intensive care unit and coronary care unit often have forms to suit their particular patient populations.

Ancillary Forms

Ancillary data are typically collected by practitioners other than physicians and nurses, with the exception of patient and family teaching and case and staff conferences in which a wide variety of clinicians may participate.

Electrocardiographic Reports

The electrocardiograph records the electrical activity of the heart. The ECG is the graphic tracing produced by plotting these waves against time on a continuous paper roll or as a computer view. The report contains the cardiologist's signed interpretation and may include the tracing. When tracings are not provided, they are stored in the laboratory for reference.

Laboratory Reports

Laboratory reports detail analysis or examination of blood, urine, stool, and other body substances. The medical laboratory may be within the facility or one that is used on a contractual basis. The laboratory usually provides the results of urinalysis and blood chemistry and hematology, microbiology, and serology reports. Tests should be completed and reported promptly. A report identifies the date, time, test, results, and the reference values for the test's normal range. Reports are usually computer generated and may be printed on standard-sized pages or on small slips designed to be taped on mounting sheets. Cumulative reports may be provided, which reduce the bulk of the chart. In an electronic view laboratory results can be profiled over time and presented in graphic format. When blood banking is done, the American Association of Blood Banks has particular requirements detailed in its Technical Manual.

Radiology and Imaging Reports

Radiology reports describe diagnostic or therapeutic services. Diagnostic procedures include modalities such as radiography, nuclear medicine, computed tomography, magnetic resonance imaging, and ultrasonography, which create an image that can be visualized. On a form similar to that used for the consultation, the upper portion notes the attending physician's request for the study and specifies the diagnostic question and area to be examined. A physician, usually a radiologist, interprets the image and adds an impression at the bottom of the form. The report is typically dictated and transcribed. Both physicians authenticate their respective sections. In a computerized view the image can be viewed online, and a portion of the image can be enlarged for detailed visualization if necessary. Where films are used, they may be stored in the department that produced them. Computer reports and images are typically part of the hospital clinical information system. Where images are digitized, they are typically stored in a specialized computerized system called a picture archiving and communication system (PACS), which also facilitates consultations via telemedicine.

Radiation Therapy

Therapeutic radiology services more closely resemble the consultation process. They are major procedures that require a special consent. A treatment plan is written; each treatment is reported, including the amount of radiation given for each dose, and a summary is provided. The therapeutic radiologist signs each report.

Therapeutic Services

Therapies (e.g., physical, occupational, respiratory, speech, dietary) include assessment and treatment plans designed to restore patient function. The therapist documents the services, including the patient's response, and signs the report or progress notes. Care plans are updated as needed, and a summary may be completed at the end of the episode of care. Notes are objective and goal-oriented. TJC has documentation requirements for each of these services, particularly as they relate to rehabilitative care.[5]

Discharge Forms

A variety of forms are used to plan for and facilitate a smooth transition from one site of care to another or to home.

Discharge and Interval Summary

The discharge and interval summary, or clinical résumé, concisely reviews the patient's course. It is typically associated with admissions, but it may be provided in other care settings. The summary begins with the reason for admission and includes chronological descriptions of significant findings from examinations, tests, procedures, and therapies performed, along with the patient's response. Details regarding discharge are also recorded, including the condition on discharge related to the condition on admission and follow-up instructions specifying medications, level of physical activity, diet, follow-up care, and patient teaching. Because the discharge summary is frequently referred to, standard terminology is essential, and abbreviations and ambiguous terms such as *improved* should be diligently avoided. All relevant diagnoses established by the time of discharge and all operative procedures performed should be recorded in standard terminology that indicates topography and etiologic factors as necessary. When final diagnoses and procedures are listed on more than one form, attention must be paid to their agreement. In special cases, a final progress note may substitute for a discharge summary. Patients admitted for less than 48 hours with minor problems, uncomplicated deliveries, and normal neonates are examples. The discharge summary should be written or dictated immediately after discharge and authenticated.

Patient and Family Teaching and Participation

Evidence of patient and family teaching and understanding has become increasingly important as more treatments become available for patients and families to implement at home. Lifestyle changes are also appropriate topics for teaching. A wide variety of practitioners engage in patient and family teaching along the continuum of care. Regardless of the profession or the setting, the teaching and the redemonstration of understanding should be described. If any preprinted material is provided, it should also be noted and a copy kept on file in the HIM department or an online repository if it should be necessary to interpret the record. Some segments of health care require documentation of family participation in planning, goal setting, and carrying out of lifestyle changes, therapies, or other activities.

Case Management and Social Service Record

Case managers coordinate care and resources across settings to reduce costs while improving quality of health care and achieve desired outcomes. Case management records contain data on the patient's background, social information, and problems identified by the patient, family, and case manager. The case manager has access to a great deal of sensitive personal information in addition to private medical information. The formal record includes a plan of action, progress notes, and a discharge note.

Discharge Planning and Follow-Up

A discharge plan is begun at the time of admission or initiation of services; it gives a general assessment of plans to maintain continuity after this episode of care. This may represent transfer from acute care to long-term care, initiation of home health care, or provision of one or several available community services. Any agencies to be used should be identified. Social Services often coordinates the plan, which includes both medical and financial arrangements and considers the family's needs as well as those of the patient.

SELF-ASSESSMENT QUIZ

7. What is the role of users in the development of the health record?
8. Are there required forms or views for the health record?
9. What are good sources to use when designing forms and views?
10. Research nursing diagnoses, and compare and contrast them with medical diagnoses.
11. Research medical staff bylaws, rules, and regulations related to health records.

Documentation Guidelines

Although practitioners are trained to document patient care during their education, organizations should provide training in their specific policies, procedures, and systems. These efforts support communication, continuity of care, patient safety, and overall high-quality patient care. In addition, because the patient record is also the facility's business record, such efforts will support compliance with federal and state regulations and accreditation, professional practice, and legal standards. It is often said, "If it isn't documented, it wasn't

BOX 4-2 Standard Content of Record

Centers for Medicare and Medicaid Services Standards
The medical record must contain information to justify the admission and continued hospitalization, support the diagnosis, and describe the patient's progress and response to medications and services.

http://www.gpo.gov/fdsys/pkg/CFR-2011-title42-vol5/pdf/CFR-2011-title42-vol5-sec482-24.pdf. Accessed March 27, 2014.

done." Ultimately, the individual practitioners are responsible for the quality of their entries, including authentication.

Paper forms and computer views provide the structure for the documentation of patient care activities. Although they support a complete and quality record, they do not guarantee it. The system and the individuals who document in the clinical record contribute to the quality of the content of the record. If the health record is to fulfill its unique roles for the patient, providers, as a legal record, for researchers and education, the content must be of high quality.

The CMS Standard for Content of the Medical Record is provided in Box 4-2. This overall goal of documentation is also included in the TJC standards. Table 4-6 presents some essential entry guidelines. Chapter 6 includes a description of data quality characteristics for EHRs.

General

The patient's name and other key identifying data must be on all pages of the record and on a computer view. The author's identity can be authenticated as described subsequently and must include credentials to indicate his or her role in the patient's care. Authors must only document their own interactions for the patient and avoid charting for others because they are legally responsible for both their care and their entries. In some care environments, one individual may be designated to draft the treatment plan on the basis of the input of several team members. One or more team members may sign the plan. Using the appropriate form or view facilitates others' finding the information in the record. Forms and views also help remind practitioners of care elements and essential documentation.

Entries should include the date and time and should be charted as close to the time of care as possible. Notes should never be written in anticipation of care being provided because other events may intervene, creating errors in the sequence of events. Descriptions are best understood when they are specific and exact and include the use of standard terms spelled correctly. Although accuracy and clarity are essential, notes do not require complete sentences. In most care settings, notes are written in a concise style. The word *patient* is not routinely required because it is understood to be the patient's chart.

Abbreviations and Symbols

The use of abbreviations, acronyms, and symbols saves substantial time for practitioners. They also pose significant risks of being misunderstood either through poor handwriting or the fact that many have more than one meaning. HCOs

TABLE 4-6 Health Record Entry Documentation

General Guidelines

- Identify the patient: name and number on all new pages added to the chart.
- Identify the author: signed with an initial, last name, and credentials.
- Document only the author's care, never anyone else's.
- Use the proper form or view: this aids communication by structuring the chart.
- Complete all items: to ensure completion of all content.
- Include date and time: to relate observations and activities to each other.
- Are timely: recorded shortly after, and never before, completing patient care.
- Are specific: record patient behavior and complaints in specific terms.
- Are exact: noting time, effect, and results of all procedures, avoiding ditto marks.
- Are concise: recording all necessary information and nothing else; avoid meaningless phrases, the word *patient,* and complete sentences.
- Spell correctly, use standard terms and symbols.
- Abbreviations: use only approved and safe abbreviations.

Paper-Based Records

- Are legible: ensuring that other members of the care team can read the entries.
- Use black ink: ensures the best photocopies, faxes, and document imaging.
- Leave no blank lines: draw a line through the center of an empty line to prevent charting by someone else in the area signed.
- Chart omissions as a new entry: never backdate or add to prior entries.
- Never obscure entries: draw a line through any mistake and write "error" or "mistaken entry" above it. Erasures, white out, and heavy mark-outs create doubt when the record is needed by other users.

should establish policies and maintain an official abbreviation list approved by the organization and, if appropriate, the medical staff, for use in patient care documentation. When more than one definition exists, only one should be approved, with the preferred approach being to avoid the abbreviation entirely. Research by the IOM published in 2000 focused the attention of the public and health professionals on a variety of patient safety issues.[6] In response, TJC established national patient safety goals, which include prohibiting the use of "dangerous" abbreviations, acronyms, and symbols in patient records. These abbreviations, acronyms, and symbols have caused confusion or problems in their handwritten form. The minimum "do not use" list includes such items as avoiding "U" for unit, which can be mistaken for 0, 4, or cc. Spelling out "unit" is preferred.

? DID YOU KNOW?

Acronyms are created from the first letter of several words where "acr/o" is for extremity or the extreme first letter and "-nym" is for name. They are typically capitalized.

Authentication

Authentication identifies the author of an entry in the patient record and that the entry has been verified or validated by the author. Only the author can authenticate an entry. Organizational policy, consistent with law and regulation, may also require some entries by non-LIPs to be authenticated by an LIP as well. If any of the information is in disagreement, additions or corrections should be made before authentication. In some settings, such as when interdisciplinary care plans exist, multiple authors may be included. TJC requires that a minimum of the following four documents be authenticated: H&Ps, operative reports, consultations, and discharge summaries.[5]

There are several methods for authentication. Medical staff bylaws, rules, and regulations as well as federal and state laws should be consulted regarding their use. In a paper-based environment, practitioners may sign with their first initials, last names, and credentials or disciplines, with full names being preferred if similar names exist. Initials may be used when there is a legend available in the record providing the full signature and the related initials. The use of signature stamps typically requires the owner to sign a statement that only he or she will use the stamp. Because of their high potential for abuse, signature stamps should be discouraged. Electronic authentication may include an e-mail signature, digitized image of a signature, a unique logon and personal identification number, unique biometric identifier (such as a fingerprint), or digital signature using encryption. These technologies are discussed further in later chapters.

Paper-Based Records

Several historic charting challenges, such as legibility and author identification, are substantially resolved by the use of EHRs. When paper records are still used, practitioners should be encouraged to write legibly and to use black ink, which promotes good-quality photocopying, faxing, and scanning or document imaging. No blank lines should remain between entries, where others can chart. Any omissions should be charted as new entries and marked as such. When errors occur, corrections should be made with a single line so as not to obscure the entry. A notation such as "mistaken entry" or "error" should be added and initialed and the corrected documentation entered. See further discussion of corrections and amendments in the chapters on EHRs and legal aspects.

Format Types

The CMS Meaningful Use program includes financial incentives to encourage HCOs to progress along the migration path to a full EHR. While some HCOs have migrated entirely to an EHR, others are in various hybrid states and some remain paper-based. The sequence of the paper-based health record is referred to as its format. As with forms in general, there are no directives on which format to use. Organizations are free to design their own as long as the format chosen is standardized. The reference that defines the organization's standard sequence of pages to be followed in each record is called a chart order. There may be a different order for records during care and after discharge. With implementation of the EHR, the order of the paper will cease to be an issue; however, there will be times when the content of the EHR will be printed out and require an organizing format.

As part of its responsibility to ensure communication among practitioners, the medical staff participates with representatives of other departments on the hospital's information management or medical record committee. This committee should approve forms to be used in the clinical record as well as the organizing format. There are three common formats: source oriented, problem oriented, and integrated.

Source-Oriented Medical Record

The most common paper-based health record format is source oriented, meaning that the record is organized into sections according to the practitioners who are the source of both the treatment and the data collection. Within each section, sheets are arranged in chronological order, perhaps with some divisions by episodes of care. During admissions, the current episode is typically kept at the nursing unit in reverse chronological order with the most recent materials on the top. The trend is to keep the record in this order rather than commit the staff time to reversing the chart. If a record is kept in the same order during and after care, it may also be referred to as "universal" chart order. An advantage of standardized source-oriented records is the speed with which an individual sheet can be located. The major disadvantage is lack of a clear picture of the patient's problems and how each department is contributing to their resolution.

Problem-Oriented Medical Record

The problem-oriented medical record (POMR) was developed by Dr. Lawrence L. Weed in the 1960s in response to the major deficiency in the source-oriented format—lack of a clear picture of the patient's problems. The POMR system focuses on the documentation of a logical, organized plan of clinical thought by practitioners. The system has four parts: a database, problem list, initial plan, and progress notes. The database was an early MDS similar to those in place today. The problem list is a dynamic document showing titles, numbers, and dates of problems, and it serves as a table of contents of the record. The problem is stated at the level of the physician's current understanding and modified as further data accumulate. Problems may be initial symptoms or well-defined diagnoses. The problems are past and present and social, financial, and demographic as well as medical. The initial plans describe what will be done to investigate or treat each problem. Plans refer to the problem number and can be of three types: the need to collect more decision-making information, therapy (e.g., medications, treatments), and patient education. Progress notes are written in a distinctive style according to the acronym SOAP, translated as shown in

TABLE 4-7	Progress Note Elements: Problem-Oriented Medical Record

S = *Subjective,* which records the patient's statement of the problem

O = *Objective,* which records what the practitioner identifies through the history, physical examination, and diagnostic tests

A = *Assessment,* which combines the subjective and objective into a conclusion

P = *Plan,* or what approach is going to be taken to resolve the problem

 SELF-ASSESSMENT QUIZ

12. Who is ultimately responsible for the documentation in the patient record?
13. Identify the overall criteria required by CMS for medical record content.
14. Identify the benefits and risks of using abbreviations, acronyms, and symbols.
15. For both paper-based and electronic records, identify two ways authors can authenticate entries.

Table 4-7. SOAP notes are also numbered to correspond to the problems. The discharge summary is considered a special progress note.

Weed suggested that forms be designed to support the numbering and tracking of problems. He was also an early advocate of a team approach, encouraging all practitioners participating in the patient's care to document sequentially in the progress notes. Each practitioner would contribute as appropriate to his or her training, licensure, and understanding of the problem. The major advantage of the POMR is that it creates a holistic picture of the patient and his or her care. Although it does not guarantee quality care, it provides an excellent communication and evaluation tool that highlights the thinking process. The major disadvantage is the time and commitment needed on the part of the practitioners to implement and maintain the system. With the exception of the SOAP style of progress notes and the problem list, the full system has not been widely accepted for use with the paper-based health record. Components of the system, such as the problem list and SOAP notes, are often used in ambulatory settings. Behavioral health transformed the problem list into a list of goals and objectives that serves the same function as a problem list. Behavioral health may use a modification of SOAP notes that combines the "S" and "O" into "Data," resulting in DAP—Data, Assessment, and Plan—to structure progress notes. The POMR is finding renewed support in the EHR model because of its logical approach to organizing data.

Integrated Medical Record

The integrated record is strictly chronological without any divisions by source. This format keeps the episode of care clearly defined by date, which is an advantage when the flow of care is being considered. The major disadvantage is that information from the same source, such as laboratory data, is not easily compared. Some chart order arrangements integrate selected types of forms, such as progress notes, and keep others, such as radiology reports, by source. Integrated progress notes resemble the team approach of the POMR, which provides a more holistic view of the patient. If progress notes are integrated, paper forms can be designed to easily find and track the notes of a particular category of practitioner.

DESIGN AND CONTROL OF PAPER FORMS AND COMPUTER VIEWS AND TEMPLATES

When forms or computer views (information on screens) and templates are well designed and controlled, they enhance technology by providing a smooth link in the communication process. They permit recording of varying data without recopying constant information. This reduces clerical work, decreases the number of errors, and increases efficiency. When they are well designed, they assist in actual direct patient care. Many of the principles of design of forms or views apply to both paper and computer forms. Templates and some specific guidelines for computer formats are also discussed in Chapter 6.

As with data collection and technology, form or view design should emphasize the needs of users. It is the responsibility of each health care facility to develop its own forms or views. Accrediting and regulatory bodies such as TJC and CMS and standards organizations such as ASTM do not recommend particular forms or views with which to collect their required data elements, nor do professional organizations such as AHIMA and AHDI. When developing forms or views, the designer can refer to health information books, journals, and newsletters, including those noted in the chapter references, and can consult professional colleagues in similar facilities for ideas. For smaller practices, vendors can be a resource. In some geographic areas, several facilities have formally joined together and adopted basic health record forms and views that are acceptable to the medical staffs of each facility. This saves the time of health care providers who practice at more than one site and facilitates the paper or electronic interchange necessary to care for patients and carry out the business of each facility. It also permits administrative cost savings through bulk purchasing and reduced programming charges. Such strategies are also common in corporate facilities, where core forms or views are designed for all the facilities, and local facilities design their own additions according to guidelines that have been provided.

With the transition from the paper-based record to the electronic record, paper forms will decline. However, there are other business purposes for which good form designs are helpful and HIM professionals should be prepared to guide their design and production.

Forms or Views Team

The management of forms or views is a collaborative process. Members of the forms or views team include representatives from the following services:

- HIM
- Patient care services
- Quality improvement
- Information systems
- Materials management
- Others as needed

The HIM professional plays a leadership role by providing knowledge of rules and regulations related to health record content, medical science, computer applications, the flow of data throughout the organization, and the information needs of the health care delivery system. The forms or views design and control process also benefits from the involvement of an information systems manager who is responsible for computer input and output, a materials or purchasing manager who is responsible for inventory and ordering paper forms, a patient care professional who represents clinical needs, a quality improvement (QI) professional to provide input regarding forms or views created to address quality issues, and others as needed. The team's charge may be to work on administrative and patient information applications and to become involved in the selection of data collection technology. The team forwards its patient-related recommendations to the clinical information committee for approval, and its administrative recommendations follow the organizational chain of command.

General Design Principles

Needs of Users

The needs of both internal and external users must be considered when designing forms or views. It is important to remember that users are not only the patient and providers, but also the organization's administrative, financial, and legal staff. External users collect data from many locations, and the data are combined or aggregated. These may be local, state, and federal agencies and other planning and research groups. Collecting enough of the right type of data to satisfy this range of users means clearly defining the purpose of the form or view.

Purpose of the Form or View

Patient record forms serve many purposes. They standardize, identify and instruct, facilitate documentation and decision making, and promote consistency in data collection, reporting, and interpretation. Forms identify patients and practitioners and instruct them step by step in what data items to gather, where to obtain them, and how to record them. Good instructions, when followed, facilitate complete and accurate documentation, which is the foundation of effective decision making.

H&P forms provide good examples of these purposes. When standardized, all elements of the history, ROS, and physical examination (as listed in the ASTM standard) are collected. Both the patient and the practitioner are identified with names and unique numbers either electronically or manually. The patient may follow a set of instructions on paper or computer to provide his or her medical history. The provider then follows a set of instructions when performing the ROS and proceeding with the physical examination. The documentation thus collected is the foundation on which the patient and practitioner can make decisions and take action regarding lifestyle changes, diagnostic testing, medications, or other treatments. At the close of an encounter, a return appointment is frequently scheduled, which assigns responsibility to both the patient and the practitioner for follow-up. Thus the H&P form or view has structured the majority of the communication between the patient and the practitioner and continues to communicate with other users as the need arises.

Selection and Sequencing of Items

When the purpose of the form or view is established, the next step is to construct a list or grid of required data to ensure the collection of all essential items and the elimination of unnecessary or redundant items. Effective and efficient sequencing of the form or view should follow the traditional pattern—from left to right and top to bottom—permitting a continuous operation whether reading, writing, or entering data on the computer. The flow should be logical and take into consideration the order of data collection or transfer. In addition, numbering items makes references to both items and written instructions on completion of forms faster and easier.

Standard Terminology, Abbreviations, and Format

Often, large numbers of people within an organization use each form or view, and with the expansion of the EHR this number increases. Effective communication therefore depends on the use of terminology that is understood by all. Use of standard terminology, when available, is recommended. For example, standard definitions for commonly collected data items published by ASTM are described later in this chapter. When standard definitions are not available, the form or view should supply the definition. Standard definitions are particularly important when linked databases are used.

Words, numbers, and abbreviations should be standardized as well. For example, users need to know whether hyphens should be included when entering Social Security numbers (SSNs). They also need instructions on how many digits to use for patient record numbers and how to enter coded data. Abbreviations have great appeal for health care providers because they save both reading time and entry time. Their major liability is misunderstanding. Caregivers depend on understanding the record to provide quality care. Administrative, legal, licensure, accreditation, and personal uses also depend on a clear understanding of the record. As mentioned earlier, any abbreviations permitted in the patient record must be understood by all.

Another aspect of form or view design that promotes consistency is the development of a master format or template. The placement of data in the same sequence on similar forms or views with similar layouts facilitates rapid entry and retrieval. Consistent location of patient identification and unique identification number are an example.

Instructions

Instructions should briefly identify who should complete the data items and should also provide additional guidance as necessary. Computer views typically provide this information on introductory screens and as needed throughout data entry. Paper forms usually separate the instructions from the data entry spaces and place them at the top. The identification and distribution of copies also need to be specified. If the instructions need to be more extensive, they can be printed on the back, on a separate sheet, or in an administrative manual. If any of these alternatives are used, reference to the location of instructions should be made on the face of the form.

Simplification

With such a host of users, purposes, technologies, terms, and formats, it is easy to feel overwhelmed by the complexity. The last general consideration is to attempt to keep forms or views simple. Forms or views should be created only when there is an established need that is not being adequately handled by an existing form or view or when revision is impractical. The purpose of a form or view management program is to ensure that each tool has a desired purpose, that only necessary forms or views are maintained, and that all forms or views are documented and available. Simplification provides considerable savings in time, effort, and materials.

Paper Forms Design and Production

When the health care facility uses paper forms for data collection, discussion with a printer can provide basic information and help avoid costly mistakes. The development of a standardized guide, such as the example shown in Figure 4-4 developed by one health care facility, also helps to ensure satisfactory results. The major segments of a paper form are the header and footer, introduction and instructions, and body and close. A guide, called a *chart order,* is also necessary to standardize the assembly sequence of various documents within the paper health record.

Header and Footer

The title and subtitle (if any) identify the form and are typically positioned at the top as a header. In facilities that bind their records at the top, it is easier to locate the title if it appears at the bottom. Form titles should appear in the same font and font size on each form. Forms for external use should include the facility name, address, phone number, and perhaps a logo. Any code that is required for scanning technology should appear as part of the header. The footer contains information about the form, such as the control number, edition date, and page numbers or letters, usually at the left. This location enables reference information to be visible in most types of bindings and makes it easier to locate forms in the stockroom. Forms that have multiple pages or that are printed on both sides should carry a footer on each page. This assists printing, completion, and insertion in the patient record. The edition date is particularly important in ensuring that only the current version of the form is used and that obsolete versions are destroyed. Also included in the header or footer is a place to imprint the patient's name and health record number. There should be a place to imprint the patient's name and number on all pages of a multipage form or on each side of double-sided forms.

Introduction and Instructions

The introduction should explain the purpose of the form. The title is often sufficient, but occasionally patients and others outside the organization may need a subtitle and an additional explanation to understand the form's intent to complete it appropriately. The history form to be completed by the patient is an example.

Body and Close

The body contains the main content of the form, and the close provides the space for authenticating or approving signatures. The documentation method and the data item to be completed should determine the appropriate size of entry space to be drawn on the form. The amount of information a form can contain is significantly affected by spacing. For example, computer-printed or typewritten words require $\frac{1}{16}$-inch vertical height, whereas handwritten words require $\frac{1}{3}$-inch. When multiple-copy forms, such as carbon or no-carbon-required (NCR) packs are used, more space may be needed for handwritten material because of the need to increase handwriting pressure, which frequently results in larger handwriting size.

Fonts

Type styles should be well chosen and contribute to readability. Items of similar importance should be equal in size and type, and the number of different fonts used should be few. Italics and boldface characters should be used to maintain the effect of emphasis only. Style considerations may include the requirement to use a specified font type that is identified with the name and logo of the organization.

Barcodes and Optical Character Recognition

Forms may include machine-readable representations of data. One example, indicated on the upper left of Figure 4-4, is optical character recognition (OCR). Another is a barcode, which is made up by varying the widths and spacings of parallel lines. Either of these technologies can be used to identify forms for scanning and retrieval. Barcodes are used in other health care applications for patient identification, medication administration, and processing laboratory specimens.

Rules and Lines

Rules are vertical or horizontal lines that structure the form. They may vary in style but serve to divide the form into logical sections and to direct data entry length and location. If several people have areas to complete, the data sets each person is to document should be presented in the order of

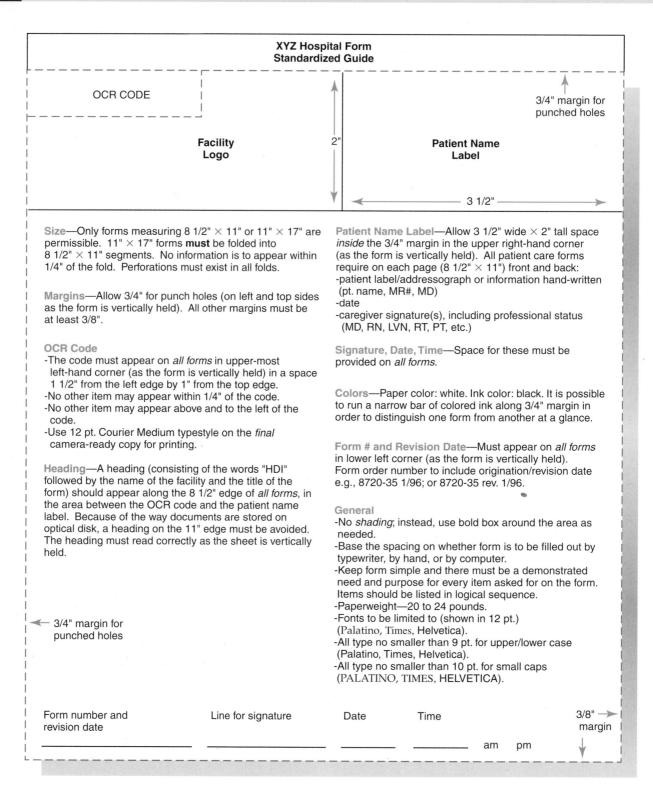

FIGURE 4-4 Vertical forms guide.

completion. Heavy lines can help to separate sections of the form visually. Horizontal lines on forms are desirable for long sections of the forms that are handwritten. Examples are forms for handwritten progress notes and physicians' orders. Rules are often used to create smaller sections or boxes for data on a form, such as the top section of the admission/discharge record (face sheet). Vertical and

horizontal rules should be aligned as much as possible to make the form less "busy" visually. Box titles or captions should be located to the upper left of the boxes in small font sizes. Check boxes or lines (sometimes called *ballot boxes*) are other time-savers that conserve space and improve legibility. When check boxes or lines are used, there should be consistency throughout the form whether the boxes or lines are to the immediate left or immediate right of the caption. These should be aligned vertically when appropriate. The box or line to check should be very close to the caption so that the person performing the documentation checks the correct line or box.

Borders

Rules that frame a section are called *borders*. Borders are preferable to screening or shading, which often causes indistinct electronic copies and transmissions. Some sections may be intentionally obscured or blacked out when, for confidentiality, data items are not desired on every copy of a form. Borders around an entire form create a margin. Margins provide visual appeal as well as being important for printing. For example, a space of ¾ inch may be necessary for punched holes, and allowances may be needed for printing equipment. Forms that are to be typed should have at least a ½-inch margin at the bottom to avoid paper slippage in the platen when typing near the bottom of the page.

Production Considerations

If data are to be entered on a computer screen or view and then printed on a preprinted paper form (e.g., billing form, patient care plan form), refer to the vendor or machine specifications for correct data placement. If the form is not designed appropriately, data will not be printed in the exact locations required on the form. If data entry on a form is to be done by typewriter, the spacing and alignments should be carefully designed to avoid constant readjustment of the forms in the machine while typing. Forms to be completed by handwriting need adequate space. Discussing such specifications with a printer or the purchasing department is important in all aspects of form design.

Beyond design guidelines, paper forms require some production considerations. The master is the original from which copies are produced. Masters may be designed and produced internally by desktop publishing software or advanced word processing techniques and a high-resolution laser printer. This approach is quick, easy, and cost-effective, particularly when photocopying is the method of duplication. When more elaborate and formal printing is desired, the master should be created by a professional typesetter. In either case, the master should be carefully proofread before reproduction.

Physical building of the form refers to its size and special properties. Using standard-sized paper, such as 8½ × 11 inches, keeps costs low and facilitates copying and filing. When double-sided forms are used, it is important to include the word "over" because of the need to turn them over when photocopying, microfilming, or scanning. Oversized forms involve similar special copying considerations because they require reduction or other special handling. Undersized forms that are to be pasted, in a shingled manner, onto health record forms should be avoided because of extra time needed for chart preparation when photocopying, scanning, or filming.

Multipart forms require planning to provide sufficient copies and construction with carbon sheets, carbon spots, or NCR paper. This packet of pages creates a forms set that is precollated and prefastened with a perforated stub. The advantages of multipart forms include standardization; having to write data only once, which reduces mistakes; and being able to provide quick, inexpensive copies. The disadvantages include the limited number of copies that these forms can create. Although copies in carbon packs are easier to read and more copies can be made per original than NCR copies, the carbon paper between the copies must be removed, which creates waste. Ink smears on copies and hands frequently result when tearing the carbon sets apart. NCR copies, although cleaner, are difficult to read, especially the copies beyond two or three in the set, and the ink can fade with time. Photocopies of NCR copies are nearly impossible to read. Extra copies that are created and not used in multipart forms diminish any original savings and produce additional waste.

Forms may be produced as individual form sets or as a continuous-feed strip. Forms may also be prepared as unit sets consisting of single forms glued along one edge to create a pad. Paper has many features, including weight grade, grain, and finish. These aspects combine to affect the form's suitability, durability, and permanence. Suitability reflects how easy the paper is to read and write on (e.g., does the ink smear because it is too grainy?), durability concerns how well a form stands up to handling, and permanence reflects how long the paper lasts in hard copy. It is extremely important that the paper's weight is suitable for use with copiers, facsimile machines, and scanning equipment. A weight of 20 to 24 pounds is recommended for health records. For electronic, environmental, and cost reasons, white paper is recommended. If color is necessary, a tinted border may be used. The ink should be a standard black because this type reproduces best and should meet scanning specifications. The use of additional text colors should be limited because it adds to the cost of the form.

Duplicating methods include in-house preparation and commercial printing. In-house preparation entails the creation of the master and reproduction, most commonly by photocopying. Because this method is expensive, it is most suitable for a trial period or when only a small quantity of forms is needed. The same in-house master can be used for offset printing and is more cost-effective for large quantities. The commercial printer is also best for providing value-added features, such as hole punching, perforating, collating, carbonizing, and prenumbering, which can be done in conjunction with the printing process. (See the forms design activity in the supplements.)

Computer View/Screen Format Design

Computer views share the following general design features with paper forms:

- Needs of user
- Purpose of view
- Selection and sequencing of essential data items
- Standardization of terminology, abbreviations, and formats

FIGURE 4-5 Sample master patient index-view. Elsevier © 2014. SimChart for the Medical Office® (www.evolve.elsevier.com).

- Provision of instructions
- Attention to simplification

There are profound differences as well. The computer view refers to the screen format for both data entry and monitor output. Figure 4-5 illustrates a sample MPI computer view. The power of database management systems allows tremendous flexibility in which views are created for data capture and data displays, including still and moving images and sound as well as text and graphs—all in living color. Computer views require menus of alternatives to be developed and screen or window formats that may include spots to touch with a finger or light pen. It is helpful to remember that standards such as those of ASTM are only a foundation from which to begin the process of selecting data items. Once captured, the data elements may be retrieved in new configurations to meet the needs of different user groups. For example, a physician may want to view graphs that show the trends of laboratory data along with a menu of therapy options with costs, supported by a reference from a linked database. A social worker developing a discharge plan may select a summary of the patient's functional level, living arrangements, and insurance benefits to compare with services provided and prices charged by local home health care providers. This flexibility lends to both the promise and the problems of designing computer views.

Online System Interface

A person entering or viewing data encounters computer logic at the boundary where users and computers meet online—the system interface. Good interface design helps make this interaction user-friendly while reducing errors. Windows is the most common interface format, in which each window can show information drawn from a different source or database table. In some situations, systems can run separate applications in independent windows. Figure 4-6 shows such a graphical user interface (GUI), with tabs and a tool bar at the top. Well-designed screen views or forms for data entry make it possible to:

- Organize the data entry fields in logical format.
- Include field edits.
- Include passwords to add, delete, or modify data.
- Allow simultaneous entry or updating in many tables at one time.
- Include brief instructions on the screens or provide more lengthy help screens.
- Make the screens attractive through the use of color, lines, borders, and so on.
- Use default values in a field to eliminate the need to key repeated data between entries (e.g., the date field could be automatically set up to add today's date without the need to key the characters).
- Allow automatic sequential numbering (e.g., accession register numbers).
- Show data on the screen from a different table when the key field is entered (e.g., for the MPI screen form, when the doctor's number is entered, the doctor's name, address, and so on can automatically appear on the screen).
- Develop or customize menus or submenus to add, delete, or change data.

Windows-style interfaces provide menus that pull down from choices shown on a tool bar at the top of the screen. A menu is an important component of a computer view because it is central to ease of navigation. Therefore a carefully constructed sequence of menus is part of a comprehensive design. Windows interfaces are used not only on personal computers, but also on mainframe and minicomputer systems.

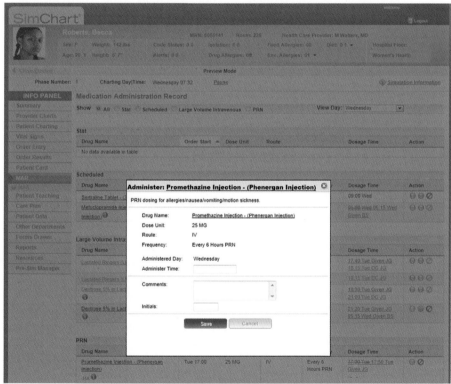

FIGURE 4-6 Graphical user interface. Arrow is pointing to tool bar. Elsevier © 2014. SimChart for the Medical Office® (www.evolve.elsevier.com).

Other Display Features

In comparison to an 8½ × 11-inch sheet of paper, the computer page or view offers a wide variety of options from viewing multiple windows to using dual monitors, some with very large screens. The number of characters per line and number of lines per view vary among monitors and software, many of which allow the user to change the size of the view. With smaller screens or mobile devices, more views are required to collect an equivalent amount of data. The advantages are that segments of a paper form completed by different practitioners can be separated for individual attention. The fact that the EHR completes part of the view with stored data is also a major advantage. Text displays can be customized with different background and font colors. Color coding text and menus can be helpful to distinguish special features, such as instructions. Blinking may be added to characters or words to attract the user's attention, and scrolling moves the screen up or down a line or page at a time. As with paper forms, special features should be kept to a minimum to enhance their emphasis and simplify the view.

General Control Principles

View identification is key to control. If the view does not have a name or number, reference to that view is subject to a great deal of misunderstanding. As mentioned, paper forms should contain a control number on each page, and computer views should be identified on the screen or in the system's written documentation. Users should not develop or customize their own data entry views without approval of their supervisors or form or view management team. Although substantial advantages of view customization are flexibility and the related user satisfaction, it is not without its disadvantages. The need to ensure that all data elements are collected, that an audit trail of views is available for legal purposes, and that confidentiality is maintained requires that standardization programs, procedural guidelines, and input and output controls be developed.

Computer systems also involve cost considerations. The paper output from the EHR system can vary from a simple printout of data entered to volumes of daily and summary reports. In all, the volume can easily exceed that generated in a paper health record environment. The output can be programmed to happen automatically or can be requested by use of report generators, and it can easily become overwhelming. To control output as well as information overload and its associated costs and confidentiality risks, the form or view management team must include the paper output in its scope of concerns.

Forms and Views Summary

Well-designed forms or views facilitate work by guiding the user through data entry, interpretation, and validation. They also contribute to the quantity and quality of work performed. A continuing process of review and revision maximizes the benefits by clarifying ambiguities and collecting only necessary data items, which allows time to be devoted to other activities. Other chapters of this text explore the range of issues related to data analysis, evaluation, use, and access.

 SELF-ASSESSMENT QUIZ

16. Who should be included in the forms and views design team?
17. Are there required forms, views, or formats for the health record? What are good sources?
18. Research, then compare and contrast the chart order from various facilities.
19. In addition to the health record, what other HIM functions benefit from good forms and views design?

HEALTH RECORD FLOW AND PROCESSING

The patient health record begins with the patient's arrival at admission or registration and is developed with the forms and documentation guidelines described previously. Figure 4-7 illustrates the model flow of the inpatient record in both the document-based and database environments. Currently a wide variety of hybrid versions of record systems exist. After admission, the MPI/EMPI is queried for the patient's unique personal identifier number. The MPI/EMPI is the most essential HIM tool in an organization that numbers its records because it is the bridge between the patient and the record number. Extensive guidance is given by AHIMA in the development and maintenance of the MPI. During and after patient care, key reports such as the H&P are dictated, transcribed, and added to the patient chart. These reports and other documentation are completed and authenticated. After patient discharge, the paper record is forwarded to the HIM department for retrospective completion. Assembly is the arrangement of the chart in the designated chart order. Quantitative and qualitative analyses are described later. Diagnoses and procedures are coded and abstracted for reimbursement and statistics. When complete, the chart is archived in the permanent file. Migration to a database model for the EHR and for record processing is increasingly providing numerous advantages, including facilitating the provision of records from previous episodes of care, more rapid inclusion of dictated and transcribed reports, promotion of authentication at the time of care, and more rapid completion and abstracting. Chapter 6 provides additional insight into the advantages of the EHR.

Medical Transcription

Several of the key reports in the health record are routinely dictated by the provider, including the H&P, operative report, consultation, and discharge summary in acute care. Other dictated reports may include pathology, radiology and diagnostic imaging, and progress notes. After providers dictate the report, the content is retrieved by medical transcriptionists who use word processing software or "Dragon" voice recognition software in which dictated words appear in a document, which is then edited by the transcriptionist or document editor to create the completed document for authentication and inclusion in the original health record. As organizations move increasingly toward the EHR, providers are using voice recognition technology to dictate reports for editing to facilitate timely electronic access. The format of reports is included in the responsibilities of the forms, views, and templates design team.

Transcription is a core function in the flow of health record information in many organizations and requires specific management attention. As we have seen in the previous discussion, several important reports have accreditation and regulatory time frames for completion (for example, availability of the H&P on the chart within 24 hours). Providers

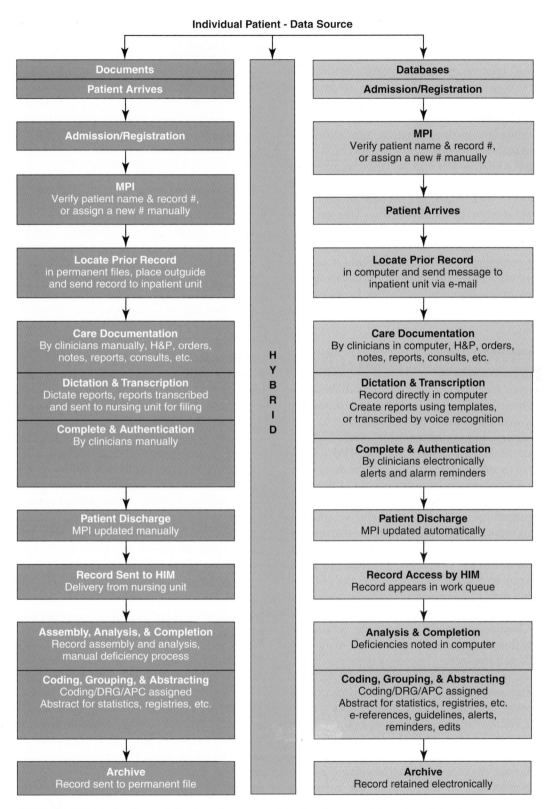

FIGURE 4-7 Model flow of the inpatient record in the document-based and database environments. A wide variety of hybrid versions may exist that combine documents and databases. *APC*; *DRG,* diagnosis-related group; *HIM,* health information management; *H&P,* history and physical examination; *MPI,* master patient/person index.

depend on a prompt turnaround time for patient care. Because slow turnaround time for reports may compromise patient care, delay record completion, and affect the ability to meet compliance objectives, management processes must be put in place and closely monitored. Resources are available from the AHDI. The next section addresses additional record completion requirements.

Transcriptionists are medical language specialists who bring important skills to the HIM team. Certification is available through the AHDI, which also provides resources for management (http://www.ahdionline.org). Staffing may be provided internally with employees on site or at home, through contract services, or by outsourcing. Transcription systems must be purchased and interfaced with other computer systems. Dictation is increasingly digital and may include voice recognition software. Transcription is accomplished by use of word processing software, including special references. These management and technology issues are discussed in other chapters.

METHODS TO ENSURE DATA QUALITY

HIM professionals have always been concerned about the quality of information in both primary and secondary health records and have used various methods to help ensure the accuracy and completeness of these records. Data quality activities are a priority for the HIM professional because of the many users and uses of the data; these functions have a sharper focus with the advent of the EHR because the model changes from ensuring data quality through documentation audits and retrospective completion of missing reports to designing systems that ensure data quality at the point of service and then monitoring the effectiveness of these systems. TJC's current approach to continuing record review is consistent with the philosophy of expecting data to be recorded concurrent with the patient care event and monitoring to see that it happens. In The Joint Commission model, the facility determines what should be monitored and uses a sample of records or data to track performance.

The accuracy of data depends on the manual or computer information system design for collecting, recording, storing, processing, accessing, and displaying data and on the ability and follow-through of the people involved in each phase of these activities. One crucial way to ensure the accuracy of data is to develop systems that ensure accuracy and timeliness of documentation at the point of care, to monitor the output, and to take appropriate corrective action when needed.

Before the QI study approach to assessing data quality is discussed, it is helpful to review the concepts of record content review and retrospective record completion activities related to that content because historically that process was one of the primary methods to obtain missing data and authentications. It was also the basis for TJC's record deficiency standards (Table 4-8).

TABLE 4-8	The Joint Commission and Delinquent Medical Records

The presence of a complete medical record for each patient is highly valued by TJC. Three EPs for acute care are of particular importance.

- The hospital defines a complete record and the time frame within which the record much be completed after discharge, not to exceed 30 days after discharge.
- The hospital measures medical record delinquency at regular intervals, no less frequently than every 3 months.
- The number of delinquent records is greater than 50% of the average number of discharged patients per quarter, over the previous 12 months.
- Failure to meet the criteria is grounds for Conditional Accreditation if the total number of delinquent medical records averaged over the 12 months before survey is greater than or equal to twice the average monthly patient discharge rate.

EP, Element of performance; *TJC,* The Joint Commission.
From The Joint Commission: *Comprehensive accreditation manual for hospitals (CAMH), scoring guidelines,* Chicago, 2013, The Joint Commission.

The presence of a complete medical record for each patient is highly valued by TJC. Three elements of performance for acute care are of particular importance:

- The hospital defines a complete record and the time frame within which the record must be completed after discharge, not to exceed 30 days after discharge.
- The hospital measures medical record delinquency at regular intervals, no less frequently than every 3 months.
- If the number of delinquent records is greater than 50% of the average number of discharged patients per quarter over the previous 12 months, verify the context. Failure to meet the criteria is grounds for conditional accreditation if the total number of delinquent medical records averaged over the 12 months before the survey is greater than or equal to twice the average monthly patient discharge rate.[5]

Record Content Review and Retrospective Completion

The review of patient records for documentation accuracy and completeness has always been a functional role of the HIM department staff in all types of health care facilities. This review has been necessary because of the variety of sources of patient record information and the large number of entries made by different professionals in the patient's record on a daily basis. If the health care provider has a busy day or if internal systems for ensuring the presence of required content or authentications are not adequate, documentation may be inadvertently omitted or inaccurate.

The thoroughness and method of this evaluation have evolved over time in an attempt to meet licensure, certification, and accreditation standards for completion and timeliness of documentation. In the past, the HIM department in an inpatient, long-term care, or home health setting used a traditional approach and performed a detailed review, or quantitative analysis, of all predischarge or postdischarge patient records for the presence of required reports and authentications and then obtained the signature or reports retrospectively, often weeks or months after the event. Although the quality of the data within the reports was not evaluated, the analyses did help to ensure the eventual presence of authentications and categories of data required by the standard-setting agencies. The usefulness and legal value of these late reports and signatures, however, were doubtful.

The related process of statistical analysis, or abstracting, is performed to select specific data items from medical records for clinical and administrative decision making. Uses range from billing and case-mix analysis to selection of cases for quality review. Data sets, discussed later in this chapter, identify the core data items and their definitions. Statistical analysis also uses nomenclatures and classification systems, indexes and registers, and statistical methods. These topics are discussed in separate chapters.

In the traditional retrospective data collection process, after the patient's paper record has been received in the HIM department on discharge from a health care facility, clerical staff assemble the record forms in a prescribed order (or leave the recording in the "universal" order) and then review all records for missing authentications and reports. Although categories of information reviewed vary with each facility, those typically checked include the following:

- Listings of principal and secondary diagnoses on discharge
- Presence of discharge summaries, history, physical reports, and operative or procedure reports

In addition, forms are checked to see whether there is correct patient identification on every page (front and back) and if all physician reports, progress notes, and orders are authenticated by the appropriate resident or attending physician. Some facilities may review for the presence of other reports and authorizations. Documentation review may be performed at the nursing unit while the patient is still active. If the record is incomplete, a deficiency slip is prepared by the analyst that itemizes missing documentation or signatures (Figure 4-8). Pages are flagged with colored tabs at the location of missing signatures, and appropriate HIM department procedures are followed to obtain these from the physician or other providers.

The method used to assist physicians in record completion after patient discharge varies by facility and includes either a manual or a computer system of physician notification, record location tracking, and administrative reporting. One copy of the deficiency slip is usually attached to the record. The incomplete record is either placed in a designated record completion area or interfiled in the main record storage area.

If the retrospective completion process is in use at the facility, it usually has a requirement that providers complete reports and records according to the time frame specified in organization policies and procedures, and in the medical staff bylaws, rules, and regulations. The requirements in policies and procedures are based on good professional practice, laws and regulations, and accreditation standards. When an incomplete record has not been finished within the time specified, it is termed a delinquent record. Most hospitals have some type of physician sanction when delinquent records exist. Some may impose fines on the basis of the number of delinquent records. Others may temporarily place a physician on a suspension or no-admissions list until delinquent records are completed. In this instance, physicians may not admit patients or arrange surgery for unscheduled patients unless authorization is received from the chief of staff or designated hospital administrator.

Because of the seriousness of the sanctions for both the physician and the hospital, and the amount of resources used in a paper environment, it is extremely important that the detailed retrospective completion process be reviewed to determine whether it should continue. The HIM professional should take the lead in encouraging the facility to evaluate this process because this is not a value-added activity related to quality data, and it is an expensive activity for the facility. If the medical staff, hospital administration, and legal counsel deem it important to continue detailed deficiency analysis in a paper-based environment, then policies and procedures must be specific. For example, if the procedure for obtaining signatures retrospectively is to continue, then the review should be done on a predischarge basis to obtain the signatures as close to data entry as possible. Only orders that the medical staff consider potentially hazardous to the patient as outlined in the medical staff's rules and regulations should be checked for authentication. Only key reports should be monitored to determine whether they are present with follow-up as appropriate. They include the H&P, operative reports, consultations, pathology reports, radiology reports, and discharge summary. Although some of these reports may be received after patient discharge and are of questionable value to the hospital at that point, they are still helpful to follow-up facilities that are treating the patient, which rely on the data in these reports. The reports would be more valuable, however, if they were sent to them at the time of patient transfer to the facility or organization.

DATA QUALITY MONITORING METHODS AND SOLUTIONS

If the database system is developed to allow data quality capture and reporting and if point-of-care systems are designed to capture data correctly, the next step is to monitor data in patient records and secondary reporting systems to determine possible quality problems so that corrective action can be taken when necessary.

Quality Assessment and Improvement Study of Patient Record Documentation

One method to evaluate data quality is to do a QI study of a sample of paper or computerized patient records that assesses the presence of reports and authentications and the quality of the information documented in the entries.

| Patient Name: _____   MR# _____   Admission Date: _____ |

Name of Report	Attending Physician	Physician/Practitioner #2	Physician/Practitioner #3
Inpatient Face Sheet	Complete – Sign No abbreviations		
Discharge Summary	Dictate – Sign		
History & Physical	Dictate – Sign		
Consultation Report		Dictate – Sign	Dictate – Sign
Progress Note: Admit	Document Date Sign		
Progress Note: Daily	Document Date Sign	Document Date Sign	Document Date Sign
Progress Note: Discharge	Document Date Sign		
Physician/Provider Orders	Document Date Sign	Document Date Sign	Document Date Sign
Discharge Order	Document Date Sign		
Operative Report	Dictate Sign	Dictate Sign	Dictate Sign
Anesthesia Report	Document/Sign	Document/Sign	Document/Sign
Pathology Report		Dictate Sign	Dictate Sign
Radiology Report		Dictate Sign	Dictate Sign
Other	Document Date Sign	Document Date Sign	Document Date Sign
Other	Document Dictate Date Sign	Document Dictate Date Sign	Document Dictate Date Sign

Instructions: Review the patient record, identify the physicians/practitioners, and circle the deficiency requiring completion. Form number and date

FIGURE 4-8 Inpatient Quantitative Analysis Deficiency slip.

The purpose is not to obtain data retrospectively but to monitor the adequacy of current systems and to make changes in the information system when needed.

Quantitative Analysis

Performing a quantitative analysis means ensuring the following:

- Patient identification on every paper form (front and back) and screen is correct.
- All necessary authorizations or consents are present and signed or authenticated by the patient or legal representative, including those for general agreement, specific procedures, photographs, experimental treatment, advance directives, and autopsy.
- Documented diagnoses POA, principal diagnosis on discharge, secondary diagnoses, and procedures are present in the appropriate form or location within the record. This information is completed and authenticated by the physician or authorized clinician.
- Discharge summary is present, when required, and authenticated.
- H&P are present, documented within the time frame required by appropriate regulations, and authenticated as appropriate.
- Consultation report is present and authenticated when a consultation request appears in the listing of physician or practitioner orders.
- All diagnostic tests ordered by the physician or practitioner are present and authenticated by comparing physician orders, financial bill, and the test reports documented in the patient's health record.
- An admitting progress note, a discharge progress note, and an appropriate number of notes (frequency depends on the type of case or HCO) documented by physicians or clinicians throughout the patient's care process are present.
- Each physician or practitioner order entered into the record is authenticated. An admitting and a discharge physician or practitioner order is present. Orders are present for all consultations, diagnostic tests, and procedures when these reports are found in the record.
- Operative, procedure, or therapy reports are present and authenticated when orders, consent forms, or other documentation in the record indicates that they were performed.
- A pathology report is present and authenticated when the operative report indicates that tissue was removed.
- Preoperative, operative, and postoperative anesthesia reports are present and authenticated.
- Nursing or ancillary health professionals' reports and notes are present and authenticated.
- Reports required for patients treated in specialized units, such as those for patients receiving care in the obstetrics unit, neonatal nursery, or mental health or rehabilitation units, are present and authenticated.
- Preliminary and final autopsy reports on patients who have died at the facility are present and authenticated.

The amount of detailed checking varies by facility according to the nature of the QI study, type of HCO, and facility policy.

Qualitative Analysis

A qualitative analysis involves the following checks:

- Review for obvious documentation inconsistencies related to diagnoses found on admission forms, physical examination, operative and pathology reports, care plans, and discharge summary.
- Analyze the record to determine whether documentation written by various health care providers for one patient reflects consistency.
- Compare the patient's pharmacy drug profile or medical orders with the MAR to determine consistency.
- Review an inpatient record to determine whether it reflects the general location of the patient at all times or whether serious time gaps exist. Times noted on nursing documentation indicating when the patient left the unit and returned to it can be used as the reference point for this type of study.
- Determine whether the patient record reflects the progression of care, including the symptoms, diagnoses, tests, treatments, reasons for the treatments, results, patient education, location of patient after discharge, and follow-up plans.
- Interview the patient or family. Review recorded patient demographic information and medical history with the patient several hours or days after admission to determine completeness and accuracy. A patient may be too physically ill or mentally confused at admission or the family may be too preoccupied with the patient to provide valid data.
- Compare written instructions to the patient that are documented in the record with the patient's or family's understanding of those instructions. Ask the patient or family to repeat instructions to verify consistency.
- Review for other documentation as determined by the individual facility.

The results are presented to the appropriate medical or clinical staff committee for appropriate follow-up.

Legal Analysis

A legal analysis consists of checking for the following:

- Entries are documented in ink if a paper record or recorded on other legally recognized media, such as microfilm or a disk. The entries are legible and timely.
- If gaps in documentation appear on handwritten pages, such as progress notes, orders, or nurses' notes, a line is drawn through this area to prevent future tampering.
- Entries are authenticated by the person who made the observation or who conducted the test or treatment.
- If regulations, standards, or hospital policy requires an attending physician to complete a report and if the report is written by a resident, the report should reflect authentication by both persons. Examples are physical examinations, consultations, and operative reports.

- Errors in documentation are corrected in a legal manner. Amendments include alteration of the health information by modification, correction, addition, or deletion or by documentation in the wrong record. All amendments should be made in an explicit and timely manner. For paper records, a single line is drawn through the error, the phrase *error in entry* or synonymous words are written, the new information is inserted, and the corrected entry is dated and authenticated by the person making the change. This process leaves the change in view whether it is a modification, a correction, or a deletion. Amended entries should be readily identifiable to readers, with the original entry retained and linked to the amendment. For computerized records, policies and procedures must be established to track the process accurately from error identification or request for amendment through the completion of the amendment or its possible denial. ASTM Standard 2017-99 addresses amendments in a computerized health information system. See Chapter 6 for additional discussion of amendments in an EHR.
- No misfiled documents are present.

Special Concerns of Alternative Care Settings

The HIM professional must design a flexible approach to ensuring data quality that considers the type of health care facility, its data requirements, level of technology available, type of health care providers who are the major sources of documentation, types of common documentation problems, and results related to missing documentation (e.g., loss of revenue). Whether retrospective documentation should occur is a decision to be made by the facility administrator, medical staff or medical director, and legal counsel with advice from the HIM professional. However, accuracy of documentation at the point of care should be emphasized and quality studies of samples of clinical records are appropriate.

Clinical Staff Activities Related to Data Quality

Medical Record Committee

Responsibility for the timeliness and accuracy of patient records is shared by the clinicians providing care and the organization's staff members who design and support the record system. The committee is often composed of representatives of the medical staff, administration, HIM department, nursing, and other departments or services. Together they develop policies related to analysis of patient records for documentation deficiencies, including items to review, frequency, and types of penalties for incomplete reports. The committee also coordinates activities with clinical staff departments and other medical staff groups related to clinical documentation, such as QI committees and credentialing committees. If no separate medical record committee exists, these functions are carried out by other committees. For example, in a hospital setting with an open medical staff, relevant documentation policies developed by the medical record committee, such as loss of admitting privileges for incomplete records, are adopted by the medical staff as a whole and incorporated in medical staff regulations.

Continuing Record Reviews

Hospital medical records should be reviewed on a continuing basis at the point of care and based on organization-defined indicators that address the presence, timeliness, readability (whether handwritten or printed), quality, consistency clarity, accuracy, completeness, and authentication of data and information contained within the record.[5]

In describing the continuing record review process at her hospital, Lewis[7] indicates that a review for documentation refers to the "completeness, adequacy, appropriateness, accuracy, and quality of documentation rather than to the quality of clinical care." A detailed documentation review of a representative sample (5%) of the health records is completed by her hospital's HIM staff, physician reviewers, and nursing staff. HIM personnel review the record for the presence of specified content in reports. For example, the operative report for each surgery is reviewed to determine the presence of a description of the findings, technical approach used, specimens removed, preoperative diagnosis, postoperative diagnosis, surgical indications, estimated blood loss, and detailed description of the procedure performed. Other reports in the record that are reviewed for the presence of content by the HIM staff include the H&P, anesthesia report, discharge summary, consultations, and progress notes.

Lewis[7] further describes the review by the physicians, which relates to the quality of specified content. For example, the physician reads and indicates whether the H&P is adequate to meet requirements, whether the discharge summary has adequate medical information to provide continuity of care, whether progress notes adequately reflect the patient's course in the hospital and are sufficient to permit continuity of care, and so on. Nursing staff review the adequacy of nursing documentation.

Simple check-off review forms have been developed for record analysis. The completed evaluation forms are reviewed by the HIM professional, summarized in report format, and presented to the medical record committee for review and action.

The ability to perform accurate health record reviews for the quality of patient care is affected by the accuracy and completeness of the documentation describing the patient's health history, diagnostic and therapeutic care, examination and test results, and status. For example, ORYX, TJC's performance measurement and improvement initiative first implemented in 1997, moved the accreditation process from a "snapshot" once every 3 years to a continuous QI process. ORYX for hospitals, also known as the *National Hospital Quality Measures,* required hospitals to collect and transmit data on key patient care, treatment, and service issues. Examples of current measures include pneumonia, heart failure, and children's asthma care. The more recent tracer method, which applies to all accredited facilities, places increased emphasis on open medical record review at the point of care.

The HIM director must be familiar with the requirements for all documentation indicators. TJC continually updates its approach to quality reviews. For the most current information, check its website (http://www.jointcommission.org/). TJC and other initiatives are discussed in Chapter 12.

The success of these systems depends on the presence of required information in the health record. Careful planning is needed to develop data systems to meet these requirements. It is crucial that staff members who perform QI studies and those who report results of core measures work jointly with the HIM professional to design the data collection processes and refer documentation problems to the appropriate medical staff committee or other committee and the HIM professional for resolution.

Clinical Documentation Improvement

The recognition of the high volume and complexity of health record data along with the value of accurate clinical documentation for patient safety, quality, and reimbursement, has led to the development of clinical documentation improvement (CDI) programs. Clinical documentation specialists (CDSs) have additional training in documentation rules and regulations, and in opportunities for improvement, and conduct concurrent record review. Credentialing is available through the AHIMA. Initial efforts focused on Medicare-compliant documentation of the principal diagnosis, complications, and comorbidities before discharge to improve reimbursement and quality scores. Initiatives related to hospital-acquired conditions and POA reporting have increased the importance of this role. With their extensive understanding of the health care delivery system and detailed knowledge of coding and related topics, HIM professionals are well suited to this role.[8]

Organization Structure That Encourages Data Quality

The Joint Commission Information Management Standards

TJC's *Comprehensive Accreditation Manual for Hospitals* (CAMH) chapter titled "Information Management" promotes coordination of activities that relate to the acquisition, analysis, and reporting of information within the health care facility.

TJC's standards require the following:
- Institution-wide planning and design of information management processes
- Confidentiality, security, and integrity of information
- Uniform data definitions and methods of data capture
- Education and training in principles of information management by decision makers as well as those who generate, collect, and analyze data and information
- Timely, accurate transmission of data in standardized formats when possible
- Integration and reporting of data with linkages of patient-care and non–patient-care data across departments and care modes over time

- Detailed list of patient-specific data
- Aggregate data from the entire institution
- Incorporation of knowledge-based information, including the library, formulary, and poison control information, in the information management systems plan
- Contributions to and use of external reference databases

AHIMA actively participated in the development of this Joint Commission standard.

Information Resources Management Committee

Although many HCOs have an information resources management committee (also called *management information system committee, health information systems committee,* or *data quality council*) to coordinate automation activities, not all are truly successful because of the lack of adequate leadership, competition between departments, lack of a mission, and so on. TJC requires coordination of activities, and its information management standard can help to focus more centralized planning within a facility.[5] The HIM and information system departments must work closely together to meet TJC information management standards. A chief information officer (CIO) and a chief technology officer (CTO) are management positions in some HCOs. The information resources management committee, with the assistance of the CIO and CTO, assist with hardware and software selections, approve systems to ensure the quality of computer data input activities, ensure the inventory of facility databases and the preparation of data dictionaries, approve the frequency and distribution of computer reports, and approve systems to ensure report accuracy.

Information Governance

Information is increasingly being viewed as a strategic resource. In this era of big data as well as cloud, mobile, and social computing, information assets are growing faster than many organizations can manage within their current structures. Legal cases requiring e-discovery have focused additional attention on risk management. In response to these trends, information governance (IG) structures have begun to emerge. IG expands traditional records management best practices to create a holistic approach to managing enterprise information across all phases of the information life cycle. Data governance, by comparison, focuses on the individual data elements at the operational level. IG focuses on the enterprise level and data as a business asset.

Gartner is a leading information technology research and advisory company (http://www.gartner.com). Their online *IT Glossary* includes the definition of IG shown in Box 4-3. Gartner recommends processes, roles, standards, and metrics to ensure the effective and efficient use of information. They stress accountability, rather than coercion, to encourage right behavior.

As with other data-related initiatives, IG benefits from the participation of a wide variety of stakeholders. Although IT departments own the systems used to create, store, and secure information, it is the users who know the value and

BOX 4-3   Information Governance

Information governance is the specification of decision rights and an accountability framework to encourage desirable behavior in the valuation, creation, storage, use, archival, and deletion of information. It includes the processes, roles, standards, and metrics that ensure the effective and efficient use of information in enabling an organization to achieve its goals.

Gartner *IT Glossary*. http://www.gartner.com/it-glossary/information-governance. Accessed November 27, 2013.

what needs to be saved. Compliance and risk management add additional levels of complexity. There may be a single committee in smaller organizations, whereas large health systems may have separate committees for administration and clinical information as well as infrastructure. Regardless of the type and number of committees, the goal is to create an information accountability structure and culture that minimizes costs, manages risks, and maximizes value.

The electronic discovery reference model was created in 2005 to address the lack of standards in e-discovery. It has evolved into an industry community of more than 250 organizations and 900 experts (http://www.edrm.net). Their Information Governance Reference Model (IGRM) version 3 (Figure 4-9) provides an informative graphic illustrating information as an asset linked to duty and value. To quote

their final report, "The IGRM is a tool that reinforces and illustrates the inter-connectivity of people and processes required for effective information governance." HIM professionals can gain insight from their framework.

Activity

View this slideshow as an example of an executive summary on the importance of information governance in managing risks, reducing costs, and maximizing the value of information. http://www.slideshare.net/norwiz/information-governance-26272383.

Characteristics of Data Quality

As the health record continues the migration path from paper-based to a hybrid environment, to the fully implemented EHR, definitions of quality must become increasingly precise.

Definitions

The term *quality* has several meanings according to the dictionary. The following definitions are especially pertinent to the HIM professional:
1. A degree of excellence of a thing
2. A required character or property that belongs to a thing's essential nature

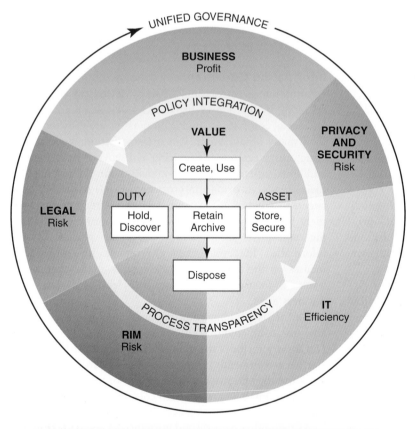

FIGURE 4-9 Information Governance Reference Model (IGRM) V. 3.0

Duty:	Value:	Asset:
Legal obligation for specific information	Utility or business purpose of specific information	Specific container of information

TABLE 4-9   Characteristics of Data Quality

Accessibility: Data items should be easily obtainable and legal to collect.

Accuracy: Data are the correct values and are valid.

Comprehensiveness: All required data items are included. Ensure that the entire scope of the data is collected, and document intentional limitations.

Consistency: The value of the data should be reliable and the same across applications.

Currency: The data should be up to date. A datum value is up to date if it is current for a specific point in time. It is outdated if it was current at some preceding time yet incorrect at a later time.

Definition: Clear definitions should be provided so that current and future data users will know what the data mean. Each data element should have clear meaning and acceptable values.

Granularity: The attributes and values of data should be defined at the correct level of detail.

Precision: Data values should be just large enough to support the application or process.

Relevancy: The data are meaningful to the performance of the process or application for which they are collected.

Timeliness: Timeliness is determined by how the data are being used and their context.

The expression *data quality* suggests the correctness of data. When reference is made to the "qualities of data," however, the characteristics or attributes that make up data or factual information are implied (Table 4-9). Both concepts are integral in the development of health information systems and the subsequent monitoring of data to ensure that the information produced is accurate and dependable.

The quality of data is the outcome of data quality management (DQM). DQM skills and roles are not new to HIM professionals. To illustrate them, the AHIMA first published "Practice Brief: Data Quality Management Model" in 1998 with an updated version in 2012.[9] A checklist to assess DQM efforts is included. The DQM functions involve continuous data QI throughout the enterprise and include data application, collection, analysis, and warehousing. The practice brief includes a graphic of the DQM domains as they relate to the characteristics of data integrity and examples of each characteristic within each domain. The model is generic and adaptable to any care setting and for any application. It is a tool or model for HIM professionals to make the transition into organization or entity-wide DQM roles. For the purpose of this chapter, the 10 characteristics and their relationship to data collection are provided. The full practice brief should be consulted for further details.

Accessibility

Data items should be easily obtainable and legal to collect. When the data collection instrument is developed, methods to obtain needed data and ensure that the best, least costly method is selected should be used. The amount of accessible data may be increased through system interfaces and integration of systems. For example, the best and easiest method to obtain demographic information may be to obtain it from an existing system. Another method may be to assign data collection by the expertise of each team member. For example, the admission staff collects demographic data, the nursing staff collects symptoms, and the HIM staff assigns codes. Team members should be assigned accordingly.

Accuracy

Data are the correct values, and they are valid. In data collection, ensuring accuracy involves appropriate education and training and timely and appropriate communication of data definitions to those who collect data. The data represent what was intended or defined by their official source, are objective or unbiased, and comply with known standards. For example, data accuracy helps ensure that if a patient's sex is female, it is accurately recorded as female and not male.

Comprehensiveness

All required data items are included. Ensure that the entire scope of the data is collected and document intentional limitations. Cost-effective comprehensive data collection may be achieved by interface with or download from other automated systems. Data definition and data precision affect comprehensive data collection (see these characteristics in the following subsections).

Consistency

The value of the data should be reliable and the same across applications. In data collection, the use of data definitions, extensive training, standardized data collection (procedures, rules, edits, and process), and integrated or interfaced systems facilitates consistency.

Currency

The data should be up to date. A datum is up to date if it is current for a specific point in time. It is outdated if it was current at some preceding time yet incorrect at a later time. Data definitions change or are modified over time. These should be documented so that current and future users know what the data mean. These changes should be communicated in a timely manner to those collecting data and to the end users.

Data Definition

Clear definitions should be provided so that current and future data users know what the data mean. Each data element should have clear meaning and acceptable values. Clear, concise data definitions facilitate accurate data collection. For example, the definition of patient disposition may be "the patient's anticipated location or status after release or discharge." Acceptable values for this data element should be defined. The instrument of collection should include data definitions and ensure that data integrity characteristics are managed.

Granularity

The attributes and values of data should be defined at the correct level of detail. Collect data at the appropriate level of detail or granularity. For example, the temperature of 100° F may be recorded. The granularity for recording outdoor temperatures is different from that for recording patient temperatures. If patient Jane Doe's temperature is 100° F, does that mean 99.6° F or 100.4° F? Appropriate granularity for this application dictates that the data need to be recorded to the first decimal point, whereas appropriate granularity for recording outdoor temperatures may not require it.

Precision

Data values should be just large enough to support the application or process. To collect data precise enough for the application, acceptable values or value ranges for each data item must be defined. For example, values for age may include a four-digit year of birth or may use age categories for some uses, that is, a patient satisfaction survey.

Relevance

Relevance means that the data are meaningful to the performance of the process or application for which they are collected. To better ensure relevance, a pilot of the data collection instrument should be completed to validate its use. A "parallel" test may also be appropriate, completing the new or revised instrument and the current process simultaneously. Results should be communicated to those collecting data and to the end users. Changes should be facilitated or negotiated as needed across disciplines or users.

Timeliness

Timeliness is determined by how the data are being used and their context. Timely data collection is a function of the process and collection instrument.

Data Integrity

There is a major focus on data integrity because of the increased interest in data exchange and data mapping.

Integrity is the property that data are true to the source and have not been altered or destroyed in an unauthorized manner or by unauthorized users, the extent to which data are complete, accurate, consistent, and timely.

It is a security principle that protects information from being modified or otherwise corrupted either maliciously or accidentally. In addition, data are identically maintained during any operation, such as transfer, storage, and retrieval. For example, integrity can be threatened by hardware problems, power outages, and disk crashes, but most often integrity is threatened by application software or viruses. In a database program, data integrity can be threatened if two users are allowed to update the same item or record at the same time. Record or file locking, where only a single user is allowed access to a given record at any one point in time, is one method of ensuring data integrity. In a paper-based system, the integrity of the clinical record system could be at risk when an organization has individuals or departments that keep a "shadow record" or a record at their location in addition to the legal record of the organization. The data from the shadow record may not be incorporated into the legal record of the organization.

DATA NEEDS ACROSS THE HEALTH CARE CONTINUUM

Having explored the general concepts of data collection, we now investigate the specific applications along the health care continuum. As the health care delivery system has diversified, the number of providers and locations with which a patient will interact over a lifetime has multiplied. The following major areas of care are typically identified:

- Acute care
- Ambulatory care (including emergency care and public health)
- Long-term care (including rehabilitation)
- Home health care (including hospice)
- Behavioral health care

Efforts such as those by the NCVHS have taken on the challenge of establishing standard definitions for data elements to enhance the effectiveness and efficiency of electronic data interchange (EDI). Initiatives have been intentionally designed to incorporate the requirements of various previously existing content directives, such as TJC standards; government regulations, including the CMS CoPs for Medicare; and MDSs.

Minimum Data Sets

The purpose of all MDSs, as with the core health data elements, is to promote comparability and compatibility of data by using standard data items with uniform definitions. Although the data items are recommended as a common core, they do not constitute a complete record. In light of the data item definitions provided earlier, their presentation in the following sections has been abbreviated, and only special areas of interest have been highlighted. When any standard or data set is applied, it is important to refer to the most recent edition of the data set. MDSs exist for ambulatory care, acute care, long-term care, and home care. In situations in which an MDS is not available, such as behavioral health, it is appropriate to use core data elements and other data sets as guides.

Acute Care

Acute care, which is provided to hospital inpatients, has the longest history of regulation and accreditation. Hospitals may be small rural community facilities, large urban tertiary care centers, or designed to address the needs of specific patient populations. Acute care was the focus of the early phases of the prospective payment system, which provided incentives to reduce the lengths of stay and contain costs. This mandate has been successful in achieving its goal, with inpatient acute care admissions continuing to decline. As a result, ambulatory care, long-term care, and home health care have all been substantially affected. Because of the resulting change in how patients receive their care, the severity of illness and the intensity of service in acute care hospitals have increased. Because the length of stay in acute care sites is reduced, sicker patients are also being treated in long-term care and home health programs. Although acute care is facing many challenges, it has the advantage of being centralized, with a staff that is sophisticated and well controlled and that has the longest history of documenting patient care.

Data Needs

Acute care hospitals function for three shifts, 7 days a week, every week of the year (sometimes referred to as 24/7/365), and they collect a great deal of highly technical data. The federal CMS CoPs detail the content of the inpatient record expected in hospitals that serve Medicare and Medicaid patients, as does the TJC CAMH Record of Care, Treatment, and Services (RC) standard and state licensing regulations. Most of the basic forms and data described are included in the inpatient record. The MDS that applies in the inpatient hospital segment of the delivery system is the UHDDS.

Uniform Hospital Discharge Data Set

The UHDDS was promulgated by the secretary of the Department of Health, Education, and Welfare in 1974 as a minimum, common core of data on individual hospital discharges in the Medicare and Medicaid programs.[10] As with other MDSs, the purpose was to improve uniformity and comparability of data. The UHDDS has undergone several revisions and is under the direction of the NCVHS of the DHHS. The UHDDS contains the following 20 items and is not segmented. Again, details are limited, and the most current edition should be consulted.

1. Personal identification
2. Date of birth (month, day, and year)
3. Sex
4. Race and ethnicity
5. Residence (usual residence, full address, and zip code [nine-digit zip code, if available])
6. Hospital identification number (Three options are given for this institutional number, with the Medicare provider number as the recommended choice. The federal tax identification number or the American Hospital Association number is preferred to creating a new number.)
7. Admission date (month, day, and year)
8. Type of admission (scheduled or unscheduled)
9. Discharge date (month, day, and year)
10. Attending physician identification (unique physician identification number [UPIN])
11. Operating physician identification (UPIN)
12. Principal diagnosis (the condition established after study to be chiefly responsible for occasioning the admission of the patient to the hospital for care)
13. Other diagnoses (Includes all conditions that coexist at the time of admission or that develop subsequently that affect the treatment received or the length of stay. Diagnoses that relate to an earlier episode and have no bearing on the current hospital stay are excluded.)
14. Qualifier for other diagnoses (A qualifier is given for each diagnosis coded under "other diagnoses" to indicate whether the onset of the diagnosis preceded or followed admission to the hospital. The option "uncertain" is permitted.)
15. External cause-of-injury code (Hospitals should complete this item whenever there is a diagnosis of an injury, poisoning, or adverse effect.)
16. Birth weight of neonate
17. Procedures and dates
    a. All significant procedures are to be reported. A significant procedure is one that (1) is surgical in nature, (2) carries a procedural risk, (3) carries an anesthetic risk, or (4) requires specialized training.
    b. The date of each significant procedure must be reported.
    c. When multiple procedures are reported, the principal procedure is designated. The principal procedure is one that was performed for definitive treatment rather than one performed for diagnostic or exploratory purposes or was necessary to take care of a complication. If two procedures appear to be principal, then the one most related to the principal diagnosis is selected as the principal procedure.
    d. The UPIN of the person performing the principal procedure must be reported.
18. Disposition of the patient
    a. Discharged home (not to home health service)
    b. Discharged to acute care hospital
    c. Discharged to nursing facility
    d. Discharged to home to be under the care of a home health service
    e. Discharged to other health care facility
    f. Left AMA
    g. Alive, other; or alive, not stated
    h. Died
19. Patient's expected source of payment
    a. Primary source
    b. Other source
20. Total charges (List all charges billed by the hospital for this hospitalization. Professional charges for individual patient care by physicians are excluded.)

Special Forms and Views

Most acute care forms have been described previously, although, as mentioned earlier, they are typically more elaborate than those for other sites of care. Of particular note are time frames related to the H&P.

History and Physical Examination

If an H&P was performed within a week before admission, such as in the office of a physician staff member, then a durable, legible copy of this report may be added to the record with any interval changes documented. When the patient is readmitted within 30 days for the same or a related problem, an interval H&P may be completed if the original is readily available.

Issues in Data Collection and Quality

Acute care has the advantage of a long history of improving documentation and data collection. Emphasis on data collection has increased since the implementation of the prospective payment system. Mandates to decrease lengths of stay have required that more data be collected before admission and that data be readily available to expedite treatment. Trends toward ambulatory and home health care have resulted in admissions being limited to the most severely ill patients receiving the most intensive services. Quality issues have been described previously.

Ambulatory Care

Four major trends since the mid-1980s have contributed to the shift away from acute inpatient care toward ambulatory care:

- *Technology* has provided the opportunity for many diagnostic tests, therapies, and surgeries to be done in the outpatient setting. Outpatient surgery visits accounted for approximately 10% of surgeries in 1980, approximately 50% of all surgery visits in 1996, and are projected to approach 75% in the next decade.
- *Reimbursement incentives* provided by government, third-party payers, and business, including prospective payment, encourage the use of this more cost-effective segment of the delivery system. Data from the American Hospital Association show that revenues from outpatient services have doubled from approximately 20% in 1980 to 40% in 2008.
- *Managed care* focuses on the primary care physician as the coordinator (or gatekeeper) of the patient's care, selecting other providers and care sites according to the patient's needs. Use of outpatient services is emphasized and often required to achieve the cost-saving objectives of managed care. The Affordable Care Act and incentives to create patient-centered medical homes will continue this trend.
- *Consumerism,* which has increased since the mid-1960s, has also encouraged the expansion of this alternative to inpatient treatment primarily because of accessibility and convenience.

Ambulatory care, or outpatient care, has emerged as the centerpiece of the U.S. health care delivery system. Physicians' offices and clinics, including public health, are the most frequently used and most familiar care sites. Patients may be referred to other sites, including urgent care centers, diagnostic centers, free-standing surgery centers, and specialty care centers, for dialysis, physical therapy, and radiation therapy. Hospitals, in addition to providing acute inpatient care, offer the following types of ambulatory care:

- Ancillary services, such as laboratory and diagnostic imaging
- An organized outpatient department, which may include both primary care and specialty clinics
- Ambulatory surgery centers (ASCs)
- Emergency department (ED)

Multiple delivery sites and entry points for ambulatory care create unique operational challenges for hospitals. In addition, the definition of ambulatory care within a given facility is continually evolving as hospitals expand these services to keep pace with technologic advances.

Data Needs

As noted in the NCVHS core health data elements and as we will see in the EHR in Chapter 6, the patient record is designed around a core header or demographic segment collected at the outset of care and updated as needed. This reemphasizes the centrality of ambulatory care to both the data collection and patient care processes. TJC's *Comprehensive Accreditation Manual for Ambulatory Care* details the content of the outpatient record in the RC standard. In addition to the CMS CoPs and TJC requirements, it is important to investigate other accrediting bodies such as the NCQA and the AAAHC as well as any state regulations that specify record content. The MDS that applies in this segment of the delivery system is the Uniform Ambulatory Care Data Set (UACDS). A more recent addition is the Data Elements for Emergency Departments (DEEDS).

Uniform Ambulatory Care Data Set

The NCVHS approved the UACDS in 1989.[11] This data set was the product of collaboration between its Subcommittee on Ambulatory Care Statistics and the Interagency Task Force of the DHHS. The task force was charged with surveying the data needs of the DHHS agencies, and the subcommittee considered the applicability of the data set to the wider health care delivery system, including other agencies; private providers, practitioners, and payers; and researchers. Providers are encouraged to record all items in the individual patient's record, although some may be located in billing records. When this is the case, the ability to link data from separate sources is an important requirement. The data set includes segments that describe the patient, the provider, and the encounter. Most items are required; some are optional. Detail of items is limited, given the core health data elements definitions stated previously. As with all MDSs, the most current edition should be consulted.

Segment 1: Patient Data Items
1. Personal identification (including name and number)
2. Residence (usual residence, full address, and zip code)
3. Date of birth (month, day, and year)
4. Sex
5. Race and ethnic background
6. Living arrangement and marital status (optional)
   a. Alone

b. With spouse (alternate: with spouse or unrelated partner)

c. With children

d. With parent or guardian

e. With relative other than spouse, children, or parents

f. With nonrelatives

g. Unknown

Multiple responses can be made to this item because of living arrangements that are a combination of spouse, children, parents, and nonrelatives.

In those data systems that choose to collect marital status in lieu of or in addition to living arrangement, the following categories should be used:

Marital status

a. Married—A person currently married. Classify common law marriage as married.

b. Never married—A person who has never been married or whose only marriages have been annulled.

c. Widowed—A person widowed and not remarried.

d. Divorced—A person divorced and not remarried.

e. Separated—A person legally separated or otherwise absent from spouse.

f. Unknown.

Longitudinal studies will have the opportunity to study transitions from one type of living arrangement or marital status to another.

Segment 2: Provider Data Items

An individual provider has been defined as a health care professional who delivers services or is professionally responsible for services delivered to a patient, who is exercising independent judgment in the care of the patient, and who is not under the immediate supervision of another health care professional. An encounter is defined as a professional contact between a patient and a provider during which services are delivered.

The following characteristics should be collected for the provider of record for each encounter. The user may decide to collect the additional provider data element, discussed earlier under definitions, for the provider who initiated the encounter (if different from the provider who delivered or was responsible for the services delivered). If such a decision is made, consideration will also have to be given to the necessary identification elements required for this item.

7. Provider identification (name and UPIN)

8. Location or address

9. Profession

This is the profession in which the provider is currently engaged and includes physicians (physicians and osteopaths), dentists (doctors of dental surgery and dental medicine), other licensed or certified health care professionals, and other health care providers. The specialty should be listed.

Segment 3: Encounter Data Items

10. Date, place or site, and address of encounter, if different from item 08

a. Date of encounter: month, day, and year

b. Place or site of encounter (A list of 29 places of encounter is provided; examples include office, home, and hospital outpatient.)

c. Address of facility where services were rendered if different from item 08

11. Patient's reason for encounter (optional)

Describe all conditions that require evaluation or treatment or management at the time of the encounter as designated by the provider. It is recommended that the standard coding convention for this purpose should be the widely used *International Classification of Diseases* (ICD) and, in the United States, its clinical modification (i.e., ICD-9-CM or ICD-10-CM), with all codes available for use. This approach should accommodate the coding of symptoms, ill-defined conditions, and the problems when a firm diagnosis has not been established.

The condition that should be listed first is the diagnosis, problem, symptom, or reason for encounter shown in the patient record to be chiefly responsible for the ambulatory care services provided during the encounter. List additional codes that describe any coexisting conditions. Do not code diagnoses documented as "probable," "suspected," or "questionable," or "rule out" as if they were established. Rather, code the condition or symptom to the highest degree of certainty for that encounter.

12. Services

Describe all diagnostic services of any type, including history, physical examination, laboratory, radiography, and others performed that are pertinent to the patient's reasons for the encounter; all therapeutic services performed at the time of the encounter; and all preventive services and procedures performed at the time of the encounter. Also, describe to the extent possible the provision to the patient of drugs and biologicals, supplies, appliances, and equipment.

The diagnostic, therapeutic, and preventive services rendered in connection with the encounter should be captured where they are provided. The CMS's Healthcare Common Procedure Coding System, which is based on the Current Procedural Terminology for physician services and has been augmented for nonphysician services, is the most inclusive coding system for fostering uniformity in reporting these services.

13. Disposition

This is the provider's statement of the next step in the care of the patient. As many categories as apply should be reported. At a minimum, the following classification is suggested:

a. No follow-up planned

b. Follow-up planned

(1) Return anticipated as necessary but not scheduled

(2) Return to the current provider at a specific date

(3) Telephone follow-up

(4) Returned to referring provider

(5) Referred to other individual provider

(6) Referred to other provider for consultation

(7) Referred to an adjunctive provider agency

(8) Transferred to other individual provider

(9) Admit to acute care hospital

(10) Admit to residential health care facility

(11) Other

14. Patient's expected sources of payment

Related to E1384-07, Segment 3, Financial. Eleven source categories are provided—for example, self-insured, insurance companies, workers' compensation, and government programs, including Medicare, Medicaid, and others.

   a. Primary source

   b. Secondary source

   c. Other sources

   d. Payment mechanism (related to this service)

      (1) Fee-for-service

      (2) Health maintenance organization or prepaid plan

      (3) Unknown or unidentified

15. Total charges

List all charges for procedures and services rendered to the patient during this encounter. This includes a technical component or facility fee when billed separately from the professional component.

Data Elements for Emergency Department Systems

The National Center for Injury Prevention and Control (NCIPC) is coordinating a national effort to develop uniform specifications for data entered in ED patient records. The initial product is DEEDS. These recommendations are intended for use by individuals and organizations responsible for maintaining record systems in 24-hour, hospital-based EDs throughout the United States. If the data definitions, coding conventions, and other recommended specifications are widely adopted, then incompatibilities in ED records can be substantially reduced. Further, because the recommendations incorporate national standards for EDI, implementation of DEEDS in EHR systems can facilitate communication and integration with other automated information systems. NCIPC plans to coordinate a multidisciplinary evaluation of DEEDS after its initial release seeking to improve this first set of recommendations. DEEDS is composed of eight sections:

Section 1: Patient Identification Data

Section 2: Facility and Practitioner Identification Data

Section 3: ED Payment Data

Section 4: ED Arrival and First Assessment Data

Section 5: ED History and Physical Examination Data

Section 6: ED Procedure and Results Data

Section 7: ED Medication Data

Section 8: ED Disposition and Diagnosis Data

Special Forms and Views

Problem List

Ambulatory care is the one setting in which the problem list from the POMR has become a standard requirement. Symptoms and diagnoses are listed as Dr. Weed designed, with allergies, medications, significant surgeries, and perhaps any durable medical equipment that the provider has supplied.

Encounter Record

As defined in ASTM Standard E1384-07, an encounter is a professional contact between a patient and a provider during which services are delivered. The recording of ambulatory care encounters, with the exception of emergency care, is often done on a single form with minimum structure and used by all medical providers. Rubber stamps or stickers may be used to prompt for data items or serve as alerts. The CMS CoPs for hospitals note the following standard when describing outpatient documentation: Enough information about the patient must be included to ensure continuity of care, including the following:

- Medical history
- Physical findings
- Laboratory and diagnostic test results
- Diagnosis
- Treatment record

TJC has the following requirements:

- Identification
- Relevant history of the illness or injury and physical findings
- Diagnostic and therapeutic orders
- Clinical observations, including results of treatment
- Reports of procedures, tests, and results
- Diagnostic impression
- Patient disposition and any pertinent instructions given for follow-up care
- Immunization record
- Allergy history
- Growth charts for pediatric patients
- Referral information to and from agencies

In addition, procedures and outpatient surgeries must be documented in a manner similar to that described under General Forms and Views.

Emergency Record

No form benefits more from efficient design than the emergency record. Data collection may begin with an ambulance service picking up the patient in the community. Vital signs, history of the current illness, monitoring of the patient's condition, and any procedures performed are documented on a prehospital care report, also known as a *run report*. If the problem resolves or the patient dies, this is the complete record of care. If the patient is transferred to a hospital ED, a copy of this record may be attached or necessary information abstracted onto the hospital form. The CMS CoPs for hospitals require the following data items:

- Identification
- History of the disease or injury
- Physical findings
- Laboratory and radiology reports, if needed
- Diagnosis
- Treatment
- Disposition of the case

The responsible physician signs the record. TJC specifies that the following items be included:

- Identification
- Time and means of arrival

- History of current illness or injury
- Physical findings and vital signs
- Emergency care given before arrival
- Diagnostic and therapeutic orders
- Reports of procedures, tests, and results
- Clinical observations, including results of treatment
- Diagnostic impression
- Conclusion at the termination of treatment, including final disposition, patient's condition at discharge, and any instructions given to the patient or family for follow-up care
- Patient leaving AMA

Items are usually recorded on a single form divided into appropriate segments. A form is completed for each emergency encounter, with the original kept by the provider. A copy may be sent to the patient's physician. If additional resources are needed in the area of emergency and trauma information, other resources deal with emergency transport data in ASTM standards, the DEEDS data work, and trauma registry efforts.

Issues in Data Collection and Quality

Maintaining continuity of care across multiple providers and practitioners delivering a wide scope of services is one of the most challenging aspects of ambulatory care. The potential for the EHR to transform this exchange of information into a truly dynamic process will have profound advantages for providers, practitioners, and, particularly, patients. Incentives, such as Meaningful Use, and HITECH workforce training of HIT professionals have accelerated the migration to the EHR. Because the record may develop over a long period, organization is important so that essential data can be located easily and not overlooked. All encounters, including those over the telephone or perhaps online, must be documented. Specificity is often a problem inherent to ambulatory care when diagnoses are in the process of being clarified. Change in ambulatory care reimbursement to a prospective payment system has required increasing detail in encounter records. Surgical reports have often omitted such items as length and size of lesions excised and wounds repaired; a description of the layers of fascia, muscle, and skin involved in a repair; and wound debridement for major infections or contaminations.

An outpatient clinic or a physician's office has data requirements and documentation practices for records similar to but different from those of an acute care hospital. A continuous QI approach for documentation review may be more appropriate than would a continuing daily record review on all patient visits. Many ASCs use the same manual or automated systems to monitor data quality, as do acute inpatient facilities.

Stopwatch studies of physician outpatient clinic activities have shown that 50% of the physician's day is spent on direct patient care activities related to patient interviews, examinations, and procedures, and the other half of the time is spent on "housekeeping" activities including reviewing records, documenting records, dictating reports, and reviewing radiology issues and results. To allow more patient appointments to occur during the day, an important revenue consideration, it is crucial for the HIM professional to evaluate current practices of the physician, review the clinic office system and organizational structure, and modify the information system to help improve physician efficiency.

For example, a clinic may find that if a physician documented in the visit note what he or she planned to do at the patient's next visit, the nurses or medical assistants could review the record the day before the next appointment and would know how to prepare the examination or treatment room for that visit and which supplies were needed for that encounter. Encouraging the physician to document orders rather than give verbal orders increases patient safety by decreasing the chance for error by the office staff. Physicians may resort to verbal orders because documentation time may be excessive. The HIM professional should identify the nature of the problem, evaluate the current system, and find solutions to the problem. Improved efficiency of documentation of orders might be accomplished by using simple check-off paper forms or by having physicians input data directly into the computer.

Surveys and focused interviews with physicians and the clinic staff can determine their satisfaction with the current system, their ideas, and their needs, how they would like to use computers in their practice, the type of computer training they would like, and their satisfaction with transcription and other systems.

Long-Term Care

Integral to cost containment is the concern over the effect of the tremendous growth in the older adult population. The Bureau of the Census has projected a doubling of the 65-years-or-older age group between 1980 and 2020 with an even more rapid increase in the 85-years-or-older age group. The reimbursement incentives that cause shorter lengths of stay in acute care facilities result in the discharge of patients with more complex problems to long-term care facilities.

Data Needs

Lengths of stay in long-term care facilities may extend from months through years. A great deal of routine data is collected, which typically accumulates into multiple volumes. The CMS CoPs detail the content of the long-term care record, as does TJC's *Comprehensive Accreditation Manual for Long-Term Care* RC standard. The MDS that applies to this segment of the delivery system is the Minimum Data Set for Long-Term Care Facility Resident Assessment, version 3.[9] As with all MDSs, the most current edition should be consulted.

MDS 3.0: Minimum Data Set for Long-Term Care Facility Resident Assessment Instrument

This MDS is under the direction of the NCVHS and shares the purpose of increasing uniformity and comparability of data. The MDS was originally developed in 1980, with Version 2 in the late 1990s, and Version 3.0 beginning in 2010 with a focus on improving the data quality from 2.0, particularly accuracy and reliability. As with other MDSs, the current edition should be consulted. The MDS 3.0 is divided into alphabetic sections provided here. The items that follow represent the Full Assessment Form. There is also a follow-up assessment version.

Section A: Identification Information
Section B: Hearing, Speech, and Vision
Section C: Cognitive Patterns
Section D: Mood
Section E: Behavior
Section F: Preferences for Customary Routine and Activities
Section G: Functional Status
Section H: Bladder and Bowel
Section I: Active Diagnoses
Section J: Health Conditions
Section K: Swallowing/Nutritional Status
Section L: Oral/Dental Status
Section M: Skin Conditions
Section N: Medications
Section O: Special Treatments, Procedures, and Programs
Section P: Restraints
Section Q: Participation in Assessment and Goal Setting
Section R (not used)
Section S: Reserved
Section T: (not used)
Section U: (not used)
Section V: Care Area Assessment (CAA) Summary
Section W: (not used)
Section X: Correction Request
Section Y: (not used)
Section Z: Assessment Administration

Special Forms and Views

The long-term residential care record is similar to the acute care record in that it is also a record of an admission to a facility. Differences include a longer record, which typically needs to be thinned during the length of stay, and the emphasis on nursing care. Details of functional capacity, activities of daily living (ADLs), nutrition, bowel and bladder habits, and medication interactions also take on prominence.

Pharmacy Consultation

Because most older adults take multiple medications, a pharmacy consultation is required to review for potential drug interactions, discrepancies in medications ordered versus those given, and any recommended changes. The consultation may appear on the physician's order sheet, in the progress notes, or on its own sheet and it should be documented monthly.

Transfer or Referral Form

When a resident is admitted to a facility, a transfer form provided by the hospital, physician, or other facility should accompany the patient or follow immediately. The form facilitates the continuity of care and should include the following:
- Reason for admission
- Diagnosis

- Current medical information
- Rehabilitative potential

The physician should certify the level of care required and the anticipated length of stay. The form should also contain the following administrative data:
- Identification (resident's UPIN)
- Names of the transferring and receiving institutions
- Date of transfer
- Diagnoses
- Physician's and any nurse's report

When patients are routinely transferred between facilities, it is common to have a transfer agreement signed by both institutions. This formalizes and facilitates the continuing exchange of information whenever patients move between the institutions. Transfers between long-term care facilities are also possible.

Issues in Data Collection and Quality

Long-term care facilities have had to adjust to the extensive MDS. Many have computerized these data and have benefited from the alerts and alarms and the automatic generation of the patient care plan. The update intervals are also automatically identified. One particular difficulty in documenting long-term care is that the patient's status may change more slowly or in smaller increments. Practitioners need to be encouraged to be continuously attentive to even small changes in patient status and reflect them in the patient's record.

Long-term care records are created for patients or residents who stay at a nursing facility for months or years. Because documentation requirements vary significantly from those for acute inpatient settings, many of the traditional acute care inpatient record documentation review systems need to be modified to meet the needs of the long-term care industry. Quantitative and qualitative reviews are usually done within 1 to 2 days after admission and then periodically at least every 30 to 60 days and again at discharge. Quality assessment and assurance worksheet forms can also be developed to check documentation for specific topics.

Long-Term Subacute Care

Changes in both technology and reimbursement incentives has seen the rise of long-term subacute care (LTSC). LTSC provides comprehensive inpatient care for patients who have had an acute illness, injury, or exacerbation of a disease process. It is goal-oriented care rendered immediately after or instead of acute hospitalization for treatment of active complex conditions or for administration of technically complex treatments. Subacute care is generally more intensive than traditional nursing home care and less intensive than acute care.

Rehabilitation

Rehabilitation facilities vary widely in type from infant development to spinal cord injury, from chronic pain management to vocational evaluation. The range of services is equally extensive, from prosthetics to patient advocacy, from ADLs to audiology. Matching the patient's needs to the type of facility and its services is an important case management function. When the facility has been selected, the patient is registered or admitted and oriented. During this screening process, the patient is assessed and the interdisciplinary patient care plan developed. Any services that need to be referred are arranged.

The CARF has developed standards requiring that a single record be maintained for any patient and that it include the following:

- Identification data
- Pertinent history
- Diagnosis of disability
- Rehabilitation problems, goals, and prognosis
- Reports of assessments and individual program planning
- Reports from referring sources and service referrals
- Reports from outside consultations and laboratory, radiology, orthotic, and prosthetic services
- Designation of a manager for the patient's program
- Evidence of the patient's or family's participation in decision making
- Evaluation reports from each service
- Reports of staff conferences
- Patient's total program plan
- Plans from each service
- Signed and dated service and progress reports
- Correspondence pertinent to the patient
- Release forms
- Discharge report
- Follow-up reports

Inpatient Rehabilitation Facility Patient Assessment Instrument

The Medicare Inpatient Rehabilitation Facility Patient Assessment Instrument (IRF-PAI) is used to gather data to determine the payment for each Medicare Part A fee-for-service patient admitted to an inpatient rehabilitation unit or hospital. IRF-PAI data items address the physical, cognitive, functional, and psychosocial status of patients. A copy of this instrument can be found on the Evolve website.

Issues in Data Collection and Quality

In rehabilitation, it is common for departments to keep raw patient data, such as attendance, which are summarized for the record. Maintaining a comprehensive unit record must therefore be closely monitored for compliance with standards.

Home Health Care

Home health care describes services provided to the patient in his or her place of residence. Like ambulatory care, home health has been the recipient of both increased patient volume and regulatory attention as incentives have been provided to find alternatives to acute care. Advances in technology have added momentum to the home care movement with the

availability of infusion for antibiotic therapy and chemotherapy, total parenteral nutrition, respiratory care (including ventilators), and other high-technology treatments. A nurse manager typically coordinates a case on the basis of the attending physician's orders. Health care analysts predict an increase in the number, regulation, and sophistication of home care services and agencies.

Regulations for home health care are more limited than for acute or long-term care and substantially follow the CMS CoPs for Medicare-certified home health agencies. The focus is on collecting the following data to complete the standard CMS forms:

- Home health certification and plan of treatment
- Medical update and patient information
- Plan of treatment
- Medical update and patient information addendum
- Home health agency intermediary medical information report

To be Medicare certified, an agency must provide skilled nursing care and at least one of the following therapeutic services: physical, speech, or occupational therapy; medical social services; or home health aide services. The CMS classifies home health agencies into the following categories:

- Hospital or provider based
- Proprietary
- Private nonprofit
- Government (state or local health and welfare departments)
- Voluntary nonprofit (Visiting Nurses Association)

Data Needs

TJC's *Comprehensive Accreditation Manual for Home Care* provides RC standards for both home care and hospice. In addition, the National League for Nursing has an accreditation program. The National Homecare Council represents and accredits agencies that provide homemaker and home health aide services and includes some record-keeping guidelines.

Outcome and Assessment Information Set

In January 1999, final regulations were published implementing a data set for home health care, titled the Outcome and Assessment Information Set (OASIS).[12] It was an outcome of the Omnibus Budget Reconciliation Act of 1987, which mandated that Medicare monitor the quality of home health care and services with a standardized, reproducible assessment instrument. There are versions for start of care, transfer, follow-up, and discharge. A new version, called OASIS-C, was implemented in 2010 to better align with MDS 3.0 for long-term care and CARE as part of a larger effort to standardize assessment and quality measurement across postacute health care settings.

A standard definition of a home care visit or length of stay has yet to be developed. For the purpose of Medicare reimbursement, each encounter with a health care practitioner is a visit; for example, if the nurse and the respiratory therapist both see the patient on the same day, two visits are counted. The MDS that follows represents the start-of-care version.

The main segments are presented here. As with the other data sets, there is additional detail and the current version should be consulted.

- Patient Tracking Items
- Clinical Record Items
- Patient History and Diagnoses
- Living Arrangements
- Sensory Status
- Integumentary Status
- Respiratory Status
- Cardiac Status
- Elimination Status
- Neuro/Emotional/Behavioral Status
- ADLs/Instrumental ADLs
- Medications
- Care Management
- Therapy Need and Plan of Care
- Emergent Care
- Data Collected at Transfer/Discharge

Special Forms and Views

The central coordinating tool in the home care record is the interdisciplinary patient care plan. A summary should be provided for the attending physician at least every 60 days. When the patient is discharged from a particular service, a service summary is written, followed by an overall discharge summary at the termination of care. Most of the documentation is done by nurses and therapists. If the care is provided through a hospital, the home care record should be combined with the inpatient unit record.

Service Agreement

The patient or guardian should sign a service agreement that outlines the services to be provided, the times services are to be provided, the charges, and the parties responsible for payment.

Issues in Data Collection and Quality

One of the major challenges in home care is that a significant part of the record may remain in the home for documentation by practitioners representing various disciplines who provide care at intervals. Returning these portions of the record to the agency needs attention as one aspect of coordinating a team diverse in specialty and location. The record in the home should also contain the name of the agency, the people to contact along with their telephone numbers, patient or family instructions for care, a list of medications with potential adverse effects, and emergency instructions. The presence of this information in the home should be documented in the agency record. Training in patient record practices may also need special attention. Because the staff is not centralized, well-designed policies and procedures and initial orientation and follow-up sessions are important. Homemakers, companions, and family members may need to be instructed on how to record data.

Home health records pose special problems related to record documentation systems. Laptops and other computerized systems are being implemented, but although some of these records remain paper-based, these problems will continue because the patient is not located at the health care facility when treatment is rendered. The typical flow of documentation received concerning the home health patient's agency begins with the initial referring information obtained by telephone or facsimile (fax) from the transferring health care facility or physician. Copies of the referring facility's H&P report, discharge summary, and transfer form are critical at this point. A clinician is assigned to the patient, and the referring information must be available to the nurse or therapist before the first home visit. The clinician verifies demographic and reimbursement information with the patient on the first visit, and signed patient consent-for-care forms are obtained. Subsequent information is recorded in the patient's home, clinician's car or home, agency office, or other location by the clinician. The documentation includes the following:

- Assessments
- Plans of treatment
- Progress notes (one note per visit is required)
- Clinician discharge summary

This information is brought to the agency's HIM department at a later time (often several days later) for incorporation in the patient record. The original patient record must not leave the office to avoid the possibility of tampering or loss and so that it is available for others who need access to the record, such as other clinicians involved in the case and clinical supervisors. Therefore the nurse or therapist relies on copies of original records that are maintained at home or in the car, preferably in a locked briefcase when not stored at the clinician's office desk. The nurse or therapist may not visit the office every day, which may create problems in terms of record access and updating of the original record by the clinician. Paper record systems in home health agencies not only pose system problems but also have the potential to create major problems related to loss of confidentiality.

Designing a method of documentation review for a paper record system is difficult at best. Abraham[13] has written an excellent discussion of client record review guidelines and procedures. The first review should be done within 10 days of patient admission to the home health agency. The record should be reviewed for the following:

- Receipt of information from transferring facilities (correct and complete referral information)
- Presence and authentication of assessment documents by all professional disciplines involved in the case
- Plans of treatment and other reports
- Signed consent-for-care forms from the patient

Every 30 to 60 days while the patient is still active and again at discharge, the record should be reviewed to make sure the following are present:

- Team case conference notes
- Updated and signed plans of treatment and orders from physicians
- Home health aide supervisory visit notes by a nurse or therapist
- Clinician discharge summary and other reports
- Authenticated progress notes for each visit made by the clinician

An example of a state-mandated clinical record review form from Wisconsin is provided in Figure 4-10. The figure shows

DEPARTMENT OF HEALTH SERVICES
Division of Quality Assurance
F-62680 (Rev. 04/09)

STATE OF WISCONSIN
DHS 133, Wis. Admin. Code
Page 1 of 3

HOME HEALTH AGENCY
CLINICAL RECORD REVIEW

Name – Patient		Start of Care	Patient ID Number
Date of Review	Surveyor Number	Agency License Number	Pay Source	☐ Open ☐ Closed

Tag	DHS 133	Regulation	Yes	No	NA
141	.08(2)(a)	Patient Rights – Written acknowledgement of acceptance. *Waived for federally certified agencies.*			
149	.08(3)	Complaint Form F-62069			
150	.09	**ACCEPTANCE AND DISCHARGE**			
152	.09(2)	**SERVICE AGREEMENT** - Signed with services, fees, and charges identified			
153	.09(3)(a)1.	**DISCHARGE OF PATIENT** – Written Notice			
154	.09(3)(a)2.a	Non-payment			
155	.09(3)(a)2.b	Unable to provide care			
156	.09(3)(a)3.a	Staff safety compromised			
157	.09(3)(a)3.b	Physician orders discharge			
158	.09(3)(a)3.c.	No longer needs home health care			
159	.09(3)(a)4.	Copy in patient record			
160	.09(3)(a)5.a	Reason for discharge			
161	.09(3)(a)5.b	Patient right to file complaint			
162	.09(3)(b)	Discharge summary within 30 days			
168	.11	**REFERRALS** – Appropriate referrals made			
169	.12	**COORDINATION WITH OTHER PROVIDERS**			
		Conferences with other agency providers			
		Appropriate referrals made			
231	.21	**MEDICAL RECORDS**			
237	.21(5)(a)	CONTENT – Record must include the following: Patient ID information			
238	.21(5)(b)	Appropriate (hospital) information			
239	.21(5)(c)	Patient evaluation and assessment			
240	.21(5)(d)	Plan of Care			
241	.21(5)(e)	Physician orders			
242	.21(5)(f)	Medication list and patient instructions			
243	.21(5)(g)	Progress notes with services, condition, and progress			
244	.21(5)(h)	Summaries of review of Plan of Care			
245	.21(5)(i)	Discharge summary within 30 days			
246	.21(6)	Form of entries			
		Entries are legible.			
		Entries are permanently recorded.			
		Entries are authenticated with name and title.			
	.20	**PLAN OF CARE**			
224	.20(1)	Requirement: Plan developed within 72 hours in consultation with physician, patient, and contractual providers.			
		Plan signed within 20 working days			
225	.20(2)(a)	Contents: Goals Measurable – time specific with benchmark dates			
226	.20(2)(b)	Plan of Care complete and accurate (includes Methods / Discipline)			
227	.20(3)	Review of plan – MD review at least every 60 days			
		MD notified of changes in condition			
229	.20(4)	Physician Orders - Drugs and treatments provided per order			
		T.O. signed by MD within 20 days			

FIGURE 4-10 Home Health Agency Clinical Record Review, State of Wisconsin, Department of Health Services, Division of Quality Assurance. (http://www.dhs.wisconsin.gov/forms1/f6/f62680.pdf)

the initial portion of the review. The full form can be viewed online or on the Evolve website.

Third-party payers require a progress note for each visit billed. If the note is not present, the agency could lose revenue for that visit. This last item is difficult to review because the patient is usually not visited every day. Therefore a method needs to be devised to match the date of each billed visit with the presence of a progress note. In many agencies, this is a complex problem because thousands of patient visits may be made each month. Many agencies have daily or weekly individual employee service records, sometimes referred to as "itineraries," on which the clinician documents each patient visit. This form is sent to the business office, which uses it as the data source for billing third-party payers and as an employee time card. Many agencies require that the clinician attach the individual progress notes to these handwritten service records and bring them to the HIM department. The HIM department staff members record the receipt of these progress notes by comparing them with each visit noted on the service record. They follow through on missing documentation with the clinician before the final monthly bill is submitted to the third-party payer by the business office. Other agencies bill directly from the progress notes and do no further checking. Some agencies perform random review only, comparing bills with patient records to assess accuracy. A paper clinical record system is cumbersome for home health agencies, not only for the clinicians but also for the HIM department staff. To ensure data quality, it is imperative that the HIM professional understand and evaluate the agency's current system of data collection and make changes as necessary. The increased use of secure mobile computing has reduced some of these challenges by enabling practitioners to download the records for their schedule of visits and upload their documentation at the end of their workday. Review by supervisors and the HIM department is also facilitated.

Continuity Assessment Record Evaluation

The **continuity assessment record evaluation** (CARE) Item Set is a framework for a standard set of items for Medicare beneficiaries at acute discharge and measures changes in severity and other outcomes for Medicare postacute care patients in inpatient rehabilitation facilities, long-term care hospitals, skilled nursing facilities, and home health care. CARE has been developed as a requirement of the Deficit Reduction Act of 2005 to develop a Medicare Payment Reform Demonstration. Both core and supplemental items are included. B-CARE is a streamlined version being considered for use within the Bundled Payments for Care Improvement Initiative. While CARE and B-CARE are in their developmental stages, they demonstrate the trend toward standardizing data items and facilitating analysis across care settings.

Hospice

Hospice care provides supportive services for terminally ill patients, their families, and significant others. Psychosocial support and spiritual support are central to this type of care, and only palliative medical attention is provided. In addition to the interdisciplinary team of health care providers, volunteers contribute in important ways to patient care. Hospice services are frequently provided in the home. A primary caregiver, who may be a relative or friend, is identified. Home care or an inpatient admission may occur for symptomatic management, but no life-prolonging measures are undertaken. Hospice is a philosophy of care more than a location. A unique feature of hospice care is that not only the patient but also the family or significant other are provided services. The family or significant other may receive after care for as long as 1 year after the death, depending on the need.

The following data are required by TJC RC hospice standards:

- Identification
- All pertinent diagnoses
- Prognosis
- Designation of an attending physician
- Designation of the family member or person to be notified in the event of an emergency or death

An interdisciplinary patient care plan is the foundation of the record. Both a physical and a psychosocial assessment are required. The physical assessment describes functional capacity, acute or chronic pain, and other physical symptoms and their management. The psychosocial assessment of the patient and the family includes spiritual needs. As in other care settings, updating of the care plan is continual. A review of the care plan is required every 30 days and must be documented. A summary of care is prepared and should include information on the coordination of transfer from the hospital to home care and when the patient dies. The Medicare CoPs closely follow the TJC standards. A specific addition relates to following the hospice patient care plan even when inpatient services are provided. Medicare reimburses hospices at four levels: routine home care, continuous home care, inpatient respite care, and general inpatient care. Data collected should justify the level of care provided. The National Hospice Organization is a resource for data collection guidelines.

Hospice is more specific in defining its episodes than home care is. The first episode of care begins with the patient's or family's admission to the hospice program and ends when the patient is transferred, is discharged, or dies. This episode includes all services provided, regardless of the setting. The second episode of care begins with the patient's death and the transition of the family or significant other on the next day into bereavement care, and ends when the survivors are discharged, perhaps as much as 1 year later.

? DID YOU KNOW?

The words *hospice* and *hospital* have their roots in the words *hospitality* and *host.*

Special Forms

If the hospice care is provided by a hospital or home care agency, the completed record should be filed with other records of the patient. Forms documenting spiritual needs and responses, pain assessment and management, and bereavement are particularly important in the hospice setting.

Issues in Data Collection and Quality

Like home care, hospice employs a diverse team of people in various locations. Coordination and training are among the most important concerns. Hospice records usually reflect the characteristics of the facility or agency that maintains the hospice program. The hospice program often uses forms that are the same as or similar to those of the facility as a whole, and it uses many of the same record completion review procedures. Many hospices are affiliated with home health agencies or long-term care facilities, and their records reflect those systems. Abraham provides forms, record content requirements, and procedures unique to hospice programs.[13]

Behavioral Health

Behavioral health provides services in a variety of settings to individuals who have an array of problems from mental health to chemical dependency. The individuals served may be developmentally disabled, older adults, children, homeless, in prison, or working and struggling with emotional issues. The effect of mental illness on health and productivity is often profoundly underrecognized. It is estimated that in technologically developed countries, such as the United States, mental illness equals heart disease and cancer as a cause of disability.[14] Behavioral health services are traditionally not recognized by payers as equal to physical health problems, although mental health is achieving parity through legislation at the federal level and in a number of states that require health insurance to cover behavioral health care. Some individuals are treated for their behavioral health problem by their medical provider; others are treated by specialists in the mental health or chemical dependency services. Behavioral health services work closely with primary care medical providers. Two unique features of behavioral health are close monitoring of the patient's legal status and additional attention to confidentiality. Legal requirements must be carefully reviewed when planning and managing patient information. Organizations may provide inpatient or outpatient care and adult, child, and adolescent care.

Data Needs

Behavioral health programs are regulated by various state and federal requirements, including the CMS CoPs. Organizations may be accredited by TJC using the *Comprehensive Accreditation Manual for Behavioral Health Care* standards or by CARF, which accredits the full spectrum of behavioral health programs, including mental health, chemical dependency, housing, and employment services. There is currently no MDS, but data collection resembles patterns previously described for inpatient or outpatient care. A preliminary treatment plan is required on admission to programs. The initial assessment must be completed within 72 hours if an individual is admitted to a psychiatric hospital or detoxification facility. Physical examinations are required in inpatient and residential programs. A detailed initial assessment or intake is typically completed on an individual who registers for outpatient treatment in a behavioral health organization. Record content expectations are contained in state and federal laws and regulations as well as standards of the accrediting bodies. Progress notes may use the "DAP" format—data, assessment, plan.

Special Forms and Views

The previously explained forms and views apply to behavioral health care, with some additions. An interdisciplinary care plan is a core expectation in most programs. This care plan may be goal or recovery oriented. It describes what the individual will do to achieve certain objectives as well as how the care team will support the process. Issues of patients' rights receive particular attention in behavioral health care because of its potentially restrictive nature. Patients and guardians must be informed of their rights, and whenever a patient's rights are denied, justification must be documented. When the reason for the denial is no longer present, rights must be restored.

Although not part of the clinical record, incident and accident reports are of particular importance.

Comprehensive Initial Assessment

In addition to basic assessment features, the patient's legal status is assessed, and social, recreational, and vocational assessments are included. This assessment is typically conducted by a mental health professional.

Psychiatric History and Diagnosis Report

In addition to the detailed initial assessment, a psychiatrist evaluates the individual on admission to an inpatient facility. Outpatient organizations also determine the need for a psychiatrist's evaluation or consultation.

Special Assessments

When there is concern about suicide, a lethality assessment is performed. Additional assessments such as a cultural assessment are useful and performed as appropriate. Although physical health is not the primary focus, behavioral health may recommend that a client get a physical examination, a nutritional assessment, or a dental examination. When treatments such as seclusion, restraint, or electroconvulsive therapy are considered in an inpatient or residential setting, an additional assessment is required. Seclusion, restraint, and electroconvulsive therapy must be closely monitored because of the risk to the individual involved.

Deescalation, Restraint, and Seclusion

When a client is disruptive, the least restrictive attempts at control are attempted first. In a behavioral health environment, staff are trained in deescalation techniques. If the client continues to disrupt the inpatient or residential therapeutic environment, seclusion may be considered. If this is unsuccessful, restraint may be used. Restraint and seclusion should be used only to protect the client and others and to avoid damage to the facility. In an outpatient environment, staff seldom use restraint, tending more toward a deescalation model. However, if a client's behavior is endangering himself or herself or others, staff may call the police.

If either restraint or seclusion is chosen as a treatment procedure, the assessment with justification, implementation, monitoring, and termination of restraint or seclusion must be carefully documented. As mentioned, a physician must assess the client and provide a clinical justification and attempt to manage the client by use of less-restrictive measures. An order is then written that is to last no longer than 24 hours. Staff are to monitor the client every 15 minutes. If restraint or seclusion should be required in an emergency, trained staff may proceed, with a phone order from the physician for continuation. In any event, when restraint or seclusion is considered necessary for longer than 24 hours, the head of the professional staff should be informed and the case reviewed.

Electroconvulsive and Other Therapies

Electroconvulsive therapy, psychosurgery, behavior modification using painful stimuli, and experimental treatment, although not frequently used, are other areas of behavioral health treatment in which extreme care must be exercised and documentation meticulously recorded. Special consents must be signed by the client or guardian. Other therapies that may be used include therapeutic passes and behavior modification contracts. If either of these is used, any agreements with and response from the client should be included in the record.

Issues in Data Collection and Quality

Historically, behavioral health care has been difficult to quantify, and records have relied almost exclusively on narrative description, with the exception of diagnoses, procedures, services, and medications ordered. The need for quantifiable measures has been addressed through behavioral severity scales and global assessment of function scales to assess clients. As in other care settings, it remains important that practitioners document as clearly and objectively as possible.

Personal Health Record

The IOM found that "When patients see multiple providers in different settings, none of whom have access to complete (health) information, it becomes easier for things to go wrong."[6] Each health care provider maintains his or her own separate patient records for patients treated. This means that health information is fragmented among the many individual and organizational providers where the patient has received care, which can lead to an incomplete story about a patient's health. What is needed is a way to coordinate the documentation among all the clinical stakeholders in a patient's care. One obvious coordinator is the patient. The patient can coordinate his or her own care using the PHR.

Data Needs

As we have seen throughout this chapter, a wide variety of health record documents are created in multiple care settings. The PHR is not a substitute for the legal record kept by providers. Patients collect copies of pertinent documents from their various providers. They may also add information on personal wellness activities such as exercise and diet as well as other items such as medication instructions.

Special Forms and Views

A PHR is a combination of copies of documents generated by providers and additional information gathered by patients or

their caregivers. AHIMA's consumer-information website (http://www.myPHR.com) provides forms and a list of recommended content. Some examples include:

- Personal identification, including name and birth date
- People to contact in case of emergency
- Names, addresses, and phone numbers of your physician, dentist, and specialists
- Health insurance information
- Living wills, advance directives, or medical power of attorney
- Organ donor authorization
- A list and dates of significant illnesses and surgical procedures
- Current medications and dosages
- Immunizations and their dates
- Allergies or sensitivities to drugs or materials, such as latex
- Important events, dates, and hereditary conditions in one's family history
- Results from a recent physical examination
- Opinions of specialists
- Important tests results; eye and dental records
- Correspondence between patient and providers
- Current educational materials (or appropriate web links) relating to one's health
- Any information an individual wants to include about his or her health, such as exercise regimen, any herbal medications taken, and any counseling received

In addition, personal family history may also provide insights.

Issues in Data Collection and Quality

Because individuals select the items to include and control access and use of their PHR, the record may not be comprehensive or current. It is important for patients to bring their PHR to their appointments and for providers to review items carefully, including content and dates. A variety of formats are available, including file folders, binders, CDs, USB drives, and so on. In addition, commercial companies have started to offer online services through which patients can upload their information and approve access by others. Recognizing the importance of electronic access and information to patients, some providers and MCOs are creating patient portals that allow patients to make appointments, leave messages, review their laboratory results, and so on. Although related, they are not a true PHR, which is controlled by the patient. HIM professionals have an important, emerging role in assisting consumers with the creation and maintenance of a PHR for themselves and others for whom they have responsibility. AHIMA provides a variety of resources.[15]

SELF-ASSESSMENT QUIZ

20. How do forms and views differ among the sites of care?
21. How do the data sets differ across the sites of care?
22. What is the value of creating and maintaining a PHR?

PATIENT-CENTERED CARE

In their landmark report, *Crossing the Quality Chasm: A New Health System for the 21st Century* (2001), the IOM focused on six "Aims for Improvement," including care that is safe, effective, patient-centered, timely, efficient, and equitable[16]. Although patient safety has received significant attention, patient-centered care has become a priority more recently.

Patient-Centered Medical Home

The concept of a medical home was first proposed in the 1960s, but did not gain momentum until 2007 when four physician practices developed a common model of the patient-centered medical home (PCMH). Their model is organized around seven principles stating that primary care is patient-centered, comprehensive, team-based, coordinated, accessible, and focused on quality and safety. It has become a widely accepted model for how holistic primary care should be organized and delivered.

Of particular importance to HIM professionals and the health record is the element of coordination, which emphasizes that care is organized across all elements of the health care system. The EHRs and HIEs are key to accomplishing this coordination as is the standardization of data elements.

Patient Portal

A patient portal is a secure web-based system that provides patients convenient 24-hour access to personal health information from anywhere with an Internet connection. Using a secure username and password, patients can view health information such as laboratory results, medications, immunizations, and so on. Patients can then add these documents to their PHR. Options may also include the ability to make appointments, pay bills, and communicate with practitioners. Chapter 6 further explores this emerging technology and its relationship to the EHR. Patient portals are hosted by health care providers (who may contract with a vendor who has a business associate agreement with the provider) and are protected under HIPAA. The portal belongs to the health care provider.

ELECTRONIC HEALTH RECORD INITIATIVES

As patient records migrate from paper-based to EHR systems, they build on a foundation of sound record practice described here, including the focus on the needs of users, data collection standards, and efficient record management and reporting. Chapter 6 explores EHRs, their structure, challenges, and the profound opportunities for improvement in patient care, health care delivery, and research.

SUMMARY AND MANAGEMENT ISSUES

Health care decisions may make the difference between life and death for patients and between success and bankruptcy for providers. There is little room for error. Timely and accurate information is needed to make these decisions with the highest possible degree of confidence. A prerequisite to such quality information and decision making is quality data. Data items that are well defined, selected, and collected make efficient use of human and computer processing resources and produce valuable information. Awareness of the needs of users, the flow of data throughout the facility, and the health care delivery system, as well as standards and content directives, positions the HIM manager at the hub of the health care decision-making process.

CHAPTER REVIEW

1. Why are good data essential to sound decision making, both clinical and business related?

2. What are the five unique roles of a health record?

3. What is similar and what is different about the records in the following care settings: inpatient, ambulatory, home care, hospice, behavioral health, long-term care, and rehabilitation?

4. Who uses health records? Give an example of a use for each user.

5. What is the purpose of standard data sets in health care? List at least three examples and discuss.

6. What are some principles associated with data collection and organization?

7. Have we been successful in standardizing the health record in any care setting? Discuss your answer.

8. Why do some organizations use paper records? Do you see paper as temporary in today's health care environment?

9. Why should everyone consider creating either a paper or electronic PHR for themselves and, if appropriate, their family members?

10. As patient-centered care is more widely implemented, how do you envision health record practice evolving?

REFERENCES

1. Ackoff RL: From data to wisdom, *J Appl Systems Anal* 16:3–9, 1989.
2. ASTM International: *E1384-07: Standard practice for content and structure of the electronic health record, section 4.2.1,* Philadelphia, 2013, ASTM International.
3. American Health Information Management Association: Fundamentals of the legal health record and designated record set, *J AHIMA* 82(2), 2011, Expanded online version http://library.ahima.org/xpedio/groups/public/documents/ahima/bok1_048604.hcsp?dDocName=bok1_048604.
4. Department of Health and Human Services: *Core health data elements: report of the National Committee on Vital and Health Statistics,* 1996. http://aspe.hhs.gov/datacncl/ncvhsr1.htm (Accessed 22.02.10).
5. The Joint Commission: *Comprehensive accreditation manual for hospitals: the official handbook,* ed 2014, Oak Brook, IL, 2013, Joint Commission Resources
6. Kohn LT, Corrigan JM, Donaldson MS, editors: To err is human—building a safer health system. In *Committee on Quality of Health Care in America,* Washington, DC, 2000, Institute of Medicine, National Academy Press. http://www.nap.edu/catalog/9728.html (Accessed 13.03.10).
7. Lewis KS: Medical record review for clinical pertinence, *Top Health Rec Manage* 12:52–59, 1991.
8. *The uniform hospital discharge data set,* Washington, DC, 1974, Department of Health, Education, and Welfare.
9. *Long term health care: minimum data set: Report of the National Committee on Vital and Health Statistics,* Washington, DC, 1998, Department of Health and Human Services.
10. Department of Health and Human Services: *The uniform ambulatory care data set. Report of the National Committee on Vital and Health Statistics and Its Interagency Task Force in the Uniform Ambulatory Care Data Set,* Washington, DC, 1989, Department of Health and Human Services.
11. American Health Information Management Association: Data quality management model (updated), *J AHIMA* 83(7):62–67, 2012.
12. *Outcome and assessment information set (OASIS),* Washington, DC, 1999, Department of Health and Human Services.
13. Abraham PR: *Documentation and reimbursement for home care and hospice programs,* Chicago, 2001, American Health Information Management Association.
14. *Healthy People 2010:* http://www.healthypeople.gov/Document/pdf/Volume2/18Mental.pdf (Accessed 13.03.10).
15. Wolter J, editor: *The personal health record,* Chicago, 2009, American Health Information Management Association.
16. IOM (Institute of Medicine): *Crossing the quality chasm: A new health system for the 21st century,* Washington, DC, 2001, National Academy Press.

DATA ACCESS AND RETENTION

Mary Alice Hanken

(e) Student Study Guide activities for this chapter are available on the Evolve Learning Resources site for this textbook. Please visit http://evolve.elsevier.com/Abdelhak.

CHAPTER CONTENTS

OBJECTIVES

After reading this chapter, the reader will be able to do the following:
✓ Define key words.
✓ Describe the various numbering systems for health information.
✓ Compare and contrast the filing options for the paper record.
✓ Compare and contrast scanning of records versus commercial storage and identify when each method is desirable.

✓ Identify key milestones in a file conversion.
✓ Identify considerations important to the selection of file folders.
✓ Describe the benefits of color coding to any of the filing methods.
✓ Describe how an automated record-tracking system can be developed and implemented.
✓ Identify how bar code technology interacts with an automated record-tracking system.

✓ Explain how the statute of limitations pertains to record retention.

✓ Describe the different hardware options available when designing an automated data access and retention program.

✓ List the necessary components of a scanning system and the various cost factors involved in implementing a scanning system.

✓ Identify possible steps in the implementation of an optical imaging system.

✓ Describe why electronic storage of data is a prerequisite to the successful implementation of the electronic health record.

✓ Examine a current storage and retrieval system and determine alternative solutions to solve identified problems.

✓ Prepare strategies for planning and implementing solutions to information system problems.

KEY WORDS

Active record	Encounter	Outguide	Serial-unit numbering
Alphabetical identification	File guide	Picture archiving and	Statute of limitations
Bar code device	Inactive record	communication system	Symbology
Centralized filing	Master patient index	Requisition	Terminal digit filing
Color coding	Numerical identification	Retention period	Unit numbering
Decentralized filing	Optical character recognition	Scanner	Voice recognition
Disaster recovery	Outcard	Serial numbering	

ABBREVIATIONS

AHIMA American Health Information Management Association
ASCR Association of Specialists in Cleaning and Restoration
CPI Corporate Person Index
ED Emergency Department
EDM Electronic Document Management
EHR Electronic Health Record
HIE Health Information Exchange
HIPAA Health Insurance Portability and Accountability Act
HIM Health Information Management
HIT Health Information Technology

LHR Legal Health Record
MFD Multifunctional Device
MPI Master Patient Index
eMPI Electronic Master Patient Index
OCR Optical Character Recognition
PACS Picture Archiving and Communication System
PC Personal Computer
PPI Pixels per Inch
RFID Radiofrequency Identification
UPC Universal Product Code

ACCESS AND RETENTION OF HEALTH INFORMATION

Health care is information dependent and cannot be provided efficiently without facts regarding the patient's past and current conditions. Various systems are necessary to ensure that the information is available where and when it is needed for patient care at a reasonable cost.

The patient record provides the data to establish the who, what, when, where, and how of patient care. It is the documentation of everything that takes place during the provision of health care. These data are maintained to provide better quality health care, to support billing accuracy, to minimize litigation losses, to comply with applicable laws and regulations, and to aid in medical research efforts. Retaining the data so that they are available for use in the future is a major concern of all health information professionals.

This chapter describes various ways in which patients' health information can be accessed and retained. The discussion begins with the paper record and progresses to electronic document management (EDM) to the electronic health record (EHR). Additional discussion of health information processes associated with the EHR are found in other chapters.

The role of the health information professional is to evaluate past and current methods and current and future needs and to select the best system to meet those needs. This may involve converting to new filing methods or filing media, maintaining current systems more efficiently, or making decisions regarding the destruction of nonuseful material. In addition, health information professionals must keep their knowledge of technologies current so that plans can be made to keep the data retention program current with the technology. Just as an IBM 286 personal computer (PC) with a 5¼-inch disk drive is not current technology today, the state of the art today may no longer be usable or accessible for data retrieval in the next 5 to 10 years. *Data access* and *retention* mean ensuring that no data are lost to technology obsolescence. Every effort must be made to ensure that, as technology advances, either the old technology is maintained to ensure access or the new technology can access the old data.

The health information professional's knowledge of information management consists of more than information systems concerning the formal patient record. Information management knowledge can easily be applied to other areas as well, such as radiology image storage, human resource management, and administrative records. No other field of study within the health care arena provides information management background, although each discipline maintains patient health care records. Wise facility managers use the health information professional as an in-house consultant to these other areas to improve overall facility efficiency. Therefore the concepts covered in this chapter present ways of accessing and retaining information, regardless of the scope, size, or shape of the information or storage media involved.

ACCESS AND RETENTION OF PAPER-BASED RECORDS

Although there is an active transition occurring in our profession to the paperless record, health care facilities may still be using paper-based methods or they may maintain a substantial portion of their patient records in a paper-based format or receive paper from other entities. The first portion of this chapter discusses maintenance and filing of the paper-based format of the patient record and methods of identifying the record.

Record Identification

Alphabetical Identification

Identifying the record by patient name, called alphabetical identification, is the most basic identification system used in health care. Although it sounds simple, the system can be more difficult to maintain than it appears.

In maintaining an alphabetical identification system, the correct patient name is the vital piece of information. All patient names, both first and last, must be spelled accurately to be sure that the record can be located in the future. All name changes must be indicated on the patient record folder in a paper-based system, creating a cross-reference for the previous location in the file. Alphabetical identification systems can be maintained without a separate master patient index (MPI) because the records themselves form a large patient index. If a separate index is used, cross-referencing of name changes must also be completed in the index; this requires extra work.

An advantage of the alphabetical identification system is that the record can be located using information obtained directly from the patient. The disadvantage of the system is the complex spelling of many names and the frequency with which individuals change their names. In addition, not everyone knows instinctively how to file names alphabetically. To achieve the consistency needed for successful future retrieval, the record maintenance staff must be taught the filing rules adopted by the facility and reference them while completing their work.

Numerical Identification

An alternative method of identification is to use a number to identify the patient record; this is called numerical identification. Assigning a number to a patient record requires the use of the MPI, which contains a minimum of the patient name and the patient identification number. Additional data elements to be included in this index are covered later in this chapter. In the manual version of this identification system, the MPI cards are filed alphabetically and referenced to find the patient identification number. In an automated format, a computerized database serves as the MPI. The computer file is searched for the required name or a similar combination of letters. The correct name is determined, and the associated identification number is displayed on the computer screen.

The manual version of this method has some of the same problems as the alphabetical filing of patient records. The computerized version provides the added advantages of allowing access to the identification number by multiple users at one time and consistently sorting the database in the same way for each user. The computer also allows searching by one or more elements to identify an individual (last name, birth date, medical record number, etc.). The computer also provides the flexibility of producing reports in both alphabetical and numerical order.

Methods of Numbering

A number identification system can be designed in several ways. *Serial, unit,* and hybrid *serial-unit numbering* are discussed here.

Serial Numbering

Serial numbering is a system of number assignment in which a patient receives a number for each encounter at the facility. The patient could have multiple numbers, all of which require entry onto the manual index card or maintenance in the computerized database. This method has a higher supply cost because each encounter at the facility requires the use of a new file folder on a paper-based system. Each new folder is filed in a different location, requiring the searching of multiple locations to retrieve one patient's entire record, a time-consuming process. Serial numbering can be used effectively when the patient return rate is low or the population served is transient.

Unit Numbering

To avoid the extra effort of assigning a new number for each encounter and the searching of multiple locations for record folders, the unit numbering system was developed. In the unit numbering system, each patient receives an identification number at the first encounter and retains that number throughout all contacts with the facility. With this numbering system, a facility can easily create a unit record for the patient, filed in one location in the file in a paper-based system.[1] Labor costs are reduced because the number is entered into the MPI only once, and supply costs are lower because the same folder is used for all encounters except when the number of encounters exceeds the storage capability of the folder, thus resulting in additional folders. The unit numbering system is the most popular system for both paper-based records and EHRs.

Technically, any number could be chosen as the unit number identifier, but most facilities prefer to assign numbers sequentially, starting with the number 1. Although the individual's social security number has sometimes been used as the unit number, its use is discouraged because of privacy, security, and identity theft issues.

In a variation of the unit numbering system, a number is assigned to a family rather than to an individual. This numbering system is common in community health centers that treat a family as a unit. This approach allows common identification of a family unit, even if the family members have different last names. If this method is chosen, consideration must be given to assigning each family member his or her own identifier as an additional number and giving the person his or her own folder in a paper-based system.

Serial-Unit Numbering

In an attempt to combine the ease of number assignment from serial numbering and the unit record concept from unit numbering, the serial-unit numbering method was developed. Numbers are assigned serially, but as each new encounter takes place, all the former records in a paper-based system are brought forward to the most recently assigned record number and filed together as a unit in the same folder. Typically, the previously used folders remain in place and a note is placed on or in the folder noting the newly assigned number.

Table 5-1 shows a comparison of these three numbering systems. In the future, the concept of a unique (unit) identifier for each patient for a lifetime will become more attractive. Some form of unique identifier can provide the common link for all the information contained in the multiple computerized databases of information maintained on individual patients.

Organizations are very diligent about keeping their master patient/person index clean. Any concerns about duplicate number assignment in a unit numbering system are addressed quickly (one person with more than one number). Another issue that is sometimes present in a unit number system is number sharing (more than one person is assigned to the same number). This type of clean up of numbering systems is needed in both paper-based and electronic systems.

We do not yet have agreement on a unique health care number for each individual in the United States. Each organization is able to assign its own identification number to an individual. As organizations merge or align themselves and as we move into health information exchanges (HIEs), there are reasons to again address the concepts of a master person/patient index. Because each organization can assign its own person or patient ID number, the master person/patient index at the enterprise or regional level may contain several "unit" identification numbers. In organizational mergers the master person/patient index may be called the *enterprise level index* and contain the person or patient identification number for each organization. As HIEs emerge we are seeking ways to be sure of the identity of the subject of the information to be exchanged. This has renewed interest in unique health care numbers for individuals and the coordination of master person/patient indices.

✅ SELF-ASSESSMENT QUIZ

1. Name the different types of record identification.
2. What are different types of numerical identification?
   a. Serial
   b. Unit
   c. Hybrid serial-unit numbering
   d. All of the above

Filing Equipment

Making a decision about how to store paper-based patient records and other record-related material is a situation that all health information professionals usually face at some point in their careers. Although sales personnel are trained to assist in the decision-making process, it is helpful to know the advantages and disadvantages of the different types of storage equipment before the process begins. Table 5-2 compares the available types of storage equipment according to physical description, strengths, weaknesses, and facility types where they are best suited. Figure 5-1 shows an aerial view of open shelves and compressible units. Most large health care facilities start a computer-based EHR system and go forward with computer-based storage, leaving a legacy of paper-based records to manage either until the required time for retention has expired or, for some research facilities, forever.

The International Fire Safety Code and state fire codes provide guidance related to aisles and exits. The fire safety codes require that certain minimum allowances be made

---

TABLE 5-1 Numbering Systems		
System	Number Assignment	Filing Concepts
Serial numbering	A new number is assigned for each encounter.	Each record is filed separately using the number that has been assigned for that visit.
Unit numbering	One number is assigned at the first encounter and used for all future encounters.	The record is filed using the unit number.
Serial-unit numbering	A new number is assigned for each encounter.	The record containing each number is brought forward and filed using the newest number assigned.

TABLE 5-2 Comparison of Different Types of Storage Equipment

Equipment	Physical Description	Strengths	Weaknesses	Best Suited For
Filing cabinets	Three to five drawers, vertical or lateral arrangement	Can be purchased as a fireproof cabinet. Can be purchased with locks. Protects records from the environment	Requires dedicated aisle space. Difficult and time consuming to open each drawer. Can open only one drawer at a time	Small facilities. Dirty environments. High fire dangers. Low file activity requiring high security
Open-shelf files	Five to eight shelves with full access to the front (similar to bookshelves)	Easy access to any part of the shelves and multiple shelves at a time. Can accommodate multiple workers at one time	Requires a 36-inch dedicated aisle between shelving units. Records open to the environment	High-volume files with multiple file maintenance workers. Relatively clean environments with sufficient space for aisles. Works well in a clinic facility for active records and in hospitals for outpatient records
Motorized revolving units	Shelves move around central spine like a Ferris wheel with records carried on bucket shelves; run by a motor	Little aisle space needed. All work is at one height level. Records can be covered and locked	Must be carefully loaded and unloaded in a balanced manner or it will not run. Motor or power failure causes record unavailability. High initial cost, maintenance contract costs	Limited space with low file activity and one primary file maintenance worker. Dirty environments
Compressible units	Open-shelf files that move in parallel lines to form an aisle opening. Motor-assisted movement or hand cranked	Saves space of unused aisles. Easy access to shelf currently opened to the aisle. One dedicated aisle required	Time needed to locate where the access aisle is needed and to open the mechanism to the aisle. Limited number of aisles. Mechanical failure causes record unavailability. Maintenance contract costs	Limited space with low to medium file activity and two to three files maintenance workers. Works well in a hospital facility for inpatient records or inactive records

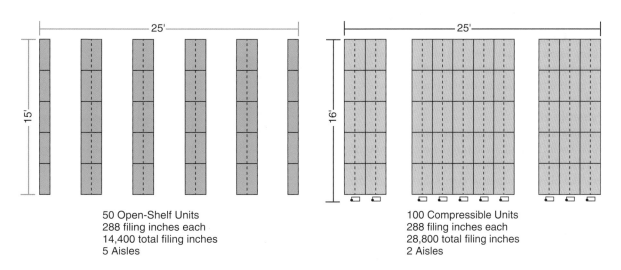

50 Open-Shelf Units
288 filing inches each
14,400 total filing inches
5 Aisles

100 Compressible Units
288 filing inches each
28,800 total filing inches
2 Aisles

FIGURE 5-1 Overhead view of open-shelf and compressible units.

for aisles. Typically, the minimum aisle width varies from 28 inches to 36 inches. These aisles and exit paths must be kept clear of any clutter or protrusions into the space. Wheelchair access minimum is 30 inches. The code has information guidance based on the typical occupancy and use of the space. Access the national code at http://www.nfpa.org/codes-and-standards (verified 2/13/14).

Filing Cabinets
Vertical filing cabinets are the traditional type of drawer files seen in many offices. They vary in height, width, depth, and number of drawers. These cabinets are specifically constructed to hold cards, letter files, and legal files, or they can be constructed as a combination of card file drawers and larger drawers.

Lateral filing cabinets are also available. The file drawers in a lateral filing cabinet open from the long side, and the entire cabinet resembles a chest of drawers. Because these cabinets have drawers that are not deep, they are well suited to narrow spaces, such as along walls. or as room dividers.

Both vertical and lateral filing cabinets are available with two to five drawers and can be purchased with special fireproof wall and drawer construction or with locks. Although they protect records from the environment, considerable effort is required to open each drawer when filing or retrieving a record. These files are best suited to small settings such as physician practices or nursing homes in which record retrieval is limited and performed by one or two people.

Open-Shelf Files

Open-shelf files resemble bookshelves and provide ready access to records without having to open any drawers. They are available with five to eight shelves per section and they are usually adjustable to accommodate different heights of folders. Adjustable shelf dividers help support the file folders on the shelves. The files, which require a dedicated 36-inch aisle, leave records open to the environment. Open-shelf files are the storage equipment of choice for high-volume file rooms in which many people require simultaneous access to the shelves, such as in clinics and hospitals.

Motorized Revolving Units

The motorized revolving file contains shelves that rotate around a central spine like a Ferris wheel. The records are placed on a shelf similar to an open shelf or on a bucket shelf in a lateral file. Files must be loaded or unloaded from the machine in a balanced manner, just as passengers are alternately loaded onto and off a Ferris wheel. If the load is unbalanced, the machine stops to avoid damaging the internal mechanism. These files are best suited to small facilities in which record retrieval is limited and performed by one person, such as solo physician or dental practices.

Compressible Units

These movable-aisle systems, or compressible units, are similar to open-shelf files but are mounted on tracks secured to the floor. The shelf units move on the tracks, and the operator opens the file at the appropriate place to create the aisle where needed. They are available in both manual and motor-assisted models. Although this type of filing equipment saves considerable floor space, access to files is limited because only one or two aisles can be created at a time. Compressible units are best suited to files with low to medium file activity with only a few people working in the files at one time. In the electronic style (motorized) models, electrical wiring is necessary. Electrical models are priced more intensively but may save greater time and labor, thus increasing staff productivity overall. The pros and cons of each option on the basis of the staffing levels and physical constraints must be considered before shelving decisions can be made. They may solve some space issues for health information departments.

 SELF-ASSESSMENT QUIZ

3. What is the most common type of paper filing system used in large health care organizations?
   a. Open-shelf files
   b. Vertical filing cabinets
   c. Compressed units
   d. Motorized revolving units

Space Management

Centralized and Decentralized Files

Facilities can use a centralized or a decentralized filing method for paper-based records. In centralized filing, there is a single location for all records created throughout the facility. This centralized file location is staffed by specialized personnel who provide records that have been requested by authorized users.

In the decentralized filing method, parts of the record are filed in different locations in the facility. Outpatient and emergency departments (EDs) may file their active records in their own departments. In clinic facilities, decentralized records may be created when specialty departments maintain their own records. Table 5-3 shows the advantages and disadvantages of the centralized and decentralized record management alternatives.

SELF-ASSESSMENT QUIZ

4. True or False. In the decentralized filing method, parts of the record are filed in different locations in a facility.

TABLE 5-3	Comparison of Centralized and Decentralized Paper-Based Record Management Alternatives
Centralized Files	**Decentralized Files**
Overall supply costs are lower.	Supply costs for storage equipment and multiple folders are increased.
High level of security with record control is easy to maintain.	Record control is more difficult to maintain.
Standardized procedures for file maintenance can be developed.	File format can be flexible to meet the unique needs of the patient and providers.
Specialized staff can be trained to perform file maintenance as their primary duty.	File maintenance staff are harder to train consistently, and file maintenance may be a low priority for staff with other duties.
Consist supervision is available for file maintenance staff.	Supervision is provided by department staff in the area where the records are located.

Filing Methods

Designing a numbering and filing system within a facility is a major responsibility, and the decisions can affect other functions in the facility. Understanding each of the options is important. Although the term *filing* does not connote a high degree of professionalism, the efficient management of records in any format requires managing an important asset of the organization. The health information professional serves as an in-house consultant to the organization for numbering, filing, and record management.

Alphabetical Filing

How to Use

An alphabetical identification system and the alphabetical filing method must be used together. The alphabetical filing method starts with last names that begin with A and continues through all the names, ending with Z. For records of patients with identical last names, the first name and then the middle initial are used to determine the exact filing order. When first names are a single initial or no middle initial is given, the rule of nothing before something is used to determine filing order. Each name (last, first, middle) or the corresponding initial is treated as a group when filing. A single-initial name is the shortest name possible and would be filed first. The file would look like this:

1. Henri, Martha
2. Henry, J
3. Henry, J T
4. Henry, John T
5. Henry, Judy
6. Henry, Judy R

Specific alphabetical filing rules are shown in Box 5-1.

Names that contain nonalphabetical characters, capitals, or spaces, such as *O'Dell, McCallum,* and *Van Braun* often cause variations in filing accuracy. Add to this the complexity of numerical modifiers such as *Sr, Jr,* and *III.* Each facility should maintain consistency in filing by deciding how special filing situations are to be handled, documenting the correct order, and referencing the documentation as the filing process is completed.

Space Planning

Letters of the alphabet appear in any given volume of records with an average frequency. These frequencies can be used to predict the percentage of file space that should be allowed for each letter of the alphabet (Box 5-2).

File Guides

File guides are used to aid in the filing process. These guides list the letter of the alphabet and any vowel subdivisions within the main letter category, such as *Da, De, Di, Do,* and *Du,* all within the main letter category of D.

Benefits and Considerations

Alphabetical filing systems work well for facilities with fewer than 5000 paper-based records, a stable patient population, and little or no computerization. They may not work well

BOX 5-1 Alphabetical Filing Guide

1. Use the last name first and then the first name followed by the middle name or initial according to strict alphabetical order.
2. If there are two or more identical last name and first name combinations, use the middle name to determine the order. If the middle name is the same or no middle initial is given, use the birth date, filing the oldest patient first. (This may occur when father and son have the same name.)
3. Names with prefixes (*O', D', Mc, Mac, Von,* etc.) are filed as if there was no apostrophe or space (*O'Brien* is filed as *OBrien*).
4. Hyphenated names are filed as if there was no hyphen (*Mayberry-Quinn* is filed as *MayberryQuinn*).
5. If an initial is given instead of a first or middle name, use the "nothing before something" rule to file *J T Henry* before *John T Henry.* If you are using a searchable database, double check that *J T Henry* is not the same individual as *John T Henry.*
6. Do not abbreviate names in alphabetical filing. However, if the name is abbreviated and you cannot check the database to confirm the full name (i.e., *Wm* is *William*) file it as it is spelled (*Wm* is *W-M*).
7. Do not include seniority designations (Sr, Jr) or titles (MD, PhD) in alphabetical filing. If found, do not use in determining file order. Computer databases can accommodate prefixes and suffixes, and this information may be useful for other purposes.
8. Computer systems may vary in their search capabilities; however, partial name searches typically bring up several names from which to select the correct name. Alphabetical filing rules may also provide options. If the system allows double last names to be entered then it may allow both the inclusion of a dash as in *Kitt-Young* or allow both names to appear separately as *Kitt Young.* In this instance an example of the filing might be: *Kitt Young, Andrew; Kitter, Daniel; Kitter, Margaret; Kitt-Young, Samuel.* Another example of use of two last names not combined for filing is: *Al Aassi, Andrew; Al Abuddi, Sam; Al Asad, William; Alani, Tamera; Alameda, George.* Typically the abbreviation *St* is spelled out. Filing for this might be: *Saint Martin, Edward; Saint Martin, Jessie; Saintplant, Kirk.*

BOX 5-2 Alphabetical Frequency Distribution

A 3.2%	M 9.3%
B 9.7%	N 1.7%
C 8.0%	O 1.3%
D 4.9%	P 4.5%
E 2.2%	Q 0.2%
F 3.8%	R 4.8%
G 4.9%	S 10.2%
H 7.8%	T 3.4%
I 0.4%	U 0.4%
J 2.6%	V 1.0%
K 3.6%	W 6.8%
L 4.5%	X, Y, Z 0.8%

in ethnically homogeneous areas in which last names are frequently repeated.

Straight Numerical Filing

How to Use

Facilities that have more than 5000 paper-based records, have frequently changing populations, or have become computerized usually assign numbers to their patients. They may choose to file their records in straight numerical or sequential order, a basic system that starts with a record of the lowest number value and ends with a record of the highest number value. New records are always added at the end of the number series, concentrating most of the filing activity in one area of the file. Accountability for filing accuracy is harder to track when most of the record maintenance staff is focused in one area of the files.

File Guides

File guides are used in this system to help the eye determine the change in digits. If the folders are thick, file guides should be placed every 100 records. If the folders are thin, one guide for every 1000 records may be sufficient.

Space Planning

To plan space adequately for a straight numerical filing system, consideration should be given to thinking of the file room as a circle. As inactive records are removed from the lower-numbered areas, these areas can be consolidated forward, creating additional room for the end of the number series to grow into. This method is far easier than moving the entire contents of the file area back to the starting point whenever the end of the number series has come to the end of the filing space. Inactive records are also discussed under record management later in this chapter.

Terminal Digit Filing

How to Use

The terminal digit filing method is based on a patient identification number that is divided into three parts. Most facilities use a minimum of six digits (filling any unused digits on the left for numbers lower than 100,000 with zeros), and other facilities use the terminal digit method with numbers as large as a nine-digit number.

See the following example of a standard six-digit identification number.

Example of a Standard Six-Digit Identification Number

12	34	56
Tertiary digits	Secondary digits	Primary (or terminal) digits

The number (12-34-56) is read from left to right for identification purposes and from right to left (from the terminal end) for terminal digit filing purposes. To understand the filing concepts, it is best to visualize the file layout in a terminal digit system. If the file room has 100 sections of filing equipment, each would contain the records labeled with one of the 100 possible primary digit combinations (from 00 to 99). Using the preceding example, the 56 section would be further visually subdivided into 100 possible locations for records. Record number 12-34-56 would be in the thirty-fourth subdivision (secondary digits of 34), or approximately one third of the way into primary section 56. Within the thirty-fourth subdivision, records are filed in straight numeric order by the

tertiary digits. In this example, the record is number 12, following record 11 and preceding record 13. File sections 56 and 57 would look like this:

11-34-56
12-34-56
13-34-56 . . . to 99-34-56, with the next folder being
00-35-56
01-35-56 . . . until 99-99-56 is reached, with the next folder being
00-00-57
01-00-57 and so on.

The steps in finding record 12-34-56 are as follow:
1. Go to section 56.
2. Within section 56, go to the subdivision of 34s.
3. The record is the twelfth record in subdivision 34 if all records are present.

The same concepts used in our monetary system, 100 pennies in a $1 bill and 100 dollar bills in a $100 bill, apply here. In this system, the pennies are records.

File Guides

File guides are used to mark primary digit sections in small, paper-based file systems. In larger file systems, each group of 10 secondary digits is guided, in addition to the primary digit sections.

Space planning is easiest in a terminal digit system. Because new numbers assigned sequentially are evenly distributed among all 100 filing sections, the file grows evenly. Time has shown that records become inactive at a relatively even rate of distribution, allowing the file to increase or decrease evenly in size. This system also allows those who work in the file area to be distributed more evenly and perhaps assigned responsibility for a section of the file area because the activity is not focused in one section of the filing space.

Space Planning

To determine the size of each primary section in a new file area in a paper-based system, calculate the available inches of filing space by measuring the lengths of the actual shelves or drawers available. Divide the total number of inches of filing space by 100. The result is the number of inches of filing space to allow for each primary digit combination. Remember to start allocating space for number 00, not 01. This may leave considerable space between primary sections but saves the time of shifting the records later as the file grows. Theoretically a terminal digit filing system would grow equally and take up an equal amount of space per terminal digit. Realistically, however, they may not grow equally. For this reason, it is important to not plan to fill up the shelving to full capacity. Filing units should be purchased in multiples of 5, such as 5 units (or cabinets), 25 units, 50 units, or 100 units, if space permits. This allows each terminal digit number to reside in an area of a filing unit. If 50 units of storage space are purchased, two terminal digit numbers are placed in that shelving unit or cabinet. Table 5-4 compares the advantages and disadvantages of straight numerical filing and terminal digit filing.

TABLE 5-4	Characteristics of Straight Numerical Filing and Terminal Digit Filing for Paper-Based Record Systems			
Straight Numerical	**Sample Order**	**Terminal Digit**	**Sample Order**	
Training period is short.	29160	Training period is slightly longer.	24-29-04	
File grows at the end of the number series, requiring backshifting.	30158 101412	File grows evenly throughout 100 sections—no backshifting required.	25-29-04 10-14-12	
Inactive records are pulled from one general area.	107412 107643	Inactive records are purged evenly throughout the 100 sections.	49-32-12 10-74-12	
File staff is "bunched" in the highest numbers, causing less accountability for filing accuracy.	107644 123456 242904	Work is evenly distributed throughout the 100 sections, causing accountability for accuracy in that section.	10-76-43 10-76-44 12-34-56	
Number is dealt with as a whole, causing mental fatigue, transpositions, and misfiles.	252904 493212	Number is dealt with in two-digit pairs, easing mental fatigue and causing fewer transpositions and misfiles.	03-01-58 02-91-60	

SELF-ASSESSMENT QUIZ

5. Which of the following are filing methods (select all that apply):
   a. Alphabetical
   b. Straight numerical
   c. Terminal digit
6. In the following example, identify the tertiary digits: 15-33-64

Master Patient Index

The MPI is the key to locating the patient record in any filing or computer system. It identifies all patients who have been treated by the facility and lists the number associated with the name. The index can be maintained manually or as part of a computerized system. In either case, the MPI should be maintained permanently.[1] Most health care MPIs are electronic databases (eMPIs). They typically serve a health care organization or a group of health care organizations that form an enterprise system. As health care moves forward with data exchange, the MPI is key to correctly identifying patients and supporting the exchange of health information. At the 2012-2013 House of Delegates of the American Health Information Management Association (AHIMA), the House passed a resolution on "Managing the Master Patient Index in a Healthcare Environment." The purpose of the resolution is "to emphasize the importance of accurate identification of individuals contained in a master patient (person) index in a healthcare environment."[2] The MPI is the building block that will allow the accurate exchange of information across a continuum of care. It is essential that identity integrity is preserved to appropriately link an individual's information. The MPI is often a component of a Registration/Admission/ Discharge/Transfer computer application and may be referred to as *Reg/ADT*. This is often a front-end component of an EHR system.

Content

The MPI should contain enough demographic data to readily identify the patient and his or her record. There are usually two levels to the MPI. The first is the demographic level, which contains information about the patient that usually remains consistent from visit to visit and does not reflect episode-specific data. The second, or episode level, reflects visit or account information that varies by the date of service. The content of the MPI usually includes the following:

Demographic Level
1. Full name (last, first, and middle) (plus suffixes and prefixes)
2. Patient sex
3. Race
4. Ethnicity
5. Patient date of birth
6. Patient identification number: Medical record or unit number (a lifetime number that follows the patient throughout all visits in this health care system)
7. Other cross-reference numbers or names (previous names, maiden name, or alias)
8. Other demographics that represent the patient at the time of encounter: address, phone numbers, Social Security number, guarantor, and so on
9. Facility ID

Visit Level (Episode of Care)
1. Specific account or episode numbers
2. Encounter dates (i.e., admission and discharge)
3. Service type
4. Location of service
5. Admitting diagnosis or encounter diagnosis
6. Attending physician name and primary provider
7. Facility ID

Additional data elements recommended for an enterprise or expanded MPI include:
1. Place of birth
2. Advance directive
3. Power of attorney for health care
4. Organ donor status
5. Emergency contact information
6. Master problem list[3]

In most settings the MPI is an electronic database that serves many purposes. It is the link to other databases and, if an organization has a numerically filed, paper-based record system, the MPI is the key to record location. It is also used for report routing, statistics, and historical identification of activity within the facility. It is not intended to be used as a marketing or community database. Episodes of care must be unique, must reflect only individual occurrences, and must not be combined for the purpose of combined billing. Gaps in recurring care, unless identified through other means, must be separated by use of individual accounts.

Alias names are not recommended for use in an MPI because they must eventually be cross-referenced to the actual name and may draw more attention to the individual than is necessary in a health care setting. As an alternative, appropriate security controls and flags indicating not to display information where not needed by those directly involved in the care should be used. Figure 5-2 is a sample alias policy and waiver form for the MPI. In a computer-based system the health care organization may offer an individual other options such as putting an individual's record into a sensitive or secure status and restricting and auditing access to the record.

Patient Waiver for Use of an Alias

Philosophy: This facility believes mechanisms should be available to provide an extra level of online security access in extraordinary circumstances. This facility also believes that this mechanism should provide for long-term integrity of the patient data and master patient index as well as continuity of care, and thus should be administered according to detailed procedures that help support confidentiality as well as validity of information.

General Security:
1. All patient information is protected by general release of information policies and is available only on a need to know basis within the scope of work or with appropriate patient or legal guardian authorizations.
2. All behavioral medicine patients are protected with an extra level of computer access security based on the patient type utilized within the hospital information system upon patient registration.

Extraordinary Circumstances:
1. Typically, an individual requesting use of an alias makes contact with a facility staff member.
2. Staff notifies supervisor or appropriate charge person.
3. Supervisor is to evaluate request against the following criteria for validity:
    a) Is patient a VIP requiring anonymity due to public notoriety?
    b) Is patient's safety or care endangered if identity is revealed? (i.e., criminal, victim of rape, incest, or other abuse)
    c) Has physician ordered, and patient agreed, to use of an alias?
4. If request is received outside of Patient Registration and falls into approved criteria, supervisor is to notify Patient Registration Charge Person to initiate the alias process.

5. **Registration Procedure:**
    a) Patient is to sign waiver for use of an alias form. Alias will not be used unless the patient signs the waiver.
    b) Patient is registered for this episode of care using legal name (may or may not already exist in the MPI) in order to originate or use correct unit number (MRN).
    c) Patient signs all consent/authorization and other legal forms throughout the episode care using his or her legal name.
    d) After registration is complete, registrar will change legal name within the computer system to the alias of the patient's choice as documented on the waiver form. Legal name will be retained as an alias within the system during the current episode of care.
    e) The face sheet will be sent to the unit supervisor with the original of the alias waiver form. These are to be retained as a permanent part of the medical record.

6. **Discharge Procedure:**
    a) On the day of discharge, immediately prior to the actual discharge, the supervisor on the discharging nursing unit will notify the Patient Registration Charge Person of the impending discharge.
    b) Patient Registration will change the alias back to the patient's legal name, now retaining the alias as a previous name in the computer system. It is important to do this prior to discharge to ensure billing will occur correctly.

FIGURE 5-2 Patient waiver for use of an alias. *MPI,* Master patient index; *MRN,* medical record number.

Continued

Waiver for Use of an Alias

You have requested to use an alias (pseudonym) while you are a patient. When using an alias, certain consequences may occur. Although an alias may superficially help protect your confidentiality to a higher level, it may also actually draw attention to your presence in the facility, due to the number of steps necessary to implement a pseudonym. Therefore, we ask that you read the following information and give your consent to the use of the alias you have chosen.

I understand:

1. My insurance company may not verify coverage using an alias. I will provide the facility with my legal name and sign all the paperwork using my legal name for billing as well as medical consent purposes. I will be liable for any bills my insurance company refuses to pay because of the use of an alias.

2. Information I provide about next of kin will not be changed to an alias.

3. Previous medical information or information provided by other health care providers may not be readily available if I choose to use an alias. I understand if I do not use the same alias each time I choose an alias, my medical records may not be recognized and retrieved in a timely manner to assist with my care.

4. My alias will be returned to my legal name within the computer system after my episode of care is completed. My alias name will be cross-referenced to my legal name at that time.

5. Portions of my medical record will contain both my legal name and alias name depending on when the results are printed.

6. The pharmacy and other ancillary areas of the facility may not be able to release prescriptions and results to me while I am using an alias, unless proper identification of my legal name is available.

Legal name is: (print) _____

Alias name is: (print) _____

Signature of patient/legal guardian _____ Date _____

Witness Signature _____

FIGURE 5-2, cont'd

Creation of the Index

If an electronic system is not available, a manual MPI can be maintained according to alphabetical filing rules (see Box 5-1), keeping in mind the need for consistency in filing. Computerized indexes must have the same consistency and careful data entry.

Whether manual or computerized, hyphenated names present a challenge in the MPI because they are retrieved differently from the same two names combined without a hyphen. In most computerized systems, hyphens are excluded from the name. Also, prefix names entered without a space (such as McDonald) are retrieved separately from those entered with a space (Mc Donald). When numbers are assigned in a unit numbering system, these database retrieval problems can cause the patient to be incorrectly assigned an additional number. New MPIs should be entered consistently, and continuing indexes should be verified for possible problems with inconsistent data entry. Figure 5-3 shows a sample basic MPI screen for a facility that uses unit numbering.

Policies and procedures must be set up to ensure MPI data validity. The MPI is generally originated on patient scheduling or registration; maintained or added to during the course of clinical care; and validated, updated, and maintained by health information professionals. Duplicate number assignment can result in the need to merge visits, which must include updating any and all corresponding reports, records,

Name: Smith, John James	MR#: 12-34-56
DOB: 03-03-1936	SS#: 294-55-3235*
Sex: M	

Dates of Admission: 01-10-84	Discharge: 01-15-84
06-05-91	06-07-91
10-20-94	10-26-94

* Social Security numbers are obtained voluntarily from patients

FIGURE 5-3 Master patient index screen. *MR*, Medical record; *SS*, Social Security.

and databases in a health care facility (paper and electronic) for consistency. Figure 5-4 shows sample MPI creation policy and procedure guidelines. Many facilities engage in a daily reconciliation and validity checking process for the MPI to ensure that duplications and errors are cleansed. Others use specialized software designed to screen and identify existing or possible discrepancies at the time of creation of the MPI or afterward in a batch mode. This area of the profession has become so specialized that today companies have been established to handle MPI maintenance, elimination of duplication, and general overall validation.

Backup of the MPI is extremely important because this is a primary index for record retrieval functions in a paper-based clinical record system and an important component of an EHR system. Backup files must be available for staff during computer system downtime. The backup files in an EHR environment provide at least the basic information about the patients and individuals being provided services during a computer downtime. In a paper-based environment the MPI is the index to finding the records in a numerical filing system.

The use of corporate or enterprise-wide identification numbers is popular so that patients can be identified to the demographic level within a health care system. This usage also allows such entities to continue to use a separate and unique numbering system without losing the ability to identify shared patient information within the corporation (Box 5-3). However, care must be taken when working within a corporate health system not to merge the MPI, unless there is also a way to unmerge the same index in case of separation of entities within a system. If multiple facilities are serviced through one index, such as in a multihospital system, the index should indicate the facility in which the admission or encounter occurred.

Records Management Issues

File Folders

Until the day that all records are computerized, the folder that contains patient information is important for anyone who has responsibility for the record. Many facilities may use the paper patient record as a historical document well into the future. The file folder is the most fundamental

element of record management. The folder should be viewed as a tool for protecting documents and managing information. For this reason, it is important to be aware of the difference that choosing the right folder can make. All these considerations also apply to the management of other records that are housed in file folders. Considerations in folder size and design are as follows:

- Standard folders for patient records are 9½ inches high and 12¼ inches wide.
- Standard folders are manila but other color choices are available; typically up to 12 colors are available.
- Reinforced top and extended side panels are important when there is a high rate of record retrieval from the file.
- Folder bottoms should be scored (manufactured with indented lines that assist in creating straight folds) to allow the folder to accommodate a patient record of average size for the facility. Consider the average number of pages per discharged record, the number of annual outpatient encounters,[2] or both when estimating the average record size. Also consider whether the facility provides any services that are long term in nature (e.g., oncology, dialysis) or creates especially large records for documenting complex care, such as neonatal intensive care records. High-volume ambulatory practices can also produce a large amount of paper documentation.
- The thickness of the folder should be appropriate for the expected rate of use, with the understanding that heavier folders cost proportionately more. The two standard thicknesses are 11 point and 14 point, with 14 point being heavier and more durable. Manila stock is also available in 13, 14, 15, 18, and 20 points. Of these, 11-, 14-, and 15-point stock are the most commonly used. Please note: *Point* and *weight* are different. Point measures thickness (a point measure is equal to $\frac{1}{1000}$ inch or 0.001″). Weight measures density (measured by weighing 1000 sheets of sized paper stock). To determine the correct weight, consider the following:
  - The number of pages expected to be protected and filed in the average folder
  - The specific retention period of the paper record
  - The average number of times the folder will be removed from the shelf in its lifetime of use (the wear-and-tear factor)

If the wear-and-tear factor is low or the retention period for the paper folder is projected to be short (2 to 3 years), the 11-point folder is adequate. If the paper record is expected to be used for 3 or more years, the 14-point folder is a wiser investment.

There are two basic configurations of folders: end tab configuration and top tab configuration. End tab is primarily used for open-shelf file systems. Top tab configuration is primarily used in pull-drawer filing systems. Folders can be purchased with or without fasteners, and the fasteners can be applied in various positions within the folder to aid in organizing the data to best meet the facility's needs. Additionally, reinforced extended tabs add to the longevity of the folder. However, reinforced extended tabs may not be the best

Master Patient Index Creation Policy and Procedure

Philosophy: A computerized Master Patient Index (MPI) is a legal record to be maintained permanently for all patient episodes of care. These episodes are identified by a unique unit number (also known as medical record number [MRN]) and account numbers for each case or series of care. Maintenance of an accurate and timely master patient index is essential to the operations of the facility. Patient Registration areas are responsible for the accuracy of the information entered into the computer system upon registration or pre-registration. Clinical/Ancillary areas are responsible for the data integrity during patient care that is required to accurately reflect activity. Health Information Management will facilitate revisions needed after patient discharge to maintain data validity.

I. Master Patient Index Creation Guidelines

A. Upon registration, only legal names shall be entered into the computer system unless specific policy dictates otherwise.
   1. Verify with proof of identification (preferably Driver's License) at the time of registration whenever possible.
   2. Nicknames or alias is not to be used unless there is a risk to patient safety. (See Alias Policy and Procedure.) In the rare circumstance that an alias is utilized, appropriate Alias Waiver will be utilized.
   3. Do not use punctuation, spaces, or symbols in a name. Hyphenated names are to be entered as a single continuous name without a hyphen.
   4. Enter middle name only if entire name as listed on legal ID fits in designated space. Otherwise, use middle initial only.
   5. Do not use title (religious, medical, etc.)
B. Check for previous name or numbers (which must be done at EACH REGISTRATION).
   1. Check the Master Patient Index by entering last name and first initial.
   2. Use birth date, address, mother's maiden name, and/or social security number as an additional check.
   3. Use phonetic search if no name is found.
   4. Never enter middle initial or middle name when searching the MPI for purposes of registration.
   5. Verify with the patient or family member that no other name may have been given when registering previously.
C. Unidentified patients:
   1. Until accurate information can be obtained:
      a. Females should be entered as Doe, Jane with a birth date of January 1 of the current year.
      b. Males should be entered as Doe, John with a birth date of January 1 of the current year.
      c. If multiple Does are entered, the middle initial should be entered in alphabetical order (i.e., Doe, John A).
      d. Trauma patients are entered as TRAUMA, ###### (# representing the number they are given in a trauma situation).
   2. Social security number should be entered as all zeros for unidentified cases.
D. Newborn babies are to be entered upon birth as "Last name, Baby boy". (or Baby girl) (i.e., Jones, Baby boy)

II. Demographic Data Changes

A. Incorrect patient name:
   1. If patient has been registered under a previous name which is not the legal name (but is a name the patient may have given at the time of the previous registration), correct the previous name. Only the legal name should be retained.
   2. If a patient has been registered under a previous name which was the legal name previously (i.e., the maiden name), both names are to be retained. Keeping a previous name creates an alias.
   3. If a patient has been registered under a previous name that has an incorrect spelling, correct the previous name. Do not retain the incorrectly spelled name.

FIGURE 5-4 Master patient index creation policy and procedure.

Continued

4. For newborns, adjust the permanent name from the original. Newborns will be changed from "Last name, Baby boy" format to the "Last name, First name" format without retaining an alias. However, for newborns whose legal name is different from that given at registration and/or different from the mother's name, two name changes will be required. First, from baby to given first name, which does not require an alias, and second, upon registration (with the updated first name) to legal name appearing on the birth certificate, which will require an alias to be retained.

Example A: Jones, Baby boy (name change without alias retention) to Jones, Michael

Example B: Jones, Michael (name change with alias retention) to Smith, Michael

III. Duplicate Unit (Medical Record) Number

A. If one or more duplicate unit numbers are discovered:

  1. Register the patient's new account under the earliest (oldest or lowest number) in the system. This is the "correct" number.

  2. Notify HIM of the duplicate number by completing the duplicate unit number report form. A copy will also be given to the Patient Registration Manager. Items to be recorded include:

    a. Patient Correct/Legal Name

    b. Date of Birth (DOB)

    c. Correct (original) Unit Number

    d. Wrong Unit Number (duplicate)

    e. Last Account Number created in incorrect unit number

    f. Registrar Initials

  3. All patient records, centrally or de-centrally stored, and applicable databases will be reconciled by managing departments to concur with correct and cross-referenced unit numbers.

  4. If patient is registered under another patient's unit number, transfer account from one unit number to the other.

B. If one or more duplicate unit numbers are discovered when the record is being processed:

  1. Complete the Patient Data Validity and Correction Form and route to the manager.

C. Correct Inpatient/Outpatient Records and Databases after the unit numbers have been merged:

  1. Obtain report of daily MPI merging activity.

  2. Locate the record using the invalid unit number.

  3. If the record is in the permanent file:

    a. Cross out the invalid number on the facesheet and document (in red) the valid number.

    b. Update the letter color labels if necessary.

    c. If the patient has had previous admissions under the valid unit number, file the record under that valid number.

    d. If the patient has not had previous admissions, update the folder to reflect the valid unit number and patient name, file in correct terminal digit location.

  4. If the record is anywhere outside of permanent file:

    a. Cross out the invalid unit number and patient name on the facesheet and document (in red) the valid number.

    b. Update the letter color labels if necessary.

    c. Return the record to the proper location.

    d. Notify the Incomplete Record Area staff of the merge so that proper updating in the Deficiency System is made if the record is incomplete.

FIGURE 5-4, cont'd

course of action when you consider adding year bands, color-coded labels, or computer-generated labels on the extended tab.

Color Coding

Using color coding to designate certain letters or digits helps to prevent misfiles and aids in rapid storage and retrieval.

Color can also provide an easy way to distribute workload and make sorting of folders much easier.

Differently colored folders can be used to designate changes in primary digits of a terminal digit system. Color bars designating letters or digits can be preprinted on the folder or added by using adhesive labels. The color bars may have both a color designation and a position

BOX 5-3 Case Study: MPI Software Cleans Up and Prevents Duplicate Medical Record Numbers

This case study concerns how two hospitals with a combined total of nearly 40,000 inpatient discharges and 185,000 outpatient visits a year with different information technology and different data fields came together beginning with a corporate person index (CPI). The challenge was to implement a common CPI for two hospitals while performing a data integrity improvement of each of the existing master patient indexes (MPIs). The target date for completion was 2 months.

The health information department was assigned responsibility for identifying "duplicate" patients in the CPI between the two facilities and updating the respective separate MPIs to reflect the most current information. The process began with a traditional deterministic search method to identify duplicates within each facility's MPI.

The following elements were researched in an exact deterministic match on all elements:
- Last name, first name
- Social Security number
- Date of birth

The problem with this method is that it is not possible to detect duplicates caused by errors in name spelling or number transposition. Also, there is no easy way to cross-reference merged duplicate numbers.

After a year of manual clean-up effort and more than $60,000 in manpower, time had run out. When the two hospitals' MPIs were loaded into the CPI, another 78,000 duplicates occurred within the CPI. An immediate and cost-effective solution had to be found. At that point the director of patient financial services recommended using a computerized process that searched the MPI files by using algorithms. Because time was of the essence, a product and a vendor who had an immediate solution had to be selected. A vendor was selected to install electronic clean-up software. The vendor accomplished the installation and had the software operating in less than 3 months.

The software was able to identify duplicates by using the following:
- Phonetic search
- Deterministic search
- Probabilistic algorithms that rank the information from 100 to 1 as a probable duplicate record number

In addition, the software used name normalization, address normalization, and a stoplight method of highlighting potential duplicate data fields, thus expediting the process of duplicate number decisions by the clerical clean-up team.

At the time the two hospitals decided to embark on this partnership, there was a multidisciplinary conversion team formed that included all ancillary departments, patient financial services, the internal audit manager, computer services, and medical records. The high volume of duplicates affected the ancillary departments. In addition, as the clean-up was occurring, the health information department became frustrated that duplicates continued to occur as a result of new duplicates being generated every day during registration.

In addition to the conversion team, a registration team was formed. This team worked with the director of health information management (HIM) and the health information support manager responsible for making recommendations about decision rules for the clean-up process. The decision rules regarding which medical record number would "survive" as the permanent number was a collaborative effort among the vendor experts, computer services, and the health information professionals. The registration team worked on data element standardization between the two facilities so the data element *sex*, for example, was *F* for *female* in both sites and *M* for *male* versus using *b* for *boy* and *g* for *girl*. The MPI team started with the highest probabilistic matches because the team was simultaneously cleaning the MPI and the CPI. However, as the clean-up project continued, it was apparent that new duplicates

continued to be created every day. The director of the health information department felt that the project value was mitigated without "up-front" (at the time of registration) prevention of new duplicate numbers. This viewpoint was strongly supported by the ancillary departments. The blood bank, for example, was very supportive of duplicate prevention software. As a result of the team support, the hospital elected to add up-front duplicate prevention software.

Unfortunately, the problem of duplicate medical record and guarantor numbers in health care provider settings is not unique. What makes this case study interesting is that the electronic solution of the 78,000 CPI duplicates was completed in less than 4 months. Today the MPI remains very clean with a computer "refresh" run every 6 months. The computerized refresh presents only duplicate numbers that have been issued since the last refresh and does not present duplicates that have been rejected as "not a duplicate."

Definitions

1. *Corporate person index (CPI):* A person index that contains person names and medical record numbers for multiple facilities. Person names may be the patient or guarantor of the account
2. *Cross-reference:* Archive of numbers file that, when created electronically, allows all numbers that pertain to the same patient to be filed together in the cross-reference
3. *Deterministic:* Able to establish an association between two files by searching for an exact match against a set of given criteria (e.g., medical record number) (AHIMA Practice Brief: Fundamentals of Building a MPI/Enterprise MPI, 2010 available at www.AHIMA.org)
4. *False positive:* If a record is reported as a duplicate but on review is determined not to be a duplicate and is rejected, careful attention has to be given as to where in the 100 to 1 probabilistic scoring the majority of these occur
5. *Merge:* Once the patient number that is to survive is selected, the computer electronically merges data from nonsurvivor (retiree) encounters together with the survivor number, therefore providing continuity of patient information
6. *Name normalization:* A process that links common names such as *William, Billy,* and *Bill* together under one name
7. *Pairing rule:* A data element field or fields used as a key by the scoring algorithm for identifying potential duplicates
8. *Phonetic file:* A system to file and find names without regard to vowels; used to locate names that sound alike but are not spelled the same way
9. *Probabilistic:* Capability or linking of data elements that compensate for discrepancies by using all the information recorded in two files and attach a weighted value for matching discrepancies (*AHIMA Practice Brief*, November 1997)
10. *Refresh:* Computer capability to locate all new person or patient numbers issued since the last update, excluding those designated as "not a duplicate" during the earlier number clean-up efforts; to "refresh" the file is to bring out all legitimate duplicates created since the last time the process was refreshed
11. *Retiree:* The duplicate patient number that is determined to be sent to an archive cross-reference list and not to be used for further patient care
12. *Scoring:* Weighted or probabilistic algorithm for quantifying the relative validity of a potential duplicate
13. *Street normalization:* A table that brings "Berkshire St." and "Berkshire Street" together
14. *Survivor:* The duplicate patient number that is selected to remain in the active file and that will be used in new encounters

(Courtesy MediBase and Mary Mike Pavoni, RHIA, FAHIMA.)

designation. If either the color or the position on the folder is incorrect when it is placed in the file, it indicates a misfile.

Employees working in a color-coding environment should be tested by the human resources department to ensure that candidates for working in the file room are not color blind.

Record Security

Patient records should be stored in an area or a room that can be locked to prevent inadvertent loss, tampering, or other unauthorized use. The area can be secured by the traditional lock-and-key method or with a computerized access panel that operates by activating the correct key combination. The computerized access panel has the advantage of being easily updated with a new code if a security problem is noted, rather than by attempting to physically locate all the keys. The Health Insurance Portability and Accountability Act (HIPAA) and organizational policies typically permit access on a need basis only. Security of computerized records is discussed in Chapter 8, Technology, Applications, and Security.

Storage of Inactive Records

An organization may determine how to keep frequently needed paper-based files accessible. One perspective is to define files as active and inactive on the basis of the health care activity of the patient. Active records are stored in a location commonly referred to as the *active files*. Activity is determined by the frequency of encounters with the typical patient and the amount of filing space that is conveniently located. For example, if a patient has not received treatment or had other activity associated with the record for more than 5 years, then the record could be declared inactive. The organization decides the period of time associated with the definition of active record. Inactive records do not need to be as readily available but do need to be accessible when they are needed. For example, one hospital has limited space for its paper-based clinical records and can only maintain approximately 1 year's worth of records on site. Records stored off site are accessible through a contract delivery and storage service that provides twice-a-day and on-call deliveries to the hospital.

Alternate Location

Two options are available to store inactive records no longer in high demand without changing the records to another format or medium. One option is to store records in an organized filing system located in another area of the facility. Another option is to use the services of a commercial storage company.

Commercial Storage

Commercial storage companies store different types of records but may specialize in highly confidential records, such as legal or patient records. As a minimum, the commercial storage company should have the following:

- Business associate agreements compliant with HIPAA rules and regulations

- HIPAA-acceptable confidentiality policies and statements signed by their employees
- Acceptable references from health care facilities or similar business facilities
- Insurance coverage for loss, damage, personal injury, and workers' compensation
- Record return guarantee by either faxed or electronic transmission
- Reasonable retrieval fees
- No surrender fee (cost to remove all the records from storage)
- Quality control in both storage and retrieval methods

Other items to be included in contract discussions with commercial storage companies are the "hidden," or seldom thought of, questions, such as the following:

- Who pulls the files from the current storage system (who pays for it)?
- Who completes the list of what is to be stored (who pays for it)?
- Exactly when does the custody of the record change over to the storage company (whose insurance is paying for it)?
- What are the billing terms (yearly, monthly, as used)?
- What price increases to expect and frequency of these increase over the life of the contract?

Each possible storage company should be screened to evaluate its overall costs and services provided. Investigate other alternatives discussed in this chapter when developing a long-term storage and retrieval system. Calculate the costs for all options in accordance with the facility retention policy or over a minimum of 10 years to provide adequate comparison of the costs.

File Conversion to Terminal Digit System

Existing alphabetical and straight numerical paper-based filing methods often do not meet the needs of growing facilities. Increased filing efficiency is usually sought by converting existing systems to numeric identification and the terminal digit filing method. Conversion sounds intimidating, but it does not need to be if thorough planning takes place. Conversion concepts can apply to moving the contents of a department or file room to a new location (see Box 5-4). If it is decided to convert to a new filing system, consider taking a picture of the file area before beginning the process to be able to visually show the success afterward.

Planning Process

Make as many changes as possible before the actual conversion. If the files are being converted from an alphabetical arrangement to a straight numerical or terminal digit arrangement, they need to have numbers assigned to them and an index must be created. If a computer system is already in use, a patient number field must be available to store the numbers. Either assign the numbers and enter them into the computer or have the computer complete the number assignment process.

BOX 5-4 — File Space Conversion Checklist

1. _____ Take "before" pictures.
2. _____ Develop a chart of project timelines and post it.
3. _____ Purge the records if not all are to be converted.
4. _____ Assign numbers to record, if necessary, and create an index.
5. _____ Apply color coding or bar code labels, if necessary.
6. _____ Schedule an actual conversion date.
7. _____ Hold a project meeting with the staff.
8. _____ Complete test trials to determine average times.
9. _____ Complete an estimated count of the records to be converted.
10. _____ Calculate staff needs and obtain staffing commitments.
11. _____ Assign team leaders, project teams, and duties.
12. _____ Hold a project meeting with the staff.
13. _____ Train the staff in the terminal digit system; take "field trips" as necessary.
14. _____ Take "halfway" pictures (with color-coded labels out of order).
15. _____ Alert and train the clinical staff about conversion.
16. _____ Hold a project meeting with the staff to establish ground rules for the conversion weekend.
17. _____ Order food for breaks and meals and tables and carts for sorting.
18. _____ Determine and label new terminal digit section placement in the file.
19. _____ Organize the chart return day for 1 day before conversion.
20. _____ Locate a secure area, with keys, for personal belongings.
21. _____ Receive delivery of tables and carts.
22. _____ Actual conversion takes place.
23. _____ Take "after" pictures (with labels in order).

Before filing systems are converted, the following steps should be taken:

1. Be sure that all record management applications have been thoroughly explored, giving equal consideration to imaging and scanning or EDM. Software, hardware, file supplies, and employee costs are all factors in the equation. If the decision is to continue using paper-based records and to do a conversion to a new filing system, then proceed with this plan.
2. Change to new folders. In converting to an automated record-tracking system, some manufacturers can manufacture file folders with bar codes already printed or embedded on the folder, thus saving time and money.
3. Apply color coding or other labels to ease the re-sorting process during the conversion.
4. Purge the files not being converted so that the fewest records possible need to be moved.

Schedule the conversion during an off-peak time for the facility, such as during the slower summer months. The move should be scheduled for a weekend from Friday at 5:00 pm to Monday at 8:00 am.[4] Trial tests should be made with a small number of records to determine the time it takes to complete each phase of the conversion work, with an average time per unit of work being multiplied by the estimated number of work units to be completed. Allow for 10% fatigue time when converting patient record folders. Schedule enough workers to complete the conversion on the basis of the number of hours available and the average times calculated from the trial tests.

Develop a visual display of the project timelines. Post the chart in a prominent place in the department, and educate all staff members about their roles in adhering to the conversion timeline. Hold as many preparatory meetings as necessary to make the staff feel comfortable with the conversion.[2] Take "before" pictures of the file room area before the conversion starts.

Train all staff to a working comfort level. Inform employees about the theory behind terminal digit filing, train them in its use, and have the employees practice the methods.[5] Considering that most file system conversions incorporate new folders, color-coded applications, and possibly computer interface, ask your vendors to assist in providing a small mock file room for practice purposes and other hardware applications necessary to train staff. Check the work of each employee to determine the employee's understanding of the terminal digit system. Also, educate the remainder of the facility staff and the medical staff about the changes that will be taking place in the department to increase their understanding.[5] Answer their questions, reassure them that service will not be interrupted during the conversion, and enlist their cooperation during the conversion period.

Have sufficient staff and supplies available for the conversion. Use department staff and supplement them with other workers as necessary. Order folding tables for sorting and transportation carts from a rental company, or borrow them from another facility.[5]

Conversion Process

There are four project phases in the conversion, each requiring a team leader assignment:

1. Transport the records to the sort area and back to file.
2. Rough-sort into 10 terminal digit sections (e.g., 00-09, 10-19).
3. Secondary-sort into 00, 01, 02, and so on.
4. Fine-sort into strict terminal digit order on the file shelves.

Begin the conversion by removing records from the areas prelabeled as section 00 and section 50. Remove an equal number of records from the areas that will hold each terminal digit section. This minimizes the number of records that must be off the shelves at any given time and provides a place to put records as soon as they are sorted. Team 1 transports the records to the sort area and back to the file. Team 2 rough-sorts the records onto sorting tables (or boxes on chairs), and Team 3 does an intermediate-sort into 00, 01, 02, and so on. To minimize back injury from lifting, have employees avoid placing records on the floor or lower than waist height. Use carts to transport all records.

When sufficient records are available in any given primary section where shelving is available, Team 1 transports the records back to the shelving area and places them on the appropriate shelf. Team 4 then fine-sorts the records into strict terminal digit order. Continue this process until all records have been rough-sorted and returned to the file in their primary section. At that time, Teams 2 and 3 become fine sorters with Team 4, and Team 1 assists in any shifting of files necessary within primary sections.

Teams should be scheduled in 8-hour shifts, all taking breaks and lunches together.[5] The facility food service or an outside catering service should prepare meals and break refreshments for the team staff. A secured, lockable area where personal belongings can be stored should be provided.[4] Throughout the process, expect the unexpected and adjust plans as necessary.

When the process is complete, take "after" pictures of the finished product. Tell of your success and hold an open house for the facility.[4] Today, many organizations publish an in-house newspaper for its staff and employees. This is a great vehicle to share your success and recognize those who assisted in the process. And finally, do not forget to send thank-you messages to all participants.

Record Tracking

Regardless of how paper-based records are filed within the facility, one of the biggest concerns is knowing where a record is when it is needed. For a record management system to be efficient, there must be some method of tracking the current location of a patient record.

Manual Record-Tracking Systems

Manual record-tracking systems are the most common, with use of outguides and requisitions as their basic tools.

Outguides

An outguide is a plastic folder used in place of a record when the record has been removed from the files. It can be thought of as a placeholder. Outguides usually contain two separate see-through pockets, one to hold the requisition slip and one to hold any loose papers to be filed in the record that accumulate while the record is out of file.

Requisitions

A requisition is somewhat like an IOU. It is an acknowledgment that someone has taken a record and intends to return it.[6] **Figure 5-5** shows a typical paper patient record requisition slip. Part 1 of the requisition slip is placed in the outguide as the record is removed from the file. Parts 2 and 3 travel with the record as a routing slip. Part 2 can be used by the requester as a transfer notice if the requester forwards the record to another location. Notification of a record transfer is important to obtain but can be especially difficult to obtain in a manual system. The notices are usually slips of paper that can easily be lost in transit. The transfer notices that do make their way to the file area should be given a higher priority than the retrieval of records. Filing the transfer notices first ensures that the most current location for every record is known before retrieval is attempted. Facilities with computerized registration and appointment systems can typically generate requisition slips that print out in the location where the record is filed. These systems typically also print lists of records to be pulled for appointments.

Manual record-tracking systems should also be able to determine when the record has been purged, or thinned, from the active files and either moved to an alternative storage site or converted to another medium, such as digitally scanned. Outcards listing the new location or medium should be used for this purpose.[6] An outcard differs from an outguide in that outcards are usually cardboard to allow the patient name and record number to be written directly on them. Outcards stay in the file permanently to tell the new location of the paper record or the new medium to which it has been transferred.

Record Retrieval Steps

The steps in retrieving a paper-based record in a manual system are typically as follows:

1. Receive the request for a record.
2. Verify the name and number of the record.
3. Place the requisition slip in an outguide.
4. Locate the record on the shelf.
5. Put the outguide on the shelf and remove the record.
6. Forward the record to the requester.

When the record returns, refile it on the shelf and remove the outguide, placing any loose filing material in the outguide into the file itself.

FIGURE 5-5 Requisition slip.

Patient Number: _____

Patient Name: _____

Date of Request: _____ Time Needed: _____

Requestor: _____

Transferred to: _____

Number of Volumes sent: _____ Date: _____

1 | Routing Slip

2 | Transfer Notice

3 | Requisition Slip for Outguide

Color coding methods can also be applied to the use of outguides. Two common methods of color coding outguides are assigning colors for specific request reasons or assigning colors to a specific retrieval time period. Using unique colors for different request reasons alerts the staff to immediately check another location, such as the release of information area or the physicians' incomplete area.

When assigning colors to a specific retrieval period, some departments use a differently colored outguide every week on a 4-week rotating cycle. As a new week begins, the outguides from the past 4 weeks (four different colors) are counted. All outguides older than 3 weeks are checked and updated with the new location. This provides a constant file review process for records out of file longer than 4 weeks. Other similar plans can be used to track records according to specific facility needs.

A sufficient supply of outguides is important to a record-tracking system. Past activity levels can help determine the quantity of outguides to have on hand. Be sure that the outguide pockets are large enough to accommodate both the requisition slip and any loose papers. Filing loose papers in the outguide allows the staff to forward information to a requester if the record is unavailable and allows the record to be updated immediately when it returns to the file.

Although these manual system procedures are typical, this tracking system is not without certain disadvantages, including the following:

- Time lags in updating record locations[7]
- Extra time needed to file transfer notices to keep record locations current
- Illegibility of many handwritten requests[7]
- Difficulty in prioritizing workload
- High frustration levels of staff whose work is crisis oriented[7]
- Dissatisfaction of record requesters with service

Automated Record-Tracking Systems

Software Considerations

Automated record-tracking systems were developed to address the concerns just listed. An automated record-tracking system is a database that stores the current and past locations of the record. The automated system is similar to both inventory control software that is used in manufacturing to track parts and tracking systems used by the U.S. Postal Service, UPS, FedEx, and others. The fact that the system is automated does not mean that outguides and requisition slips are forgotten. Outguides can still aid in the refiling process and hold loose papers. However, organizations have been known to forward loose documents to the holder of record for filing. Requisition slips identify the name and number associated with the outguide. Once the record is retrieved, the outguide is no longer considered the source of information on the record location. The tracking system holds the information about all record requests and transfers.[8] It is possible, therefore, to run various reports that assist the health information professional in managing records wherever they are located.

The tracking system is often linked to other facility systems to avoid duplication of effort. For example, linking the tracking database to the MPI eliminates the need for this second database to contain large amounts of patient demographic information. It is also efficient to link the record-tracking database to a patient scheduling system to allow automatic transfer of requests for appointment records.[9] Linking the system to a record deficiency system gives an added advantage of knowing which records need to be returned for completion.

Having an online request-for-records feature speeds the request process and produces legible requisitions with complete and accurate information with each printing. This feature also allows the tracking software to prioritize the requests according to date and time of need and whether the request is for direct patient care. This feature significantly decreases the need for telephone requests for records and frees the staff to spend time retrieving records rather than answering the telephone. Printers are used to printing requisitions and are placed in the file area near where the records are located.

An automated record-tracking system should be able to produce both management reports and statistical reports (Box 5-5).

Data Entry Capabilities

Automated systems work extremely well when integrated with bar code technology to speed the data entry process. Bar code labels can be applied to existing folders in preparation for converting to a bar code system or as an enhancement to a current record-tracking system to increase productivity.

BOX 5-5

Software Requirements of an Automated Record-Tracking System for Paper-Based Records

Dictionary driven, user definable
- Reasons for requests
- Out-of-file locations

Reporting capabilities

Management reports
- Appointment listings
- Unsatisfied requests listings
- Location listings (for use during downtime)
- Overdue listings by user-defined time frames
- Out-of-file listings by location
- Inactive record listings by alternative storage site or medium

Statistical reports
- Total scheduled appointments and percentage satisfied
- Total walk-in appointments and percentage satisfied
- Total stat requests and percentage satisfied
- Total requests for each out-of-file location and percentage satisfied
- Grand total of all requests and percentage satisfied
- Total records refilled
- Total records retrieved from inactive storage and other media

Bar codes have been used in health information departments since the 1980s. The Health Industry Bar Code Council, which was formed in 1984, approved a particular bar code symbology specifically for use in health care: code 39. The symbology of a bar code means the way the lines and spaces in the bar code are arranged. Code 39 was selected for its variable length, accuracy, and flexibility.[10] Materials management was initially the first area in the hospital to use bar codes because the early bar codes were associated with products supplied to hospitals. Materials management, radiology, and food service all use the same standard bar code to track supplies, radiology films, and meals, respectively. The bar code symbology for record folders contains at least two pieces of information: the patient number and the volume number of the record. If other information is needed, it is usually retrieved by online access to the MPI or other database.

When a bar code is read, the software receives the characters as if they were entered by way of the keyboard and it processes the information in the same way. This is the same as the process used in a grocery store scanner that reads the universal product codes (UPC) from canned and packaged products. If the UPC is unreadable, the cashier enters the number on the keypad. Also see Chapter 8, Technology, Applications, and Security, for information on bar coding.

 DID YOU KNOW?

In 1952 Joseph Woodland and Bernard Silver received the first patent for their invention, the barcode. They developed the concept at the request of a food chain store owner who was looking for a method to automatically read product information during checkout. By 1970, a company named Logicon, Inc. wrote the Universal Grocery Products Identification Code, which eventually evolved into the UPC, invented in 1973 by George Laurer. The first product to have a bar code was a packet of Wrigley's Gum.

Hardware Needs

Programmable color laser printers can be purchased that can print a strip label for the side of the folder that contains the patient's name and identification number, the bar code, and the color code bars. This method ensures that records are labeled uniformly and that the labeling process is completed with the least amount of hardware and supplies.

Bar code scanners are available in two types: contact and noncontact.[11] A contact scanner is sometimes referred to as a *light pen* or *wand* and must come in contact with the bar code to read its contents. Noncontact scanners can be handheld or fixed. Department store cashiers frequently use handheld scanning "guns" to read product labels. Fixed scanners, such as grocery store scanners, read labels that are passed over or under them.

Even with all the automated assistance, the ultimate success or failure of an automated record-tracking system still depends on proper training, commitment of all staff to use it consistently, and the system's ease of use.

Entering all data contained in previous paper records would be an extremely costly project, and therefore these records need to be tracked until they are no longer useful or until the majority of historical information is entered into the EHR.

Record Retention

Health information professionals are frequently asked questions about how long to keep patient records. There is no universal answer to the question. Several factors need to be considered.

Federal Statutes and Regulations

The federal government has a number of laws and regulations related to record retention. Depending on the type of organization, the health care facility may be subject to one or more federal laws and regulations. For example, Department of Veterans Affairs hospitals are expected to keep their patient records 75 years from the date of last activity. Hospitals and other types of health care organizations can check federal requirements related to participation in certain programs and the length of time records should be retained to prove that services were provided in case there is a billing or payment review some years after the service is rendered.

State Statutes and Regulations

State law provides concrete guidance on record retention. The state laws should be referenced individually to obtain the most current information related to retention requirements. State laws may be specific to the type of organization, such as hospital, boarding home, psychiatric hospital, or behavioral health clinic. In 2002 and in 2011 the AHIMA reviewed record retention requirements and recommended categorical timelines as guidance in the absence of a particular law. The document also reviewed federal laws and state laws on retention of records. For example, Washington State requires hospitals to keep patient records a minimum of 10 years after discharge. If the patient is a minor at the time of discharge the record must be kept until the age of majority plus 3 years or 10 years, whichever is longer (RCW 70.41.190). Washington law also requires that a record be kept at least 1 year after a request for information from the record (RCW 70.02.160). The statute of limitations in each state should be considered when determining a retention policy. The statute of limitations determines the period in which a legal action can be brought against an organization for injury, improper care, or breach of contract.[12] In most states the statute of limitations begins at the time of the event or at the age of majority if the patient was treated as a minor. In some states the time for bringing certain actions begins when the individual discovers the problem (i.e., a surgical instrument left during a procedure). For example, if the typical period of time is 8 years and that period has expired, the individual is given 1 additional year in which to bring an action (RCW 4.16.350).

In February 2008 AHIMA published E-Discovery Policies: Retention, Storage and Destruction of Paper and Electronic Health Information and Records which can be used in conjunction with the original 2002 publication. (Available at www.AHIMA.org.)

Organizational Needs

Institutional policy is another source to be considered. Because the organization maintains the record for the benefit of the patient, the physician, and the health care organization, it is the responsibility of the organization to keep the record for the use of all three parties.[13] Organizations usually require that information in an MPI be kept permanently. Ideally, key elements of the patient record would be maintained indefinitely. Although this is the best policy, it may not be possible from a financial or other practical standpoint. Because computer storage issues have changed and no longer drive retention decisions, it is possible to retain large amounts of clinical data, reorganize it into useful segments, and rethink retention practices.

An organization should also consider the rate of patient readmission and the level of commitment to research and education in the final decision on retention. An organization with a high readmission rate will find its own records extremely valuable in the future care of the patient. Longitudinal studies conducted in research facilities are difficult to complete if short retention periods are chosen for patient records.

Different types of medical organizations may have different retention requirements. In some states the record retention for long-term care facilities is 5 years. In other states free-standing ambulatory settings or physician practices may not have record retention regulations or statutes. Therefore it is incumbent on the health information management (HIM) professional to research existing statutes, regulations, professional practices, and organizational needs to recommend an appropriate course of action.

Retention Schedule

Once a facility makes the decision about which records to keep and for how long, a record retention schedule should be developed and approved by the facility attorney, facility compliance officer, malpractice liability insurance carrier, and board of directors. The schedule should list all medical and business records and should address retention and destruction of both original records and copies of records.[12] For hospital settings, the American Hospital Association recommends retaining records for a minimum of 10 years.[13] When destruction is determined to be appropriate and no federal or state laws preclude this guidance, then a minimum retention schedule should be as follows:

- If the patient was older than the age of majority when treated, 10 years.
- If the patient was a minor when treated, several years past the age of majority depending on the statute of limitations in the state.
- If federal or state laws require longer retention periods, then the federal or state laws or regulations should be followed. Records involved in an investigation or in litigation should never be destroyed, even if they are due for destruction according to the retention schedule.[12]

- If an organization is reviewing an EHR system for retention and future use by clinicians and patients, there are reference documents related to longitudinal health records and continuity of care documents that provide guidance related to the most useful long-term data to retain related to patient care. Various research, public health, and quality improvement programs have additional data recommendations for retention of certain data, perhaps for extended periods.

As a general recommendation, the following information should be retained permanently in some format, even if the remainder of the record is destroyed:

- Dates of admission, discharge, and encounters
- Physician names
- Diagnoses and procedures
- History and physical reports
- Operative and pathologic reports
- Discharge summaries[1]

Destruction

Destruction of records should take place only after approval by the facility administration, facility attorney, malpractice liability insurance carrier, and board of directors. Complete details of all records destroyed must be kept indefinitely. A manifest including all patient record numbers and patient names should be created as the records are purged or removed from the files. The destruction process, either by shredding or by incineration, should take place in the presence of two witnesses who both sign a destruction letter with the date and method of destruction that has the complete manifest as a referenced attachment. If only components of records are being destroyed, the destruction records must be clear about which components were destroyed.

The AHIMA issued a practice brief on the subject of health information retention in 2013. It outlines legal and regulatory requirements, accreditation requirements, and recommendations. This practice brief and others are available online by visiting the AHIMA website at www.ahima.org.

Destruction of electronic records and protected health information may include not only consideration of the legal patient record, but also other devices and media that store patient data. Many of these devices are updated and upgraded from time to time, making them obsolete or no longer needed. These devices and media include computer tapes, hard drives, DVDs, flash drives, copiers, fax machines, and so on. Planning for the consistent, reasonable destruction of these devices and media are vital in the electronic environment. A variety of methods are used to destroy the data. Methods are selected based on the type of equipment and media and include shredding, pulverizing, and degaussing. Companies specialize in the destruction of electronic information. A business associate agreement should outline the company's process, safeguards, and responsibilities (HIPAA privacy rule 45 Code of Federal Regulation Parts 160 and 164). A detailed record of destruction must be retained by the organization.

Facility Closure

Special considerations are necessary regarding record retention when a facility closes, either by sale or by dissolution of a physician practice. The two major considerations are protecting the confidentiality of patient information and ensuring the availability of the information for patient care.[14] In planning for a facility or provider's closure of a practice, both federal and state laws should be consulted.

If the facility is sold to another provider of health care services, the records are usually considered an asset of the sale because they provide a considerable marketing advantage to the new owner and are exempt from federal law that restricts the sale of protected health information. If the buyer is not a health care provider, records should not be considered assets of the sale and other arrangements should be made. To ensure that patients are aware of what is happening to their information, a series of notices should be published on the facility or provider's website and in local newspapers, and other reasonable means should be used to inform patients and interested parties of the planned date of closure and new location of the records. Patients can be encouraged to request a copy of their record or key components of their record prior to planned closure. The facility or individual provider can then contract with another health care provider, the facility attorney, or a commercial storage company to assume responsibility for the records and provide information to authorized requesters in the future. Other considerations should be evaluated such as scanning the records. Scanning may be less expensive than a long-term storage solution. As a last option, the state department of health may assume responsibility for the records. In any case, every effort should be made to ensure that all records are complete as of the date of transfer.

AHIMA issued a practice brief on the subject of protecting patient health information after a facility closure in November 2011. This brief is available online by visiting the AHIMA website at www.ahima.org.

The Legal Health Record Definition

Work by a task force of the AHIMA related to defining the legal health record (LHR) can be found at www.ahima.org. A group of HIM professionals continues to discuss this topic and provide guidelines for hospitals on how to create an individualized definition of the LHR for their facilities. This legal record reflects the documentation of the health care services provided by the organization. With the recent proliferation of different modes of digital input and output of record text, images, and other forms of documentation, it is difficult to determine what is truly part of the "legal" record versus a byproduct of the patient care process not considered part of that legal output. Also some documents may, for convenience, be kept with the record but not considered part of the legal record. There are practical considerations with today's technology that make it unlikely that a single repository could be created to house all varieties and types of documentation created, so the LHR must be defined in each organization.

Once a multidisciplinary team completes a full forms, computer views (paper and electronic), and database inventory, the subset identified as the LHR can be confirmed. When records are stored in a paperless format, that subset defined as the legal record can be parsed out or printed on demand to created the episodic version of the health record that will be used for that facility's LHR document of care. From a management perspective, this allows a "wrapper" to be put around the health record that is both reasonable and manageable.

Disaster Planning

Disaster planning is carried out in every health care organization. Part of that process typically organizes in ways that allows the health care community to continue to provide necessary services in its area or to plan to transfer patients to other areas. The United States has experienced major natural disasters, and it is very clear that planning and preparation are needed. A core component of providing health care is the provision and exchange of health information.

In August 2012 Hurricane Isaac hit Louisiana on the seventh anniversary of Hurricane Katrina. These natural disasters tested the ability of the region and of the United States to care for and share health information about displaced patient populations. The Southeast Regional Health Information Technology (HIT)–Health Information Exchange (HIE) Collaboration addressed these issues through a consortium that includes Alabama, Arkansas, Florida, Georgia, Louisiana, and Texas. The report of the consortium was published in July 2012. The group is working to translate their recommendations into practice. The consortium acknowledges the legal issues, especially those associated with the privacy of health information; however, to meet extraordinary needs and circumstances to provide health care and exchange health information more efficiently during a disaster, the group made the recommendations listed in Box 5-6 and encourages other states and regions to consider incorporating these recommendations into their disaster planning.

The Department of Health and Human Services also provides information on disaster planning and the use of health information. Their information includes a decision tool that applies HIPAA privacy rules to the likely actions to be taken during a disaster (Figure 5-6).

As HIE capabilities increase at the state and regional levels, disaster planning and coordinated responses should include the element of basic health information to support care in a disaster. HIM professionals can join their local and state planning groups to assist in identifying key data useful in providing care in a disaster and how to make that data available when and where it is needed. Consideration can be given to using the Continuity of Care standard document as a starting point.

Disaster Recovery

Disasters can result from fire, broken pipes, blocked drains, malfunctioning equipment, environmental storms, and floods. Water is a frequent culprit in the destruction of paper

BOX 5-6   Southeast Regional HIT-HIE Collaboration Recommendations

The recommendations of the Southeast Regional Health Information Technology (HIT)–Health Information Exchange (HIE) Collaboration are:

1. Understand the state's disaster response policies and align with the state agency designated for Emergency Support Function #8 (Public Health and Medical Services) before a disaster occurs.
2. Develop standard procedures approved by relevant public and private stakeholders to share electronic health information across state lines before a disaster occurs.
3. Consider enacting the Mutual Aid Memorandum of Understanding to establish a waiver of liability for the release of records when an emergency is declared and to default state privacy and security laws to existing Health Insurance Portability and Accountability rules in a disaster. States should also consider using the Data Use and Reciprocal Support Agreement to address and expedite patient privacy, security, and health data-sharing concerns.
4. Assess the state's availability of public and private health information sources and the ability to electronically share the data using health information exchanges and other health data-sharing entities.
5. Consider a phased approach to establishing interstate electronic health information sharing capabilities.[15]

records, causing them to become soaked and possibly contaminated with pollutants, such as sewage.

As with most things, planning ahead can make all the difference in the ability to restore records and media to a more usable form. Preparation for disaster recovery includes investigating a local or regional restoration specialist. Property insurance carriers are a good source of qualified referrals. In addition, most qualified restoration specialists are members of the Association of Specialists in Cleaning and Restoration, International (ASCR). The ASCR website (www.ascr.org) states that when large quantities of paper records are water damaged, they should be frozen as soon as possible to prevent mold or mildew from forming and to prevent swelling and rippling of the paper. Smaller volumes of wet records, such as 10 average-sized records or fewer, can be air dried by separating the pages and exposing them to the air. Restoration vendors can freeze the records while other options are being considered.

If the volume of wet paper records is too great to freeze immediately, changing the environment of the location will help retard mold or mildew development. The heat should be turned off and the air conditioning used to bring the temperature of the room as low as possible under 70° F and to reduce the humidity to below 60%. Fans can be used to help circulate cool, dry air, and wet-dry vacuums can be used to remove water trapped in carpet or standing on floors. Wet records can be dried with a vacuum thermal drying process. A vacuum is created inside a special chamber, a source of heat is introduced, and the records are dried at temperatures above 32° F.[16] This method may cause more rippling of dried pages than other methods.

Freezing the paper records provides two other alternatives for restoration—freezer drying and vacuum freezer

drying. In either case, restoration specialists want to know what types of paper are included within the wet records. They need to be especially careful with coated paper, such as the paper used for electrocardiograms and other medical tracings. This paper tends to stick together more than traditional bond paper. Photographs contained within the record should be dried separately by a photograph conservator.

Freezer drying of wet paper removes water by vaporizing the ice crystals without melting them and may take several weeks to several months to complete. Vacuum freeze drying involves the use of specialized equipment. A vacuum is created, a source of heat is introduced, and the records are dried at temperatures below 32° F. The process may take only a few weeks because the vacuum process speeds the overall drying time, just as pressure cooking speeds the overall cooking time for food.

Another method of preparation for a disaster is to minimize the potential for water damage from malfunctioning sprinkler systems or sprinklers that are activated during small fires. Staff should be trained to know where the sprinkler shutoff valves are and to turn them off as soon as any danger has passed. An appropriate tool kit should be kept in the area of the fire extinguisher.

If records are maintained in an electronic format, a disaster plan is also necessary. Some of the same issues of protection from the elements are true with the hardware, software, and data storage components of electronic record systems. The advantage in electronic systems is that backups can be kept at an off-site or remote location. If a fire or other disaster strikes one location, the other location may not be harmed. Also electronic data storage is often protected in special vaults created for this purpose. Another advantage is that moving the electronically stored data out of harm's way is typically easier because it involves moving a much smaller set of media.

? DID YOU KNOW?

Several organizations provide suggestions regarding disaster planning for health care organizations. AHIMA offers a Disaster Planning and Recovery Toolkit which incorporates records management, disclosure of health information, and confidentiality of health records. It also includes sample contingency plans, checklists, and forms.

The Joint Commission requires disaster planning in its standards related to emergency management. The standards require organizations to identify potential emergencies and develop a customized plan that covers mitigation, preparedness, response, and recovery. The plan must also address command structures and backup communications systems, among other issues. They offer the free guide, "Surge Hospitals: Providing Safe Care in Emergencies," which provides lessons learned from hospitals affected by hurricanes. They also offer the free guide "Standing Together: An Emergency Management Planning Guide for America's Communities."

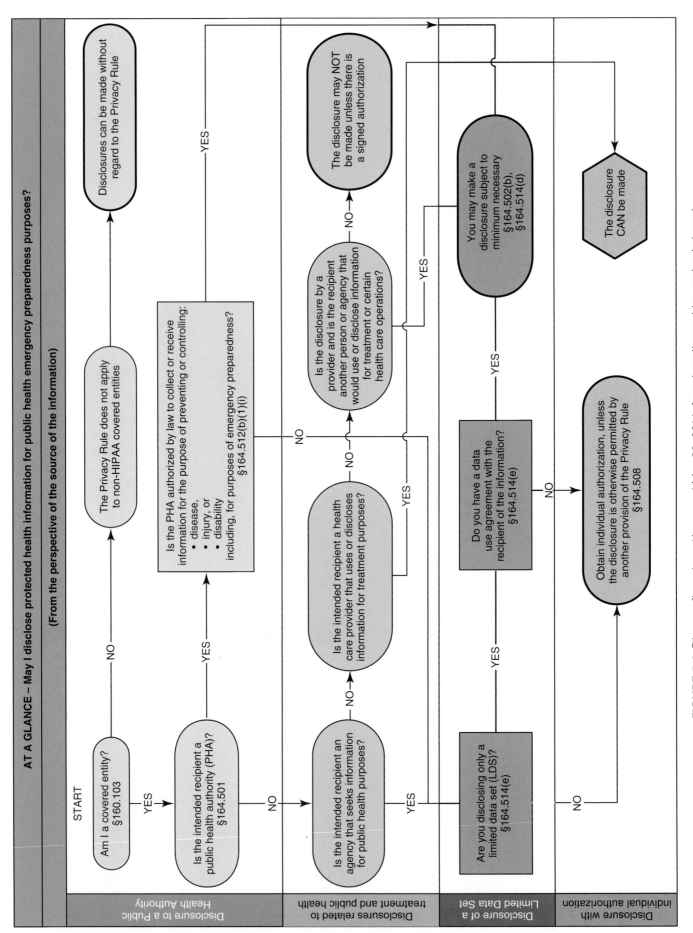

FIGURE 5-6 Disaster flow chart. (Accessed May 22, 2014, from http://www.hhs.gov/ocr/privacy/hipaa/understanding/special/emergency/decisiontool.html.)

TECHNOLOGY IN ACCESS AND RETENTION

Data access and retention rely on information technology to collect, store, manage, and transmit health information. The following briefly reviews examples in these areas and illustrates their roles in automating the processes of data access and retention.

Input, Output, and Storage Devices

Data can be collected automatically from other computer systems or can be entered through a data entry process. Biomedical devices such as automated electrocardiogram systems and patient monitoring systems convert data from one form to another and transmit the data to a database. PCs, optical scanning devices, tablets, phones, cards with embedded chips, and other devices are operated by users to capture and enter data into computer systems. Computers can receive input directly from remote computers through communications networks. Many of these devices can also be used to access and store data.

Radiofrequency Identification

Radiofrequency identification (RFID) is a process in which a tiny microchip is attached to or embedded in an item (i.e., a clinical record folder in this case or an ID card) to assist in tracking the object. Similar to a bar code, this tag can be embedded with information that allows a user to know the location of a device. However, it is more reliable than a bar code system because it does not rely on manual intervention (scanning or checking in and out of locations) to update the location. Instead, the RFID chip acts as a sensor in which the various frequency receiving devices can "track" the location of the microchip as it travels throughout a facility, providing instantaneous "update" information through a computer network.[17] Chapter 8, Technology, Applications, and Security, provides additional information on technology used in health care.

Document Imaging Devices

One approach to developing an EHR is to use document imaging as a way to capture and store text-based information. Records are stored in digital format. The records can be indexed and organized for access and retrieval. These types of systems serve many types of record systems (e.g., human resources, health care, accounting). Some health care organizations have already initiated this process as a strategic step in moving toward a fully EHR. In these organizations, patient record forms are scanned and indexed as soon as they are sent to the HIM department. For some organizations scanning is an adjunct to the EHR system. The organization may choose to scan certain documents (e.g., consent forms signed by the patient or external records). Other organizations may

choose scanning as their primary tool. For example, in a hospital when the discharge record for an inpatient stay has been scanned either as a freestanding scanned record or combined as a portion of an electronic record system, all functions needed to process the discharge record, such as quality review, coding, data abstraction, and others, can be done through a workstation that provides the capability to retrieve the entire record. This offers relatively fast processing and retrieval capability available through onsite and remote workstations.

As a data input approach, document imaging builds an effective bridge to the next generation of information processing by familiarizing providers with the general technology and the capability to retrieve needed information electronically in multiple locations. Through workstations and other access devices, health care providers can access records of previous visits. With the technology of multimedia, many health care organizations are combining the use of digital imaging/scanning storage systems with electronic data systems to provide an EHR.

Voice Recognition

Voice recognition is considered by many to be a key to automation of the patient record. It offers an efficient means for many practitioners to incorporate data capture into their normal routines. When the health care team works with many patients throughout the day, the methods used to capture the necessary clinical and service information must be easy to use. How do busy practitioners incorporate working with a computer into daily activities in ways that conserve time? For many, the possibility of voice recognition offers the greatest promise. This technology has grown phenomenally over the past 10 years, and it continues to grow. Effective uses were noted in ED, radiology, and surgical pathologic applications in the late 1980s; however, speed was generally slow and the vocabulary was limited. The systems have improved significantly and are being employed in hospitals behind the scenes to speed transcription of documents such as history and physical records, operative reports, and discharge summaries. The transcriptionist is presented with a partially completed document and then proceeds to edit by listening to the dictation. Alternatively, the health care provider dictates using the appropriate software and the dictated words appear on his or her computer screen for editing.

Compatibility with existing software, expansion of vocabulary, techniques for establishing computer recognition of the user's voice, and cost are issues that require review. However, voice recognition systems have improved. In one example, the use and benefits of an automated speech recognition application were explored for nursing documentation in a hospital. The system allowed nurses to create patient documentation by speaking directly to a microphone connected to a PC. There was little or no use of a keyboard. Linked directly to a hospital information system, this application provided immediate retrieval and a hard copy. This hospital acquired three voice systems that contained 10,000-word, speaker-independent vocabularies. (*Speaker-independent* refers to the ability of the system to recognize words regardless of who speaks.)

Nurses in two target areas, the ED and surgery, were selected as domain experts and worked with the developers to set up a nursing documentation care plan. The user spoke a few "trigger" words into the system to call up much longer phrases that were then entered into the text. For instance, a trigger word allowed the nurse to express complex observations by using several key words or phrases, thereby saving significant nursing documentation time and still capturing patient data efficiently. In this case, just 12 words triggered the system to create a 44-word passage that completely, accurately, and in accordance with standardized guidelines described the nursing assessment for a particular patient.[18] Radiologists in an academic medical center who were given sufficient training in voice recognition software use were able to reduce the turnaround time for producing radiology reports. The average report turnaround time for the department prior to using voice recognition software was 28 hours. After 9 months of use the average turnaround time for reports was 12.7 hours. Participants who created the reports concurrent with the image review benefited most from the use of voice recognition software.[19] Continuous voice recognition and extensive vocabularies assist in data capture and retrieval and will grow quickly.

Computer-Assisted Coding Tools

Computer-assisted coding tools encompass several different types of technologies available to HIM departments to help automate the coding process in health care facilities. These tools can be as simple as an embedded link between text and codes in a table (more commonly referred to as *structured text coding*) or as complex as logic-based tools that interpret and translate different syntax combinations into code sets (known as *natural language processing*). Most commonly used today in simpler documentation settings (e.g., physician clinics, ambulatory care, radiology tests), computer-assisted coding tools have evolved from the use of a pure encoder as a logic- or dictionary-style assist tool to one that actually can replace portions of coding automatically, and save the work of performing all of the coding manually (documentation to coder–translator to coding system generator) to one in which electronic documentation is reviewed solely by the software program and generates a code. This process, without human intervention, is helpful in generating a code that can then be verified by a coder. For example, codes that are closely linked to procedures billed through a chargemaster that is carefully constructed and is kept up to date helps to generate codes for review and verification. (Refer to Chapter 18, Revenue Cycle and Financial Management, for a discussion of the chargemaster.) Computer-assisted coding has great potential in helping to screen and process repetitive and simple documentation for coding and allowing the coding staff to focus more of its time on complex coding. Coding staff can also use

preliminary output as a first phase in quality checking and editing of coding output. The use of computer-assisted coding software may help improve the consistency of coding, and the use of this type of software is expected to grow as more of the patient record components are computerized.

AUTOMATED ACCESS AND RETENTION OF RECORDS

Automated data access and retention can be divided into two main branches—image-based and scanned records and electronic records. These two subjects are covered in the remainder of this chapter.

Electronic Document Management

Storing paper records in an onsite storage area or with a commercial storage company seems like an economic alternative to having crowded active files readily available. The alternative site approach should be compared with converting the records to another medium. It could free up space for patient care services, it could allow the documents to be accessed remotely, and it could have a reasonable payback period. If an organization has an entirely paper record system, paper volumes have likely increased. Even hybrid systems in transition from paper to an EHR still tend to have paper. Additionally, there is an expectation that access to the clinical record should be easy and fast.

An early approach to document management was to microfilm or miniaturize paper documents. *Micrographics* is the formal name for the process of creating miniature pictures on film, commonly referred to as *microfilm*. Micrographics was first used commercially by the banking industry in the 1920s as a solution for the growing volume of canceled checks that banks needed to store.[4] The microfilming process was used for years in health care for storage of patient records, and many facilities routinely microfilmed their inactive records after a certain period. Microfilmed images are small negative photographs of the original documents that cannot be read with the unaided human eye. These photographs must be magnified for viewing by special reading devices. Many hospitals still have microfilmed records in their storage areas. Microfilm solved the storage space issues but it was not easily accessible when and where needed.

Therefore EDM systems have become popular technology for HIM use. This is the method of digitizing paper-based and electronic documentation into secure electronic storage.

Electronic Health Records and Electronic Document Management

As the EHR and its definition mature, it is easier to differentiate between an EHR system and EDM system. In the EHR model, data become part of an electronic database or repository of data, which assists practitioners in documenting care, determining trends in information such as laboratory results, and in manipulating the data into various formats. An EDM system provides a method for capturing document images in an archival manner. The EDM can be linked to or embedded in an EHR system. Like an EHR system, an EDM system provides easy access and enhancements to workflow processing. An EHR database typically does not have the ability to capture handwritten or externally received paper documents. Most facilities have 40% to 70% of records captured electronically, with the remainder handwritten (e.g., consent forms). Although these numbers are changing as providers of care become more automated with computerized physician order entry and other EHR tools, paper is still used for a number of the handwritten forms included in a patient record. Therefore many EHR systems combine electronic data and images. EHR systems and their components, development, and selection are also discussed in Chapter 6. In a hybrid approach, an organization may choose to keep a paper file area for handwritten forms, forms with signatures, and paper forms received from external sources to accompany its EHR database or combine an EDM system with its EHR system.

EDM System Components

Scanner

A scanner converts the images on paper into digital images. Dot patterns, called *bitmaps,* are created in the same pattern as the dots in the paper image, much as in today's fax technology. The scanner itself looks like a copier, with an automatic document feeder, a flatbed, or both. Scanner quality is rated in pixels per inch (PPI): the higher the PPI, the higher the resolution and the clearer the document. Most scanners read in only paper-based images, but some special scanners can read in microfilm images.[20]

Certain multifunctional devices (MFDs) are able to serve as any combination of scanner, photocopier, fax, or printer output device. A picture archiving and communication system (PACS) provides rapid access to digitized film images for radiology applications and it can help eliminate the cost of film processing and storage. Currently, because of the pixel quality required and storage size limitation, few systems archive film, voice, or video images with other paper documents. As storage becomes less of an issue, archiving decisions related to other media will change.

Many scanners can accommodate double-sided scanning and can adjust to colored and variously sized source documents. Some have the ability to scan color images and photographs from the document to the screen. The PC attached to the scanner is used not only for indexing but also for quality review of the image database.

The health information professional should be aware of the speed at which a scanner can scan documents into the system. Scanner speed is rated in pages per minute. When considering a scanner purchase, actual speed should be determined by using sample forms from the current files. The speed of the scanner determines, in large part, the labor involved in placing documents in the system because work can proceed only as fast as the scanner can go. High-speed scanners are available, reliable, and expensive. Two high-speed scanners may be sufficient to meet the needs of a large hospital. In some cases, scanning may be done concurrently at the time and site where the document is being produced (e.g., a nursing unit). At other times, it may make more sense to scan the document at the end of care in a centralized location. The scanner should be equipped with an image-enhancement feature that adjusts the density and contrast of an image automatically. This eliminates the need to stop the scanner to adjust these settings manually. The scanner is usually attached to a PC, where the images can be viewed as they are being scanned. The most time-consuming components of this process are usually preparing the documents to scan and performing a quality review of the scanned documents. For example, if documents are received from an external source they may not have the patient's correct medical record number or identification number on each page of the document. The preparation stage includes looking up and verifying the medical record number and placing it on each page. For some organizations bar codes are used for the medical record number and the document type. The bar codes are preprinted on the forms or labels or are created and placed on the forms prior to scanning.

Quality review is essential as well because the intent is typically to destroy the paper documents once the digitized images are made part of the patient record. Scanned documents may be stored in a temporary file until copied into a permanent EDM or EHR. This is a quality control function that allows rescanning of images that are poor quality or otherwise incorrect before the images become permanent or filed into a patient record. Many organizations keep the paper documents only as long as needed to be reasonably sure the scanning process was completed successfully.

In the scanning process, the images are indexed. The index is in a database format and allows the documents in the imaging system to be retrieved easily. The information can be indexed by patient name, medical record number, form type, or other identifying information. With multiple cross-indexes, the chance of a document being lost in the computer system is rare. Determining which fields to index the individual records by is the most important part of planning a scanning installation. For example, portions of the record may be indexed separately, such as the discharge summary and operative report. Some facilities regularly index the physician number, diagnosis codes, and procedure codes associated with the encounter. This indexing step can be valuable if there is a need to locate a particular report quickly without having to search through the entire record database. The disadvantage of complex indexing is the time consumed in completing the process. Some companies provide web-based services that place scanned documents directly into an active archive system, which is then managed remotely.

Optical Character Recognition

Optical character recognition (OCR) is an automated option that helps decrease the cost of indexing by speeding up the entry process. This indexing method recognizes alphabetical or numerical characters and their position, and creates the index from these codes. Documents must be redesigned into standard formats that are readable by the equipment if this indexing method is to be effective. Some digital systems also read typed characters embedded in a document so a scanned document can be searched for key words. Accuracy rates can vary, especially if characters are hand entered (as in scores on a patient questionnaire), and more intensive quality checks after scanning may be necessary.

Bar Code Readers

Bar codes can be used in a variety of ways in imaging systems to automate indexing of documents and files. Patient demographics (e.g., name, account number, date of birth) can be placed on a label or laser-printed form or folder to identify the case. Individual pages of the record may have a bar code imprint that identifies the form type or number. This number can be programmed to correlate with a specific section of the imaged file so that presorting or manual indexing is not necessary. Each page may be date stamped or have the imprint of patient identification on it so that individual loose or late reports may be easily entered into the system after scanning.

Digital Document Imaging

Imaging capability and technology will continue to change and offer more options. A significant change was the ability to scan documents into multiple formats, store these documents in digital format, and easily retrieve the documents or words stored in the documents. In addition, the use of this technology has become more affordable. Organizations now have the option of setting up full imaging management resources internally or contracting with companies that use a secure website to process images and then provide access to scanned documents.

Database Software

One of the most important components of any system is the imaging system software. This part of the system determines the practicality and appropriateness of the system for the environment. As with other software, there are proprietary systems and open, or public domain, systems. A proprietary system is owned or copyrighted by an individual or a business and is available for use only through purchase or by permission of the owner. In open systems, the specifications are made public to encourage third-party vendors to develop add-on products for them. These systems are designed to incorporate all kinds of devices, regardless of the manufacturer or model, that can use the same communications facilities and protocols.

System Benefits and Advantages

Space Savings

The simplest and easiest-to-implement use of an EDM system is as a storage and archival system to replace inactive paper-based records. Although this provides a great space savings, similar to the space saving by use of micrographics, it does not use the technology of EDM to the fullest extent or provide the dollar savings of a true imaging solution that uses workflow applications.

Work Flow Applications

Many work flow applications built into imaging software (and EHR systems) foster improved processes to reduce labor costs in a health information or other department and provide better access to records.[21] Some examples are:

1. Incomplete processing. Records need to be minimally assembled, and only portions requiring manual scanning and indexing need to be placed in sequential order. Analysis of deficiencies may be assigned automatically from an order-entry system or during the scanning portion. Application software may be able to provide "color-coded" flagging of items needing authentication, and with the availability of online incomplete lists within the network, the need for an incomplete paper record staging area is eliminated.

2. Correspondence and release of information. Records may be requested online; reviewed by HIM staff; and sent to requesters by printed, faxed, or electronic (onscreen) output. This application is excellent to speed internal reviews, and some external customers such as insurance companies and other providers of health care may be able to accept electronic documents.

3. Coding and abstracting. Online access can make coding a function that can be decentralized by including home-based staffing. A patient can be seen in one facility, records created, and then the records coded or quality audited at another physically distant location or facility. Access to the previous record assists in coding validity, and diagnosis-related group optimization and reduced accounts receivable days become a byproduct of better access. Cancer registry follow-up becomes easier, and records that need to be completed by physicians are simultaneously available and are not delayed by the coding process.

4. File and retrieval. Permanent file and study retrieval or refile are virtually eliminated when all records are part of the EDM system. During temporary holding of records, which takes place for a certain period to assess quality, paper records can be maintained as a back up.

Loose report scanning is reduced and simplified, and misfiles are reduced. Back scanning is usually not done except for the case of readmissions or special needs, but staff must be allocated for previous record retrieval if any paper records exist. Table 5-5 and Table 5-6 show sample workflow changes for the physician record completion and patient readmission processes in EDM and EHR systems. Uses of these databases can extend to workflow to support clinical activities as well. For example, a notification can be built into the system to notify a clinician when a report is scanned into the system. The notified clinican can then view the report and could mark the report as reviewed.

TABLE 5-5   Sample Workflow Changes: Physician Record Completion

Paper Record System	EDM or EHR System
Physician deficiency identified	Physician deficiency identified (potentially automated with link to order entry system)
Record flows through processing (up to 1 week delay)	Records immediately available for online completion
Physician calls for records	Automated audit trails
Records retrieved (30% refile rate)	
Work completed	
Deficiencies updated	
Record refiled	

EDM, Electronic document management; EHR, electronic health record.

TABLE 5-6   Sample Workflow Changes: Patient Readmission and Review of Previous Record

Paper Record System	EDM or EHR System
Provider request	Provider access record
Health information staff retrieves*	Record reviewed online
Record outguided	Automated audit trails
Unit called to pick up or health information staff delivers	
Paper record received on unit	
Record picked up after discharge	
Record refiled and outguides reconciled	
Chart tracking system updated	

EDM, Electronic document management; EHR, electronic health record.
*Separate subprocess of search and retrieval if out of file.

Productivity Gains

EDM (scanning) and EHR (database) systems can dramatically decrease the amount of time spent moving records from one location to another. The tasks of retrieving, assembling, transporting, and filing paper-based records are eliminated. Telephone calls to initiate record searches and requests to copy records on the photocopy machine are also eliminated. By deleting these paper-based steps from the record management process and replacing them with an automated retrieval system such as imaging or EHRs, the facility realizes several important advantages.

One advantage is 24-hour access to records by authorized users, without clerical staff assistance and with a considerable reduction in retrieval time. There are also no lost or misplaced documents to be searched for, and the documents maintain their long-term quality for future use. An additional advantage is the opportunity to use available work hours to complete other tasks, such as monitoring documentation patterns and performing quality studies.

Increased Use of Computer Technology

The use of imaging and more advanced technology encourages the use of computer technology. To retrieve an image, the user must use a workstation, and the workstation displays a familiar-looking document, much like the paper document that has always been used. This familiarity enhances user acceptance of optical images or other technologic advances that are computer generated, such as laboratory values and transcription output. These systems help prepare the user for future information technologies that are completely computer based.

Multiuser Simultaneous Access

One of the greatest benefits of an EDM system and an EHR system are that they offer multiuser access to the same information at the same time—something that neither paper-based nor microfilmed records can provide. With an EDM system, many people, including coders, physicians, social workers, nurses, and others, can view the same information at the same time because each is viewing a copy of the image. The result is greater efficiency by eliminating the waiting time for the record before they can perform their functions. A physician treating a patient in the ED can view a record from the patient's recent visit to the hospital at the same time that administrative users are viewing it. This has a positive effect on the quality of care that can be provided and is extremely valuable when facilities provide care across a variety of settings and sites or have a large number of outpatient encounters.

Online Availability of Information

An EDM system and an EHR system can create an online record for patients as they are admitted. The system can incorporate data from different sources as the information is created electronically at multiple points in the hospital (e.g., registration, laboratory, pharmacy, rehabilitation, radiology). The images and data are compiled into one record, maintained digitally during hospitalization, and viewed by many users while the patient is being treated.

System Security and Confidentiality

System security is maintained because images and data stored in the EDM and EHR systems can be viewed only by use of access codes with passwords. Access to clinical records and data can be controlled by the organization's security measures. This use of access control makes the EDM and EHR systems more secure than paper-based or microfilm systems.

User-specific retrieval of information can be implemented to increase security. Individual users can receive only the portions of the record that are required for their assigned duties (role-based security). Physicians can view only cases that their facility numbers have been associated with (physician of record). A physician's billing staff can view only demographics and insurance data for patients whose records carry the physician's facility number. Other user-specific retrieval specifications can be developed to increase security, such as audit trails to review emergency access to cases that were outside the scope of the previous clinician of record.

Database Retrieval

The EDM software and EHR software can perform database searches for specific information. In the EDM system data that has been indexed can be searched. If the diagnosis and procedure codes were indexed, the imaging software can serve as the MPI, disease index, operative index, and physician index that were traditionally done manually or in an abstracting system. After a database search for a specific diagnosis is performed, the software displays the list of patients with that diagnosis and can organize their records for review or retrieval. Similar functionality and more capability is available in EHR systems.

Evaluating EDM System Requirements

When the need for an alternative solution to a storage, retrieval, and workflow application system has been recognized as a stand-alone system or as part of an EHR system, the health information professional will obtain approval from the appropriate level of authority in the facility to evaluate possible alternatives, typically enlisting a team of stakeholders.

Analyze Problems and Conceptualize Solutions

As system requirements are being determined, the current problems must be analyzed and appropriate solutions conceptualized. All proposed automated systems must solve the major problems identified in the current system, not merely add costs.[22] If the proposed system can solve problems without creating long-term additional ones, the system should be developed in detail, including the following:

- Identifying new or different tasks that affect work flow for the new system
- Determining the current volume of work and the projected volume of each task to be completed in the new system
- Determining whether the skill levels of the staff need to be adjusted to a higher or lower level in the new system
- Developing productivity targets
- Identifying tasks that could be completed during off hours or off site
- Interviewing potential system users in the facility to obtain their view of the current system, its problems, and their future needs
- Designing a diagram of the processes in the new system for explanation and training purposes
- Determining equipment needs and specifications
- Use approaches illustrated in other chapters for the cost comparison of paper-based record storage and scanning systems. Other chapters also contain analysis tools to assist in the decision process.

EDM Implementation Strategies

Phasing in the New System

There is no perfect or universal method for phasing in a new system. Some sources suggest that the initial place to start is the outpatient area or ED of the hospital or online patient records at admission.

Others suggest that a scanning system could be initiated by scanning inpatient discharge charts the day after discharge. Scanning systems need to interface with current electronic systems. A scanning system is often an adjunct to an EHR or part of a transition to an EHR system. Regardless of where the implementation starts, forms should be redesigned or evaluated for design purposes. When a scanning system is implemented, forms should include bar codes for automatic indexing as soon as possible. The process of inventorying forms and providing bar codes on the forms takes time and should be initiated well in advance of the implementation if bar codes are to be used. The bar codes should be placed in exactly the same location on every form and provide sufficient information to identify the patient, the form type, and the date of the documentation contained on the page. Many EHR systems also use a scanning component to handle forms received from external sources and some handwritten forms such as consent forms.

Staff training is also essential.

Redefining Jobs and Skills

The introduction of an EDM or an EHR system results in the need for internal change in the health information department more than in any other department of the facility. The department staff needs to learn as much as possible about the new technology before it is implemented and should help in the redesign of staff job functions. Positions will probably not be eliminated with the initial implementation of the system. Employees should be reassured that staffing duties will be changed but not eliminated. Any eventual staffing decreases that might be realized can be handled through transfers, formal retraining, or attrition.

Legal Considerations

Each state can specify whether business records reproduced by a particular medium are admissible as evidence, but not all have addressed the issue of scanning. As business practices evolve into a more electronic environment, patient records in a variety of mediums are being recognized.

When states address business records as evidence, the Federal Rules of Evidence, Rule 803(6) of the Uniform Rules of Evidence, or the Uniform Photographic Copies of Business and Public Records Act is used as their basis. The facility's legal counsel should be consulted for an opinion if state statutes are unavailable or unclear. This is an excellent reason why HIM professionals need to help the facility define its LHR.

KEY CONCEPTS

- Paper-based records are still present in health care today, although it is widely recognized that paper is not the best medium for all situations. Digitally scanned records and electronically stored data are two alternatives to paper-based records.
- Records are identified by two methods—alphabetical identification and numerical identification. Alphabetical

identification uses the patient's name as the identifier for the record, and numerical identification uses a number, typically assigned by the facility.[23]

- Paper records are stored in different types of equipment. Filing cabinets work well for small files; compressible files work well for medium and moderately active files; and open-shelf files work well for large, active files.

- Filing systems can be either centralized or decentralized and use one of the three common filing methods: alphabetical filing, straight numerical filing, or terminal digit filing.

- File folders for paper records should be chosen after considering the size of the average record, the usage rate of the record, and the type of filing equipment used to store the record. Filing efficiency can be enhanced by choosing colored folders or by adding color coding to a plain folder.

- Manual record-tracking systems use outguides, requisitions, and transfer notices as their primary tools. Outguides mark the spot from which a record was removed; requisitions list the patient identifiers and requester; transfer notices alert the file personnel that a record has been moved to a new location.

- Automated record-tracking systems hold the requisition and transfer information in a database. They allow computerized requesting of records and online inquiry regarding the current record location.

- Paper-based systems require large amounts of storage space. As records become less actively used, the format or medium is often changed to reduce the storage space they require. Image-based systems are considered an acceptable alternative. Paper records may also be moved to off-site storage facilities.

- A scanning (EDM) system and an EHR system can be costly, but the cost can be justified by considering the space savings, productivity gains, multiuser access, online availability of information, and increased system security.

- The legality of scanned and fully electronic records as admissible evidence in court is determined differently in each state, and opinions should be obtained from the facility attorney.

- Retention and retrieval of records in various formats must be part of the initial planning for any system. Although scanning and electronic record systems provide reasonable means to store and organize patient records, the HIM manager must continually balance access, retrieval, and retention schedules to make the stored information available over time in a manner that meets the needs of the patients, the organization, and other users. Constantly changing technology creates retrieval challenges. Technology in use today may not be in use 5, 10, or 20 years from now, so continual planning for data access, retrieval, and mapping as systems change and are upgraded is critical.[24]

REFERENCES

1. Skurka M: *Health information management in hospitals: principles and organization for health record services,* Chicago, 1994, American Hospital Publishing.
2. Managing the master patient index in a healthcare environment: Resolution adopted at 2012-2013 AHIMA House of Delegates (http://library.ahima.org/xpedio/groups/public/documents/ahima/bok1_049789.hcsp?dDocName=bok1_049789).
3. Fundamentals for building a master patient index/enterprise master patient index, *AHIMA Practice Brief,* 2010 (http://library.ahima.org/xpedio/groups/secure/documents/ahima/bok1_048389.hcsp?dDocName=bok1_048389).
4. Estep B, Kirk R: Relocating a medical record department: "A moving experience," *J Am Med Rec Assoc* 57:22, 1986.
5. Bertrand M: Moving a medical record department: a case study, *Top Health Rec Manag* 6:65, 1985.
6. Johnson M, Kallaus W: *Records management,* Cincinnati, 1982, Southwestern Publishing.
7. Allen B, Barr C: The impact of automated medical record tracking systems on the ability to reduce staff—A research study, *J Am Health Inform Manage Assoc* 64:74, 1993.
8. Greenberg SP, Larsen EJ: An automated medical record ordering and tracking system at the Cleveland Clinic Foundation, *Med Rec News* 50:31–37, 1979.
9. Glass B, Mitchell S: The ambulatory care medical record: an administrative nightmare, *J Med Group Manage* 39:60, 1992.
10. Lach J, Longe K: Bar coding and the medical record manager, *J Am Med Records Assoc* 58:24, 1987.
11. Majerowicz A: Selection and implementation of a bar code–based record management system in ambulatory care, *J Am Med Records Assoc* 61:29, 1990.
12. American Health Information Management Association: Practice brief: retention and destruction of health information (2013): AHIMA.org.
13. American Hospital Association: *Preservation of medical records in health care institutions,* Chicago, 1990, American Hospital Association Institutional Practices Committee.
14. *Protecting patient information after a closure, AHIMA Practice Brief,* Chicago, 2011, American Health Information Management Association.
15. ONC State Health Policy Consortium Project: Health information exchange in disaster preparedness and response. Southeast Regional HIT-HIE Collaboration Final Reports, July 2012, RTI International, Research Triangle Park, NC.
16. Buchanan S: *Emergency management—Drying wet books and records,* North Andover, 1994, Northeast Documentation Conservation Center.
17. Coustasse A, Tomblin S, Slack C: Impact of radio frequency identification (RFID) technology on the hospital supply chain: a literature review, *Perspect Health Inf Manag Fall* 1–17, 2013.
18. Trofino J: Voice recognition technology applied to nursing documentation, *Healthc Inform Manag Syst Soc* 7:42, 1993.
19. Krishnaraj A, Lee JK, Laws SA, Carwford TJ: Voice recognition software: effect on radiology report turnaround time at an academic medical center, *Am J Roentgengenol* 195(1):194–197, 2010.
20. McLendon K: Optical disk imaging—Tomorrow's technology today for medical records, *J Am Med Records Assoc* 61:32, 1990.
21. Rhodes H, Dougherty M: Practice brief. Document imaging as a bridge to the EHR, *J AHIMA* 74:56A–56G, 2003.
22. Kahl K, Casey D: How to evaluate and implement office automation, *J Am Med Records Assoc* 55:20, 1984.
23. AHIMA e-HIM Work Group on Regional Health Information Organizations (RHIOs): using the SSN as a patient identifier, *J AHIMA* 77:56A–56D, 2006.
24. Kohn D: When the writ hits the fan, *J AHIMA* 75:40–44, 2004.

6 CHAPTER

ELECTRONIC HEALTH RECORD SYSTEMS

Gretchen F. Murphy • Susan Helbig

ⓔ Student Study Guide activities for this chapter are available on the Evolve Learning Resources site for this textbook. Please visit http://evolve.elsevier.com/Abdelhak.

CHAPTER CONTENTS

OBJECTIVES

After reading this chapter, the reader will be able to do the following:

✓ Define key words.
✓ Describe electronic health records in various care settings.
✓ Explain how improving the quality of patient care links to electronic health records.
✓ Build a case for electronic health records as central components in integrated and networked systems.
✓ Discuss how personal health records can be linked to electronic health record systems.
✓ Review the progress in electronic health record development.
✓ Explain the role of enterprise systems in integrated electronic health record systems.
✓ Illustrate patient safety improvements.
✓ Explain how progress in electronic health record implementation is measured through levels and stages.
✓ Describe key functions, requirements, and expectations for electronic health records.
✓ Relate accreditation and regulatory requirements to electronic health record systems
✓ Describe **health informatics** standards and their general effect on health information technology and electronic health record systems.

✓ Explain how the certification process (Commission on Certification of Health Information Technology) affects electronic health record products and the health care industry.
✓ Contrast clinician and other user needs in an electronic health record environment.
✓ Describe technical building blocks and illustrate information system components.
✓ Discuss document, data, and information concepts for health information systems and electronic health records.
✓ Contrast roles and functions of clinical data repositories and data warehouses.
✓ Explain the role of scanning and scanned documents as a key element of enterprise electronic health record systems.
✓ Discuss the role of systems migration in meeting electronic health record goals
✓ Illustrate how legacy systems and new application developments offer a migration path to developing enterprise electronic health record systems.
✓ Explain health information management business processes and changes in the electronic health record environment.

✓ Develop an understanding of transition management in planning and implementing new technology required.

✓ Identify common health information management operational issues in a hybrid and electronic health record environment.

✓ Identify resources and strategies needed by health information management professionals to lead and participate in electronic health record projects.

✓ Describe the obstacles encountered in progressing toward electronic health records.

✓ Define and characterize interoperability for health information technology and electronic health records.

✓ Illustrate how informatics standards lead to assessment of "meaningful use" of electronic health record systems.

KEY WORDS

Authentication
Biomedical device
Clinical data repository
Classification system
Computer-based patient record
Confidentiality
Data

Data interface standards
Data security
Data warehouses
Electronic health record
Health care information
Health informatics
Information

Infrastructure
Knowledge
Multimedia
Natural language processing
Patient record
Patient record system

Registration—admission, discharge, and transfer
Script-based systems
Template
Text processing
Vocabularies

ABBREVIATIONS

AHIMA American Health Information Management Association
AMIA American Medical Informatics Association
ARRA American Recovery and Reinvestment Act
ASTM American Society for Testing and Materials
CCHIT Commission on Certification of Health Information Technology
CCD Continuity of Care Document
CCR Continuity of care record
CDR Clinical data repository
CDS Clinical decision support
CHI Clinical Health Informatics
CIM Clinical Information Management
CPOE Computerized physician order entry
CPR Computer-based patient record
CPRS Computerized patient record system
CPT Current Procedural Terminology
DGI Drummond Group, Inc.
ECG Electrocardiogram
EHR Electronic health record
FDA Federal Drug Administration
FOIA Freedom of Information Act
HIE Health information exchange
HIM Health information management
HIMSS Health Information Management Systems Society
HIPAA Healthcare Insurance Portability and Accountability Act
HIT Health information technology

HITECH Health Information Technology for Economic and Clinical Health (Act)
HL7 Health Level 7
HMO Health maintenance organization
ICD *International Classification of Diseases*
IOM Institute of Medicine
LHR Legal health record
LOINC Logical Observation Identifier Name Code
MDDS Medical device data system
MIS Medical Information Section
MPI Master patient index
NLM National Library of Medicine
ONCHIT Office of the National Coordinator for Health Information Technology
PACS Picture archiving and communication system
PHR Personal health record
PIV Personal identification verification
PMR Perpetual medical record
Reg-ADT Registration—admission, discharge, transfer
SDO Standard development organization
SNOMED-CT Systematized Nomenclature of Medicine—Clinical Terms
SSN Social Security number
VLER Virtual lifetime electronic record
XML Extensible markup language

ELECTRONIC HEALTH RECORDS: THE CASE FOR QUALITY AND CHANGE

In its 2013 report to Congress on the adoption of health information technology (HIT), the Office of the National Coordinator for Health Information Technology (ONCHIT) lays out the broad progress and value of HIT and related efforts to advance health information exchange (HIE), and sets the framework for the role that **electronic health records (EHRs)** play:

Health IT [information technology] comprises technologies—from electronic health records (EHRs) and personal health records (PHRs) to remote monitoring devices and mobile health applications—that can collect, sort, and transmit health information. By enabling health information to be used more effectively and efficiently throughout our health system, health IT has the potential to empower providers and patients; make health care and the health systems more transparent; enhance the study of care delivery and payment systems; and drive substantial improvements in care, efficiency and population health.[1]

The underlying foundation of the electronic health record creates the map of individual and collective care provided to populations. The pace of commitment to adoption of the EHR continues to accelerate and more institutions are achieving industry benchmarks in EHR systems. Along with steady growth, analysis and research on EHR benefits and concerns is also emerging, and this research is enough to entice and to give pause to the work ahead because EHRs face multiple challenges. It is important to study the EHR today to build on its strengths and resolve its limitations. Some organizations have come a long way in achieving EHRs as they are defined today. Today, the term *qualified electronic health record* means an electronic record of health-related **information** on an individual that does the following:

1. includes patient demographic and clinical health information, such as medical history and problem lists; and
2. has the capacity—
   a. to provide clinical decision support (CDS)
   b. to support physician order entry
   c. to capture and query information relevant to health care quality
   d. to exchange electronic health information with, and integrate such information from other sources[2]

In this chapter, we explore the qualified EHR in detail and the processes to maintain it. The first half of the chapter focuses on EHR progress, including defining, discussing, justifying, and characterizing EHR systems among institutional enterprise systems and system users generally, and explaining their role beyond the organizations. The second half of the chapter focuses on the management role of health information management (HIM) practitioners and the specific health information business functions they direct within the industry.

So we begin with a snapshot of the complexity of EHR systems, and their role in information governance and health care generally. We review their development, progress, and emerging models. From an enterprise systems framework, the flow of health information is featured. Systems migration and links to EHRs and commercial products are considered, followed by a stepwise look at EHR definitions, standards, content, functions, and **infrastructure**. Discussion of the legal health record (LHR), the PHR, and the EHR as it develops in a health care setting contributes ideas on how EHR systems could expand to better serve various customers. Tying evaluation to the national focus on meaningful use of EHRs underscores the progress made. New challenges in HIE are discussed.

The second half of the chapter addresses health informatics and HIM practice in today's systems' environment. This features the computerized patient record system at the Veterans' Administration of Puget Sound in Seattle, an awarding-winning advanced EHR system supported by a nearly virtual health information department. Practitioner case studies illustrate challenges and solutions. The chapter concludes with a look at progress of practitioners in the field, including benefits and challenges, and presents strategies health informatics and health information managers need to meet current and future demands in the rapidly changing environment.

Analysts interested in understanding the pace of EHR advancement have projected development and adoption patterns for many years. The Health Information Management Systems Society (HIMSS) EMR adoption model trends in hospitals illustrates how functions and capabilities build on each layer of development leading to an advanced system. In Figure 6-1, notice how the applications evolve and

FIGURE 6-1 Hospital electronic health record adoption levels of implementation. *CCD*, Continuity of Care Document; *CDR*, clinical data repository; *CDS*, clinical decision support; *CDSS*, clinical decision support system; *CPOE*, computerized physician order entry; *ED*, emergency department; *EMR*, electronic medical record; *HIE*, health information exchange; *HIMSS*, Health Information Management Systems Society; *PACS*, picture archiving and communication system. *Q2*, second quarter; *Q3*, third quarter; *R-PACS*, radiology picture archiving and communication system. (HIMSS Web Site).

	US EMR Adoption Model[SM]		
Stage	**Cumulative Capabilities**	**2013 Q2**	**2013 Q3**
Stage 7	Complete EMR; CCD transactions to share data; Data warehousing; Data continuity with ED, ambulatory, OP	2.1%	2.2%
Stage 6	Physician documentation (structured templates), full CDSS (variance and compliance), full R-PACS	10.0%	11.1%
Stage 5	Closed loop medication administration	18.7%	20.9%
Stage 4	CPOE, Clinical Decision Support (clinical protocols)	14.6%	15.1%
Stage 3	Nursing/clinical documentation (flow sheets), CDSS (error checking), PACS available outside radiology	34.5%	31.9%
Stage 2	CDR, Controlled medical vacabulary, CDS, may have document imaging; HIE capable	9.0%	8.4%
Stage 1	Ancillaries - Lab, Rad, Pharmacy - All installed	3.8%	3.5%
Stage 0	All three ancillaries not installed	7.2%	6.9%
Data from HIMSS Analytics™ Data base © 2014		N = 5,439	N = 5,437

electronic information increases for the users as organizations achieve more comprehensive EHR capabilities. The Office of the National Coordinator for Health Information Technology reports that by 2012, 44% of nonfederal acute care hospitals had implemented certified EHR technology. The percent of hospitals with certified EHRs increased by 18% between 2011 and 2012.[3] By 2012, the HIMSS analytics report notes that stages 5 and 6 grew by 80% and stage 7 by 66%.[3]

And hospitals are not alone in their progress. Ambulatory care EHR systems are also advancing steadily. By 2012 nearly three quarters (72%) of office-based physicians adopted EHR systems and 4 out of 10 (40%) adopted basic EHRs with advanced capabilities.[3] Table 6-1 lists the components of the basic functions of EHR systems in ambulatory care settings. Notice that many features are consistent with hospital EHR features described by the HIMSS analytics model in Figure 6-1. Table 6-2 is a summary of combined and detailed requirements and standards for certified EHRs today.

TABLE 6-1 Ambulatory Electronic Health Record Basic Systems

Electronic Health Record Basic System Functionality 72% of Office Based Systems

Patient demographic information

Patient history and follow-up

Patient problem list

Physician clinical notes

Comprehensive list of medications and allergies

Computerized orders for prescriptions

Viewing laboratory results

Viewing imaging results

Electronic Health Record System with Added Functionality to Meet Meaningful Use Objectives 27% of Office Based Systems

Patient demographic information

Patient history

Patient problem list

Clinical notes

Comprehensive list of medications an allergies

Prescription order entry

Recording and charting vital signs

Recording patient smoking status

Reminders for guideline-based interventions or screening tests AND warnings of drug interactions or contraindications provided

Reporting clinical quality measures to federal or state agencies (such as CMS or Medicaid)

Providing patients with electronic copy of their health information

Providing patients with clinical summaries for each visit

CMS, Centers for Medicare and Medicaid Services.
Hsiao, Chun-Ju and Hing, Esther, Use and characteristics of electronic health record systems among office-based physician practices: United States, 2001-2012, *NCHS Data Brief,* Centers for Disease Control and Prevention, Number 111, December 2012.

Notice the requirements include specific content and functions of EHRs, including those for eligible providers in ambulatory care, and eligible hospitals, including critical access hospitals. These requirements specify individual federal standards that apply to each item. This criteria is driven by the need to ensure that EHRs are used meaningfully in their setting. Today, EHR applications are certified by a federally approved certification body. The Drummond Group, Inc., (DGI) and the Commission on Certification of Health Information Technology (CCHIT) are examples. These criteria compose the fully functional ambulatory EHR featured in this table. The certification organizations exert a growing influence on institutions and vendors as the industry grows. They certify EHR products against specific criteria for functionality. Common components of hospitals and ambulatory sites are evident in the figure and tables presented. The EHR picture is coming together for individual health care organizations.

With the passage of the Health Information Technology for Economic and Clinical Health (HITECH) Act as part of the American Recovery and Reinvestment Act (ARRA) legislation in 2009, with its specific attention to advancing EHRs, federal dollars are dedicated to expanding EHR use in physician offices and more. And monies are set aside to help build technical infrastructure to enable providers and patients to exchange information across sites.[4] This has resulted in major changes for providers as they launch EHR applications and seek to demonstrate using them in meaningful ways.

Yet significant challenges continue, and we are a long way from EHR products that are easy to install and fully functional, with interoperability that can truly take the place of the paper record systems that still litter health care institutions around the country. HIM now and in the future requires knowledge of enterprise and EHR systems, organizational leadership, understanding of data and interoperability requirements, and change management skills to advance the implementation of quality EHR systems. Today there are many systems on the market and some are making significant gains in market share. Yet these systems do not easily talk to one another. Until we accept and apply standardized terminology, definitions, **templates**, and tools, we do not have a national commitment to an EHR system that is easily used and understood by everyone in the U.S. health care arena. EHR systems and various non-core data found in ancillary systems will keep us from truly being connected for years to come.

EVOLVING PATIENT RECORDS

Chapter 4 features **patient records** in primarily paper and hybrid record systems; this chapter focuses on the evolving status of EHR systems and their effect on the care delivery process and on health informatics and HIM. As the technology, standards, and meaningful use expectations develop and deepen, bridging data from enterprise to provider practice to individual patient PHRs in real time is a major challenge for

TABLE 6-2 Summary of Electronic Health Record Certification Criteria for Eligible Providers and Hospitals

General Criteria for Eligible Providers and Eligible Hospitals	Ambulatory Eligible Provider Settings	Hospital Settings—Eligible Hospitals and Critical Access Hospitals
Computerized provider order entry		
Demographics		+ Date and preliminary cause of death
Vital signs, body mass index, and growth charts		
Clinical decision support		
Drug–drug, drug allergy interaction checks		
Smoking status		
Patient list creation—sort by date and time, based on at least one combination of categories	Include patient communication preferences	
Patient-specific education resources		
Transitions of Care—Receive, display and incorporate transitions of care/referral summaries		
Transitions of Care—Create and transmit transition of care/referral summaries		
Problem list		
Medication list	Over multiple encounters	For duration of hospitalization
Medication allergy list	Over multiple encounters	For duration of hospitalization
	Electronic prescribing	Electronic medication administration record
Clinical information reconciliation		
Incorporate laboratory tests and values/results		
Security Requirements • Authentication, access control and authorization • Auditable events and tamper resistance • Audit reports • Amendments • Automatic log-off • Emergency access		
End-user device encryption	View, download, and transmit to third party	View, download, and transmit t to third party
Message Integrity	Clinical summary	Transmission to public health agencies
Optional—Accounting of disclosures	Secure messaging to patients	Transmission of reportable laboratory tests and values/results
Immunization information		Transmission to public health agencies
Transmission to immunization registries		Advance directives
Electronic notes		Electronic prescribing
Image results	Transmission to public health agencies—syndromic surveillance	Drug formulary checks
Family health history	Optional—cancer case information	Transmission of electronic laboratory tests and values/results to ambulatory providers
Clinical quality measures—capture and export		
Clinical quality measures—import and calculate		
Clinical quality measures—electronic submission		
Data portability		

Federal Register, 2014 Edition EHR Certification Criteria 45 CFR 170.314.

information users. And demands for interoperability will advance HIE more broadly. How? Identifying and harmonizing data definitions among disparate systems, mapping the flow of information, and expediting its seamless movement across settings is the foundation for a national health information highway. What is clear today is the steady development and deployment of technology in health care organizations with the EHR central to that effort.

Even before EHR systems are acquired, incremental changes occur as patient record components are processed, maintained, and provided electronically. Institutions offer their clinicians online access to transcribed documents. Providers admit their patients to hospitals using online links from their offices. Provider offices scan and transmit patient record content to support referrals. In addition, disparate systems and products are linked to form parts of an EHR system. One hospital may have a **registration—admission, discharge, transfer** administrative system; laboratory; and a radiology imaging system. Online diagnostic applications and laboratory, electrocardiogram (ECG), and radiology results may be posted for online viewing in another location. Many organizations are in transition with one or more pieces of an EHR in place. As the industry experiences positive feedback from EHR systems with improved access to patient information, streamlined services, and links among provider offices, hospitals, and specialty services, more hospitals and other health care organizations become willing to invest in EHRs to acquire capabilities far beyond those found in paper record systems.

Health informatics and HIM professionals are already managing various transitions to fully implemented EHR systems; these professionals understand how new technology fundamentally changes what happens on a daily basis and in the longer term. They meet professional responsibilities as they change in the EHR environment, and are now managing system initiatives and relevant life cycle activities. They broker health record data, and help patients participate in their own health management processes through enterprise patient portals to their provider organization's health records and through PHRs available in a variety of formats.

QUESTIONS AS GUIDES TO THE CHAPTER

In guiding the discussion through this chapter, overarching questions provide a framework to understand the momentum toward EHRs, describe EHRs, explain their components, and examine how they operate within the health care system. The challenges faced for those managing the culture, cost, and changes to EHRs are considered. We need to understand EHR systems from the *what, why, how,* and *where* perspectives. Here are questions to guide our discussion through this chapter:

- What are the current and emerging roles of the patient record in HIT, and do industry advances contribute to or hold back EHR systems?
- How do enterprise information and systems support or hinder EHR implementation?
- What is the case for advocating change from paper and hybrid patient records to a fully implemented EHR to advance quality in health care?
- What key definitions and concepts provide the framework for change?
- Are standards supporting the advancement of systems, especially standards related to exchange of data, interoperability, and data content?
- What are EHR systems and how do they work?

- How does the record itself change and evolve in the electronic environment?
- How do technical infrastructure, data requirements, and operations workflow fit in EHR systems, and what is the role of IT migration paths in achieving EHR success?
- How are EHRs evaluated?
- What brings health informatics together with HIM?
- How must HIM business processes change in the EHR environment?
- How have HIM professionals managed specific challenges?
- How are organizational policies and procedures being updated to guide EHR users and systems?
- How can health information professionals lead and participate in EHR transition work?
- What industry and operational challenges affect EHR planning, implementation, and benefits assessment?

THE PAPER PATIENT RECORD DRAWBACKS

As described in the previous chapter, the patient record is the principal repository for information concerning a patient's health care, uniquely representing patients and serving as a dynamic resource for the health care industry. Over time, it paints a longitudinal picture of health problems and services for individuals and, collectively, for the industry itself. It has grown into a complex, data-intensive series of documents organized to support both clinical and administrative needs, sometimes composed of multiple volumes of paper files.

The limitations of paper records continue to present problems. By its very nature, the paper record cannot meet the needs of complex care environments, and its use is becoming unrealistic in the presence of pressures to control operational costs and deliver information effectively. As a physical entity, the record is found in a single location for a single use and is restricted to one user at a time. The nature of information collected on patients through diagnostic tests and bedside monitoring devices alone has evolved into new and more sophisticated ways of gathering, presenting and archiving **data**. Clinicians want access to quickly act on various test results to meet the clinical needs of patients. The complexity of the health care delivery process in managed care and integrated delivery systems underscores the need for effective health information systems to meet both care and care coordination requirements.

The style and completeness of documentation in patient records varies from one setting to another. And this is also true of documentation in an EHR. Many traditional paper record entries rely on open-ended narrative as do various reports, progress notes, and so on, in an EHR. It can be difficult in many paper systems to easily identify what facts are missing. There is no easy way to check for data and information inconsistencies in paper records. EHRs can be built to do this. In paper records, the data cannot be rearranged for display in alternative formats that might help view data relationships in new ways. The record is limited to the fundamental chronological flow of information. Caregivers and researchers must page through thick documents to connect related information from many and often diverse locations. The paper record's weaknesses in understandability, legibility, chronology, and data organization are difficult if not impossible to overcome. In contrast, when using technology to access the information in the record, diverse information is available in the patient snapshot screen display as shown in Figure 6-2.

Health care needs data in aggregate form to understand the effectiveness of care. Health services research needs aggregate data for evaluation of cost and quality. Although a considerable amount of data is available through national and regional public databases, these data have limitations. EHR systems offer new resources to both internal and external studies of patient care, and early research on the effects is promising. Examples of quality improvements include documented decreases in medication errors with the implementation of computerized provider order entry and improved patient engagement with access to their medical information.[5] Information technology buttresses the rationale for focusing on the EHR to meet quality and cost objectives.

Patients and providers want the patient record to function beyond a basic data repository. And yet there are very few EHR systems in hospitals that have a complete data repository. These continue to develop. Adding efficient decision support tools, for example, will help organizations and clinicians meet patient safety improvement goals. Consumers who experience the convenience of online prescription refills, test results, and appointment scheduling are enjoying a more effective health care experience. As practice settings produce an electronic summary of the patient visit, the sense of better, more organized care is settling in. Furthermore, consumers appreciate the 24-hour access to their health information as their health provider works to meet their unique health care needs.[6]

Although the technical capability exists to send documents and images produced by external resources such as radiologists to other care settings, special study programs, and education, the technical standards, business framework, and policies lag behind. One reason for this is that unlimited information in such varied formats is difficult to manage in a system in which the users expect almost immediate response time. As technology offers more **multimedia** capacity for voice, data, image, and video, and faster electronic transmission of data, this is changing. Multimedia capacity will allow incorporation of additional information on patients from internal and external sources.

FIGURE 6-2 Electronic health record patient snapshot screen. Elsevier 2014. SimChart for the Medical Office® (www.evolve.elsevier.com).

With ongoing advances in technology and compelling evidence of practical benefits in HIT, the past several years have seen major changes. Although still rooted in paper-based models, the medical record is rapidly changing. In many settings, it has moved to a hybrid paper and electronic format or to a fully electronic format. Today **patient record systems** may store data electronically through online systems, maintain clinical data repositories, use links to diagnostic applications for ongoing information, and combine these elements with scanned copies of paper images so that users can access the entire record through secure devices.

The challenge to the industry is twofold. First, the information contained in patient records continues to expand in content and form to include text; wave forms; imaging studies such as chest films acquired, stored, and displayed in digital form; monitoring data such as vascular pressures, ventilator, and heart monitoring data; videos; and more.[7] Second, the technology that enables making that content available for health care team members across care settings through interoperability resources is becoming a realistic option in more environments.[5] Chapter 4 outlined a substantial list of uses and users of the patient record. As the source and record of individual care that provides the aggregate data needed to assess care effectiveness, the EHR must meet past, current, and future demands. As the migration to electronic records proceeds, users need to be able to rely on a hybrid record system to meet their needs while working toward a fully electronic system that can provide additional data and capabilities. Those who manage EHRs need to build skills that support uses of the record for traditional purposes and for more sophisticated quality and research monitoring of health care processes and events such as more timely clinical outcomes research. Building reliance on EHRs to support syndromic surveillance for public health purposes will grow the capability to identify emerging health syndromes that offer faster response and serve the public more effectively. Eventually, the full implementation of EHRs and HIEs will transform individual patient data and health information into knowledge and wisdom resources that help manage the health of our many communities across the United States.

SELF-ASSESSMENT QUIZ

1. How has federal legislation contributed to the adoption of EHRs in provider offices?
2. How do EHRs address the limitations of paper records?
3. What role do EHR systems play in meeting the health care and health services research needed to understand the effectiveness of care and evaluate cost and quality of care?

ELECTRONIC HEALTH RECORDS TODAY

Patient safety concerns, a national focus on HIT, health services quality, paper record shortcomings, and cost containment demands strengthen the historical drivers to EHR adoption. National debates and reports are shining a spotlight on health care facts that call for correction and for using technology more effectively. Among six trends noted by the Gartner Research Group on Information Technology, "A 50% growth in healthcare software investment could enable clinicians to cut the level of preventable deaths by half in 2013."[8] This prediction made in 2005 reflects the gathering energy for applying technology to the health care process. By 2012, Kern and colleagues reported on a study to determine the effect of EHRs on ambulatory quality in a community-based setting in which EHR use was associated with a higher quality of care.[9]

Patient Safety and Data

During the 2000s, the Institute of Medicine (IOM) issued a series of critical reports on the nation's health care on the basis of a concerted, continuing effort focused on a 1996 initiative to assess and improve the nation's quality of care. In a key report, "To Err Is Human: Building a Safer Health System," the authors cite between 44,000 and 98,000 U.S. deaths per year caused by medical errors.[10] In the follow-up report, "Crossing the Quality Chasm: A New Health System for the 21st Century," the authors call for better systems and better data.[11] We continue to work on the goals set forth in these landmark reports.

Following these reports, endorsements for industry investment in EHRs and better information sharing grew substantially. Industry leaders, professional organizations, and payers added their perspectives. Notable work by the Markle Foundation's public–private collaborative Connecting for Health and the Leapfrog Group invested in partnerships with government, industry, health care, and consumers expanded the discussion and strengthened the drive to focus on patient safety through improving the health information needs for the country. The Markle Foundation works to advance consumer acceptance and use of technology resources in health care and fosters opportunities for consumers to learn about their options with PHRs as a critical measure. The Leapfrog Group monitors patient safety through hospital surveys and produces reports that bring transparency to the public.[12,13]

Substantial progress in hospital EHR systems such as the Veterans' Administration computerized patient record system and the Kaiser system offer evidence that care can be improved and become more efficient when these systems are used.[14] With data availability improved through their EHR and specialized registries, the Kaiser system demonstrated patient safety improvements through combining the technology with new care team measures to reduce cardiac deaths by 73%.[15]

The Geisinger Clinic, an integrated delivery system serving a population of 2.5 million members, demonstrated returns on innovation over ambulatory services and a fully implemented hospital EHR by emphasizing collaboration of clinical, operational, payer, and selected patients to identify which care model will offer the most value. The team links redesign of the care process, improving the clinical workflow, and key process steps within the EHR with the decision support system and patient engagement, and calls for metrics to monitor progress.[16] So industry leaders in EHR technology generate major energy as HIT grows rapidly across the country.

National Progress on Health Information Technology

In April 2004 President George W. Bush called for "the majority of Americans to have interoperable electronic health records within 10 years," named a national coordinator for HIT, and established the ONCHIT.[17] The first national coordinator, Dr. David Brailer, delivered a critical new strategic framework and set four goals still targeted today:

- Inform clinical practice by providing incentives for EHR adoption, reducing risk, and promoting diffusion in underserved areas.
- Interconnect clinicians through regional collaborations and networks and coordinating federal health information systems.
- Personalize care by encouraging PHRs, enhancing informed consumer choice for clinicians and services, and promoting telehealth systems.
- Improve population health by unifying public health surveillance architectures for interoperability, streamlining quality and health status monitoring, and accelerating research.

Creation and diffusion of EHRs, interconnecting clinicians and care sites for sharing patient information, using technology tools to support and remind clinicians about care and safety matters, and charging the American consumers with adopting PHRs are key elements for advancing information technology in health care. With more comprehensive technology support and improved health surveillance, health status monitoring and research can advance rapidly.[18]

In February 2009 President Obama signed the HITECH Act. This legislation provided 17.2 billion dollars to providers to move ahead on EHR adoption. This program uses incentives through the Medicare and Medicaid programs. It served to jumpstart EHR initiatives for many who would not otherwise act.[4] The initiative addressed support for providers to acquire technology, establishment of regional extension centers, and workforce retraining to improve the technological skill set in the industry and support eligible practitioners in acquiring and implementing EHR systems.[4] See Chapter 3 for more information on the national efforts to increase the application of information technology to **health care information**.

Emerging Models and Alliances

Changes in health services delivery, particularly new funding models, drive the expansion of integrated delivery systems. Around the country large hospital systems are forming alliances with nearby hospitals and incorporating ambulatory group practices into their systems. These new partnerships and collaborations call for increasing more efficient access to and use of patient information. The industry is engaged in implementing EHRs as essential components of their business models.

EHRs have already contributed improvements in delivering health services, from streamlined work flows to better communications, care coordination of services, and referrals for which critical patient information is immediately available to the care team. Increasing adoption requires the capacity to initiate change effectively, moving from paper-based and scattered information systems environments to fully integrated interconnectivity and functioning institutional EHRs. Ideally, as organizations recognize the value of EHR systems, they will also recognize the value of standards applied to both data content and data exchange.

Health informatics and HIM professionals play a pivotal role in advancing the transition to EHRs as they are challenged to understand, lead, and manage a transition between paper and electronic media, and ensure the quality and availability of patient data in a changing environment. Many are already working in a fully electronic environment. The HIMSS Analytics report for 2012 notes the progress of major health information electronic business functions.[19] The goals set for health care in the new millennium are ambitious. HIM professionals work side by side with medical and clinical informatics colleagues as electronic HIM, also referred to as *applied health informatics,* brings us to the collective objectives of improved patient care and improved health information systems.

For health informatics, "science that deals with health information, its structure acquisition, and uses," the foundation role of EHRs is a clearly stated goal.[20] The infrastructure, hardware, software, communications, and building block systems required to implement EHR systems are better understood today, although the vision of the potential of electronic health information systems continues to evolve. Today's view draws on a synergistic reality. In larger organizations such as hospitals and integrated delivery systems, current EHR systems typically pull data from multiple applications such as diagnostic systems and data capture applications, organize it, store it in a clinical repository, link applications with interface engines, perform data integration, manage communications, incorporate physician order entry and decision support functions, and provide workstation navigational tools to establish a functional EHR system. This suite of applications and tools may be unique to health care organizations. Recall Figure 6-1 and Table 6-2 at the beginning of the chapter to consider the complexity of these systems.

The health care environment is also exploring how to move to an integrated delivery and information system that respects individual privacy rights. More than ever, we understand the need for longitudinal information to support individual patient treatments to achieve better outcomes and to better manage unique population health needs. HIT initiatives are influenced by government and payers. The Health Insurance Portability and Accountability Act (HIPAA) legislation that mandated electronic claims processing through standard transactions and code sets is an excellent example of a government initiative that resulted in improved health care business processes.

As organizations acquire and refine administrative and clinical systems, the pressure is on for health care organizations to use their information systems to deliver data for more efficient operation of daily business activities, demonstrate cost effectiveness through work and data flow improvements, and standardize communications. They must also define and deliver data as an organizational resource through clinical data repositories; and provide patient data to a growing number of authorized users within and beyond the organizations. They need to offer streamlined data capture, particularly for use by direct care providers. The emphasis is on interoperability, networks, and the infrastructure needed to enable linkages within and beyond organizations to community, regional, and national data systems. Information systems must be capable of efficient connectivity so that the data can be collected and used by repositories and warehouses to provide timely, accurate, and increasingly comprehensive views of an individual's EHR individually and by population. And they must do all of this while maintaining effective security measures. More detailed discussion of the technical architecture and applications that serve as a foundation for EHR systems can be found in Chapter 8.

✅ SELF-ASSESSMENT QUIZ

4. The Leapfrog Group, Markle Foundation, and the IOM have influenced the developments and perceptions of EHR systems and HIT in general.
5. Describe strategies for advancing information technology in health care.
6. Using the ideas discussed and additional resources, design or prepare a two-page outline, paper, or presentation for an institutional leadership conference that will be used as an introduction to a planning session for an EHR.

ENTERPRISE SYSTEMS AND ELECTRONIC HEALTH RECORDS

Viewing the Health Information Flow throughout Enterprise Systems

As noted in the discussion on information governance, the EHR today draws in and feeds the overall information flow in the enterprise. Information technology reflects the patient care experience beginning with administrative systems such as registration and appointment scheduling through clinical systems to financial systems for billing and claims processing. The relevant data is extracted and then aggregated into data warehouses to support clinical and business analytics for the organization. Beyond the organization, mandatory and collaborative reporting is done to meet legal and research needs. For those who administer EHR systems, understanding the enterprise structure of information is essential. The principle of *capture once and use many* applies to mapping how individual data is collected for multiple purposes across the enterprise. The data is defined in enterprise systems to ensure that accuracy and timeliness goals are met. Not only is information needed on what health information is maintained in in specific enterprise systems, but careful attention to establishing user authorization for access to specific systems is also needed. The patient record—even when electronic—is also the business record for the organization and must support clinical, administrative, and financial requirements needed to deliver health services. Figure 6-3 illustrates a health information map across enterprise systems.

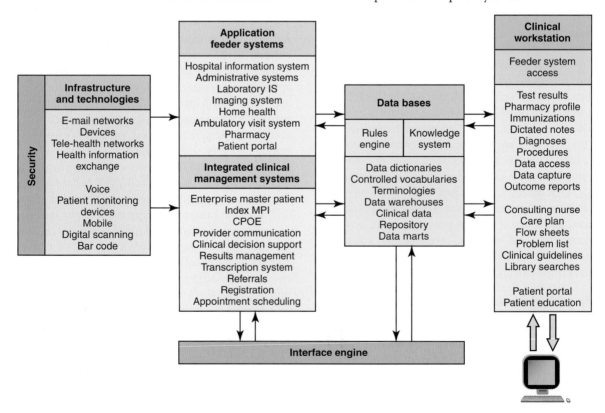

FIGURE 6-3 Health information mapped across enterprise systems. *CPOE,* Computerized physician order entry; *IS,* ***; *MPI,* master patient index.

Understanding the Role of Systems Migrations

Organizational migration benchmarks consist of the planned implementation sequence and timing for adding applications to be acquired in building toward the comprehensive EHR environment. These migration plans are established as organizations map out the building blocks of IT applications that yield increasing content and technology resources on the way toward achieving the optimal HIT goals. Figure 6-4 illustrates a migration plan for an integrated delivery system. Sophisticated planning is needed to build on existing legacy systems, identify replacement systems, and select new applications that become interfaced or integrated to produce the EHR system. There are options to consider.

Some organizations have selected one vendor's integrated product; some have elected to combine multiple vendors. Other organizations have adopted preliminary strategies for increasing automation in a stepwise manner along a selected migration path, moving toward integration at some point in the future. In these cases, the premise is that there is time to take some key steps and wait to adopt a single-focus direction. The advantages of working with one vendor are speed of implementation and tight integration of applications. The downside is that the vendor may not have the best functionalities for all applications needed by the organization and the organization is tied to this particular vendor. A number of vendors offer EHR software and include multimedia functionality in their products. For many hospitals and other health care organizations, a single vendor may be the best approach. Organizations often rely on a vendor's history, experience, and support of the necessary interfaces to existing applications in their organizations in making purchase decisions.

For other settings, the decision may be made to adopt a "best of breed" approach so that individual departments or services may adopt the application that offers the most benefits in their area, and rely on interfaces and interface engines to collect data from the specific area and make it available for access for direct care purposes in an organized presentation layer. If this is the choice, then the organization must plan

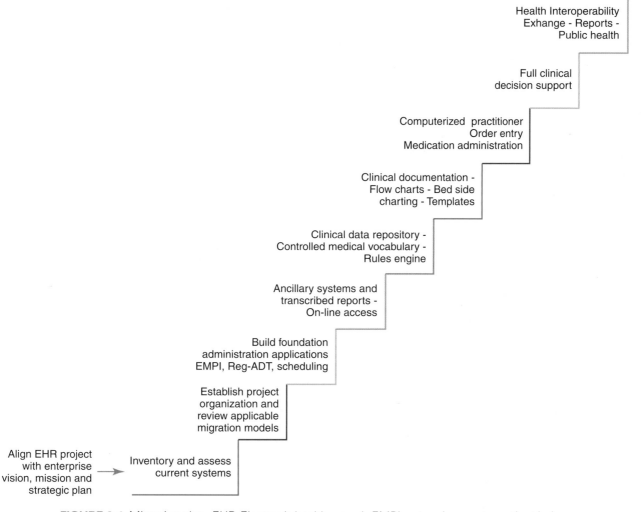

FIGURE 6-4 Migration plan. *EHR,* Electronic health record; *EMPI,* enterprise master patient index; *Reg-ADT,* registration—admission, discharge, transfer.

and budget for ongoing interface resources, not just an initial interface.

Many EHR vendors recruit and hire experienced health information professionals in positions ranging from design consultants to vice presidents. With HIM subject matter expertise and **knowledge** in place, these EHR product developers have access to HIM experts who design or advise on how their products can be used from the patient record management perspective and what features can be incorporated into the product. Historically, health information professionals have made steady gains in leading efforts to transform the paper record content into electronic formats in a stepwise fashion. Online storage, access to transcribed reports, and links to other legacy systems such as the laboratory and the pharmacy offered a rudimentary view into an EHR system capability. As organizations are able to offer safe authorized access to ancillary applications through today's workstations, tablets, and smart phones, patient data use and subsequent demand for more data will focus the energy toward EHRs.

There are, of course, management issues concerning the volume and organization of data in large-scale organizational efforts to implement an EHR system. As yet, no commercial vendor can deliver all the components of an EHR system with the consistent strength to produce the EHR as it is envisioned today. Most organizations and vendors acknowledge the value of an integrated system, but producing an integrated system that does everything well is difficult. In acknowledgement of the more common approach to use legacy systems and build and link applications, one approach is to combine the data from legacy systems and new applications within a single organization—data transferred from diverse applications (perhaps running on different computer platforms)—and reorganize the data into a clinical data repository (CDR). Developing a data repository offers organizations the ability to establish the database and provide access to patient data normally contained in patient records. This repository is designed to deliver the longitudinal collection of data about individuals to providers, have some capability for reporting, and have some patient record functionality in offering information for direct care. In cases in which the EHR products on the market still do not offer data extractions capabilities that meet data analytics needs, this approach is also used to provide additional data warehouses where the data is structured for supporting analytics.

? DID YOU KNOW?

The Veterans' Administration computerized patient record system, as well as the Kaiser Foundation, New York Presbyterian Hospital, and many others enjoy significant progress in EHR developments. These organizations are notable for their inclusion of key elements of the **computer-based patient record** (CPR) goal articulated in the previous decade. These organizations represent evidence of real progress toward the goal of a full EHR system.[5]

Enterprise Systems Links to Electronic Health Records

Registration and appointment scheduling systems serve as the initiation of patient information into electronic systems for hospitals and ambulatory settings. The initial set of patient demographic information commences the record for all subsequent actions from the initial set of provider's orders to the receiving departments such as the laboratory, radiology, and pharmacy, who will act on the order and begin their action by verifying the patient demographic essentials. When providers order medications, the EHR system links to drug–drug interaction protocols and the drug formulary used by the hospital. In turn, the approved order links to the medication administration record that tracks the nurse giving the medication to the patient. In turn, a bar code identification bracelet that was created at admission or registration is now used to verify the correct patient identity and to ensure the right patient is receiving the right medication at the right time. Thus the CDS function that oversees the order entry medication links to the EHR system.

In the ambulatory environment, the patient receives a summary of the visit that compiles the reason for making the appointment and the physician's progress notes on the visit. The summary may also check to see what preventive tests need to be addressed and add them to the summary list so the patient sees that a mammogram or an influenza vaccine needs to be scheduled. What are other examples of enterprise system links to EHRs? The reality is that health information extends through the enterprise systems to both feed and receive data from the EHR.

Integrating Medical Devices into the Electronic Health Record

It is crucial for excellent patient care for the care team to have all needed and reliable data about an individual patient displayed at the point of care in that patient's EHR. Timely, meaningful biomedical information enables clinicians to make real-time clinical decisions within the clinical workflow itself. There are, however, many key diagnostic and treatment devices generating patient-specific health care data that are not yet necessarily part of an organization's EHR system. These types of devices include cardiac output monitors, defibrillators, electrocardiographs, fetal monitors, infant incubators, infusion pumps, intelligent medical device hubs, interactive infusion pumps, physiologic monitors, ventilators, and vital signs monitors, as well as many other current and emerging devices. Medical device connectivity includes patient data that is collected at home as well as in a hospital or other care site. Patient home-generated data can include vital signs such as blood pressure, weight, and blood glucose.[21]

According to a 2010 HIMSS Analytics report, only one third of hospitals are presently interfacing key medical devices at their organizations with their EHR.[21] In 2011 an article from *Medical Device Integration* reported the general impression from chief medical informatics officers and chief nursing informatics officers is that attaining a complete electronic record is not possible unless data generated from various medical devices is included. Additionally, transitioning to meaningful use for health care organizations includes capturing comprehensive data from individual medical devices for better use by clinicians and to encourage interactions between patients and providers.[22]

What is a medical device? The Federal and Drug Administration (FDA) defines a medical device as:

an instrument, apparatus, implement, machine, contrivance, implant, in vitro reagent, or other similar or related article, including a component part, or accessory which is:

- *recognized in the official National Formulary, or the United States Pharmacopoeia, or any supplement to them,*
- *intended for use in the diagnosis of disease or other conditions, or in the cure, mitigation, treatment, or prevention of disease, in man or other animals, or*
- *intended to affect the structure or any function of the body of man or other animals, and which does not achieve any of its primary intended purposes through chemical action within or on the body of man or other animals and which is not dependent upon being metabolized for the achievement of any of its primary intended purposes.*[23]

The FDA then classifies medical devices based on risks associated with the device. Devices are classified into one of three categories: Class I, Class II and Class III:

- Class I devices are deemed to be low risk and are therefore subject to the least regulatory controls. For example, dental floss is classified as Class I device.
- Class II devices are higher risk devices than Class I and require greater regulatory controls to provide reasonable assurance of the device's safety and effectiveness. For example, condoms are classified as Class II devices.
- Class III devices are generally the highest risk devices and are therefore subject to the highest level of regulatory control. Class III devices must typically be approved by FDA before they are marketed. For example, replacement heart valves are classified as Class III devices.

These devices provide various measurements that help staff diagnose and treat a disease or condition. When integrated into an organization's EHR system, the data can be viewed across the continuum of care. Medical devices can be portable or fixed. Sometimes the device is at the patient's bedside such as a blood pressure meter; sometimes the patient is taken to the device such as an x-ray. Staff can and do manually enter blood pressure and other vital signs into the EHR but there may be transcription errors. Sometimes reports from medical devices are simply scanned and indexed as part of the EHR.

Medical device connectivity is not, however, about the connection. It is about workflow automation between the medical device and the EHR. A medical device must be able to export data in a digital form through a port or must have a network connection located within the device itself. A server or centralized computer aggregates data from an organization's medical devices. It may perform additional tasks such as converting units of measure, relabeling data, storing data in temporary databases, or providing users a way to review, validate, and edit this acquired data before it is pushed into the EHR.

Some organizations use a medical device data system (MDDS). An MDDS is able to transfer, store, or display medical device data. It can also convert data into specific formats within preset specifications.[24] An MDDS, however, cannot control or alter functions of any medical device. At present, it is considered a Class I device by the FDA.

The value of medical device integration is the same value of implementing an EHR in the first place. The organization intends to optimize quality of care by increasing accuracy, timeliness, and access to health care documentation across the continuum of care so that any authorized user can see that data in real time and the data can be leveraged for real-time clinical support.

SELF-ASSESSMENT QUIZ

7. Trace the patient experience through the enterprise systems. What serves as the initiation of patient information into electronic systems for hospitals and ambulatory settings?
8. The FDA classifies medical devices into three categories. Which category is high risk?
9. Why would an EHR system that includes at-home monitoring of patients with chronic diseases such as diabetes increase patient engagement and ultimately quality of care?
10. How would a hospital choose which medical devices to integrate into its EHR? And how would HIM expertise assist the hospital in making these choices?

DEFINITIONS FRAMEWORK

The key to understanding the components involved in advancing EHRs in the industry is acquiring a firm understanding of the larger picture as well as the interconnected elements and systems that come to compose an EHR in an individual setting. The HITECH legislation launched a national initiative that calls for applying technology to improve patient care, health care processes, cost, and benefits. Consider the definitions for *HIT, LHR, EHRs, PHRs, designated record set,* and the role of *metadata.* Like a multifaceted engine, these elements are coming together to create a national synergy.

Health Information Technology

The overarching framework for viewing EHRs is HIT. HIT has been described as "hardware, software, integrated technologies or related licenses, intellectual property, upgrades, or packaged solutions sold as services that are designed for or support the use by health care entities or patients for the electronic creation, maintenance, access, or exchange of health information."[25] Another definition of HIT is "the area of IT involving the design, development, creation, use and maintenance of information systems for the healthcare industry. Automated and interoperable healthcare information systems are expected to lower costs, improve efficiency and reduce error, while also providing better consumer care and service." These examples reflect the breadth of challenges faced in achieving effective information technology in and across organizations. The ONCHIT was established by President Bush, and its role expanded through the ARRA legislation in 2009. The ONCHIT established the national certification and program for EHRs, and Medicare and Medicaid established the incentive program to ensure that implemented EHR systems would be used in a meaningful way. The ONCHIT is responsible for setting the standards, implementation specifications, and certification criteria for EHR technology. Thus the collaborative HIT incentive program was established for providers and hospitals to meet the national agenda. To begin at the beginning is to start with reviewing the definition of the *LHR*.

Legal Health Record

As more and more data historically contained in paper patient records are stored in databases and as data are available in multimedia formats, the boundaries between patient record data and other patient data types are changing. What constitutes the health record? Does it include the same historical content in a new format? Are there new data that will simply reside in electronic systems but never become part of the "official" patient record? For example, a pharmacy record of patient prescriptions, including who processed the prescription, may reside in the pharmacy system and be available for viewing online through the pharmacy system, but that information is not included in the paper record. Are there parts of the record that are dynamic and change over time, such as a problem list or various patient alerts such as a behavioral issue or a do not resuscitate order? An American Health Information Management Association (AHIMA) task force appointed to study the issues about the LHR published the results in an AHIMA practice brief.[26] The "legal record" is the record that would be released or disclosed if an organization received a request for a copy of a patient record. In reality, each organization today needs to identify what is included in its "legal medical record." Understandably, it may differ with different health care organizations according to laws, standards, and the health care services provided in each. The legal record in a behavioral health facility reflects the unique health information and services provided in that setting, and may differ from a regional rehabilitation center. The AHIMA task force report guides the decision process for an organization. More discussion of the release or disclosure of information is found in Chapter 15. Typically, each organization evaluates the legitimacy of the request, what data are actually needed, whether the patient has authorized release, and other factors when responding to a request for a copy of a patient record or specific information from an EHR. It is important to recognize, however, that any record, data, or information that is generated and maintained in the normal course of any organization's business can be obtained by a subpoena or court order.

AHIMA's working definition of an LHR is "the documentation of the healthcare services provided to an individual during any aspect of healthcare delivery in any type of healthcare organization. It is consumer or patient centric. The LHR contains individually identifiable data, stored on any medium, and collected and directly used in documenting healthcare provided or health status." Of course, the organization must also explicitly identify the source systems in which the information originates. Organizational policies specify the legal record definition in their setting, which fully defines the content from origin to placement and maintenance in the record. Policies also designate data stewards responsible for representing the information and ensuring that the information meets regulatory compliance requirements.[26]

The LHR meets acceptable laws and standards, records care in any health-related setting, may physically exist in multiple mediums, and is the legal business record generated by the health care organization at the time of service to a patient. In issuing this practice brief, AHIMA affirms previous concepts of the record as a business record of the health services provided, accommodates hybrid record models, acknowledges the breadth of data involved in providing care, and recognizes the increasing scope of media for storage.

Hybrid records are the norm in the majority of health care settings. As previously discussed in Chapter 4, hybrid records are a combination of paper records and data stored in electronic systems. If a particular document is stored in both media (paper and electronic), the organization should determine which of the formats it is recognizing as its "legal documentation." For example, if the organization has both a paper copy and an electronic copy of an operative report, the copy that is signed (authenticated) is traditionally considered the legal copy. There is no reason to sign both paper and electronic reports of the same document; the organization, of course, must retain the record that is authenticated. Electronic signatures and handwritten signatures are acceptable for the legal record. Policies and procedures establish the organizational decisions in hybrid record systems to determine which documents, in which format, constitute the legal patient record for an individual organization.

Laws, regulations, and practice principles must be examined and perhaps changed in some states to better describe the legal medical record in an electronic environment. Table 6-3 shows the AHIMA legal health record description by type of content.[26] The AHIMA practice brief illustrates how an organization can use policies and procedures to identify the source systems in which some of the record is stored electronically. Source systems might be laboratory information systems, pharmacy systems, or imaging systems, as well

TABLE 6-3 Data and Documents to be Considered Part of the Record

Advance directives	Nursing assessments
Allergy records	Operative and procedure reports
Alerts and reminders (see "Alerts, Reminders, and Pop-Ups," earlier in chapter)	Orders for treatment including diagnostic tests for laboratory and radiology
Analog and digital patient photographs for identification purposes only	Pathology reports
Anesthesia records	Patient-submitted documentation
Care plans	Patient education or teaching documents
Consent forms for care, treatment, research	Patient identifiers (medical record number)
Consultation reports	Photographs (digital and analog)
Diagnostic images	Sticky notes and annotations containing patient–provider or provider–provider communications regarding care or treatment of specific patients
Discharge instructions	Practice guidelines or protocols and clinical pathways that embed patient data
Discharge summaries	Problem lists
E-mail messages containing patient–provider or provider–provider communications notes regarding care or treatment of specific patients*	Progress notes and documentation (multidisciplinary, excluding psychotherapy)
Emergency department records	Psychology and psychiatric assessments and summaries (excluding psychotherapy notes)
Fetal monitoring strips from which interpretations are derived	Records received from another health care provider who was relied on to provide health care to the patient (see "Continuing Care Records," earlier in chapter)
Functional status assessments	Research records of tests and treatments[7]
Graphic records	Respiratory therapy, physical therapy, speech therapy, and occupational therapy records
History and physical examination records	Results of tests and studies from laboratory and radiology
Immunization records	Standing orders
Instant messages containing patient–provider or provider–provider communications[†]	Telephone messages containing patient–provider or provider–provider communications regarding care or treatment of specific patients
Intake and output records	Telephone orders
Medication administration records	Trauma tapes
Medication orders	Verbal orders
Medication profiles	Waveforms such as ECGs and electromyograms from which interpretations are derived
Minimum data sets (MDS, OASIS, IRF, PAI)	Any other information required by the Medicare Conditions of Participation, state provider licensure statutes or rules, or by any third-party payer as a condition of reimbursement

*Washington State Pilot Health Record Bank Project: www.microsoft.com/en-us/download/details.aspx?id=16357. Accessed August 30, 2014.
[†]Halamika, John: Life as a Healthcare CIOP, The Massachusetts A Hoc HIE Workgroup, June 16, 2010: cmio.wordpress.com/2010/06/16/the-geek-on-massachusetts-hie. Accessed August 30, 2014.
Hoyt, John et al: Industry Report: 2012 Annual Report to the U.S., Hospital IT Market, HIMSS and HIMMS Analytics, 2013.
American Health Information Management Association, update: Guidelines for defining the legal health record for disclosure purposes: library.ahima.org/xpedio/groups/public/documents/ahima/bok1_048604. Accessed August 30, 2014.

as data or information generated by one or more of the medical devices discussed earlier in this chapter. Table 6-4 illustrates how hybrid health records systems identify the content of the record using the source systems such as transcription, laboratory, radiology, pharmacy, and more. No matter what EHR transition status an organization is in at any particular moment, HIM staff must ensure that the organization has a complete medical record. This means changing business processes to accommodate electronic source systems that maintain original care documentation to ensure that the LHR can be provided as a complete entity for care and business purposes.

TABLE 6-4   Defining Hybrid Records—Paper to Source Systems Illustrated

Patient Record Report	Media	Source Systems
Admission history and physical examination	Paper	Transcription
Physician orders	Paper	Paper record
Clinical laboratory results	Electronic	Laboratory information system
Radiology reports	Electronic	Radiology information system
Medication records	Electronic	Bedside documentation system
Preoperative progress notes	Paper	Paper record
Progress notes	Paper	Paper record
Consents	Electronic	Optical scanning system

Electronic Health Records

EHRs were initially defined from a national perspective by an IOM committee in 1991. At that time, the committee's charge was to examine the current state of medical record systems, identify impediments and ways to overcome them, develop a research agenda, and develop a plan for improved medical record systems. They were also charged to recommend policies and other strategies to achieve the improvements.

Noting that patient record systems could be part of hospital information systems, medical information systems, or a type of clinical information system, they proposed the term *computer-based patient record* (CPR) to define the entity they envisioned.[27]

Table 6-5 lists key definitions for EHRs and related concepts. The original ideas continue to live in subsequent definitions.[28] Definitions over time have maintained basic concepts and have been expressed in more or less detail. These definitions continue to evolve as more is learned.

The term *electronic health record* has the broadest interpretation as a record of all types of care to prevent and treat illness. Ideally, the record is maintained over a long period in a manner accessible to caregivers, the patient, and others who

TABLE 6-5   Key Definitions

Electronic Health Record

The Electronic Health Record (EHR) is a longitudinal electronic record of patient health information produced by encounters in one or more care settings. Included in this information are patient demographics, progress notes, problems, medications, vital signs, past medical history, immunizations, laboratory data, and radiology reports. The EHR system automates and streamlines the clinician's workflow. The EHR has the ability to independently generate a complete record of a clinical patient encounter, and possesses sufficient data granularity to support clinical decision support, quality management, clinical reporting, and interoperability.

Electronic Medical Record

An electronic record of health-related information on an individual that can be created, gathered, managed, and consulted by authorized clinicians and staff within one health care organization.

Electronic Health Record

An electronic record of health-related information on an individual that conforms to nationally recognized interoperability standards and that can be created, managed, and consulted by authorized clinicians and staff across more than one health care organization.

Personal Health Record

An electronic record of health-related information on an individual that conforms to nationally recognized interoperability standards and that can be drawn from multiple sources while being managed, shared, and controlled by the individual.

Legal Health Record (LHR)

The LHR is the documentation of the health care services provided to an individual in any aspect of health care delivery by a health care provider organization. The LHR is individually identifiable data, in any medium, collected and directly used in and/or documenting health care or health status.

Electronic Health Record

The Electronic Health Record is a secure, real-time, point-of-care, patient-centric information resource for clinicians. The EHR aids clinicians' decision-making by providing access to patient health record information where and when they need it and by incorporating evidence-based decision support. The EHR automates and streamlines the clinician's workflow, closing loops in communication and response that result in delays or gaps in care. The EHR also supports the collection of data for uses other than direct clinical care, such as billing, quality management, outcomes reporting, resource planning, and public health disease surveillance and reporting.

Guidelines for Defining the Health Record for Legal Purposes, American Health Information Management Association, 2005.
Health Information Management Systems Society: *HIMSS Definition 1.0, 2003.*
HIMSS Electronic Health Record Association Definitional Model and Application Process, March 2009: http://www.himssehra.org/docs/EHRVA_application.pdf. Accessed July 1, 2014.
National Alliance for Health Information Technology: Report to the Office of the National Coordinator for Health Information Technology on Defining Key Health Information Technology Terms, April 28, 2008.

need access to specific information or to aggregate information to prevent illness and improve future treatment.

Today's EHRs are being designed for large hospitals, group and single practices in ambulatory care, long-term care, behavioral health, home health, and hospice settings. Increasingly, EHRs are implemented in integrated delivery systems that contain multiple levels of care delivery. In all these settings, the basic content of patient records is becoming part of one or more electronic databases. As the capability to exchange data across settings grows, coordination of care can be achieved and cost and quality benefits expand. And the clinicians that use EHRs will be able to access and manage their patients' needs in less time and with better and more complete data. Still, innovation is required to create EHR features that invite clinicians and other users to engage and use EHR tools.

An EHR works best if the users can access a large, easy-to-read screen and sophisticated navigational tools. The screen shown in Figure 6-5 illustrates an institutional EHR opening navigational screen used by physicians seeking information on their patients in a hospital setting. Clinicians must be able to access, retrieve, and capture data from a variety of sources and point-of-care settings and make use of available clinical and technological tools that make information readily available and improves health services workflow. Practice management modules that support a specific health care documentation function for individual disciplines or departments, such as surgery, radiology, or laboratory, and access to decision support and expert system tools are components that the clinician must be able to easily retrieve and view from their workstations. EHR systems are complex in complex work environments and straightforward in single-user

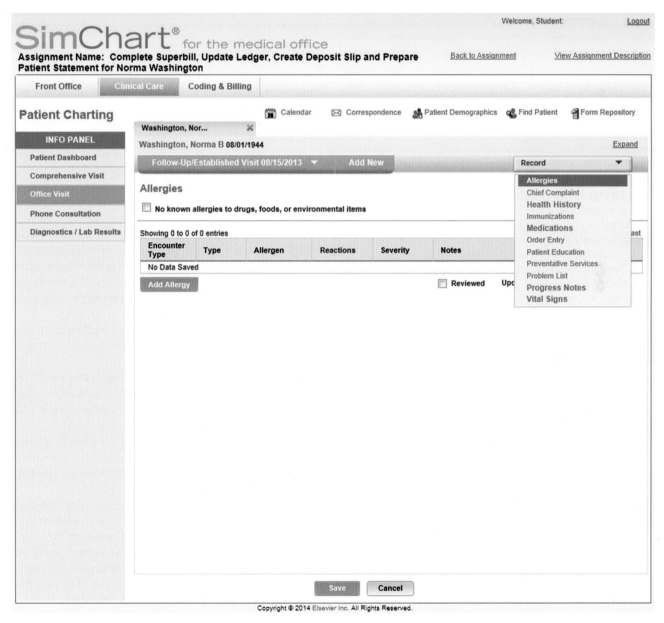

FIGURE 6-5 Workstation navigation screen. Elsevier 2014. SimChart for the Medical Office® (www.evolve.elsevier.com).

environments. In line with patient record access rights and known benefits in which patients are more engaged in their own health care experiences, more organizations are opening patient portals for individuals to access parts of their EHR. For example, The Department of Veterans Affairs offers a patient portal called "My Health eVet" that allows patients to navigate to information and on-line functions (https://www.myhealth.va.gov/index.html).[29]

The breadth of information brought together on behalf of patients and the technology required to access and use it within EHR systems is clearly beyond the historical view of patient records as a set of data to be collected on paper forms during the care process.

Personal Health Record

The IOM has found, "When patients see multiple providers in different settings, none of whom have access to complete [health] information, it becomes easier for things to go wrong."[30] Each health care provider maintains his or her own separate patient records for patients treated. This means that health information is fragmented among the many individual and organizational providers where the patient has received care, which can lead to an incomplete story about a patient's health. What is needed is a way to coordinate the documentation among all the clinical stakeholders in a patient's care. One obvious coordinator is the patient. The tool a patient needs to do this is called the *personal health record* (PHR).

Through an AHIMA workgroup established in 2004, AHIMA published a definition of an electronic PHR:

The personal health record is an electronic, lifelong resource of health information needed by individuals to make health decisions. Individuals own and manage the information in the PHR, which comes from healthcare providers and the individual. The PHR is maintained in a secure and private environment, with the individual determining rights of access. The PHR does not replace the legal record of any provider.[31]

In April 2009 the National Alliance for Health Information Technology published a consensus definition for a PHR. They define the PHR as "an electronic record of health-related information on an individual that conforms to nationally recognized interoperability standards and that can be drawn from multiple sources while being managed, shared, and controlled by the individual."[32] This definition clearly reinforces the work done by AHIMA and adds the focus on interoperability.

Key considerations for the health information manager in an organizationally controlled PHR is the PHR's format and content, privacy, access and control, maintenance and security, and interoperability. Ideally, such a PHR does the following:

- Eases the transition from paper to electronic record keeping.
- Allows the patient to refill prescriptions electronically.
- Addresses health literacy skills (reading and writing) in the context of language and culture.
- Is designed so that interfaces are patient friendly.
- Can custom-tailor views.
- Enables information sharing among patient and providers.

- Is portable and remains with the patient.
- Helps organize personal health information.
- Assists patients with decision making, wellness, self-care plans, and patient safety alerts.

In fact, PHR proponents believe that patients who keep their own complete, updated, and easily accessible health records are taking a more active role in their own health care and participate in shared decision making with their physicians. As consumers, patients need to carefully consider where to store their PHR and how to evaluate PHR vendors, especially in relation to the privacy and **confidentiality** afforded (or not) by the vendor. The growth of the internet combined with easy access to huge amounts of health information has led to the concept of consumer health informatics: "the branch of medical informatics that analyzes consumers' needs for information; studies and implements methods for making information accessible to consumers; and models and integrates consumers' preferences into medical information systems."[33] A patient could decide to use a portion of the PHR to organize health information gleaned from the Internet.

PHRs can be stored on paper or electronically. If patients, including ourselves, keep medical records at all, they are still likely to be paper copies of various reports from family practitioners, obstetrician-gynecologists, and so forth. PHRs can also be maintained in a PC or tablet device; the patient can type in specific health information such as glucose levels tracked at home, or scanned copies of medical record reports and office visit summaries can be provided by the practitioner. There are web-based PHR products in which the patient's information is securely stored on a web server and is accessible through an Internet connection. Various portable devices (flash drives, personal digital assistants, smartcards, etc.) can be used in connection with other PHR solutions. Figure 6-6 illustrates a PHR linked to care sites.

To promulgate adoption of PHRs, AHIMA developed a community-based public education campaign with several objectives:

- Increase public awareness and understanding of the issues surrounding personal health information and health records.
- Provide individuals with the information they need to better manage their personal health information and to encourage them to maintain a PHR to improve the quality of care they receive.
- Create greater public awareness of the HIM professional and the important role HIM professionals play in effective management of personal health information needed to deliver quality health care to the public.[34]

Individual health care organizations have developed patient portals so that patients can have electronic access to views of their EHR in that care environment. It is important to note that even though PHRs and patient portal technologies offer important improvements in methods patients use to collect and maintain information in a PHR, significant issues remain. Patient privacy concerns, the ability to send or receive PHR information electronically, and timeliness and completeness of the information contained in the PHR are all issues that need further work and oversight. The effect

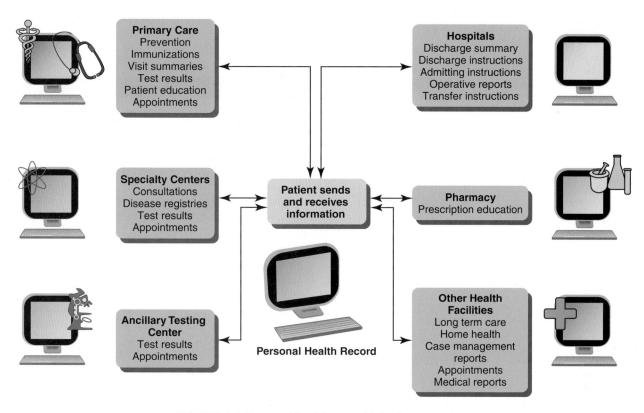

FIGURE 6-6 Personal health record linked to care sites.

of the PHR systems in the overall health information and individual patient's health status and care coordination will merit research. Their potential to link provider EHR systems merits extensive study.

Designated Record Set

The Healthcare Insurance Portability and Accountability Act (HIPAA) is an important federal law that reinforces the privacy protection given to individually identifiable health data created and held by health care organizations and other groups designated in the law. The administrative simplification portion of the HIPAA legislation uses the term *designated record set*. Designated record sets are defined in a manner that covers all types of organizations that maintain health information. For health organizations that provide health services, the patient and billing records are the typical records addressed by HIPAA. Third-party payers and other organizations also maintain records about the individual's enrollment, payment, claims adjudication, or case management records that are used in whole or part to make decisions about the patient.[35] This record set will vary on the basis of the requestor and the requestor's rights and needs because another component of HIPAA provides that the minimum amount of data necessary to accomplish a request for information should be released. The law specifies much more detail about its application. The primary purpose of HIPAA privacy regulations is to protect the privacy of individually identifiable information. Because organizations determine their designated record set, they also address the hybrid record status in their institutions and determine the best

sources for assembling specific data into the record set. AHIMA publishes guidelines on designated record sets that institutions can use as they establish through policy and procedures what constitutes the designated record set for their organization. AHIMA's Table 6-6 illustrates the difference between a designated record set and the LHR.

SELF-ASSESSMENT QUIZ

11. Explain why the LHR might be defined differently in different health care settings.
12. Both electronic signatures and handwritten signatures are acceptable for the legal record.
13. How does a PHR work with partners to improve patient record practices?
14. Using information from this chapter and other resources, prepare a chart that describes the views an attending physician, nurse, and coder might use in looking at the EHR for an individual patient.

HOW HEALTH CARE STANDARDS GUIDE ELECTRONIC HEALTH RECORDS

Standards Development and the Electronic Health Record

Many organizations develop or assist in the development and publication of health care standards that play a role in the progress toward EHR systems. This chapter discusses the American Society for Testing and Materials (ASTM), Health Level 7 (HL7), HIPAA, Logical Observation Identifier Name

TABLE 6-6 Designated Record Set Versus The Legal Health Record
This Side by Side Comparison Demonstrates the Differences Between the Two Sets of Information, as well as Their Purposes.

	Designated Record Set	Legal Health Record
Definition	A group of records maintained by or for a covered entity that is the medical and billing records about individuals; enrollment, payment, claims adjudication, and case or medical management record systems maintained by or for a health plan; information used in whole or in part by or for the HIPAA-covered entity to make decisions about individuals.	The business record generated at or for a health care organization. It is the record that would be released upon receipt of a request. The legal health record is the officially declared record of health care services provided to an individual delivered by a provider.
Purpose	Used to clarify the access and amendment standards in the HIPAA privacy rule, which provide that individuals generally have the right to inspect and obtain a copy of protected health information in the designated record set.	The official business record of health care services delivered by the entity for regulatory and disclosure purposes.
Content	Defined in organizational policy and required by the HIPAA privacy rule. The content of the designated record set includes medical and billing records of covered providers; enrollment, payment, claims, and case information of a health plan; and information used in whole or in part by or for the covered entity to make decisions about individuals.	Defined in organizational policy and can include individually identifiable data in any medium collected and directly used in documenting health care services or health status. It excludes administrative, derived, and aggregate data.
Uses	Supports individual HIPAA right of access and amendment.	Provides a record of health status as well as documentation of care for reimbursement, quality management, research, and public health purposes; facilitates business decision-making and education of healthcare practitioners as well as the legal needs of the healthcare organization.

HIPAA, Health Insurance Portability and Accountability Act.
AHIMA. Mary Beth Haugen, MS, RHIA, Anne Tegen, MHA, RHIA, HRM, Diana Warner, MS, RHIA, CHPS, "Fundamentals of the Legal Health Record and Designated Record Set" library.ahima.org/xpedio/groups/public/documents/ahima/bok1_048604. All accessed on August 30, 2014.

Code (LOINC), and AHIMA. It is important for those working in health informatics fields to become familiar with the various standard-setting organizations that focus on the EHR and to become aware of the similarities and differences. The reality is that standards bodies such as the Joint Commission, HL7, and ASTM often develop the initial standards initiatives that are then adopted as regulatory standards after they have been tried in the marketplace. Today the federal government plays a leading role in ensuring that EHR products are consistently designed and meet national standards. Eligible providers, hospital, and other ambulatory and long-term or specialized care organizations can identify certified HIT.

The ONCHIT approves testing and certifications to oversee the quality of HIT products. Vendors submit their product for testing and certification to assure the customers that the product meets standards, implementation, and certification criteria that has been adopted by the HHS. A key example of this process is the work of the approved oversight body CCHIT.

Commission on Certification of Health Information Technology

The CCHIT publishes standards for ambulatory care practice and inpatient EHRs according to increasing expectations of functionality. It reviews vendor EHR packages to certify how well the application meets published CCHIT standards. Of

particular note, the CCHIT benchmarks increase in functionality expectations each year, and vendor applications can measure the level of certification by the year certified.[36] It serves as a conduit for eligible professionals and hospitals to monitor certification requirements that affect their situation. In addition, it maintains postings of the certification status for vendor EHR applications. Today's certification requirements encompass the content required in EHRs along with the functionality that describes how that content is organized, captured, accessed, and used. Standards for maintaining security and measures to monitor secure practices are included as well. Foundation work from HL7 served as a primary resource for establishing certification requirements for EHR products. Health informatics and information management practitioners juggle a growing stable of standards from standards development organizations (SDOs) to accreditation standards relevant to health care organizations along with the federal certification standards for EHRs.

Health Insurance Portability and Accountability Act

HIPAA was established to streamline the designated business processes in billing and claims, and to define standards for privacy and security of an individual's personal health information so that health information systems and their various customers would handle it appropriately. HIPAA security standards are part of the national requirements for certified

EHRs and specify provisions that need to be incorporated into certified health record applications. By mapping our privacy provisions for managing personal health information within systems and governing those to access and retrieve information, HIPAA lays out the framework for major functions in systems, including designating how information is protected through basic tools such as managed user authorization and monitoring tools and encryption applied to secure messaging. Today's federal standards interconnect EHR features and security policies, procedures, and audit requirements. HIPAA legislation continues to tighten up standards to ensure privacy and security, and sets guidelines for business associates of health care organizations to comply with them as well.

Key Health Care Standards Organizations

Health informatics standards have been evolving over decades. SDOs have focused on specific areas of interest as they sought to bring standards into place to solve specific problems.

For example, individuals interested in establishing standard names for laboratory tests so information could be reasonably and consistently used and shared worked on developing the standard LOINCs. Other individuals worked on standards in billing and claims ultimately leading to the provisions in the HIPAA previously mentioned. Still other organizations focused on standards for security or health record content or pharmacy. The combined work of standards organizations continues to move the industry forward toward the goals of establishing consistency of information within systems and organizations that can enable a higher quality of data, more trustworthiness of the data, and, ultimately, the capacity to transmit information on behalf of patients that will be viewed by the data receiver with the understanding of the information. It can be a business challenge for those who seek to innovate products that serve their customers to be motivated to collaborate through using standards in their products. Today's health industry demands are changing that dynamic as federal legislation specifies certification of products that meet standard criteria and have the capability to meet the patient's health care needs across organizations. SDOs are coming together and collaborating to meet both industry and business goals. Of these, several merit attention.

American Society of Testing and Materials

The AHIMA has published guides on the content of patient records and professional practice standards for a number of clinical settings. It has also supported the formal development of voluntary standards for EHRs by working with the ASTM, a national standards development body. The ASTM was formed more than 90 years ago to develop industrial standards. More recently, a section of ASTM has developed in health care informatics. Committees are formed and revised as this effort evolves. Examples include E 1384–07 Standard Practice for Content and Structure of the Electronic Health Record (EHR), E1762–95 Standard Guide for Authentication of Healthcare Information (Reapproved 2003), E 2017–99 (Reapproved 2005) Standard Guide for Amendments to

Health Information, and E1714–00 Standard Guide for Properties of a Universal Healthcare Identifier.[37]

An ASTM standard is a published guide that defines and describes how business processes or data are to be managed consistently. The standard may specify how a computer application should be designed or how data elements are to be defined. Standards are also written as guides—for example, a guide for a software development process. Standards offer models for adoption and, in some cases, a specific blueprint to be followed.

The data elements contained in the standard E1384–07, Standard Practice for Content and Structure of the Electronic Health Record (EHR), are based on research on the common data sets of interest in health care (e.g., Uniform Hospital Discharge Data Set, Uniform Ambulatory Care Data Set) and on new or missing elements needed to fully describe the health record of a person over a lifetime. The standard applies to all types of health care services throughout the continuum of care.[38] When there are agreed upon universal content definitions, the content of data transferred between two facilities is clear, even if one of the facilities uses an alias term. An alias term would translate back into the formal term and definition. For example, if the formal term is *patient identifier* or *number*, a facility could choose to call the patient identifier a *medical record number*. *Medical record number* would then be an alias term for *patient identifier*. The electronic data interchange at a meaningful content level requires the use of common data definitions.

As with The Joint Commission standards, ASTM standards are voluntary. They are developed through a consensus process and improved through feedback from users. Reviews are conducted frequently to verify the validity of published standards. In 1991 the ASTM published the initial version of standard (E1384) as a guide to the content and format of an EHR. This standard was revised in 1998 and 2002 and reapproved in 2007. Readers interested in obtaining a current version of the full standard should contact ASTM.[39]

An example of an EHR standards developed through the ASTM standards development process is ASTM E1384–07 Content Guide for the Electronic Health Record applies to all types of health care services, including those given in acute care hospitals, nursing homes, skilled nursing facilities, home health care, and specialty care environments as well as ambulatory care. The principles are shown in Table 6-7. The standard applies to both short-term contacts (e.g., emergency department services and emergency medical service units) and long-term contacts (e.g., primary care physicians and other health care providers with long-term patients).

The standard delineates the components and content of the patient record and includes definitions that conform to standard nomenclature. It is divided into segments that are grouped within or around an entity that organizes them into broad categories, such as patient, provider, problem, or observation. These broad groups are another way of depicting data in object-oriented view. Each data element contained in the standard is mapped to a code set that is defined in the companion standards for E1633 Coded Values

TABLE 6-7 Purposes of the Standard Guide for Description for Content and Structure of the Electronic Health Record (e1384)

- To identify content and logical structure of an EHR consistent with current acknowledged patient record content
- To explain the relationship of data coming from diverse source systems (e.g., clinical laboratory information management systems, order entry systems, pharmacy information management systems, dictation systems) and the data stored in the EHR as the primary repository for information from various sources.
- To provide a common vocabulary for those developing, purchasing, and implementing EHR systems
- To describe examples of a variety of views by which the logical data structure might be accessed or displayed to accomplish various functions
- To provide a common vocabulary for those developing, purchasing, and implementing HER systems.
- To map the content to selected relevant biomedical and health informatics standards.

for Content and Structure of Electronic Health Records. A more complete description of the ASTM 1384 Standard can be seen in the website.[38]

Health Level 7

One of the major SDOs, HL7 is working closely with the AHIMA and other organizations on the functional capabilities of the EHR. In 2004 HL7 published a draft standard for trial use for EHR systems to guide the work in designing and developing EHR systems and to offer a resource to the health care industry. This standard proposes more than 125 functions.[40] It organizes the functions into three main components: direct care, supportive, and information infrastructure. Figure 6-7 illustrates how these functions are connected; note the scope of content and the traditional patient record forms titles. The direct care section addresses care delivery functions. The supportive section addresses functionality for administrative and financial requirements related to care delivery. The information infrastructure section addresses the information infrastructure and technical capabilities needed to support the care process.

The HL7 standard identifies health record information and management in the purpose statement: "Manage EHR information across EHR-S applications by ensuring that clinical information entered by providers is a valid representation of clinical notes; and is accurate and complete according to clinical rules and tracking amendments to clinical documents. Ensure that information entered by or on behalf of the patient is accurately represented." This standard is suitable for multiple care settings and reinforces the overriding objective for validity, accuracy, and completion of the clinical content within an appropriate legal context.

The direct care management functions of the HL7 standard include provision for health information capture, management, and review that addresses health record content. Care plans; guidelines, protocols, and patient education; medication ordering and management; orders, referrals, and results management; consents and directives; and decision support are addressed in this standard. Although this standard is revised with ongoing use, it offers specific details and describes products that should be available through EHR systems. For example, the standard describes a series of lists (problem list and others) that should be routine components of an EHR. It provides enough explanation of technical capabilities that system developers can be guided on specific features and provides the foundation for the CCHIT, the DGI, and others to set benchmark functionality for EHR applications.

Table 6-8 illustrates the relationship between components in the HL7 standard and the CCHIT certification requirements.

ASTM and HL7 Collaborative Work

ASTM continues to contribute to current EHR development. As previously discussed, ASTM has a number of standards related to the development and use of EHRs. The ASTM Standard on Electronic Health Record Content and Structure (E1384) and Coded Values for Content and Structure of Electronic Health Records (E1633) focuses on the overall data contained in the patient record and offers guidance to data models and dictionaries associated with EHRs, whereas the HL7 standard adds technical system "how to" to the picture. An excellent example of a collaborative product is the continuity of care record (CCR).

In a joint effort with the Massachusetts Medical Society, the HIMSS, the American Academy of Family Physicians, the American Academy of Pediatrics and participating vendors, the ASTM developed a CCR standards that called for exchanging information to support coordination of care. This standard was subsequently mapped to the HL7's clinical document architecture and renamed the *Continuity of Care*

Direct Care	Information Infrastructure
• DC.1 Care Management • DC.2 Clinical Decision Support • DC.3 Operations Management and Communication	• IN.1 Security • IN.2 Health Record Information and Management • IN.3 Registry and Directory Services • IN.4 Standard Terminologies and Terminology Services
Supportive	• IN.5 Standards-based Interoperability
• S.1 Clinical Support • S.2 Measurement, Analysis, Research and Reports • S.3 Administrative and Financial	• IN.6 Business Rules and Management • IN.7 Workflow Management

Source: HL7 2007

FIGURE 6-7 Health Level 7 (HL7) Draft Standard—Trial Use.

TABLE 6-8	HL7 and CCHIT EHR Content Comparison		
	EHR Function	HL7	CCHIT
Organize patient data	Patient demographics	X	X
	Clinical/encounter notes	X	X
	Medical history	X	X
	Record patient-specific information	X	X
	Patient consent	X	X
	Generate reports	X	X
	Advance directives		
Compile lists	Medication lists	X	X
	Allergy lists	X	X
	Problem/diagnoses lists	X	X
Receive and display information	Laboratory test results	X	X
	Radiology results	X	X
	Radiology imaging results	X	X
	Capture external clinical documents	X	X
Order entry (CPOE)	Electronic prescribing	X	X
	Reorder prescriptions	X	X
	Laboratory order entry	X	2010
	Radiology order entry	X	2010
Decision support	Reminders for care activities	X	X
	Dosing calculator	X	X
	Preventative services	X	X
	Drug alerts	X	X
	Disease or chronic care management	X	2010
	Knowledge resources	X	X
	Clinical guidelines		
Communication and connectivity	Electronic referrals	X	X
	Clinical messaging/e-mail	X	X
	Medical devices	X	X
Administrative and billing support	Scheduling management	X	X
	Eligibility information	X	X
	Electronic billing/integration with practice billing system	X	X
	Drug formularies	X	X
	Clinical task assignment and routing		
Other	Immunization tracking	X	X
	Public health reporting	X	2010
	Patient support	X	X

CCHIT, Commission on Certification of Health Information Technology; *CPOE,* computerized physician order entry; *EHR,* electronic health record; *HL7,* Health Level 7. Measurement of the Utilization of an Installed EHR. www.healthcareitnews.com/...care-document-approved-hl7-endorsed-hitsp. Accessed February 14, 2007.
Dullabh P. et al: White Paper prepared for U.S. Department of Health and Human Services, National Opinion Research Center, NORC, and the University of Chicago, June, 2009, Appendix C.

Document (CCD). It is designed for transmission of referral information between health care providers and is a practical tool today.[41] The CCD provides a standard format for exchanging demographics, problem list, medications, laboratory information, and allergies. This has value for provider organizations and could also play a significant role in transferring information from provider organizations to PHRs. The Department of Health and Human Services adopted this standard in 2008, thereby endorsing a national format for exchanging health information.[42] The SDOs' resources are valuable to vendors, health care organizations, and HIM professionals as they develop the functional requirements for their organization in preparation for acquiring an EHR system and evaluating the capabilities of EHR systems on the market.

Often data from like or similar activities are placed together (e.g., computer screen formats, paper forms). In the paper-based health record, forms are created to allow documentation of similar activities on one form or a related series of forms. For example, inpatient nursing activities may be recorded in one section of the record on a series of related forms. As the activities of care and the methods for delivering care change, the forms are redesigned. Once recorded on paper, the data are static and cannot easily be reorganized or integrated with other data. Data entered using the computer screen format can be manipulated and reorganized. It is important to recognize that if new data are created or used differently, then the data items must be defined and promulgated within the organization's policies.

If you conceptualize the data required to describe the activities of health care as data elements not tied to a paper form, you can begin to think of the patient data as a database. A database must be well organized and contain all the data elements necessary to describe the health care process. It is much more flexible in the ways data can be organized, reorganized, and retrieved to give various views of the data or to show trends. For example, the data, or view, needed by admitting staff is not the same view as that needed by the laboratory staff to carry out their responsibilities. A clinician may want to see the trend of blood glucose test results from the past 3 days mapped to insulin dose, meals, and activity. The data in a database can be extracted and reorganized to provide this view both as raw data and as a graph.

Major effort is being invested in developing data models for health care. The natural result of these data models is the databases needed to describe and carry out health care activities. One of the major components is the EHR. This record in its final evolution is a sophisticated database. To help arrive at the EHR, those in the field must agree on definitions of terms and content. Although it is possible to create crosswalks between systems and to use alternative or alias terms, it is still essential that there is basic agreement on content definitions. For example, if HIM professionals are exchanging authorized data for a patient and the request is for "Medical Alerts–Allergy Section," then the data to be transferred should be retrievable and translatable into a message standard format, but most important, the content must be any known allergies to medication, food, or other substances for this patient.

The early IOM work that establishes the framework of EHR system was expanded by health informatics standards development work. Follow-up work on HL-7 standards included the IOM functions within the Draft Standards for Trial Use initially published in 2004, which served as foundation for the CCHIT certification of EHR products discussed earlier in this chapter.[43]

Logical Observation Identifiers Names and Codes

The LOINC is a universal code system used for identifying laboratory and clinical observations. It has been part of the functionality expectations for clinical laboratory systems and is anticipated for use with EHR systems.

LOINC uses standardized terms including clinical terms such as blood pressure and laboratory test names, and has standardized terms for all kinds of observations and measurements that can be used when health information is exchanged. It covers laboratory and related diagnostic test names and results and also can represent clinical facts within the record. It works with partner standards to make up a message that needs to communicate the laboratory test results from the laboratory system to a diagnostic test results application. Think of the HL7 exchange standard as supplying the wagon to carry the message and the LOINC code to be used to describe the clinical observation or test result riding in the wagon. When these standards are used, the senders and receivers could then work with a consistent representation of a specific laboratory test, clinical observation, or other standardized term. Just as other standards, the LOINC standard is in ongoing development. It plays an important role for EHR systems as the national standards for certified EHR systems require that laboratory test results use the LOINC system. When used consistently, the LOINC standard can enable exchange of electronic health data from many independent systems. These codes can be used to evaluate aggregate data as well. LOINC offers a user's guide to guide individuals working with the LOINC standard.[44]

People across the United States and many other countries use LOINC to meet health data exchange goals.

RxNorm

Just as attention is given to the standardization of laboratory and clinical observation naming, standards to support medications and pharmacies also play a significant role in evolving systems. The RxNorm standard provides a consistent naming system for drugs and also serves as a tool that supports the interoperation between drug terminologies and pharmacy knowledge base systems. The National Library of Medicine (NLM) creates and maintains the RxNorm standard. As noted in the NLM website, the role that RxNorm performs is to provide normalized names and unique identifiers to be applied to both brand name and generic drugs.[45] This allows consistent naming and exchanging of information. By using this standard, hospitals, clinics, pharmacies, and other organizations can pass information from one system to another. The significance of this standard is notable. Medications are a critical element of patient information. Just as the LOINC standard is called for in certified EHR systems, the RxNorm standard is required in the e-prescribing function in ambulatory EHRs.

A broad picture of standards associated with EHRs includes the examples discussed so far and many others. Standards influence how we design these new EHR systems and, more importantly, how we judge their effectiveness. Use these as a guide to measure and assess considerations about specific EHR systems. See Table 6-9 for an illustration of HIT standards organizations.

TABLE 6-9   Health Care Informatics Standards and Electronic Health Records

Standard	Standards Organization	Purpose	How Standard Contributes to EHR Systems
Data Exchange/Messaging Messaging Standards Version 2 and 3 (HL7 V2.X3 and V3)	Health Level Seven www.hl7.org	Electronic message formats for clinical, financial, and administrative data. V2 is common in commercially available software. V3 was launched in January 2005.	Establishes standard message format and "envelope" through which data can be exchanged from one computer system to another. Can be used to support interoperability among applications that may send data to an EHR system.
Digital Imaging and Communications in Medicine (DICOM)	National Electronics Manufacturers Association www.nema.org	Format for communicating radiology images and data	Allows information from imaging devices to be accessed and viewed through EHR system.
National Council for Prescription Drug Programs (NCPDP)	National Council for Prescription Drug Programs www.ncpdp.org	Structure for transmitting prescription requests and fulfillment	Provides standard protocol for sending prescription information between provider EHR applications to pharmacies for billing and claims.
Accredited Standards Committee X12 (ANSI ASC X12)	American National Standards Institute (ANSI), Accredited Standards Committee www.x12.org/x12org/index.cfm	Electronic messages for claims, eligibility, and payments	Allows EHR system clinical and administrative data (e.g., diagnostic codes) to be organized for standardized eligibility, claims, and payment purposes.
Institute of Electrical and Electronics Engineers (IEEE) 1073	Institute of Electrical and Electronics Engineers Standards Association standards.ieee.org/sa/sa-view.html	Messages for medical device communications	Connects patient data from medical devices such as patient monitors and ventilators, offers practitioners to view those data on applications linked to or part of EHR systems.

TABLE 6-9 Health Care Informatics Standards and Electronic Health Records—cont'd

Standard	Standards Organization	Purpose	How Standard Contributes to EHR Systems
Terminology			
International Classification of Diseases, ninth edition (ICD-9)	World Health Organization www.who.int/en	Diagnosis and disease codes commonly used in billing and claims; version 9 is often used in United States for billing and reimbursement	ICD9-CM codes are assigned on the basis of clinical content and health services documented in EHR systems to meet research and financial needs.
Logical Observation Identifiers names and Codes (LONIC)	Regenstrief Institute for Health Care www.lonic.org	Concept-based terminology for laboratory orders and results	Provides standard terminology for laboratory test names and results that can be used in EHR systems.
Systematized Nomenclature of Medicine—Clinical Terms (SNOMED-CT)	College of American Pathologists www.cap.org	Mapping clinical concepts with standard descriptive terms	Provides electronically supported nomenclature representation of patient clinical data in EHR systems. Codes offer the most granular representation of concepts.
Unified Medical Language System (UMLS)	National Library of Medicine www.nim.org	Database of 100 medical terminologies with concept mapping tools	Allows EHR system (program) to understand meaning of the language of biomedicine and health.
Document			
Continuity of Care Record (CCR)	ASTM International, E31 Committee on Health Informatics www.astm.org	Document format that gives snapshot of patient's core data and recent encounter (allergies, medications, treatment, care plan) and makes it available to next caregiver	Defines core set of clinical data for continuity of care purposes and sets XML standards for data organization of clinical content for electronic data exchange.
Clinical Document Architecture (CDA)	Health Level 7 www.hl7.org	Standard exchange model for clinical documents such as discharge summaries and progress	Provides model to use for document formats for specific clinical documents to be maintained in EHR systems and used when sending and receiving clinical documents notes. Formally known as *patient record architecture.*
Clinical Document Type Definitions (ASTM 2183-02) (ASTM 2182-02)	ASTM International, E31 Committee on Health Informatics www.astm.org	Provides standard specification for XML document type definitions that match electronic document requirements in health care industry (e.g., patient history, discharge summary)	Provides tools to represent clinical data using XML to organize document content and enable web browser to access information. Provides specifications to organize and apply tags to content Document Type Definition (DTD) in health care documents to represent content for data exchange purposes.
Content and Structure of Electronic Health Records (ASTM E1384, ASTM E1633)	ASTM International, Committee on Health Informatics www.astm.org	Describes content to be included in her; content descriptions range from data elements (defined) to documents	Provides comprehensive data content model to serve as a resource for EHR systems, including data element dictionaries and coded data guidelines and definition of longitudinal content with minimum data set specified.
EHR Systems: Draft Standards for Trial Use (HL7: DSTU)	Health Level Seven www.hl7.org	Proposed comprehensive functionality for EHR systems; includes health data	Offers draft model of EHR system functions that can assist organizations planning for EHR in determining basic requirements to be considered.
Infrastructure/Policy			
Information Access Privilege (ASTM E1986-98)	ASTM International, Committee on Health Informatics www.astm.org	Standard guide for access privilege for EHR, including emergency setting	Provides comprehensive model to use for information access privilege by health workers.

Continued

| TABLE 6-9 | Health Care Informatics Standards and Electronic Health Records—cont'd | | | |

Standard	Standards Organization	Purpose	How Standard Contributes to EHR Systems
Authentication and Electronic Signature (ASTM E 1762-03) (ASTM E 1985-00) (ASTM E 2084-00)	ASTM International, Committee on Health Informatics www.astm.org	Standards guides for establishing and managing authentication and electronic signature	Provide guidelines for policy and procedures and business rules for user requirements for designing/selecting electronic mechanisms to enable authentication and electronic signatures for EHR systems.
Audit and Disclosure Logs (ASTM E 2147-01)	ASTM International, Committee on Health Informatics www.astm.org	Describes specifications for audit trials in manual and EHR environment	Provides structures of information disclosure logs/audit trails.
Amendments to Electronic Health Information (ASTM E 2017-99)	ASTM International, Committee on Health Informatics www.astm.org	Addresses criteria for amending individually identifiable health information	Serves as a basis for policy development and user requirements for processing amendments in EHR systems.

EHR, Electronic health record; *XML*, extensible markup language.

SELF-ASSESSMENT QUIZ

15. HIPAA was established to do which of the following:
    a. Streamline the designated business processes in billing and claims
    b. Define standards for privacy and security of personal health information
    c. Both a and b
16. True or False? ASTM standards are voluntary.
17. Access standards and a government website. Compile a profile of relevant standards that should be considered by a large ambulatory group practice planning an EHR acquisition. Explain why these standards apply.
18. Standardize data elements. Give three to five examples of patient data that need to be standardized or harmonized if disparate organizations are going to exchange patient information. Provide your rationale.

WHAT ARE ELECTRONIC HEALTH RECORD SYSTEMS AND HOW DO THEY WORK?

Electronic Health Record Systems and Their Functions

EHR systems can be one-system applications, as seen in a small practice environment, as well as a group of integrated systems that contain all the elements required or a suite of systems that are linked together to provide all the functions needed. In truth, the evolving EHR functions noted in the beginning of the chapter in the definition of a qualified EHR illustrate the multiapplication and systems integrated view. EHRs need to be built at an enterprise level and connect to and from multiple integrated systems, both internal and external, to meet the needs of the population. Consistent descriptions of key functions help build collective expectations of what such systems need to do. In 2003 the IOM issued a report, "Key Capabilities of an EHR System," calling for basic functions or applications to be included in EHR systems; this report reinforced the view that EHR systems were a series of linked applications or functions. These overview functions are:

- Health information and data—central repository for patients' data from a variety of sources
- Results management—from diagnostic tests
- Order entry and management—order tests and prescribe medications and treatments
- Decision support—help clinicians manage care through evidence-based guidelines
- Electronic communication and connectivity—communicate among providers and resources to coordinate care
- Patient support—offer education for the patients
- Administrative processes—better scheduling and billing
- Reporting and population health management—report infections disease, support epidemiology research[30]

This list of functions or applications builds on the initial concepts of an EHR system and includes the scope of capabilities ranging from health data to connectivity and resource availability, regardless of where or how these components originate. Multiple functions happen through multiple, linked applications. Take another look at Table 6-2, which features the parts and functions of qualified EHR summary of requirements for certified EHR systems to see how these concepts are evolving into practical directives. The following list of applications feature more specific capabilities of EHR systems as an expansion of the IOM list. Adapted from Amatayakul's sample list of applications that can be mapped to the CCHIT requirements, the following list presents a broad array of applications and functions that benchmark experience has shown to be EHR system components. An enterprise EHR system today may be composed of cohesive linked applications and include the following:

- Registration—admission, discharge, transfer, administrative applications
- Patient financial services
- Order communications/results retrieval systems that allow staff to enter orders from paper records and view the status of the orders and the ancillary diagnostic results

- Departmental clinical applications—laboratory, radiology and imaging, pharmacy, dietary, surgery, pulmonary diagnostics, and cardiology
- Specialty clinical applications—intensive care, emergency department, perioperative and surgical, oncology
- Smart peripherals—medicine dispensing devices, robotics, monitoring equipment, etc.
- Computerized physician order entry (CPOE) systems designed for providers to enter orders online with capability to link to advice that can be used in the care process
- Results management—diagnostic test results and feedback
- Data repositories that collect and store data from feeder systems and deliver patient record information to users through workstations
- Point of care charting to capture continuing documentation that replaces traditional paper-based progress notes and, depending on the scope of the documentation capture, transcribed documents
- Document scanning and imaging systems that capture paper documents and capture and store diagnostic images (enterprise document management system)
- Clinical messaging systems that streamline communication between providers, providers and systems, and patients and providers often through web browser style–user workstations
- Provider-patient portals that use the Internet to enable patients to access their health information, communicate with their providers, and arrange for health services such as appointments and prescription renewals
- CDS systems that link patient data to medical knowledge resources and offer feedback directly to clinicians responsible for patient care
- PHRs that are maintained by the patients in electronic form that can be authorized for access by the patient's provider and to which data can be electronically sent by the provider
- Population health reporting that serves epidemiology and research
- Electronic medication administration record and bar code identification - automates processes of hospital medication administration
- Clinical data warehouse
- HIE provisions[43]

Figure 6-8 illustrates how the components of an EHR system link together and are accessed through a user workstation. Notice the breadth of systems that contribute to the working EHR. Not only are traditional administrative systems such as

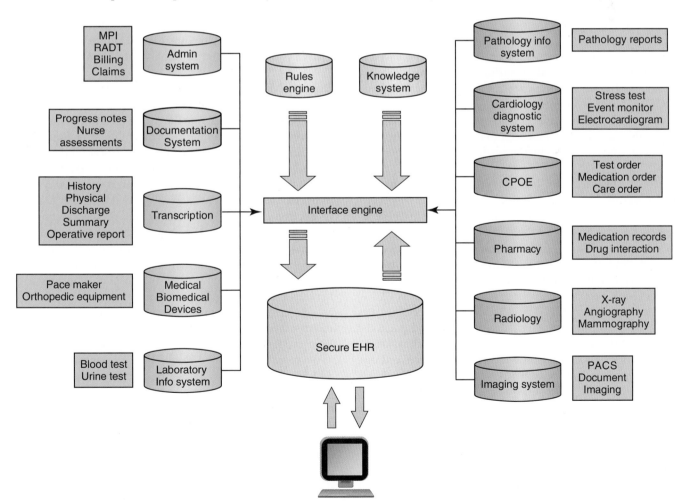

FIGURE 6-8 Components of electronic health record (EHR) systems and workstations in a hospital setting. *CPOE,* Computerized physician order entry; *MPI,* master patient index; *PACS,* picture archiving and communication system; *RADT,* registration—admission, discharge, transfer.

the master patient index and the registration—admission, discharge, transfer (Reg-ADT) administrative applications providing data, the diagnostic testing data resources are extensive. Laboratory results, pathology reports, picture archiving and communication systems (PACS), ECGs, and echocardiograms are online. **Biomedical devices** are online as well. Historical and persistently paper documents, such as patient consents and advance directives, are captured in document imaging systems that can be viewed through EHR workstations. Systems are available that allow the clinician, patient, and witness to complete informed consents and advance directives using a digital pen to affix a signature. As technology enables health care enterprises to better support linked care delivery, single large systems that manage hospitals, ambulatory care, long-term care, and home health services through building interoperable capability among them will emerge.

How Health Data is Entered, Accessed, and Retrieved for Care
Electronic Health Record System Functions and Patient Record Development
In Figure 4-7, the process of assembling the patient record, gathering the physical components of the record, is linked to the patient care process. In an EHR environment, the patient record supports the same care process but may look different. For example, when a patient arrives for health services in an organization where an EHR has been in place for some time, the patient's historical health record data are maintained in an electronic form that can be accessed and searched for prior information. With historical data available electronically, only updated and new information is needed to begin the care process. It is useful to understand just how the patient record comes together through electronic components.

Patient Registration, Identity Management, and Admission
Patients who are admitted for care in a hospital or in an outpatient setting begin with the fundamental registration function, which is directly linked to the institutional master patient (or person) index. This administrative application combines demographic data captured in the registration (master patient index [MPI]) application with administrative census (ADT) applications in hospitals. The Reg-ADT application initiates or updates basic demographic data, establishes and tracks the location or service of the patient, and feeds data to other systems such as billing or the laboratory. In ambulatory care settings, demographic data collected by the registration application is also shared with appointment scheduling applications to arrange patient appointments and referral functions as the patient's individual care process is established and carried out.

Ordering and Documentation at Admission to Hospitals and Residential Settings
Once admitted to a hospital or other type of residential or structured care program, patient care continues through an order entry or CPOE application. The order entry and management capability streamlines the fundamental workflow of the care process, allows orders to be monitored electronically,

and links them to the ordered test results for online viewing. Think of this capability as the initial foundation of online orders and results. The more advanced version of order entry, CPOE, is more powerful and includes linking patient data to intelligence options such as a patient-specific allergy alert or drug–drug interactions. CPOE enables physicians and other independent practitioners to enter their own orders online with links to decision support so that feedback on the order can be provided and any appropriate changes made at that point. HIMSS Analytics cites that CPOE has grown more than 10% between 2011 and 2012.[3] The objective is to improve the quality of care and to make health care safer. An example of decision support is linking an order for medication to an individual patient's health data and a pharmacy system's resources on drug allergies or drug contraindications. An immediate feedback alert to the ordering physician allows the order to be modified and an alternative medication selected. Similarly, the CPOE function in outpatient settings focuses on ordering diagnostic tests, treatment modalities, referrals, and prescriptions. The value in streamlining these functions and yielding fewer medication ordering errors cannot be understated. Figure 6-9 depicts an order entry screen in a CPOE system.

History and physical examinations and nursing assessments are performed at admission. The documentation of these services may use a combination of dictation or voice activation applications or direct data capture so that information is organized and available for online viewing.

Results Management—Diagnostic Tests to Transcribed Documents
Providing online "results" to the care team is one of the major components in developing EHR capability. This function is often an early step in an EHR migration process and provides immediate benefits to busy practitioners. Results review allows the care team to view ancillary test results and other information items such as transcribed documents that are in electronic form. Test results in this review function are presented in a "look up" fashion with the information shown in a mode similar to how test results are presented in paper mode. In many cases, information may be looked up through secure web access from outside the hospital. The advent of handheld devices holds promise for even more flexible access. As increased access offers more information to the clinicians, the need to be able to "act" on the information calls for more flexibility in the software.

In more sophisticated results management applications, additional functionality allows the care team to access a specific patient's test results, radiology images, transcribed reports, and other information, and view them online with additional features. There may be the capability to flag the most recent findings, highlight out-of-range or contrast alternative test results, or view data in historical patterns or other formats, often in graphic displays. In these cases, depending on the state of adoption of the electronically stored patient data, test results may be printed out and added to paper records or stored electronically.[30] In some patient portal applications, test results are available for patient viewing with the same graphics options so they can track

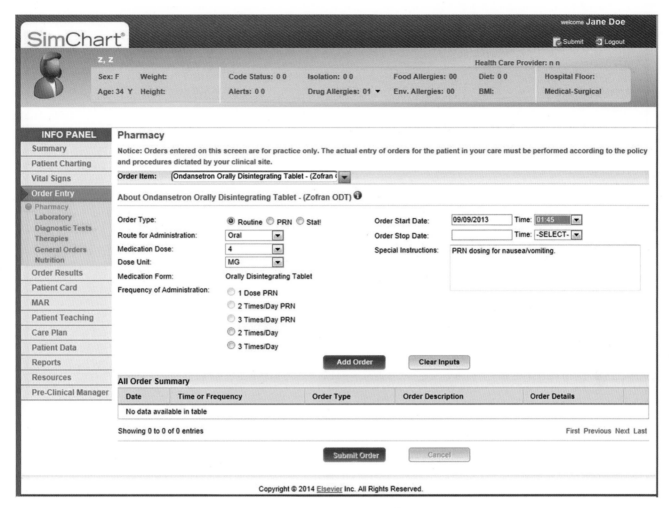

FIGURE 6-9 Order entry screen. Elsevier 2014. SimChart® (www.evolve.elsevier.com).

information on their health status as well. The navigation options available to clinicians as they review results enables more streamlined care management. Figure 6-10 shows how a results management screen display can offer immediate options for the clinician.[46]

Communication Links

Electronic communication and connectivity through networks is used to link applications together for data access and exchange purposes. Providers and administrative staff use electronic communication for clinical and administrative purposes to support the care team and expedite messages needed to clarify orders or discuss results. Few organizations can imagine functioning efficiently today without the benefit of e-mail and other communication mechanisms. The same is true for the health care environment. Attention is needed to ensure that patient privacy is maintained. Encryption, a more affordable tool today, and a key element of certified EHR technology, is an important tool for health care organizations to meet their security goals. Even e-mail has a more affordable encryption and security options that can protect patient privacy and still allow streamlined communication among the care team that may be using the organization's intranet or the internet.

Online Documentation

As a hospitalization or an encounter progresses, clinicians use workstations with EHR software navigational tools to document care and services online. Vital signs, medication administration, assessments, treatment and care plan notes, and structured and free text progress notes replace hand-written notes.

Clinicians may use free text or "unstructured" data to enter information directly online or may continue to dictate their notes directly or with voice-activated dictation. They may use structured data entry in which they draw from standard phrases or pick lists and pull-down menus to help guide the entry and ensure that complete information is included. These data "tools" make use of predefined text scripts, lists, and terminology, and help guide the documentation. In some settings, scribes are used to assist clinicians in documenting their notes into the EHR application. Depending on the organization's policies, both the scribe and the clinician–author authenticate the note. Scribes are valuable in training and support functions as new online documentation applications are implemented. Specialized templates also help organize the data for both the author and eventual readers. The template is structured to improve ease for both access and data capture. It can provide a means of breaking narrative into

Laboratory Results - Arterial Blood Gases

	Result		Reference Range
pH	7.22		7.35 to 7.45
Partial Pressure of Oxygen (Po2)	72	mm Hg	80 to 100 mm Hg
Bicarbonate (HCO3)	28	mEq/L	21 to 28 mEq/L
Partial Pressure of Carbon Dioxide (Pco2)	50	mm Hg	35 to 45 mm Hg
O2 Saturation		Percent (%)	Adult: 95% to 100 % Elderly: 95%
O2 Content		Percent (%)	15 to 22 vol %
Base Excess		mEq/L	0 2 mEq/L

Save   Close

FIGURE 6-10 Results management screen. Elsevier 2014. SimChart® (www.evolve.elsevier.com).

several smaller recognized segments. It may also draw from data already collected and allow the clinician to modify and complete information. HL7 has a Templates Special Interest Group that focuses on various standards to address templates such as the CCR, referral and consult reports, and order sets that represent common groupings of orders so that consistency in content and interoperability can be achieved.[47] This promotes more complete recording of required information such as smoking status, body mass index, and immunization status. Workstation design also can help support accuracy, completeness, and access of data. Especially when the clinician is collecting and entering the data in the presence of the patient, ergonomic design is important to support the clinician–patient interaction. Figure 6-11 is an example of a template used for data capture in an ambulatory care system.

Evidence from EHR systems that have been implemented in hospital and ambulatory care settings provide helpful suggestions for future planning. The EHR team at the Geisinger Clinic (50 locations) stresses the value of simplicity as the "heart of clarity and the single most important usability guideline" for workstation design. Noting that the design must help the clinician to focus rapidly on the most relevant information and be mindful of how clinicians use patient information, the team emphasized that this is key to realizing workflow improvement.[16] For those clinicians who use the

EHR to educate patients about their health care while their patients are sitting with them, the workstation must be large and flexible enough to permit easy viewing by the patient.

Over the course of a hospitalization, administrative data, orders, test results, transcribed reports, and patient care documentation applications are used to assemble the information so that clinicians may access and manage data through electronic means. Patient care coordination and the care team's workflow improve when readily available data that provides up-to-the-minute information to the clinicians at the bedside and through workstations at their offices and through approved hand-held devices. These tools strengthen more consistent information use and improve efficiency in the care process.

Similar information coordination is needed in outpatient and other care settings. In the ambulatory setting, for example, certified EHR products provide a visit summary designed to summarize the visit and instructions to the patient provided at the end of each visit. Visit summaries are practical resources for patients and providers that can be incorporated into PHRs that the patient maintains at home. More and more institutions are encouraging patients to access their health information online and, in some chronic disease situations, the online record system assists the clinician and the patient in monitoring key indicators that the patient reports by e-mail. In fact, by 2006 74% of Americans reported they

FIGURE 6-11 Ambulatory care clinic notes template. Elsevier 2014. SimChart for the Medical Office® (www.evolve.elsevier.com)

wanted to go beyond self-care and e-mail their physicians. Patients want to access test results, the ability to refill and renew prescriptions, check on referrals, report monitoring of chronic disease tracking measures, and learn how to help manage their own health.[48] The better informed patient is a stronger member of his or her own health care team.

Clinical Decision Support Systems

Decision support systems are integral components of EHR systems. This is the component that offers direct intervention in the care process and has the power to improve the process as it works hand in hand with CPOE for diagnostic tests, medications, and procedures because it can provide immediate feedback to the planned action. Decision support applications use rules engines to program the logic that links patient data with clinical guidelines, disease-specific protocols, and expert systems to provide alerts and reminders directly to clinicians through the EHR workstation. As systems designed for acute

and ambulatory care, these modules are capable of numerous functions, including providing drug interaction, alerts, clinical practice guidelines for particular chronic diseases, knowledge resources prompts, and reminders for health maintenance.[49] CDS criteria detailed in the required standards for EHR technology provides direction for evidence-based decision support interventions, referential requirements, and technological configuration. The goal is inform the provider as he or she plans and orders care for the patient. The Committee on Patient Safety and Health Information and Technology Board on Health Care Services states,

> *Potential benefits could be reductions in*
> - *Relative risk of medication errors*
> - *Risk of toxic drug levels*
> - *Time to therapeutic stabilization*
> - *Management errors of resuscitating patients in adult trauma centers*
> - *Prescriptions of nonpreferred medications.*[49]

Of course the alerts bring effective notices to clinicians to note adverse conditions. Yet despite these potential benefits, there can be problems with the system as well. The drug–drug interaction alerts may differ—some may be more effective than others. And the care team must deal with how they override alerts to be sure critical cases are addressed.

The alerts and reminders may be e-mail messages with a high-priority indicator such as a medication contraindication alert or a clinical messaging application designed to send information to a physician's electronic inbox or a pop-up reminder that is generated when a physician signs on to the system. Handheld devices also serve as a conduit for sending messages to the clinician about significant alerts about patients. Patient safety improvements are well documented when the care process has the benefit of these resources.[50] Figure 6-12 illustrates how decision support operates.

The benefit in quality and cost for EHRs are heavily based on the CDS component. In a 2009 report of a research study of 41 acute care hospitals across Texas, each 10-point increase in decision support system integration was associated with a 16% reduction in complication rates and a 15% lower rate of in-hospital deaths.[51] Drug–drug interaction alerts offer valuable safety options to providers and patients, and are a driving motivation for moving EHRs to include the CDS component.

Even with the value added, however, many physicians experience problems using the drug interaction alert, and many find the amount and frequency of alerts to be intrusive. Selecting the right balance is a challenge and may need to be tailored by practice style. Other physicians found that the information was not helpful, leading to slowdowns in workflow. Some organizations allow physicians flexibility in how they use the CDS function. In fact, allowing EHR users to set the level of CDS interaction is a certification-required functionality. This means that individual physicians can set their own thresholds even at the individual patient level, and thereby need to monitor the CDS activity and outcomes in a systematic way.

System Capabilities

The range of EHR systems from single-practice ambulatory vendor products to large, complex institutional systems in health maintenance organizations (HMOs), hospitals, and integrated delivery system settings reflects a common core of functions, but there is often a wide variation in the functions offered by different vendors.

In cases in which EHR system vendors market products that include only selected modules, they partner with the customer to link those modules with existing legacy systems. To illustrate, a product collects data from existing legacy administrative applications such as hospital and clinic Reg-ADT systems and ancillary systems, and then combines and maintains it with historical patient health data within a CDR for rapid retrieval through a workstation. As noted in Figure 6-13, the workstation serves as a window to all the contributing applications that send data to the repository. The EHR system products designed for large hospital and integrated delivery settings have been in place for some time and their core functions are reasonably stable and their system support is reliable. Large delivery systems may use an EHR product along with individual department products. Departmental applications for intensive care units, emergency departments, and diagnostic applications may have their own applications with unique functions that are not available through established EHR system modules. These cases require attention to interfaces and, if possible, data integration capability to bring the information together for more seamless access by clinicians. These are challenges for all aspects of managing the information. In other settings, simpler solutions may still meet the organization's needs.

EHR systems have also advanced in alternative care areas beyond acute and ambulatory care. Although there are a limited number of long-term EHR system vendors serving the market compared with those serving hospitals and larger HMOs and ambulatory centers, progress has been made in long-term, behavioral health, and home health applications.

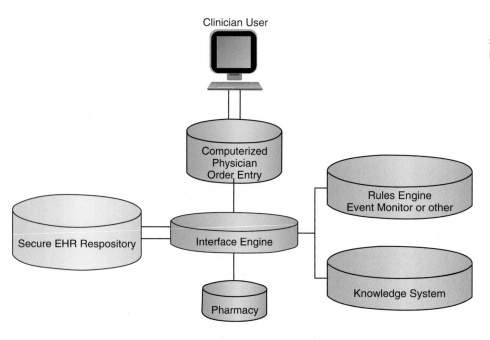

FIGURE 6-12 Decision support system schematic. *EHR,* Electronic health record.

FIGURE 6-13 Workstation schematic—data view.

Clinical data repository

Data access	Practice tools and data capture	Advice and reporting
Test results	Computerized physician order entry	Alerts
Medications	Problem list	Reminders
Allergies	Clinical data capture	Internal/external guidelines
Transcribed reports	Templates	Library searches
Encounter data	Consult advice	Standard reporting
Hospital data	Flow sheets	Ad hoc reporting
Outside facilities data	Patient car plan	Outcome reporting
Provider communication	Consulting nurse	
Patient communication		
Specialized registries		
Referrals		

These vendors often look to user groups to provide feedback and to influence product upgrades. This is less the case in other environments. Many smaller vendors still come and go in the marketplace, a fact that does not encourage provider's investments in EHR systems.

Once components are in place and an EHR system is acquired or under development, how do individuals use it? What does such an EHR system actually do? Regardless of the care setting and the EHR system, users must perform basic processes on data, including the ability to:

- Access health record data and documents through a variety of patient and health information systems in the organization.
- Order tests and treatments electronically.
- Retrieve and capture data through well-designed workstations with PC, tablet, smart phones and other emerging electronic tools.
- Use communication and network technology to access applications and communicate with peers and patients.
- Apply readily available CDS tools and references while engaging in the care process.
- Adhere to required security mechanisms.
- Use whatever HIE systems that are in place.
- Support external reporting and research.

With industry benchmarks, consolidation of a more consistent definition of the components of EHR systems, and evidence of the value of advancing information technology in health care, progress is visible. This decade confirms there is more energy and momentum to develop and implement EHR systems.

SELF-ASSESSMENT QUIZ

19. Compare and contrast online documentation methods. Research the role of transcription when organizations implement online documentation.
20. Describe the role CDS plays in validating the value of EHRs, and illustrate your description with examples and research findings.

HOW DO TECHNICAL INFRASTRUCTURE, DATA REQUIREMENTS, AND OPERATIONS WORKFLOW FIT IN EHR SYSTEMS?

Technical Infrastructure and Data Requirements

Technical infrastructure refers to the technology architecture required to maintain systems. Technology infrastructure includes the hardware, software, network, and communication resources required as underpinning to an EHR system. Of course, enough workstations must be deployed across the organizations so that user access is facilitated. And with the increasing use of mobile devices, workstation functions must be delivered in new ways. Analogous to a transportation infrastructure, voice, data, image, and video need adequate size transport (networks) to get the job done. Chapter 8 details how infrastructure fits together to support health information systems, their functions, and interoperability. What is important to note is that infrastructure provides the foundation to link legacy systems with new applications and must be robust enough to handle "industrial strength" secure data processing, storage, and widespread access and retrieval. Both internal and external requirements to meet HIE objectives must be considered within this context.

Data Requirements for the Electronic Health Record

Along with the technology infrastructure, data requirements must be addressed in migrating to an EHR environment. Data elements themselves can be viewed as the raw material of information systems. Users require data that are transformed into information and then into knowledge. Van Bemmel and Musen noted that a patient or a biologic process generates data, which are observed by the clinician with subsequent information derived from interpretation. Uninterpreted data elements are given to the problem solver. This can include data as elementary as age, pulse rate, test result, diagnostic code, height, and weight.[52]

On the other hand, information refers to a collection of data that contains meaning when data are processed, resulting in a display or report containing information. In this context, data and information can be stored in a permanent, accessible database. The EHR, stored or accessible online, includes data and information resulting from the analysis and processing of other data. For example, results reported from laboratory tests and presented through a computer workstation flow sheet provide time-oriented information to the provider of care.

Knowledge is defined as the "formalization of the relationships among elements of information and data."[53] That is, new data or information can be inferred from the data and information already present. For example, test results (data) can be organized into a diabetic care management flow sheet (information) and a clinician can assess that a patient's condition has undergone a change (knowledge). Perhaps the most easily understood description of knowledge in this context is the use of rules that are applied to the data and information that enable providers to apply medical judgment to the care processes.

Covey noted that the "contents" of EHRs and health information systems can be expressed as data types or as data elements.[53] Table 6-10 lists the variety of data types required in patient record systems. Data types should be presented in ways that provide information when comparisons, trends, and confirmation of differential diagnostic investigations are sought by clinical providers. If we understand the role of data types more clearly, we can better comprehend the complexity of moving from data to information to knowledge. Significant thought must be given to transforming data into information for the purposes of medical knowledge. The ability to collect, organize, analyze, retrieve, and present data electronically by computers in a meaningful way extends and expands the discriminating capacity and problem-solving abilities of providers and the value of EHRs. In fact, EHR

systems themselves can provide usage reports on which functions are actually being used. The system may also be able to identify missing content or reports using an electronic auditing methodology.

Data interface standards such as those developed by X12 and HL7 SDOs, vocabulary dictionaries, and interface engines are used to transfer data between systems. Sometimes data are translated or reformatted as required. HIPAA legislation imposed standards on the data exchange of billing data. Certain coding systems and an X12 schema for data transfer are required. The intent of this change is to reduce the administrative costs associated with the billing process. In some cases, data are transferred to external partners. These include other health care organizations that may use HIE to share information on patients for coordination of care such as health record banks. In other cases, data may be sent to business-oriented entities such as insurance companies, third party payers, or the U.S. clearinghouse for billing that processes the billing data. The data definitions and codes need to be standardized to provide useful data.

Terminologies and the Electronic Health Record

To establish EHR systems with predictable data requires standardized terminologies, **vocabularies**, that are used to represent concepts and to communicate them, including symptoms, diagnoses, procedures, and health status. A *terminology* is a set of terms representing the system of concepts of a particular subject or field. A controlled medical terminology is a coded vocabulary of medical concepts and expressions used in health care. *Controlled* refers to managing the content to ensure it remains structurally sound, biomedically accurate, and consistent with current practice.[53] Code systems require information to be represented in a preestablished, recognized system. Examples are the Systematized Nomenclature of Medicine—Clinical Terms (SNOMED-CT) and the *International Classification of Diseases,* ninth edition, Clinical Modification (ICD-9-CM) and ICD-10. Some code systems are nomenclatures or defined systems for naming. The SNOMED-CT is the most widely used nomenclature system in healthcare.[43] Other code systems are classification systems. **Classification systems** organize like entities or conditions. ICD-10 is an example of a classification system. See Chapter 7 for more information on terminologies and code systems.

Giannangelo presents a useful distinction for considering the role of terminologies and the EHR. Terminologies are designed to facilitate data collection at the point of care; capture the detail of diagnostic studies, history and physicals, visit notes, ancillary department information, and nursing notes; and allow the ability to send and receive medical data in an understandable and predictable manner. Classification systems focus on collecting and reporting basic health statistics, to ensure quality data for an organizational database for accurate clinical and statistical data for research and outcomes analysis, and to provide data used in payment systems and for mandatory public health reporting.[54]

TABLE 6-10	Data Types Required for Electronic Health Records
Data Type	Examples
Text	Hospital discharge, summary, history and physical examination, narrative operative reports
Numbers	ICD-9-CM codes CPT codes Blood pressure value recording
Voice	Stored dictation accessed by phone or personal computer. voice recognition or radiology dictation films
Image	Radiology film, document image
Video	Echocardiogram
Drawings	Drawing of burn distribution on body surface
Signal	Electroencephalogram or ECG tracings

CPT, Current Procedural Terminology; *ECG,* electrocardiogram; *ICD,* International Classification of Diseases.

Coded data are exemplified by the use of standard coding systems such as the ICD-9-CM, ICD10, and Current Procedural Terminology (CPT). Specific to EHRs is the National Committee on Vital and Health Statistics–approved core set of terminologies for patient medical record information. They chose SNOMED-CT, which works behind the scenes to code the content of the electronic record, the LOINC used for representing laboratory data for ordering and naming specific test results, Accredited Standards Committee X-12-N (ASC) standards for claims attachments, RxNorm for clinical drugs for communication to retail pharmacies for e-prescribing, and the Universal Medical Device Nomenclature System, a standard international nomenclature and computer coding system used to facilitate identifying, processing, filing, storing, retrieving, transferring, and communicating data about medical devices.[54]

They also noted the value of additional code systems such as established nursing terminologies that represent nursing concepts. A health care organization is likely using multiple coding systems in its efforts to organize and communicate its computerized data. Coded data have the advantage of consistency of expression for diagnoses, procedures, laboratory tests, drugs, and so on. Yet because of the strengths and weaknesses in these systems, none completely addresses the clarity and precision required to capture and represent all clinical facts contained in patient records. The NLM project to establish the Unified Medical Language System is an ambitious attempt to bring together diverse coding schemes with general medical terms to create a vast thesaurus linking together more than 100 terminologies and related clinical terms to assist diverse users.

Many health information system developers spend significant energy improving coding systems used for claims processing, billing, and epidemiologic factors, and to track quality improvement outcomes and research efforts. These efforts are focused on using ICD-9-CM and ICD-10. SNOMED-CT, a nomenclature, is identified as having the most potential to handle the complex data representation required in EHRs. Unlike codes assigned by individuals working from the information in the record, the SNOMED-CT is designed to be embedded in a EHR system and to code the clinical language used in the EHR in the background, thereby capturing the information in great detail. Problem list statements can be represented in SNOMED-CT. This functionality lays the groundwork for further technological improvement by using **natural language processing** to abstract the SNOMED-CT codes and then to crosswalk these codes to ICD-9-CM, ICD-10-CM, and CPT.

Advocates believe that strong terminologies or coding schemes are essential components of health information systems and that the fastest way to establish and secure consistent data from health care organizations is through standard terminologies. There continues to be national and international interest in identifying an "ideal" terminology or system to secure accurate, efficient data capture from the care delivery experience that accurately represents the clinical concepts. Coding systems are critical to capturing and processing clinical data consistently. Terminologies and code systems are used to represent information in a predictable, consistent, and reproducible manner.[54] ICD, SNOMED-CT, and LOINC address part of the problem but do not fully support current models of thinking used by all types of clinicians involved in collecting data as part of their roles in the care delivery process.

A major component of the patient record in most organizations is unstructured text. This is the most natural medium of expression and, to date, best represents the thinking and conclusions of those planning and delivering care. In fact, the majority of the content of paper records is narrative text. Because of this, the potential value of technology for natural language processing is well recognized. Giannangelo states,

> *Medicine needs a system based on an architecture that can capture medical data in natural language form, structure it in alternative ways and retrieve it through queries that allow users to retrieve and display information in multiple forms including conversion into standard codes as well as natural language expressions.* **Text processing** *may be defined as the computerized processing of natural language.*[54]

This is a far more sophisticated endeavor than searching text by key words, a process well known in library research today. Text processing requires comprehensiveness and completeness of content such that a given domain of medicine is adequately represented. Natural language processing for cardiology, for instance, would need to include all the terms and expressions used by cardiologists in their models of thinking. Symptoms, related medical terms, and specific cardiology expressions (including semantic linkages and relationships) would all be required elements.

Script-based systems, an alternative form of structured text, combine key words and scripts. A script may be a predesigned expression that represents information about consequences of care processes. Scanning for key words invokes a particular script. The script itself then serves as a building block for the remainder of the text-processing event. It may act as a template that specifies necessary components and the properties required. Medical transcriptionists apply a similar concept when they develop and maintain stored phrases that can be invoked to assemble reports such as history and physical examinations quickly. This allows single key words to be indexed to longer medical expressions. Physician dictation, for instance, is significantly streamlined when such tools are used. For example, a radiologist dictating a radiology report may state "normal 3" to indicate to the transcriptionist that this text is already programmed into the transcriptionist's software to mean "normal chest x-ray." It is incumbent on the HIM professional to ensure that these kinds of preprogrammed texts are agreed on by those involved and included in the organization's policies.

Newer approaches to handling narrative text organize the text in a consistent manner and establish standard tags to label the text. Standard generalized markup language, hypertext markup language, and extensible markup language (XML) are used to organize the data within documents by displaying information in standard ways to allow users to launch from key words in one document to other documents. Transcribed reports are then organized according to predetermined formats that can be labeled and retrieved for manipulation.[46] Chapter 8 offers additional detail on these topics.

✓ SELF-ASSESSMENT QUIZ

21. Explain why unstructured text continues to add value to the content of EHRs.

Clinical Data Repositories

CDRs are a core component of EHR systems. A CDR is a real-time database that consolidates data from a variety of clinical sources to present a unified view of a single patient. It offers a comprehensive source for storage and retrieval of relevant clinical information needed for patient care. Payne describes the CDR as a "database that is optimized for storing and viewing clinical information sent over interfaces from departmental systems."[55] It allows clinicians to use workstation tools to search and view data that originates from other applications and retrieve data for a single patient. CDRs use relational databases to store the data and match relevant data contained in the repository by using a rules engine to implement the protocols for CDS. Typical data types sent to a CDR include clinical laboratory test results, patient demographics, pharmacy information, radiology reports and images, pathology reports, hospital admission, discharge and transfer dates, ICD-9 codes, discharge summaries, and progress notes. Notice that a CDR may contain both data values (e.g., laboratory data) and text (e.g., progress notes). CDRs are designed to deliver the individual patient's information to the care team through a clinical workstation. It is at the workstation itself where the content and presentation capability takes over to provide views and functions that assist the end user.[55] Although organizations look to data warehouses for strategic business analysis needs and sophisticated reporting options not always found in older generation CDRs, newer CDRs offer more data manipulation and reporting options. For example, at Sound Mental Health in Seattle, Washington, clinicians and administrators can access the EHRs Report Center for population and program data, especially when using transaction data.

Data can also be presented in a series of clinical views or profiles designed to deliver the EHR content to users. Golob characterized the purposes of a **clinical data repository** as follows:[56]

- Provides easy access to patient information for providers and demonstrates time saved over paper record use.
- Expedites results reporting through customizable displays.
- Provides quick and easy access to longitudinal patient data for an individual patient.
- Supports a common user interface for accessing patient information, usually through a workstation.
- Provides information in a comprehensive, integrated manner rather than by departmental orientation.
- Provides an easy vehicle for applying population management for the prospective clinical planning needed today.
- Supports monitoring and analysis of patient care outcomes.

Although CDRs are varied as a practical resource for these purposes, the reality is that the data needs for analytics are less well served by the CDR.

How Health Data Are Extracted for Analysis

It is important to note that a CDR is not a data warehouse. Shortliffe notes the importance of making the distinction between them. The CDR serves the needs of day-to-day operations, whereas a data warehouse serves longer term business and clinical needs of the organization and often uses summarized data over several years.[57] The data warehouse is a database that provides access to data that has been aggregated for analysis purposes. In fact, Wager points out that the underlying structure of a data warehouse is designed so data can be extracted by time, location, services, and so on, and may allow data to be retrieved and organized into data marts or grouped data sets.[58] A variety of analysis tools are used to enable greater detail. For instance, an analyst could view the number of hip replacement surgeries that were performed by year, by month, or by day. In another case, clinic visit numbers can be viewed by primary care providers within an enterprise, then in a specific network, then by providers in individual clinics within the network. So, in addition to a CDR, health care organizations also establish information (or data) warehouses that receive clinical data from transactions systems such as a pharmacy system or a radiology system, reorganizes the data or information, and then combines it with other organizational data from administrative and financial systems to enable the types of sophisticated queries needed. **Data warehouses** provide functionality for decision support using multiple files, databases, and internal and external data. They are usually designed for read-only access and can accommodate simple and complex queries with the capability of data mining. It is important to understand that the terms *data repository* and *data warehouse* are now often being used interchangeably as technology improves its ability to process larger and larger amounts of information more efficiently. Some health care organizations are generating special data collections from their EHRs to support more sophisticated analysis of essential clinical and business performance information.

State and other data systems that require data from hospitals or participating organizations are examples of data repositories that act like data warehouses. In fact, the advances made in community-based health information systems have relied on the original principles and benefits of the repository approach. Its ability to provide data and information across institutional settings makes the repository or warehouse valuable to participating providers. Even organizations taking a slower approach to acquiring an EHR in their institutional settings may already be involved in community-based health information through their participation in state data systems or, more recently, repositories associated with HIE programs.

The Role of Patient Data, Public Health, and Research

Public health reporting has long been a component of managing patient records to meet customer needs. Mandatory reporting for infectious diseases, abstracting for special purposes registries, and collecting standard information on hospital discharges are typically sent to local and state health departments for the purpose of meeting the collective needs of the community public health. Statewide immunization registries and cancer registries are examples. Consistently collected data enables more effective preventive measures to be developed and implemented. Planning for efficient data reporting for such needs requires reliable and trustworthy methods and timely attention to collecting the data. With the advent of the EHR, the technology has opened the door to more efficient and accurate data abstracting from patient records and strengthened the processes used to serve public health. Furthermore, the HITECH act incorporates details into the expectations of EHRs. The certification criteria for both providers and hospitals calls for capability to electronically transmit data to meet public health goals and explicitly identifies immunization reporting as well. Certified EHRs must develop and maintain effective HIE capability that will be used to transmit relevant information to extended care sites as well as to reporting agencies. But the anticipated improvements do not stop there. More is expected.

Syndromic surveillance is the process of monitoring data that can identify when specific epidemiologic syndromes initially appear. Monitoring information that can offer early detection alerts of outbreaks of health problems is a key goal for EHR systems. Being able to quickly identify instances of food poisoning, new strains of influenza, and other community-based health issues will advance the public health response capability to meet these health challenges. So the collective goals for public health become more attainable.

The use and users of patient records can be better served at multiple levels when technology is employed effectively.

The Public Health Informatics Standards Consortium identified extensive additional data uses to improve the health of citizens with the implementation of EHR systems. The benefits to individual patients and to society as a whole through improved process and better public health surveillance are well documented.[59] Public health, which provides both direct clinical services and community services, can be a powerful tool to accomplish changes in the overall health of the population. To achieve such goals requires an integrated information system to provide accurate, understandable information for policymakers, community leaders, health plans, and health care providers. Public health practitioners and advocates are sharing their experiences with standardizing immunization information systems, public health laboratory information systems, vital registration and disease surveillance information systems, and integrating these systems into electronic EHR-based regional HIEs. HIM professionals have the knowledge and skills to support the data and information systems of the public health system, and can contribute to the overall health and well being of the entire population.

With the advent of more sophisticated ways to extract data from EHRs, researchers have more options for identifying data. From an era when coded data provided the primary foundation for identifying candidate cases, the use of natural language processing and more sophisticated code systems generate more accurate case identification and follow-up.

The EHR capability to collect and store clinical information longitudinally is creating a rich resource from which researchers can investigate care outcomes using more complete information, another benefit for the public and the industry as a whole.

HOW ARE ELECTRONIC HEALTH RECORD SYSTEMS EVALUATED?

Health Care and Health Services Evaluation Overview

In considering evaluation of EHRs, researchers are looking at a broader picture—that of the effect and value of HIT within the health care delivery system overall. Because the patient record is a primary business record that documents the care provided and the results of that care, it provides core information to the evaluation process. Coded data that represents diagnoses and procedures for individual patients is collected and organized so that it can be drawn from the record for analysis against various criteria that target the clinical and business outcomes for the enterprise and for specific products and services. As EHR systems have moved right along within the industry, the key question is whether these systems deliver information efficiently to the health care team and meet the overall administrative and financial requirements for the organization. Ball and colleagues point out major metrics to be used in determining the business case.[60] A summary of these metrics include:

- Cost savings and cost avoidance
- Improved staff and processes productivity
- Clinical quality improvement and medical outcome improvement
- Improved satisfaction (customer, physician, patient, and employee)

Cost Savings, Cost Avoidance, and Return on Investment

Implementing EHR systems will save some costs and add efficiency to organizational patient services. In addition to the obvious, such as eliminating paper supplies and the clerical staff needed to process paper records, reducing transcription costs, and eliminating copy service, a business case for adopting EHRs can be made from a broader perspective. However, eliminating clerical staff may mean hiring a smaller, more skilled staff of health information technicians and specialists who perform the ongoing tasks needed to manage a robust EHR system. Additionally, the overall cost of an EHR implementation and ongoing system maintenance may well outweigh the cost of clerical staff and other line items.

In addition, data availability, provider productivity, service efficiency, and operational savings can be measured. Evidence mounts that benefits of EHR systems can be realized, although not all of the known benefits can be tied to metrics. Cost benefit has become an effective resource to the future of EHRs. The Veterans' Administration realized $3 billion in net benefits for their investment in HIT, including their computerized patient record system (CPRS).[61] So if EHRs have such demonstrated potential, why is it taking so long? The reality is that EHRs are complex, multifaceted, and interrelated systems that need to meet variable customer needs. There isn't a "right size fits all" solution, but there are common functions and expectations.

Improved Staff and Processes Productivity

Improved productivity is based on a foundation of workflow analysis and improvement. The advent of EHR components such as CPOE illustrates streamlining the care process. *Workflow* refers to the sequence of tasks that need to be done to complete a process. Improvements in provider order entry can affect workflow speed and overall processing. Using an e-mail or a secure messaging application to communicate with patients can streamline provider–patient communication. Medication administration improvements generated through integrating provider order entry, pharmacy drug checks, and delivery of medication, and integration with patient identification bar code application can result in improved workflow. When planning for implementing EHRs, workflow analysis helps identify the overall processes into component tasks, specify who performs the task, and determine the appropriate business rules for each task. These, in turn, are used to determine how the applications within the EHR system such as provider order entry can improve the processes by streamlining the tasks and improving the business rule applications. The California Healthcare Foundation cites key success factors for performing workflow analysis to support EHR implementation:

1. Bring together a multidisciplinary team.
2. Make sure the process analysis—a written narrative of a process map—includes a review by staff who actually do the work.
3. Don't rely on the vendor for workflow analysis.
4. Assign responsibility for the task by appointing a project manager, data steward, or other point person.

They point out that the most important workflow to analyze and understand is the patient step-by-step process for their experience working through their health care visit or encounter.[62] Understanding how a new system will actually work in the care environment will not happen unless the details that flow from the processes that derive from that experience and related operations are thoroughly analyzed. To improve productivity, the processes must be identified, documented, and measured both before and after the EHR implementation. Analysis of these processes not only provides the foundation for improving them in readiness for implementing a new system, but also provides the basis for determining productivity gains when they are in place.

Another opportunity that comes with implementing EHR systems is to improve and streamline care protocols as attention is directed to CDS processes. These are the backbone of the CDS functions and evidence has shown that improvements can be made in these areas as well. So have workflows improved? Does attention to them make a difference in measuring productivity outcomes? There are well-documented examples of improved quality through productivity. The following are cited in post–EHR implementation settings. EHRs have resulted in the following improvements:

- Streamlined major processes within the orders operations reduce order entry from initiation through completion.
- System alerts prompt nursing staff to complete tasks on time.
- Medication processes overall are more streamlined.
- Evidence-based alerts reduce provider time.
- Illegible orders have been reduced.
- Nurse time on direct patient care is increased.
- CPOE allows faster physician ordering of tests, procedures, and medications.
- Centralized, electronic scheduling reduces time spent on patient scheduling.[5]
- Improved patient engagement as patients experience access to their records and electronic communication with their providers in managing chronic diseases.

Clinical Quality Improvement and Medical Outcome Improvement

As already noted early in this chapter, studies are showing improved quality with EHR systems. The very fact that EHRs bring identifiable patient information to the care team providers on demand and offer legible and up to date information on the patient's condition provide the welcomed first step in improving the quality of care through immediately available patient information. Additional resources are cited about the Kaiser EHR experience that leverage system functionality to provide drug–drug interaction, health maintenance reminders, best practice alerts, dose restrictions for specific drugs, and after-visit summary reports for patients afford necessary tools for health care providers to meet quality goals and patient safety targets.[5] Quality improvements have been demonstrated across settings. Carilion Roanoke Memorial Hospital cites quality improvements such as an EHR "workbench" that creates reports with trends and benchmarks to be shared with quality groups in the organization. Nursing dashboards provides tracking features to nurses when time-sensitive care processes are imminent.[5] Documentation on improvements in managing chronic disease patients via EHR structured progress notes cited early in the chapter are another example. We celebrate the examples of better outcomes and care improvements and care management. The goals for health informatics and information management practitioners to work to foster and maintain quality health information through systems and manage the business processes required to see that the systems contain accurate, timely, and complete health information remains an ongoing challenge. The models are changing, and effective oversight, assessment, and application of change management strategies can be found in both positive and negative experiences. How happy are the customers of the EHR?

Do physician, patients, and employees celebrate the benefits or are they challenged by the differences?

Improved Customer Satisfaction: Providers, Patients, Employees

Although it is a major adjustment for physicians, nurses, and other direct care providers to use EHRs, their satisfaction ranges. Providers may accept and endorse the product. They may grudgingly accept it as a benefit to the patient although costing more of the provider's time. Some don't yet see the benefits.

Here is where system design features can be tailored to support the provider care processes. From establishing templates for capturing direct entry provider notes to incorporating voice activation that streamlines transcription processes, the technology affects the caregiver's day to day experience. For those growing up in the technology age, working directly in the EHR system may be an easy transition. For those who have little experience with the technology resources in other aspects of their lives, changing their work habits to work directly with the computer is a significant challenge. The reality is that while health care is adjusting to the EHR, it is adjusting to an electronic representation of paper records. Innovation in design of access and retrieval of clinical information is needed to transform the way the information is used in the EHRs of tomorrow. For patients, satisfaction is evolving.

Some patients appreciate the ability to access their information through their provider portals to see laboratory results, order prescription refills, and schedule appointments. Other patients are not as comfortable with the technology and may not yet experience direct benefits in this way, but may recognize that their physician has all their information available when they are seen in the physician's office. For others, there is some concern about the privacy and security of their information.

Employee experience and satisfaction depends on their role in the organization. Some staff embrace the technology whole heartedly and welcome the changes it brings. For instance, appointment scheduling systems and bar code systems may streamline and make work more accurate for some. For others, the new system may take more time to complete routine tasks. They may need to learn new systems and processes and may find that the ongoing changes are not trustworthy. As HIM practitioners work to lead and participate in advancing EHR systems in their organization, their efforts on working with knowledgeable staff to fully understand workflow analysis and propose updates associated with system design and implementation will be important to employee satisfaction in adjusting to changes. For all of these customers, their experience and opinions are tied to the effectiveness of training and the availability of resources to help guide them through change. Still, even with optimal experiences in EHR implementation, it is also true that unintended consequences have occurred through EHR systems.

Electronic Health Records Progress: Unintended Consequences

Unintended consequences have occurred with EHRs. Institutions may fail to achieve anticipated cost benefits. There may be failure to incorporate leadership and key areas in the process so that effective life cycle management from planning through implementation may not happen. And there may be failure to understand the sheer complexity of EHRs and their influence on the organization.

Functional problems can also occur when:
- Screen directions are confusing.
- A provider documents or places an order in the wrong record.
- Medication errors occur because of overreliance on outdated lists of formularies.
- A wrong item is selected from a pick list.
- Copy/paste tools are used poorly.
- Exceptions to standard care path protocols are not recognized.
- Staff rely too heavily on the computer to complete essential communication tasks.
- Templates are used incorrectly.

Just as we are celebrating benefits that are discovered in the research on EHR system outcomes, researchers are also noting the problems that are surfacing. The American Medical Informatics Association (AMIA) published a set of guiding principles and recommendations that focus on critical usability issues that adversely affect patient safety. They call for establishing standardized use cases for use in EHR systems and the development of a core set of measures for adverse events to assess the incidence for analysis and correction. They recommend research and promotion of best practices for safe implementation of EHRs. For national policy purposes, AMIA recommends that the ONC standardization and interoperability across EHR systems should take account of usability concerns and that an adverse event reporting system for HIT and voluntary HIT event reporting be established. And they cite the need to develop and disseminate an educational campaign on the safe and effective use of EHRs to bring increased attention to issues and concerns.[63]

Vendor Collaboration

As health care organizations work with EHR systems and identify issues with customer satisfaction, vendors become involved in incorporating satisfaction issues into their ongoing upgrades. Product satisfaction becomes a negotiation and a matter for future decisions in the important area of HIT. Product user groups become a valued resource for the vendors and for contracted health care organizations in collaborating their customer findings and soliciting improvements to systems and applications. It becomes a practical matter to set aside time for key users to participate in user groups and the ongoing oversight and management of EHRs will require constant attention to validate and adjust priorities for vendor attention as implementation shifts into operations. In these instances, vendors are partners for change.

INDUSTRY-WIDE GOALS TO USE ELECTRONIC HEALTH RECORDS EFFECTIVELY

What Are Meaningful Use Requirements and How Do They Work?

It isn't enough to acquire and install EHR systems. It is important that providers and organizations make "meaningful use" of them to be deemed effective. The ARRA established financial incentives to stimulate adoption of EHRs and required that providers select certified EHR products and that "meaningful use" be made of them. Meaningful use is using certified EHR technology to:

Improve quality, safety, efficiency and reduce disparities.
Engage patients and their families in their health care.
Improve care coordination.
Improve population and public health.
Maintain privacy and security of patient information.[64]

Meaningful use includes using a certified EHR in three broad areas:

- Use in a meaningful manner (e.g., collect data, order medications)
- Use to provide electronic HIE for quality of care
- Participate in reporting quality of care measures[65]

As a measure of the scope required to achieve these critical strategies, seven principles for meaningful use and qualification or certification of EHRs were established. These principles call out the role of HIT from investment to critical assessment, and tie information resources to the role of the users of the technology. They specify tangible timelines and underscore the need and value of metrics to measure progress. Finally, they tie the progress in HIT to consumers and reinforce the need to accomplish these goals without sacrificing patient privacy. Details on these principles are shown in Table 6–11.[66]

In April 2009 HIMSS published a definition for *meaningful use* that called for the requirements to be introduced and staged for incremental stringency. Their work called for the definition to include four attributes:

1. A functional EHR certified by the Certification Commission for Healthcare Information Technology
2. Electronic exchange of standardized patient data with clinical and administrative stakeholders using the Healthcare Information Technology Standards Panel's interoperability specifications and Integrating the Healthcare Enterprise's frameworks
3. CDS providing clinicians with clinical knowledge and intelligently filtered patient information to enhance patient care
4. Capabilities to support process and care measurement that drive improvements in patient safety, quality outcomes, and cost reductions[65]

They also stressed staged implementation and endorsed coordinated harmonized standards for recommended specific phases over a 5-year period. Although the goals to advance certified EHR systems that are used in a

TABLE 6-11 Foundational Principles for Meaningful Use

Prioritize "measures that matter" for health improvement—measures that demonstrate improved health outcomes and greater cost-effectiveness.

Be operationally feasible for 2011 and beyond for a broad range of providers, vendors, and the Centers for Medicare and Medicaid Services. This will mean a phased approach with expectations and rigor of methods becoming more precise and exacting over time. The approach will account for variability in the capacity and capabilities of systems and providers while improving the usefulness, integrity, and comparability of information over time.

Leverage existing quality reporting efforts if they meet these criteria and work in alignment toward meaningful use goals.

Implement processes that will proactively improve data quality and data integrity over time.

Minimize unnecessary burden and cost by enabling reporting of "measures that matter" as a byproduct of using qualified health information technology. Providers should be able to demonstrate meaningful use without significant additional overhead and effort.

Give providers timely access to the quality and cost information they need to improve care. Demonstrating meaningful use should help providers and patients improve health and health outcomes, and not just be a time-consuming administrative data reporting or documentation exercise.

Demonstrating Meaningful Use of Health IT for 2011 and Beyond Collaborative Comment *Markle Foundation, Center for American Progress (CAP), Engelberg Center for Health Care Reform at Brookings* December 4, 2009. http://www.markle.org/publications/862-demonstrating-meaningful-use-health-it-2011-and-beyond

meaningful and measureable way are focused as a necessary achievement, the counterweight is the recognition that the pace of change and expectations of clinicians to learn and use these systems effectively requires a careful consideration and appreciation of the time needed to effect significant cultural change.

Incentive Program for Meaningful Use

The Medicare and Medicaid EHR incentive program is designed to engage providers to move forward with EHRs and demonstrate that they are using them in a meaningful way. Providers and organizations that meet this objective receive reimbursement to help offset the cost of their experience.

To do this, the incentive program mapped out a series of objectives, criteria, and measures to confirm objectives are met.

This program has progressed in stages and is designed to increase the sophistication and capability of the implemented systems through each state. Table 6-12 compares and contrasts target objectives by stages and includes the criteria to be measured to ensure that the objectives are being met. And additional resources are available for organizations

TABLE 6-12 Meaningful Use Stage 1 Illustration.

EP	EH	Meaningful Use 42 CFR 495.6(j)-(m) Stage 2 Objective	Meaningful Use 42 CFR 495.6(j)-(m) Stage 2 Measure	2014 Edition EHR Certification Criteria 45 CFR 170.314	Standards
CORE EP	EH	Use CPOE for medication, laboratory and radiology orders directly entered by any licensed healthcare professional who can enter orders into the medical record per State, local and professional guidelines.	More than 60% of medication, 30% of laboratory, and 30% of radiology orders created by the EP or authorized providers of the EH'S or CAH'S inpatient or emergency department (POS 21 or 23) during the EHR reporting period are recorded using CPOE. *Exclusions apply: see CMS rule for details	§170.314(a)(1) Computerized provider order entry. Enable a user to electronically record, change, and access the following order types, at a minimum: (i) Medications; (ii) Laboratory; and (iii) Radiology/imaging.	

CORE
EP
		EPs: Record the following demographics:
		• Preferred language
		• Sex
		• Race
		• Ethnicity
		• Data of birth.
			More than 80% of all unique patients seen by the EP or admitted to the EH's or CAH'S inpatient or emergency department (POS 21 or 23) during the EHR reporting period have demographics recorded as structured data.	§170.314(a)(3)
				
				Demographics.
				(i) Enable a user to electronically record, change, and access patient demographic data including preferred language, sex, race, ethnicity, and date of birth.
				   A. Enable race and ethnicity to be recorded in accordance with the standard specified in § 170.207(f) and whether a patient declines to specify race and/or ethnicity.
				   B. Enable preferred language to be recorded in accordance with the standard specified in § 170.207(g) and whether a patient declines to specify a preferred language.
				(ii) Inpatient setting only. Enable a user to electronically record, change, and access preliminary cause of death in the event of a mortality.
					▪ § 170.207(f) – OMB standards for Maintaining, Collecting, and Presenting Federal Data on Race and Ethnicity, Statistical Policy Directive No. 15, Oct 30, 1997.
					▪ § 170.207(g) – ISO 639-2 alpha-3 codes limited to those that also have a corresponding alpha-2 code in ISO 639-1.

CORE	EH	EHs/CAHs: Record the following demographics: • Preferred language • Sex • Race • Ethnicity • Date of birth • Date and preliminary cause of death in the event of mortality in the EH or CAH.			
CORE EP	EH	Record and chart changes in vital signs: • Height/length • Weight • Blood pressure (BP) (age 3+) • Calculate and display BMI • Plot and display growth charts for children 0–20 years, including BMI.	More than 80% for all unique patients seen by the EP or admitted to the EH'S or CAH'S inpatient or emergency department (POS 21 or 23) during the EHR reporting period have BP (for patients age 3+ only) and height/length and weight (for all ages) recorded as structured data. *Exclusions apply: see CMS rule for details	§ 170.314(a)(4) Vital signs, body mass index, and growth charts. (i) Vital signs. Enable a user to electronically record, change, and access, at a minimum, a patient's height/length, weight, and blood pressure. Height/length, weight, and blood pressure must be recorded in numerical values only. (ii) Calculate body mass index. Automatically calculate and electronically display body mass index based on a patient's height and weight. (iii) Optional – Plot and display growth charts. Plot and electronically display, upon request, growth charts for patients.	

http://healthit.gov/sites/default/files/meaningfulusetablesseries1_110112.pdf

and professionals working to achieve meaningful use goals in their organizations.

The Center for Medicare and Medicaid Services also provide a series of specification sheets through their website to support the customer. These include information on the following:

Meeting the measure for each objective
How to calculate the numerator and denominator for each objective
How to qualify for an exclusion to an objective
Definitions of terms that clarify objective requirements
Requirements for attesting to each measure[65]

By offering an incentive for eligible providers and organizations to prepare for the technology requirements in their future, the government offered a carrot. A stick will be applied in the form of reducing payments for the care of federally insured patients whose care information is not transferred electronically. This will occur starting in 2015.

Meaningful use has advanced the work for EHRs in supporting eligible providers and organizations to acquire and install EHRs. Making sure they meet the standards is an ongoing process.

Functionality of EHR systems must support the exchange of information to support coordination of care. As systems mature and the industry provides the technology and resources, the coordination of care and the capacity to draw data from the systems to collect and report on data quality is growing as well.

WHAT ARE THE REQUIREMENTS AND CHALLENGES OF HEALTH INFORMATION EXCHANGE

Securing National Goals for Health Information Exchange

The goal of readily available health information has been in place for many years. The industry has worked to transfer information between facilities and provide referral information when patients move from primary care to specialty care. This involved written documents and copies of hospital discharge reports when patients were transferred to long-term care settings, and the use of fax machines in recent years. In the age of increasing presence of EHRs, making patient health information available electronically is widely viewed as critical to realizing quality and efficiency improvements from the large investment in EHRs. When providers must treat patients with insufficient information, they are forced to repeat diagnostic tests and potentially delay treatment. Of course this means higher costs as well. Making health information available across settings in a timely and easy-to-access fashion has largely remained an unmet goal. It is no surprise that HIE has been incorporated into the HITECH legislation and made a key priority. In fact, almost $600 million in funding was made available to states to help them work on HIE solutions that fit their communities.[67] Specific state HIE progress and strategic plans can be found on the State HIE Cooperative Agreement Program website.[67]

So is there progress on this front? First, a look at examples of functioning HIEs is in order. Then a look at the business case issues clarifies some of the continuing barriers to accomplishing this goal.

Health Information Exchange Model Profiles

HIE occurs when individual health care organizations arrange to exchange clinical data with unaffiliated organizations such as with physician practices in the area. In a 2013 report on HIT in the United States, the Robert Wood Johnson Foundation reported on a surveys on HIE activity that identified 322 organizations that were potentially involved.[67] Types of organizations actually participating in operational exchange included hospitals, ambulatory practices, independent laboratories and radiology services, payers, public health departments, and independent pharmacies. Among these, the top two types of data exchanged were test results (82%) and summary care records (79%). Other types in order of frequency were discharge summaries (66%), clinical summaries (61%), ambulatory problem lists (56%), and public health reports (30%).[67]

So how did the actual exchange take place? The most common model was one in which participants could query a partner to access information on a specific patient, providing an on-demand practicality. This requires that specific providers, such as in an emergency department, know about and use this model.

The second most common model is one in which the organizations holding the data send it to scheduled partners such as community physicians. In this case, the information is sent to partners and the on-demand needs, such as in the emergency department, go unmet.

Another model is an "end to end" integration model that automatically sends the data to an EHR. A more sophisticated model, this requires an electronic system and may be used along with the two previous models that allow users with only Internet access to view data.[68]

More recently, an approach that uses a point-to-point transport through a secure, inexpensive connection is Direct. Direct is promoted by the federal government and provides for data to be moved to partners in a planned schedule. This is viewed as a less expensive solution that may be expandable.[65]

Making and Maintaining the Business Case

The meaningful use requirement has certainly driven the business case for many. National data notes that 2362 (75%) of hospital service areas in the United States had an operational HIE.[65] Of course the purpose here is to enable providers to use and reuse health information for caring for patients beyond their environment to achieve quality and cost goals. Historically, it has been difficult to maintain a business case for HIE because financial sustainability has been a key barrier. In addition, potential participants are concerned about patient privacy and security, lack of funding, competitive advantage, technical and operational capabilities, and accurately linking patient data.[69] EHR provisions that include technical capabilities that support HIE opportunities may help address some of these barriers. The solutions go beyond technical and operational processes, and require that institutional policy and compliance targets be met and a changing of the culture so that providers expect to have and use information exchanged from the larger care team.

 SELF-ASSESSMENT QUIZ

22. Using the previous discussion on PHRs, research additional sites on PHRs and patient or consumer portals. Prepare a two-page report or visual that contrasts these approaches to patient access and management of their personal health information and discuss how each links or can link to EHRs. Gather your own personal history and significant medical data and create your own PHR.
23. Prepare a position paper on web-based PHRs versus institution-based patient portals. Which do you recommend and why?

CHANGING ELECTRONIC HEALTH RECORD TECHNOLOGY

Changes in the Role and Scope of the Health Information Management Professional

Management Questions and Moving to the Virtual Department

The patient and his or her information are the center of the health care delivery system. Without patients, the health care system would not exist; without a health care system of some type, patients would not come to be listened to, examined, tested, diagnosed, and treated. Whenever a patient and provider interact within the health care delivery system, whether the communication is clinical or administrative in nature, face to face, on the telephone, or conducted by use of a new technology, such as telehealth, information is set down in a record to preserve knowledge of what happened. Documentation in the record is the patient's health information, which means different things to different people depending on the context in which it is being used or discussed. Original health information, created during an interaction between a patient and a health care professional, has a life cycle of its own and often goes through many permutations before it is filed and complete. During the course of a lifetime, a person's health records are created and maintained in many different settings, for example, the hospital where they were born, the clinics and physician offices where they were treated, schools, the military, and so forth. Technological innovations are radically altering the processes that are used to collect, process, store, and retrieve health information. The health record itself, at one time simply a collection of various documents stored in a manila folder, is also in the midst of a major transformation.

Because health information and health record processes and technologies are changing, traditional HIM professional management of both an individual patient's health record

and multiple health records is shifting as well. Standards, laws, and regulations are being modified to reflect changes in technology and processes. What are not changing are the basic reasons that health information is recorded and the core documentation principles.

To understand the evolving health record, one must understand the types of health information content that make up a health record, the modalities used to capture the content, and the processes used to manage each. All these elements are undergoing a major change and will continue to do so. As the elements change and evolve, so will the HIM roles. It is incumbent on current and emerging HIM leaders to envision the new EHR reality and make a conscious choice to assist in the transition from manual, paper-bound departments to a mature organization-wide EHR.

The AHIMA Data Quality Management Model presented in Chapter 4 is an excellent description of key dimensions of data quality that professionals reference in their HIM practice in both paper and EHR systems. In the EHR environment, there are additional considerations in how these and other quality measures are described.

Documentation Principles

Recall the basic purpose of recording health information is simply to preserve what went on between the patient and the provider. How and what clinicians document in the health record is based on their original training, their experiences as residents or trainees working under attending physicians or preceptor guidance, reimbursement requirements, and the type of training they have received from HIM documentation specialists. In addition, documentation principles are derived from accreditation standards, clinical specialty societies, and state licensing bodies. Federal laws, reimbursement guidelines, and clinical coding organizations advise or mandate certain aspects of clinical documentation. It is critical to understand that the standards remain the same for both manual records and EHRs; it does not matter how the information is captured or how it is reported.

Unique Patient Identification

The documentation and data must always be linked to the correct patient's identification (usually at least the patient's name and unique identification number) at the time of capturing information, generating reports, and accessing the information. The system should provide linkage between the different identities of the same patient, identification of potential duplicate numbers of the same patient, and a method to merge and correct them and distinguish between patients with similar names.

Legibility

Documentation, including signatures, must be legible (i.e., it must be easily readable). If not legible, documentation becomes a major patient safety issue. Orders can be misunderstood, medications or dosages may be misread, and patient care can be compromised. An EHR in which all documentation is entered directly through keyboarding or is transcribed and uploaded to the system is, of course, legible. A scanned handwritten document, however, is really only as legible as the original handwriting. Yes, in many systems, one can magnify portions of the scanned document, but this is an extra step that takes time and should not be considered a normal practice.

Accuracy

Information throughout a report and the record itself needs to be accurate and consistent, and not contradict itself.

Completeness

The document and record must be complete according to standards adhered to by the organization. What content is required for a particular health care intervention (e.g., what are the required elements of a history and physical? an operative report? an informed consent? an authorization for disclosure? an initial assessment outpatient note? a transfer summary? a discharge summary? etc.)? If there is an addendum to the document, can it be retrieved with the original document? Is an addendum clearly marked for the reader? Accrediting bodies, regulatory bodies, clinician specialty, and organizational policies and reimbursement rules drive the content considered necessary.

Timeliness

Timeliness of documentation is linked to accurate documentation. Individual documents in the record must be created in a timely manner, again according to standards used by the organization. If documentation is created too distant from the patient care encounter, the accuracy of the documentation can be questioned. Because a clinician is treating many patients every day, it is difficult to believe he or she can remember enough detail to fully record the encounter if it is not done soon after the encounter. Timely documentation is key for the continuum of care when another provider who needs information from previous encounters sees the patient. In an EHR, timeliness tracking is an inherent process of the computer where the documentation is taking place. In the paper world, time is often left out when handwriting a note.

Integrity

Integrity in a health record means data or the content in an order or a text document such as a history and physical examination, operative report, progress note, discharge summary, laboratory result, and so forth has not been altered or destroyed in an unauthorized manner.[70] In the paper world, any changes in an original document or report were accomplished by drawing a line through the erroneous entry, handwriting the changes, and then dating and initialing the entries. When one enters a hybrid entry in an electronic environment, health record integrity becomes a significantly larger issue, one in which the HIM professional is uniquely qualified to set policy and business processes that ensure the organization's EHR

integrity. Content integrity is coupled with both document authentication and security. (See Chapter 8 for a discussion on security.) Health record integrity management requires an exquisite understanding of the various, authorized ways in which document content may be changed.

Authentication

Each entry in the health record must identify who (or what in the case of machines) created the entry or document and who is responsible for its accuracy, timeliness, and completion. Its author must authenticate each entry or document. **Authentication** is the process of identifying the source of health record entries by attaching a handwritten signature, the author's initials, or an electronic signature. In a paper system, *authentication* means a legible, handwritten signature.

In an electronic system, the electronic signature must ensure that the signed document was not modified after the signature was affixed. Additionally, the electronic signature must ensure that only the signer could have created a signature. This requirement is called *nonrepudiation*. After the signature has been affixed, any change in the document's information must cause the signature verification process to detect that the information has been changed. This ensures the integrity of the author's content and prevents others from altering the information. Some systems guarantee document integrity by "locking" the document after the electronic signature has been affixed. To display a change, therefore, the same or different author must write an addendum to the original document that requires an electronic signature as well with the same functionalities.

Privacy, Confidentiality, and Security

Health information must adhere to federal and state laws to protect both the patient and the organization. This is discussed in more detail in previous chapters.

Although core documentation principles remain basically the same in both paper and electronic formats, how they are defined or implemented within a specific organization may vary, depending on the organization's process in implementing an EHR system. For example, authentication on a paper document could mean a physical signature by a physician, appended by his or her professional degree, MD, and specialty, cardiology. In an electronic document, a standard (or organizational policy) might also require a provider identification number as well. Each of these elements can be defined somewhat differently depending on a standard, law, reimbursement requirement, and so forth, as well as the organization in which the clinician is practicing. The Joint Commission has core documentation standards, many of which are found in the chapters on records of care, treatment, and services their various manuals. Certain other documentation standards are found in the chapters covering provision of care, treatment and services, national patient safety goals, and the information management chapters.[71] These standards are often revised; it is important, therefore, to stay abreast of changes by visiting the Joint Commission website on a regular basis.

✓ SELF-ASSESSMENT QUIZ

24. Go to The Joint Commission (THC) website at www.jointcommission.org. Notice TJC standards are not available on this website.
    - How can you find out about specific standards, including those for health records and health information management?
    - Click on the Standards FAQs which brings you to a list of manuals. How many types of organizations can be accredited/certified by TJC?
    - Familiarize yourself with other aspects of TJC by clicking on the banner topics across the top.
    - Use the Search box to find the Medical Records Statistics Form which is used by hospitals. What is the standard for delinquent medical records?

THE PHYSICAL PAST

Many health care organizations are just beginning to emerge from a manual, paper health record system. In this type of manual, paper-based system, health information is stored as various types of paper documents in manila folders, the health record, each of which identifies the patient, usually with a unique patient medical record number. The documents may include computer-generated registration information, handwritten or transcribed clinical documents, various kinds of laboratory results and reports, and administrative and medical correspondence from other health care providers.

The systems are physical; the health records (the "charts") are stored on shelves in various types of file rooms or on racks on inpatient wards. Managing physical chart movement is a major HIM function in a traditional paper-based health record system. The charts must be physically moved from place to place and each movement tracked with some sort of manual or computerized tracking system. Knowing where each chart is at all times is critical because various authorized users of the chart may need it at the same time. Only one person can use/view the chart at one time. For example, a clinician wants the chart to finish dictating his discharge summary. An HIM coder needs the chart to code the chart to meet the billing deadline. A HIM release of information (ROI) technician needs the chart to release information to another outside provider. And, of course, if the patient is presenting for care, the chart must be provided to the clinician, preferably in advance of the encounter.

Individual documents, loose reports, must be manually filed one by one in the correct patient record. If the record is not in the file room, then the file clerk must drop file reports in an outguide that is placed in the location where the health record will be returned.

In a traditional, manual environment, most HIM functions and provider/patient interactions are totally dependent on having the hard copy health record to perform their tasks. For that matter, the organization is also dependent on a well-managed paper health record system that requires the health record to be physically present for the reader to access and use the information contained in it. And, the documents must be filed accurately and include all up-to-date information. HIM managers of paper health record systems are under tremendous pressures to ensure record availability and completeness, especially in large organizations that have active, ambulatory care with more than 2500 scheduled and unscheduled visits each day. How well a traditional HIM department functions is predicated, to a large part, on the efficient and effective management of the file unit.

THE EMERGING PRESENT

As organizations leave a mostly manual, paper-based environment, they are entering a hybrid health information world where some parts of the health record itself and some of its processes may be manual or electronic. The HIM professional must view himself or herself as a change master and develop the skill to conceive, construct, and convert current behavior into a new, living organizational reality.[72] This means clearly understanding current HIM practices from clinical documentation to management of HIM functions at all levels. Almost all medium and large health care organizations generate or store some part of health information in an electronic format. (See Chapter 9 for a discussion of health information systems.) Many of the business processes that are managed by HIM are actually systems themselves. As Scholtes[73] describes, *system* refers to interactions and interdependencies on a large scale; *processes* refer to components of the system. Processes have purposes and functions of their own, but by themselves processes cannot accomplish the purpose of a system. When viewing an HIM department in an organization, we are looking at a complex social system and a technical system consisting of several subsystems and processes. The health record system is but one interacting, interdependent part of the larger system. When an organization or a section of an organization begins to move from a paper to a hybrid environment, the changes may be uncomfortable for all levels of staff. This is a normal reaction to change and it is important for the HIM professional to understand this about one's self as well as for clerks, coders, transcriptionists, administrators, nurses, physicians, and so forth. Planning in as much detail as possible is critical. In fact, it is important to visualize the eventual positive outcomes and then work backward to identify the necessary tasks. Project management is a necessary skill for anyone who is working in a hybrid system going to a total EHR system.

Although the business processes that a HIM department manages may differ in sequencing in various organizations, the flow described in Chapter 4 provides a high-level flow diagram typical of HIM processes. Using somewhat different terminology, following are some common information processes that support clinical activities that need to be evaluated as an organization moves into a hybrid environment.

✓ SELF-ASSESSMENT QUIZ

25. Assume an organization is in a hybrid EHR environment and allows its clinicians to dictate operative reports, radiology reports, pathology reports, and discharge summaries. The organization has a CDR that provides views for these reports as well as laboratory reports and patient demographics. Explain why coding after discharge is likely to be accomplished more quickly in the hybrid environment than when the organization was paper-based.

Patient Identity Management

Although the operational unit that handles patient registration and admissions ordinarily performs the daily operational tasks of registering and admitting a patient, it is the HIM department that carries out quality control reconciliation processes when duplicate names or numbers appear. This may mean correcting the MPI entries of one or more patients or tracking down document and data in both paper and electronic systems to ensure that the patient's information is flowing correctly from one system to the other. In a paper health record system, HIM staff members often physically correct patient identity information by hand on every single page of the record. In an EHR, however, corrections may be done by keyboarding changes without necessarily accessing a paper document. Three linking methods may used to determine the correct patient.

One method compares records on selected data elements, usually name, birth date, social security number (SSN), or sex. Exact match and deterministic linking are examples. In an exact match, all specified data elements must be identical. With a deterministic method, specified data elements must be an exact match or a partial match. Partial matches can include substring matches (e.g., first three letters of the last name or last four numbers of the SSN) or phonetic matches (e.g., Soundex).

An intermediate method enhances exact match and deterministic tools with additional logic and arbitrary or subjective scoring systems, including subjective weighting, ad hoc weighting, fuzzy logic, and rules-based algorithms. With this type of method, the health care organization assigns a value to key patient identifying attributes such as the last name, first name, date of birth, and so forth.

The most advanced set of identity management tools for matching records relies on mathematical theory. Mathematical algorithms are used to supplement or enhance the tools available in the basic and intermediate methods. Probabilistic, bipartite graph theory and mathematical modeling, machine learning, and neural networks are examples of advanced matching tools.[74] Only when the MPI is in an electronic form can these more sophisticated matching techniques be used.

Providing Prior Information

After a patient arrives for care, either as a scheduled or unscheduled admission or visit, or after registration and admitting staff has verified the patient's identity, HIM is responsible for providing previous health records to the caregivers. In a totally manual environment, this means pulling the record from the file unit and most likely delivering it to the inpatient unit or outpatient location where the patient will be seen. The organization may have some of the patient's previous administrative and clinical information stored electronically. Or the organization may store the information both in the hard copy health record and in a computerized repository. The information may include the patient's demographics, transcribed reports such as previous history and physical examinations, radiology reports, "final" laboratory reports, allergies, discharge summaries, and a problem list. Depending on the organization's practices and EHR implementation strategy, these reports may be available for viewing at workstations and for reading as printed, paper documents that are filed in the hard copy health record. In most cases, HIM is responsible for physically moving the health record to the needed location. In some cases, HIM is also responsible along with the IT department to ensure that all of the documents that are stored electronically are indeed complete and viewable.

Who Is Authorized to Make Entries in the Health Record?

Who can actually write in the health record must be clearly defined in the organization's policy. The Joint Commission's long-standing policy called for only authorized individuals to make entries in the medical record. In a paper world, this was not too difficult a task. A simple list of the type of staff allowed to document was often enough. In a more electronic environment, however, one cannot simply go to a computer and document care. One needs specific privileges, menus, or functions to access the computer system and document and electronically sign the entry. One needs to think out very clearly who and why certain types of staff are "authorized" (to use The Joint Commission terminology) to document in the record. This policy is one that needs to be fully discussed and approved by the organization's medical record committee. Depending on the type of entry (notes, orders, administrative information, etc.), different policies will need to be developed. Appendix A is a sample policy directed toward staff who write progress notes in the health record.[74]

DOCUMENTING CARE

Clinicians document care by several different methods:
- Handwriting
- Speech
- Direct input
- Document imaging
- Device capture
- Clinical imaging

✓ SELF-ASSESSMENT QUIZ

26. Why would an organization with an EHR need to have policies defining who is authorized to write in the record?

Handwriting

In a paper-based system or a document imaging system that digitizes (scans) documents, the most common way to document care is to handwrite it on medical record forms that have been approved by the organization's medical record forms (sub)committee. The HIM director or designee often chairs the forms committee to ensure that forms design meets clinical documentation needs and content criteria. Handwriting is known by all clinicians, is an easy way to document, and can be signed by the author at the time of recording. It has its pitfalls in that it may not be readable, and other than digitizing the document, it cannot be integrated into an EHR system by reusing all or some of its information in other notes. A controlled vocabulary is not really possible because the author uses terminology that he or she is most familiar with. To determine whether handwritten documentation meets accreditation or a legal, billing, and organizational requirement obliges HIM and an interdisciplinary team to manually audit documentation note by note. In an inpatient setting, clinicians may handwrite history and physical examinations, progress notes, and orders. A paper-based system requires the HIM department to actively manage the folders and forms that make up the manual health record.

Speech

Speech is the second most common way to document care. It is known as *dictation and transcription.* Dictation and transcription is a dual process that combines both information capture and report generation. Physicians dictate clinical information, and medical transcriptionists convert this verbal information into written information. The transcribed products are formatted into reports such as history and physical examinations, operative reports, consultation reports, radiology reports, emergency department reports, discharge summaries, and so forth. As the document is being generated, medical transcriptionists transcribe, edit, and format it so that it is ready for review and authentication by the author. Macros or templates may be used during the process.

Speech is also captured for automatic transcription by speech recognition software. After the recognition process is completed, either the author or a medical transcriptionist edits it.

The transcribed output can be printed and authenticated with a "wet" signature (handwritten) on a paper document or it can retained in electronic form and authenticated with an electronic signature. HIM must establish business processes that track incomplete documents (i.e., those documents lacking the author's signature). Transcription is a costly process in terms of needed hardware and software and because there are not enough trained, expert medical transcriptionists available. In the traditional dictation–transcription process, there is lag time between dictation and the time when the report becomes available for viewing in either paper or electronic form. HIM business processes require monitoring of the status of dictated and transcribed reports to meet certain organizational standards.

HIM business processes that manage transcribed output change when the output is no longer printed and physically sent to another location (e.g., an operative report sent to an inpatient unit) or physically filed in the hard copy health record. With paper-based output, processes are designed to send and track the "original" document to the physician for wet signing. Copies of authenticated or unauthenticated documents, depending on the organization's policies and procedures, may also be sent to the billing office, to referring providers, to other designated clinicians within the organization, and so forth. Paper output processes often require printing an envelope, stuffing it with the report and mailing it. Managing printed, transcribed reports is a labor-intensive process.

The organization may decide to no longer print reports for internal needs and store them instead in a document repository that may or may not be part of an EHR system. No longer printing documents is a major decision that will affect all users of the health record. When this decision is made, policies and processes need to be created that support this change. For example, will the organization allow online viewing of unauthenticated reports? If so, how will the organization ensure that no changes are made to the report before the electronic signature? Will an electronic signature lock the report's content? What process will alert a clinician that he or she needs to electronically sign reports? How, for that matter, will HIM track electronic incomplete documents? How will the billing office know when a report is available for its use? How will the organization control printing reports outside the HIM department? Or does the organization control where reports are printed? How will the organization protect the confidentiality of the information if reports are printed in various locations? When printing is allowed, who is responsible for printing and ensuring that printed documents with identifying health information are secured? For example, are printed documents shredded at the point of printing when no longer needed? Or are they placed in a specialized, secure container for confidential documents?

These are examples of the kind of technical questions HIM professionals must ask themselves as they migrate from manual to hybrid electronic systems. It is a challenge to identify and understand, as much as possible, the interests and purposes of the interacting, interdependent components of the organization's systems.

The human aspect of such a major change as ceasing to print documents to hard copy cannot be ignored. It is no small thing to require users to view the health record online rather than read and turn pages in a hard copy record. In the beginning, until they become comfortable with viewing online, it will take longer for users to find and use what they need in the record

Direct Input

Direct input means care documentation is accomplished by clinician keyboarding, clicking a mouse, or touching a screen. The information can be entered as free text as in handwritten notes or it can be entered using templates.

(Templates are discussed in greater detail in a later section in this chapter.) Just as with handwritten notes, authentication can be accomplished immediately after completing the documentation. This means there is no lag time to wait for authentication. When clinicians directly enter their documentation into the computer, the HIM role changes to one of assisting the clinician at the point of documentation. It is important to realize that in the early 2000 decade, there are four generations of workers in the health care field. Those in older generations do not always easily use a computer keyboard nor find their way intuitively around computer functionality. One of the HIM roles and therefore necessary processes is the ability to provide adult education classes and one-on-one tutorials for clinicians using direct input. Direct input of notes and orders plunges the organization onto the path of a fully functioning EHR system. It is necessary for HIM staff specialists to fully understand the clinical processes that clinicians go through and how care documentation can be integrated into care processes. Teaching clinicians the intricacies of documenting in an EHR means the HIM specialist needs to pay compassionate attention to the learning needs and constraints of each trainee.

Document Imaging

Document imaging (or document digitizing) involves prepping, scanning, indexing, and performing quality control on paper documents that are being entered into a computer system. Paper documents, created through handwriting or transcription, can be transferred into digital form with image scanning, optical recognition, or a combination of the two. The ability to easily identify and retrieve individual documents depends on indexing that must be precise, unalterable, and correct. Document imaging requires HIM to develop processes for each of it steps. Document imaging is discussed in more detail in Chapter 5.

Device Capture

As discussed previously, device capture is a process by which a system captures health information directly from a medical device such as an ECG, thermometer, or ventilator. The machine-generated information must be read and interpreted by a clinician and validated. In the paper world, the output from a medical device may or may not have been filed in the paper chart. Fetal monitoring strips are an example of output that is normally filed in the hard copy chart. With an EHR and an appropriate interface, these types of output can be stored and viewed electronically.

Clinical Imaging

Clinical imaging involves data capture using photography or various imaging devices used in conjunction with diagnostic testing such as radiology, magnetic resonance imaging, and so forth. If the organization defines photographs as being part of the (legal) health record, then the HIM department must develop processes to ensure that the photographs are filed in the hard copy record. As the EHR develops and it becomes possible to attach digital photographs to electronic notes, then HIM must work with the medical photography unit and units who routinely take photographs (e.g., dermatology) to develop consistent processes to ensure uploading to the EHR. The ability of clinicians besides radiologists to view radiographic images on screen affects the radiology file unit in much the same way it does in the medical record file unit. Clerks are no longer needed to file films in folders and pull them when needed by radiologists. There is no more film, only digitized images that can be viewed from local and remote workstations.

It is important to realize that an EHR may consist of discrete data fields, images, and text documents.

Copying and Pasting

The electronic function of copying and pasting is a powerful tool that can, when used appropriately, increase a clinician's documentation efficiency. *Copy and paste* refers to duplicating selected text or graphics and inserting it in another location, leaving the original unchanged. Copying and pasting from other areas of the EHR must, however, be done with caution. Clinical, financial, and legal problems may result when text is copied in a manner that implies the author or someone else obtained historical information, performed an examination, or documented a plan of care when the author or someone else did not personally do it. When organizations begin implementing an EHR, they do not always understand the ramifications of inappropriate copying and pasting. Copying information does not always assist the reader and often makes the documents longer, making the chart more difficult and time consuming to read. It behooves the organization to set clear policy guidelines as to what is and is not appropriate copying and pasting practices.[75] For example, the organization might provide guidelines similar to those in Box 6-1. The organization's medical record committee should include a way to monitor this type of policy. Be warned that monitoring copying and pasting is difficult unless the EHR system itself was designed to track the use of copying and pasting.

BOX 6-1	Sample Copy and Paste Guidelines

- Plagiarized data in the health record is prohibited. Make sure to attribute the content you are copying to whoever originally wrote it. Using quotation marks around the copied data is acceptable.
- Never copy the electronic signature block from one note into another note (e.g., a nurse must never copy the content or information that a physician has written).
- Never copy data or information that identifies a health care provider as involved in care that the health care provider is not involved in (e.g., the results of a physical examination done by someone else).
- Do not copy entire laboratory findings, radiology reports, and other information verbatim into a note. Data copied into a note needs to be specific and pertinent to the care provided during that specific encounter.
- Do not reenter previously recorded data.
- Authors are responsible and liable for the content of copied items within the notes they authenticate.

Storage and Retention

Storage and retention of health records and health information is a major management challenge for the HIM department whether the records are physical, electronic, or a combination. Traditionally, HIM professionals were and are responsible for the department's filing systems, policies, and procedures; that they comply with federal and state regulations and accepted standards of practice; and that they meet the clinical and administrative needs of the organization. Filing, storage, retention, and destruction of health records and health information all require policies and procedures. Unless a new health care facility opens "paperless," using an EHR, where there is no need for physical storage of hard copy health records, the HIM professional must manage the physical storage of hard copy health records. The first consideration is to ensure that hard copy records can be retrieved and delivered in a timely manner for patient care or other authorized purposes. AHIMA's Practice Brief: Retention of Health Information recommends excellent guidelines for establishing retention schedules for all media including paper, images, optical disk, microfilm, and CD-ROM.[76] Although operational responsibility may be redelegated to the information technology department when the records are stored electronically, it is still HIM's role to ensure that the organization's retention and destruction policies follow state and federal laws and accreditation requirements.

Because health records and health information are increasingly stored in various types of media, it is also crucial that HIM be a strong advocate for ensuring that patient information is retrievable in a reasonable amount of time. For example, if older health information is only available on imaging platters, will the organization be able to retrieve the information when that technology is no longer current? If health information is written to tape, how fast can HIT find the specific information that is being requested? HIM professionals must stay current on evolving storage technologies and must be ever vigilant to ensure that historical health information is retrievable as needed.

Thinning Records

In a paper-based health record environment, when a patient has a long inpatient stay and remains an inpatient, nursing services may ask HIM staff to thin paper records because nursing has run out of physical space on the inpatient units to store all of the data and documents that have been generated during a specific patient's stay. Once again, this is a manual process that HIM performs using guidelines developed by the HIM department in conjunction with nursing services. The thinned portions of the records are returned to the main file room and are filed in the appropriate location. In an EHR, the process of thinning records on an inpatient unit does not exist. If the organization is still in an early transition to a hybrid environment, the nursing unit may still be printing orders, progress notes, and other results, and may need to shred them after they are no longer needed. All the information still resides in the EHR's clinical repository.

Coding

After a patient is discharged (or sometimes during the hospitalization itself), the HIM department codes the inpatient stay, which may include both facility and professional coding, involving at least two different coding systems. Even in organizations with a paper-based health record, most use an encoding software system to assist professional coders with their tasks of coding and grouping diagnoses and procedures. In a paper-based system, however, it is incumbent for HIM to have streamlined processes in place to acquire the hard copy record as soon as possible after discharge so that coding and therefore billing can take place. There is tremendous pressure on HIM directors to quickly and accurately complete coding so that billing can occur and the organization can receive its payment. In a paper-based system, this is no easy thing to accomplish because the chart may not be complete when it is received in the department and "loose paper" can continue to trickle into the department for some time. When the organization implements an EHR for inpatients, coders can perform their tasks without reading the hard copy chart. This is a major change for the coders because they will not be using the physical chart to read the documentation. They will read and code online. Processes will need to change. No longer will a supervisor be able to simply look at the number of charts needing coding by date of discharge; there can be a computer work queue that coders access to find the next case to code. When the entire inpatient episode is online either through an EHR or because everything is part of a document imaging system, it is possible to move the coders offsite either to a different location, to their homes, or to an outsourcing vendor who may have coders in many geographic locations. To do this requires clear policies and procedures as to how the work is accomplished, what kind of workstations are needed, how they will be maintained and updated, and security procedures to protect the confidentiality of the information, and so forth.

Health Record Review

Health care organizations should design and implement a health record review program as part of their site's overall information management, performance measurement, and quality management systems. The health care record review program will need to continually change and improve as regulations and accreditation standards evolve to meet increasing demands for accountability. Health record reviews meet many requirements, including mandatory reporting for regulatory and accreditation and for performance monitoring, record completion, and quality improvement. The HIM role in the design and deployment of a health record review program is a vital part of the umbrella of information management.[77-79]

In setting up or modifying an already existing health record review function, an important guiding principle is to incorporate all health record review activities into one encompassing, integrated health record review program, even if the program crosses organizational boundaries. All staff involved in any aspect of the health record review program need to understand the scope of review activities to minimize redundant reviews and conflicting data definitions.

At the heart of this review is documentation analysis of various aspects of the health record. Sometimes organizations use the term *abstracting* to refer to the actual collection of data from the health record. Traditionally, HIM staff and others in the organization such as quality managers, utilization review coordinators, and cancer registry staff, and so forth, reviewed individual records against certain criteria. It was and still is, for the most part, a manual process. The Joint Commission has always included standards that incorporate some type of continuing health record review. Since January 1, 2004, however, The Joint Commission is no longer prescriptive. Instead, the patient specific information standards in the 2010 Hospital Manual RC.01.01.01 through RC.02.03.07 (2010) require an organization to demonstrate and report evidence of standards compliance.[80] To know how well the organization is doing on information management and other standards, the organization needs to collect and analyze data. Consider the following:

- What health record content and standards need monitoring?
- What are current organizational priorities, accrediting, or regulatory agencies?
- Of these priorities, what areas lend themselves to health record review? What performance measures provide information to make a difference in how the organization is doing, if it is meeting its goals, if its customers are satisfied, if processes are in control, or if and where improvements are needed?
- What aspects of care and documentation need or require 100% monitoring or review?
- What aspects require periodic monitoring, how often, and what sampling methods may be used? What is an appropriate sampling size? Note: The most recent Joint Commission accreditation manual presents required sampling sizes for demonstrating compliance.[80]
- How frequently should each review be conducted or reported?
- Where can data collection, analysis, and display make a difference? How much realistically can be done?
- What "canned" reports or automated data are available?
- Who are collaborative stakeholders?
- Who are the organization's executives who are responsible to ensure that a review process is in place?
- Which clinical staff members are willing to champion the review process?
- Who already conducts or could participate in health record reviews? Usually one thinks of HIM and quality management data analysts. There are others who could also perform this type of review: department managers, administrative staff, business managers, clinicians, and so on.
- What would motivate stakeholders to participate in such a program?
- Who decides when and what to collect?
- Who creates and maintains the data dictionaries? (Yes, these are indeed needed!)

Reporting Structure

What reporting structure makes sense in the organization? Remember, it is important to provide the entire organization with a "picture" of how well the organization is performing and the areas needing improvement. It is also important to report results to leaders who will be able to understand the importance of the data and who will plan appropriate action.

Data Presentation

Data should be presented in such a way that information and trends can be readily understood. Graphical displays should always include a narrative description of what is being measured, including the standards; what the data mean; where, when, and how they were collected; a summary of findings; recommendations for improvement; and when and how the changes are being followed up, including a date for re-review.

Types of Review

As mentioned previously, health record review topics are left up to the discretion of the individual health care organization. The Joint Commission does, however, require that health records are to be reviewed "on an ongoing basis at the point of care." They further state that the review is based on "hospital-defined indicators that address the presence, timeliness, readability (whether handwritten or printed), quality, consistency, clarity, accuracy, completeness, and authentication of data and information contained within the record."[80]

Focused reviews, special projects, and documentation improvement activities may all give rise to health record criteria or health record reviews. HIM may be charged with coordinating or performing these reviews. Again, it is important to use consistent data definitions and prevent wasted time through redundant reviews. It may be that data previously collected can be analyzed from a different viewpoint to meet a new need. For example, data collected to track health record delinquency can also be used to pinpoint the timeliness of documentation.

Record Completion Process

In this process, tracking is done primarily for the presence, timeliness, and authentication of health record documentation.

Performance Improvement Plans

Whatever group is receiving a health record review report should be responsible for planning or delegating actions for implementation, when required.

Reports

As mentioned previously, the data collection process is still manual except in those organizations that have a health data repository. If some or all health record data are collected electronically as discrete fields during the documentation process, then it may be possible to use data mining tools to identify patterns or exceptions. If text documents such as the history and physical examinations, progress notes, and so forth are not in discrete fields, most likely a health record analyst will need to read the health record and abstract necessary information. There are electronic data collection tools designed specifically to collect and report on this type of data. Or an organization can decide to build its own tool. Following are examples that used an electronic data collection tool built and maintained by an HIM specialist. Microsoft Access was used to take advantage of its automated data tabulation and extraction functionality. Forms used to collect data are created and completed in an Access database (Figures 6-14 through 6-16).

SELF-ASSESSMENT QUIZ

27. Beyond accreditation requirements, why are structured medical record review programs necessary for health care organizations? What skills do HIM professionals provide to developing and managing such programs?

Release of Information

Once the health record is stored in an electronic format, the release-of-information function processes change dramatically over time. The electronically stored record can be either a true EHR or it can simply be a scanned health record. The term *over time* is important to understand. When requests for information come to HIM, they often include requests

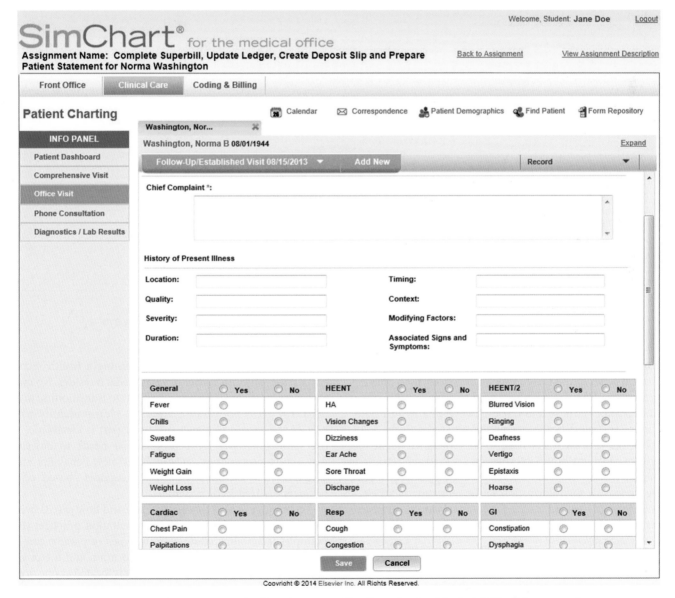

FIGURE 6-14 Sample report A. Elsevier 2014. SimChart for the Medical Office® (www.evolve.elsevier.com).

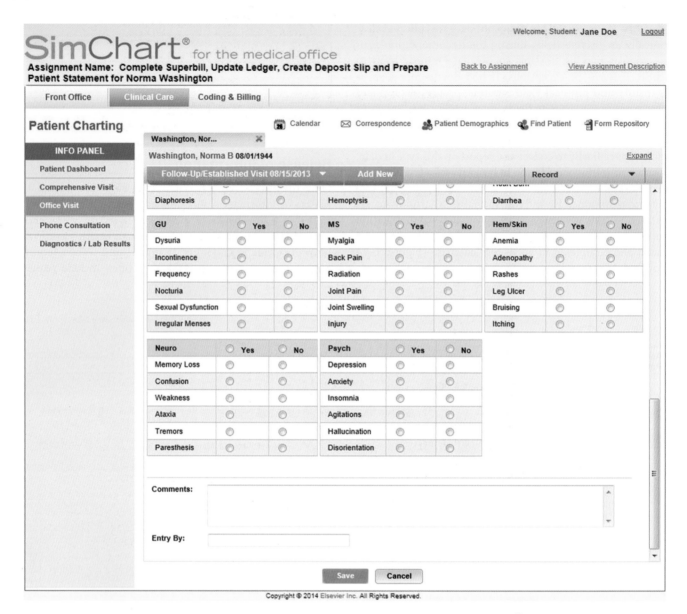

FIGURE 6-15 Sample report B. Elsevier 2014. SimChart for the Medical Office® (www.evolve. elsevier.com).

for older documents. Those documents may be contained in historical paper health records or in a previously used imaging system. The HIM processes will need to address both paper and electronic retrieval and tracking while in a hybrid state. As more and more health information is stored in the EHR system, the processes will need to be redesigned to fit the media in which the health information is stored and retrieved. When all the information retrieved is electronic, it is also possible to provide the information to the requestor in an electronic format such as a CD, DVD, or electronic transfer. This is already the practice in some organizations.

The Future Now

Management of EHRs is already changing the HIM professional's role in how an individual record is created, maintained, and retrieved. Recall that the purposes and

principles for generating and maintaining a health record remain the same, no matter in what media it resides. No matter where an organization is in relation to transitioning to an EHR, the HIM professional needs to clearly identify what part of the record is paper and what part is electronic. At the same time, the HIM professional needs to envision new action possibilities—new policies, new behaviors, new patterns, new methods, new HIM services—based on a reconceptualized EHR system.

Technology is also changing where and how care is being provided, which often affects documentation practices. For example, technology allows certain types of patient care to be set up when the patient is in one location and the physician is in another. Often, the physician is located at one organization and the patient is located at another organization. The physician can interview the patient through live computer video; there may be another clinician, such as a

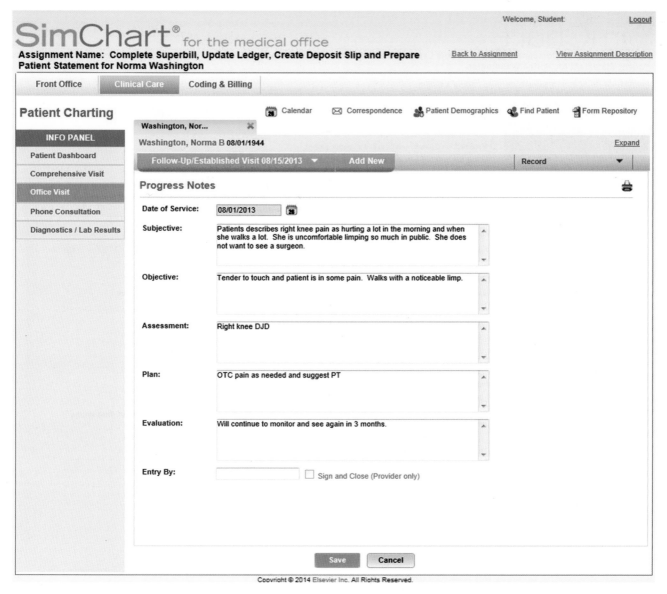

Copyright © 2014 Elsevier Inc. All Rights Reserved.

FIGURE 6-16—Cont'd

registered nurse, who may take the patient's vital signs or perform certain procedures under the direct supervision of the physician through the computer monitor. If there is a provider at both locations, then documentation occurs at both locations, either on paper or by the computer. This technology and care is called *telehealth*. Such a scenario presents a creative challenge for health information staff to develop processes to ensure that documentation and coding standards are met as well as privacy, confidentiality, and security requirements. A similar scenario called *telemonitoring* occurs when the patient has monitoring equipment installed in his or her home and communicates with the health care provider by telephone or computer on scheduled and as-needed times. The documentation may be "fed" to the organization's EHR system and a health care professional such as a nurse may monitor it at scheduled times. Or, if the home monitoring system is not interfaced with the organizations, the nurse may document pertinent information gleaned from the stand-alone system on either paper forms or in the organization's computer system. As in the first scenario, there will need to be policies and documentation processes that are agreed on and followed.

NEEDED CHANGES IN ORGANIZATION POLICIES AND BUSINESS RULES REGARDING ELECTRONIC HEALTH RECORD USERS AND SYSTEMS

Policies

It is critical that an organization's policies be rewritten to reflect changes occurring during the transition from manual to hybrid and, ultimately, to a total EHR system. ABC Hospital's overarching policy description (Box 6-2) of its health record makes this point very clearly. Notice the goal is to "standardize the record." Standardization, an oft-stated aim

FIGURE 6-16 Sample report. Elsevier 2014. SimChart for the Medical Office® (www.evolve.elsevier.com).

BOX 6-2 **Sample Health Record Policy**

ABC Hospital

Health Record Policy

ABC's health record consists of the EHR, scanned documents, and the paper record, combined. Existing policies and procedures pertaining to paper health records apply to computer-generated medical records, including but not limited to, health record delinquencies and deficiencies, responsibility for the accuracy, and authority to make entries and changes in the medical record.

The goal is to standardize the record in relation to its content, creation, maintenance, management, and processing, including quality measures. Electronically stored or printed health information is subject to the same medical and legal requirements as handwritten information in the health record.

EHR, Electronic health record.

---

of EHRs, is an ambitious goal. To accomplish this requires looking at how to normalize documentation for many types of clinicians who learned observation and documentation techniques at different colleges, universities, and training grounds, and who have differing subject matter expertise. Even in the paper world, organizations attempted standardization through the forms committee that had authority to approve or disapprove medical record forms. The forms committee is often a subcommittee of the organization's medical record committee. In the hybrid and electronic worlds, this function becomes critical if the organization decides to use templates to guide documentation of text documents such as an history and physical examination, various types of progress notes, operative reports, discharge summaries, and so forth. Again, it is important to state who has the authority over template design and construction (Box 6-3).

BOX 6-3 **Example of a Health Record Steering Committee Policy**

ABC Hospital

Health Record Steering Committee

The Health Record Steering Committee (HRSC) is responsible for overseeing the contents and quality of the health record. Membership includes the Associate Chief of Staff for Clinical Information Management, the Director of Health Information Management, Clinical Application Coordinators or Health Information Specialists, clinical staff, and other representatives as appointed by the Chief of Staff. The HRSC is co-chaired by the Associate Chief of Staff for Clinical Information Management and the Director of Health Information Management. Subcommittees may be created to address specific issues or needs.

Business Rules

Besides policies, organizations must create business rules. In a paper world, procedures implemented policies. In a hybrid and electronic world, both procedures and business rules implement policies. Policies, procedures, and computer business rules must be in concert with the organization's medical staff bylaws and rules and regulations if the organization has an organized medical staff. Business rules are:

- Prescribed statements
- Usually written as computer procedures, sets of conditions, or formulas
- Useful to define what roles certain or individuals are allowed to carry out.

For example, documentation business rules (Box 6-4) might address the following:

- Who can read entries in the EHR
- Who can write specific or all clinical documents
- Who can dictate documents
- Who can sign documents
- When a co-signature is required
- Who can edit a document and when
- Who can change (amend) a medical record entry
- When a document can be viewed
- Who can retract documents
- Who can scan documents

It is important that the HIM professional be closely involved in writing or reviewing all business rules that affect health record documentation to be sure they accurately reflect the organization's policies. For example, well-written policies, procedures, and computer business rules ensure that only authorized individuals can document in the health record.

Versioning

EHR systems save different iterations of the same document. It is important to save different versions because care decisions can be made at any point when the document is viewable. When are documents viewable? Depending on a specific EHR system, there may or may not be multiple version functionality. This means that once a document is edited, previous versions may or may not be available. It is critical for the HIM professional to understand whether versioning capability exists, at what point change versions are saved, and who can view previous versions. See Box 6-5 for a case study.

Templates

Template design and management is an emerging need in any kind of EHR and requires exquisite attention to detail and a thorough understanding of health record content requirements. It is critical, therefore, for health information specialists to step forward and acquire this skill for whatever EHR system is being implemented in the organization in which he or she is working. Both computer and aesthetic considerations drive template formats, dependent, again, on the system being implemented. A template is a pattern used in CPRs to capture data in a structured manner; it may contain both text and data objects.[81] Templates can be used for progress notes, consultation requests and reports, history and physical examinations, operative reports, and discharges summaries—any document that requires textual health information. There may be different types of templates used by the EHR system from simple plain text templates tools to dialogue and reminder templates. For example, reminder template content may satisfy a clinical reminder such as a diabetic foot examination or a flu shot. It is important for health information specialists to learn the terminology and requirements of whatever system they are working in. Before requesting a new or edited template, there are certain considerations:

BOX 6-4 **Example of Forms Policy**

ABC Hospital

Health Records Forms

All health record forms (paper and electronic templates), overprinting, assembly, and use thereof are under the surveillance and control of the Medical Record Committee. All requests for new health record documents, including templates, must be reviewed by the Health Information Management Director/designee to ensure compliance with policy before submission to the committee for approval. Repetitive fill-in data are the only data authorized to be overprinted on forms approved for use.

BOX 6-5 **Case Study for Discussion**

- Resident signed a dictated discharge summary that included a diagnosis of "CA Chest" (which is what the transcriptionist heard).
- The discharge summary document was viewable by others at this time.
- The attending physician edited and cosigned the summary with a corrected diagnosis of "CHF."
- Which version of the discharge summary was used for what decisions?
- It is critical to address when a document is viewable on the basis of the electronic health record system's capability.

- Does similar content already exist in another template? If yes, can the other template be deactivated?
- Is there some type of mandate for this template?
- Does the proposed content meet required standards (e.g., The Joint Commission, Commission on Accreditation of Rehabilitation Facilities, organizational policies)?

Templates have format requirements that are driven by whatever template software is being used. Template guidelines should require basic grammar requirements that help ensure that a reader understands the content in the template-generated document:

- Is consistent tense used throughout the template?
- Are pronouns consistent?
- Are abbreviations spelled out the first time used?
- Are periods used only after a full sentence and not after a term or phrase?
- Has everything been spell checked?

Because the ultimate purpose of any documentation is to inform the reader about the care encounter, template builders need to remember that many different types of people, users, may read the note. Users become accustomed to their own view of the health record. A view is simply how the reader sees the information on the workstation screen. It is important, therefore, to assist readers in finding information quickly. Proper template design can aid the reader by considering the following:

- Group information into small, manageable units. A manageable unit is one consisting or approximately seven to nine pieces of information.
- Group similar information together.
- After information is organized, provide a label or header for each unit of information.
- For similar subject matter, use similar words, formats, organizations, and sequences.
- Put what the reader needs where the reader needs it.

Titles

Closely aligned with templates are document titles. Before the introduction of word processing to health care organizations in the 1980s, most forms were preprinted and there was very little modification of a form's title. A progress note was a progress note, no matter who wrote on it. An orders form was an orders form. Often, these forms were color coded to make it easy for a reader to find the type of information he or she needed to read or to document. With the introduction of word processing, however, this changed. It was possible to easily create new forms and new titles. Forms "control" began to slip away from the forms committee as various clinical entities in the health care organization decided on new forms that would make their documenting responsibilities easier. They did not always think about the reader who needed to find this information. With word processing, printing is typically on white paper without colored borders. It was not uncommon for a teaching hospital to have more than 1800 different document titles! In the electronic world, it is just as important to consider how a reader of the health record finds needed information. If there are too many titles, the same problem exists. Titles must also come under the oversight of the medical record committee or its forms and template subcommittee.

Electronic Record Maintenance

Besides template design and management, other individual record management functions are different in the electronic world. One of the key functions requiring HIM expertise is managing and performing correction of erroneous documents. The EHR demands a precision that is more detailed than in a manual health record. The stated purposes, therefore, must be elucidated in a policy document. (See Box 6-6 for an example.)

The HIM director and the health record committee need to clearly define all of the terms contained in this type of policy. Depending on the system and policies, following are examples of terms needing definition[39]:

- An *addendum* for a correction must be written by the document's author and includes additional information from the source document. *Addendum* is not to be confused with an *amendment,* which, by definition, is something that the patient requests.
- To *reassign* a document means to change the encounter or patient to which the document is attached.
- To *remove* means to erase the document or a data field within a document as if it never existed. Depending on the system, this action may require a programmer.
- To *retract* an erroneous document means the content is shielded from general view. Viewing is limited to only certain users (e.g., the HIM director).
- To *delete* a document can occur only for unsigned documents that have never been viewed except by the author. The date, time, title of documents, author, and content are completely erased from the system. Notice the difference in definitions between removal and deletion.

ABC's policy document might state the following:

To preserve health record integrity, erroneously entered notes will not be deleted from the database. Depending on the individual case, erroneous notes may be corrected by adding an addendum or by retracting or rescinding the information.

Errors occur in the electronic record for a variety of reasons, some of which include the following:

BOX 6-6 Sample from an Electronic Health Record Document

. . . from an ABC Hospital policy document—document correction:
To protect patients while preserving a complete record of their care, this section establishes procedures to identify when it is appropriate to (1) write an addendum, rescind, reassign, retract, or delete erroneously entered electronic text documents, including progress notes, discharge summaries, surgery reports, addenda, images, and so forth, and to identify when it is appropriate to (2) rescind documents from active use that are no longer applicable, including advance care directives, alerts regarding allergies, adverse reactions, warnings, and agreements to participate in research, and so forth.

ASTM International: http://www.astm.org/. Accessed July 1, 2014.

- A document is created on the wrong patient (e.g., the clinician mistyped the medical record number by one digit).
- A signed document is linked to the wrong clinic visit (e.g., a transcribed document is being signed by the clinician who dictated it and chooses an earlier visit to link the transcribed document to).
- A document has an incorrect designated cosigner (when resident documentation requires an attending physician's signature) (e.g., the resident added the current month's attending physician rather than last month's attending physician when the document was originally written, or Dr. Jones was scheduled to be the attending surgeon but was sick the day of surgery and now Dr. Smith is the correct attending surgeon).
- The wrong title is used and the document's author wishes to change the title (e.g., a note by the emergency department staff was titled "Urgent Care Note" but should have been titled "Employee Health Note." Employee Health Notes raise other issues about privacy and the correct location of the data.).
- A signed consultation report is linked to the wrong consultation request or not attached to a consultation request at all. In an EHR the consultation report should be linked to the request that generated the encounter (e.g., an outpatient, nonurgent consultation was requested of a cardiologist. The patient was subsequently admitted and an urgent cardiac consultation is requested and completed. However, the inpatient report gets attached to the outpatient request, meaning the hospital team may not be notified of the results and the results would show up as part of the outpatient record instead of the inpatient record. Of course, if the result was abnormal or critical result, most often a phone call would be made to the attending physician.).
- Signed document is for the correct patient but the text is so egregiously in error that an addendum to the document will not be clear to a reader (e.g., in an operative report, the surgeon dictates left knee when in fact it is the right knee on which the surgery was performed. Or in an emergency department note, "patient reports taking codeine for pain" as opposed to "patient reports using cocaine for pain").

In addition to policy statements, procedures need to be identified for each of the policies, including who is responsible for carrying out the procedures.

Completion and Authentication

The traditional HIM role of monitoring the completion and authentication of key documents in the medical record does not go away in the electronic environment. Depending on the EHR system installed, there may be electronic tools to identify, sort, and alert clinicians who need to complete their documentation. In the paper world with stand-alone departmental systems, the HIM staff would physically identify what signatures and documents were missing from the discharged patient's record. Staff would generate letters on a monthly basis and send them to physicians. With an organization-wide health information system, it is possible to alert the affected clinicians within a secure electronic e-mail system or when they sign onto the EHR system. Reports may still need to manually be rolled up from spreadsheets or databases. In an even more sophisticated environment with standardized document titles, it may be possible for the EHR system to perform almost real-time monitoring and alerts for documentation needs. For example, if a patient is admitted and there is no history and physical examination in the record within 8 hours of admission, the system could automatically page the identified HIM staff to contact the responsible clinician's office or the system could directly page the admitting clinician. It is possible to design reports and graphs that are automatically generated by clinical services and individual clinicians. As mentioned previously, this function may be subsumed in an organizational health record review program.

Printing

The HIM professional must seriously consider the printing issues in an EHR environment. Does the EHR system support printing functionality? Most of these systems are not designed to produce paper. When printing from an EHR, the volume of paper increases by at least 25% and even much more if only one side of the paper is printed. When a document is printed, it must be in a format that is understandable by the reader. Often, because the systems were not designed for printing, printed output is not useful for the reader. For example, when printing progress notes, the program may simply run them together, making it difficult for the eye to find the particular needed notes. HIM professionals who have implemented EHR systems strongly discourage printing electronic data and documents and recommend from the very beginning of any EHR implementation project that the concept of "no printing" be discussed and a transition date be set to go "no printing." In the meantime, decide whether the print functionality can be restricted by role description. If "print screen" is an option in the system, can it be controlled? Decide who can print, why printing a document is necessary, and what and when a user can print. Decide who is authorized to print the entire medical record and if there will be designated areas for printing. For example, HIM could be authorized to print documentation for release of information, transfer of records, and archiving records. Be sure to consider privacy issues of printed documents whether printing in one's own organization or printing remotely.

There needs to be accountability for printing. If possible, the user name and ID should be printed on each document. Use caution, however, with printing the user's name. The organization's name and location should also be on each page of the printed document. There should be a statement in the document footer or header that reads, "If document received in error, please contact the corporate privacy officer at XXX-XXXX."

Decide on a strategy on how to stop routine printing. For example:

- Make sure there are enough workstations for viewing.
- Mandate computer entry for all staff through official committees.

- Phase printing out and electronic entry in. Remember, however, they are asynchronous because they are phased in and out at different rates.
- Identify when there are enough documents in the system to stop printing.
- Make sure users know where to find the information in the her.
- Publicize what you are doing broadly. Make sure both staff and patients are aware as changes are being planned.

- Decide when you can routinely stop delivery of the hard copy chart. This can be phased in by location depending on receptivity of the staff.
- Continue to educate.
- Publicize and celebrate milestones.

Recognize that a print function will be required and that there should be some planning related to printing documents in readable formats. Box 6-7 shows a snapshot of how one health care organization migrated to the EHR.

BOX 6-7   **Benchmark Data—Department of Veterans Affairs: Puget Sound Health care System's Transition to an Electronic Health Record**

The Way We Were

Up until the late 1990s, this hospital had a limited hybrid environment. Basically, laboratory and radiology reports were electronic but still filed in the hard copy chart. All other documentation was either handwritten or transcribed, "wet signed"/handwritten and filed in the hard copy chart. In the 1990s, the paper record included the following:

- Progress notes
- Physician orders
- Consultations
- Medication flow sheets
- Discharge summaries
- Other flow sheets
- Printed laboratory reports
- Consents
- Printed x-ray reports
- Printed ECGs
- Printed pathology reports
- Diagnostic studies
- Procedure reports

As in any hybrid system, the paper chart was pulled for scheduled and unscheduled appointments and admissions, for coding, for quality review, for utilization review, and so forth. Some processes had to wait until the record could be "corralled" long enough to complete the work. Even with an excellent chart tracking system, charts were available to clinic appointments only 95% of the time, and when other processes such as coding required the chart, it may have been taken before the record was coded, necessitating another retrieval and use of staff time. Filing documents into the paper record was difficult because the records were constantly moving into and out of the medical record file unit. If a clinician wanted the most up-to-date information and requested the hard copy chart, it was often not available because the filing was waiting for the chart to remain long enough in the unit for filing to occur.

What We Decided

In the mid-1990s, much discussion focused on what the organization needed from a health record system. Availability was one of the key identified needs. Other major needs included saving space (decreasing the amount of paper in the chart and the physical size of the file area), ease of clinician documentation and timeliness of document completion, readability (making documents more consistent in their formats), and legibility. Clinicians clearly stated a preference to refer to only one source for each type of information, meaning they did not want to look in the computer and in the paper chart for laboratory results or progress notes and so forth. The organization decided that an EHR implementation was required to meet the identified major needs. It was recognized that this required a substantial investment of resources into technology, hardware, software, hiring specialized staff, as well as an enormous educational effort for every level of clinical and administrative staff.

What We Did

Starting in about 1995, clinician order entry was mandated for all inpatient orders and was allowed for any outpatient order. **To require clinician direct order entry at the beginning of an EHR implementation is unusual for most EHR implementations.** The decision was largely driven by patient safety and the need to get the clinicians on board. Pharmacy was another advocate for direct order entry for prescriptions. With direct order entry, prescriptions could be filled faster because pharmacists would no longer need to contact clinicians because of legibility issues for both the actual prescription and the prescriber. Physician order entry resulted in fewer erroneous or duplicate tests and allowed near real-time electronic results reporting back to the ordering physician, who knew the results were ready because he or she received an electronic alert. Despite some resistance, the transition went quickly and fairly smoothly and resulted in a clinician base that was beginning to be comfortable using a computer to input and receive clinical information about their patient. By mid-1997, radiology and laboratory results, orders, and order results were available online.

In 1997, we decided to expand the use of the EHR and established a rough time frame to phase in various components. Beginning almost immediately, all discharge summaries for inpatient stays more than 48 hours were required to be either direct entered or dictated, transcribed, and uploaded to the EHR. Stays less than 48 hours could still be handwritten on a special form. The mandated use of electronic progress notes was phased in by one clinical service at a time and by one inpatient ward at a time. At this point, outpatient use was voluntary, and some clinicians chose to directly enter their progress notes in the clinics.

In 1998, the decision was made to stop printing radiology and laboratory results because clinicians were used to viewing the results on the computer screen. This meant the file unit no longer had to file these voluminous reports. HIM, however, was still delivering hard copy charts to both inpatient units and clinics. As stated earlier, clinicians had always wanted "one-stop shopping" for reviewing patient history. At this point, HIM was still printing every progress note and filing it in the paper chart. In fact, we continued printing and filing until 1999.

By January 1999, all levels and types of clinicians on all inpatient units were using electronic progress notes and orders. This meant they both entered data through the EHR and viewed the information on computer screens. At this point, inpatient orders and progress notes ceased being printed daily but were still being printed at discharge and filed in the paper chart because there was a clinical concern that there be hard copy documentation if the computer system went down.

Continued

BOX 6-7 Benchmark Data—Department of Veterans Affairs: Puget Sound Health care System's Transition to an Electronic Health Record—cont'd

To address the very real patient safety issue of what to do when there was computer down time, scheduled or unscheduled, the organization came up with a creative idea. Each inpatient unit, the emergency department, and several outpatient areas were issued special "downtime computers." These devices had dedicated power supplies and memories robust enough to accept regular downloads several times an hour for all current inpatients (on inpatient units) and all scheduled outpatients for the previous day, the current day, and the next day (in the emergency department and outpatient areas). A summary document is created for each patient and includes a variety of components: the last three discharge summaries, the past 7 days' progress notes for inpatients, the past year of outpatient progress notes for outpatients, current medication lists, problem lists, laboratory and radiology results, and so forth. The system rolls up the components, creates the summary document, and pushes all of the summaries to each downtime computer.

Meanwhile, in the outpatient arena, a similar phased approach was being implemented beginning in mid-1998. Primary Care volunteered to be the pilot. By June 2000, all outpatient clinics were required to enter progress notes directly into the computer. Initial assessments were allowed to be dictated, transcribed, and uploaded; all other notes were required to be entered directly.

By June 2000, it was recognized that no one was referring to the hard copy chart for inpatient orders or notes. Therefore all printing ceased for inpatient cases. In the outpatient setting, many clinicians felt they needed a 2-year history before they could give up the hard copy chart. HIM negotiated halting printing on a specialty-by-specialty basis and stopped printing outpatient progress notes in July 2000 and began phasing out chart deliveries 6 months later, again, specialty by specialty. By 2004, only the eye clinic still required paper charts because of the eye drawings and non-computerized testing equipment where handwritten results were used. The eye testing equipment could not be interfaced into the EHR. In 2005, however, new eye testing equipment was purchased that allowed direct entry into the EHR of these important tests.

During 2003, the organization began scanning selected documents, including advance directives, power of attorney for general and health care, and certain financial records. Because of the phased in use of electronic notes, it was decided not to back-scan previous health record documentation. Without a robust, precise indexing system designed for easy, efficient retrieval of imaged documents by the end users, it is very difficult and time consuming to locate and retrieve the needed scanned images. Any scanned documentation was viewable on the same clinical workstations.

By June 2000, a mandate stated that any clinical documentation that could be entered into the EHR had to be done electronically. By June 2001, anything that was in the EHR was no longer printed for inclusion in the paper record. There were, however, certain exemptions granted by the Medical Record Steering Committee that allowed handwritten documentation, either because of software limitations or staffing issues. Also, because of software limitations, medication and intensive care unit flow sheets remained handwritten.

Paper Chart Status—2006

Throughout 2006, the organization continued to mandate the use of the EHR exclusively where possible. HIM received some loose filing for inclusion in the paper chart including:

- Intensive care unit and certain other flow sheets
- Hand drawings
- Outside documents

When requested by physicians, HIM staff scanned and indexed outside documents including discharge summaries, consultation reports, operative reports and other clinical documents.

- "Downtime" documents (i.e., any handwritten documents created during a downtime)
- Consents

During this time, we were still phasing in an online patient consent program in which the patient, the clinician, and witness sign online.

EHR Status—2010

By the beginning of 2010, Puget Sound's medical record and radiology file rooms had both been closed for 4 years. Because VA Puget Sound is a federal organization, medical records are governed by federal retention requirements. These requirements state that medical records remain on site at the hospital for 3 years after the last patient encounter and then are sent to a federal records archival center for another 72 years. These records, however, are often called back for one or more reasons.

One of the innovative processes the HIM department at Puget Sound developed was to identify those documents most likely to be recalled and scan and index them. This process is an enhancement to an older (no longer mandated) Veterans' Health Administration requirement for a perpetual medical record (PMR). PMRs were specific documents on individual patients from certain episodes of care and selected administrative documents that were maintained at the facility after retirement of the medical record. Every time a paper medical record is recalled from archives means there is a cost to the hospital. After identifying these key documents, HIM staff looked through every individual paper medical record being prepared for archiving and pulled specific documents from the record. As mentioned previously, these documents were then scanned and indexed in the appropriate patient's EHR. Did this take a lot of time? Was this staff resource intensive? Yes, to both questions. But the result was to reduce the amount of time and resources that would have been spent in the years to come when these documents are needed. Creating a PMR saved the hospital approximately $50,000 over the past 4 years since the file rooms were closed. Additionally, scanned documents combined with those in the EHR means most release of information requests are fulfilled on the same day as the request. There is no need to wait several weeks for records to be recalled from the archives.

In 2010, two remaining types of paper records were still being maintained by HIM. One type was the radiation oncology record that had never previously been filed in the HIM medical record and had been stored separately in the oncology area until 2007, at which time they were brought to the HIM department for filing and maintenance. In 2010, they could not be scanned because of their size and because they contained printed radiologic images that could not be scanned to clinical standards. The other type of record was the dental record that included dental x-rays. HIM storage of dental records was phased out in July 2010 because of two activities: all older dental progress notes had been completely scanned into the EHR and all on-site dental x-rays were sent to the dental department for filing. Because Puget Sound now has a dental electronic record that includes digitized images that are automatically transferred with the reports to the EHR, older films are being phased out.

Continued

BOX 6-7	Benchmark Data—Department of Veterans Affairs: Puget Sound Health care System's Transition to an Electronic Health Record—cont'd

EHR Status—2013

By the middle of 2013, VA Puget Sound's EHR was more comprehensive, using newer technology including both nonportable and portable mobile devices to collect patient care information that is either electronically or manually uploaded into the EHR system. For example:

- There is now a wireless network installed in the main hospital building, which allows provider outpatient documentation and accompanying clinical codes to be captured by a data vendor product, which is then imported into the EHR system.
- Various radiology devices, echocardiograms devices, vascular images (Doppler studies), and vitals telehealth carts all use the wireless network to upload patient documentation into the EHR.
- Cardiac catheter images will soon be able to be loaded directly into the radiology PACS.
- ECGs are kept on a separate server until authenticated by the cardiologist; then a technician manually loads the image and the report into the EHR.
- In the operating room, an electronic anesthesia system takes information directly from the patient; data is then manually uploaded as a PDF to the EHR.
- An outside cardiology company, Holter, sends imaged reports to a Puget Sound secure website. A Puget Sound ECG technician moves the images and reports to secure drives where the cardiologist signs on, reviews the entire Holter ECG report, writes a summary report and signs it electronically. The ECG technician then imports the whole imaged report and attaches it to the cardiologist-authenticated summary report.
- If a VA patient is at home and has been set up for remote monitoring, blood pressure monitors, blood sugar monitor, or pacemakers (internal defibrillator devices), a camera for wound surveillance allows VA nurses to interact with patients using a telephone or computer.
- Using a personal identification verification (PIV) card rather than a wet signature on a paper script, Puget Sound providers can now use e-prescribing for needed narcotics for their patients. Before this could happen, it had to be approved by both the FDA and the VA's national Office of Information and Technology. The provider must have a card reader to use this technology. If a physician is prescribing at home and has a card reader, it no longer makes a difference as to what is being prescribed. In general, the PIV badge improves staff identification by a computer and the ability to get into specific programs.
- Clinical reminders now include diabetes foot and eye examinations and rechecks for diabetics with blood pressure above a certain level, as well as many others such as the annual flu shot, pneumonia vaccine, colon cancer screening, depression screening, and posttraumatic stress syndrome screening.

In addition to external paper medical records received by Puget Sound that must be scanned and indexed, in late 2013 certain internal paper medical record documents are sent to HIM for scanning and indexing. These include handwritten, patient-generated health questionnaires, flow sheets, any patient wet-signed discharge instructions, inpatient valuables, belongings and patient-carried medications, certain mental health agreements between a patient and physician, and advance care directives on a VA-developed form. Also, when there is a computer downtime, clinicians can choose to write their progress notes on paper; these are also scanned and indexed in the VistA Imaging system. (This happens infrequently.)

There are still EHR problems that require collaboration among clinicians, the information technology department, administration, HIM experts, and sometimes vendors to come up with workable solutions. For example, interfaces are often required to move information from vendor medical devices that are separate from the EHR; writing these interfaces is expensive and time consuming. It is also still a time-intensive process to design, program, test, and revise new templates. An EHR cannot create the documentation for clinicians. It can make documentation easier and faster, but the clinician is still responsible to create the document, make sure it is accurate and complete and then to authenticate it. A good EHR allows documentation templates to be used; by increasing the number and robustness of these templates, overall documentation can be enhanced, especially in light of the impending implementation of ICD-10-CM.

Besides continuing to improve the EHR to make it more functionally friendly for clinicians, there are projects that the VA and Puget Sound have been working on for some time:

- MyHealtheVet, the VA's award-winning online PHR has a mission to improve health care for all veterans by providing one-stop online access to better manage health, make informed health decision, and store important health and military history information. Veterans are now able to view their information within 7 days of their visit or discharge.
- The virtual lifetime electronic record (VLER) is a free and voluntary program that shares parts of a veteran's health record between the Department of Veterans' Affairs, the Department of Defense and selected private health care providers over a secure network known as the Nationwide Health Information Network. This is important because many veterans receive a portion of their health care from non-VA health care providers. This program will reduce the need for patients to carry records among health care providers. The parts of the record that will be shared include a list of health problems, allergies, medications, vital signs, immunizations, laboratory tests, and some notes.

Status—2014

During the past 30 years, Puget Sound's medical record department has evolved from a traditional, manual, paper-based department to a hybrid department with certain electronic record elements to a fully functioning, robust EHR system used throughout its hospitals, clinics, and all clinical programs. It began its journey as the Medical Information Section (MIS):

- 1984 MIS reports to the Business Office.
- 1989 Coding reports to Quality Assurance under Chief of Staff.
- 1991 MIS disbanded; functions relocated to other services.
- 1996 MIS reconstituted, including coding; now called HIM services; reports to the Business Office.
- 1998 HIM now reports to chief information officer and Information Services Section (ISS).
- 2007 HIM and Clinical Information Management (CIM) merge into new Service Line (SL), still called *ISS;* former HIM chief named SL director; reports to chief operations officer.
- 2009 Privacy and Freedom of Information Act (FOIA) officer placed directly under chief executive officer.
- 2010 ISS name changed to Clinical and Health Informatics (CHI).
- 2013 Privacy and FOIA Officer placed back under CHI

Continued

BOX 6-7	Benchmark Data—Department of Veterans Affairs: Puget Sound Health care System's Transition to an Electronic Health Record—cont'd

CHI includes all of the traditional HIM functions: scanning and indexing, coding, release of information, dictation and transcription, health record and health data review, and data management. Its span of control and influence also encompasses clinical information management (those who provide services to clinicians regarding anything to do with the EHR), MyHealtheVet, VLER, Telehealth, Privacy, FOIA, and the facility's records management program.

CHI is at the forefront of making quality improvement changes, not only in HIM but in the clinical workflows and business processes where so much health information is created. HIM and CIM work collaboratively with clinicians to develop and improve on the templates that are key to clinician productivity.

Puget Sound's EHR journey is not yet complete; in fact, it will never be complete. It began in the 1990s as a discussion of major needs and goals regarding clinical information:

- Availability
- Saving space
- Ease of clinical documentation and timeliness of completion
- Readability
- One source for all clinical information

These goals have long been accomplished with one exception as discussed previously: an EHR cannot actually create clinical documentation. During this EHR journey, the organization has seen that the EHR can do so much more than originally envisioned. Clinicians, CHI staff, administrators, general staff, and vendors have all learned to see, expect, and ask much more from the EHR. This technology begets newer technology, fresh perspectives, and excitement from those who work with it. The EHR has and will continue to transform how patient care is delivered.

Lessons Learned

- The HIM Director and key HIM staff must be involved in the early discussions and planning for an EHR implementation to ensure that information and documentation principles are considered in the design. It is far more difficult to make a change in an implemented system than to design it in the first place.
- Regular, scheduled downtime (for system maintenance, updates, patching, etc.) decreases the amount of unscheduled downtime and allows staff to plan and become familiar with downtime contingency processes.
- Although not discussed in the case, a strong clinical champion is absolutely the most important element in a successful implementation.
- A strong, collegial HIM director who can work with the clinical champion, executive leadership, and clinical and administrative staff is also key to a successful implementation. Building trust and maintaining positive relationships throughout the organization is necessary for optimal results.
- Clearly define milestones when objectives will be met are necessary.
- Celebrate successes often; publicize them, especially when others have made the success happen!
- Be open to change and protect the integrity of the health record in whatever forms or stage it happens to be at any specific moment.
- Remember, plans change as implementation progresses; be flexible and adapt to what the organization needs.

Special thanks to Sean Longosky, VA Puget Sound Director, Clinical and Health Information and to Terry Liljencrantz, VA Puget Sound Records Manager.

VIRTUAL HEALTH INFORMATION MANAGEMENT DEPARTMENT

The "future now" means living and working as if the future EHR is already here. What might this mean to a traditional HIM department that is bound by physical constraints because the business processes must take place near where the physical, paper record is located? If the organization is transitioning to a hybrid or EHR status and business processes will no longer be tied to the paper, physical record, the HIM department must consider the possibility of a virtual HIM department—one where many HIM business processes are conducted outside the physical organization. If the file room will soon only reside in computer servers, if coding and transcription are done from home, if one can have meetings by phone or Internet, what are the challenges HIM professionals must address as we migrate to different and more sophisticated technologies for supporting patient care documentation?

HOW DO INDUSTRY CHALLENGES AFFECT ELECTRONIC HEALTH RECORD PLANNING, IMPLEMENTATION, AND BENEFITS REALIZATION?

Selected Milestones

To achieve the benefits sought in the health information systems and associated EHRs discussed in this chapter, the health care industry must address a number of challenges. These include:

- Cost requirements to get EHR system projects under way
- Technology infrastructure requirements and customer expectations
- Legislation that lags behind the uses of technology
- Privacy and security concerns
- Inadequate progress in health informatics standards
- The culture of changes in healthcare

Cost Issues

Capital requirements and on-going high maintenance costs are the primary barrier to EHR acquisition and implementation. Costs associated with EHRs continue to present the most significant challenge to the industry. The basic cost of the EHR products is just the beginning. In addition to the cost of the products, project development and management, vendor selection, consultants, system implementation, interfaces and networks, and training need to be considered. It isn't surprising that a 2009 report in the *New England Journal of Medicine* reported only 1.5% of U.S. hospitals have a comprehensive EHR and 7.6% have a basic version. And few definitive studies exist that provide useful information on economic benefits for those that are in place. In fact, it has been pointed out that evaluating components of EHRs will produce conflicting results.[82] By 2013 HIMSS Analytics reported that by 2011, the number of hospitals at level 7 had grown to 66. By 2012 a record number of 40 hospitals had reached the EMR Adoption Model stage 7.[83]

Once the system is in place, value opportunities of the EHR stem from several attributes. Among them are:

- Enhanced knowledge asset for clinical and administrative purposes
- Standard descriptive nomenclature
- Utilization review– and quality assurance–driven rules
- Storage of discrete clinical data with expanded opportunities for users
- Improved care process driven by information availability
- CPOE
- CDS
- Interdisciplinary, fully integrated critical paths
- Integrated medication cycle with potential for improving patient safety
- Alerts and reminders for the care process and health services
- Protocols (care algorithms)
- Improved documentation
- Improved operational processes from the care cycle to information management
- Instant records access for clinical and administrative purposes
- Faster claims processing
- Coding efficiencies
- Revenue cycle enhancements
- Enhanced medical management
- Support for strategy
- Customer satisfaction—patients, clinicians and administrative staff
- Administrative decision support
- Patient safety
- Support for strategic initiatives[84]

Still, there has been progress. Although studies are few, there is evidence emerging that some components in EHRs are proving to be cost beneficial. As noted in a 2009 research report of Texas hospitals' use of EHRs, per-patient hospital costs were reduced by $538 for each 10-point increase in the integration of computerized decision support systems into the clinical care process. In that same study, researchers found that per-patient costs were reduced by $110 for each 10-point increase in electronic reporting of test results.[85]

Along with the results from this study, the earlier example from the Geisinger Clinic experience points out the value of innovation in revising operational and clinical processes that advance innovation and improve the health care experience.[6]

This list and the examples offer a view into the range of potential cost benefit. Also, the list includes some basics that aid HIM managers and others to advance the case for EHRs for their organizations within an issues document or a white paper. Facts about operational workflow from existing and anticipated viewpoints can incorporate benchmark data for decision making and contribute to the strategic planning process when organizations mount institutional initiatives for acquiring EHR systems.

Infrastructure Requirements

As already discussed in this chapter, fundamental infrastructure is essential to EHR developments. The computing power must be established with appropriate technology and tools so that the users can readily access the information across applications in efficient ways. The enterprise information technology strategy dictates the potential for all systems. Customers expect access and easy navigation to crucial health information. The care team relies on sufficient resources to aid daily care activities as well as an option to use handheld and other devices to access their patient's information. The research by Jha and his team found that time-saving upgrades of calling up laboratory results onscreen had been implemented by 75% of the hospitals surveyed, illustrating that implementing online access to laboratory results is a powerful benefit.[82]

As efforts advance to strengthen data capture at the point of care, workstations (stationary or mobile) need to be accessible by those who direct care from internal, mobile, and external sites. As data repositories grow and access to expert systems and research expands, the customer expects that the necessary infrastructure will move and deliver data and images—not to mention video—at a credible speed. Continuous assessment and expansion of the technology infrastructure go hand in hand with EHR developments. The infrastructure required for EHR systems depends on upfront investment, continuing support, and a tolerance for adding emerging technological tools. The challenge for HIE has been targeted by the federal government who issued contracts to health care organizations and business entities to build HIE capability. The ARRA legislation calls for interoperability as a requirement to demonstrate meaningful use of EHR systems.[4]

Laws and Progress

In addition to managing institutional requirements needed to meet federal regulations for EHRs, there are state-by-state variations in laws related to EHR systems that will need attention. Electronic signature, format, retention, and e-discovery are examples. In most states general business laws recognize the use of computerized records and digital signatures. The storage methods used for EHR systems vary. Tools in place that access EHR historical content may be quite different as the technology evolves. In addition to meeting external compliance requirements, providing longitudinal data across multiple provider sites is needed. Because of some state laws and the concern about the long-term accessibility of digital data, many organizations feel compelled to retain paper record printouts of EHRs.

The focus on developing the EHR system has been primarily from a clinical and billing perspective of getting the data into the system and meeting short-term use requirements. Easy access to data over long periods requires much more planning and maintenance. In fact, longitudinal EHRs can be enterprise assets in which analysis and research benefits yield improvements in understanding the health care environment as well as the health status of the population. In addition to these basic business aspects, federal and state laws also involve privacy and security of personal health information.

Privacy and Security

Privacy and security are continuing topics of discussion and the subjects of state and national legislation. If the goal is to implement EHRs to reach national goals, EHR systems need to protect the privacy of patient data, provide appropriate access, and use recognized data security measures.[86] This is not entirely a "systems" issue. Providing a secure and confidential system involves people. Many of the measures that will ensure patient confidentiality and security are embedded in commitments from the people who handle health information. These individuals must be trained, know the constraints on the use of health information, and be subject to penalty for misuse of the information. HIM professionals have always been part of the health care system's effort to protect the confidentiality and security of health information. In today's environment, HIM professionals often have more comprehensive roles in enterprise privacy and security oversight. The privacy and security standards in the HIPAA legislation of 1996 and the ARRA legislation of 2009 reinforced this activity. And individual state laws also address the matter.

Privacy is the right of individuals to control disclosure of their personal information. Confidentiality is an ethical and a legal concept endorsed by health professionals to meet the expectation of patients that their information, when provided to an authorized user, will not be redisclosed or misused. Data security refers to the technical and procedural methods by which access to confidential information is controlled and managed. Laws frequently guide how confidentiality and privacy concepts are applied. Incorporating these concepts into policies for health information systems and the EHR brings new challenges. Access to health information within and organizational context is based on users'

legitimate need to know to perform their jobs. Providers restrict access to specific applications or elements of patient health information according to the requesting individuals' role in the organization and audit or verify that individuals stay within the boundaries of appropriate use.

Within organizations, on the operations side, health information professionals are typically responsible for overseeing confidentiality matters and updating organizational policies and procedures. Many of these policies and procedures have their roots in paper-based systems and need to be updated. The privacy polices need to be supported by the technical systems design. Comprehensive system and physical security tools are in place in most organizations. (See Chapter 8 for additional discussion of security measures.) The goal is to have sufficient protection from unauthorized or inadvertent access, disclosure, modification, or destruction. As more data become available in electronic format, more users will want access from a wider variety of locations with relative ease. The access and use will need to protect an individual's privacy by use of approaches that apply people and system security measures. To manage the confidentiality and **data security** needs in health information systems effectively, we need to establish the following:

- Institutional oversight groups to recommend policies, approve procedures, and recommend appropriate access and management strategies
- Operational policies and procedures, including confidentiality statements signed by all staff
- Thorough education programs for all health facility staff on confidentiality and data security responsibility and accountability
- Individual user identification for all staff based on their role in the organizations and keyed to their "need to know" to perform their job functions
- Individual passwords, key cards, and biometric or other means for precise registering of system access
- Monitoring and audit capability for access tracking and follow-up
- Management reports on access and potential confidentiality breaches for line managers to use in supervising staff
- Human resources policies to manage the consequences when staff breach confidentiality

Health Care Information Standards and Interoperability

The role of standards in the health information system environment cannot be overemphasized. Standards are agreed-on conventions for using terms, code schemes, and processes used to establish information system requirements and processes, and to designate technical specifications. In health care, advances are continuing as discussed earlier in the chapter. As standards continue to bring consistent data and interoperability capability, health informatics and information management professionals will play an ongoing role. Partners including The Joint Commission and other accrediting bodies, the federal government, ASTM, HL7, Digital Imaging and Communications in Medicine, Institute of Electrical and Electronics Engineers, and other standards development groups will be in the game. Coding systems are standards. Computer systems that use common data definitions recognized throughout a particular industry are using standards.

The goals haven't changed. To meet consistent and reliable access to longitudinal health care information on patients, we must agree on the following:

- A vocabulary so that the meaning of terms can be trusted and that information can be compared among institutions
- Conventions to be used to transmit data from one computer system to another to meet interoperability requirements
- Communications protocols if an electronic superhighway is to be achieved for the health care industry
- Technical security standards to be used within the information infrastructure if the American public is to accept the technology benefits inherent in patient data automation

Work on developing standards for these areas has been under way for more than 30 years in voluntary standard setting groups and the federal government discussed in this and other chapters in this text. Thoughtful planners, clinicians, and systems developers have recognized that agreements on standards would be essential to successful advancement of interconnected systems. Although individual system developers build and market individual systems that meet the needs of one or more organizations, it is clear that compelling forces such as health care reform, technology imperatives, market advantage, cost containment, and the changing nature of health care delivery itself demand that standards development be pursued cooperatively rather than competitively. Both the federal government and private sector recognize the value of standards.

The standards initiatives have been reinforced through HIPAA and, more recently, the ARRA legislation. This legislation called for standards methods to transmit codes for billing and claims. The Medicare drug legislation requires standards for transmitting prescription data electronically with use of National Council on Prescription Drug Programs standards. Table 6-5 features key standards associated with EHR systems, their source development organization, and their general purpose. Figure 6-17 illustrates the relationship between exchange standards and the EHR.

Challenge to Health Information Professionals

Sustaining quality through transition to a true EHR is the continuing challenge. Mastering the future requires a solid "feet on the ground" understanding of how the basic information processing activities function in health delivery settings in both paper and hybrid environments and the capacity to track, anticipate, and plan for the future reality.

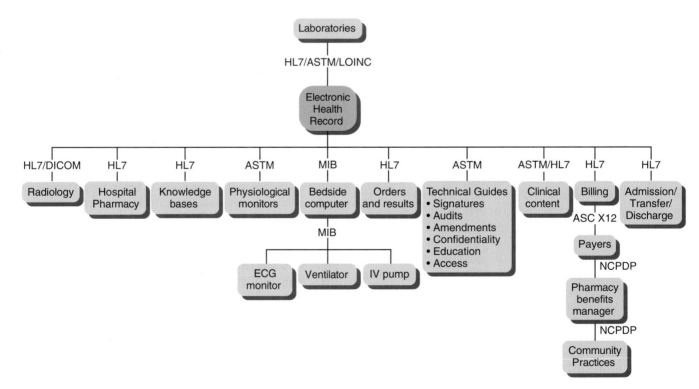

FIGURE 6-17 Data exchange standards and the electronic health record. *ASC X 12*, ***; *ASTM*, American Society for Testing and Materials; *DICOM*, Digital Imaging and Communications in Media; *ECG*, electrocardiogram; *HL7*, Health Level 7; *IV*, intravenous; *LOINC*, Logical Observation Identifier Name Code; *MIB*, ***; *NCPDP*, National Council on Prescription Drug Programs.

What actions need to be taken to both advance the EHR initiatives in individual organizations and maintain fundamental quality in patient data and data systems fundamental to day-to-day operations? Further, how can health information interoperability be planned and executed as more EHRs are in place? As a future HIM professional, consider what strategies you will choose and commit to as you embark in leadership and team initiatives on various transition projects on the way to an EHR.

1. Build on the professional competencies identified within our professional community. Strive to achieve skills in leadership in information governance, enterprise team administration, domain expertise, health information data steward, team-based collaborative skills, and, if interested, more detailed aspects of the technology side. The challenges are many, and there are good options.

2. Build and maintain your knowledge. Educate yourself and your health care organizations, practitioners, and consumers to prepare for enterprise EHRs. Recognize and acquire a solid understanding of EHR systems as enterprise-level systems, their capabilities, the benefits and challenges realized so far, and the laws and standards that affect them and track the intentions of industry leaders and the environmental scan on EHR progress across the delivery spectrum. Study the pathways anticipated to accomplish meaningful use of the EHR in health care organizations. Health care is increasing the use of technology in everyday operations and adapting innovative ways for those in health care organizations to communicate with their peers, their practitioners, and their patients.

3. Embrace consumer informatics and work with consumers to coordinate their health information needs through technology, already happening through secure portals where they can access their own medical records. Develop policies and methods to transfer their information to PHR products as well. Meaningful use requirements call for better patient engagement. As this occurs, providers can rely on up-to-the-minute data and research to communicate with patients. We will foster a different kind of patient—one who can function as a stronger member of the health care team.

SELF-ASSESSMENT QUIZ

28. Prepare a communication plan for educating staff and consumers about planned service changes to take effect as an EHR system is implemented in your organization. Access web-based resources to supplement information in this chapter.

4. Upgrade organizational policies and procedures to redefine the patient record and move from a paper record to the new EHR system. This work is modeled at national and state association levels as well as within individual institutions. Hybrid "how to's" offer road maps and recommend concrete measures to support the hybrid to electronic developments. Plan for multimedia patient health information to grow in a clinically designated "virtual" record. This helps formalize the data system's content as part of the patient record. Use established e-HIM recommendations and insights in addressing this preparation.

5. Recommend, coordinate, and participate in programs that stage EHR-related development within information systems master plans that sponsor EHR systems as an enterprise-level initiative. This endorses the concept of a unifying principle. Research and conceptualize how EHR systems come online and identify how migration master plans work. Benchmarks are available to help identify examples. Learn about them. Some of these go hand in hand to cover the most return on investment and, at the same time, extend value added to multiple customers.

6. Actively support revised legal frameworks so that federal and state legislation allows the transition from paper to electronic media to occur. State laws are in the process of being realigned with federal requirements in these areas. Promulgate the new federal definition of qualified EHRs to clinicians and staff. New definitions of the legal patient record, accepted changes in storage requirements, and automated authentication techniques are all needed to advance the work. Legislation on digital signatures paved the way to electronic authentication at a new level.[87]

SELF-ASSESSMENT QUIZ

29. Revise existing policies on health information disclosure for a community hospital based on your review of legislative provisions and guidelines.

7. Lead and participate in reengineering current user processes. We need to prepare the operational workflow for change. We have learned that simply installing computer systems for existing business processes fails to realize the benefits. Business processes, the way we move patients through appointment, check-in, care, and follow-up, must be reexamined. Along with other business processes, track the data flows in detail. These workflows require careful review to see whether there are more efficient ways to accomplish them. This applies to the way we organize and use the patient record content and formats. The notion of continuously improving our business processes to be sure that the best methods are in place fits in with the quality management philosophy and principles. We can expect to reengineer patient-related care processes; update the processes used to capture, document, and transfer the resulting health information; and design better ways to use this information. Reengineering means fundamental rethinking and transforming business processes to achieve dramatic performance improvements with radical redesign. Cost, quality, service, and speed of operations can be improved. Considering

that providers are expected to incorporate new technology in direct care practices, examining how data capture and retrieval can occur most efficiently, particularly across functional processes and departments, can lead to better alternatives.

8. As the EHR moves into place, move from change management to administrative management. Incorporate a thorough knowledge of the effect of change on the workforce into administrative direction and oversight from a top-down approach. We know that technology affects organizational culture, including structure and design. It changes work flows and brings in new job designs and responsibilities. Some functions go away entirely. Staff requires new skills and knowledge to perform their work. Worker motivation and incentives call for new communications and operations policies and procedures to build the kind of strong teamwork required to absorb change. Human resources personnel are strategic partners for all managers in the long-term change agent tasks, and new skills are required for managers as well as workers. Assembling and participating in strong teams are essential. HIM professionals are already assuming leadership roles with project management requirements. An EHR project is mapped out in Figure 6-18. Consider the AMIA and AHIMA competencies required for individuals to work with EHRs as a guide.[88]

SUMMARY

Transformation marks the current state of patient record systems and requires HIM professionals to apply theories and practices to parallel realities. Determining the future reality and recognizing the pathway to reach it is a fascinating and challenging task. The fundamental change involved in moving from paper record systems under one operational unit to EHR systems that expand operational boundaries and enable enterprise-wide patient information to be used, processed, protected, and resourced opens the door to expanded professional influence and responsibilities. To understand what the future looks like and how it may function—along with issues and barriers that must be considered—is essential. This chapter addressed the what, why, where, when, and how aspects of the future and proposed concrete steps to manage the transition from paper to electronic records. Given the changing boundaries and professional challenges required today, more complex roles have been described to prepare for leadership and teamwork in EHR projects of all kinds. When "at the table" as EHR systems projects are planned and implemented, the required set of working tools include knowledge of EHR systems and their functions, assessment, and syntheses of benchmark experiences; alternative "maps" of successful migration paths

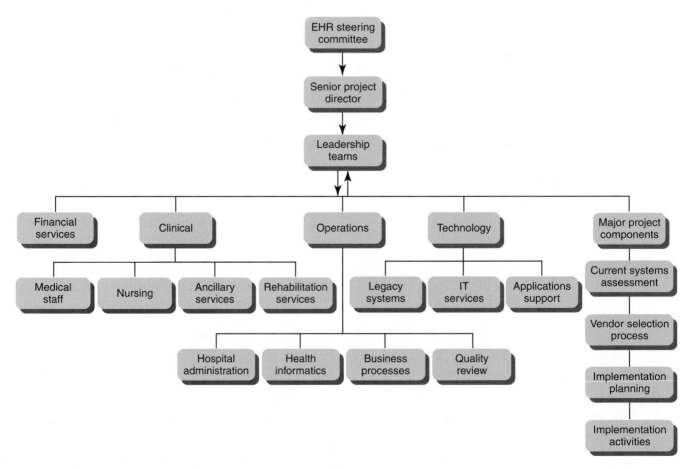

FIGURE 6-18 Electronic health record (EHR) project map. *IT,* Information technology.

for EHR systems; change management principles and skills understanding; and facts about costs and clear details of how the EHR system components meet the patient care and patient record business processes from hybrid to electronic cases. The virtual HIM department has been characterized as an example of emerging business processes. The gathering energy to improve health information from

individual practices from practitioners to comprehensive health care settings within an expanding national health information infrastructure is well underway. Health information demands from those who provide health care and those who receive it will be met. Your challenge as an HIM professional is to seize the transition opportunity to help build and improve our nation's EHR systems.

CHAPTER REVIEW

1. Describe current and emerging roles of the patient record in HIT today.

2. Explain the relationship of enterprise information systems and EHR systems.

3. Why are standards an essential component of HIT and EHR systems?

4. Prepare a flowchart to contrast and illustrate how EHR systems work in a hospital settings versus in an ambulatory setting.

5. You have recently been hired as a HIM specialist by a community hospital to implement the ICD-10 coding system within the HIM department. Using the VA case study in Box 6-7 and implementation information presented in the chapter, identify the steps you will take as you plan your first 6 months at work.

6. Select three VA business processes mentioned in the case study and describe how they changed over time as the EHR system was implemented at VA Puget Sound.

7. Explain how HIM professionals, subject matter experts in the HIM domain, can and should collaborate with information technology specialists when introducing and applying specific EHR standards in their work environment.

REFERENCES

1. Office of the National Coordinator for Health Information Technology (ONC): Update on the Adoption of Health Information Technology and Related Efforts to Facilitate the Electronic Use and Exchange of Health Information: Report to Congress, June 2013. www.ilhitrec.org/ilhitrec/pdf/ONCSummaryCongress_July2013.pdf. http://healthit.gov/sites/default/files/rtc_adoption_of_healthit_and_relatedefforts.pdf. Accessed August 30, 2014.
2. *Federal Register:* 45 CPR 170 Subpart B.
3. Annual report to the U.S. hospital IT market, HIMSS Analytics, 2012. http://apps.himss.org/foundation/docs/2013HIMSSAnnualReport Dorenfest.pdf
4. American Recovery and Reinvestment Act of 2009.
5. Silow-Carroll S, Edwards JN, Rodin D: Using electronic health records to improve quality and efficiency: the experiences of leading hospitals, *Commonwealth Func Pub* Report number 1608 17:29–38, 2012.
6. Gardner E: Electronic health records gaining acceptance, *Huffpost Health Living:* http://www.huffingtonpost.com/2012/09/04/electronic-health-records-medical_n_1855589.html. Accessed July 24, 2013.
7. Payne T, editor: *Practical guide to clinical computing systems: design, operations and infrastructure,* London, 2008, Elsevier.
8. Gartner: Gartner identifies six IT trends that will have a significant impact on people, businesses and the IT industry, press release: www.gartner.com/press_releases/asset_140599_11.html. Accessed April 13, 2010.
9. Kern L, et al: Electronic health records and ambulatory quality of care, *J Gen Intern Med* 28(4):496–503, 2013.
10. *Institute of Medicine Committee on Quality of Health Care in America: To err is human: building a safer health system,* Washington D.C., 1999, National Academy Press.
11. Briere R, editor: *Crossing the quality chasm: a new health system for the 21st century,* Committee on Quality of Health Care in America, Institute of Medicine, Washington, DC, 2001, National Academy Press.
12. Markle Foundation releases blue button video to show promise and potential of consumers access to their own health information, *Markle:* http://www.markle.org/news-events/media-releases/markle-foundation-releases-blue-button-video-show-promise-and-potential-c. Accessed August 30, 2014.
13. Mobley E, Heckman S: Latest hospital safety scores show incremental progress in patient safety, *Leapfrog Group* May 8, 2013, http://www.leapfroggroup.org/policy_leadership/leapfrog_news/5033815. Accessed July 24, 2013.
14. Stires D: Technology has transformed the VA, *Fortune* May 11, 2006, http://archive.fortune.com/magazines/fortune/fortune_archive/2006/05/15/8376846/index.htm. Accessed April 5, 2010.
15. Kahn R: Kaiser Permanente pilot reduces cardiac deaths by 73%, *Kaiser Permanente News Center* March 27, 2009. www.ihi.org/.../Publications/DecadeofHealthInformationTechnology.aspx
16. Paulus RA, Davis K, Steele G: Continuous innovation in health care: implications of the Geisinger experience, *Health Aff* 27(5):1235–1245, 2008.
17. Brailer DJ: The decade of health information technology, delivering consumer-centric and information-rich health care: framework for strategic action, *Letter accompanying the report to Secretary T G Thompson* July 21, 2004. http://www.himssanalytics.org/docs/medicaldevices_landscape.pdf
18. Office of the National Coordinator for Health Information Technology: www.healthit.gov. Accessed April 5, 2010.
19. Annual report to the U.S. hospital IT market, *HIMSS Analytics,* 2012. http://www.himssanalytics.org/docs/medicaldevices_landscape.pdf. Accessed September 1, 2014.
20. Stead WW: The challenge to health informatics for 1999-2000, *J Am Med Inform Assoc* 6:88–89, 1999.
21. Medical devices landscape, current and future adoption, integration with EMRs and connectivity, HIMSS Analytics, sponsored by Lantronix, December 1, 2010.
22. Medical device integration: *CMIO and CNO perspectives,* HIMSS Analytics, *Sponsored by Capsule Tech, Inc, November 2011:* www.capsuletech.com. Accessed August 2013.
23. U.S. Food and Drug Administration: www.FDA.gov. http://www.himssanalytics.org/research/AssetDetail.aspx?pubid=79251&tid=130. Accessed January 9, 2014.

24. DiDonato S: Integrating medical equipment with electronic health records: www.hfmmagazine.com.

25. Public Health Service Act Health Information Technology and Quality, Section 3000: 3001(c)(5): http://www.hipaasurvivalguide.com/public-health-service-act/text.php. Accessed August 2, 2013.

26. American Health Information Management Association: Fundamentals of the legal health record and designated record set, *J AHIMA* 82(2)2011, http://Library.ahima.org/xpedio/groups/public/documents/ahima/bok1_048604.hcsp?dDocName=048604. Accessed July 1, 2014.

27. Dick RS, Steen EB, editors: *The computer-based patient record: an essential technology for health care,* Washington, DC, 1991, National Academy Press.

28. Report to the Office of the National Coordinator for Health Information Technology on Defining Key Health Information Technology Terms, National Alliance for Health Information Technology, April, 2008. http://www.nacua.org/documents/HealthInfoTechTerms.pdf

29. My Healthy Vet program. https://www.myhealth.va.gov?index.html.

30. Tang P, Coye M, BE, et al: Letter report: key capabilities of an electronic health record system, *Committee on Data Standards for Patient Safety, Institute of Medicine* 2003, http://www.nap.edu/openbook.php?isbn=NI000427.

31. American Health Information Management Association e-HIM Personal Health Record Work Group: The role of the personal health record in the EHR, *J AHIMA* 76:64A–64D, 2005.

32. The Definitions Project: http://www.healthcare-informatics.com/news-item/nahit-releases-hit-definitions. Accessed January 7, 2014.

33. Eysenbach G: Consumer health informatics, *BMJ* 320:1713–1716, 2000.

34. Dimick C: The great PHRontier, *J AHIMA* 79(6):25–28, 2008.

35. Health Insurance Portability and Accountability Act of Administrative Simplification, 1996: http://www.cms.gov/Regulations-and-Guidance/HIPAA-Administrative-Simplification/HIPAAGenInfo/index.html?redirect=/HIPAAGenInfo. Accessed January 9, 2014.

36. Scott DiDonato: Certification Commission for Health Information Technology: www.cchit.org. Accessed July 1, 2014.

37. Health Informatics Standards E 1384–07 Standard Practice for Content and Structure of Electronic Health Record, E1762–95 Standard Guide for Authentication of Healthcare Information–2003, E2017, Standard Guide for Amendments to Health Information, *ASTM Standard,* 14.01, West Conshohocken, PA, 2008, American Society for Testing and Materials.

38. Standard Guide for Content and Structure of Electronic Health Records, E1384-07, *ASTM Standards* 14.01, West Conshohocken, PA, 2009, American Society for Testing and Materials.

39. ASTM International: www.astm.org. Accessed July 1, 2014.

40. Dickinson G, Fischetti L, Heard S, editors: *HL7 EHR system functional model draft standards for trial use,* Ann Arbor, MI, 2004, HL7 Inc.

41. Unlocking the power of health information, *Health Level Seven International Proceedings,* www.hl7.org/documentcenter/public/.../HL7_TWITTER_20100224.pdf.

42. Continuity of care document is approved by HL7, endorsed by HITSP: http://www.healthcareitnews.com/news/continuity-care-document-approved-hl7-endorsed-hitsp. Accessed January 9, 2014.

43. Amatayakul MK: *Electronic health records, a practical guide for professionals and organizations,* ed 5, Chicago, 2013, American Health Information Management Association.

44. McDonald C, Huff S, et al: *Logical Observation Identifiers Names and Codes (LOINC) users guide, 1995-2013:* 1995-2013, Regenstrief Institute, Inc. and the Logical Observation Identifiers Names and Codes (LOINC) Committee www.loinc.org. Accessed August 2, 2013.

45. U.S. National Library of Medicine National Institutes of Health: Unified Medical Language Systems (UMLS), RxNorm overview: http://www.nlm.nih.gov/research/umls/rsnorm/overview.html. Accessed August 2, 2013.

46. Murphy GM, Hanken MA, Waters K: *Electronic health records: changing the vision,* Philadelphia, 1999, WB Saunders.

47. HL7 Clinical Templates Work Group: http://www.hl7.org/Special/committees/template/products.cfm. Accessed January 9, 2014.

48. Cummings J: *Few patients use or have access to online services for communicating with their doctors, but most would like to,* Harris Interactive Health Care Poll, *September 22, 2006.*

49. *Institute of Medicine Committee on Patient Safety and Health Information Technology Board on Health Care Services, 2012: Health IT and patient safety: building safer systems for better care,* 2012, National Academies Press. http://iom.edu/Reports/2011/Health-IT-and-Patient-Safety-Building-Safer-Systems-for-Better-Care.aspx

50. *Patient safety and the EHR,* Presented at the Second Annual Northwest Conference on Patient Safety, SeaTac, WA.

51. Dullabh P, Moiduddin A, Babalola E: White paper: measurement of the utilization of an installed EHR: prepared for the U.S. Department of Health and Human Services, NORC and the University of Chicago, June, 2009, Appendix C. http://aspe.hhs.gov/sp/reports/2009/ehrutil/index.shtml. Accessed January 9, 2014.

52. Van Bemmel JH, Musen MA, editors: *Handbook of medical informatics,* Houghten, The Netherlands, 1997, Springer.

53. Covey HD: The digital hostage takers syndrome: reflections on the computer-based patient record, *Manag Care Q* 1:60, 1993.

54. Giannangelo K, editor: *Healthcare code sets, clinical terminologies, and classification systems,* Chicago, 2006, American Health Information Management Association.

55. Payne T: *Practical guide to clinical computing systems: design, operations, and infrastructure,* San Diego, 2008, Elsevier.

56. Golob R: Securing a bridge to the CPR: clinical data repositories, *Health Informatics J* 11:50, 1994.

57. Medical informatics—computer applications in health care and biomedicine. Shortliffe EH, Perreault LE, editors: ed 2, New York, 2000, Springer.

58. Wager KA, Lee FW, Glaser JP: *Managing health care information systems—a practical approach for health care executives,* San Francisco, 2013, Jossey-Bass.

59. Caeser C, Claudio Y, Carmor K, et al: *Ad hoc task force on electronic health record–public health (EHR-PH): report to the HL7's electronic health record special interest group [white paper],* Baltimore, 2004, Public Health Informatics Data Standards Consortium.

60. Healthcare, information management systems. Ball MF, Weaver CA, Keil JM, editors: ed 3, New York, 2004, Springer.

61. Byrne CM, et al: The value from investments in health information technology at the U.S. Department of Veterans Affairs, *Health Aff* 29 (4):629–638, 2010.http://content.healthaffairs.org/cgi/content/full/29/4/629. Accessed January 11, 2014.

62. Kushinka SA: Workflow analysis: *EHR deployment techniques,* California Healthcare Foundation Issue Brief, *January 2011:* http://www.chcf.org/publications/2010/03/ehr-deployment-techniques#ixzz3C6nmXTOd. Accessed January 9, 2014.

63. Middleton B. Bloomrosen M. Dente M.A, et al: *Enhancing patient safety and quality of care by improving the usability of electronic health record systems: recommendations from AMIA Board position paper.* http://jamia.bmj.com/content/early/2013/01/24/amiajnl-2012-001458.

64. Achieving the health IT objectives of the American Recovery and Reinvestment Act—a framework for meaningful use and certified or qualified EHRs, April 2009: *Markle Foundation Connecting for Health,* April 2009, http://www.markle.org/publications/403-achieving-health-it-objectives-american-recovery-and-reinvestment-act. Accessed April 5, 2010.

65. Meaningful use: http://www.cms.gov/Regulations-and-Guidance/Legislation/EHRIncentivePrograms/index.html?redirect=/ehrincentiveprograms/.

66. http://www.cms.gov/regulations-and-guidance/Legislation/EHR/IncentiveProgram/MeaningfulUse. Accessed January 14, 2014.

67. *Health information technology in the United States: better information systems for better care 2013,* Robert Wood Johnson Annual Report.

68. Handler GT, Holtmeier R, Metzger J, et al: HIMSS electronic health record definitional model, version 1.0, EHR definition, attributes and essential requirements, version 1.0, Chicago, 2003, Health Information Management Systems Society.

69. Using electronic health records to improve quality and efficiency. the experiences of leading hospitals, *The Commonwealth Fund* July 2012.

70. Murphy GF, Hanken MA, Waters K: *Electronic health records, changing the vision,* Philadelphia, 1999, WB Saunders.

71. The Joint Commission, 2013: http://www.jointcommission.org/.

72. Kanter RM: *The change masters,* New York, 1983, Simon & Shuster.

73. Scholtes PR: *The leader's handbook,* New York, 1998, McGraw-Hill.

74. Fernandes L, O'Connor M: The future of patient identification, *J AHIMA* 77(1):36–38, 40, 2006.

75. Hammond KW, Helbig ST, et al: Are electronic medical records trustworthy? Observations on copying, pasting and duplication. In *Proceedings of American Medical Informatics Association Symposium,* 2003, pp. 269-273, Bethesda, MD.

76. American Health Information Management Association: *Practice brief: retention of health information,* Chicago, 2002, American Health Information Management Association.

77. Clark JS: *Information management, the compliance guide to the JCAHO standards,* ed 4, Marblehead, MA, 2004, HCPro.

78. Pinder RS, Osborne FH: *Automate ongoing records review,* Oakbrook, IL, 2002, Opus Communications/HCPro.

79. Spath PL: *Fundamentals of health care quality management,* Forrest Grove, OR, 2000, Brown-Spath & Associates.

80. Joint Commission on Accreditation of Healthcare Organizations: *Comprehensive accreditation manual for hospitals: the official handbook,* Chicago, 2006, Joint Commission on Accreditation of Health Care Organizations.

81. Heller T, Aanes D: *Unleashing the power of personal templates, class 240,* 2005, VHA eHealth University. www.vehu.med.va.gov, Accessed August 21, 2006.

82. Jha AK, et al: Use of electronic health records in U.S. hospitals, *N Engl J Med* 360:1628–1638, 2009.

83. Healthcare provides network solutions, barriers and challenges, HIMSS. Analytics, May 2012. http://www.himssanalytics.org/research/AssetDetail.aspx?pubid=82090&tid=127. Accessed January 14, 2014.

84. National health information exchange survey shows increased activity, cost savings, positive impact on physician practices: eHealth Initiative releases results from 2009 survey on health information exchange: http://www.ehidc.org/upcoming-events/78-2013-hie-survey-results. Accessed January 11, 2014.

85. Gever J.: Electronic Health Records with Decision Support Can Save Big Bucks: http:www.medpagetoday.com/PracticeManagement/Information Technology/12597. Accessed January 11, 2014.

86. American Society for Testing, Materials: *ASTM 1869 standard guide for confidentiality, privacy, access and data security principles for health information including electronic health records, 1999:* West Conshohocken, PA, 1999, American Society for Testing and Materials. http://www.astm.org/Standards/E1869.htm

87. 2008 *HIMSS Analytics ambulatory healthcare IT survey, final report,* October, 2008.

88. Crocker Janice, et al: Physician Practice Check-Up: Assessing a Practice's Readiness for Electronic Health Records, *J AHIMA* Vol. 80, No. 8, August, 2009 p. 20–24.

CHAPTER 7

CLASSIFICATION SYSTEMS, CLINICAL VOCABULARIES, AND TERMINOLOGY

Marsha C. Steele

e Student Study Guide activities for this chapter are available on the Evolve Learning Resources site for this textbook. Please visit http://evolve.elsevier.com/Abdelhak.

CHAPTER CONTENTS

Derivations of the *International Classification of Diseases*
  Diagnostic and Statistical Manual of Mental Disorders
  International Classification of Diseases for Oncology
  Current Procedural Terminology
  Healthcare Common Procedure Coding System

Diagnosis-Related Groups and MS-DRGs
Adaptation of Administrative Terminologies
Going Forward
Chapter Review
References

KEY WORDS

Application terminology
ASC-X12N
Backward mapping
Classification system
Clinical document ontology
Clinical interface terminology
Clinical terminology
Clinical Terms Version 3
Code
Code set
Controlled clinical reference
  terminology
Controlled vocabulary
CPT
Data mapping

Desiderata
Document naming nomenclature
DRGs
DSM
EDI
Federal medication terminologies
Forward mapping
GEM
Granularity
HACs
HCPCS
Hierarchical relationships
Health Insurance Portability and
  Accountability Act

Interoperability—basic, functional,
  semantic
IPPS
Location code
LOINC
Mapping
MeSH
Metathesaurus
NDCs
NDF-RT
NIC
NOC
Nomenclature
Omaha System
Ontology

RELMA
RXCUI
RxNorm
Semantic network
SPECIALIST lexicon
Standardized terminology
Structured data
Template
Terminology
Thesaurus
Transaction standards
UMDNS
UMLS
Vocabulary

ABBREVIATIONS

AHCPR   Agency for Health Care Policy and Research
AHIMA   American Health Information Management Association
AMA   American Medical Association
ANA   American Nurses Association
CC   Complication or Comorbidity
CDA   Clinical Document Archives
CDC   Centers for Disease Control and Prevention
CHI   Consolidated Health Informatics
CINAHL   Cumulative Index of Nursing and Allied Health Literature
CIS   Commercial Information System
CM   Clinical Modification
CMS   Centers for Medicare and Medicaid Services
CPOE   Computer Physician/Provider Order Entry
CPRS   Computerized Patient Record System
CPT   Current Procedural Terminology
CUI   Concept Unique Identifier
DHHS   Department of Health and Human Services
DRG   Diagnosis-related Group
DSM   *Diagnostic and Statistical Manual of Mental Disorders*
EHR   Electronic Health Record
FDA   Food and Drug Administration
FMTs   Federal Medication Terminologies
GAF   Global Assessment of Functioning
GEM   General Equivalence Mapping
HAC   Hospital-acquired Condition
HCPCS   Healthcare Common Procedure Coding System
HIM   Health Information Management
HIPAA   Health Insurance Portability and Accountability Act
HITSP   Health Information Technology Standards Panel
HL7   Health Level 7
ICD-9   *International Classification of Diseases,* Ninth Revision
ICD-9-CM   *International Classification of Diseases,* Ninth Revision,
  Clinical Modification

ICD-10   *International Classification of Diseases,* Tenth Revision
ICD-10-PCS   *International Classification of Diseases,* Tenth Revision,
  Procedural Coding System
ICD-O   *International Classification of Diseases for Oncology*
ICNP   International Classification of Nursing Practice
IHTSDO   International Health Terminology Standards Development
  Organization
IPPS   Inpatient Prospective Payment System
LOINC   Logical Observation Identifiers Names and Codes
MCC   Major Complication or Comorbidity
MeSH   Medical Subject Headings
MS-DRG   Medicare Severity-Adjusted Drug-Related Group
NANDA   North American Nursing Diagnosis Association
NCHS   National Center for Health Statistics
NCVHS   National Committee on Vital and Health Statistics
NDC   National Drug Codes
NDF-RT   National Drug File–Reference Terminology
NEC   Not Elsewhere Classified
NIC   Nursing Interventions Classification
NLM   National Library of Medicine
NOC   Nursing Outcomes Classification
ONCHIT   Office of the National Coordinator of Health Information
  Technology
PCS   Procedural Coding System
PMRI   Patient Medical Record Information
PNDS   Perioperative Nursing Data Set
POA   Present on Admission
RBRVS   Resource Based Relative Value Scale
RELMA   Regenstrief LOINC Mapping Assistant
SDO   Standards Development Organization
SNODENT   Systematized Nomenclature of Dentistry
SNOMED CT   Systematized Nomenclature of Medicine,
  Clinical Terms

SNOMED RT   Systematized Nomenclature of Medicine, Reference Terminology
TJC   The Joint Commission
UMDNS   Universal Medical Device Nomenclature System

UMLS   Unified Medical Language System
VA   Department of Veterans Affairs
VHA   Veterans Health Administration
WHO   World Health Organization

THE CHALLENGE OF CLINICAL COMMUNICATIONS AND INFORMATION EXCHANGE

In any health care environment, we rely on a variety of systems and applications to register a patient, identify the payer and the provider, capture the patient's history and findings of the physical, communicate the orders and plan, track diagnostics and test results, record vital signs and inputs from monitoring devices, do the assessments, provide the treatment and care, document the response to care, and so on. You may recognize the system applications by the functional names of various processes such as the master patient or person index; admission, discharge, and transfer; order entry results management; and communications systems, to name a few. The most common communication need is between the clinician and ancillary departments, and among other members of the health care team. The complexity of communications accelerates with the need to share these communications between systems in different health care settings, between clinical sources such as electronic health records (EHRs) and research databases, and with sharing patient information with other health care institutions or regional health information exchanges.[1] Health care is a long way from having a true longitudinal patient record with the ability to track episodes of care across providers throughout the patient's lifetime. Every aspect of health care depends on information. We must be able to create and exchange health information with ease and flexibility to enter information as demanded by clinicians, while at the same time managing its costs, maximizing its benefits, and protecting its security.

Interoperability and Shared Terminologies

Interoperability means the "ability to communicate and exchange data accurately, effectively, securely, and consistently with different information technology systems, software applications, and networks in various settings, and exchange data such that clinical or operational purpose and meaning of the data are preserved and unaltered."[2]

At the application level, *interoperability* means the capacity of an authenticated user to access and transmit or receive and exchange usable information with others. At the systems level, it means the ability of different information systems and software applications to communicate and exchange data accurately, effectively, and consistently. It includes the ability to use the information that has been exchanged. On an expanded level, it means the ability of health information systems to work together within and across organizational boundaries and disparate systems to other authorized entities in real time.[3]

The U.S. National Committee on Vital and Health Statistics (NCVHS) describes three levels of interoperability:

1. **Basic interoperability** allows a message from one computer to be received by another, but does not require the receiving computer to be able to interpret the data. This might be viewed as technical connectivity. It is analogous to putting a letter in an envelope and mailing it. The letter gets from the sender to the recipient. It does not matter what is in the envelope.
2. **Functional interoperability** defines the format of messages. This ensures messages between computers can be interpreted at the level of the data fields, so that the data can pass from a structured field in one system to a comparably structured field in another. Neither system, however, has understanding of the meaning of the data within the fields.[4] This is similar to e-mail in that the format is agreed on with To/From/Subject/Message. Like basic interoperability, technical connectivity is achieved and must follow a standard format, but the system is not trying to understand the meaning of the message.
3. **Semantic interoperability** provides common interpretability, that is, information within the data fields can be used intelligently.[5] It has the ability to allow information to be understood by shared systems. This level of interoperability depends on the degree of agreement of data terminology and its quality. An example of this is found at Methodist University Hospital in Memphis, Tennessee, where they use robots in their pharmacy. Because they use semantic interoperability, various fields mean the same thing across systems. This enables the computerized physician/provider order entry (CPOE) information to be "understood" by the robots.

The system uses customized operating software, advanced robotics, and pharmacy system middleware to automate pharmacy orders. The robot is able to measure, compound, and fill medication orders. It can apply patient-specific barcode labels, do compliance checks, and keep records. The robot can fill up to 600 doses per hour with precision, thereby increasing patient safety and reducing medication errors. The robot can also package daily doses for specific patients, remove expired drugs from inventory, and mix and fill intravenous syringes.[6]

The Health Level 7 (HL7) EHR Interoperability Work Group stated that "interoperability is not a quality or qualification, but rather a noun describing a relationship between systems."[1] Interoperability is not simply a successful transfer of information from one system to another in the correct format. To understand interoperability more fully, we must pursue the notion of semantics to ensure the preservation of the "meaning" of the message. This means that we must also employ *shared terminologies and definitions*. "In health care, semantic operability, or shared terminology, is as important as system interoperability, or shared functions, and must occur in order to achieve the maximum benefit to use the information that has been exchanged. Interoperability is one of the most critical concepts confronting the adoption and implementation of enhanced electronic information technologies into our national healthcare infrastructure."[7] Clinical data in health information systems need to be recorded at the appropriate level of detail. It must remain consistent over time and across boundaries and be able to be transmitted without any loss of meaning or accuracy. Without the use of semantic interoperability and shared terminologies, the potential for errors can increase, and data reliability and validity can be reduced.[8]

Putting Terminologies in a Framework

Structured versus Unstructured Text

In Chapter 6, Murphy and Helbig build a contextual framework for understanding how terminologies and classifications are used in EHR systems. For EHR systems to produce predictable data, they require standardized

terminologies to represent concepts and to communicate them effectively and in the manner intended. Clinicians document in the EHR in a variety of ways. They may use free text or "unstructured" data to enter information directly online or may continue to dictate their notes directly or with voice-activated dictation. Figure 7-1 illustrates an order form used to enter unstructured text directly online.[9]

Clinicians often enter documentation using a combination of free text and structured data. Structured data entry allows users to draw from standard phrases or pick lists and pull-down menus to help guide the entry and ensure that complete information is included. These data "tools" make use of predefined text scripts, lists, and terminology.

Figure 7-2 illustrates the ability to type free text or unstructured data to indicate the reason for the request when ordering a consultation. Pick lists also appear on the consult order to prompt the use of standardized data to name and direct the order to the appropriate service or specialty. Other structured data needed for the consult order include selections to indicate urgency, inpatient or outpatient service, and the location where the consultation will take place.[10]

In addition to documenting in the patient record, standardized text can be used to look up information, as shown

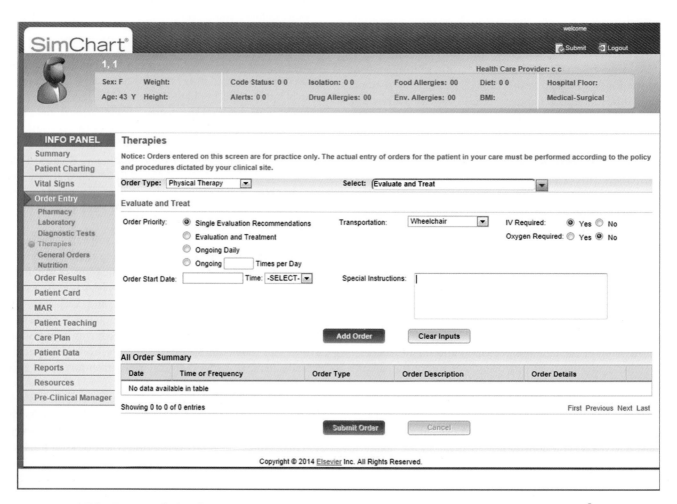

FIGURE 7-1 Order form to enter unstructured or free text. Elsevier © 2014. SimChart® (www.evolve.elsevier.com).

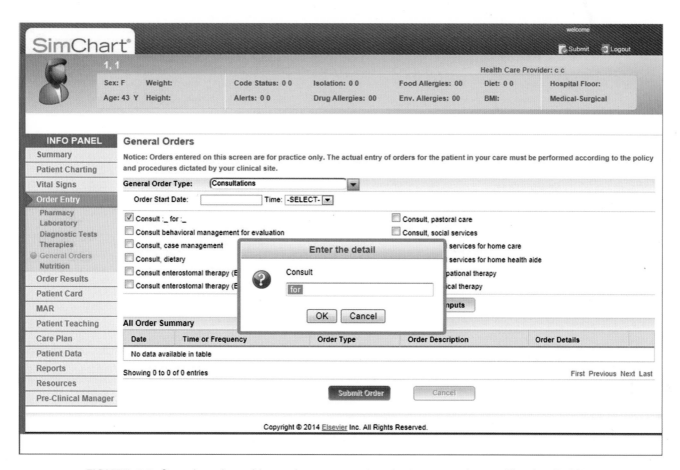

FIGURE 7-2 Consult order with combo structured and unstructured text. Elsevier © 2014. SimChart® (www.evolve.elsevier.com).

in Figure 7-3. Selecting a laboratory test from the pick list on the left results in the description of the test being displayed on the right and indicates the tests that are included in the laboratory panel.

In some settings, templates are used to guide entries and facilitate data capture.[9] A **template** is constructed like an electronic form and guides the user to enter specific content. The template has a combination of drop-down lists and areas for entering free text that are visible to the person documenting the note. The template becomes transparent to the reader as the system will pull the structured and free text into a note that reads like a narrative report. You can select desired items from the pick lists and preview how they will read in the note. In designing the template, the service requesting it must reach consensus and decide which phrases and content are the most clinically appropriate and reflect the most natural expression of the provider. The order of the content should also follow the natural work-flow process used by the clinician. Figure 7-4 shows patient instructions for genitourinary assessment created via a template.

Standardized Terminology

Regardless of the tools employed, standardized terminologies are needed to represent concepts and to communicate them accurately. The terms and concepts used to create clinical documentation for symptoms, diagnoses, procedures, test findings, health status, problem lists, and plans in the EHR need to be interpreted and understood by persons authorized to access that information in the same way that the author wanted it to be represented, exchanged, and interpreted. Uniform definitions are necessary to convey accurate and useful information consistently. This is especially important when information is shared and exchanged. In health care, semantic interoperability, or shared terminology, is as important as systems interoperability, or shared functions, and must occur to achieve maximum benefit to use the information.[1]

The adoption of a single common medical language to meet all information needs is not practical. Although there are many excellent and robust clinical terminologies available, each terminology differs in purpose, scope, and granularity. Terminologies used to enter and capture clinical documentation in the health record must also be interoperable with subsystems, such as the laboratory or pharmacy. Standardized terminology and structured clinical data enable computer processing and are a prerequisite for interoperability, sharing, and exchanging health care information.[11] A balance must be sought to find terminologies that offer the level of detail and ease of use that clinicians need to provide and document care, achieve semantic

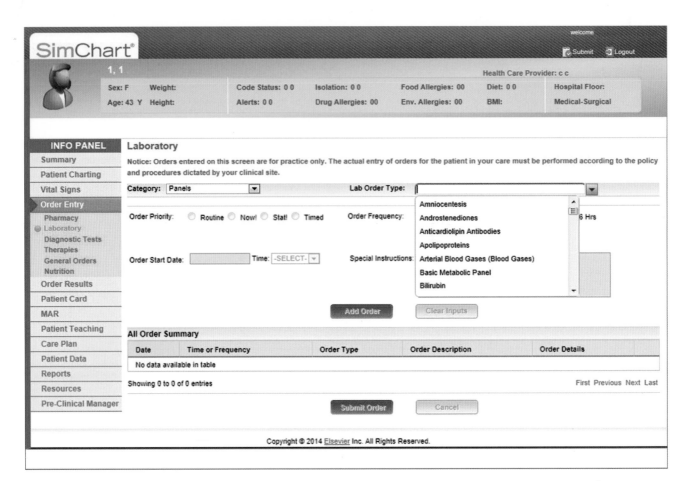

FIGURE 7-3 Laboratory test pick list with branching content. Elsevier © 2014. SimChart® (www.evolve.elsevier.com).

interoperability, and work with the messaging and exchange infrastructure within the EHR and across systems. A standard EHR and a national health information infrastructure require the use of standardized medical language and terminologies to transmit clinical data across diverse information systems.[12]

eHealth: Standardized Terminology

The World Health Organization's (WHO) report *eHealth: Standardized Terminology* underscores the importance of a terminology that ensures that information exchanged between different users will be faithfully understood and reliably used. Content standards, independent of technical standards, must reflect the most advanced scientific understanding of terms and concepts and adhere to the best available knowledge-representation principles.[13] Today's health care environment is experiencing an explosion of knowledge that requires standardization to collect, store, archive, retrieve, process, analyze, and exchange vast amounts of health data. Agreed-on definitions and the usage of terms and concepts underpin the reliability and accuracy of the health information that we collect, whether it is about a single patient or about many patients aggregated into statistics and reports.

Standardized terminology is the key to integration and to managing the complexities of moving from data to knowledge for the purposes of medical knowledge and improving patient care.

The ability to move data to knowledge has significant implications. An individual provider can document the condition and care provided to one patient. These problems and treatments are then coded. These data can then be aggregated and grouped with similar conditions and treatments. After the data are grouped, we can look at the similarities and differences in the problems, as well as the successes and failures in the treatment, to enable us to learn something. If this grouping never happens, it is up to individual care providers to learn from their own patient base—and the immediate group with whom they share information—likely a less effective and slower process. Knowledge is the collective information, understanding, and experience that gives individuals the power to learn from this collective experience and make informed decisions to improve care.

Basic Understanding of Terms
Advocates believe that strong terminologies or coding schemes are essential components of health information systems and that the fastest way to establish and secure consistent data from health care organizations is through standard

FIGURE 7-4 Template preview of pick list for basic nursing care and genitourinary assessment. Elsevier © 2014. SimChart® (www.evolve.elsevier.com).

(Continued)

terminologies. There continues to be national and international interest in identifying "ideal" terminologies to secure accurate and efficient data capture from the care delivery experience to accurately represent clinical concepts.

Health information management (HIM) professionals play an important role in helping health care organizations achieve the benefits of health information technology. David Brailer, MD, PhD, the first national coordinator for health information technology, noted that HIM professionals know what to do with records, how they flow through the systems, who uses them, who has access to them, and how to release information appropriately. With expertise in health information, data standards, coding, documentation, EHR functionality, and business processes in a variety of health care settings, health information managers serve as advocates and subject matter experts. They help to resolve a wide range of health information technology issues from data standardization to privacy. To be effective in this evolving role, HIM professionals must understand the uses and limitations of different health care terminologies and be able to assist in the selection of appropriate terminologies for use with EHR systems.

Vocabulary

A **vocabulary** typically means all the terms that are recognized for communication within a domain; it is a collection of words or phrases.

A **controlled vocabulary** means that the terms within the vocabulary are carefully selected for their inclusion; terms outside that boundary are not included. You already use controlled vocabularies in everyday activities. The Yellow Pages makes use

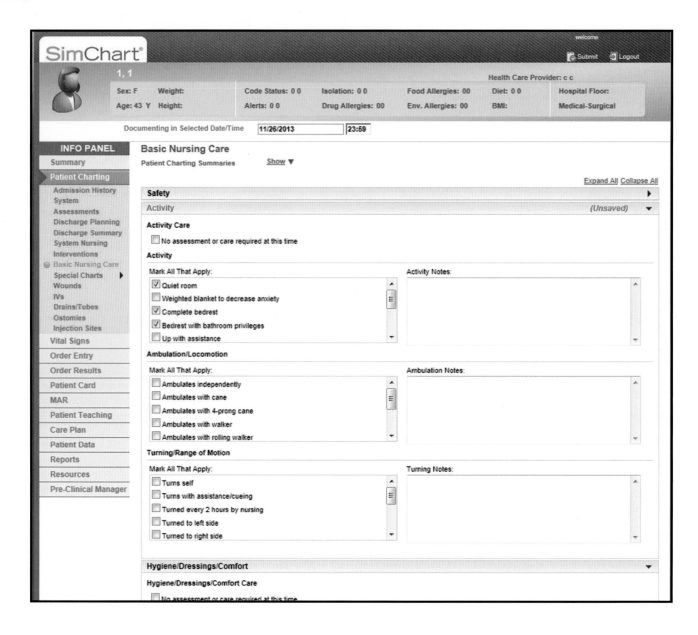

FIGURE 7-4—CONT'D

of a controlled vocabulary. If you look up "doctors," you will be redirected to "See Physicians & Surgeons," using the preferred terminology rather than the vernacular. In a controlled vocabulary, a list of approved terms has been enumerated explicitly. Two rules are generally followed: (1) if the same term is commonly used to mean different concepts in different contexts, then its name is explicitly qualified to resolve the ambiguity; (2) if multiple terms are used to mean the same thing, one of the terms is identified as the preferred term, and the others are listed as synonyms.[14] The Dental Informatics Online Community provides these examples: white spots or tooth decay will be mapped to the preferred term "DENTAL CARIES." Similarly, oral cancer or mouth tumor will be mapped to the preferred term "MOUTH NEOPLASMS."[15] The most standard controlled medical vocabularies used for coding patient information are ICD-9-CM, SNOMED, LOINC, UMLS, and READ

(see the list of abbreviations at the beginning of this chapter for the full name of these vocabularies). They are discussed in further detail in this chapter.

Terminology

A terminology generally means a set of terms representing the system of *concepts* of a particular subject or field. When used in health care, a terminology is a set of terms that describe health concepts. In contrast to a vocabulary, a terminology includes a prescribed set of terms authorized for a specific use. For example, Current Procedural Terminology (CPT) is used for reporting diagnostic and therapeutic procedures and other services performed by physicians.[16] CPT is intended for use for administrative and reimbursement purposes. Generally, procedures are lumped into categories.

TABLE 7-1	CPT Codes for Liver Transplantation	
Donor Hepatectomy	**Recipient Liver Transplant**
47133 Donor hepatectomy from cadaver donor	47135 Liver allotransplantation; partial or whole; from cadaver or living donor, any age
47140 Donor hepatectomy from living donor; left segment only	47136 Liver allotransplantation; heterotopic, partial or whole; from cadaver or living donor, any age
47141 Donor hepatectomy from living donor; total left lobectomy	
47142 Donor hepatectomy from living donor; right total lobectomy	

The CPT codes dealing with liver transplantation in Table 7-1 demonstrate concepts to distinguish between the donor and the recipient, the segment of the liver used, whether the specimen came from a living or cadaver donor, or is from the same species.[17]

A clinical terminology is used to represent the information in a health record, whether it is in paper or electronic form. It is composed of standardized terms, concepts, and their synonyms. Clinical terminologies are used to record patient findings, circumstances, events, and interventions with sufficient detail to support clinical care, decision support, outcomes research, and quality improvement. They are used for many tasks, from simple archiving and retrieval of medical information to complex clinical decision support and data sharing between systems. Clinical terminologies can be efficiently mapped to broader classifications for administrative, regulatory, oversight, and fiscal requirements.[18] Clinical terminologies provide a way to input clinical data into a health record and support the transmission of patient data across information systems.[19]

Terminologies have been developed to represent diseases, procedures, interventions, medications, devices, anatomy, functional status, demographics, and other types of information. Classifications, code sets, vocabularies, and nomenclatures all come under the umbrella of *terminology*.

Classification System

A classification system is a scheme for grouping similar things in a logical way on the basis of common characteristics. It is a system that is clinically descriptive and arranges or organizes like or related entities.[20] Items are grouped according to type or class within an organized system. Libraries organize their collections using the Dewey Decimal System. It, too, is a classification system. Like classifications we use in health care, it must be updated to include new topics and discoveries. The Dewey Decimal System maps to the Library of Congress Subject Headings and to Medical Subject Headings (MeSH) to organize medical literature. Classification systems vary in their level of detail; some offer very general groupings, whereas others allow more detailed groupings and subgroupings, enabling the user to capture a greater degree of specificity (a level of detail), or **granularity**, of data. As an example, ICD-9-CM contains 17,000 codes, whereas ICD-10-CM and ICD-10-PCS code sets have more than 155,000 codes. This improved granularity greatly assists in identifying medical conditions and procedures with high precision. There is only one code for angiography in ICD-9. In contrast, ICD-10 provides 1170 coded descriptions that can identify the location of the blockage and the device used for the procedure. You can move from a highly granular code set to a more generalized one without disrupting the integrity of the codes; however, if you move from a generalized code set to a more specific one, it is difficult to achieve the level of granularity required. As with paint, you can put two specific colors together in one bucket, but it is almost impossible to separate them back into the original colors they once were.

When used in health care, a classification system groups together similar diseases and procedures and organizes related entities for easy retrieval. It groups clinical conditions and procedures into manageable, predetermined categories for external reporting purposes, including reimbursement for health care services and statistical data analysis, such as epidemiologic analysis or trending of disease incidence. Because the main purpose of a classification is statistical analysis and reporting, this type of system is intentionally limited to a relatively small number of mutually exclusive categories. To support statistical reporting needs, classifications use a complex system of conventions, instructional notes, and reporting rules. However, they are not as comprehensive as terminologies because classifications are not intended to represent the complete clinical content of the health record. They are not designed for primary clinical documentation of care at the point of care.[13]

Essentially, terminologies and nomenclatures are more *granular* than classifications, because a classification categorizes and aggregates clinical concepts rather than supports detailed descriptions of distinct clinical concepts. A classification provides the ability to aggregate the terms in a reference terminology for administrative purposes. Because a classification aggregates or classifies clinical terms, it is also considered a type of clinical terminology and may be referred to as an *administrative, aggregate,* or *reporting terminology*.[13] Some examples of classification systems are included in Box 7-1.

BOX 7-1	Examples of Classification Systems

The International Classification for Nursing Practice (ICNP)
The International Classification of Diseases—Oncology (ICD-O)
The International Classification of Diseases, Ninth Revision, Clinical Modification (ICD-9-CM)
The International Classification of Diseases, Tenth Revision, Clinical Modification (ICD-10-CM)
The International Classification of Function, Disability, and Health (ICF)
The International Classification of Impairments, Disabilities, and Handicaps (ICIDH)
The International Classification of Primary Care (ICPC)

TABLE 7-2	Universal Medical Device Nomenclature System Codes	
UMDNS Code	**UMDNS Term English**	
16421	Trocars, Suprapubic	
16422	Cannulae, Nasal	
16424	Capsules, Dental Amalgam	
16425	Sponge Carriers, Endoscopic	
16426	Carvers, Dental Amalgam	
16427	Carvers, Dental Wax	
16428	Tissue Cassettes	
16429	Catheters, Cholangiography	
16430	Catheters, Anesthetic Conduction	
16431	Catheters, Intrauterine	
16432	Catheters, Nasopharyngeal	
16433	Catheters, Peritoneal	

TABLE 7-3	SNOMED CT Naming Structure Mapping to Relationships
Type of Relationship	**Manifestation**
"IS" a relationship between concepts	**Pain** in the **hand** Pain + hand
Finding site relationship	Injury to the **thumb**
Laterality of site relationship	Injury to the **thumb** of the **left hand**
Causative relationship	Injury by **staphylococcus**
Associated morphology relationship	**Foreign body** (metal shard) under nail
Severity relationship	**Severe** pain

Nomenclature

A **nomenclature** is a naming convention or systematic listing of names that have been assigned according to preestablished rules.

An example of a nomenclature is the Universal Medical Device Nomenclature System (**UMDNS**). It is a proprietary, standardized, and controlled international nomenclature and coding system for medical devices that has been adopted by more than 90 countries and more than 5000 institutions. Table 7-2 shows a section of UMDNS codes and the device term.[21] This nomenclature is discussed later in the chapter.

There is often overlap between the terms *nomenclature* and *vocabulary*. For example, the Systematized Nomenclature of Medicine, Clinical Terms (SNOMED CT) is both a vocabulary and a nomenclature. There is a naming structure in SNOMED that maps relationships. It contains more than 311,000 active concepts and approximately 1,360,000 links or semantic relationships between SNOMED CT concepts.[22] Let's look at a patient who has severe thumb pain because of an infection under his nail (Table 7-3).

Compare the table with the diagrammatic representation (Figure 7-5) offered by the International Health Terminology Standards Development Organization (IHTSDO).[23]

Codes

A **code** is a unique identifier assigned to a specific term, description, or concept. A list of codes and the terms or descriptions with which they are associated is known as a **code set**. In some code sets, the codes serve as a kind of shorthand—or a way of conveying meaning with a minimum of complexity. For example, in the fourth edition of the CPT, developed by the American Medical Association (AMA), codes between 80048 and 89356 are all related to pathologic and laboratory practices.

Compositional grammar mapped to diagrammatic representation
53057004:363698007=(76505004:272741003=7771000),272141005=24484000

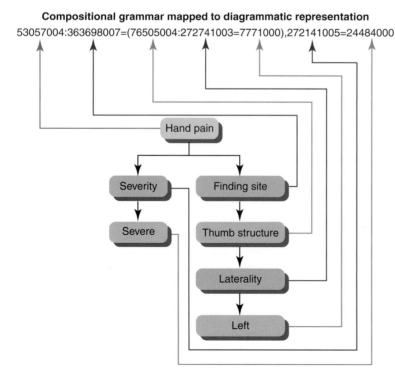

FIGURE 7-5 Diagrammatic representation of severe pain in left thumb. (From *International Health Terminology Standards Development:* http://www.ihtsdo.org/publications/fileadmin/user_upload/Docs_01/Recourses/Introducing_SNOMED_CT/SNOMED_CT_Basics, IHTSDO_Taping_Aug08.pdf. Accessed March 22, 2010.)

In HIM, *coding* commonly refers to the selection of alphanumeric codes to represent diseases, procedures, and supplies used in the delivery of health care and the assessment of the quality of care. As an example, CPT Category II codes are often used to code services that support performance measures and approved clinical treatment protocols. Statistical analysis may be based on formulae such as these:

CPT II Code: All patients with chest x-ray performed
– –
ICD-9-CM code: All patients with diagnosis of community acquired bacterial pneumonia
CPT II Code: All patients with pulmonary rehab exercise training
– –
ICD-9-CM code: All patients with diagnosis of COPD ICD-9-CM code, dyspnea CPT II code 01019F (dyspnea assessed and present)

Administrative coding may be done manually by using code books and other reference sources or with the assistance of electronic tools.[24]

However, when used in the broader context of EHRs, *coding* (or *encoding*) refers to the assignment of unique identifiers to the terms within a particular clinical terminology. Rather than being assigned manually, codes are assigned according to some predetermined algorithm, usually without any manual intervention. In a well-designed terminology, no meaning can be discerned from a code itself; it is simply a unique identifier that represents a more detailed description, concept, or term. The codes themselves remain unknown to most users. When a user selects a term to use, the associated code is stored electronically. These codes are used to transmit health data from one electronic system to another for analysis, aggregation, or use at the point of care.[25]

As an example, location codes enable systems to identify the source from which data originate. A facility may have 15 different locations or "location codes." These code numbers do not have meaning but make the data easier to handle. The users do not have to enter the codes and are unaware that that a unique identifier is being used.

Codes provide a more concise and efficient means to store and transmit detailed information than free text does. Reliance on free text information limits our ability to aggregate and compare information from different sources and presents challenges to the designers of advanced EHR tools. With encoded data, information can be displayed in a form that human beings can read, understand, and store in a form that computers can exchange and manipulate. Clinical terminologies that use codes to represent detailed concepts provide a way to combine the expressiveness and flexibility of free text information with the clarity and computability of encoded information.[26]

Classifications and terminologies are used with code sets to define and classify individual health terms. They serve as a way to relate terms to one another so that they are easily and consistently understood by users. Classifications arrange related terms for easy retrieval, whereas vocabularies are sets of specialized terms that facilitate precise communication by eliminating ambiguity. A coding classification system groups related terms or conditions together into classes. For this reason, classification systems have less granularity and specificity than nomenclatures. Nomenclatures use precise naming conventions to represent a term or condition in more detail. A coding system with more specificity can be more readily converted to one that groups or classifies, whereas once grouped, the detail is lost, and it is more difficult to revert back with accuracy.

As an example, ICD-9 has only one code for angioplasty, a procedure for widening a narrowed or obstructed artery; ICD-10 offers 1170 codes with a granularity that pinpoints the location of the blockage and the device used for each procedure. Similarly, ICD-9 does not have codes to distinguish laterality; ICD-10 has codes that allow the identification of the left or right side. These are just some of the differences between these coding systems. When comparing the 17,000 codes in ICD-9 to the more than 155,000 codes in ICD-10, it is easy to understand the concept of granularity and data loss if reverting back to ICD-9 from ICD-10. Important classifications include ICD-9-CM, ICD-10, ICD-10-CM/PCS, and ICF. Important terminologies include LOINC and SNOMED. There are subtle differences among vocabularies, nomenclatures, terminologies, and classifications.

Administrative Terminologies

Administrative terminologies are classification and coding systems that are primarily designed to support the administrative, financial, and regulatory functions associated with patient care. They serve as the primary communication tool between those providing services and those paying for those services. They are also used by providers, payers, researchers, governmental agencies, and others to create secondary statistical reports as well as facilitate the activities that follow:

- Measuring the quality, safety, and efficacy of care
- Managing care and disease processes
- Tracking public health and risks
- Providing data to consumers regarding costs and outcomes of treatment options
- Payment system design and processing of claims for reimbursement
- Research, epidemiologic studies, and clinical trials
- Designing health care delivery systems and monitoring resource utilization
- Identifying fraudulent practices
- Setting health policy[27]

Clinical Terminologies

Clinical terminologies are those designed to represent the information in the patient record, whether in paper or electronic form. When clinical terminologies are used, much of the ambiguity inherent in natural language can be eliminated because the definitions, concepts, and relationships that represent the concepts have been predetermined. Human readers can easily interpret narrative information and automatically add context that helps them interpret that information. In reviewing another clinician's progress note about a patient, for example, a physician might recall a previous conversation that was not documented in the record, think about practices at the other hospital where the patient had been treated, or even consider who wrote the note to capture subtleties that a computer might miss.

In contrast, computers are quite literal in their interpretation of data. A classic example of this is illustrated by the sentence, "Baby swallows fly." This sentence could be interpreted in different ways, depending on whether the verb in the sentence is *swallows* or *fly* and on whether *baby* is a noun or an adjective.

Health data can also be ambiguous. The word *cold,* for example, can refer to many different things, including temperature, mood, illness, and influenza. For example, a patient might report to her physician that she has a cold or that she feels cold all the time. If the letters *COLD* were transmitted from one provider to another as part of the patient's medical record, the recipient might wonder whether the patient had chronic obstructive lung disease unless additional information were provided to clarify the use of the term. When clinical terminologies are used, much of the ambiguity inherent in natural language can be eliminated.

A controlled medical terminology or controlled clinical reference terminology is a coded vocabulary of medical concepts and expressions used in health care. It is concept-based and allows for the complex organization and aggregation of clinical information. The term *controlled* refers to managing the content to ensure that it remains structurally sound, biomedically accurate, and consistent with current practice. It facilitates the use of standardized terminology and the collection of structured data when creating EHRs. An example of a controlled reference terminology is SNOMED CT. It allows a variety of practitioners to use multiple terms to express the same concept. The system inserts an *interpretive layer* of semantics between the term entered by the user and the underlying database to better represent the original intention of the terms of the user. This helps others to understand the entry made by the author in the way it should be interpreted[14] (Box 7-2).

BOX 7-2   Interpretive Layer for Semantic Concept

For example, consider the concept *gastric ulcer:*
- The "finding site" = "gastric mucosa" is a *necessary* condition for "gastric ulcer."
  - This is true because all gastric ulcers necessarily involve the "gastric mucosa."
- The definition "morphology" = "ulcer" and "finding site" = "stomach structure" is a *sufficient* definition for "gastric ulcer."
  - This is true because any ulcer in a stomach structure is a "gastric ulcer."
- Therefore an assertion that a person has an "ulcer" with finding site "stomach" is *sufficient* to imply that they have a "gastric ulcer."
  - Because a gastric ulcer *necessarily* involves the "gastric mucosa," it should be possible to deduce that a person with an "ulcer" with findings site "stomach" has a disorder with a site of "gastric mucosa."

CLINICAL TERMINOLOGIES

Desirable Characteristics of Clinical Terminologies

In 1998, a medical informaticist named James Cimino, MD, identified 12 desiderata, or desirable characteristics, that would make clinical terminologies more useful.[28] These desiderata have since gained broad acceptance and are now considered the fundamental principles for the development and integration of clinical terminologies. The 12 characteristics are as follows:

Content
The usefulness of a given terminology is largely determined by its content. There must be a formal method for adding content when gaps in content coverage are discovered.

Concept Orientation
Each terminology should have a concept orientation—that is, each term should correspond to a single concept and that concept should have a single, coherent meaning. A given concept may be interpreted differently when used in different contexts; for example, a condition recorded under the personal history of a patient may have different implications than the same condition recorded under family history.

Concept Permanence
Concept permanence means that once a concept has been created within a terminology, its meaning cannot change and it cannot be deleted. The preferred name of the concept can change, or the concept may be deemed inactive, but its meaning must remain fixed as long as the terminology is in use. Concept permanence helps prevent the users from misinterpreting historical data.

Nonsemantic Concept Identifier
There must be a nonsemantic concept identifier associated with each term. This means that an identifier does not carry any meaning in itself and does not indicate the hierarchical position of the term it represents.

Polyhierarchy
Many terminologies are arranged hierarchically. A hierarchical structure can help users locate concepts, group related concepts, and add context. It is not necessary to have a single hierarchy; in fact, polyhierarchy is necessary to support different users and uses of the same terminology (e.g., SNOMED accomplishes polyhierarchy through the use of "is-a" relationships).

Formal Definitions
Formal definitions are those that follow a formal structure, that is, definitions that are represented in a form that can be manipulated by a computer, as opposed to narrative text definitions intended for human readers. These definitions can be expressed through the use of "is-a" relationships connecting concepts in a vocabulary.

In Figure 7-6, the concept "Coronary Atherosclerosis" can be defined with an "is-a" link to the concept "Arteriosclerotic Vascular Disease" and a "site" relationship to "coronary artery."

Reject "Not Elsewhere Classified"

Not elsewhere classified (NEC) terms are used to collect concepts that are not covered elsewhere in a terminology. Because NEC terms are defined by exclusion, their meaning can change every time a new concept is added to the terminology.

Multiple Granularities

Granularity refers to the degree of specificity and refinement of a term. Different users are likely to require different levels of granularity. Terminologies that include multiple granularities of the same content can support many more users than those with a single level of granularity.

Multiple Consistent Views

Multiple consistent views are required to support the different views of the vocabulary depending on the utility. Cimino states that polyhierarchical terminologies with multiple levels of granularity must not permit inconsistent views of a single concept.[28]

Context Representation

A well-designed terminology must allow for context representation. It should include formal, explicit information about how concepts are to be used.[28] This means that there is a "grammar" that can be used to manipulate data and that there is also context-specific information about what is "sensible to say." For example, it would be sensible to see the word *rupture* used in relation to *appendicitis* but not to the term *eyebrow*. The ability to represent context is essential to avoid the misinterpretation of health data.[29]

Graceful Evolution

The structure and content of a terminology must change over time to reflect scientific advances, administrative changes, and other relevant factors. There must be a formal method for adding content to the terminology so that it does

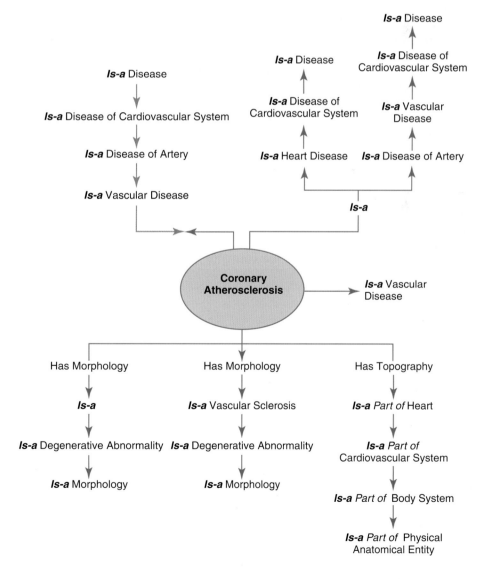

FIGURE 7-6 The concept of coronary atherosclerosis. (From SNOMED RT®, a previous edition of SNOMED CT® from the College of American Pathologists.)

not become obsolete as the field of medicine evolves, and all changes should be described and documented in detail.

Recognized Redundancy

Redundancy is a characteristic of language. Redundancy occurs within a terminology when there is more than one term with the same meaning. This is desirable as long as the redundancy is recognized. Recognized redundancy means that terms with the same meaning are treated as synonyms and are represented by the same identifying code. Ideally, these redundant entries map to the same concept; for example, *myocardial infarction* and *heart attack* are synonyms and should be treated as though they represent the same concept.

On the basis of experience in implementing a clinical terminology for Kaiser Permanente, Campbell identified six additional desirable characteristics.[30,31]

Copyrighted and Licensed

The terminology should be licensed, copyrighted, and maintained by a single organization to prevent local modifications that might make the data incomparable across disparate sites, systems, or organizations.

Commercial Information System Vendor-Neutral

The design of the terminology should not give any advantage to a particular commercial information system (CIS) vendor. This will ensure that the terminology is available nationally (or internationally), prevent limits on its use for profit reasons, and protect the terminology from events that adversely affect a vendor. ICD-9, CPT, and SNOMED are all vendor neutral.

Scientifically Valid

The terminology should be understandable, reproducible, useful, and reflective of the current understanding of science.

Well Maintained

There must be a central authority responsible for keeping the terminology current and for providing rapid response to new terms. ICD is updated on a regular basis. The ICD-9-CM Coordination and Maintenance Committee reviews proposals to update ICD-9-CM; changes are effective October 1 each year.

Self-Sustaining

The terminology should be supported by public or endowment funding or by license fees to cover development and support costs.

Scalable Infrastructure and Process Control

Tools and processes used to maintain the terminology should be scalable to the number of users so that timely maintenance is not jeopardized.

Table 7-4 from "Interface Terminologies: Facilitating Direct Entry of Clinical Data into Electronic Health Record Systems" demonstrates desired attributes for a controlled medical terminology.[32]

INTERFACE TERMINOLOGIES

Interface or application terminologies are designed to support efficient structured clinical documentation into EHR system interfaces and computerized note capture tools. They

---

TABLE 7-4 Some Desired Attributes for a Controlled Medical Terminology, as Represented in Cimino,[81] Chute et al.,[18] and the International Organization for Standardization Technical Specifications for Terminologies[81]

Terminology Attribute	Cimino	Chute et al.	ISO
Statement of purpose, scope, and comprehensiveness			x
Complete coverage of domain-specific content	x	x	x
Use of concepts rather than terms, phrases, and words (concept orientation)	x		x
Concepts do not change with time, view, or use (concept consistency*)	x		x
Concepts must evolve with change in knowledge	x	x	x
Concepts identified through nonsense identifiers (context-free identifier)	x	x	x
Representation if concept context consistently from multiple hierarchies	x	x	x
Concepts have single explicit formal definitions	x	x	x
Support for multiple levels of concept detail	x	x	x
Methods, or absence of, to identify duplication, ambiguity, and synonymy	x	x	x
Synonyms uniquely identified and appropriately mapped to relevant concepts	x	x	x
Support for compositionality to create concepts at multiple levels of detail	x	x	x
Language independence		x	
Integration with other terminologies		x	x
Mapping to administrative terminologies		x	x

*Includes the concepts "multiple consistent views" and "concept permanence."

help users view categorical data by providing common collo-quial terms as synonyms and enable natural language text generation. They are used to present preselected subsets or pick lists to end users to facilitate data entry and standardization when documenting in the EHR. The terms in the pick lists are generally selected from a reference terminology.[33] Figure 7-7 demonstrates the use of preselected subsets to facilitate data entry.[10]

A clinical interface terminology is a systematic collection of health care–related phrases that supports clinician entry of patient-related information into computer programs. Interface terminologies also facilitate display of computer-stored patient information to clinician users as simple human-readable text. Thus interface terminologies "provide the interface" between the clinician's own conceptualizations of patient descriptors and the more structured, coded internal data elements used by specific clinical computer programs. Interface terminologies allow users to interact easily with concepts through common colloquial terms and synonyms.

An example of how interface terminologies can support provider entry of patient information into computer programs and display it can be found in the illustration of a reminder dialog. At the time of the patient encounter, the provider needs to store actions for follow-up. These follow-up reminders can be customized to the condition of the patient and the specialty of the physician, who then uses a check box to select the actions for follow-up that the patient needs. Each check can open more detail if the icon is selected. Future follow-up actions can be set to send reminder messages in the future, such as to get a flu shot each fall or tetanus shot every 10 years. When the follow-up activity has taken place and the patient has received the services, the system facilitates entering a description of what has occurred.

Copyright © 2014 Elsevier Inc. All Rights Reserved.

FIGURE 7-7 Interface terminologies translate language into structured representations. Elsevier © 2014. SimChart® (www.evolve.elsevier.com).

BOX 7-3

Interface Terminologies—From Natural Language to Structured Representation

Frontal and lateral views of chest compared to previous examination of 6/20/2010. *Cardiomegaly* is present with *pulmonary vascular congestion,* not significantly changed compared with the previous examination. A new, more focal opacity is seen in region of right middle lobe. *Bilateral* small *pleural effusions* are seen increased on left.

EHR systems depend on interface terminologies for successful implementation in clinical settings because such terminologies provide the translation from the individual clinician's own natural language expressions into the more structured representations required by application programs. This enables unlocking clinical data from narrative reports. Box 7-3 demonstrates the use of an interface to capture information from unstructured natural language to a structured representation.

Interface terminologies have three classes depending on the intended use or task:

1. *Interface* supports a user-friendly structured data entry interface.
2. *Processing* optimizes natural language processing.
3. *Reference* enables storage, retrieval, and analysis of clinical data.[34]

Clinical interface terminologies have been used for problem list entry, clinical documentation in EHRs, text generation, CPOE with decision support, and diagnostic expert programs.

MAPPING

Data mapping is the process of creating data element mappings between semantic and representational terms residing in two distinct data models. Data mapping is used as a first step in data integration which involves combining terms residing in different sources and to provide users with a unified view of these data. Semantic mapping is analogous to an auto-connect feature that looks up a term and its synonyms. It is a way of graphically representing concepts by constructing a semantic map and identifying ideas and how they fit together. The aim is to explain precisely a subset of real information to improve communication with precision. For example, if the source system lists "LAST NAME" and the destination system lists "SUR NAME," the mapping will recognize that these data elements are synonyms. There are limitations, however, in that mapping is only able to find exact matches. Metadata must be used to indicate that these two distinct terms are indeed synonyms.

In the future, tools based on semantic web languages will make data mapping a more automatic process for improved retrieval and navigation of health information by using search engine methodology to infer synonyms and semantic relationships.[35]

General Equivalence Mappings

The Centers for Medicare and Medicaid Services (CMS) and the Centers for Disease Control and Prevention (CDC) created the national version of the general equivalence mappings (GEMs) to ensure that consistency in national data is maintained. CMS and CDC will maintain the GEMs for at least 3 years beyond October 1, 2014, which is the compliance date for implementation of ICD-10-CM and ICD-10-PCS. The GEMs are a comprehensive translation dictionary that can be used to convert, accurately and effectively, any ICD-9-CM–based application or data to ICD-10-CM or PCS, including data for tracking quality, recording morbidity and mortality, and calculating reimbursement. The GEMs can be used to convert large applications with a high degree of complexity and still preserve the essential logic of the application.

The GEMs are a bidirectional tool that can be used to convert applications and data from ICD-9-CM to ICD-10-CM/ PCS and vice versa. Mapping from ICD-10-CM and PCS codes back to ICD-9-CM codes is referred to as backward mapping. Backward mapping is used to map a newer code set to an older code set. Mapping from ICD-9-CM codes to ICD-10-CM and PCS codes is referred to as forward mapping. Forward mapping maps from an older code set to a newer code set.

Caution should be used in using GEMs, because they are not a simple one-to-one crosswalk. ICD-10 is much more specific than ICD-9 and contains many more codes (Box 7-4).

Additionally, ICD-10 contains new and additional concepts that have no predecessor in ICD-9. In some cases, one ICD-10 procedure code may have many ICD-9 codes. Conversely, one ICD-9 code many have multiple ICD-10 codes. There is different content in the GEM for each direction. The GEMs work by linking a code in the source system to all valid alternatives in the target code set. Box 7-5 indicates why we need GEMs by showing one ICD-9 diagnosis code with its associated multiple ICD-10 codes, which provide much more specificity. To correctly use this level of specificity, there must also be more detail in the clinical documentation to support the selected codes.[36]

The GEMs are complete for all the mapping possibilities, as well as when there are new concepts in ICD-10-CM or PCS that are not found in ICD-9-CM. All ICD-9-CM codes and all ICD-10-CM and PCS codes are included in the GEMs. A breakdown of the GEMs follows for diagnosis and procedure codes:

All ICD-10-CM codes are in the ICD-10-CM to ICD-9-CM GEM.

All ICD-9-CM diagnosis codes are in the ICD-9-CM to ICD-10-CM GEM.

BOX 7-4 **ICD-9 to ICD-10 Coding**

Diagnoses	Procedures
ICD-9-CM 14,025 codes	ICD-9-CM 3824 codes
ICD-10-CM 68,069 codes	ICD-10-PCS 72,589 codes

BOX 7-5 ## Why We Need General Equivalence Mappings

- One ICD-9 Diagnosis Code for Fracture of Midcervical section of femur, closed
  82002
  Fracture of Midcervical section of femur, closed
- Multiple codes in ICD-10
  S72031A
  Displaced midcervical fracture of right femur, initial encounter for closed fracture
  S72031G
  Displaced midcervical fracture of right femur, subsequent encounter for closed fracture with delayed healing
  S72032A
  Displaced midcervical fracture of left femur, initial encounter for closed fracture
  S72032G
  Displaced midcervical fracture of left femur, subsequent encounter for closed fracture with delayed healing
  S72033A
  Displaced midcervical fracture of unspecified femur, initial encounter for closed fracture
  S72033G
  Displaced midcervical fracture of unspecified femur, subsequent encounter for closed fracture with delayed healing
  S72034A
  Nondisplaced midcervical fracture of right femur, initial encounter for closed fracture
  S72034G
  Nondisplaced midcervical fracture of right femur, subsequent encounter for closed fracture with delayed healing
  S72035A
  Nondisplaced midcervical fracture of left femur, initial encounter for closed fracture
  S72035G
  Nondisplaced midcervical fracture of left femur, subsequent encounter for closed fracture with delayed healing
  S72036A
  Nondisplaced midcervical fracture of unspecified femur, initial encounter for closed fracture
  S72036G
  Nondisplaced midcervical fracture of unspecified femur, subsequent encounter for closed fracture with delayed healing

Centers for Medicare and Medicaid Services: *ICD-10-CM/PCS* implementation and general equivalence mappings (crosswalks) overview: http://www.cms.gov/ICD10/downloads/7ICD-10_Implementation_and_GEM_Overview_Presentation.pdf. Accessed March 31, 2010.

All ICD-10-PCS codes are in the ICD-10-PCS to ICD-9-CM GEM.

All ICD-9-CM procedure codes are in the ICD-9-CM to ICD-10-PCS GEM.

The Role of the Unified Medical Language System and Mapping

No single terminology is appropriate for all uses or meets the needs of all users. A great deal of work is under way to define appropriate uses of available health care terminologies and the relationships between them. The U.S. National Library of Medicine (NLM) has developed the Unified Medical Language System (UMLS) to bring together diverse coding schemes with multiple terminologies. UMLS is a valuable resource for interrelating terminologies by supporting mappings and cross-references among them. It connects scores of vocabularies, classifications, and other sources by concept, allowing users to map data from one terminology to another. Mapping is useful for retaining the value of historical data when migrating to newer database formats and terminology versions (e.g., migration from ICD-9 to ICD-10). Mapping also enables users to use data for multiple purposes without having to capture the data in multiple formats.

The UMLS is a large, multipurpose, and multilingual vocabulary database that contains information about biomedical and health-related concepts, their various names, and the relationships among them. It is built from the electronic versions of many thesauri; classifications; code sets; and lists of controlled terms used in patient care, health services billing, public health statistics, indexing and cataloging biomedical literature, and basic, clinical, and health services research. The NLM states that the purpose of UMLS is to facilitate the development of computer systems that behave as if they "understand" the meaning of the language of biomedicine and health. It contains more than 1 million biomedical concepts from more than 100 source vocabularies, and more than 5 million terms organized by meaning into concepts and assigned to a unique identifier.

The UMLS, begun in 1986, uses one identification code to represent the same concept from different vocabulary sources. As an example, mapping between the NLM's medical subject headings and ICD-9 or ICD-10 would enable an EHR to use this link to generate an automated literature search based on a patient's ICD-9 or ICD-10 diagnosis code, and allow the treating physician to retrieve relevant literature through a MeSH-based query to NLM's PubMed system. The UMLS is a compendium (a concise yet comprehensive body of knowledge) of more than 100 controlled vocabularies and classifications in the biomedical sciences. It overcomes the challenges imposed by the variety of ways that the same concepts are expressed by different people and different computer systems. UMLS supports the conversion of terms from one controlled vocabulary to another to enable information exchange among different clinical databases and systems. UMLS provides a mapping structure among these vocabularies and thus allows one to translate among the various terminology systems. UMLS may also be viewed as a comprehensive thesaurus (a work that lists words grouped together according to similar meaning) and ontology (a formal representation of a set of concepts within a domain and the relationships within those concepts). Ontologies are used as a form of knowledge representation and have a shared vocabulary of biomedical concepts. UMLS further provides facilities for natural language processing. It is intended to be used mainly by developers of systems in medical informatics (Figure 7-8).

UMLS consists of the following components:

- Metathesaurus, the core database of the UMLS, is a collection of concepts and terms from the various controlled

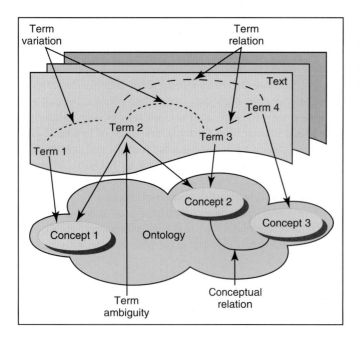

FIGURE 7-8 The relationships of terms to concepts within an ontology. (From Spasic I, Ananiadou S, McNaught J, Kumar A: Text mining and ontologies in biomedicine: making sense of raw text, Briefings in Bioinformatics Date of revised form: June 7, 2005.)

vocabularies and their relationships. It is organized by concepts that are linked to corresponding concepts in various source vocabularies. It comprises more than 1 million biomedical concepts and 5 million concept names.

- **Semantic network** is a set of categories and relationships that are being used to classify and relate the entries in the metathesaurus. Each concept in the metathesaurus is assigned to semantic types, and relationships are determined. Each semantic type is assigned an identifier, definition, examples, and relationships. The semantic network is, in a sense, a catalog of these types and relationships.
- **SPECIALIST Lexicon** is a database of lexicographic information for use in natural language processing. The lexicon includes more than 200,000 items and identifies their spelling, form, and structure, as well as how they are put together to create meaning. The lexicon is used in natural language processing applications.
- A number of supporting software tools are also included.

Figure 7-9 is an illustration of how concepts are organized in UMLS. Medical vocabulary terms are grouped as synonyms. These synonyms are clustered, and then the concepts of the terms are organized across vocabularies. The concepts are categorized, edited, and identified as concepts in UMLS.

The UMLS was designed and is maintained by the NLM. It is updated quarterly and may be used for free. The project was initiated in 1986 by Donald A. B. Lindberg, MD, then the director of the NLM (see Figure 7-9).[37]

UNDERSTANDING TERMINOLOGIES

Coded data have the advantage of consistency of expression for diagnoses, procedures, laboratory tests, drugs, and so on. However, because of the strengths and weaknesses in these systems, none possesses the full clarity and precision required to capture and represent all clinical facts contained in patient records.

The terminology issue became confused a few years ago when several terminologies were declared national standards for transmission of data. In 2003 the U.S. NCVHS and the U.S. government's multiagency Consolidated Health Informatics (CHI) council recommended a *core set of terminologies* as standards for representing aspects of patient record information. As a continuation of its Health Insurance Portability and Accountability Act (HIPAA) mandate, NCVHS assessed clinical terminology standards for the Patient Medical Record Initiative. The NCVHS Subcommittee on Standards and Security completed a detailed evaluation of 38 care terminologies and classification systems to support the electronic medical record. Ten terminologies met all of the essential criteria defined according to sound medical informatics practices. The NCVHS recommended a of "core set" of the Initiative's terminology standards.

It should be noted that at the time the core set of terminologies was identified, none of them was designed for use by clinicians at the point of care, and none was adopted for that use. The contribution and value of each one is not in dispute. It simply illustrates that terminologies are designed for different purposes.[38] We cannot expect a single controlled vocabulary to describe patient care; to populate aggregated data sets for management purposes; to capture the processes of care in messages; and to capture, store, and retrieve patient information.[39] Although many terminologies have been developed, no single terminology has been accepted as a universal standard for the representation of clinical concepts.[32] A health care organization is likely using multiple coding systems in its efforts to organize and communicate its computerized data.

Exploring the Core Set of Terminologies

Under HIPAA, the NCVHS was charged with assessing existing terminologies to define the scope of patient medical record information (PMRI) and determine selection criteria

FIGURE 7-9 Terms for Addison's disease and concepts.

for terminologies that could capture this information. NCVHS concluded that no single terminology would provide adequate domain coverage for PMRI. In November 2003 NCVHS recommended that a "core set" of terminologies be adopted as a national standard. The core set includes the minimum set of terminologies that (1) are adequate to cover the scope of PMRI and (2) meet essential technical criteria to serve as reference terminologies for PMRI.

The core set of PMRI terminologies recommended by NCVHS includes the following:

- SNOMED CT—Systemized Nomenclature of Medicine, Clinical Terms works behind the scenes to code the content of the electronic record
- LOINC—the logical observation identifiers names and codes used for representing laboratory data for ordering and naming specific test results
- RxNorm—for clinical drugs for communication to retail pharmacies for e-prescribing along with several federal drug terminologies

- The representations of the mechanism of action and physiologic effect of drugs from National Drug File–Reference Terminology (NDF-RT)
- Ingredient name, manufactured dosage form, and package type from the Food and Drug Administration (FDA) National Drug Codes (NDCs)
  - Accredited Standards Committee (ASC) X12N standards for claims attachments
  - UMDNS

The NCVHS also noted the value of additional code systems such as established nursing terminologies that represent nursing concepts. Each of these core terminologies is now discussed.[40]

The Role of IHTSDO and SNOMED-CT

The IHTSDO is an international, not-for-profit organization based in Denmark. IHTSDO owns and administers the rights to SNOMED CT and other health terminologies and related standards.

SNOMED CT intellectual property rights were transferred to the SNOMED Standards Development Organization in the formal creation of the IHTSDO.

> The purpose of IHTSDO is to develop, maintain, promote and enable the uptake and correct use of its terminology products in health systems, services and products around the world. The IHTSDO seeks to improve the health of humanity by fostering the development and use of suitable standardized clinical terminologies, notably SNOMED CT, in order to support safe, accurate, and effective exchange of clinical and related health information. The focus is on enabling the implementation of semantically accurate health records that are interoperable.[41]

SNOMED CT was originally created by the College of American Pathologists by combining SNOMED RT and a computer-based nomenclature and classification known as Clinical Terms Version 3, formerly known as Read Codes Version 3, which was created on behalf of the UK Department of Health and is a Crown copyright.

SNOMED has been refined and expanded for more than 4 decades, and it is now considered to be the most comprehensive, multilingual clinical health care terminology in the world. SNOMED CT aims to improve patient care by developing systems to record health care encounters accurately and by building and facilitating communication and interoperability in electronic health data exchange.

SNOMED CT is a coding system, controlled vocabulary, classifications system, clinical reference terminology, and thesaurus. As a clinical reference terminology, SNOMED CT is an example of a standardized terminology that can be used as the foundation for EHRs and other applications. It contains more than 310,000 unique concepts and more than 1.3 million links or relationships between them that

ensure that information is captured consistently, accurately, and reliably across the health system (Table 7-5).[42]

Some descriptions are provided to explain their attributes (Box 7-6).[43]

The SNOMED CT core terminology offers a consistent language for capturing, sharing, and aggregating health data

TABLE 7-5 Frequency Distribution of 18 Top-Level Concepts in SNOMED CT

Top Level Concepts	Frequency
Attribute	991
Body structure	30652
Clinical finding	95605
Context-dependent categories	3649
Environments and geographic locations	1620
Events	87
Observable entity	7274
Organism	25026
Pharmaceutical/biologic product	16867
Physical force	199
Physical object	4201
Procedure	46066
Qualifier value	8134
Social context	4896
Special concept	178
Specimen	1053
Staging and scales	1098
Substance	22267

BOX 7-6 Explanation of Attributes of Top Concepts in SNOMED CT

Procedure/intervention includes all purposeful activities performed in the provision of health care.

Finding/disorder groups together concepts that result from an assessment or judgment.

Measurable/observable entity includes observable functions such as "vision" as well as things that can be measured such as "hemoglobin level."

Social/administrative concept aggregates concepts from the CTV3 "administrative statuses" and "administrative values" hierarchies as well as concepts from the SNOMED RT "social context" hierarchy.

Body structure includes anatomic concepts as well as abnormal body structures, including the "morphologic abnormality" concept.

Organism includes all organisms, including micoorganisms and infectious agents (including prions, fungi, plants, and animals).

Substance includes chemicals, drugs, proteins, and functional categories of substance as well as structural and state-based categories, such as liquid, solid, gas, etc.

Physical object includes natural and manmade objects, including devices and materials.

Physical force includes motion, friction, gravity, electricity, magnetism, sound, radiation, thermal forces (heat and cold), humidity, air

pressure, and other categories mainly directed at categorizing mechanisms of injury.

Event is a category that includes occurrences that result in injury (accidents, falls, etc.) and excludes procedures and interventions.

Environment/geographic location lists types of environments as well as named locations such as countries, states, or regions.

Specimen lists entities that are obtained for examination or analysis, usually from the body of a patient.

Context-dependent category distinguishes concepts that have precoordinated *context*, that is, information that fundamentally changes the type of thing it is associated with. For example, "family history of" is context because it modifies "myocardial infarction"; the resulting "family history of myocardial infarction" is no longer a type of heart disease. Other examples of contextual modifiers include "absence of," "at risk of," and so on.

Attribute lists the concepts that are used as *defining attributes* or *qualifying attributes*, that is, the middle element of the object-attribute-value triple that describes all SNOMED CT relationships.

Qualifier value categorizes the remaining concepts (those that have not been listed in the foregoing categories) that are used as the *value* of the object-attribute-value triples.

BOX 7-7

Concept Representation and Unique Identifiers for Myocardial Infarction

Example:

Some of the descriptions associated with ConceptID 22298006:

- Fully Specified Name: Myocardial infarction (disorder)
- DescriptionID 751689013
- Preferred term: Myocardial infarction
- DescriptionID 37436014
- Synonym: Cardiac infarction
- DescriptionID 34772013
- Synonym: Heart attack
- DescriptionID 37443015
- Synonym: Infarction of heart
- DescriptionID 37441018

Each of these descriptions has a unique DescriptionID, and all are associated with a single Concept (and the single ConceptID 22298006).

across specialties and sites of care. It is based on concepts. Each concept represents a unit of thought or meaning and is labeled with a computer-readable unique identifier. Box 7-7 provides a sample of terms and symptoms associated with myocardial infarction. Note a unique identifier is provided with each term and grouped with ConceptID 22298006: Myocardial Infarction (MI).[44]

The phrases in human language used to describe the concept are called *descriptions* or *synonyms*. Each concept has one or more descriptions linked to it. SNOMED provides a rich set of logical interrelationships between concepts. Through the use of these relationships, computer-readable definitions of medical concepts can be provided. These definitions greatly enhance the value of the data collected, allowing it to be searched, retrieved, reused, or analyzed in a variety of ways.

Hierarchical relationships define specific concepts as children of more general concepts. For example, *appendicitis* is defined as a kind of "inflammatory disorder of the intestine." In this way, hierarchical relationships provide links to related information about the concept. This example shows that appendicitis also represents a part of the body and has a morphologic characteristic of inflammation (Figure 7-10).

In medicine, there are many ways to state the same concept. By linking synonyms to a single concept, SNOMED CT allows computer systems to recognize the common meaning of synonymous terms. Description logic assists in providing a complete and full definition. There are several types of relationships. Review Figure 7-6, which illustrates a more detailed representation of the "is-a" relationships of the diagnosis of coronary atherosclerosis.

One of the greatest strengths of SNOMED is that it was designed with electronic systems in mind. In addition to EHR applications, SNOMED CT is being used for problem lists, intensive care unit monitoring, decision support applications, alerts and reminders, patient care assessments, data collection at the point of care, medical research studies, clinical trials, disease surveillance, and image indexing. It is used in quality and public health reporting of infectious diseases, cancer, and biosurveillance. SNOMED CT enables patients and providers to describe an individual's health and care with true fidelity to the clinical status while maintaining the integrity of the information of both human and machine readability. The ability to capture, store, and exchange health information with this precision improves patient safety and consumer services.

As of July 2009, the core terminology contained more than 308,000 active health care concepts with formal logic based definitions, organized into hierarchies. It contains more than 791,000 active English-language descriptions to extend flexibility in expressing clinical concepts. It also provides more than 951,000 logically defining relationships that enable consistency of data retrieval and analysis.[45] SNOMED CT has gained broad popularity and use. It is even available in an iPhone and TouchPad in an app called Snomobile and a free browser named Snoflake.

SNOMED CT works to provide links to other classification and coding schemes in the United States and around the world. These links are called *cross-maps*. Mapping

Semantic Definition

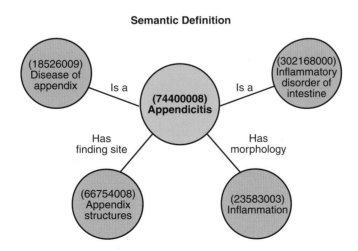

FIGURE 7-10 SNOMED CT appendicitis. (From the College of American Pathologists.)

enables users to use data for multiple purposes without having to capture the data in multiple formats. Mapping is valuable for retaining the value of historical data when migrating to newer database formats and terminology versions. SNOMED has also integrated various domain-specific vocabularies into its terminology such as the nursing vocabularies, laboratory LOINCs, and Systematized Nomenclature of Dentistry (SNODENT).[46] SNOMED has been mapped to other clinical terminologies, including LOINC, ICD-9, ICD-10, and ICD-O. Additional maps are under development. Mapping enables streamlining data capture and facilitating billing, health reporting, and statistical analysis. A single SNOMED CT concept may require one or more target codes in ICD-9-CM to fully represent the SNOMED CT concept as shown in the mapping algorithm in Table 7-6.[47]

When data links are accurate, data can be reused and fewer errors occur. The mapping resources include simple many-to-one tables, such as SNOMED to ICD-O3 topography, more complicated lists of alternatives (to ICD-9 or ICD-10), OPCS-4 classification of interventions, and nursing classification systems (Perioperative Nursing Data Set [PNDS], Nursing Interventions Classification [NIC], Nursing Outcomes Classification [NOC], and North American Nursing Diagnosis Association [NANDA]).[48,49]

In the United States, the HIT Standards Committee has endorsed the use of SNOMED CT for physician clinical observations by 2015. ICD-9 and ICD-10 are classifications created for billing and mortality purposes and are not suitable in the long term for denoting physician observations in an EHR. In 2010, providers had to use ICD-9 or SNOMED CT to qualify for federal recovery bonuses, and in 2014 they must use ICD-10 or SNOMED CT. This is part of the CMS "meaningful use" regulation with which providers must comply to qualify for bonuses for using EHR systems.[50]

Logical Observation Identifiers Names and Codes

LOINC is another example of a terminology designed for use in EHR systems.[51] It is a system of 36,000 concepts used to represent laboratory and clinical measurements, survey questions, clinical documents, and diagnostic reports. The concepts include names, codes, and synonyms. LOINC was designed to facilitate the exchange and aggregation of results—such as blood hemoglobin, serum potassium, and vital signs—for clinical care, outcomes management, and research.

The LOINC database and supporting documentation are maintained by the Regenstrief Institute,[52] with funding by the NLM, John A. Hartford Foundation of New York, and the Agency for Health Care Policy and Research (AHCPR) and through a grant and cooperative agreement from the CDC.

Regenstrief LOINC Mapping Assistant (RELMA) is the tool used to view and search the LOINC database. The purpose of the database is to facilitate the exchange of results for clinical care, outcomes management, and research. Presently, most laboratories and clinical services use HL7 to send from their reporting systems to their patient care systems. HL7 enables this exchange. However, the results in these messages are identified by local code values. The patient care systems may not be able to understand and file the results properly, unless these facilities adopt the laboratory's codes. This is problematic when multiple sources are used. The other alternative is to invest in mapping each code from the laboratories to their own internal codes. LOINC codes are universal identifiers for laboratory and other clinical observations that solve this problem.[53] The power of LOINC is in the ability to facilitate the exchange of information between health care entities. LOINC has expanded beyond the laboratory realm to include clinical measurements, assessments, and clinical document references. The clinical portion of LOINC includes vital signs, hemodynamics, intake and output, electrocardiogram, obstetrical ultrasound, cardiac echo, urologic imaging, gastroendoscopic procedures, pulmonary ventilator management, and other clinical observations and survey instruments such as the Glasgow coma score, patient health questionaire-9 depression scale, and the CMS-required patient assessment instruments. Examples of LOINC order set names and their descriptions appear in Table 7-7.[54]

Dr. Stan Huff and his colleagues at Intermountain Health Care in Salt Lake City used LOINC to establish an information model to capture the data necessary to treat patients undergoing organ transplantation effectively. The model enables them to record not only information about the patient but information about the donor as well. It is a reusable model for circumstances when it is necessary to refer to one patient's data from another patient's EHR, as is necessary in situations such as transplants and mother–child relationships.[55]

TABLE 7-6 SNOMED CT Mapping Algorithm to ICD-9-CM

SNOMED CT		Map Option	Map Group	Map Category	Map Advice	Target Code
25412000	Diabetic retinal microaneurysm (disorder)	1	1	11	Otherwise	250.50 diabetes with ophthalmic manifestations type II or unspecified type
		1	2	11	Otherwise	362.01 background diabetic retinopathy

TABLE 7-7 | LOINC Order Sets and Descriptions

LOINC_NUM	LOINC Fully Specified Name	Description
24358-4	Hemogram panel:-:Pt:Bld:Qn	HCT & HGB & WBC & RBC & Indices
24359-2	Hemogram & differential panel:-:Pt:Bld:Qn	Hemogram & Differential count
24361-8	Hemogram, platelets, & differential panel:-:Pt:Bld:Qn	Hemogram & Differential & Platelets
24317-0	Hemogram & platelet panel:-:Pt:Bld:Qn	HCT & HGB & WBC & RBC & Indices & Platelets
24388-6	Gas panel:-:Pt:Bld:Qn	pH & PO_2 & PCO_2 on blood without specifying whether arterial, venous, or other source. The report would usually include an observation about the inspired O_2 sent along with the report. It may include a variety of other patient characteristics sent by the requester and a variety of computed variables.
24366-0	Gas panel:-:Pt:BldA:Qn	pH & PO_2 & PCO_2 on arterial blood. The report would usually include an observation about the inspired O_2 sent along with the report. It may include a variety of other patient characteristics sent by the requester and a variety of computed variables.
24339-4	Gas panel:-:Pt:BldV:Qn	pH & PO_2 & PCO_2 on venous blood. The report would usually include an observation about the inspired O_2 sent along with the report. It may include a variety of other patient characteristics sent by the requester and a variety of computed variables.
29274-8	Vital signs measurement: Find: PT^Patient^Multi	Diastolic blood pressure & systolic blood pressure & pulse rate & respiratory rate
24357-6	UA dipstick panel:-:Pt:Urine-	Urinalysis dipstick results. Usually includes glucose, bilirubin, estimate of leukocytes, estimate of RBCs, estimate of bacteria, pH, specific gravity. However, we do not make distinctions about the exact set of measures on the dipstick. The ordering clinician will not necessarily know what particular dipstick is being used and is not able to or interested in making those distinctions.
29756-6	Bacterial susceptibility panel:-:Pt:Isolate:OrdQn	Would include susceptibility results for the antibiotics relevant to the isolates and kind of culture.

HCT, Hematocrit; *HGB,* hemoglobin; *O_2,* oxygen; *PCO_2,* partial pressure of carbon dioxide; *pH,* hydrogen ion concentration; *PO_2,* partial pressure of oxygen; *RBC,* red blood (cell) count; *WBC,* white blood (cell) count.

The LOINC document naming nomenclature contains five axes: subject matter domain, role, setting, service, and document type. A standard title is created by combining a term from each axis into a composite title. Not all axes are required to create a valid document title; some may be left blank as long as the correct order is maintained.

There is now what is known as clinical document ontologies, a formalized naming and coding of document types. In a study conducted in the University Hospital of Munster, Germany, a tertiary care center with 1500 beds,

1.3 million documents were studied. The documents were mapped to LOINC. For 937 of the documents, an LOINC code was identified that could be assigned to the documents, HL7's clinical document architecture (CDA) provides a framework for the exchange of documents. HL7's CDA recommends the use of LOINC codes for clinical documents. Work continues to be done to name and code documents. You can see the 45 unique LOINC codes (Table 7-8) that were identified and assigned in this study.[56]

TABLE 7-8 | LOINC Document Title Codes

LOINC Codes	Text	Count
11502	Laboratory report. Total	518141
11528	Study. total (radiology)	185686
34106	discharge summarization note (hospital)	91873
51851	administrative note (generic)	69188
34764	consultation note (General Medicine)	43859
11488	consultation note (generic)	40330
53242	charge ticket or encounter form attachment	36516
51897	Health Care associated infection report	28632
33720	Blood bank consult	23595

Continued

TABLE 7-8 LOINC Document Title Codes—cont'd

LOINC Codes	Text	Count
34130	subsequent evaluation note (hospital)	12468
18751	Study report (endoscopy)	11403
18746	Study report (colonoscopy)	9909
11526	Study report (pathology)	9305
11504	surgical operation note (generic)	8829
34104	consultation note (hospital)	8738
29750	Neonatal Intensive Care records	5744
18757	Study report (Radnuc)	5695
34133	summarization of episode note (generic)	5538
51847	assessment Plan note (generic)	5462
11492	history and physical note (hospital)	3848
18759	Study report (Respiratory system)	3413
34861	evaluation and management note (Diabetology)	3318
29751	Critical Care records	2959
34112	evaluation and management note (inpatient)	2919
11522	Study report (cardiac echo)	2789
15508	labor and delivery records	1804
28570	procedure note (generic)	1773
18729	urinalysis studies	1629
34807	consultation note (ophthalmology)	1578
34761	consultation note (gastroenterology)	1534
34109	evaluation and management note (generic)	1474
34806	evaluation and management note (oncology)	1244
11524	Study report (EKG)	1212
34752	evaluation and management note (cardiology)	1175
34905	evaluation and management note (neurology)	671
52072	non-emergency transportation attachment	605
28568	visit note (Emergency Department)	505
34103	consultation note (pulmonary)	485
34878	evaluation and management note (Emergency Medicine)	412
34796	evaluation and management note (nephrology)	387
52063	prescription for durable medical equipment attachment	243
34782	evaluation and management note (Infectious Diseases)	177
34759	evaluation and management note (dermatology)	137
34824	consultation note (physical therapy)	52
34876	pre-operative evaluation and management note (Surgery)	33

HIS, Hospital information systems; *LOINC*, logical observation identifiers names and codes.
Dugas M, Thun S, Frankewitsch T, Keitmann K: LOINC codes for hospital information systems: documents: a case study, *J Am Info Assoc* 16:400-403, 2009. http://dx.doi.org/10.1197/jamiaM2882.

Example: Use of LOINC for VA Note Titles

Virtually all clinical documents created by Veterans Affairs (VA) providers are stored in VistA; as a result, patient records containing hundreds or thousands of notes are becoming common. As of December 2005, VistA systems contained nearly 779 million progress notes, discharge summaries, and reports; 1.54 billion orders; and almost 425 million images. More than 577,000 new clinical documents, 906,000 orders, and 608,000 images are added each work day—a wealth of information for the clinician. As the volume of online information increases, the task of finding a specific note or report can be difficult, particularly when different clinicians and sites assign different names to similar documents. In using the Computerized Patient Record System (CPRS), a graphical interface to the information in VistA, clinicians use an onscreen menu to select a document based on its title. However, the readability of document titles varied widely from site to site and from author to author. Titles such as *UR 67CD (T) (K)*, *CIH/STAR II CONSUL*, or *PATIENT HEALTH EDU POINT AND CLICK*, for example, might be clear to the author but are difficult for other users to decipher. Users were often frustrated with the time required to find relevant notes among hundreds of irregularly structured titles.

To speed the retrieval of clinical information, a team of VA clinicians, developers, terminologists, and HIM professionals collaborated to establish standard conventions for naming and transmitting clinical documents created in VistA.

After researching existing LOINC and HL7 standards, the team extracted 156,000 document titles from 128 site-based databases, analyzed every term within the extracted titles, and categorized them in accordance with LOINC naming standards and HL7 messaging standards. The LOINC document naming nomenclature contains five axes: subject matter domain, role, setting, service, and document type. A standard title is created by combining a term from each axis into a composite title. Not all axes are required to create a valid document title; some may be left blank as long as the correct order is maintained. The use of standardized note titles will make it easier for users to find relevant clinical documents and to transfer and incorporate documents created at other VA and non-VA sites. To minimize disruption at the local level, VA facilities were not required to rename clinical documents already stored in VistA. Instead, the titles of existing documents are mapped to the new standard title format before the documents are transmitted to a national clinical repository, where they are accessible to providers throughout VA.

LOINC has a website that offers free downloads of LOINC, user's guides, and online training, in addition to a tutorial on clinical document naming. Check out http://loinc.org. Another site has a free SNOMED browser to look up clinical terms at www.snoflake.co.uk.

RxNorm

RxNorm is a standardized nomenclature for clinical drugs and drug delivery devices produced by the NLM. RxNorm's standard names for clinical drugs and drug delivery devices are linked to the various names of drugs present in many different controlled vocabularies within the UMLS Metathesaurus. These connections facilitate interoperability among computerized systems that record or process data dealing with clinical drugs. This standardized nomenclature serves as a means for determining when names from different source vocabularies are synonymous (at an appropriate level of abstraction), and can thereby share data efficiently at the appropriate level. The goal of RxNorm is to enable various systems using different drug nomenclatures to exchange and share data efficiently and avoid ambiguity. RxNorm preserves the meanings, concept names, and relationships from its source vocabularies.

Like the UMLS Metathesaurus, RxNorm is organized by concept. Figure 7-11 shows relationships among RxNorm drug entities to determine a concept.[57]

A concept is a collection of names identical in meaning at a specified level of abstraction. It enables strings of characters from disparate sources to be taken to the name of things that are the same. To do this, the concept is assigned an RxNorm concept unique identifier (**RXCUI**). If two drug names share the same concept, RxNorm assigns the preferred name and a concept unique identifier (CUI). The RXCUI always designates the same concept, no matter the source, the form of the name, or in what table it is found. All drugs whose names map to the same RXCUI are taken to be the same drug. They must be identical as to ingredients, strengths, and dose forms. An RxNorm clinical drug name reflects the active ingredients, strengths, and dose form for that drug. When any of these elements vary, a new RxNorm drug name is created as a separate concept. Conversely, drugs that differ in any of these particulars are conceptually distinct and will have different CUIs. An RxNorm name should exist for every strength and dose of every available combination of clinically significant ingredients.[58]

National Drug Code, RxNorm, and UMLS Metathesaurus

The NDC system was originally established as part of an out-of-hospital drug reimbursement program under Medicare but has since expanded in scope. The NCD system is currently mandated by HIPAA as the standard medical data code set for reporting drugs and biologics for retail pharmacy transactions. The NDC is owned by the FDA and distributed by the Department of Health and Human Services (DHHS) and is sometimes referred to as the *FDA-NDCs*. Drugs administered in health care settings are reported under HIPAA billing transactions. The NDC and Healthcare Common Procedure Coding System (**HCPCS**) drug codes are used for outpatient reimbursement of facility, physician, and pharmaceutical (chemotherapy and injectable) services.[21] The NDC directory lists more than 100,000 prescription drugs and selected over-the-counter drugs.

NDC uses a unique, 10-digit, three-segment number to identify drug products:

- The first segment identifies *the vendor* participating in the manufacture, packaging, or distribution of the drug.
- The second segment includes the product codes for *generic composition, specific strength, formulation*, and *dosage form*.
- The third segment is used to indicate *package size* and *types*.

This drug code is used as a universal product identifier for human drugs. The NDC Directory is organized by product trade name, NDC number, dosage form, routes of administration, active ingredients, strength, package size and type, major drug class, and FDA approval application number. The use of the NDC provides the FDA with a

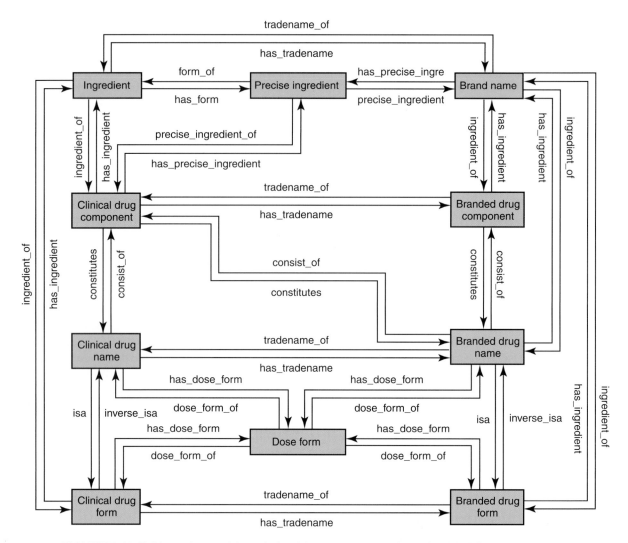

FIGURE 7-11 RxNorm drug entities relationships to concepts. (From PubMed Central: Using the RxNorm web services API for quality assurance purposes, *AMIA Annual Symposium Proc* 591-595, 2008: http://www.ncbi.nlm.nih.gov/pmc/articles/PMC2656097.)

Drug Coding Systems Working Together

RxNorm obtains NDCs from the Veterans Health Administration (VHA), the FDA, the CMS, the Multum Lexicon, and Gold Standard. NDCs are listed as attributes asserted by the

significant tool for reporting, monitoring, and sending out recalls of products identified as causing safety risks to the public (Box 7-8).

source vocabulary. RxNorm will assert what is believed to be the correct association with NDC codes. There are differences between the NDC codes and those used in RxNorm because there is not a one-to-one relationship between the NDC codes and RxNorm forms. One RxNorm form may have many different NDC codes. This is because RxNorm is concept based, whereas NDC codes include specificity down to the package size. A conflict resolution process is used to resolve issues when identified. Instances such as these furnish RxNorm with an important quality assurance opportunity.

When conflicts arise between sources, other means of obtaining information about the drug may be used to determine the correct NDC. It is important that resolutions are reached to avoid potential patient safety problems. The representation of the relationships between drugs from various sources, including their ingredients, strength, and dose forms, is essential in providing the structure to support CPOE, e-prescribing, and health information exchange.

BOX 7-8	National Drug Code Use and Structure

Food and Drug Administration National Drug Code used in product marketing and distribution to describe product presentation and formulation.

Required 10-digit, three-segment number separated by hyphens field that identifies the labeler, product, and trade package size.

RxNorm and the UMLS Metathesaurus

The full set of RxNorm files is included in UMLS Metathesaurus. Unlike the NDCs, the UMLS CUIs and RxNorm RXCUIs should have a one-to-one relationship. The Drug Listing Act of 1972 requires drug firms to provide the FDA with a current list of all drugs manufactured, prepared, propagated, compounded, or processed for commercial distribution. All drug notices received by the FDA are then coded to identify the drug by its vendor, its strength, formulation, and dosage form, and its packaging. The UMLS Metathesaurus as a whole is updated two to three times a year, but RxNorm is available as a full update on a monthly basis. In addition, a weekly update containing data from Daily Med and newly approved drugs is available weekly. Between releases of the UMLS, RxNorm update files are available through the UMLS Knowledge Source Server.

The National Drug File–Reference Terminology

The NDF-RT is produced by the VHA and is an extension of the VHA National Drug File (NDF). The NDF-RT is used for modeling drug characteristics including ingredients, chemical structure, dose form, physiologic effect, mechanism of action, pharmacokinetics, and related diseases. It combines the NDF hierarchical drug classification with a multicategory reference model. The Metathesaurus representation of NDF-RT includes only concepts above the "Packaged Product" level. Some attributes of concepts at this level have been attached to the parent product level concept. NDF-RT is updated monthly.

The graph in (Figure 7-12) illustrates the FDA, VA, and NLM drug information integration into the Metathesaurus.[59]

Table 7-9 can be searched via the NDC database to drill down to the profile of a particular drug.

Federal Medication Terminologies

The Federal Medication interagency collaboration is organizing a set of standard, comprehensive Federal Medication Terminologies (FMTs) that will be freely available in its aim to improve the exchange and public availability of medication information and support health information technology interoperability. It is hoped that this effort will provide access to a common language for communicating medication information, processes for maintaining terminologies, and an infrastructure for sharing that information (Figure 7-13).

The initial FMT set has been endorsed by the U.S. federal standards agencies, including the NCVHS, CHI, the

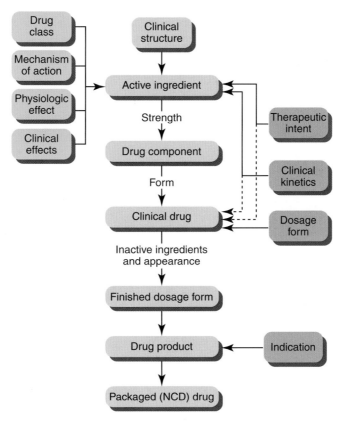

FIGURE 7-12 Drug terminologies working together. *NCD,* National coverage determination. (From Amatayakul M, Lazarus SS: PowerPoint Presentation: Hospitals and Health Systems: Negotiating the ROI for CPOE/e-Prescribing, Slide adapted from U.S. government drug terminology, Randy Levin, MD, April 14, 2004: http://www.ehcca.com/presentations/hitsummit1/7_06_2.ppt.)

TABLE 7-9 Searching National Drug Codes

ndc_code	brand_description	main_mul	Route_description	dose_form	product_streng	drug_id	active_ingredi	Strength_nu	strength_num	Obsolete_date
4569458900	Baycol	6406	oral	tablet	0.3 mg	d04140	cerivastatin sod	0.3	milligram(s)	8/7/2001
4569486100	Baycol	7025	oral	tablet	0.4 mg	d04140	cerivastatin sod	0.4	milligram(s)	8/7/2001
0026288351	Baycol	6405	oral	tablet	0.2 mg	d04140	cerivastatin sod	0.2	milligram(s)	8/7/2001
0026288569	Baycol	7025	oral	tablet	0.4 mg	d04140	cerivastatin sod	0.4	milligram(s)	8/7/2001
0026288486	Baycol	6406	oral	tablet	0.3 mg	d04140	cerivastatin sod	0.3	milligram(s)	8/7/2001
0026288586	Baycol	7025	oral	tablet	0.4 mg	d04140	cerivastatin sod	0.4	milligram(s)	8/7/2001
0026288551	Baycol	7025	oral	tablet	0.4 mg	d04140	cerivastatin sod	0.4	milligram(s)	8/7/2001
0026288451	Baycol	6406	oral	tablet	0.3 mg	d04140	cerivastatin sod	0.3	milligram(s)	8/7/2001
0026288386	Baycol	6405	oral	tablet	0.2 mg	d04140	cerivastatin sod	0.2	milligram(s)	8/7/2001
0026288686	Baycol	7748	oral	tablet	0.8 mg	d04140	cerivastatin sod	0.8	milligram(s)	8/7/2001
0026288669	Baycol	7748	oral	tablet	0.8 mg	d04140	cerivastatin sod	0.8	milligram(s)	8/7/2001
2843010117	Bayer Aspirin	5464	oral	tablet	325 mg	d00170	aspirin	325	milligram(s)	
2843020233	Bayer Aspirin	5465	oral	tablet	500 mg	d00170	aspirin	500	milligram(s)	
2843020234	Bayer Aspirin	5465	oral	tablet	500 mg	d00170	aspirin	500	milligram(s)	
2843020235	Bayer Aspirin	5465	oral	tablet	500 mg	d00170	aspirin	500	milligram(s)	
2843010112	Bayer Aspirin	5464	oral	tablet	325 mg	d00170	aspirin	325	milligram(s)	
2843019188	Bayer Aspirin	5467	oral	tablet	650 mg	d00170	aspirin	650	milligram(s)	
2843033336	Bayer Aspirin	5464	oral	tablet	325 mg	d00170	aspirin	325	milligram(s)	
2843033337	Bayer Aspirin	5464	oral	tablet	325 mg	d00170	aspirin	325	milligram(s)	
2843010118	Bayer Aspirin	5464	oral	tablet	325 mg	d00170	aspirin	325	milligram(s)	
2843010110	Bayer Aspirin	5464	oral	tablet	325 mg	d00170	aspirin	325	milligram(s)	
2843010106	Bayer Aspirin	5464	oral	tablet	325 mg	d00170	aspirin	325	milligram(s)	
2843010239	Bayer Aspirin	546	oral	tablet	325 mg	d00170	aspirin	325	milligram(s)	
2843010220	Bayer Aspirin	5464	oral	tablet	325 mg	d00170	aspirin	325	milligram(s)	
2843010181	Bayer Aspirin	5464	oral	tablet	325 mg	d00170	aspirin	325	milligram(s)	
2843010120	Bayer Aspirin	5464	oral	tablet	325 mg	d00170	aspirin	325	milligram(s)	
2843010113	Bayer Aspirin	5464	oral	tablet	325 mg	d00170	aspirin	325	milligram(s)	
2843010238	Bayer Aspirin	5464	oral	tablet	325 mg	d00170	aspirin	325	milligram(s)	
2843010111	Bayer Aspirin	5464	oral	tablet	325 mg	d00170	aspirin	325	milligram(s)	
2843010762	Bayer Aspirin PM Extr	6008	oral	tablet	500 mg–25 mg	d04155	aspirin	500	milligram(s)	

FIGURE 7-13 Federal medication terminologies components. *NCIt,*; *NDC,* national drug codes; *NDF-RT,* national drug file–reference terminology; *UNIs,* (From http://evs.nci.nih.gov/ftp1/FMT/FMT%20FHA%20Presentation.ppt.)

FMT Support to Health IT Systems

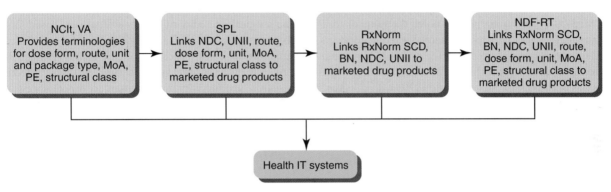

FIGURE 7-14 Federal medication terminologies that support health information technology (IT) systems. *BN,* Brand name; *FMT,* federal medication terminologies; *MoA,* mechanism of action; *NCIt; NDC,* national drug codes; *PE,* pharmacokinetic effect; *SCD,* semantic clinical drug; *SPL,* structured product labeling; *UNII,* unique ingredient identifier; *VA,* Veterans Affairs. (From http://evs.nci.nih.gov/ftp1/FMT/FMT%20FHA%20Presentation.ppt.)

Healthcare Information Technology Standards Panel (HITSP), and the Office of the National Coordinator for Health Information Technology (ONCHIT).[60]

The FMT Web Portal is accessible at http://www.cancer.gov/cancertopics/terminologyresources/FMT (Figure 7-14; Box 7-9).

Universal Medical Device Nomenclature System

The UMDNS is a proprietary, standardized, and controlled international nomenclature and coding system for medical devices. It has been adopted by many nations and is available in several languages. The U.S. NLM has incorporated UMDNS into UMLS.

The purpose of UMDNS is to facilitate identifying, processing, filing, storing, retrieving, transferring, and communicating data about medical devices, clinical laboratory equipment and in vitro diagnostics, disposables and supplies, hospital furniture, and instruments used to test clinical equipment. The nomenclature is used in applications ranging from hospital inventory and work-order controls to national agency medical device regulatory systems, from e-commerce and procurement to medical device databases. UMDNS is limited to International Medical Device codes and UMDNS codes.

UMDNS contains nearly 7500 unique medical device concepts and definitions (preferred terms), along with an additional 8000 entry terms to facilitate classifying of biomedical information. It contains explicit relationships among the

BOX 7-9	Federal Medications Terminologies Terms Defined
NDF-RT	National Drug File–Reference Terminology
SCD	semantic clinical drug
BN	brand name
NDC	National Drug Code
PE	pharmacokinetic effect
UNII	unique ingredient identifier
MoA	mechanism of action
RoA	route of administration
NCIt	National Cancer Institute thesaurus; terminologies for dose form, route, unit, and package type, MoA, PE, and structural class
SPL	structured product labeling; an American National Standards Institute-accredited Health Level 7 standard for the exchange of product information on approved prescription drug products

(Federal Medical Terminologies Standards supported by SPL include the National Library of Medicine, RxNorm SCD, RxNorm BN.)

nearly 15,500 terms, including hierarchical relationships (e.g., parent-child terms), synonymous relations, and relationships among related devices (e.g., component devices vs. the overall system).[61] Medical device codes are used to track approved medical devices, their descriptions, product safety, and their manufacturers.

Table 7-2 shows an example of terminology used for medical devices. It comes from the database maintained by the FDA. The table shows the results of a query of product defects that have resulted in death and have been recalled.

Nursing Terminologies

Under HIPAA, the National Committee on Vital and Health Statistics assessed clinical terminology standards for the Patient Medical Record Initiative and noted the value of additional nursing terminologies to represented nursing concepts. Nursing terminologies are necessary for nurses to document their effect on patient care in EHRs. Work on nursing terminologies has been ongoing since the late 1970s with the greatest thrust occurring in the 1990s.[39] The use of a standardized nursing language, along with advances in information technology, can enhance nursing efficiency, accuracy, and effectiveness and significantly improve patient care. Outcomes can be validated and linked to specific nursing care interventions. However, although great strides have been made, the consistent use of a standardized nursing terminology is still minimal in both the clinical and nursing academic settings.[62]

The American Nursing Association (ANA) has formally recognized the following nursing terminologies (Table 7-10).[63] Note the terminologies that are integrated with UMLS and SNOMED CT.

The ANA developed nursing classification themes to describe the nursing process, document nursing care, and facilitate aggregation of data for comparisons at the local, regional, national, and international levels. Two notable nursing classification systems include the NIC and the NOC. NIC and NOC are comprehensive, research-based, standardized systems used to classify the interventions that nurses perform and outcome evaluations based on those interventions.[64,65] NIC and NOC are useful for clinical documentation, communication of care across settings, integration of data across systems and settings, effectiveness research, productivity measurement, competency evaluation, reimbursement, and curriculum design. NIC and NOC can be used in all settings (from acute care intensive care units, to home care, to hospice, to primary care) and all specialties (from critical care to ambulatory and long-term care). Both

TABLE 7-10   Nursing Terminologies

ANA Recognized Terminologies	Terminology URL	Nursing Process Within Terminology	Date Recognized by the ANA	Integrated Within Other Terminologies
CCC Clinical Care Classification	http://www.sabacare.com/	Diagnoses, Interventions, and Outcomes	1992	HL7, UMLS, SNOMED CT
ICNP International Classification of Nursing Practice	http://www.icn.ch/icnp.htm	Diagnoses, Interventions, and Outcomes	Not referenced in June 2008	NLM-UMLS
NANDA NANDA International	http://www.nanda.org	Nursing Diagnoses	1992	NLM-UMLS, SNOMED CT, PNDS, HL7, NIDSEC
NIC Nursing Intervention Classification	http://www.nursing.uiowa.edu/cncce/nursing-interventions-classification-overview	Interventions	1992	NLM-UMLS, SNOMED CT, HL7, NIDSEC, ABC Codes
NOC Nursing Outcome Classification	http://www.nursing.uiowa.edu/cncce/nursing-outcomes-classification-overview	Outcomes Indicators	1998	NLM-UMLS, SNOMED CT, HL7, NIDSEC
Omaha System	http://www.omahasystem.org	Problem Classification Scheme Intervention Scheme Problem Rating Scale for Outcomes	1992	NLM-UMLS, SNOMED CT, HL7, NIDSEC, LOINC, ABC Codes
PNDS Perioperative Nursing Data Set	http://www.aorn.org/PNDS/	Diagnoses, Interventions, and Outcomes	1999	NLM-UMLS, SNOMED CT, HL7
SNOMED CT Systematic Nomenclature of Medicine, Clinical Terms	http://www.ihtsdo.org/snomed-ct/	Assessment Concepts, Diagnoses, Interventions, and Outcomes	2002	NLM-UMLS

ANA, American Nurses Association; HL7, Health Level 7; LOINC, Logical Observation Identifiers Names and Codes; NIDSEC, ***; NLM, National Library of Medicine; PNDS, Perioperative Nursing Data Set; SNOMED CT, Systematized Nomenclature of Medicine, Clinical Terms; UMLS, Unified Medical Language System.

NIC and NOC have been registered in HL7 and have been mapped to SNOMED.

Differences in NIC and NOC

NOC is focused on *outcomes*. NOC is a three-level classification system currently composed of 7 domains, 29 outcome classes, and 260 outcomes. An outcome is a measurable individual, family, or community state, behavior, or perception that is measured along a continuum and is responsive to nursing interventions. Although the entire classification describes the domain of nursing, some of the interventions in the classification are also performed by other providers. Each outcome is associated with varying quantities of indicators. Each indicator is given a score on 1 of 17, 5-point Likert-type scales. This structure allows for measurement and comparison at any point along a continuum. It is possible to follow patient outcomes for an extended period. Examples of outcomes influenced by nursing interventions include Ambulation, Caregiver Emotional Health, Mobility Level, Nutritional Status, and Cognitive Orientation.[66]

NIC is focused on *interventions*. Interventions are included for direct care and in health promotion. Although most of the interventions are for use with individuals, many are for use with families on behalf of patients (e.g., Family Integrity Promotion), and some are for use with entire communities (e.g., Environmental Management: Community). Indirect care interventions (e.g., Supply Management) are also included. Each intervention, as it appears in the classification, is listed with a label name, a definition, a set of activities to carry out the intervention, and background readings. NIC can be used by other nonphysician providers to describe their treatments. NIC is recognized by The Joint Commission (JCAHO) as one nursing classification system that can be used to meet the standard on uniform data. Both NIC and NOC are registered in HL7 and have been mapped to SNOMED.

Omaha System

The Omaha System was one of the first taxonomies or terminologies recognized by ANA. It is a research-based, comprehensive, and standardized taxonomy designed to enhance practice, documentation, and information management. It consists of three relational, reliable, and valid components: (1) the Problem Classification Scheme (client assessment), (2) the Intervention Scheme (service delivery), and (3) the Problem Rating Scale for Outcomes (client change/evaluation). Initial adopters included home care, public health, and school health practice settings and some educators in the United States. Omaha System terms and definitions are not held under copyright and so are available for use without permission. However, the source of the terms, definitions, and codes must accompany their use. Other sections of the new book are held under copyright. The Omaha System is integrated into the NLMS Metasaurus, ABC Codes, LOINC, and SNOMED CT. It is registered by HL7. It is being mapped to the International

Classification of Nursing Practice (ICNP).[67] The Problem Classification Scheme (nursing diagnosis) is organized into four levels:

Level 1: Domain	There are four general domain areas: Environmental, Psychosocial, Physiological, Health-Related Behaviors.
Level 2: Problems	There are 42 specific health-related concerns.
Level 3: Modifiers	Types of problem are Actual, Potential, Health Promotion Client Type: Individual, Family, Community.
Level 4: Signs and Symptoms	Evidence of a patient problem exists.

Example of Omaha System Within Domains and Sample Problems

Level 1	Level 2
Environment	Income, Sanitation
Psychosocial	Mental Health, Grieving, Abuse
Physiological	Hearing, Vision, Speech, Circulation
Health Behavior	Nutrition, Medication Regimen

International Classification for Nursing Practice

The ICNP is produced and owned by the International Council of Nurses. ICNP is a unified nursing language system for describing nursing practice. It is designed to facilitate the development of cross-mapping between local terms and other terminologies, and to establish international standards for describing and comparing nursing practice. Its elements are used to represent nursing diagnoses, nursing actions, and nursing outcomes. It is based on a multiaxial model that includes focus, judgment, time, location, means, action, and client. Through cross-mapping, INCP can be used along with existing terminologies to develop new vocabularies, and to identify relationships between concepts and vocabularies. Furthermore, translations are available in more than 15 languages. ICNP is integrated into UMLS Metathesaurus and is updated every 2 years.[68]

The Nursing terminologies and data sets NIC, NOC, the Omaha System (for home care, public health, and community health), and ICNP have been mapped to SNOMED CT, integrated in LOINC, and are included in the NLM Metathesaurus for Unified Medical Language and the Cumulative Index of Nursing and Allied Health Literature (CINAHL) (Figure 7-15).

Terminologies Used at Point of Care

Giannangelo presents a useful distinction for considering the role of terminologies and the EHR. Terminologies are designed to facilitate data collection at the point of care; capture the detail of diagnostic studies, history and physicals, visit notes, ancillary department information, and nursing notes; and allow the ability to send and receive medical data in an understandable and predictable manner. The definition offered by Giannangelo is, "A set of standardized terms and their synonyms that record patient findings, circumstances,

FIGURE 7-15 The relationships among the electronic health record, the terminologies, and the data repository. (From Lundberg C, Warren J, Brokel J, et al: Selecting a standardized terminology for the electronic health record that reveals the impact of nursing on patient care. *Online J Nurs Inform* 12, June 2008: http://ojni.org/12_2/lundberg.pdf.)

events, and interventions with sufficient detail to support clinical care, decision support, outcome research, and quality improvement."[69] For this reason, these are often referred to as *clinical terminologies*. Clinical terminologies that use codes to represent detailed concepts provide a way to combine the expressiveness and flexibility of free text information with the clarity and computability of encoded information.[70]

SNOMED CT is an example of a clinical terminology used to capture data at the point of care. It has been identified as having the greatest potential to handle the complex data representation required in the EHR. It is designed to be embedded in an EHR. Each term is represented as a concept that closely follows the natural thinking of clinicians. When a user selects a term to use, the associated code is stored electronically. These codes are used to transmit health data from one electronic system to another, for analysis, aggregation, or use at the point of care. With encoded data, information can be displayed in a form that human beings can understand and store in a form that computers can exchange and manipulate.

Transaction and Code Set Standards

Electronic exchanges that involve the transfer of information between parties are called *transactions,* as in the case of sending a request for reimbursement of services provided to a health insurance plan. HIPAA requires the use of transaction standards for electronic data interchange (EDI) of health care data. So far, this has been limited to transactions related to establishing health care coverage and payment for services. Covered entities must adhere to the content and format requirements of each required standard if they use electronic exchanges for claims and encounter information, payment and remittance advice, claims status, eligibility, enrollment and disenrollment, referrals and authorizations, and premium payments.

HIPAA also requires specific code sets to be used in all electronic transactions for diagnoses and procedures. The following code sets were mandated by HIPAA:
- ICD-9-CM for inpatient diagnoses and procedures are used through September 30, 2014. On October 1, 2014, ICD-10-CM replaced ICD-9-CM, Volumes 1 and 2. ICD-10-PCS replaced Volume 3 as the procedure coding system.[71]
- The reasons given for discontinuing ICD-9-CM cluster around its shortcomings. ICD-9 was published by the WHO in 1977, after which it was modified by the National Center for Health Statistics (NCHS) to gather more clinical information and capture morbidity and mortality statistics in the United States. The system is outdated. ICD-9-CM has only a limited ability to accommodate new procedures and diagnoses or new and changing medical advancements. ICD-9-CM is inadequate in the way that it places very different procedure codes into diagnosis-related group (DRG) groupings. It has not been able to accommodate new and emerging issues such as biosurveillance and pay-for-performance. Furthermore, it lacks specificity and detail and does not have codes for preventive services, new procedures, or new technology. Another limitation is that it uses terminology inconsistently.[72]
- CPT-4 for physicians' procedures are used by physicians and all health care providers other than inpatient hospitals: CPT, fifth edition (CPT-5) and the HCPCS. Inpatient hospital services procedures will be coded using ICD-10-PCS codes, which provide facility-related procedure codes suitable to inpatient environments.
- HCPCS is used for ancillary services and procedures. This code set represents items, supplies, and nonphysician services not covered by the AMA CPT-5 codes.
- NDC is used to identify the vendor, product, and package size of all medications recognized by the FDA.
- Current Dental Terminology (CDT) is used for dental services; NDC is used to code procedures, diagnoses, and drug services.[73]

HIPAA has adopted standards for unique identifiers for employers and providers that must also be used in all electronic standards for electronic data exchange of health data. Employers must have standard national numbers that identify them on transactions. The employer identification number issued by the Internal Revenue Service is to be used as the identifier for employers.

The Final Rules

The final rules were published in the Federal Register:
1. Health Insurance Reform; Modifications to the Health Insurance Portability and Accountability Act (HIPAA) Electronic Transaction Standards (74 Federal Register 3295-3328)
2. HIPAA Administrative Simplification: Modifications to Medical Data Code Set Standards to Adopt ICD-10-CM and ICD-10-PCS (74 Federal Register 3328-3362)

HIM and Commonly Used Terminologies

Classification systems focus on collecting and reporting of basic health statistics, ensuring quality data for an institutional database for accurate clinical and statistical data, and providing data used in payment systems and for mandatory public health reporting. A classification organizes and groups similar and related entities together and aggregates them under predetermined categories. They are often referred to as *administrative terminologies* as they are designed to support administrative, financial, and regulatory functions associated with health care services. They are used to produce secondary data and reports.

As clinical terminologies are used to document richer and more detailed clinical descriptions, they will replace administrative terminologies at the point of care. Administrative terminologies will continue to be used for statistical and administrative purposes.[74] Some administrative terminologies that are commonly used for administrative purposes include the ICD-10-CM, the CPT, and the HCPCS and DRGs (Figure 7-16).

International Classification of Diseases

The International Classification of Diseases (ICD) is a system used to classify inpatient and outpatient diagnoses and inpatient procedures. The foundation for ICD was established in 1893, with the development of the Bertillion Classification of Causes of Death. Although the system was initially used to classify mortality data from death certificates, it was expanded and adapted for other uses throughout the next century.

International Classification of Diseases, Ninth Revision

In 1977, the WHO published the ICD-9. In response to concerns that ICD-9 did not provide sufficient coverage for general coding and specific specialties, the NCHS initiated work to adapt ICD-9 for use in the United States. NCHS subsequently published a set of "clinical modifications" (CMs) to ICD-9, which reflected the broader use of ICD-9 in the areas of reimbursement, epidemiology, and health sciences research. In ICD-9-CM, Volume 1 contains diagnosis codes. Volume 2 is the alphabetical index for Volume 1. Volume 3 contains procedure codes. ICD-9-CM uses a hierarchical framework to describe body systems. In Volume 1, diagnosis codes contain three, four, or five numeric digits. The first three specify the disease, with the fourth digit providing additional detail. The fifth digit gives subtypes of the disease. ICD-9 uses a core classification of three-digit codes, supplemented by a fourth digit (in the first decimal place) that provides additional detail and specificity.[75,76]

The version of ICD in use in the United States until 2014 is the Ninth Revision with Clinical Modification, known as *ICD-9-CM* (Box 7-10).

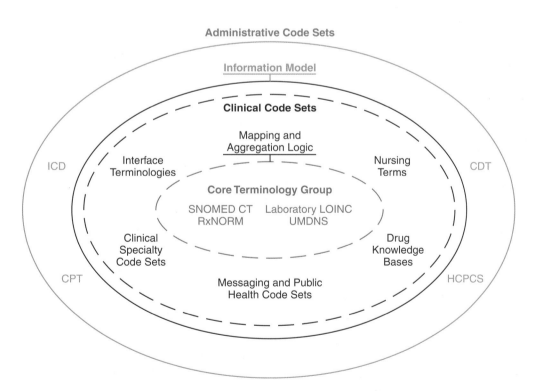

FIGURE 7-16 Administrative code sets. *CCC,* Clinical care classification; *NANDA,* North American Nursing Diagnosis Association; *NIC,* Nursing Interventions Classification; *NOC,* Nursing Outcomes Classification; *PNDS,* Perioperative Nursing Data Set. (From *Relationship of various vocabulary, terminology and classification systems. Patient safety: achieving a new standard for care.* Washington, DC, 2004, National Academic Press.)

BOX 7-10   ICD-9-CM Code Structure

Example of ICD-9-CM Codes

Diagnosis Code: xxx.xx
- First three digits specify disease
- Fourth digit gives additional detail
- Fifth digit specifies subtype of disease

Procedure Code: xx.xx
- First two digits specify anatomic region
- Last two digits specify procedure

International Classification of Diseases, Tenth Revision

In 1992, WHO published ICD-10, the tenth revision of the ICD system. (WHO no longer supports ICD-9.) The United States began to use ICD-10 to report mortality statistics to WHO in 1999. As with ICD-9, NCHS developed a CM for ICD-10 for use in the United States. ICD-10-CM contains significantly more codes and covers more content than ICD-9-CM. It also includes additional information related to ambulatory and managed care encounters, expanded injury codes, combination diagnosis–symptom codes for more concise coding, and laterality codes. Codes in ICD-10-CM are alphanumeric and can contain up to seven digits.

For example, with use of ICD-10, hemiparesis can be more specifically defined by its underlying etiologic factor of intracranial hemorrhage and the addition of a sixth digit related to the affected side of the body, as shown in the comparison between ICD-9-CM and ICD-10-CM[77] (Box 7-11).

International Classification of Diseases, Tenth Revision, Procedural Coding System

Under a contract with the CMS, 3 M Health Information Systems developed the Procedural Coding System (PCS) to replace the list of procedure codes included in ICD-9-CM. ICD-10-PCS is designed to be used for procedure coding in the inpatient hospital setting. It offers a much broader range of codes than ICD-9-CM, with room for expandability and greater specificity. ICD-9-CM is outdated and cannot adequately represent current medical practice and available medical technology. As a data capture tool, CPT does not adequately represent services provided in an inpatient hospital setting. Thus neither terminology allows hospitals to provide complete, accurate, and precise reporting of clinical care. ICD-10-PCS provides nearly 198,000 procedure codes, enabling hospitals to collect more specific information for use in patient care, benchmarking, quality assessment, research, public health reporting, strategic planning, and reimbursement.[29] Table 7-11 contrasts the format and structure of ICD-9-CM and ICD-10 CM codes. ICD-9 lacks the ability to track laterality. Box 7-12 illustrates the broad groupings used in ICD-9 as compared with greater specificity provided in ICD-10.

Although ICD-10-CM was originally targeted for release in 2001, neither the federal government nor the private sector had begun to implement ICD-10-CM or ICD-10-PCS. The NCVHS, which serves as an advisory committee to the secretary of the DHHS, recommended that the federal government make the necessary regulatory changes to require use of ICD-10-CM and ICD-10-PCS codes in the United States.[78] The American Health Information Management Association (AHIMA) endorsed the adoption and implementation of ICD-10-CM and ICD-10-PCS. DHHS announced an effective date of October 1, 2014, for ICD-10-CM compliance. In advance of that, by January 1, 2012, health care organizations were required to implement the precursory systems modifications to accommodate X12 Version 5010 and NCPCP Version D.0 for HIPAA transactions, and NCPCP Version 3.0 for pharmacy claims. Version 5010

BOX 7-11   Comparison of Hemiparesis Coded with ICD-9-CM and ICD-10-CM

ICD-9-CM	ICD-10-CM
438.2 Hemiplegia/hemiparesis	G81.00 Flaccid hemiplegia affecting unspecified side
438.21 Hemiplegia affecting dominant side due to cerebrovascular disease	G81.01 Flaccid hemiplegia affecting right dominant side
438.22 Hemiplegia affecting nondominant side due to cerebrovascular disease	G81.02 Flaccid hemiplegia affecting left dominant side
	G81.00 Flaccid hemiplegia affecting unspecified side
	G81.01 Flaccid hemiplegia affecting right dominant side
	G81.02 Flaccid hemiplegia affecting left dominant side
	G81.03 Flaccid hemiplegia affecting right nondominant side
	G81.04 Flaccid hemiplegia affecting left nondominant side
	G81.1 Spastic hemiplegia
	G81.10 Spastic hemiplegia affecting unspecified side
	G81.11 Spastic hemiplegia affecting right dominant side
	G81.12 Spastic hemiplegia affecting left dominant side
	G81.13 Spastic hemiplegia affecting right nondominant side
	G81.14 Spastic hemiplegia affecting left nondominant side
	G81.9 Hemiplegia, unspecified
	G81.90 Hemiplegia, unspecified affecting unspecified side
	G81.91 Hemiplegia, unspecified affecting right dominant side
	G81.92 Hemiplegia, unspecified affecting left dominant side
	G81.93 Hemiplegia, unspecified affecting right nondominant side

TABLE 7-11 ICD-9-CM Volumes 1 and 2 and ICD-10-CM Comparison

ICD-9-CM Diagnosis Codes	ICD-10-CM Diagnosis Codes
3-5 characters in length	3-7 characters in length
Approximately 13,000 codes	Approximately 68,000 available codes
First digit may be alpha (E or V) or numeric; digits 2-5 are numeric.	First digit is alpha; digits 2-3 are numeric; digits 4-7 are alpha or numeric.
Limited space for adding new codes	Flexible for adding new codes
Lacks detail	Very specific
Lacks laterality	Has laterality
Example: 453.41 Venous embolism and thrombosis of deep vessels of proximal lower extremity	Example: I82.411 Embolism and thrombosis of right femoral vein

ICD-10-CM Format

ICD-9-CM Vol. 3 and ICD-10-PCS Comparison

ICD-9-CM Procedure Codes	ICD-10-PCS Procedure Codes
3-4 numeric characters in length	7 alpha-numeric characters in length
Approximately 3000 codes	Approximately 87,000 available codes
Based on outdated technology	Reflects current usage of medical terminology
Limited space for adding new codes	Flexible for adding new codes
Lacks detail	Very specific
Lacks body site laterality	Has body site laterality
Generic terms for body parts	Detailed descriptions for body parts
Lacks description of methodology and approach for procedures	Provides detailed descriptions of methodology and approach for procedures
Limits DRG usage	Allows DRG definitions to better recognize new technologies and devices
Lacks precision to adequately define procedures	Precisely defines procedures with detail regarding body part, approach, any device used, and qualifying information.
Example: 47.01-Laparoscopic appendectomy	Example: 0DTJ4ZZ—Laparoscopic appendectomy

ICD-10-PCS Format

DRG, Diagnosis-related group.

accommodates ICD-10 code sets and has an earlier compliance date than ICD-10 to ensure adequate testing time for the industry. These two rules apply to all HIPAA-covered entities, including health plans, health care clearinghouses, and certain health care providers.

DID YOU KNOW?

DID YOU KNOW the World Health Organization (WHO) has scheduled ICD-11 to be presented to the World Health Assembly in May 2017?

Derivations of the *International Classification of Diseases*

Diagnostic and Statistical Manual of Mental Disorders

The *Diagnostic and Statistical Manual of Mental Disorders* (DSM), developed by the American Psychiatric Association (APA), is a derivation of ICD that is used in behavioral health settings. DSM-5 was introduced in 2014, some 18 years after DSM-IV was published in 1994 (http://www.dsm5.org). The DSM is being retitled by changing

BOX 7-12 Comparison of ICD-9-CM and ICD-10-PCS in Coding Traumatic Amputation of Foot with Laterality

ICD-9 code
896.2: Traumatic amputation of foot, complete or partial, bilateral

Comparable ICD-10 codes
Specify one of the following: S98.011: Complete traumatic amputation of right foot at ankle level, S98.021: Partial traumatic amputation of right foot at ankle level AND one of the following: S98.012: Complete traumatic amputation of left foot at ankle level, S98.022: Partial traumatic amputation of left foot at ankle level

the format of the Roman numeral designation of the edition from *DSM-IV* to *DSM-5*. It is anticipated that the APA may revise this version more frequently and label the revisions as 5.1, 5.2, and so on.

DSM-IV includes definitions and diagnostic criteria for mental disorders, with code numbers for each diagnosis.[79]

All diagnostic codes in DSM-IV are valid ICD-9-CM codes. DSM-IV systemizes psychiatric diagnosis using five axes (not all axes must be used):

Axis I   Major mental disorders, developmental disorders, and learning disabilities
Axis II Underlying pervasive or personality conditions and mental retardation
Axis III Any nonpsychiatric medical condition ("somatic")
Axis IV Social functioning and effect of symptoms
Axis V   Global Assessment of Functioning (GAF) on scale from 100 to 0
Axis I   296.23 Major Depressive Disorder, Single Episode, Severe without Psychotic Features
         305.00 Alcohol Abuse
Axis II 301.6 Dependent Personality Disorder Frequent use of denial
Axis III None
Axis IV Threat of job loss
Axis V   GAF = 53 (current)

DSM-5 has substantial changes from its previous edition. Whereas DSM-IV used a multiaxial system, DSM-5 collapses Axes I, II, and III into one axis that contains all diagnoses. As a single-axis system, it will be in alignment with the ICD by the WHO. DSM-5 will reflect new and existing mental disorders, including a section pertaining to the assessment criteria and severity scales. DSM-5 will include each of the diagnostic categories and a section on structural, cross-cutting, and general classification issues, such as dimensional measures to refine diagnosing and plans for treatment. Table 7-12 provides a comparison of criteria used for definitions of mental disorders for DSM-IV and DSM-V. DSM 5 has been mapped to ICD-10-CM. DSM 5 includes equivalent ICD-10-CM codes. New to DSM will be dimensional assessments that can be used to establish a baseline measure of severity and track changes over time. This is a step toward measurement-based care and treatment monitoring. As stated by Stein et al., "Disorders cannot be perfectly defined in necessary and sufficient detail (in mental health) and progress toward a more scientifically and more clinically useful nomenclature is possible."[80] ICD-10-CM is the HIPAA-adopted code set for HIPAA standard transactions. Organizations may use DSM 5 to formulate diagnoses or for other purposes, however, if they are billing or verifying coverage using a HIPAA transaction they will use ICD-10-CM.

ICD-CM coding systems are subject to annual updates, which may require updates in DSM 5. APA is currently using its website to publish updates and refinements to DSM 5. Some of the APA proposed changes will require changes to ICD-10-CM.

International Classification of Diseases for Oncology

The ICD for Oncology (ICD-O) is another system derived from ICD. It is used to classify neoplasms according to their site, behavior, morphologic characteristics, and how they are graded. Codes are based on the malignant neoplasm codes in

TABLE 7-12   Comparison of Criteria for Definition of a Mental Disorder DSM-IV versus DSM-5

DSM-IV	DSM-5
Features	Features
A clinically significant behavioral or psychological syndrome or pattern that occurs in an individual.	A behavioral or psychological syndrome or pattern that occurs in an individual.
Is associated with present distress (e.g., a painful symptom) or disability (i.e., impairment in one or more important areas of functioning) or with a significantly increased risk of suffering death, pain, disability, or an important loss of freedom.	The consequences of which are clinically significant distress (e.g., a painful symptom) or disability (i.e., impairment in one or more important areas of functioning).
Must not be merely an expectable and culturally sanctioned response to a particular event, for example, the death of a loved one.	Must not be merely an expectable response to common stressors and losses (for example, the loss of a loved one) or a culturally sanctioned response to a particular event (for example, trance states in religious rituals).
A manifestation of a behavioral, psychological, or biological dysfunction in the individual.	That reflects an underlying psychobiological dysfunction.
Neither deviant behavior (e.g., political, religious, or sexual) nor conflicts that are primarily between the individual and society are mental disorders unless the deviance or conflict is a symptom of a dysfunction in the individual.	That is not primarily a result of social deviance or conflicts with society.

BOX 7-13   Codes for Malignant Melanoma

ICD-O	M8720/3
ICD-10	C43
ICD-9	172.0

Like ICD, ICD-O is maintained by the World Health Organization.[16]

ICD-10. Like DSM-IV, this oncology classification is oriented on axes. There is a topography axis and a morphologic axis. The morphologic axis has five-digit codes ranging from M-8000/0 to M-9989/3. To break it down, the *M* is for *morphology*, and the first four digits indicate the specific histologic term. The fifth digit after the slash (/) is the behavior code, which indicates whether a tumor is malignant, benign, in situ, or uncertain (whether benign or malignant). A separate one-digit code is also provided for histologic grading (differentiation) (Box 7-13).

Current Procedural Terminology

CPT codes are part of the code set standard selected by HIPAA for electronic transactions. They are used to describe health care services. CPT was developed by the AMA in the 1960s to provide a uniform language for effective communication among physicians, other health care providers, patients, and third parties. CPT helped encourage the use of standard descriptors to document procedures in the medical record. CPT includes descriptive terms and the identifying codes associated with them. The first edition of CPT contained primarily surgical procedures. Subsequent editions provided an expanded set of terms and codes to represent diagnostic and therapeutic procedures used in surgery, medicine, and the specialties. The 2005 CPT update contains 8568 descriptors and codes.

Today, CPT is used extensively throughout the United States as the preferred system for coding medical, surgical, and diagnostic services. It is widely used in administrative applications for billing and reimbursement purposes. However, given the availability of CPT data, it is often used for purposes for which it was not designed—for example, as a basis for performance monitoring and measurement, for research related to professional services, and even to evaluate physician efficiency.

CPT is continually reviewed, revised, and updated to reflect changes in medical technology and clinical practice, and to accommodate new uses and users of CPT data. The current edition is CPT-5. It contains the following three sections:

1. Category I is for procedures and services.
2. Category I is new and consists of tracking codes to support performance measurement.
3. Category III is also new and includes codes to facilitate assessment of new services and procedures and other emerging technologies.

Updates to CPT are published in the fall and take effect the following January 1. CPT 2010 had significant changes from the previous year with 225 additions, 162 revisions, 77 deletions, and 27 resequenced codes (Box 7-14).

BOX 7-14   Peripheral Intravascular Stent Placement

37205	Transcatheter placement of an intravascular stent(s), (except coronary, carotid, and vertebral vessel), percutaneous; initial vessel (For radiological supervision and interpretation, use 75960)
+ 37206	Each additional vessel (List separately in addition to code for primary procedure) (Use 37206 in conjunction with 37205) (For radiological supervision and interpretation, use 75960)
75960	Transcatheter introduction of intravascular stent(s) (except coronary, carotid, and vertebral vessel), percutaneous and/or open, radiological supervision and interpretation, each vessel

American Health Information Management Association: Webinar: *Coding for peripheral vascular disease*, August 20, 2009. http://www.ahima.org/ContinuingEd/Audio/2009seminars.aspx. Accessed April 16, 2014.

Healthcare Common Procedure Coding System

CPT serves as Level I of the HCPCS, which is used to report physician services and other health care services and medical supplies, orthotic and prosthetic devices, and durable medical equipment. HCPCS Level II, also called *alphanumeric HCPCS*, consists of national codes for durable medical equipment, drugs, supplies, and services not included in Level I. Level II codes are maintained by CMS. Before 2003, HCPCS included Level III codes, which were used by Medicare carriers, fiscal intermediaries, health plans, and insurers for specific local needs. Although HCPCS Level III was virtually eliminated under HIPAA, many users still had a need for the information formerly captured through the use of Level III codes. Additional Level II codes are created and used to compensate for the loss of the Level III codes.[79] HCPCS is updated on a regular basis and providers are notified of changes as seen in Box 7-15.

Diagnosis-Related Groups and MS-DRGs

DRGs were used to categorize patients on the basis of principal and secondary diagnoses, principal and secondary procedures, age, sex, complications, discharge status, and

BOX 7-15   2010 Healthcare Common Procedure Coding System Code Update2

Urologic Supplies

Added Code

Code	Narrative
A4336	INCONTINENCE SUPPLY, URETHRAL INSERT, ANY TYPE, EACH
A4360	DISPOSABLE EXTERNAL URETHRAL CLAMP OR COMPRESSION DEVICE, WITH PAD AND/OR POUCH, EACH (*Note: Noncovered*)
A4456	ADHESIVE REMOVER, WIPES, ANY TYPE, EACH

Discontinued Code

Code	Narrative	Crosswalk to Code
A4365	ADHESIVE REMOVER WIPES, ANY TYPE, PER 50	A4456

comorbidities.[81] DRGs were designed as a way to group services and estimate costs to support prospective payment under Medicare. The basic DRG method is used by CMS for hospital payment for Medicare beneficiaries. DRGs have been widely adopted in the United States by Medicaid programs and by other third-party payers.

In October 2007, CMS implemented the most dramatic restructuring of the DRGs used in the inpatient prospective payment system (IPPS) since its inception in 1983. The new Medicare Severity-Adjusted DRG (MS-DRG) system went into effect, along with a number of other changes that affect how inpatient hospital care is paid. The new IPPS brought the number of MS-DRGs to 745 and replaced the previous schedule of 538 DRGs. The new system adjusted the DRG weights based on the severity of the patient's condition and correlates more closely with resource consumption. Unlike the previous DRG system, which used the presence or absence of a complication or comorbidity (CC), the new MS-DRGs are based on determining the severity of the illness of the patient into three categories:

1. Diagnosis with a major complication or comorbidity (MCC)
2. Diagnosis with a complication or comorbidity (CC)
3. Diagnosis without a CC or MCC

Certain conditions were excluded by CMS as CCs or MCCs.

One of the challenges that hospitals faced as a consequence of the IPPS MS-DRG system was having the level of specificity of the clinical documentation in patient records accurately reflect and determine not only the patient's severity and stage of illness, but also the consumption of resources used in the patient's care. This created opportunities for HIM professionals as clinical documentation specialists and other roles to assist providers understand how documentation issues influence reimbursement. Other issues introduced by the Deficit Reduction Act of 2005 were hospital-acquired conditions (HACs) that could have reasonably been prevented by following appropriate patient care guidelines, and conditions that were present on admission (POA). Hospitals do not receive payment for preventable conditions acquired during the patient stay. If HACs are present, the hospital is paid for the care provided during the stay but not for the care required for the HACs. CMS provided a list of conditions that it believed were preventable and would not be paid for, unless the condition was POA. Payment implications for the HACs began in October 2008. The list included 10 categories of HACs as shown in Box 7-16.

General acute hospitals must capture the POAs shown in Table 7-13 for reporting all principal and other diagnosis codes.

Adaptation of Administrative Terminologies

Terminologies developed for one purpose are often adapted or expanded to support others. For example, ICD, a system originally developed for collecting morbidity and mortality statistics, evolved into a system to support billing and reimbursement and is used for clinical research, quality improvement, and other purposes. However, not every terminology is

---

BOX 7-16   Top 10 Categories of Hospital-Acquired Conditions

1. Foreign Object Retained after Surgery
2. Air Embolism
3. Blood Incompatibility
4. Stage III and IV Pressure Ulcers
5. Falls and Trauma
   - Fractures
   - Dislocations
   - Intracranial Injuries
   - Crushing Injuries
   - Burns
   - Electric Shock
6. Manifestations of Poor Glycemic Control
   - Diabetic Ketoacidosis
   - Nonketotic Hyperosmolar Coma
   - Hypoglycemic Coma
   - Secondary Diabetes with Ketoacidosis
   - Secondary Diabetes with Hyperosmolarity
7. Catheter-Associated Urinary Tract Infection
8. Vascular Catheter-Associated Infection
9. Surgical Site Infection Following:
   - Coronary Artery Bypass Graft—Mediastinitis
     - Bariatric Surgery
     - Laparoscopic Gastric Bypass
     - Gastroenterostomy
     - Laparoscopic Gastric Restrictive Surgery
   - Orthopedic Procedures
     - Spine
     - Neck
     - Shoulder
     - Elbow
10. Deep Vein Thrombosis/Pulmonary Embolism
    - Total Knee Replacement
    - Hip Replacement

---

appropriate for every task, and terminologies designed for one purpose may not work well for others.

Simple decision-support features, such as clinical reminders to perform interventions for chronic disease, are often based on CPT and ICD-CM codes. CPT codes are used by the VA for workload capture, clinical reminders, and decision support. The presence of the ICD-CM code for diabetes mellitus can be used to prompt annual preventive interventions such as foot examinations, eye examinations, and tests for hemoglobin A1c.[82,83]

Although administrative terminologies can be used to support clinical applications, they were not designed for the primary documentation of clinical care and thus are not the most clinically relevant data sets on which to base clinical decision support.[84] Terminologies designed primarily for administrative purposes do not have the granularity of a comprehensive clinical terminology and cannot adequately capture the complexity required for advanced decision support.

Administrative data collection is often limited to billable diagnosis and procedure codes, and miscoding can compromise the validity of ICD and CPT data for clinical uses. An organization may decide only to code the first five

TABLE 7-13 CMS POA Indicator Options and Definitions

Indicator	Description	Medicare Payment
Y	Diagnosis was present at time of inpatient admission.	Payment made by Medicare, when an HAC is present
N	Diagnosis was not present at time of inpatient admission.	No payment made by Medicare, when an HAC is present
U	Documentation insufficient to determine if condition was present at the time of inpatient admission.	No payment made by Medicare, when an HAC is present
W	Clinically undetermined. Provider unable to clinically determine whether the condition was present at the time of inpatient admission.	Payment made by Medicare, when an HAC is present
1	Exempt from POA reporting. This code is the equivalent of a blank on the UB-04; however, it was determined that blanks were undesirable on Medicare claims when submitting this data via the 004010/00410A1.	Exempt from POA reporting

CMS, Centers for Medicare and Medicaid Services; *HAC,* hospital-acquired condition; *POA,* present on admission.
Coding Hospital-Acquired Conditions (Present on Admission Indicator): http://www.cms.gov/HospitalAcqCond/05_Coding.asp. Accessed May 30, 2014.

diagnoses and not to code any additional diagnoses by thinking that all of the information needed for a billing decision is contained in the first five diagnoses. The focus of this decision is reimbursement, not on establishing the most accurate clinical profile of the patient or considering other uses of the data. Even variations between inpatient and outpatient coding rules can affect the usefulness of administrative data for decision support. For example, ICD-9 coding conventions required that an inpatient admission for unconfirmed diabetes mellitus be coded. These data remain a part of a patient's EHR as an ICD-9 code even in the event that the diagnosis is later eliminated. A diabetes diagnosis may trigger a set of preventive reminders to assist clinicians in managing and improving quality of care. Populations are also tracked for quality-of-care issues, recidivism, and disease management. Reminders will continue to display erroneously as part of this patient's medical profile until they are manually deactivated. These unconfirmed diagnoses may also sit in insurance company or third-party databases and be used to make decisions.

One of the challenges facing health care is how to represent clinical data in a form that is usable for clinical decision support and data analysis. Rather than attempting to stretch the use of administrative terminologies to accommodate clinical requirements, providers are now seeking terminologies specifically designed with clinical applications in mind.[79]

Going Forward

Significant progress has been made in recent years in creating new ways to make terminologies work in a usable and transparent manner for the user. Computer-based terminology systems can have inherent constructs that are unacceptable to the user if they make clinical documentation at the point of care awkward and inhibit the natural expression and thought processes. Work must continue to develop terminologies to the satisfaction of both systems and users. It is apparent that a large number of vocabulary, coding, and classifications systems have been developed for specific purposes, and development will continue to expand and refine terminologies dedicated to meet those goals. However, the need to exchange information across disparate systems has unveiled their limitations for use to achieve true semantic interoperability as they lack consistency in coverage, granularity, and completeness. We must find ways to balance the needs of administrative and clinical demands. We need semantic interoperability that will allow clinicians to document primary clinical data using natural language that ultimately could be converted into standardized code. The push to find the "one true standard" to solve the terminology problem has diminished as new ways are found to link concepts as terminology models. There is currently lively debate focused around using concept-oriented clinical terminologies as they evolve and we learn improved ways to represent and manipulate them. Terminologies to serve specific needs cannot be built in isolation, but can now draw on important groundwork that has already been set. Linking concepts to diverse phrases in terminology systems requires scrutiny to see overlap and differences in meaning as health data are shared among systems. This requires a level of interoperability that depends on the degree of agreement of data terminology and its quality. As they are discovered, conflicts and limitations can then be addressed with further refinement and effective management.

> *Due to their inherent complexity, terminology systems will have flaws. It would be overly ambitious to expect otherwise. Thus there is a need to develop mechanisms for identifying and overcoming such flaws as they are discovered, particularly when patient safety and data integrity are at risk.*[85]

We have come a long way in being able to represent data and its intended meaning in a formal, reproducible, and useful way. Earlier work gave support for terminologies to be "concept-oriented" and listed the structural characteristics that controlled medical terminologies should have. However, desired characteristics have evolved to include both structure and purpose. There has been a need to have symbolic representation and manipulation of the terms and concepts and a push for preserving their integrity while communicating their meaning in useful and intended ways. Terminologies must be more than groupings of synonymous terms to express ideas.[86] They must be capable of conveying an understanding of their intended meaning and purpose; otherwise, we create risks in the automated reuse of data, aggregating data into summary reports, using automated inferencing in decision support, and communicating what we know about the meanings of the terms we use. Cimino has provided additional considerations for desirable characteristics of controlled terminologies that move away from structure and content and focus on their purpose and use:

1. Terminologies should support capturing what is known about the patient.
2. Terminologies should support information retrieval and allow someone returning to that information later to understand its meaning as intended by the author.

3. Terminologies should allow storage, retrieval, and transfer of information with as little information loss as possible as terminologies change over time.
4. Terminologies should support aggregation of data.
5. Terminologies should support the reuse of data.
6. Terminologies should support inferencing.[87]

Further integration into larger terminology, metathesaurus systems, and semantic webs achieve both the semantic interoperability and the ability to accommodate different representational forms, thus allowing the descriptive specificity necessary for point-of-care clinical documentation and health data to be shared and exchanged between systems.

CHAPTER REVIEW

1. Interoperability that provides intelligent use, common interpretation of the data fields is:
   a. basic interoperability
   b. semantic interoperability
   c. functional interoperability

2. A terminology generally means a set of "_____" for a particular subject or field.
   a. codes
   b. classifications
   c. concepts
   d. mappings

3. ICD-10-CM is a:
   a. controlled medical terminology
   b. nomenclature
   c. classification system
   d. mapping system

4. SNOMED began as a:
   a. pathology nomenclature
   b. medical classification of injuries
   c. medical billing system
   d. unified medical language system

5. GEMS is designed to:
   a. ensure consistency in national data
   b. ensure interoperability of HIE data
   c. link DSM to ICD-10
   d. link ICD-10 to SNOMED

6. UMLS is developed and supported by:
   a. CDC
   b. NCVHS
   c. ONC
   d. NLM

7. An example of a terminology that facilitates clinical data collections at the point of care is:
   a. CPT
   b. HCPCS
   c. SNOMED CT
   d. ICD-10-CM

8. DSM is used to:
   a. classify neoplasms
   b. group principal and secondary diagnoses
   c. describe behavioral diagnostic criteria
   d. describe traumatic injuries

9. CPT is developed by the:
   a. NCVHS
   b. AMA
   c. ONC
   d. NLM

10. The MS-DRG system contains:
    a. 0–200 DRGs
    b. 201–400 DRGs
    c. 401–600 DRGs
    d. 601–800 DRGs

REFERENCES

1. Health Level Seven EHR Interoperability Work Group: *Coming to terms: scoping interoperability for health care*, February 7, 2007. http://hln.com/assets/pdf/Coming-to-Terms-February-2007.pdf. Accessed May 28, 2014.
2. Healthcare Information and Management Systems Society: *HIMSS dictionary of healthcare information technology terms, acronyms and organizations*, Chicago, 2006, HIMSS, Taylor and Francis.
3. Amatayakul M: *Electronic health records: a practical guide for professionals and organizations*, ed 4, Chicago, 2007, American Health Information Management Association.
4. Levy B: Evolving to clinical terminology, *J Healthc Inform Manag* 18:37–43, 2004.
5. National Committee on Vital and Health Statistics: *Uniform data standards for patient medical record information: report to the secretary of the U.S. Department of Health and Human Services*. Washington, DC, 2000, U.S. Department of Health and Human Services. http://www.ncvhs.hhs.gov/hipaa000706.pdf. Accessed May 28, 2014.
6. Wilemon T: New robot fills IV prescriptions at Methodist, *Memphis Daily News* 123(219), 2008. http://www.memphisdailynews.com/news/

2008/nov/7/new-robot-fills-prescription-at-methodist/. Accessed June 30, 2014.

7. Institute of Electrical and Electronics Engineers: *Interoperability for the National Health Information Network,* 2014, ISBN 978-1-4244-2448-1. (Available through IEEE.) Accessed June 30, 2014.

8. Lundberg B: Accurate electronic patient charts—a standardized clinical language is key to success, *For the Record* 20(20):6.

9. VistA: *Computerized Patient Record System (CPRS) user guide, GUI Version,* Washington, DC, August 2009, US Department of Veterans Affairs, Office of Development, CPRS Product Line.

10. Murphy G, Helbig S: *Health information: management of a strategic resource,* ed 4, Philadelphia, 2011, Saunders Elsevier.

11. Park H, Hardiker N: Clinical terminologies: a solution for semantic interoperability, *J Korean Soc Med Inform* 15:1–11, 2009.

12. Bowman S: Coordination of SNOMED-CT and ICD-10: getting the most out of electronic health record systems, *Perspect Health Inf Manag,* 2005, Spring.

13. World Health Organization: *Executive Board, 118th Session, Provisional agenda, item 8.4, EB118/8,* Geneva, May 25, 2006, WHO.

14. InfoGrid: the web graph database. http://infogrid.org/trac/wiki/Reference/PidcockArticle. Accessed July 21, 2014.

15. Dental Informatics Online Community: *FAQ: what is controlled vocabulary?* http://www.dentalinformatics.com/learningcenter/faq_vocabulary.html#nr_5. Accessed March 30, 2010.

16. Amatayakul M: *Electronic health records: a practical guide for professionals and organizations,* ed 4, Chicago, 2007, American Health Information Association.

17. Adapted from narrative in Safian S: *The complete procedure coding book,* New York, 2009, McGraw-Hill.

18. Chute CG: Viewpoint: clinical classification and terminology: some history and current observations, *J Am Med Inform Assoc* 7:293–303, 2000.

19. Imel M: SNOMED overview. In *American Health Information Association National convention and exhibit proceedings,* 2002.

20. Giannangelo K, editor: *Healthcare code sets, clinical terminologies, and classification systems,* Chicago, 2006, American Health Information Management Association, p 110.

21. UMDNS (Universal Medical Device Nomenclature System) Code, 6212, Radiographic/fluoroscopic table systems, urological. 16213, Basins, Ear. 16214, Wheelchairs, Powered. 16215, Curtains, Cubicle. http://www.tuvamerica.com/tools/forms/UMDNS.DOC. Accessed March 15, 2010.

22. International Health Terminology Standards Development Organisation: *SNOMED CT components.* http://www.ihtsdo.org/snomed-ct/snomed-ct0/snomed-ct-components/. Accessed December 05, 2009.

23. http://www.ihtsdo.org/fileadmin/user_upload/doc/elearning.html. (provides access to several trainings including Introducing SNOMED-CT). Accesseed June 30, 2014.

24. American Health Information Management Association e-HIM Work Group on Computer-Assisted Coding: Delving into computer-assisted coding [practice brief], *J AHIMA* 75:48A–48H, 2004.

25. Case JT: Are we really communicating? Standard terminology standards in veterinary clinical pathology, *Vet Clin Pathol* 34:5–6, 2005.

26. Vardy G: Israeli coding medical information: classification versus nomenclature and implications to the Israeli medical system, *J Med Syst* 22:203–210, 1998.

27. National Committee on Vital and Health Statistics, Department of Health and Human Services: *NCVHS Reports and recommendations: 2003 to present, Report of Uniform Data Standards for Patient Medical Information,* July 2000. p. 33, http://www.ncvhs.hhs.gov/reptrecs.htm. Accessed December 21, 2006.

28. Cimino J: Desiderata for controlled medical vocabularies in the twenty-first century, *Methods Inf Med* 37:394–403, 1998.

29. Demetriades J, Kolodner R, Christopherson G: *Person-centered health records: toward healthy people,* New York, 2005, Springer Science and Business Media.

30. Campbell KE, Hochhalter B, Slaughter J, Mattison J: Enterprise issues pertaining to implementing controlled terminologies, IMIA WG 6 conference, December 1999.

31. Fenton S: *Clinical vocabularies: essential to the future of health information management,* 2004, AHIMA. http://www.ahima.org/bok. Accessed August 17, 2010.

32. Rosenbloom S, Miller R, Johnson K, et al: Facilitating direct entry of clinical data into electronic health record systems, *J Am Med Informat Assoc* 13:277–288, 2006.

33. Friedman C, Hripcsak G, Shagina L, Lui H: Representing information in patient reports using natural language processing and extensible markup language, *J Am Med Inform Assoc* 6(1):76–87, 1999.

34. Rosenbloom ST, Miller RA, Johnson KB, Elkin PL, Brown SH: Interface terminologies: facilitating direct entry of clinical data into electronic health record systems, *JAMIA* 13:277–288, 2006, http://dx.doi.org/10.1197/jamia.M1957.

35. Boulos M: A first look at HealthCyberMap, *J Technol Health Care* 12:33–41, 2004.

36. Centers for Medicare and Medicaid Services: *ICD-10-CM/PCS implementation and general equivalence mappings (crosswalks) overview (Presentation).* http://www.cms.gov/ICD10/downloads/7ICD-10_Implementation_and_GEM_Overview_Presentation.pdf. Accessed March 31, 2010.

37. US National Library of Medicine: *Unified medical language system.* http://www.nlm.nih.gov/research/umls. Accessed March 31, 2010.

38. Healthcare IT News staff: EMR: terminology key to integration (Editorial and Commentary), *Healthcare IT News,* April 5, 2005. http://www.healthcareitnews.com/news/emr-terminology-key-integration, Accessed November 12, 2010.

39. Hardiker R, Hoy D, Casey A: Standards for nursing terminology, *J Am Med Informat Assoc* 7:523–528, 2000.

40. Sujansky W, National Committee on Vital and Health Statistics Subcommittee on Standards and Security: *Scope and criteria for selection of MPRI terminologies: summary and analysis of testimony on PMRI terminology standards, Version 1,* Sept. 1, 2003. http://www.ncvhs.hhs.gov/031105rpt.pdf. Accessed Aug 05, 2010.

41. The International Health Terminology Standards Development Organisation. http://www.ihtsdo.org. Accessed December 23, 2009.

42. Chen H, Fuller S, Hersh WR, Friedman C, editors: *Medical informatics: advances in knowledge management and data mining in biomedicine,* Dusseldorf, Germany, 2005, Springer-Verlag.

43. Potamias G, editor, and the INFOBIOMED consortium partners: *Structuring European biomedical informatics to support individualised healthcare, IST-507585: state of the art on systems for data analysis,* Information Retrieval and Decision Support: Infobiomed Consortium. http://www.infobiomed.org/paginas_en/INFOBIOMED_D13_final.pdf. Accessed March 22, 2010.

44. International Health Terminology Standards Development: *SNOMED clinical terms user guide, international release, July 2007.* http://www.ihtsdo.org/fileadmin/user_upload/doc/directory.html. (select SNOMED-CT document library). Accessed June 30, 2014.

45. United States National Library of Medicine, National Institutes of Health: *SNOMED CT documentation: scope memo,* July 2009.

46. Goldberg LJ, Werner C, Eisner J, et al: The significance of SNODENT, Medical Informatics Europe (MIE 2005), Geneva, *Stud Health Technol Inform* 116:737–742, 2005.

47. http://ihtsdo.org/fileadmin/user_upload/doc/directory.html. (select Document Library, E-Learning Center for SNOMED-CT to ICD-10 CM rule based mapping). Accessed June 30, 2013.

48. Bakken S, Cimini JJ, Hripsak G: Promoting patient safety and enabling evidence-based practice through informatics, *Med Care* 42:II49–II56, 2004.

49. International Health Terminology Standards Development: *Adoption of SNOMED CT.* http://www.ihtsdo.org/snomed-ct/snomed-ct0/adoption-of-snomed-ct/. Accessed November 18, 2009.

50. Manos D: SNOMED CT will be required by 2015 for bonuses under economic recovery law, *Healthcare IT News,* August 20, 2009. http://www.healthcareitnews.com/news/snomed-ct-will-be-required-2015-bonuses-under-economic-recovery-law. Accessed Sept 10, 2010.

51. Huff SM, Rocha RA, McDonald CJ, et al: Development of the logical observation identifier names and codes (LOINC) vocabulary, *J Am Med Inform Assoc* 5:276–292, 1998.

52. Regenstrief Institute. http://www.regenstrief.org/loinc. Accessed December 5, 2009.
53. Logical Observation Identifiers Names and Codes: *History, purpose, and scope.* http://loinc.org/background. Accessed June 30, 2014.
54. *LOINC users' guide,* February 2010, Regenstrief Institute http,//loinc.org/downloads/files/LOINCManual.pdf/view. Accessed March 08, 2010.
55. Institute of Medicine: *Leadership by example: coordinating government roles in improving health care quality,* Washington, DC, 2002, National Academy Press.
56. Dugas M, Thun S, Frankewitsch T, Keitmann K: LOINC codes for hospital information systems: documents: a case study, *J Am Inform Assoc* 16:400–403, 2009.
57. Peters L, Bodenreider O: Using the RxNorm Web services API for quality assurance purposes, *AMIA Annu Symp Proc* 591–595, 2008. http://www.ncbi.nlm.nih.gov/pmc/articles/PMC2656097. Accessed March 30, 2010.
58. National Library of Medicine: *RxNorm overview.* http://www.nlm.nih.gov/research/umls/rxnorm/overview.html. Accessed November 20, 2009.
59. Nelson SJ: *Clinical vocabulary development: overview of NLM activities,* February 12, 2003. http://www.nlm.nih.gov/mesh/staffpubs_archive.html, (scroll to Nelson SJ Clinical Vocabulary Development: overview of NLM activities 2003_feb). Accessed June 30, 2013.
60. National Cancer Institute, U.S. National Institutes of Health: *Federal medication terminologies (FMT); enabling health IT interoperability,* presentation by the Federal Health Architecture Program. http://www.cancer.gov/cancertopics/terminologyresources/FMT. Accessed February 26, 2010.
61. The Emergency Care Research Institute. https://www.ecri.org/Search/Pages/SearchResults.aspx?=UMDNS. Accessed June 30, 2014.
62. Kripps B: Toward standardized nursing terminology: the next steps, *CARING Newsletter* 23(3):4–8, 2008, 15519104.
63. Lundberg C, Warren JJ, Brokel JM, et al: Selecting a standardized terminology for the electronic health record that reveals the impact of nursing on patient care, *Online J Nurs Inform* 12:1–19, 2008. http://ojni.org/12_2/lundberg.pdf. Accessed March 8, 2010.
64. Henry SB, Mead CN: Nursing classification systems: necessary but not sufficient for representing what nurses do, *J Am Med Informatics Assoc* 4:222–232, 1997.
65. American Nurses Association: *ANA recognized terminologies that support nursing practice, June 4, 2012.* http://www.nursingworld.org/npii/terminologies.htm, Accessed May 28, 2014.
66. Health Information Management Systems Society: *HIMSS standards insight: an analysis of health information standards development initiatives,* July 2003. http://www.himss.org/library/Interoperability-standards/basics. Accessed June 30, 2014.
67. *The Omaha system: solving the clinical data information puzzle.* http://www.omahasystem.org/overview.html. Accessed February 21, 2010.
68. *International Classification for Nursing Practice (ICNP) source information.* http://www.who.int/classifications/icd/adaptations/icn/en/. Accessed June 30, 2014.
69. Giannangelo K, editor: *Healthcare code sets, clinical terminologies, and classification systems,* Chicago, 2006, American Health Information Management Association, p 85.
70. Vardy G: Israeli coding medical information: classification versus nomenclature and implications to the Israeli medical system, *J Med Syst* 22:203–210, 1998.
71. *HIPAA Final Rule ICD-10: standards to adopt ICD-10CM and ICD-10-PCS,* Office of the Secretary of Health and Human Services. http://www.hipaa.com/2009/01/final-icd-10-rule. Accessed December 29, 2009.
72. Centers for Medicare and Medicaid Services: *HHS modifies HIPAA code sets (ICD-10) and electronic transactions standards* (press release), January 15, 2009, CMS Office of Public Affairs.
73. Centers for Medicare and Medicaid Services: *Transaction and code sets standards: an overview.* http://www.cms.hhs.gov/TransactionCodeSetsStands. Accessed January 24, 2010.
74. McDonald CJ, Huff SM, Suico JC, et al: LOINC, a universal standard for identifying laboratory observations: a five year update, *Clin Chem* 49:624–633, 2003.
75. *International Center for Health Statistics classification of diseases and functioning disability.* http://www.cdc.gov/nchs/icd/icf.htm. Accessed June 30, 2014.
76. Fenton S: *Clinical classification and terminologies,* Chicago, 2002, American Health Information Management Association.
77. American Academy of Procedural Coders: Roadmap to ICD-10-CM, *The Coding Edge,* February 2007.
78. Letter to the Secretary of DHHS from the Chair of the National Committee on Vital and Health Statistics, February 27, 2002.
79. Abdelhak M, Grostick S, Hanken MA, et al., editors: *Health information: management of a strategic resource,* 2 ed., Philadelphia, 2001, WB Saunders.
80. Stein DJ, Phillips KA, Bolton D, et al: What is a mental/psychiatric disorders? From DSM-IV to DSM-V, *Psychol Med* 40(1):1759–1765, 2010. http://www.ncbi.nlm.nih.gov/pmc/articles/PMC3101504/. Accessed June 30, 2014.
81. Ingenix: *DRG desk reference: the ultimate resource for improving DRG assignment,* 2007.
82. Institute of Medicine Repor: *Who will keep the public healthy: educating public health professionals for the 21st century,* Washington, DC, 2002, Committee on Educating Public Health Professionals for the 21st Century.
83. Institute of Medicine: *Letter report: key capabilities of an electronic health record system,* Washington, DC, 2003, Committee on Data Standards for Patient Safety.
84. Institute of Medicine, Committee on Enhancing Federal Healthcare Quality Programs: *Leadership by example: coordinating government roles in improving healthcare quality,* Washington, DC, 2003, National Academy Press.
85. Hardiker NR, Bakken S, Casey A, Hoy D: Formal nursing terminology systems: a means to an end, *J Biomed Inform* 35:298–305, 2002.
86. Smith B: From concepts to clinical reality: an essay on the benchmarking of biomedical terminologies, *J Biomed Inform* 39:288–298, 2006.
87. Cimino J: In defense of the desiderata, *J Biomed Inform* 39:299–306, 2006.

TECHNOLOGY, APPLICATIONS, AND SECURITY

Melissa Saul

ⓔ Student Study Guide activities for this chapter are available on the Evolve Learning Resources site for this textbook. Please visit http://evolve.elsevier.com/Abdelhak.

CHAPTER CONTENTS

OBJECTIVES

After reading this chapter, the reader will be able to do the following:
- ✓ Define key words.
- ✓ Define and describe the overall scope of health information systems.
- ✓ Discuss the evolution of information technology in health care.
- ✓ Explain the fundamental concepts of database models.
- ✓ Understand the functionality of structured query language.
- ✓ Explain how a wireless network communicates with the devices on the network.
- ✓ Characterize the differences between two-tier and three-tier architectures.
- ✓ Identify network protocols used on the Internet.
- ✓ Apply interface design principles to screen and other input devices.
- ✓ Be familiar with standards for designing web pages.
- ✓ Describe the role of an interface engine.
- ✓ Illustrate some examples of how admission, discharge, and transfer is used in a health information system.

- ✓ Understand why an organization would implement a computerized provider order entry system.
- ✓ Define scenarios in which bar code technology could be used.
- ✓ Discuss the purpose and applications of telehealth.
- ✓ Explain the authentication tools used by information systems.
- ✓ Build a case for why a firewall is necessary.
- ✓ Understand the types of malicious software.
- ✓ Define the role of the secure socket layer in Internet applications.
- ✓ Explain various techniques used to address security of health information systems.
- ✓ Discuss the benefits of an application service provider model.
- ✓ Describe the steps for building a data mart.
- ✓ Understand how data collected in a health information system can be used for business intelligence and research applications.

KEY WORDS

Applets
Application gateway
Application service provider
Application software
Ascension number
Authentication
Bandwidth
Biometric
Break glass
Business rules
Cascading style sheets
Checksum
Clinical Context Object Workgroup
Clinical decision support systems
Cloud computing
Computerized physician order entry
Data compression
Data mart
Data mining
Data repository
Database
Database management system
Database model
Decision support systems
Demilitarized zone

Denial of Service
Disaster recovery plan
Document type definition
Encryption
Ethernet
Expert system
Fiber distributed data interface
Firewall
Frames
Granularity
Graphical user interface
Grid computing
Hardware
Hierarchical
Hypertext link
Interface engine
Internet
Intranet
JAVA
Knowledge base
Local area network
Lossless
Lossy
Mainframe
Malware

Medical informatics
Microcomputers
Middleware
Mobile device
Network
Object
Object-oriented
Operating system
Order entry
Packet filter
Password aging
Phishing
Pointer
Point-of-care system
Point-to-point
Primary key
Protocols
Proxy server
Public key
Quick response code
RAID
Really Simple Syndication
Relational model
Results reporting
SAN
Servlet

Software
Software as a Service
Store and forward
Symbology
Syndromic surveillance system
Tags
Telemedicine
Templates
Thick-client
Thin-client
Three-tier
Token ring
Two-factor authentication
Two-tier
View
Virtual community
Virtual machine
Virtual private network
Voice recognition
Wi-Fi
Wi-Fi protected access
Wide area networks
Wireless
Wired equivalent privacy
XML

ABBREVIATIONS

ADT	Admission, Discharge, and Transfer
AHIMA	American Health Information Management Association
AMIA	American Medical Informatics Association
ANSI	American National Standards Institute
ASP	Application Service Provider
ASTM	American Society for Testing and Materials
ATM	Asynchronous Transfer Mode
BI	Business Intelligence
CA	Certificate Authority
CCOW	Clinical Context Object Workstation
CDC	Centers for Disease Control and Prevention
CDSS	Clinical Decision Support System
CERT	Computer Emergency Response Team
CGI	Common Gateway Interface
COBOL	Common Business-Oriented Language
CODEC	Coder/Decoder
COSTAR	Computer-Stored Ambulatory Record System
CPOE	Computerized Provider Order Entry
CPU	Central Processing Unit
CSS	Cascading Style Sheet
CT	Computed Tomographic
DARPA	Defense Advanced Research Project Agency
DBMS	Database Management System
DHHS	Department of Health and Human Services
DMZ	Demilitarized Zone
DOS	Denial of Service
DRG	Diagnosis-Related Group
DTD	Document Type Definition
EHR	Electronic Health Record
ERP	Enterprise Resource Planning
FDA	Food and Drug Administration
FDDI	Fiber-Distributed Data Interface
HDI	Health Data Initiative
HIE	Health Information Exchange
HIM	Health Information Management
HIPAA	Health Insurance Portability and Accountability Act
HIS	Health Information System
HIT	Health Information Technology
HL7	Health Level 7
HTML	Hypertext Markup Language
HTTP	Hypertext Transfer Protocol
ICD	*International Classification of Diseases*
ICU	Intensive Care Unit
IEEE	Institute of Electrical and Electronic Engineers
IETF	Internet Engineering Task Force
I/O	Input–Output
ISO	International Organization of Standardization
JVM	Java Virtual Machine
LAN	Local Area Network
Mbps	Million Bits Per Second
MPI	Master Patient Index
MUMPS	Massachusetts General Hospital Utility Multi-Programming System
NeHC	National eHealth Collaborative
ONC	Office of the National Coordinator for Health Information Technology
PC	Personal Computer
PDA	Personal Digital Assistant
PHI	Protected Health Information
QIC	Quality Improvement Council
RAID	Redundant Array of Inexpensive Disks
RBAC	Role-Based Access Control
RFID	Radio Frequency Identification Device
RSS	Really Simple Syndication
SaaS	Software as a Service
SAN	Storage Area Network
SGML	Standard Generalized Markup Language
S-HTTP	Secure Hypertext Transfer Protocol
SQL	Standard Query Language
SSID	Service Set Identifier
SSL	Secure Socket Layer
TCP/IP	Transmission Control Protocol/Internet Protocol
TDS	Technicon Data System
UX	User Experience
VPN	Virtual Private Network
W3	World Wide Web Consortium
WAN	Wide Area Networks
WEP	Wired Equivalent Privacy
WPA	Wi-Fi Protected Access
XML	Extensible Markup Language

HEALTH INFORMATION INFRASTRUCTURE, TECHNOLOGY, AND APPLICATIONS

The ideal scenario of a patient experience is one in which, on arriving at the physician's office, hospital, or another health care setting, the patient is quickly identified as someone who has been seen before. The patient's previous laboratory tests and imaging results are viewed through the web browser on a handheld device. Test results, combined with other historical and clinical data already collected into the computer system, are reviewed in minutes. If necessary, data are transferred through a network to a specialist for immediate feedback. The referring physician and the specialist view the information simultaneously while conferring by phone. New treatment is documented and automatically added to a central repository, from which the patient as well as other care providers can retrieve information in the future. Special reminders and flags that alert the physicians about special conditions that need to be investigated, such as abnormal laboratory results and new reports on patient allergies, are automatically presented when the patient's care information is retrieved. Reminders for annual immunizations and screening procedures are generated with automatic notification to the patient's e-mail address or via text message. In addition, claims for services are automatically processed through computerized systems and forwarded electronically for billing and reimbursement, and the laboratory results from the visit are posted to the patient's online personal health record. After the visit, the patient can access follow-up test results through his or her computer or mobile device. Between visits, the patient receives e-mail reminders from the physician for preventive care services. Scenarios such as this are becoming more accepted, addressing patient and provider expectations regarding health information systems (HISs), which are more generally known as *health information technology* (HIT).

We need more information in health care than ever before. We need to achieve better health care quality outcomes and cost-efficiencies in providing health services. We need to extend access to larger patient populations and health care information to more users. To meet these goals, we are applying new technology in information systems and communications to multiple business processes within the industry. Traditionally, the health care industry did not invest in technology as did other industries, such as banking or manufacturing. The soar in interest in HISs comes from several factors. In 2003 HIT became part of the federal government's initiative to improve patient safety. To accomplish this, the Office of the National Coordinator for Health Information Technology (ONC) was created to coordinate the adoption of information technology in hospitals and physician offices across the country.[1] (See Chapter 3 for more on this topic.) As part of the American Recovery and Reinvestment Act of 2009, the government has allocated $26 billion to accelerate the adoption of HIT in the United States. The Centers for Medicare and Medicaid Services with the Department of Health and Human Services (DHHS) has implemented value-based purchasing among other initiatives, which requires more attention to the quality of health care being delivered. In turn, there is also an increasing demand from health care consumers to have more efficient and improved quality of health care. The purpose of this chapter is to describe the current HIS environment, the technology used, the key clinical applications, and the data management tools available. Health information professionals need to develop a greater appreciation of the role and potential of HISs.

The term health information management system serves as an alias for many types of information systems. These include hospital information systems, clinical information systems, decision support systems, medical information systems, management information systems, home HISs, and others. The federal government's ONC defined HIT as "hardware, software, integrated technologies or related licenses, intellectual property, upgrades, or packaged solutions sold as services that are designed for or support the use by health care entities or patients for the electronic creation, maintenance, access or exchange of health information."[2]

This chapter begins with a general discussion of the current overall picture of HISs including some of their features, a review of their historical evolution, and what the typical HIS looks like today. The various technologies that support the information infrastructure are described. Computer security and the use of the Internet are discussed. Finally, the role of the health information management (HIM) professional in using these technologies analytically is presented with examples of real-life scenarios. The increased use of technology has also increased the volume, complexity, and timeliness of

health care data, or as it is known "Big Data." Although the use of "Big Data" is still in its infancy, it does show promise as a way to deliver more cost-effective and personalized treatments to patients. As health information professionals, we need to understand the environment in planning for the future.

Scope of Health Information Systems

It is important to determine the scope of an HIS as well as its components. Each of the components discussed in this chapter can be applied to almost any type of HIS. The scope includes the following:

Departmental—a system limited to a specific clinical or financial domain to serve the business functions of a department (e.g., respiratory therapy, radiology)

Intradepartmental—a system that primarily serves the business function of one department but shares information and functions with other departments (e.g., laboratory, patient scheduling)

Hospital (or site of care)–wide—a system that focuses on the integration of the various departmental systems or, in the absence of integration, may provide the primary service for a clinical area

Enterprise-wide—the system that encompasses all of the departmental systems throughout the health system, including hospitals, clinics, nursing homes, and other health facilities

External (cooperative)—a system shared among different health systems that primarily exists to report information required by regulatory agencies or as part of a health information exchange (HIE)

Components

A comprehensive HIS contains seven components:

1. Core applications such as patient scheduling and admission, discharge, and transfer (ADT) provide the central notification to the hospital of patient visits and serves as the core database for many other applications. An enterprise master patient index (MPI) is also considered a core application because it enables a single medical record number to be issued to a patient for use in all health care settings (acute, outpatient, and long-term care).

2. Business and financial systems such as patient accounting, revenue cycle management, supply chain management and payroll provide data management functions for the business activities of the organization.

3. Communications and networking applications, including web applications, transmit and manage messages among departments both within the hospital, such as nursing and ancillary areas, as well as communicating with other health care entities and third-party payers. Communications are used to notify these departments of patient admission and provide for tracking orders and results.

4. Departmental systems such as pharmacy, radiology, and laboratory are designed to manage the clinical operations and connect data to institutional databases for results

reporting, billing functions, and inclusion in the electronic health record (EHR).

5. Documentation systems are used to collect, store, and retrieve patient data. Applications in this category range from point-of-care bedside devices for capturing nursing documentation to speech recognition transcription modules that capture and store clinical reports to direct clinician entry into EHRs.

6. Reminder and advice functions assist clinicians in performing patient care activities. Such reminders can include messages to alert for significant test results, utilization criteria, and drug–drug interactions. This component includes monitoring of compliance with clinical guidelines and protocols.

7. Surveillance and related population health systems can detect and monitor disease at an earlier stage for public health surveillance. This type of system is generally referred to as **syndromic surveillance system** because it is designed to recognize outbreaks based on the symptoms and signs of infection.[3] Because the data used by syndromic surveillance systems cannot be used to establish a specific diagnosis in any particular individual, syndromic surveillance systems must be designed to detect patterns of disease in a population.

In reality, hospital information systems can be viewed along a continuum from the first three major components to acqui-

sition of all seven. Figure 8-1 is a schematic representation of the major categories in a hospital information system and examples of the components. Note that information needed at the time of registration is captured at one level and available at the next level. Components are connected through an interface engine, which is discussed in detail later. The organization relies on the HIS for daily processing activities, including patient care, research, administration, and educational initiatives.

SELF-ASSESSMENT QUIZ

1. A comprehensive HIS contains how many components?
2. Which core applications serve as the core database for other applications?
   a. Patient scheduling
   b. ADT
   c. Enterprise MPI
   d. All of the above
   e. a and b only
3. Which systems are used to collect, store, and retrieve patient data?
   a. Documentation
   b. Business and financial
   c. ADT

FIGURE 8-1 Hierarchy of health information systems. *PC,* Personal computer.

Computers in Health Care—Past and Present

Early Efforts: 1960s to 1980s

Computers were introduced into the health care arena through punch-card data processing. Early work in epidemiologic and public health applications that performed statistical analysis on the incidence, distribution, and causes of diseases in society provided the early experience with computers. Although some of the early activities were focused on decision making for physicians, many developers worked on building total information systems for hospitals. Also, during the 1960s and 1970s, significant work was undertaken by Octo Barnett at Massachusetts General Hospital in the ambulatory care environment with the development of a computer-stored ambulatory record system (COSTAR). The first patient care system that claimed to automate the patient record was initially marketed as the IBM Medical Information Systems Program in the late 1960s and sold until 1972. A number of other companies were involved in patient care information systems during this period, but only the system devised by Lockheed Aircraft, which became the Technicon Data System (TDS), survived for the next 30 years until the product was redesigned and rebranded as EHR software used for improving clinical outcomes.[4]

During the 1970s, HISs were developed in several ways. Many hospitals approached information system development by creating financial information systems and using the same system or slightly modifying the database for clinical applications. Other hospitals adopted a goal of a single integrated system that was designed to use one large database that shared its resources among departments. In contrast, other providers acquired versions of hospital information systems through departmental applications such as a clinical laboratory system to which custom features were later added. The intention was to create common data through a single shared database, but this proved difficult to achieve.[5] During this period, hospital databases were derived largely from discharge analysis of medical records. Many hospitals participated through contracts with external computer service organizations by submitting discharge abstracts to the service computer companies for processing and receiving printouts of hospital statistics. As the technology in the 1970s developed, more and more separate departments were able to acquire departmental systems that met their specific needs. Vendors began to offer packages of functions for hospital departments such as cardiology, radiology, and pharmacy. In addition, software tools emerged that reduced the mystery associated with computers, and clinicians became more interested in leading and participating in computing activities. At the end of the 1970s and into the 1980s, the introduction of the personal computer (PC) gave rise to additional empowerment and expectations of clinicians. In effect, technologic advances produced computers that were reliable, small, and low cost. Hardware became reliable and highly affordable. Computer and business communities recognized that the greatest cost involved in informatics systems development was related to the software. Software engineering emerged as a field dedicated to management of the software development process. The three major computer characteristics of the 1970s were significantly improved reliability and computing power of hardware, availability of more functional software, and reduction in cost of ownership. All this laid a strong foundation for the work to come.

Evolution of Hospital Information Systems: 1980s to Late 1990s

In the 1980s network technology emerged and expanded to enable the departmental systems that began in the previous decade to share and communicate with other systems within the organization. Demographic and associated information on patients who registered in clinics or were admitted to hospitals was now automatically sent to hospital departments so that the data could be incorporated in their database. Admission notices were communicated to dietary, housekeeping, laboratory, radiology, and other ancillary services electronically. In turn, order communications enabled physician orders to be sent from a nursing station directly to an ancillary area. In addition, significant gains were made in building computer networks that linked a variety of diverse applications together.

In 1980 Ball and Jacobs[6] described HISs at three levels. A Level I HIS included an ADT application with bed and census reporting, order entry communications, and charge capture and inquiry functions for billing purposes. A Level II HIS focused on systems that included part or most of the patient record. This provided fundamentally clinical databases and improved collection and use of clinical data within these systems. Level III described an HIS in which data were linked to knowledge bases that provided diagnostic support and actual intervention for patient care activities. In these systems, special alerts were made available that responded to specific data content and messages and notified providers through the system.

Late 1990s to 2010

The prospect for developing health care information systems that are more effective and less costly greatly improved with advances in networking and computer technology during this period. These advances include (1) the emergence of the Internet; (2) the development of reliable, scalable servers; (3) the availability of low-cost PCs, smartphones, and other mobile devices; (4) the introduction of object-oriented software such as JAVA; (5) the availability of free Internet browsers and utilities; (6) the proliferation of data management tools to end users; and (7) the government's effort in promoting a national HIT program.

2010 to Present

The growth of electronic medical records in both physician offices and health care organizations has enabled HIT to advance significantly since 2010. In 2011, 55% of doctors had at least some basic electronic medical record systems and of those, almost 75% of those installed met government standards for meaningful use, according to the Centers for Disease Control and Prevention (CDC).[7] In 2012, 44%

percent of hospitals reported having at least a basic EHR.[8] The availability of financial incentives from the federal government has greatly aided in the deployment of systems. Also, the widespread use of mobile technology has enabled patients to become more involved in their own health care. The full potential of EHRs will be fully realized when HIEs are operational. An HIE will allow for fast, accurate transmission of electronic health data between doctors, hospitals, ancillary services such as laboratories and pharmacies, and the patients themselves.

This chapter focuses on the use of these advances for health care information systems in general. Chapter 6 includes an in-depth analysis of the EHR and the effect of emerging technology on its advances.

Health Information Systems as a Critical Discipline

Health professionals from diverse backgrounds work together on medical computing in a variety of ways. Physicians, engineers, administrators, nurses, HIM professionals, software developers, and others have adopted new roles. The study of medical computing is referred to as the academic discipline of **medical informatics**. The American Medical Informatics Association (AMIA) defines *medical informatics* as "the interdisciplinary field that studies and pursues the effective uses of biomedical data, information, and knowledge for scientific inquiry, problem solving, and decision making, driven by efforts to improve human health."[9]

Postgraduate training programs are sponsored by the National Library of Medicine for physicians and other health care professionals interested in this field. Physicians usually spend several years after their residency studying medical informatics, working on developing new health care applications, and determining how biological science intersects with computer technology. In 2011 clinical informatics became a board subspecialty recognized by the American Board of Medical Specialties Medical Association. This recognition will be available to physicians who demonstrate core competencies in creating, deploying, and evaluating clinical information and decision support systems.

Today, a number of professional organizations are active in advancing the study of medical and health care informatics. The College of Health Information Management Executives, the Health Information Management Systems Society, the AMIA, and the American Health Information Management Association (AHIMA) all actively promote the advancement of HISs. The government also sponsors a private–public collaboration called the National eHealth Collaborative (NeHC). NeHC is composed of members from the government and private sector and continues to make recommendations to DHHS on how to ensure EHRs are interoperable while protecting the privacy and security of patient data.

The federal government has also gotten involved in advancing the science of health information. In 2010 the Health Data Initiative (HDI) was created by the DHHS. The purpose of the HDI is to encourage the community to use health data to develop applications to improve health. As a result, the federal government has made available greater amounts of health data free of charge to software developers and researchers to make health information more useful.

Computer Fundamentals

To deliver cost-effective and useful HIM systems, we must rely on information technology—hardware, software, and networking—to collect, store, manage, and transmit health information. The following section briefly reviews key concepts in these areas and illustrates their role in health care information systems.

Hardware

Hardware is the physical equipment of computers and computer systems. It consists of both the electronic and mechanical equipment. The computer requires a central processing unit (CPU) with capacity to hold the data being processed as well as the equipment necessary to carry out the system functions. Peripheral equipment including CD-ROMs, flash drives, and tape drives; data input devices such as PCs, tablets, and mobile devices; and output devices such as printers and scanners are also hardware. Computers come in mainframe and micro sizes. **Mainframe** machines have traditionally been used for large applications that need to support thousands of users simultaneously. Many applications can run on one mainframe. Users interact with the mainframe through terminal emulation software. The user input is transferred to the mainframe computer, where all processing occurs. **Microcomputers** are based on small microprocessing chips found in individual PCs. They are used for desktop applications such as word processing spreadsheets and database management systems (DBMSs).

Most software applications operate today in a **thin-client** environment. Thin clients have minimal or no disk space; they load their software and data from a server and then upload any data they produce back to the server. Thin clients are devices that vary from a laptop computer to a mobile device such as a smartphone or tablet. Thin-client applications are commonly called an "app" for short. Previously, software applications were **thick-client** based, requiring a desktop PC with a substantial amount of memory and disk space to perform functions that the application may require.

Increasingly, more health care organizations are taking advantage of the use of **grid computing** to maximize the use of available hardware. Grid computing is the use of a combination of computer resources from multiple administrative sites (usually other organizations) applied to a common task, which requires a great number of computer processing cycles or the need to process large amounts of data. This type of computing is distributed across large-scale cluster computers as a form of networked parallel processing. The concept is that one organization does not have to have existing resources within its own domain to perform the task but rather can have the "grid" compute the task instead. The main purpose of grid computing is to make the server infrastructure highly scalable. If more resources are needed, this is accomplished by adding more hosts to the existing grid. Grid computing is used extensively to share data and applications for collaborative research at the National Institutes of Health including the Biomedical Informatics Research Network and the Cancer Biomedical Informatics Grid. These research projects involve functions such as image analysis, data mining, and gene sequencing that are resource intensive. Each laboratory still hosts its own computers, but the grid allows the applications on the local computer to be shared by other members of the consortium.

Another hardware trend is the use of **cloud computing**. Cloud computing is similar to grid computing in that the processing power can be shared across many computers; however, the hardware is housed by a commercial vendor who specializes in cloud computer hosting. Cloud computing shifts the responsibility to install and maintain the hardware and basic computational service away from the individual laboratory (or hospital) to a cloud vendor. Cloud customers can acquire additional hardware capabilities or software applications upon request to the cloud, perhaps for a specific project. Amazon.com operates a large and popular cloud computing platform called *Amazon Elastic Compute Cloud, or EC2.*[10]

Personal Computers

A PC is a common device for data entry, management, and retrieval. PCs can be run independently or connected to an information system to enter and retrieve information. Often, the PC connects to a clinical application as a virtualized application. A virtualized application is not installed on the PC, although it is still executed as if it is. Most clinical applications that run within a hospital network are run through a virtual client and not directly on the PC. This type of implementation enables all operation and maintenance to be done remotely by the organization's technical team. It does not require a technician to visit each PC every time there is a new piece of software to install or repair. The application is fooled at runtime into believing that it is directly interfacing with the original operating system and all the resources managed by it, when in reality, it is not. All of the applications, processes, and data used are kept and run on a central server rather than on an individual desktop PC.

Smartphones and Mobile Devices

A smartphone or **mobile device** such as a tablet is a handheld device that combines computing, telecommunications, imaging, and networking features. A typical device can function as a telephone, e-mail sender and retriever, and a camera and can connect to the Internet. These devices are lightweight and can be carried in the pocket. The device can use a keyboard, a touch screen, or speech recognition for data entry. Most devices are capable of handwriting recognition so that users can write, using either their finger or a special writing instrument, to store the information in the device. Tablets are popular in collecting data directly from patients completing patient satisfaction surveys, for example.

In the health care industry, one example of the use of a mobile device is in home health organizations, in which visiting nurses use mobile devices to record visit encounter data. Another example is the use of a pen-based device to document intravenous therapy data for hospitalized patients. In both examples, the devices are used for daily tasks and are plugged into a "dock," or receiving component, that transfers the data to a larger computer system. Another example is the use of the mobile device as a resource for information. Most clinicians now have all of the standard reference books at their fingertips through the use of their mobile device. Clinical alerts and reminders are also now sent to a mobile device.

Storage

The increasing use of clinical applications in health care organizations has caused organizations to examine better solutions for the storage of data. Data retention policies often require the HIM department to store the EHR, including scanned images, radiology images, and other documentation for a definite period. Hardware redundant array of inexpensive disks (**RAID**) is a powerful and inexpensive storage solution that provides much faster disk access while completely protecting against the failure of one (or even two) disk in the physical RAID array. In the event of a physical disk failure, the RAID array is able to be reduced in size to remove the failed disk from the production line while it is being repaired. Typically, a system administrator can replace the failed drive without bringing down the array and without interruption to users. The array then rebuilds the array incorporating the new disk, and performance returns to normal. Data written on RAID is protected from physical hard drive failure.

Another type of storage solution is a storage area network (**SAN**). A SAN is a more expensive implementation of RAID hosted on a dedicated device that can accommodate large numbers of physical drives in a single array. This array presents as a single unit of space that can be subdivided as desired. SANs are fast, flexible, expandable, and robust.

Virtualization

With the increasing demand for both storage and computer servers, many organizations will implement **virtual machines** to support their health care applications. A virtual machine is a software container with an operating system and application inside. A single computer can run many virtual machines within its hardware. A virtual machine has a thin layer of software called a *hypervisor,* which separates the virtual machine from the server and dynamically allocates computing resources to each virtual machine as needed. In essence, the partitioning software is creating separate and distinct environments on a single piece of hardware. Different operating systems can run on a single server, each with its own virtual machine. This is a common implementation scenario used to test if an application can run in a Microsoft Windows environment as well as on a non-Windows computer. In the absence of a virtual machine, there would need to be two physical computers, one with a Windows operating system and the second with a non-Windows operating system, which would be much more costly than supporting one virtual machine.

If additional disk storage is needed for a specific application, an additional disk can be added to the server and incorporated into the virtual machine. When the application is no longer in need of the increased disk storage, the space can be reallocated to another application in another virtual machine on the server.

The use of virtual machines also lowers the computer cost of ownership for the organization's information systems budget. Because the number of physical computers needed is reduced, there is a decrease in the space required to house the computers as well as less power consumption and need for a separate cooling facility.

Voice Recognition

A **voice recognition** system consists of both hardware and software. It is included in this section on hardware because it is primarily an alternative to a data input device. A voice recognition system can recognize spoken words. It is an attractive technology for health care applications because it offers the most efficient means for practitioners to incorporate data capture into their normal routines. *Voice recognition* means that the computer can record information that is being said. It still does not understand what is being said, and it is important to be aware of this distinction.

This technology has grown phenomenally in recent years, particularly with continuous-speech systems. *Continuous speech* means that the user can use the system naturally and does not have to speak as slowly and distinctly as with previous systems. In its infancy these systems required an initial training session to teach the software to recognize the user's voice and dialect. Recent advances in this type of technology have removed this step. An effective use of this technology is in dictation systems. The voice recognition software is combined with templates so that the user has to speak only to complete the blank spaces in a template and not the entire document. Software for voice recognition can exist on an individual PC or be a shared application across a network. Voice recognition is offering clinicians a way to immediately dictate, sign, and produce a report independently. In other settings, voice recognition is turned on while an individual clinician dictates. The transcriptionist receives a draft document as well as the voice version and is more quickly able to complete the document and present it for signature.

SELF-ASSESSMENT QUIZ

4. Which of the following is not hardware?
   a. CD-ROM
   b. Central processing unit
   c. Desk
   d. Scanner
   e. Smartphone
5. What are the most commonly used devices for data entry, management, and retrieval?
6. What system allows clinicians a way to immediately dictate and produce a report?

Software

Software is the set of instructions required to operate computers and their applications. Software includes programs that are sets of instructions that direct actual computer operating functions, called the **operating system**, and sets of instructions used to accomplish various types of business processes, known as **application software**. Software written to process laboratory orders is application software. These instructions are combined to direct the overall functions of a given information system. The operating system directs the internal functions of the computer. It serves as the bridge to application programs. Without an operating system, each programmer would have to program all the detail involved in receiving data, displaying graphics on a screen, sending data to printers, and so forth. Operating systems contain all of the standard routine directions that handle such tasks. Operating systems act as system managers that direct the execution of programs, allocate time to multiple users, and operate the input–output (I/O) devices as well as the network communication lines. With the increase in distributed computing, most operating systems are now able to run independently of the hardware platform. An example of an operating system is UNIX. UNIX and flavors of UNIX can run on mainframes as well as workstations. UNIX is capable of running a number of powerful utility programs to support Internet applications while allowing multiuser access and file-sharing capabilities.

Mobile devices and smartphones have a different operating system than PCs and other types of computers. The two most common operating systems found on a mobile device are Android and iOS. Android was created in 2007 and is a UNIX like–based operating system that has advanced features to enable more touchscreen input and integration with other components of the device as well as being able to run more efficiently on the device battery. The operating system was designed for a handheld device and recognized the need that the user will need to conserve battery power. The operating system is licensed as open source, meaning that the software is available for download at no charge. The creators of Android encourage software developers to download the software and develop companion applications for devices running the Android operating system. iOS was created by Apple in 2007 and is available only from Apple. The operating system contains a web browser, an e-mail client, a text messaging application, and photo imaging software. The operating system, much like Android, is optimized to run on battery-powered devices with a smaller screen than found in PCs.

Programming Languages

Programming languages refer to the various sets of instructions developed to operate applications and to generate instructions themselves. Software has developed significantly since the 1980s, and the evolution of new generations of programming languages has enhanced the use and rapid development of computing power. Generally speaking, all instructions to computers are ultimately expressed in their native codes, known as *machine language*. This most basic level of programming refers to the system of codes through which the instructions are represented internally in the computer. To illustrate, a programmer writing in a computer's low-level machine language uses machine instructions (mostly all numbers) to address memory cells for storing data, accumulators to add and subtract numbers, and registers to store operands and results. Some codes represent instructions for the central processor, some codes move data from the accumulator into the main memory, some codes represent data or information about data, and some codes point to locations (addresses) in memory.

The second-generation programming languages built on machine codes by the invention of a symbolic notation called *assembly language*. Assembly language used key words to invoke sets of machine instructions instead of the numeric ones needed in the machine language. Terms such as *Add* or *Load* represented specific sets of key word machine instructions. All of the assembly languages vary by type of machine or CPU. An assembly language program is written for a specific operating system and hardware platform. It needs to be rewritten for a new operating system. It is one step closer to human language than machine language.

Third-generation programming languages extended the efficiency of programmers by offering the capability to write programs in languages that were shorter and quicker to write. They combined more and more of the machine-level instructions to accomplish their tasks. This generation of language also introduced a new capability. Some could run on different operating systems. Examples of third-generation programming languages are Formula Translator, Common Business-Oriented Language (COBOL), and C.

One third-generation programming language, Massachusetts General Hospital Utility Multi-Programming System (MUMPS), was established for specific use in health care applications. MUMPS was established in the late 1960s and is still used today in both health care and other industries. It has been renamed the *M Programming Language*. Both the Departments of Defense and Veterans Affairs have installed nationwide medical information systems using MUMPS as the primary language.[11]

Fourth-generation languages with even greater efficiencies enable programmers to use instructions at a higher level. These types of programs are commonly known as *4GL*. The concept is that program generators—sets of instructions that can be invoked as components when needed—are the foundation of the language. This allows the programmer to focus more on the logic of the program (application servers in the three-tier client server) and less on the instructions to the computer. In other words, the program generator is able to determine the lower level instructions necessary to generate the output. 4GLs were designed for powerful data manipulation and the capability of developing code that can be reused in other applications. Statistical software packages such as SAS and SPSS are considered 4GL languages. 4GLs are often proprietary to one vendor.

Databases

A **database** is a collection of stored data, typically organized into fields, records, and files. A **database management system** (DBMS) is an integrated set of programs that manages access to the database. Databases have evolved with advances of technology. The goal of the database is to represent the lowest level meaning of the data that allows users to retrieve and manipulate the data. A **database model** is a collection of logical constructs used to represent the data structure and the relationships among the data. The four major database models are:

1. Relational
2. Hierarchical
3. Network
4. Object oriented

Database Models
Relational Model

The **relational model**, the most popular database model, was developed by E. F. Codd in 1970.[12] It is designed around the concept that all data are stored in tables with relationships between the tables. A relation is created by sharing a common data element; for example, if two tables have a patient identifier, patient identifier relates those tables. How the data are physically stored is not of concern to the user. The user needs to know only what the relationships are among the entities in the database.

Figure 8-2 shows an example of three tables in a relational database used in an ambulatory clinic. The rules for a relational database used in an ambulatory clinic are as follows:

1. Each patient has only one entry in the patient table and is identified by a unique identifier.
2. Each patient has one or more entries in the visit table.
3. Each patient in the visit table is linked to the patient table by the unique identifier.

FIGURE 8-2 Sample relational database model. *DX*, Diagnosis; *ICD9-CM*, *International Classification Diseases*, ninth edition, clinical modification; *ID*, identification; *SSN*, Social Security number.

4. Each working diagnosis entry in the visit table has a lookup entry in the diagnosis master file.

The rules listed in Figure 8-2 are defined as the associations among the data. There are three types of relationships to describe associations:

1. One to many—a patient may have many visits to the ambulatory clinic, but each visit is attributed to only one patient. A patient ("one") is related to the visits ("many"). A one-to-many relationship is sometimes identified as *1:M*.

2. Many to many—a patient may have many physicians, and each physician may have many patients. A many-to-many relationship is referred to as *M:N*.

3. One to one—an *International Classification of Diseases*, ninth edition, Clinical Module (ICD-9-CM), code has only one description, and the ICD-9-CM description has only one ICD-9-CM code.

There are several reasons for choosing the relational model for this ambulatory clinic application. First, we want to store the data only once. By creating a **primary key** for the unique patient identifier, we can eliminate storing the patient's name and other demographics in the visit table. We can always join the patient and visit table by patient identifier and report the data in both tables. Second, this application requires several master or lookup tables. Lookup tables enable data translations to be stored outside the visit and patient tables. In the preceding example, the visit table contains only the visit working diagnosis code (most often an ICD-9-CM code). The diagnosis lookup table stores two fields, the ICD-9-CM code and ICD-9-CM description. Each code and description is in the diagnosis lookup table only once. In this way, the ICD-9-CM description does not have to be stored in each visit record.

Structured Query Language

Structured query language (SQL) is the relational database model's standard language. It is pronounced "see-kwell" or as separate letters: S-Q-L. It was originally designed in 1975 by IBM but has since been adopted by the American National Standards Institute (ANSI). SQL commands allow the creation and management of a database and provide a method of retrieval of data. All queries are based on the SELECT statement (see the following example of these queries).

Example of Queries Based on the SELECT Command

Using the relational database illustrated in Figure 8-2, the SQL query to list all of the visits for a patient with patient identifier 663465 is:

SELECT FROM VISIT
WHERE PATIENTID='663465';

where instructs all fields in the visit table to be printed. The output from the query would be

000000
Location
Smith
00-May-00
Working

ID	Location	Doc	Date	Working DX
663465	CMED	Smith	02-Sep-99	428.0
663465	CRHE	Jones	13-May-99	714.0

Hierarchical Model

The **hierarchical** model differs greatly from the relational model. The hierarchical model supports a treelike structure that consists of parent (or root) and child segments. Each parent segment has a child. Each child segment can have only one parent segment. However, a parent can have more than one child. A user queries the database, and the search seeks the answer from parent to child. The answer to the query is found by matching the conditions by searching downward through the tree. Retrieving involves gathering the parent record and following a **pointer** to the record in the next lower level. This model is quite effective when the queries are predetermined and pointers already identified. It is not effective for ad hoc queries or when there is information only about the data contained in the child segment. This model requires the user to understand the physical as well as the logical structure of the database. Because the logical model is replicated in the physical structure, it is difficult to change this structure. Many-to-many relationships (as described earlier) are difficult to represent in this model. It is also difficult to use the data for multiple purposes. If another type of query is needed, additional copies of the database need to be made so that the logical model can be changed to the copied database.

An example of a hierarchical database is found in hospital patient accounting systems. The system contains many patient accounts (parent) that in turn have many transactions (child). The total number of transactions is likely to be greater than 50. The rules would be:

- Each patient account (parent) has at least one transaction (child).
- Each patient account can have many transactions.
- Each transaction can be defined as a debit or credit, so that the relationship between parent and child is fixed.

A common user query would be to determine a patient's total charges. This model would easily handle that because the patient account (parent) is known. It would identify the parent and then trace the pointers to each of the transactions (child). However, it would be difficult in this model to determine all of the patients who had a specific transaction during the past year.

Network Model

The **network** model is similar to the hierarchical model except that a child can have more than one parent. In a network database, the parent is referred to as an *owner* and a child is referred to as a *member*. In other words, it supports the many-to-many relationship. It does not, as the name might suggest, refer to the physical configuration of the computer where the database resides but instead describes the logical arrangement of the data.

Object-Oriented Model

This model has experienced a surge in popularity because of the use of JAVA and other programming tools. The database is one that embraces the concept of an **object**. An **object-oriented** database is a collection of objects. Objects support encapsulation and inheritance. Encapsulation is the technique through which an object such as a patient is defined with certain characteristics. The user does not need to know how the characteristics are stored, just that the object "patient" exists and has certain attributes. Inheritance means that one object can inherit the properties of another object. For example, a physician is defined as an object with certain characteristics (a name, a specialty, an office address). A resident is defined as another object with certain characteristics with the first characteristics being those of a physician. Therefore the resident inherits the properties of the physician object. There are no primary keys in an object-oriented model. Access to data can be faster because joins are often not needed as in the relational model. This is because an object can be retrieved directly without a search, by following pointers.

Network Technology

Network technology is used within individual organizations to connect the PCs, workstations, printers, and storage devices to the organization's network and the entire outside world. It has evolved from the basic terminal to mainframe computer connection to local and wide area networks (WANs) and the client-server technology. A **local area network** (LAN) connects multiple devices together via communications and is located within a small geographic area. An example of a LAN environment is a patient scheduling system at a primary care clinic in which seven PCs are connected to a server. Each of the PCs is able to execute its own programs (e.g., word processing, spreadsheet applications) but is also able to access data and devices anywhere on the LAN. This allows all users of the LAN to share hardware such as laser printers and scanners as well as to share patient files. Users can also use the LAN to communicate with each other via e-mail or share schedule and appointment books. LANs are capable of transmitting data at a high rate, making access to the LAN resources seem transparent to the user. However, there is a limit to the number of computers that can attach to a single LAN.

The most widely used LAN network topology in use today is **Ethernet**. Developed at Xerox in 1976, Ethernet is a standard defined by the Institute of Electrical and Electronics Engineers (IEEE) as IEEE 802.3. This standard defines the transmission speed of data traveling across the LAN as either 10 million bits per second (Mbps) or 100 Mbps. The topology is designed with messages that are handled by all computers in the LAN until they reach their final destination. The disadvantage of this technology is that a failure in one segment of the network affects the entire LAN. Another type of LAN technology is **token ring**. Token ring (IEEE 802.5) means that the transmissions travel from one computer to another until they reach their final destination. This allows a single computer to

be added to or disconnected from the network without affecting the rest of the computers on the LAN. Token ring transmission speeds vary from 4 to 16 Mbps.

Wide area networks (WANs) are used for extensive, geographically larger environments. They often consist of two or more LANs connected through a telephone system, a dedicated leased line, or a satellite. The Internet is an example of a WAN. WANs are usually found in organizations that need to connect computers across an entire health care delivery system. For example, the hospital, the long-term care facility, and the physician office all have an internal LAN in their own areas, and the LAN is connected to the backbone of the WAN.

The most widely used WAN technology today is the **fiber distributed data interface** (FDDI). FDDI provides transmission at a higher rate than Ethernet or token ring. It is run with fiberoptic cable. Hundreds to thousands of smooth, clear, thin, glass fiber strands bound together form fiberoptic cables. Data are transformed into light pulses that are emitted by a laser device. Current fiberoptic technology can transmit data at speeds of up to 2.5 gigabits per second, much faster than Ethernet or token ring.

A popular type of network found in health care today is a **wireless** or **Wi-Fi** network. This type of network enables computers and other handheld devices to communicate with the Internet and other network servers without being physically connected to the network. Wireless networks use the IEEE 802.11 standard, which was ratified in September 1999. There are several versions of the 802.11 protocol in use, with the most commonly used being 802.11 g.

Each wireless network has a service set identifier (SSID). This is a code attached to all packets on a wireless network to identify each packet as part of that network. The code consists of a maximum of 32 alphanumeric characters. All wireless devices attempting to communicate with each other must share the same SSID. SSID also serves to identify uniquely a group of wireless network devices used in a given service set. For security purposes, it is important to change the default, factory-assigned SSID for each wireless network. The default SSID will identify your network location and potentially permit others to access your network.

To secure wireless networks, protocols were created to encrypt and protect wireless transmissions. One of the first protocol systems developed is the **wired equivalent privacy** (WEP) system, and it is part of the IEEE 802.11 standard. It provides an encryption scheme so that the information transmitted over a wireless network is protected as it is sent from one device to another device. Because of some weakness in the WEP protocol, **Wi-Fi protected access** (WPA) is the most popular method of securing wireless networks. Data are encrypted as they travel over the wireless network as with WEP, but the method of securing the network is greatly improved over WEP. A major improvement is the requirement that the authentication code used dynamically changes as the system is used. In previous versions, the same code was used with each transmission, and so once the code was known by the outside, the network was compromised.

Wi-Fi's greatest strength is also a weakness. Every action that is performed while connected to a wireless network is broadcast to any other network within a certain distance. Therefore it is important to secure each wireless network with encryption. Encryption is discussed in a later section in this chapter.

Wired Versus Wireless Comparison

Several **protocols** are available for communicating across networks. A protocol is a specification or algorithm for how data are to be exchanged. It is similar to the telephone system, which expects an area code as part of the phone number. Two of the more popular network protocols are transmission control protocol/Internet protocol (TCP/IP) and asynchronous transfer mode (ATM). TCP/IP is the standard protocol used to connect Internet sites. TCP/IP can run on various platforms and can connect hardware systems of different types as long as both systems support TCP/IP. It divides each piece of data that is to be sent across the network into packets, and the packets are then sent to the destination via the most available route at the time of transmission. TCP/IP allows packets to be rerouted if the network is particularly busy at one site. ATM creates a fixed path between the source and destination. The packets are of a fixed size. The benefit of this type of network is that a single packet does not overload the network, and very fast transmission is supported. It can relay images, sound, and text at high speeds. Table 8-1 illustrates the differences between wired and wireless networks.

Client–Server Platforms

The client–server architecture was developed in the early 1990s. The concept is to have most of the processing occur on the server.[13] This reduces network traffic by providing a query response rather than total file transfer. It is also referred to as **two-tier** architecture. The user interface is located on the user's desktop, and the database management application and data tables are stored on a database server. The server is a much more powerful PC or workstation than the individual desktop model. This type of architecture is found in smaller environments with fewer than 50 users.

An example of a two-tier client–server application is found in the cancer registry department. The database is located on a server. Each registrar has client software applications residing on his or her PC. When the registrar issues a query to the database, the client requests the data from the server. The server processes the request and returns the data to the client. The client machine is then responsible for the display and graphics.

There are several obstacles to implementing the two-tier architecture approach. The client software needs to be replicated on every PC on the network, which can be expensive to administer and maintain. It is difficult to change the database structure because the client software also has to be reconfigured. In addition, because it is difficult to scale up to more users, the application depth is somewhat limited.

A three-tier architecture has become popular. The **three-tier** configuration is a type of client–server architecture that has three components:
1. User interface
2. Application server
3. Database server

The difference between this configuration and the two-tier one is the introduction of the application server. The user interface is the software that runs on the user or client machine, and it can be customized to the needs of the client. The application server processes the data. The logic behind the database queries is hidden from the user. An example occurs when certain utilization review coordinators are responsible for receiving a specific set of patient claim authorizations. The logic or rules of how to process the data are included in an application server. The logic might contain items such as, "If patient is enrolled in a health maintenance organization (HMO), then display the name of both the patient and the name of the subscriber. If the patient is not enrolled in the HMO, only require that the patient's name be displayed." The database server is the physical location where the database resides and serves as the connection for the application server to process the logic.

Many health care applications that were written with the two-tier approach are being rewritten with the three-tier approach. Developers are discovering that health care requires a huge amount of application processing and that having three distinct layers to the product makes it easier to change the application piece. Changes to the application server do not have to affect the entire system. HISs need to change to reflect the changing business requirements of the industry. The choice of architecture is a critical one in deploying applications. (See the following example of developing a system for special populations.)

TABLE 8-1	Wired Versus Wireless Comparison	
	Ethernet (Wired)	Wi-Fi (Wireless)
Advantages	Very secure; reliable transfer of data; data transfer speeds up to 94 Mbps	No cables to connect to device; minimal installation costs; allows for access to the network from any location
Disadvantages	Does not permit mobility; installation costs can be high for cable routing	Extra process required to secure network; some areas may not be reachable by wireless; data transfer rates are slower than Ethernet
Cost	Network cards, cables, and labor costs of installation	Network cards (although some PCs have technology built in)

Mbps, Million bits per second; *PC*, personal computer.

Example of Home Health Care Data System

The home health division needs a system to provide case management services to its existing population as well as to identify current inpatients who may need home health services after discharge. Because the case managers are dispersed over a wide geographic region, including some in their homes, they cannot implement a system that requires a specialized PC configuration requiring daily maintenance. The database, which resides on the database server, contains all of the patient information. However, not all home health case managers need to view all of the data in the database on their PCs. Each case manager may have separate data requirements. The geriatric case managers and maternity case managers need different sets of queries and reports. These rules are commonly known as **business rules**. These are the rules that determine the user interface and database services that may be required. The business rules reside on the application server. Other items that may reside on the application server include a data retrieval engine and formulas for medication administration. Examples of business rules in this scenario are (1) display laboratory values only if they are not within the normal range, (2) require patient date of birth on input, and (3) set reminder for next month to check blood pressure.

Interface Engine

Another technology component being used in HISs is an **interface engine**. An interface engine is considered a piece of **middleware**—software and hardware that serve as a bridge between applications. An example of middleware in the previous section on client–server technology is found in a three-tier architecture model. The application server in the three-tier model is considered middleware.

An interface engine allows two applications to exchange information without having to build a customized interface for each application. Before the implementation of an interface engine, most interfaces between applications were **point to point**. *Point to point* refers to the method of connection. If the radiology system requires ADT information, then a point-to-point interface is created by the information system programmers to exchange this information between radiology and ADT. If the laboratory system requires the same ADT information, another interface is created to send ADT data to the laboratory system. The ADT data now exist in multiple copies. This is inefficient for three reasons:

1. Separate programs need to be written for both the sending and receiving applications to agree on the protocol for the transmission and define the frequency of transmissions, error handling, and so forth.
2. Duplication of data requires additional network traffic.
3. It is difficult to support and maintain because each interface requires customization and monitoring.

Figure 8-3 illustrates how an interface engine may function for an HIS. Each of the HIS applications sends data to the interface engine, which then reroutes the data to the appropriate destination. The sending or source application initiates a network connection with the interface engine usually by using the TCP/IP protocol. The interface engine can then reformat the data in a structure suitable for the target or receiving application. Reformatting might be necessary, for example, if the source application contains laboratory test codes from an outside laboratory. The target application may be expecting to receive only test codes that exist in the hospital laboratory system. The interface engine would be the translation service for both applications. Health Level 7 (HL7) transactions may be received and reformatted in the interface engine. Interface engines might also house the enterprise MPI service. The source applications from all of the various systems throughout the enterprise could route their data through the interface engine. The interface engine could reference the MPI and assign the enterprise MPI identifier to the data before the data arrive at the target application. This is an alternative to having the MPI value collected and stored within each application.

✓ SELF-ASSESSMENT QUIZ

7. What are the four database models discussed in this chapter?
   a. Relational
   b. Hierarchical
   c. Network
   d. Object oriented
   e. All of the above
8. What provides a method of retrieval for the data residing in a relational database?
   a. SQL commands
   b. SELECT
   c. Relational model
9. What is the most widely used WAN technology?

FIGURE 8-3 Interface engine example. *ADT,* Admission, discharge, transfer; *ECG,* electrocardiogram.

DESIGNING THE USER INTERFACE

The user interface or computer view refers to the screen format for both data entry and output display. The power of DBMSs allows flexibility in which views are created for data capture and data displays, including still and moving images and sound as well as text and graphs. Computer views require menus of alternatives to be developed and screen or window formats that may include a variety of input formats and output formats, including monitors, personal digital assistant (PDA) screens, mobile telephones, and so on. It is helpful to remember that standards such as those of the American Society for Testing and Materials (ASTM) are only a foundation from which to begin the process of selecting data items. Once captured, the data elements may be retrieved in new configurations to meet the needs of many different user groups. For example, a physician may want to view graphs that show the trends of laboratory data along with a menu of therapy options with costs, supported by a reference from a linked database. A social worker developing a discharge plan may select a summary of the patient's functional level, living arrangements, and insurance benefits to compare with services provided and prices charged by local home health care providers. This flexibility lends to both the promise and the problems of designing computer views.

When computer **views** (information on screens) are well designed and controlled, they enhance technology by providing a smooth link in the communication process. They permit recording of varying data without recopying constant information. This reduces clerical work, decreases the number of errors, and increases efficiency. In this section, the word view primarily refers to information on screens; however, many of the design issues associated with views also apply to paper forms. When views are well designed, they assist in actual direct patient care. For example, a well-designed nursing assessment view will enable nurses to collect the data related to the patient assessment process in the same way each time.

As with data collection and technology, user interface design should emphasize the needs of users. It is the responsibility of each health care facility to develop its own user interfaces. Accrediting and regulatory bodies such as The Joint Commission and standards organizations such as ASTM do not recommend particular views with which to collect their required data elements, nor do professional organizations such as the American Hospital Association and AHIMA. However, some standards organizations and the federal government are interested in offering templates and core documents structures in health care to facilitate the exchange of data. Large health care organizations often have enterprise-wide standards for screen displays (views and templates) so that all facilities within the organization use the same one. Before starting a project involving view redesign, it is recommended to research any existing standards or policies that may exist within your organization.

Well-designed screen views for data entry make it possible to:
- Organize the data entry fields in logical format.
- Include field edits.
- Include passwords to add, delete, or modify data.
- Allow simultaneous entry or updating in many tables at one time.
- Include brief instructions on the screens or provide more lengthy help screens.
- Make the screens easy to navigate through the use of color, lines, borders, and hyperlinks.
- Use default values in a field to eliminate the need to key repeated data between entries (e.g., the date field could be automatically set up to add today's date without the need to key the characters).
- Allow automatic sequential numbering (e.g., accession register numbers).
- Show data on the screen from a different table when the key field is entered (e.g., for the MPI screen form, when the doctor's number is entered, the doctor's name, address, and so on can automatically appear on the screen).
- Develop or customize menus or submenus to add, delete, or change data.

Furthermore, Windows-style user interfaces provide menus that pull down from choices shown on a tool bar at the top of the screen. A menu is an important component of a computer interface because it is central to ease of navigation. Therefore a carefully constructed sequence of menus is part of a comprehensive design.

User Interface Team

The creation and management of the user interface is a collaborative process. Members of the views and templates team include representatives from the following services in a hospital environment. A different environment might modify the team membership to represent its needs:
- HIM
- Information systems
- Materials management
- Patient care services
- Quality improvement
- Medical staff leadership

The HIM professional plays a leadership role by providing knowledge of rules and regulations related to health record content, the flow of data throughout the facility, and the information needs of the health care delivery system. The views or templates design and control process also benefit from the involvement of an information systems manager who is responsible for the software application that will house the view, a materials or purchasing manager who is responsible for inventory and ordering paper forms, a patient care professional who represents clinical needs, a quality improvement professional to provide input regarding views or templates created to address quality issues, and physician representatives who will be using the views. It is extremely important to have physician and other clinicians involved in this process. The team's charge may be to work on administrative and patient information applications and to become involved in the selection of data collection technology. The team forwards its patient-related recommendations to the clinical information committee for approval, and its administrative recommendations follow the organizational chain of command.

> **? DID YOU KNOW?**
>
> There has been a growing demand for professionals with experience in designing software applications and websites. This job is called a *user experience* (UX) *designer.* The UX designer can also conduct usability studies to understand how easy a system is to learn. UX professionals have a wide range of qualifications in fields such as psychology, information science, journalism, or fine arts. This profession is also suited for someone with an HIM background.

General Design Principles

Needs of Users

The needs of both internal and external users must be considered when designing views or the user interface. It is important to remember that users are not only the patient and providers, but also the administrative, financial, and legal staff of the facility. External users collect data from many locations, and the data are combined or aggregated. These may be local, state, and federal agencies and other planning and research groups. Collecting enough of the right type of data to satisfy this range of users means clearly defining the purpose of the view.

Selection and Sequencing of Items

When the purpose of the view or template is established, the next step is to construct a list or grid of required data to ensure the collection of all essential items and the elimination of unnecessary or redundant items. Effective and efficient sequencing of the view or template should follow the traditional pattern—from left to right and top to bottom—permitting a continuous operation whether reading or entering data on the computer. The flow should be logical and take into consideration the order of data collection.

Another aspect of view design that promotes consistency is the development of a master format or template. The placement of data in the same sequence on similar forms or views with similar layouts facilitates rapid entry and retrieval.

Although often overlooked, the organization should discuss how the print out from electronic views will be presented. There will be occasions when the entire EHR or major portions of the record will need to be printed to fulfill a request for information. The record may also be released electronically, but again, some plan must be in place to create a CD or other means of organizing the information.

Instructions

Instructions should briefly identify who should complete the data items and should provide any additional guidance that is necessary. Computer views typically provide this information on introductory screens and as needed throughout data entry.

Guidelines for Designing Web Pages

Designing a view or form to appear on a web page provides more flexibility and options for improved usability. Consideration of type styles, or fonts, when well chosen, contributes to readability. Items of similar importance should be equal in size and type, and the overall number of different fonts used should be low. Italics and boldface characters should be used to maintain the effect of emphasis only. Style considerations may include the requirement to use a specified font type that is identified with the name and logo of the organization.

A web-based user interface allows the form to contain **hypertext links** between documents. A hypertext link is an embedded object within the web page that enables direct access to another, related web page. Often, reference materials are not included directly on the web page but a hypertext link is available so that if the user wishes to go to the reference page website, it is only a click away.

It is important that each screen within the web application follow the same "look and feel." This includes having clear and consistent icons to let the user know where to find items on the screen. For example, it is important to have the icon to print located near the top right corner of the screen. Users expect the icon to be in that location. Second, the user should always be able to return to the home or main page of the application. The link to return to the main page should always be in the same location on the screen for each web page.

A well-designed screen will offer feedback for every required action. For example, if during data entry the user does not complete all items, there should be a message to alert the user to complete the missing information. Likewise, the screen should permit the user to undo the last action. This enables the user to feel free to navigate throughout the screen.

Users want to get information in the fewest possible steps. This means that the design of menus must be an efficient hierarchy of information to minimize steps through menu pages. Studies have shown that users prefer menus that present at least five to seven links and that they prefer a few very dense screens of choices to many layers of simplified menus. As a general rule, the screen should be designed so that the user has complete control over the system.

Screen Space

The use of **cascading style sheets** (CSS) can help the user interface optimize the use and appearance of the web page.[14] With CSS-styled pages, users can easily apply personalized formatting to web documents. A page designed using red text against a green background, for example, presents a problem for users with red-green color blindness: the contrast between text and background may not be great enough for the text to be distinguishable. If the colors are set using a style sheet, users can set their browser preferences to override settings and can apply their own style sheet to the page instead. With CSS-styled pages, users can transform web content into a format that addresses their requirements for accessibility.

A web page design should be checked to ensure that all navigation and content areas fit well within the display screen (usually 800 × 600 pixels). The use of **frames** within the web page can assist in optimizing the screen space. Frames are vertical or horizontal lines that structure the form on the screen. They may vary in style but serve to divide the form into logical sections and to direct data entry length and location. If several people have areas to complete, the data sets each person is to document should be presented in the order of completion. Different colors or shading can help to separate sections of the form visually. Horizontal frames on the screen are desirable for long sections of the forms that require free text. Vertical and horizontal frames should be aligned as much as possible to make the form less "busy" visually. Box titles or captions should be located to the upper left of the boxes in small font sizes. Check boxes (or radio buttons) and drop-down boxes are other timesavers that conserve space. When check boxes are used, there should be consistency throughout the form whether the boxes or lines are to the immediate left or immediate right of the caption. These should be aligned vertically when appropriate. The box or line to check should be close to the caption so that the person performing the documentation checks the correct line or box.

If data are to be entered on a computer screen and then printed on a preprinted paper form (e.g., billing form, patient care plan form), refer to the vendor or machine specifications for correct data placement. If the form is not designed appropriately, data will not be printed in the exact locations required on the form. Discussing such specifications with a printer or the purchasing department is important in all aspects of form design.

SELF-ASSESSMENT QUIZ

10. True or False? It is the responsibility of each health care facility to test and evaluate the user interfaces available in an information system.
11. Users of an interface include:
    a. Patient and provider
    b. Administrative staff
    c. Financial staff
    d. Legal staff
    e. All of the above

COMPUTER APPLICATIONS

In this section, several examples of administrative and clinical applications that are typical components of HISs are reviewed. Health care organizations today are heavily involved in acquiring or developing these applications and bringing them together in the EHR.

Administrative Applications

Administrative applications include those that operate the daily business functions in the organization. These typically include an MPI; an ADT system; the business functions carried out in HIM departments such as abstracting, release of information management, coding/grouping, and chart tracking; and enterprise resource planning (ERP) systems. *ERP* is the term given to a variety of applications that support materials management, general ledger, accounts payable, grants accounting, and payroll. In addition, decision support or executive information systems are considered integral to the administrative domain.

Admission, Discharge, and Transfer System

The ADT system is an example of a core administrative system. A basic module contained in both inpatient and outpatient HISs, this application collects the initial set of data that is used to establish a "record" of a new visit in all affected hospital departments, establish and update the MPI, and to modify and track the patient until discharge. It serves as an interface to almost all other departmental systems, so it is important to understand how the data are captured and stored in the database. The HL-7 standard has defined a series of transactions to identify the types of actions that can be used to create, update, or delete records from the ADT database. Some of the basic HL-7 functions that are defined for an ADT system are the following[15]:

- A01—Admit a patient
- A03—Discharge a patient
- A04—Registration
- A08—Update patient information
- A13—Cancel discharge

The ADT system houses most of the patient demographics, including financial information that will be needed to create the patient's entry into other applications. Typical data included in an ADT system are shown in Table 8-2.

In addition to basic demographic information such as name, address, and telephone number, the ADT system collects information on the patient's insurance coverage, the emergency contact for the patient, and, most often, the admitting diagnosis or chief complaint.

TABLE 8-2	Examples of Admission, Discharge, and Transfer Data
Demographics	Insurance Information	Visit Information
Patient name	Name of insured	Patient ID (medical record number)
Patient Social Security number	Relationship to patient	Attending physician
Date of birth	Primary insurance	Referring physician
Sex	Subscriber ID	Financial class
Patient address	Plan code	Admit date and time
Marital status	Secondary insurance	Discharge date and time
Patient account number	Subscriber ID	Service location
Emergency contact	Plan code	Patient visit type

ID, Identification.

The ADT system can be used to accomplish the following functions:

- Create and update the institutional MPI
- Generate census displays
- Notify transcription services of the patient's status (for report distribution)
- Indicate insurance authorization for precertification
- Pass demographic data collected on a previous visit to outpatient scheduling systems to facilitate clinic appointments
- Notify and send visit data to local applications such as cancer registries

At the point of discharge, it generates similar notification to the necessary departments so that the information for that case can be closed. Notifications initiated for new activities such as room setup and materials ordering begin when the patient is discharged. The same notice generated from ADT can activate record-tracking modules and quality monitors for follow-up action in the HIM area.

Decision Support Systems

Decision support systems are information systems designed to support planning functions of an organization. They range from simple analysis of cost per patient for specific departments or clinics to high-level strategic analysis, marketing, and policy development. They draw from multiple databases to analyze the day-to-day business activities of the organization. The data found in an administrative decision support system consist mostly of feeds from financial, ADT, and medical record abstract systems. In the last section of this chapter, an example of a decision support system is presented in the form of a data mart.

Business intelligence (BI) systems are a subset of decision support systems. A BI system extracts data from institutional databases, which are then analyzed, reorganized, and reformatted for presentation in summary format. Designed so that administrators and senior executives can view a "snapshot" of summary and trend data, these systems focus on financial "readings" that allow both summary and trend data views and the options of drilling down to detail. Some examples of reports contained in a BIS are:

- Average length of stay for the past 12 months
- Average daily census
- Average number of recovery days for accounts receivable
- Net revenue and expenses by financial class for the past two quarters
- Number of same-day surgery procedures by day for the past quarter
- List of latest patient satisfaction survey results by nursing unit
- Geographically represented map of all of the acquired physician practices

Clinical Applications

A clinical system is any system that is involved either directly or indirectly with patient care. Table 8-3 lists some of the types of clinical systems either within a department or

TABLE 8-3 Examples of Clinical Applications Found in a Health Information System

Laboratory	Radiology	Pharmacy
• Chemistry	• Diagnostic	• Orders
• Hematology	• Scanner services	• Medical administration record
• Microbiology	• Special procedures	
• Immunopathology	• Nuclear medicine	
• Blood bank		• Discharge summary
• Pathology		
• Cytology		
• Autopsy		

Cardiology	Nursing	Operating Room
• Echocardiograms	• Documentation	• Scheduling
• Electrocardiograms	• Assessments	• Resource utilization
• Nuclear cardiology	• Discharge orders	
• Cath lab	• Progress notes	• Anesthesia notes
• Cardiac rehabilitation	• Material management	

throughout the enterprise. In 2012 the Food and Drug Administration Safety Innovation Act was passed by the U.S. Congress. This Act's purpose is to make recommendations for regulatory requirements related to HIT. In particular, the Food and Drug Administration (FDA) will provide oversight to mobile applications involving imaging and digital transfers of data. Mobile applications will be assessed using the same regulatory standards that apply to other medical devices.[16]

It is important to understand the specific capabilities of each type of clinical system. This section presents results reporting, order entry, clinical decision support, and point-of-care systems as some examples. Understanding the functionality of these applications will enable us to arrive at better technologic solutions. Some of these solutions are discussed in the next section.

Results Reporting

Results reporting applications are modules designed to retrieve diagnostic test and treatment results from feeder systems such as laboratory, radiology, and other departmental settings such as transcription and present them directly on inquiry to the care provider. Results reporting modules usually include a **graphical user interface** for viewing laboratory results, electrocardiogram results, and other reports using graphics displays such as flow sheets. Results reporting is often the hospital's first attempt at providing EHR functionality or an initial comprehensive clinical information system. Implementing a successful results reporting system as the first phase of an EHR system can greatly assist in further EHR implementation. Physicians, nurses, and other care providers must see results that are timely and dependable if they are to develop an allegiance to computer-based data in general.

A results reporting system should include patient demographics (sent from the ADT system); a list of results available, usually sorted by date; and some minimal information to identify the report further. For example, it would be preferable if the first screen presented the patient's name, medical record number, attending physician, ordering physician, date of test or treatment, and a brief description of the test or treatment. It could include whether the laboratory test was done in the hematology or microbiology laboratory or whether the radiology report refers to a chest x-ray study or a computed tomographic (CT) scan.

There must also be a methodology for identifying corrected or revised results in the results reporting module. This becomes extremely important for data integrity. Remember that the results reporting module will almost replace the typical telephone call to the laboratory for a result or a paper review of a chart. Usually, most laboratory tests are stored with an **ascension number**. This is a unique identifier that identifies the specimen. Several tests can have the same ascension number because the same specimen is used to run various types of tests. However, the ascension number can be used to record the result in the results reporting system, and when a correction is received; it can overwrite the display of the previous result. Without a unique identifier, it would be difficult to identify the result that is to be modified in the results reporting system.

Order Entry

Order entry systems are designed to organize and communicate order processing functions to all personnel involved in the care of a patient. Originally driven by and connected to charge capture, they have evolved significantly and currently include order management functions, clinical event detection, and managed care initiatives support. An HIS **order entry** refers to online entry of orders for drugs, laboratory tests, and procedures, usually performed by nurses or unit clerks. Most health care organizations are implementing computerized physician (or provider) order entry (CPOE) systems, particularly for all patient orders including medication, laboratory, and radiology orders. This type of system is discussed later in this section. In most facilities, the orders are initiated at the nursing unit (usually by physicians) for diagnostic tests and treatments. The goal of the order entry system is to capture the order electronically only once.

In the interim, until the perfect world is achieved, many systems have adopted order entry systems used by nurses and unit clerks. They have been quite successful. See the following example of how an order entry system may function.

Example of Order Entry System

An order for a diagnostic radiology examination is entered through an order entry system in a hospital. The order is transmitted to the radiology system that will ultimately house the result (or report) for this test. Data noting date, time, patient demographics, and any special conditions are imported into the radiology system. The radiology system does not have to reenter any of the information that was already collected from the patient when the order was initiated. All orders for a given day may emerge on a worksheet for the radiology department personnel to follow as they set up and execute a day's schedule. Once the work is completed, the result of the test is recorded locally and then transmitted back to the ordering source so that hospital personnel can view the status of the order and either see a result directly or follow up if appropriate. The result may be a message that an examination is complete and will be available at a specified time, or it may be the actual report. At the same time, the necessary charges for services provided to the patient are captured.

Now the basic function of order entry can be extended to include order management features. For instance, some order management systems also have an "auto-complete" function that allows the user to type the first few letters of a word that matches the desired order name. The system then searches for potentially matching terms from the possible choices and provides the user with a "pick list" of order names, from which the user can select. This is a feature that is borrowed from word processing software and e-mail systems, which also have this capability. For example, typing "potass" into an order system would return a list of possible choices including "potassium."

Example of Order Management Features

An order placed for a thyroid-stimulating hormone test is received by the laboratory system and compared with data already collected for that patient. The comparison shows that the same analysis was completed recently. The system invokes a standard message to the ordering location; the unit clerk may call the physician to reconsider the need for the order. This example is one of adding intelligence to the order entry system to avoid overuse of laboratory services. In fact, the current focus on such systems is to build them so that such interventions are standard features.

Computerized Provider Order Entry

In the ideal situation, a provider would place the order via the order entry system, and a clinical decision support system (CDSS) would validate it and send it to the receiving service. If any clarification is needed, the provider can respond immediately. This is often termed a **computerized physician order entry** (CPOE) system. *CPOE* refers to a variety of computer-based systems that share the common features of automating the ordering process and that ensure standardized, legible, and complete orders. It was shown as early as 1998 that a system like this can serve as an intervention tool to prevent adverse events such as medication errors.[15]

A CPOE system functions as part of an EHR in which the user provides a login to the EHR system. The EHR system confirms that the user login is authorized to initiate and authorize patient orders. After initiating the CPOE application, a patient is selected. The user enters and modifies orders using an electronic "notepad" that holds orders but does not deliver them immediately to the ancillary department.

The user then reviews and edits the pending orders on the notepad, accepts the orders, and the order is sent to the ancillary department. There is no paper generated during this process. CPOE systems are usually designed with a hierarchical selection of orders with departments (i.e., pharmacy, radiology, laboratory) being the first level of entry. The second level of entry is the type of test or medication that needs to be ordered, such as a chemistry test or an intravenous medication. The third level of entry is the specific test or medication found in the second level. The process is designed to guide the user to make the correct selections for each order.

CPOE systems require a data dictionary that contains all of the valid ordering selections and components. Each department maintains its own data dictionary and coordinates the entries with users in other departments. For example, the data dictionary contains an entry defined as "orderable" for an intravenous medication used for pain management. The user would select this medication from the list of orderable medications. However, within the data dictionary is a listing that defines what components are found in that medication. It is the individual components that are then sent to the pharmacy for dispensing. The CPOE system should not disrupt the usual workflow of how the clinician would perform the same order on a paper form.

Benefits of CPOE include process improvement, cost efficiencies, clinical decision support, and optimization of provider time in many ways, including:

- Elimination of lost orders
- Elimination of ambiguities caused by illegible handwriting
- Check for potential drug–drug or drug–allergy interactions
- Alerts to physicians of high-cost tests and drugs before actual use
- Access to online pharmacy and laboratory reference sources

Most important, these systems can serve as an intervention tool to prevent adverse events, such as medication errors.[17]

Clinical decision support features within CPOE systems can also help clinicians with reminders for cancer screenings, vaccinations, and other types of preventive care. Many CPOE systems will contain recommended guidelines from the National Cancer Institute, the American Diabetes Association, and other groups to allow for the clinician to be reminded of the recommendations when ordering a particular test for a patient. If the guidelines are modified by the external organization, it only requires a small change within the CPOE system, thus enabling the clinician to have the most up-to-date guidelines available.

Clinical Decision Support Systems

Clinical decision support systems (CDSSs) can be characterized as systems that provide diagnostic investigation tools and clinical guideline advice to patient care providers. Most CDSSs have become part of an existing system, such as a provider order entry system described in the previous section.

Basic clinical decision support provides computerized advice regarding drug doses, routes, and frequencies; more sophisticated CDSSs can perform drug allergy checks, drug–laboratory value checks, and drug–drug interaction checks, and can provide reminders about corollary orders (e.g., prompting the user to order glucose checks after ordering insulin).

Another class of CDSS is an automated alert system. This type of system notifies providers of potential adverse events. The intent of this type of system is to signal the physician that there is a potential problem and provide an opportunity for intervention. Generally, these systems have three types of alerts: critical laboratory alerts, physiologic alerts, and medication alerts. When an alert condition is detected, an application formats a message and transmits it by phone, pager, or mobile device to the medical team. See the following example of a CDSS.

Example of a Clinical Decision Support Alerting System

Each hour, a list of patients who are receiving certain medications that are stored in the pharmacy database is queried against the laboratory system to determine whether any of these patients have abnormal laboratory values that may be caused by the use of the medications. The results of both the pharmacy and laboratory queries are then analyzed by a CDSS. Depending on the system, the physician who ordered the medication may receive an alert by pager or e-mail to log onto the HIS for a message. The idea of a decision support system is to provide guidance, not actually to make the decision in place of a physician.

Another class of decision support systems is an expert system. An **expert system** is a program that symbolically encodes concepts derived from experts in a field and uses that knowledge to provide the kind of problem analysis and advice that the expert might provide. Expert systems provide the capability to perform tasks that would be carried out by an expert in the field. The expert system is dependent on a **knowledge base** that is a collection of stored facts, heuristics, and models that can be used for problem solving. One example of an expert system is the software developed to help residents and interns move through steps designed to identify a specific diagnosis. The user is prompted to enter each of the patient's symptoms, and using the knowledge that it has already learned, the expert system suggests several working diagnoses for that patient. Identified as resources to strengthen the diagnostic investigation, evaluation, and treatment processes, these programs are seen as powerful tools for clinicians. At the same time, challenges arise in updating and maintaining the knowledge base needed for these types of systems to be successful.

Point-of-Care Systems

A **point-of-care system** is a system through which data are captured at the place where the care is provided. One of the most common examples is a bedside system designed for patient data capture. These systems are located where the patient is receiving care, such as the bedside, or they are carried around by the caregivers, such as with handheld devices. As the use of handhelds and other devices expands, more options are available for entering data while in the presence of the patient.

In bedside applications, clinicians capture information about the patient directly, often through "smart" **templates** that prompt users to enter in the information that is required for both documentation and coding. These systems are intended to minimize data entry time and to ensure consistent and legible documentation.

? DID YOU KNOW?

In 2010, the DHHS in partnership with public and private organizations began an annual meeting entitled "The Health Datapalooza." The purpose of the meeting is to promote the use of publically available health data to develop new software applications for use in improving population health and access to health services. More than 1500 data experts, technology developers, entrepreneurs, policy makers, and community advocates attend each year with representatives of more than 80 companies.

Point-of-care systems also incorporate data read from bedside monitoring devices and transmitted into the computer directly. Examples include data from ventilators, vital signs, and I/O balances. These systems can be found in intensive care units (ICUs), where a great volume of data is collected and monitored for each patient.

In an automated point-of-care system, the vital signs flow sheet, intake and output balances, fluid levels, and laboratory results are all calculated and recorded automatically on the patient's electronic chart. Table 8-4 lists some of the functions found in a point-of-care system. The tasks that can be automated in a point-of-care system include:

- Nursing assessments
- Nursing care plans
- Flow sheets
- Medication administration record
- Data collection, calculation, and recording from bedside and home-based devices such as glucose monitoring devices

TABLE 8-4 Report Functions Available in a Point-of-Care System

1. Vital sign flow sheet with an overlay of medication history
2. Vital sign flow sheet identifying all caregivers who entered data on that patient showing date and time
3. View of the medical administration record
4. Detailed view of how a patient is following a specific protocol or clinical pathway
5. View of online nursing notes

✔ SELF-ASSESSMENT QUIZ

12. In which system are most of the patient demographics housed?
13. Most health care organizations implement what type of order entry?
14. Name some of the tasks that can be automated in a point-of-care system.

EMERGING TECHNOLOGIES

Bar Coding

Bar code technology is a replacement for traditional keyboard data entry. It requires that an identifier be converted to machine-readable identifier that can be printed on or attached to an item that can be read by a scanner and fed into a computer. Bar codes have been used in other industries such as retail for many years. Health care is a more recent user of this tool. Bar codes are most commonly used in health care in medication administration, materials management, and forms processing. Often, the forms contained in the medical record contain a bar code to scan the document electronically into an optical disk system.

The application of this technology can be found in almost all departments. Examples of this include the following:

- Patient wristbands contain a bar code representing the patient identification (medical record number or name).
- Supplies used in diagnostic tests and operating room procedures that are consumed during the process can be scanned. This enables inventory tracking and charge creation.
- Radiology films and laboratory specimens contain bar codes for tracking of results delivery.
- Medications given on the nursing unit have bar codes on each dose.
- Patient invoices can have the bar code printed on the remittance portion of the bill to increase accuracy when posting patient payments.
- Medical record forms contain a bar code to indicate the type of form (i.e., progress note, order sheet, discharge summary).

The format of the bar code is determined by **symbology**. *Symbology* is the term used to describe the font in which a machine-readable code is written.[18] Bar codes have printed bars and intervening spaces that define the output. The type and number of characters encoded, the print quality, and the amount of space available for the bar code determine which symbology is most appropriate. The two most common symbologies found in health care are code 39 and code 128. Code 39 produces a long bar code, whereas code 128 produces a denser bar code that will fit in smaller areas. Code 128 is the preferred symbology for patient wristbands, pharmacy packages, blood products, and laboratory specimens.

Bar codes always start with a special character, or symbol, that tells the machine scanning that bar code to start the reading process. The Start character will also tell the reader what bar code symbology is being used. A bar code always ends with a special character, or symbol called a *Stop character,* that tells the reader that this is the end of the bar code. Some bar codes also require a **checksum**. A checksum is a special character added to the bar code. The checksum tells the bar code reader that the bar code is correct. The checksum character is read by the bar code scanner, but it is not passed along as part of the data. The checksum must be printed after the data, and before the Stop code.

Following is an example of a Code 128 bar code for a patient with medical record number 000345 that will be placed on a discharge form numbered 999.

The FDA requires all medications to have a bar code, so the pharmacy relies on them.[19] The bar code contains the national drug code; lot, control, and batch numbers; and the drug expiration date. The regulation covers most prescription drugs and certain over-the-counter drugs. The rule also requires machine-readable information on labels for containers of blood and blood components intended for transfusions.

A **quick response** (QR) **code** is an example of a two-dimensional bar code that has grown in popularity. A QR code consists of black modules (square dots) arranged in a square grid on a white background. The QR code can be read faster and contain more information than a traditional bar code. Many mobile devices have an application that can read a QR code directly from the device. This technology allows for all kinds of documents to contain the QR code and be able to be read without a specialized bar code scanner.

Radio Frequency Identification Device

A radio frequency identification device (RFID) is a chip that is embedded in a plastic wristband or card. It is a means to store a greater amount of information locally that can travel with a patient. Currently, up to one megabyte of information can be stored on an RFID chip.

RFID tags contain antennas to enable them to receive and respond to radio frequency queries from an RFID transceiver. There are three types of RFID tags: passive, semiactive, and active. A passive tag draws all of its power from the radio waves transmitted by an RFID reader. A semiactive tag uses a battery to run the microchip's circuitry but not to communicate with the RFID reader. An active tag is powered entirely by battery to send and receive RFID information.

RFID tags require a reader similar to a bar code scanner, but it can read the chip content within 20 feet. There are no line-of-sight requirements. The major advantage of the RFID chip is that it is able to have write-many capability. Therefore it is feasible for a patient's allergy information to be contained on an RFID chip, and when this information changes, the RFID can be updated. Previous technologies were not able to handle changing information.

✓ SELF-ASSESSMENT QUIZ

15. The three most common areas where bar codes are used in health care are medication administration, materials management, and _____ _____.
16. Which regulatory organization requires all medications to have a bar code?

Internet and Web Services

The **Internet** has had a tremendous effect on the availability and accessibility of health care applications. There is no one central computer that runs the Internet. Rather, the Internet is equivalent to a network of networks. The Internet began in the 1960s when researchers began experimenting with linking computers to each other through telephone lines. This research was funded by the U.S. Defense Department Advanced Research Project Agency (DARPA). As the system, known at the time as *ARPAnet,* grew in size and volume, work was done to establish a protocol to transmit data among the networked computers. This is how the TCP/IP protocol was developed.

Today the Internet is made possible through creation, testing, and implementation of Internet standards that determine how the network should function. These standards are governed by a nonprofit organization called the Internet Engineering Task Force (IETF) with oversight from the Internet Society.[20,21] This organization defines all of the technical aspects of the workings of the Internet. Further, the World Wide Web Consortium (W3; http://www.w3.org) is responsible for managing the textual standards discussed in the next section.

Fundamentals

The workings of the Internet rely on software called a *browser,* which resides on the user's PC or mobile device. Browsers are examples of client software. Examples of browser software are Microsoft Internet Explorer and Mozilla Firefox. The user of the browser does not have to know any technical details of where the data exist because the browser handles all of the connections, display features, and security. Browsers can run on almost any type of operating system. This enables programs and data that might have been created on one computer and operating system to be displayed on a different computer with a different operating system. Web browsers are often found on thin-client devices because the requirements to run a browser on the client side can be programmed to be minimal.

The Internet adheres to the TCP/IP protocol for transmission of data as discussed in the previous section. The IP component of the protocol refers to a unique network address that is assigned to each computer on the Internet. The specific algorithm assigned to the transfer of data through web browsers is the hypertext transfer protocol (HTTP).[22] HTTP determines how information is formatted and transmitted, and what action browsers take in response to commands. S-HTTP is an extension of the HTTP protocol to allow data to be sent in a secure mode. S-HTTP was developed to transmit individual messages between the browser and the server. It does not secure the entire connection, only the transmission.

Internet Tools

Several tools are available for preparing documents to be viewed through a browser. The following are three types of Internet tools.

1. HTML—hypertext markup language
2. SGML—standard generalized markup language
3. XML—extensible markup language

HTML is the most common format used for structuring documents on the web. HTML was created to give information on the web an easy-to-read screen. It is designed to structure documents and makes the content accessible through a browser. HTML is well suited for distributing information such as online references because the content is displayed following the same style each time it is accessed.[23] A word processing document posted directly to the web could not display properly any special structure such as titles, headings, and paragraphs. HTML makes use of **tags** that define the text that is contained in them. For example:

> <B>This will be bolded.</B>

is the notation used to indicate that the text following the tag is to be displayed in boldface type until the closing tag. In the following example, a bold tag is given for the heading "History and Physical." Other examples of tags are:

- <P> begins a new paragraph.
- <TITLE> puts the name of document in the title bar.
- <img src="imagefilelocation"> places an image in the document.

Following is an example of a generic history and physical report as it would appear in HTML.

Example of a Generic History and Physical Report Appearing in HTML

```
<HTML>
<HEAD>
<TITLE> ABC Physician Specialists </TITLE>
</HEAD>
<FONT SIZE=2><P ALIGN="CENTER">ABC Physi-
    cian Specialists </P>
<P ALIGN="CENTER">121 Main Street </P>
<P ALIGN="CENTER">Anytown, ZZ 12345-6789 </P>
</FONT><B><FONT FACE="Times Roman" SIZE=4>
    <P ALIGN="CENTER">History and Physical </P;>
<P> </P> </B></FONT><FONT FACE="Times
    Roman">
<P>NAME: John Doe </P>
<P>UNIT#: 123456 </P>
<P>DATE: 12/01/2013 </P>
<P>DOC: Mary Brown, M.D.</P>
</FONT><FONT SIZE=2>
<P> </P>
<P>CHIEF COMPLAINT:</P>
</HTML>
```

During a document exchange, a browser requests a document from a web server and displays the document on the user's display device. If the first document contains a link to another document, the browser retrieves and displays the linked document.

A web server may receive and process an HTML form and then initiate a program to complete a specific action. This program that runs on the web server is called a common gateway interface (CGI) program. A CGI program is usually written in a scripting language such as Perl or PHP or a programming language such as C or C++. The CGI script is stored on the HTTP server so that when an HTML document is requested, the server can tell that the file contains a program to be run rather than a document to be displayed by the browser. When the program executes, it prepares an HTML document based on the results of the CGI script. The HTML document is then sent to the browser in the usual fashion. CGI scripts are used extensively to integrate databases with the web. Figure 8-4 illustrates how a web server running the HTTP protocol with a CGI script processes a user query.

HTML does have certain limitations. First, the language lacks expandability. The set of tags that can be used to identify text and images is limited. It is not possible to create additional tags to accommodate special formatting needs. Second, HTML treats the entire document as a single representation. In other words, HTML lacks any intelligence about items or fields in the document. It can process a form but not specific data elements that exist in the form. It does not make a distinction between forms and fields. Third, it lacks the ability to validate the information in the document. For example, HTML would not be able to process directly a request to view only inpatient data. That specific request would need to be handled in the CGI script. The CGI script would include commands to prepare the HTML document to be returned to the user. The HTML document, without the CGI script, could not understand how to filter data from the document. In summary, HTML is designed mainly as a presentation tool for information; it was not designed to process information. HTML5 is the fifth revision of the HTML standard and is widely used today. It is designed to support multimedia that was not present when the initial version of HTML was created.

HTML is actually a subset of SGML. SGML is a standard governed by the International Organization for Standardization (ISO)-8879. SGML is used more frequently to manage large documents that need to be printed in different formats. It is suited for documents that have the same content but are to be formatted for different purposes. It is built with a **document type definition** (DTD), a document describing its own grammar. In other words, the DTD allows the definition of specialized document type. For example, mailing addresses might have a DTD defined for an envelope and a separate DTD defined for printing on a sheet of labels. SGML was developed in the printing industry for editing and revising documents on a typesetter. It has many features that are not applicable to web documents, which makes it somewhat difficult to use it for the web.

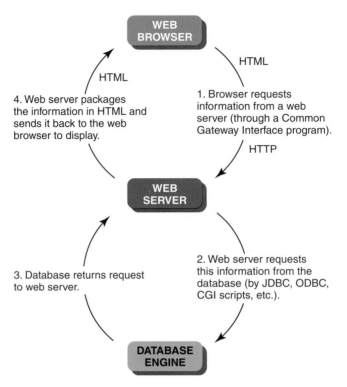

FIGURE 8-4 End user to web server request with common gateway interface (CGI) mechanism. *HTML*, Hypertext markup language; *HTTP*, hypertext transfer protocol; *JDBC*, Java database connectivity; *ODBC*, open database connectivity.

Equipped with more web functionality is **XML**, which is a language that is popular because of its advanced features.[24] XML still makes use of many of the HTML conventions but includes additional capabilities to enhance its functionality. XML is being used in the ASTM Standard for the Continuity of Care Record. This standard is intended to facilitate the transfer of certain data content between providers who are caring for a patient.

In a large EHR system with millions of patients, there is a great need for a single, easy-to-handle language capable of displaying only the patient's name and complete blood count. Likewise, this defined tag allows a result from a database query to be placed directly in the web document at the proper location. XML allows a user to define new tag and attribute names. Tags can be invented to describe the type of information that resides within the tag. This enables a search to be done within the document to find only the patient's chief complaint. Using the preceding example, the XML version:

<xml version="1.0"fi>
<LIST>
<PRACTICE____NAME>ABC Physician Specialists</PRACTICE____NAME>
<PRACTICE____ADDRESS>121 Main Street</PRACTICE____ADDRESS>
<PRACTICE____CITY>Anytown, ZZ 12345-6789</PRACTICE____CITY>
<REPORT____TYPE>History and Physical</REPORT____TYPE>
<PATIENT____NAME> John Doe</PATIENT____NAME>

<UNIT____#> 123456</UNIT____#>
<DATE> 12/01/2013</DATE>
<PHYSICIAN>: Mary Brown, M.D.</PHYSICIAN>
<CHIEF____COMPLAINT>Shortness of Breath</CHIEF____COMPLAINT>
</LIST>

JAVA

JAVA is a programming language introduced in late 1995 by Sun Microsystems, now a part of the Oracle corporation.[25] It could have been discussed in the previous section on programming languages, but its purpose is more closely related to the web. It is thought to be less complicated than the C programming language. The main objective of a JAVA program is to allow applications to be built as stand-alone programs that can be transferred across the web and run independently on a client computer. JAVA is an object-oriented language that is compiled into a universal, non-machine–dependent format. Other programming languages such as COBOL or C++ require the compiled code to reside in the native mode for a specific processor. JAVA can run on any platform; it requires only that a JAVA compiler be resident on the client. A JAVA compiler is part of the browser software. JAVA applications are referred to as "write once, run anywhere."[26]

JAVA allows programs, called **applets**, to live on top of HTML pages. Applets, which run on the client side, are more efficient than CGI scripts. CGI scripts tend to run slower as the number of users accessing a Web page increases, which puts additional burden on the web server. An applet might exist for a nursing unit to calculate the appropriate dosing for a medication given the patient's recent laboratory values. The JAVA applet is available through the user's web browser. After the user clicks on the submit button, the JAVA applet is downloaded to the user's machine temporarily and performs the calculations in real time. A device that is capable of running JAVA is also called a *Java Virtual Machine* (JVM). A network computer, as discussed in an earlier section, might be considered a JVM.

Another piece of JAVA is a **servlet** or server-side scripting. A servlet functions much like an applet but resides on the server side, not on the client. A servlet is much more efficient than a CGI script because it executes itself on the web server. It handles multiple requests simultaneously. Servlet functions by having the user's request run directly on the web server to generate dynamic HTML pages. This technology is generally used to provide interactive websites that interface to databases or other data sources. The major advantage to servlets is the ability to highly customize the web page based on the user's access rights or database queries. Examples of server side scripting languages are Active Server Pages and PHP languages.

Intranet

An **intranet** is like an Internet that runs exclusively within a network. It is accessible only by users who can be authenticated as being within a specific network. Intranets have become popular for communicating and sharing the organization's policies and procedures. For example, the corporate project tracking system might reside on the intranet so that all of the employees can update and view their project plans. The organization would not want this information available to users outside the organization. Another use would be to post the organization's employee handbook. This enables employees to have an updated reference manual with search capabilities, which would be difficult to obtain in a hard-copy form. There is no longer a need to publish and distribute these types of documents and be concerned with distributing updates to the employees.

Virtual Private Network

A **virtual private network** (VPN) is much like an intranet, but it allows users outside the network to gain access to the network through a password. It is equivalent to an access control list for a health care application. For example, a third-party payer might set up a website that contains information regarding claims processing but want it to be available only to its current providers or those with whom it has a contract. The data should be available only to authorized and authenticated users.

Another component of a VPN is a **demilitarized zone** (DMZ). This is a network area that sits between an organization's internal network and the VPN. The DMZ allows outside organizations to access the area while protecting the network from possible intrusions into the internal network. Connectivity is allowed from the internal network to the DMZ, but no access is allowed from the DMZ to the internal network. Applications using a DMZ include mail and web services as well as file transfers. Many of the out-sourced medical record transcription services use a DMZ to transfer files to and from the dictation system to the transcription system.

Web 2.0

The term *Web 2.0* became popular at a industry-sponsored conference in 2004 as a result of computer professionals looking for additional utility for the Internet.[27] Before 2004 the Internet was not a very interactive platform. Web pages had a tendency to become static and stale. Updates to web pages could only happen if the web administrator made a centralized change to the web page. Web 2.0 technology enabled new applications such as blogs, wikis, online communities, photo-sharing, and social networking. This suite of applications originally was given the global term *Web 2.0* but is now referred to as *social media*. A website running a Web 2.0 application allows its users to interact with other users or to change website content, in contrast to non-interactive websites on which users are limited to passively viewing information provided to them.

One of the more useful 2.0 tools used in health care is the adoption of **Really Simple Syndication** (RSS), which is a tool for syndicating content so that it can be appear on sites beyond the author's control. This enables a health system, for example, to have an RSS feed to the CDC website so that any updates to clinical outbreaks will automatically appear on a physician portal without having to check the CDC web page manually. Within the field of dental informatics, the National Library of Medicine in 2005 began the initiation of an online dental informatics community or "virtual community" found at www.dentalinformatics.com. **Virtual communities** can be defined as an aggregation of individuals or business partners who interact around a shared interest, where the interaction is at least partially supported or mediated by technology.[28] Communities are commonly associated with web applications that facilitate interactive information sharing, interoperability, and collaboration. Examples of Web 2.0 group collaborations include web-based communities, social-networking sites such as Facebook and Twitter, and video and photo-sharing sites.

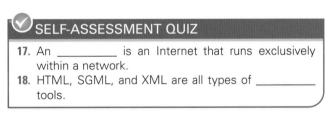

SELF-ASSESSMENT QUIZ

17. An _____ is an Internet that runs exclusively within a network.
18. HTML, SGML, and XML are all types of _____ tools.

TELEMEDICINE AND TELEHEALTH

Telehealth is "the use of telecommunications technologies to deliver health-related services and information that support patient care, administrative activities, and health education."[29] Now that physicians use e-mail to communicate with patients, and drug prescriptions and other health services are being offered on the Web, telehealth is generally used as an umbrella term to describe all the possible variations of health care services using telecommunications. The term

telemedicine more appropriately describes the delivery of clinical care via telecommunications—diagnosing, treating or following up with a patient at a distance. Telemedicine can be defined in three categories: (1) store and forward, (2) remote monitoring, and (3) interactive sessions such as videoconferencing.

Examples of telemedicine use and categories today include the following:

1. It provides the ability of a radiologist located in another region of the country to review a CT scan during off-coverage hours at a community hospital (store and forward).
2. Patient consultations of audio or video can be exchanged between the patient and the physician. This consultation will take the place of a face-to-face visit (interactive telemedicine).
3. It enables remote patient monitoring for testing blood glucoses and measuring daily weights in homebound patients (remote monitoring).
4. It provides consumer health information to patients to participate in web casts and other interactive video with experts in the field (interactive telehealth).
5. It provides continuing medical education credits for health professionals and special medical education seminars for targeted groups in remote locations (interactive telehealth).

There are broad and different types of telemedicine technologies, which can include the following:

- Facsimile
- Audio
- Still images
- Full-motion video

Telemedicine is useful for situations in which physical barriers prevent the ready transmission of information between physicians and patients. Examples of telemedicine applications occur in teleradiology, dermatology, pathology, behavioral health, and home health services. Telemedicine offers many benefits: better access for patients in rural and underserved areas, reduced travel time for health care providers, and improved techniques for medical education. In 2008 it was reported that as many as 300 hospitals nationwide, and two thirds of radiology practices appear to be using some form of teleradiology.[30]

Fundamentals

One of the requirements of a telemedicine system is appropriate **bandwidth**. Bandwidth is a measure of how much information can be transmitted simultaneously through a communication channel. It is measured in bits per second. The telemedicine system uses the available bandwidth to transmit the various forms of information that are necessary to complete the telemedicine interaction.

There are several types of telemedicine interactions, and they vary in complexity. The simplest scenario might have the optical disk system at a hospital transmit images, text, and other data to a physician at home. The physician would require little bandwidth or specialized equipment. Second, a

medical education course might be given from a hospital location to students who may be scattered throughout the region. A one-way video would enable the students to view the lecture; a two-way, real-time video would enable the students to view and participate in the lecture. The instructor could transmit sound, video, text, images, and voice to multiple classrooms simultaneously. Minimum bandwidth for this type of interaction is moderate to high.

Medical consultations are another service for telemedicine. The basic consultation could involve having a specialist review still images or video clips with text information. In this interaction, data could be transmitted on a low bandwidth because the data would be sent and then reviewed at a later time. This type of interaction is sometimes referred to as **store and forward** technology because the data are initially gathered and then sent at another time. The second type of consultation incorporates real-time telephone voice interaction in addition to the images and video clips and requires greater bandwidth. Finally, the consultation could include real-time interactive video. For example, cardiology videos such as cardiac catheterizations or echocardiograms can be reviewed. It requires significant bandwidth.

Implementation

The use of telemedicine has increased with technologic advances, but there are still a few technical and administrative issues to work through for successful implementation. One of the obstacles for use in teleradiology is the size of the images that need to be transmitted. A standard chest x-ray image is approximately a 5 megabyte file, whereas a CT scan can range in size from 150 to 1000 megabytes. Transmitting this amount of data, before data compression, could take hours to download the information.

Advances in **data compression** have greatly helped to overcome this barrier. Data compression is a mathematical technique that applies formulas to a file to produce a smaller file. Files are compressed by eliminating strings of redundant characters and replacing them with more compact symbols. If data compression is able to reproduce the original file exactly, the compression ratio is said to be **lossless**. If the compression causes some information to be lost in the translation, the compression is **lossy**. Depending on the amount of loss that the user is willing to tolerate in the output, typical compressions of 20:1 to 50:1 are possible.

Each multimedia file transmitted in a telemedicine application requires a utility that will both compress the file and decompress it on the receiving end. This is accomplished by using a mutually agreed upon coder/decoder (CODEC). The operation of a CODEC is similar to the way a modem is used to connect to a personal communicator. It translates analog transmissions into digital ones and compresses the signals.

A second obstacle is the lack of bandwidth to transmit the image itself. A typical office LAN can support transmission at 10 Mbps, but that is usually not sufficient for a telemedicine application. Most telemedicine applications need to have fiberoptic or FDDI networks in place to deliver timely and sufficient data.

Telemedicine faces several administrative barriers that are still undergoing regulatory review. The major issue today concerns the reimbursement of telemedicine services. In July 1997, Congress agreed to reimburse telemedical consultations for rural Health Personnel Shortage Areas and those done with live two-way videoconferences.[31] Partial Medicare reimbursement for telemedicine services was authorized in the Balanced Budget Act (BBA) of 1997. Reimbursement expanded in 2000 with the Benefits Improvement and Protection Act of 2000 as long as the patient resides outside of a metropolitan area. Store and forward consultations such as radiology are covered the same as services delivered when onsite. This ruling is because Medicare does not consider this service to be telemedicine as the difference is only in the location of the physician. Many home telehealth services are not currently covered by Medicare or Medicaid.

There is also an issue regarding physician licensing and medical liability. Because physicians are licensed by the state in which they practice, there is a question of what constitutes "practicing." Teleradiology companies have required that their radiologists be licensed in the states of the patients whose films they are reading, have medical-staff privileges at the patients' hospitals, and have local malpractice insurance. It is not clear whether providing telemedicine services from another state is considered practicing medicine. Physicians also need to review whether their malpractice insurance covers telemedicine services. Again, the increase in these regulatory constraints make it difficult to attract and retain qualified physicians for a telemedicine program.

Finally, there is concern regarding patient confidentiality and security. From a security standpoint, it is a concern that the networks used to transmit patient data are not secure enough or do not have the proper encryption technologies to ensure patient confidentiality.

COMPUTER SECURITY

The substantial growth in the use of software, network technology, and the Internet has made it necessary to establish policies and procedures for protecting the data. This section discusses the technical approaches that are available for data security. This section presents three topics: (1) technical components that are found in a secure information system, (2) the functionality required in an application to ensure proper data access, and (3) examples of organizational policies that can protect information systems from unauthorized use. Other examples of protecting the privacy of health information are found in Chapter 15.

The increased use of HISs has intensified both the amounts of data available electronically and the functionality to link the data to an identifiable person. The goal is to guard against inappropriate use without compromising the caregiver's "need to know." Often, the computerized version of the information is all that exists and denying access or making access impossible would have serious patient care

consequences. Most systems that have tight security also have a "**break-glass**" option that allows a user who is not typically authorized to access a certain database or individual's record with that opportunity. *Break glass* (which draws its name from breaking the glass to pull a fire alarm) refers to a quick means for a person who does not have access privileges to certain information to gain access when necessary. When the "glass is broken," an automatic review is triggered to determine why the access took place. If there is a legitimate reason for access, no problem exists, and there are no consequences to the individual who "broke the glass." There is a constant struggle for information system administrators to achieve a balance between protecting patient confidentiality and the cost of creating and implementing security mechanisms.

Costs of security can be viewed as both direct and indirect. Direct costs include the cost of purchasing and installing the security measures, which could be hardware, software, or both. In addition, there is the cost of training and staff development of employees who are responsible for ongoing maintenance. Indirect (and harder to quantify) are the costs associated with the additional training of the user population to understand the security measures, the extra time required to modify the current operating procedures, and ultimately the cost of preventing access to an authorized user by mistake.

The National Library of Medicine asked the Computer Science and Telecommunications Board of the National Research Council to examine ways to protect electronic health information. The study began in 1995 and ended with the issuance of a report in 1997.[32] Some of the key practices that the committee recommended are the following:

- Individual authentication of users
- Access controls
- Audit trails
- Disaster recovery
- Protecting of remote access points
- Protection of external electronic communication

The Health Insurance Portability and Accountability Act (HIPAA) of 1996 issued the Security Standards for the Protection of Electronic Protected Information.[33] The Security Standards were completed and promulgated after the HIPAA Privacy Standards were completed and promulgated. The Privacy Standards are supported by the Security Standards. The Security Rule became effective as of April 2003, and most covered entities needed to be in compliance by April 2005.[34] This standard lists four general rules for security:

1. Ensure the confidentiality, integrity, and availability of all electronic protected health information (PHI) the covered entity creates, receives, maintains, or transmits.
2. Protect against any reasonably anticipated threats or hazards to the security or integrity of such information.
3. Protect against any reasonably anticipated uses or disclosures of such information that are not permitted or required.
4. Ensure compliance with this regulation by its workforce.

A covered entity is defined as any group that transmits electronic PHI. This includes health plans, health care billing companies, or health care providers. HIPAA applies to all covered entities from the one-person physician office to the insurance company with thousands of employees. The Security Rule is organized into three categories: administrative safeguards, physical safeguards, and technical safeguards, containing 18 standards. The administrative safeguards require documented policies and procedures to protect electronic health information and the conduct of personnel handling this type of information. The physical safeguards relate to the protection of the physical systems, including hardware and software. The technical safeguards pertain to processes that control and monitor access to the information. Table 8-5 lists the elements of the HIPAA Security Rule.

The standards do not specify specific technology that the organization needs to implement. Instead, the regulation lists the capabilities that the organization needs to have in two categories—required or mandated and addressable or suggested. Mandated items include a risk analysis and management plan to assess and reduce potential risks and vulnerabilities, a sanction policy to handle violations of those who do not comply with the security policies, and information system activity review. It also requires that the organization have a data backup plan, a **disaster recovery plan**, and an emergency mode operation plan.

It also requires that each system have a unique identification code for each user. In some instances, organizations previously used a shared login for access to systems.

The standard requires an emergency access procedure for obtaining necessary electronic PHI during an emergency, such as if an emergency room physician's password does not function when needing to check a patient's EHR. As noted earlier, this process is called a *break-glass policy*. Systems containing primary source data (information) for treatment must develop, document, implement, and test break-glass procedures that are used in the event of an emergency requiring access to electronic information.

> ### ✓ SELF-ASSESSMENT QUIZ
>
> 19. The HIPAA Security Rule requires that all health care organizations that use PHI have the following:
>   a. Data backup plan
>   b. Disaster recovery plan
>   c. Emergency mode operations plan
>   d. Break-glass option
>   e. a, b, and c

Authentication Tools

In this section, we examine some of the authentication tools available in greater detail. **Authentication** is the process of verifying or confirming the identity of a user who is requesting access to the information. This procedure has existed for many years in medical records departments with the paper version of the medical record. The user in need of the information must present a valid form of identification to prove that he or she is entitled to receive the information. Authentication techniques must be established in electronic form just as they were for hard copies before the electronic age.

Authentication is usually based on various criteria:
1. Something that you know (password)
2. Something you have (a key, credit card)
3. Something that is a part of you (your fingerprint, DNA sequence)
4. Something indicating where you are located

Passwords
Passwords are a common part of everyday life. They exist for many types of operations from home security systems to access to library resources. Users, if not regulated or policed, tend to use common words or phrases for passwords. Passwords are sometimes shared among co-workers. However, technology can assist with certain steps to enforce proper use of passwords to keep them secure:

- Require the user to show photo identification to obtain the initial password or if the password is forgotten. Do not send passwords in the mail (electronic or postal service) or provide them over the telephone. For remote sites where providing photo identification might not be possible, a designated employee can be assigned at the site to be responsible for distributing the information to the user.
- Implement password aging on the operating system. **Password aging** is the term given to the process through which users must change their password at a specific frequency (e.g., 30 days, 90 days). This enables the passwords to remain unique and identifies users who do not log in for a certain period.

TABLE 8-5	Safeguards of the Health Insurance Portability and Accountability Act Security Rule		
	Administrative Safeguards §164.308	Physical Safeguards §164.310	Technical Safeguards §164.312
	Security management process	Facility access controls	Access control
	Assigned security responsibility	Workstation use	Audit controls
	Workforce security	Workstation security	Integrity
	Information access management	Device and media controls	Person authentication
	Security awareness and training		Transmission security
	Security incident procedures		
	Contingency plan		
	Evaluation		
	Business associate contracts		

- Install a password history file on the operating system. A password history file keeps a record of all of the previous passwords of a specific user. The physical file needs to be kept in an encrypted form so that it can be viewed only by the system utilities.
- Allow only one login per user identification at a time. The user should be allowed to log in to only one session. This helps to identify and monitor the sharing of passwords.
- Disable accounts after a maximum number of login attempts. Failed login attempts assist in identifying unauthorized uses of a password.
- Implement an automatic logout policy so that after a certain period of inactivity (e.g., 10 minutes, 30 minutes), the session is automatically disconnected from the system.

? DID YOU KNOW?

DARPA, a division within the Department of Defense, created Computer Emergency Response Team (CERT) in 1998 to coordinate communication among experts during computer security emergencies and virus threats. CERT is headquartered at Carnegie-Mellon University in Pittsburgh and has a staff of more than 150 computer security experts who develop advanced techniques for securing computer networks and provide training to government and law enforcement on how to deal with cyber threats.

Single Sign-On

Many organizations are adopting the use of single sign-on technology for their clinical applications. This technology enables the user to have one password to access multiple systems. It is common for a health care worker to have 5 to 10 usernames and passwords to access information. The goal of single sign-on is to only have one username, usually one's network sign-on plus one password.

A technique of implementing single sign-on is Clinical Context Object Workgroup (CCOW).[35] CCOW is a standard written and adopted by the HL7 group. It is vendor-independent. The clinical context refers to having the information obtained via CCOW be for the same patient. In other words, a query of John Smith's pharmacy information on the pharmacy system enables the user to obtain the laboratory results on the same John Smith. CCOW does not permit the user to view any other records on the secondary system, but only the records that belong to the same patient who was accessed during the initial query on the initial application.

Tokens or Cards

A token is the size of a credit card and displays a number that changes each minute. Each user card generates a unique sequence of numbers and, through an algorithm, assigns the user access privileges for an application. The computer system incorporates the same algorithm in its authentication mechanism. Because the holder of the user card and the number sequence is unique, the number sequence is used as the session password for that computer system. If the number being generated is seen by an outsider, it needs to be synchronous with the holder of the card. There is discussion about using

encoder rings instead of cards for the same purpose. The problem with cards is that they can be lost, stolen, or duplicated. The use of a token plus a password is called **two-factor authentication**. This authentication protocol requires two forms of authentication to access the system. This is also called *strong authentication*. A common example of this protocol is the use of a bank card to withdraw monies from an automated teller machine. The card is the physical item, and the personal identification number is something known only to the user. Deploying this technology requires that the organization's software applications have the capability to read the token sequence and the user password. Older applications are still written to accept only a user password.

Biometric Devices

A **biometric** is a unique, measurable characteristic or trait of a human being that can be used for automatic recognition or identity verification.[36] A biometric device is capable of analyzing human characteristics for security purposes. Examples are fingerprints, retinal patterns of the eye, or speech scans. The primary advantage of using these types of devices for granting access to a computer system is that it is not possible to forge identity. The disadvantages are that the device may fail and prevent an authorized user from gaining access to the system. Because device failure has such serious consequences, implementing this type of security requires around-the-clock maintenance.

Access Controls

Each information system should have the ability to control which users can access the system and what a user can view. The term used to describe this is *role-based access control* (RBAC).[37] This type of control may also be referred to as a "need to know" basis. Usually, access is granted on the basis of two criteria:
1. The role of the user
2. The permitted roles for specific information access

TABLE 8-6 Examples of Role-Based Access Controls

HOSPITAL OR PHARMACY SYSTEM				
Position	Create	Modify	View	Authorize
Pharmacist	Y	Y	Y	N
Pharmacy technician	Y	N	Y	N
Nurse	N	N	Y	N
Attending physician	N	N	Y	Y
Consulting physician	N	N	Y	N
Home health nurse	N	N	Y	N
Social worker	N	N	N	N

Y, Yes; *N*, no.

The role of the user is usually defined by position or employee status. Table 8-6 shows an example of user roles found in a hospital information system. Within the access control, there are functions to determine the types of actions each user role can have. Usually these functions include (1) access to read the data, (2) access to write to the data, (3) access to change the data, (4) access to delete the data, and (5) access to change or override the access list itself. Table 8-6 also includes the permitted roles for each of the users.

The major obstacle to this type of implementation is developing a mechanism for a role that needs access on two levels. For example, a unit nurse might need access to patients only at a certain location but on weekends might cover for the ICU nurse. The ICU nurse role is defined differently from the unit nurse role. The system needs a method to accommodate these special situations. In addition, the system should have the capability to override the standard settings in case of an emergency.

The creation and maintenance of RBAC lists are difficult tasks. It requires collaboration between information security personnel, human resources, clinical administration, and others. Some organizations have a data protection officer to oversee these activities. Maintenance items include tracking when a user has changed roles or left the institution or when the role itself needs to be modified. Some RBAC utilities can receive a data file from the organization's payroll system that can aid in identifying users who might have changed positions or left the organization. Some users may have multiple roles—for example, a physician has a particular panel of patients that she is treating, but she is also a member of the Quality Improvement Council (QIC). As a member of the QIC, she is asked to review a set of clinical records and some administrative reports. The QIC role allows access to different data and information than the role associated with her panel of patients.

 SELF-ASSESSMENT QUIZ

20. What process verifies or confirms the identity of a user who is requesting access to information?

Reporting Capabilities

It is helpful for the information system to generate reports of user activity and role-based access lists for the various applications on a periodic basis. This helps to monitor and protect the system security. ASTM has a Standard on audit trails that provides some useful ideas for auditing and creating reports. Examples of security reports are as follows.

Examples of Security Reports

1. Show all users logged in and from what location or domain.
2. Show all users who have not logged into the system in the past 3 months.
3. Show all users who have access to delete records.

4. Show all users who have tried to log in unsuccessfully more than once.
5. Show all users who are defined in the role of "pharmacist."
6. Show all changes made to the role-based access lists and by whom.

Physical Security

Most networks have a central area where the servers, terminals, modems, and so forth are stored; access to this area must be controlled and the area must be locked at all times. Access cards should be granted to employees who maintain and support this hardware. There should also be a log of all employees who have entered the area.

When disposing of outdated computers, the data that reside on the disk should be entirely cleaned off by not only deleting the information but also cleaning the data from the disk. Files can be easily undeleted if they are not wiped clean. Similarly, dispose of all diskettes, tapes, and other storage devices properly. Again, the data protection officer should be able to assist in carrying out these functions.

It is also important to keep a detailed database of the inventory and configurations of the existing hardware. This information helps in identifying missing equipment and is useful if the internal configuration has been altered. An inventory consisting mostly of mainframe computers is fairly straightforward, but tracking individual PCs in various departments is a challenge. Users can easily add to or change the PC configuration without the knowledge of the information systems personnel. It is even more difficult to track the inventory for areas such as home health or patient education when most of the users work in remote locations. It is important to develop a policy and procedure for inventory control purposes to help prevent theft.

External Controls

Firewalls

The technology used to control access to the HIS network is growing in sophistication. Most of it is controlled via a **firewall**. A firewall is a system to prevent access to a private network from the outside or limit access to the outside from within the network. Firewalls can be implemented using hardware, software, or a combination of both. The concept is basic: all data that enter or leave the organization's network must pass through the firewall. The firewall acts as a filter, providing a single point of entry to a network. Software can then analyze the incoming or outgoing data to determine whether they are appropriate and should be granted access to the network. A firewall is maintained by the system administrator, who is responsible for implementing the organization's policy on network access.

There are several types of firewall solutions:

1. **Proxy server**—intercepts all messages entering and leaving the network so that the network address is hidden. A proxy server might be installed in an organization so that all outbound network traffic is sent and controlled through a central location.

2. **Packet filter**—examines data entering or leaving and accepts or rejects the data on the basis of system-defined criteria. For example, all requests from an Internet address not associated with the organization could be denied.

3. **Application gateway**—allows only certain applications to run from outside the network. This is applicable if an organization wants to prohibit outside entities from transferring files to its network. In this instance, the file transfer service would be restricted to users defined in the firewall software configuration.

See the following example of firewall configuration and modification.

Example of Firewall Configuration and Modification

The hospital's outpatient dialysis clinic has been outsourced to a private, nonprofit organization. The organization has a computerized patient record system for the patients seen at its dialysis clinics throughout the country. The system physically resides in the corporate database at the main office in Tennessee. The patient care providers for these dialysis patients are still based at the hospital and need access to the computerized patient record in the corporate database. Currently, the dialysis organization does not allow network connections from outside the organization. To provide access to the clinical data, the system administrator at the dialysis clinic has modified the firewall configuration to accept connections from the hospital network. This type of example is common and is usually handled on a case-by-case basis.

Encryption

Encryption changes readable text into a set of different characters and numbers based on a mathematical algorithm. Computers on either end of the transmissions must have keys to encrypt the information being sent and then decrypt the text at the receiving end into the original text. One of the most popular forms of encryption is **public key.** A public key is a key that the user gives to anyone he or she wants to receive the message. Web servers often have a public key available to the requester of a web document. A private key is one that the user maintains and never gives out. Together, these two keys scramble, send, and then unscramble an encrypted transmission.

The Internet makes use of public key encryption by the use of a certificate authority (CA). A CA acts like an electronic notary public and verifies and stores the sender's public and private encryption keys. The CA issues a digital certificate or seal of authenticity to the recipient (usually the system administrator for the website). The recipient includes a reference to the digital certificate on its web server to enable encrypted communications. See the following example of use of the digital certificate.

Example of the Use of the Digital Certificate

One of the local retail pharmacies would like to receive prescription orders and refills electronically. The new web-based clinical information system in the ambulatory clinic has physician order entry capabilities, so the application is modified to include ordering to the retail pharmacy. However, the retail pharmacy needs to verify that the prescription was sent and authorized by the physician, and the physician needs to ensure that an authorized party received the order. In this scenario, the web server in the ambulatory clinic possesses the digital certificate so that the retail pharmacy is certain the order came from a trusted source. The pharmacy also accesses the web server with a password to further protect access to the system.

Internet Security

To meet the need to provide encryption for connections to the Internet, the Secure Socket Layer (SSL) protocol was initially developed by Netscape Communications Corporation.[38] Figure 8-5 illustrates how a web server enables an SSL connection. An SSL connection allows the browser and the server of the web transmission to authenticate identities and encrypt the data transfer. It ensures that the data came from the web server it is supposed to have originated from and that no one tampered with the data while being sent. Web servers that support an SSL session have a web address that starts with *https* instead of *http*. A remaining piece is left unsecured because the data are encrypted only during transmission between the two locations, and the data that reside locally on the client or server are still accessible in a nonencrypted format. HIPAA requires that all Internet transmissions containing patient data be sent using, at a minimum, SSL to protect confidentiality. SSL works by using a private key to encrypt data that are being transferred. In August 2008 version 1.2 of Transport Layer Security was released to improve on some of the features of SSL, but the basic operating principles remain the same between the two protocols.

Malicious Software Protection

HIPAA includes protection from malicious software (or **malware**) as one of the addressable components of the security regulation. The term computer virus is usually used to generalize malware, but computer viruses represent only one type of malware. Malware can be any unauthorized

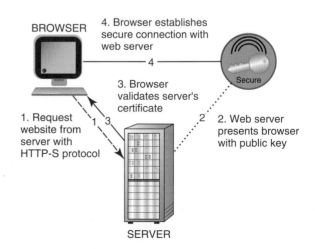

FIGURE 8-5 Example of Secure Socket Layer connection. *HTTP-S,* Secure hypertext transfer protocol.

software found in an information system. Malware attacks often interfere with the computer's functionality and may cause loss or damage to software.

Types of malware include the following:

Masqueraders—software that appears to be a part of the existing software but produces unwanted behavior. Examples of this software are Trojan horses found in e-mail messages or macros that might be run in a word processing program. A masquerader could also be someone pretending to be the authorized recipient of sensitive data but is not.

Incapacitation—the most common type of this software is a **denial of service** (DOS) attack. This occurs when the attacker overloads the targeted system by flooding it with data transmissions so that the target system becomes unavailable.

Corruption—a computer virus is an example. Corruption also occurs when software is changed to perform a malicious activity without the user's knowledge. A recent development in this area is spyware—software installed on the user's computer without his or her knowledge and that collect personal information from the computer, then sends it to an unauthorized database.

Misuse—a computer worm will deliberately install itself on a computer connected to a network. The worm will then extend itself to every other computer on that network, either promoting DOS attacks or performing unauthorized acts. Worms can be found in e-mail applications when a message is opened and automatically sends the worm to the e-mail server and then sends a second e-mail to every user listed in the mailbox directory.

It is critical that the organization have policies in place to deal with malware. Most organizations require that all computers run an antivirus software checker, which screens all incoming e-mail. Some e-mail servers also run this software.

Viruses and worms typically infiltrate a PC via e-mail attachments or files downloaded from websites. After they seize control of the computer, they can destroy critical files or disable the system. Some enable hackers to use the computer to send large volumes of spam or to attack specific websites. Viruses and worms have been known to spread by e-mailing copies of themselves to address book listings found in each PC.

Phishing is also considered a security threat. Phishing can be found in an e-mail message that appears to come from a legitimate business or organization requesting personal information such as an account number. The e-mail message contains a link to a website to submit the information. However, the website is not from the business or organization mentioned in the e-mail message but rather a site designed to capture personal identifying information. These web addresses often contain misspellings of business names or have logos or graphics similar to those of the legitimate business. After the user inputs personal information, the phishers can use this information maliciously.

Remote Hosting Models

With the emergence of the Internet as a convenient way to access information from virtually any location, many health care organizations use some type of remote hosting. This trend began in the late 1990s using **application service providers** (ASPs). An ASP is a business that provides computer-based services to customers. The application software resides on the ASP network and is accessed by users through a web browser. An ASP may offer functional services such as billing and payroll management to various types of businesses or may provide specialized services to a particular industry such as medical transcription to a physician group. The HIM professional will certainly be involved in setting up the ASP operation as it relates to confidentiality and security of the organization's information.

General guidelines for using an ASP within the organization are as follows:

- The ASP owns and operates a software application.
- The ASP owns, operates, and maintains the servers that run the application. The ASP also employs the people needed to maintain the application.
- The ASP makes the application available to customers everywhere via the Internet.
- The ASP bills for the application either on a per-use or a monthly or annual fee basis.

An ASP is an attractive option for medical transcription services. It is argued that it is more cost-efficient to have an ASP operate the transcription system than to operate an in-house system. Economies of scale can be easily achieved because the software and hardware for transcription is a fixed cost. It usually costs the same whether 5 or 50 transcriptionists are using the system. Workforce shortages in this area also enabled organizations to go outside, even to other countries, to have transcriptionists working.

An organization's website could be run as an ASP model. Many ASPs provide web hosting services that enable a customized website to reside on the ASP's web server. This scenario is correct if the organization does not have full-time staff devoted to web development or does not have the network bandwidth to support a busy website.

An advantage of an ASP is that there is a low cost to entry. There is no hardware or software to buy, and the system can be operational quickly. There is no need to hire additional personnel to get a working system. The "pay as you go" model is also attractive for smaller organizations that cannot afford a large capital expenditure. Another instance in which having an ASP would be beneficial is if the technology is highly specialized and the organization cannot support that. For example, if the technology requires a SQL database and it does not have the resources to hire a full-time SQL database administrator, it would be advantageous to have the ASP serve as the database administrator.

A disadvantage to the ASP model is that the organization is making no investment in its own capital and resources. It is similar to leasing equipment when at the end of the lease period the leased equipment needs to be returned. There is also the possibility that the ASP could go out of business on short notice, leaving users without a working system.

It is important that the HIM professional be involved in selecting and negotiating the contract with an ASP. Because the information will be residing on the ASP network, it is critical that the ASP adhere to the organization's security and privacy policies. HIPAA requires that any ASP have a business associate agreement with the organization that clearly delineates the roles and responsibilities of the ASP's handling of PHI.

An alternative to an ASP model is using **Software as a Service** (SaaS). It is an economic model more than a technology model, and functions similar to an ASP. However, with SaaS, users can also download the software application to their own web server or device to use on a subscription basis. This type of "on-demand" licensing allows the user to not have to invest resources into technology that may be used only on a sporadic basis. A use case for SaaS in HIM may be for an application that can de-identify transcription documents that may be needed for a clinical research project. Because de-identification is not a function that is needed on a daily basis, the health information department may choose to buy software for this purpose on an "as-needed" basis rather than invest in a software application that is locally hosted.

SELF-ASSESSMENT QUIZ

21. What are the types of malware?
    a. Masqueraders, incapacitation, corruption, and misuse
    b. Incapacitation and misuse
    c. Masqueraders, corruption, and misuse

DATA MANAGEMENT TECHNOLOGY

Throughout this chapter, descriptions of health care computer applications and technology have been provided. The complex nature of health care almost always ensures that data will need to be integrated from various types of information systems. It requires substantial effort to provide effective data management that is useful to the health care organization. The effort requires expertise in database management, clinical data analysis, and technology assessment.

HIM professionals have an ideal skill set for directing and managing these types of projects. These projects require understanding of the technology, database management, and health care software applications and ensuring that the data are kept securely and available only to authorized users.

This section explores two data management applications that are gaining popularity among most health care organizations: the data mart and data modeling or, as it also called, *data mining*. Using an HIS for outcomes research can be a great tool, but a problem arises when the clinicians requesting the information lack the domain knowledge required for the specific databases.[40] Establishing a data mart removes some of the mystery of using databases for the health care providers. Figure 8-6 provides an illustration of how HISs interact with a data repository or data mart. Likewise, **data mining** encourages a broad view of all data for a set of patients to explore relationships among the data that might not be readily apparent during the initial hypothesis.

Data Mart

A **data mart** is a subset of data extracted from the larger database. It is not to be confused with the **data repository**. A data repository contains all or almost all of the data in an information system. A data mart is a smaller application with a focus on a particular subject or department. A data mart has several advantages:

- The unit cost of processing and storage is less than the unit cost of processing and storage in a large database.
- The selection of a database model and technology can be tailored to the needs of a department.
- The amount of historical data and level of granularity required for the data mart can be specific to the needs of the department.

Granularity is the term given to the level of detail in the data. For example, an ICD-9-CM code has finer granularity than a diagnosis-related group (DRG). A DRG is a broad category, and ICD-9-CM provides more specificity in the data.

The data mart may contain additional information that is collected outside of the HIS. For example, it may include national or regional benchmark data to allow for comparison of data between hospitals.

Example of Creating a Data Mart

The administrator for long-term care at a large health system is interested in tracking ancillary costs for all of the skilled nursing facilities in the system. The administrator currently receives monthly reports, but they do not allow any further manipulation of the data or cannot incorporate outcomes data collected by the facility's case manager. In addition, the monthly report is not timely. The administrator would prefer weekly or perhaps daily uploads of the current data. The administrator and staff do not have the time to attend a week-long SQL class to learn how to query the data repository directly. There is also concern that the data capture methodologies for inclusion in the repository might be slightly different among the facilities. The administrator wants to be able to view the raw data and aggregate data as appropriate.

Table 8-7 contains a list of data elements that might be found in a data mart for a long-term care administrator.

Creating a Data Mart
Step 1—Define the Scope

Determine, in collaboration with the end users, what purpose the data mart will serve and, just as important, what data analysis is outside the scope of the data mart. It is important to determine these in this step so that the project does not grow over time and result in the same functionality as the data repository. For instance, determine that the data mart will contain only inpatients discharged within the past 12 months. Analysis of outpatient activity will not be within the scope of this data mart.

Step 2—Perform a Technology Assessment to Determine the Selection of the Most Appropriate Database Model and Architecture

As discussed earlier in the chapter, a relational database is the most commonly used model for data marts. This is because it is easier to add and modify the database structure, and several query language tools are already available to the end user. The architecture, however, requires some study. It needs to

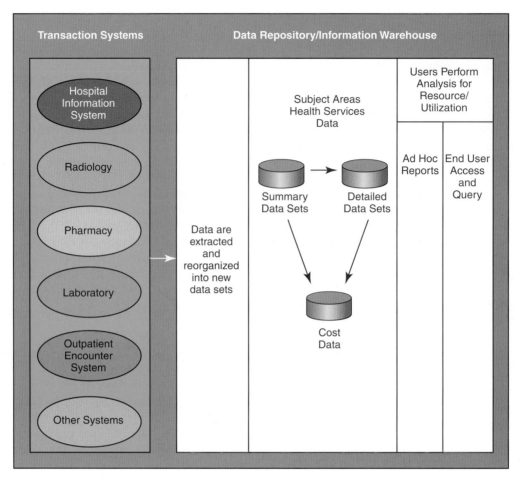

FIGURE 8-6 Feeding data for decision support. The data repository is part of an information warehouse. This approach increases the value of existing data stores and empowers end users to meet simple reporting needs through local workstations.

| TABLE 8-7 | Examples of Data Elements for a Long-Term Care Data Mart |

Cost Variables	Outcome Variables
Total cost	Mortality
Pharmacy cost	DRG
Physical therapy/speech therapy cost	LOS
Chemistry and hematology cost	Age
Medical procedures	Readmission to acute care
Room charges	Discharge disposition
Medical and surgical supplies	Ventilator-dependent

DRG, Diagnosis-related group; *LOS,* length of stay.

be determined whether it will be a small application that might be able to support a two-tier approach or whether the logic for the queries is complicated enough to warrant a three-tier approach and an application server. A hardware assessment within the user community also needs to be completed at this time. This helps to determine the parameters or size limitations that might have to be imposed on the

application. It also enables decisions to be made about whether the client software is run as a thin-client or a thick-client application.

Step 3—Identify the Data Elements and Best Source

Analyze what types of data might be available initially, and assess the data integrity. The data elements stored in the medical record discharge abstract might be more reliable and accurate than unstructured text captured on a form. It is important to document all of the decisions made at this point. It will be helpful to refer to this document as the project continues to develop.

Step 4—Develop and Run the Program for Extracting the Data Elements

This procedure should be designed to run automatically at a given interval. It might be necessary to revise the run intervals if the data elements are collected from different sources. For instance, not all of the financial data are available at the time of discharge. Several days are needed for late charges to clear. This type of special condition should be noted when determining the extract schedule. The use of Extract Transform Load software will enable this process to be automated in a repeatable fashion. Again, it is important to document and publish this as part of the project schedule.

Step 5—Perform Any Data Cleansing or Filtering

When combining data from different sources, it is usually necessary to filter the data before importing it to the data mart. The data might need to be converted to common units to support comparisons. For example, some incoming data might be expressed in hours and others for the same field expressed in minutes. Second, the end user of the data mart might not be interested in the lowest detail of data, so the data are aggregated and recoded if necessary. In a possible scenario, there are several ways to identify patients who died while in the hospital. In the data mart, there is only one field for mortality—a yes or no logical value. The data cleansing process will transform each of the coded elements in the hospital's database that represent "died" into the data mart logical value for mortality.

Step 6—Import the Data into the Data Mart

This should be established as a routine procedure. After each import, quality control programs or queries need to be executed to ensure that the import was successful.

Step 7—Train the End Users, and Solicit Feedback on Improvements or Additional Features

Using the project scope developed in Step 1, create a training plan that will cover all of the different types of users of the data mart. It is often the case that a department will designate a 'super-user' within the group to become trained on the system initially. This person will be the most familiar with system functionality and can serve as the main resource for supporting users within a department. Encourage the 'super-user' to report usability issues to the project team so that these items can be addressed during a subsequent release.

Step 8—Maintain the Data Mart and Establish a Change-Control Form

The change-control form needs to be completed when any additions, deletions, or modifications to the data mart occur. This form provides documentation to the users and assists in any alterations that need to be made in the database structure.

Data Modeling

Another technique that the computer can assist with is identifying patient subgroups, a variation of data mining for use in predictive modeling.[39] With a paper-based medical record, clinicians and other researchers were limited to analyzing the data that they knew about. For instance, an emergency room physician kept a log of patients treated for gunshot wounds. The physician's study was therefore limited to the cases that could be identified in the log.

With paper-based records and early HISs, we were focused on using data for reporting and monitoring functions. We sought to answer questions such as "How many patients received a blood transfusion?" or "What is the turnaround time for our transcribed reports?" by generating reports from a single department system. The answers to these questions, while still of interest to the operation of the hospital, are not adequate to keep pace with the changing health care marketplace. We need more information that will help us predict or simulate patient care trends rather than just report retrospective events. Health care data must now help us understand what processes will improve health care and measure successful patient outcomes.

With the increased availability of data, we can now use a software application to identify the set of patients of interest. The first step for the application to do is to use a broad definition of the study criteria, usually by ICD-9-CM code or some other structured data set. The researcher then reviews the cases and selects the final set of patients that meet the criteria. A statistical model is then constructed for the patient set and used to help locate additional cases. This cycle of modeling and classification continues until the user is satisfied that enough cases have been identified. See the following example of a computer system identifying cases of particular interest.

Example of Computer System Identifying Cases of Particular Interest

A researcher is interested in the study of complications following kidney transplantation. The researcher is interested in all of the things that happened to the patients after transplantation and wishes to determine whether any relationships exist among the patients. A query is written to identify all patients who received a kidney transplant procedure through the ICD-9-CM code (55.69). The first exclusion criterion is death on the same day as the transplantation. From the remaining cases, the computer generates a frequency distribution of the characteristics of these cases. Characteristics might include whether the patients received a certain drug, had an abnormal laboratory result, or received a blood transfusion. The researcher reviews the list and selects the characteristics that are important in identifying the proper set of patients with a complication. The data-modeling program will now restrict selection to patients meeting the revised criteria. The researcher adds characteristics to and deletes characteristics from the model after reviewing the online discharge summaries of the revised set of patients. The data-modeling program is run again to see how well the revised criteria performed in identifying the set. This cycle is repeated until an acceptable patient set is found. The model has retained the inclusion and exclusion criteria from the iterations so that, when presented with new cases, it will be able to recall lessons already learned.

✓ CHAPTER REVIEW

1. What was the first patient care system that claimed to automate the patient record?
   a. COSTAR
   b. CISCO
   c. IBM medical information systems program
   d. TDS

2. What technology connects PCs, printers, and storage devices within an organization and to the outside world?
   a. database management system
   b. network
   c. software

3. What type of network allows computers to communicate with the Internet without being physically connected to the network?

4. The use of _____ within the web page can assist in optimizing screen space.
   a. frames
   b. check boxes
   c. drop-down boxes
   d. background photos
   e. a, b, and c

5. What is often a hospital's first attempt at providing EHR functionality?

6. True or False? Outside users cannot access a VPN?

7. Which department uses bar code technology for managing its inventory and delivering supplies?
   a. accounting
   b. nursing
   c. pharmacy
   d. none of the above

8. _____ is an umbrella term that describes all possible variations of health care service using telecommunications.

9. Which identity verification device analyzes human characteristics such as fingerprints, speech scans, or eye retinal patterns?

10. Which term refers to a quick means for a person without access privileges to gain access when necessary?

11. A _____ is a system to prevent access to a private network from the outside or limit access to the outside from within the network.
    a. VPN
    b. firewall
    c. password

12. True or False? One advantage of a data mart is that the selection of a database model and technology can be tailored to the needs of the department.

REFERENCES

1. Department of Health and Human Services, Office of the National Coordinator for Health Information Technology: A record of progress on health information technology: http://www.healthit.gov/newsroom/about-onc (Accessed September 26, 2013).

2. Dick RS, Steen EB, editors: Computer-based patient record—an essential technology for health care (Institute of Medicine Report). In Washington, DC, 1997, National Academy Press, p 12.

3. Wagner MM, Moore AW, Aryel RM: Handbook of biosurveillance, Burlington, MA, 2006, Elsevier Academic Press, p. 3.

4. Eclipsys Corporation: Acute care EHR: http://www.allscripts.com/en/solutions/acute-solutions/ehr.html/. (Accessed October 2, 2013).

5. Dornfest S: History and impediments to progress in the development and implementation of the computerized patient record, Proc Health Inform Manage Syst Soc P: 84, 1993.

6. Ball MJ, Jacobs S: Hospital information systems as we enter the decade of the 80s, Proceedings of the IEEE Fourth Annual Symposium on Computer Applications in Medical Care, New York, 1980, Institute of Electrical and Electronic Engineers, p. 183.

7. Jamoon E, Beatty P, Bercovitz A, Woodwell D, Palso K, Rechsteiner E: Physician adoption of electronic health record systems: United States, NCHS Data Brief 98, January 20132011, U.S. Department of Health and Human Services, Centers for Disease Control and Prevention, National Center for Health Statistics, p. 1.

8. DesRoches CM, Charles D, Furukawa M: Progress on electronic health record adoption among US hospitals, Health Affairs (Millwood) 32(8) 2013 [Published July 9, 2013, ahead of print].

9. Kulikowski CA, Shortliffe EH, et al: AMIA Board white paper: definition of biomedical informatics and specification of core competencies for graduate education in the discipline, JAMIA 19 (6):931–938, 2012.

10. Glaser J: Cloud computing can simplify HIT infrastructure management, Healthcare Finance Management 65(8):52–55, 2011.

11. U.S. Department of Veterans Affairs: VistA monograph: http://www.va.gov/vista_monograph. (Accessed October 12, 2013).

12. Date CJ: An introduction to database systems, ed 7, Reading, MA, 2000, Addison-Wesley.

13. Sommerville I: Software engineering, 2007: ed 8, New York, 2007, Addison-Wesley, p. 271. http://www.w3.org/standards/webdesign/htmlcss#whatcss.

14. Bates DW, Leape LL, Cullen DJ, et al: Effect of computerized physician order entry and a team intervention on prevention of serious medication errors, JAMA 280:1311–1316, 1998.

15. Health Level 7: HL7 Standards: http://www.hl7.org/implement/standards/index.cfm. (Accessed October 1, 2013).

16. Guidance for Industry 21 CFR Part 11; Electronic Records, Electronic Signatures, Electronic Copies of Electronic Records: http://www.accessdata.fda.gov/scripts/cdrh/cfdocs/cfcfr/CFRSearch.cfm?CFRPart=11&showFR=1&subpartNode=21:1.0.1.1.8.3. (Accessed November 11, 2013).

17. Miller RA, Waitman LR, Chen S, Rosenbloom ST: The anatomy of decision support during inpatient care provider entry (CPOE): empirical observations from a decade of CPOE experience at Vanderbilt, J Biomed Inform 38:469–485, 2005.

18. Cummings J, Bush P, Smith D, et al: Bar-coding medication administration overview and consensus recommendations, Am J Health Syst Pharmacy 62:2626–2629, 2005.

19. Bar Code Label Requirements for Human Drug Products and Biological Products. 21 CFR Parts 201, 606, and 610 Docket No. 2002N-0204.

20. Internet Engineering Task Force: Overview of the IETF: http://www.ietf.org/about. (Accessed August 21, 2013).

21. Internet Society: Introduction to ISOC: http://www.internetsociety.org/who-we-are. (Accessed August 21, 2013).

22. Lee-Berners T: Hypertext transfer protocol design issues, 1991: http://www.w3.org/protocols/DesignIssues.html. (Accessed October 11, 2013).

23. Musciano C, Kennedy B: *HTML: the definitive guide,* ed 2, Sebastopol, CA, 1997, O'Reilly Associates.

24. W3c: Extensible Markup Language, June 16, 2013: http://www.w3.org/XML. (Accessed August 1, 2013).

25. Oracle Corporation: The Java tutorials: about the Java technology: http://docs.oracle.com/javase/tutorial/. (Accessed October 1, 2013).

26. Sun Microsystems, The Java Tutorials: About the Java Technology: http://java.sun.com/docs/books/tutorial/getStarted/intro/definition.html. Accessed September 17, 2014.

27. O'Reilly T: What is Web 2.0?: http://oreilly.com/web2/archive/what-is-web-20.html. Accessed (Accessed October 1, 2013).

28. Spallek H, Irwin JY, Schleyer T, et al: Supporting the emergence of dental informatics with an online community, *Int J Compu Dent* 10:247–264, 2007.

29. Dixon BE, Hook JM, McGowan JJ: *Using telehealth to improve quality and safety: findings from the AHRQ portfolio* (prepared by the AHRQ National Resource Center for Health IT under Contract No. 290-04-0016; AHRQ Publication No. 09-0012-EF), Rockville, MD, December 2008, Agency for Healthcare Research and Quality.

30. Steinbrook R: The age of teleradiology, *New Engl J Med* 357: 5–7, 2007.

31. American Telemedicine Association: Medicare payment of telemedicine and telehealth services, January 2013: http://www.americantelemed.org/docs/default-source/policy/medicare-payment-of-telemedicine-and-telehealth-services.pdf. (Accessed October 2, 2013).

32. Committee of Maintaining Privacy and Security in Health Care Applications of the National Information Infrastructure: *For the record protecting electronic health information,* 1997, National Academy Press. http://www.nap.edu/openbook.php?record_id=5595&page=R1.

33. Health Insurance Portability and Accountability Act of 1996, Pub L 104-191, 110 Stat. 1998 (August 21, 1996).

34. Health insurance reform: security standards 45 C.F.R. § 160, 162, 164 (2003).

35. HL7. Context Management Specifications (CCOW) V1.6 February 2011: http://www.hl7.org/implement/standards/product_brief.cfm?product_id=1. (Accessed October 1, 2013).

36. Woodward J, Horn C, Gatune J, Thomas A: *Biometrics: a look at facial recognition, 2003:* p. 1: Santa Monica, CA, 2003, Rand (Accessed 11.10.13). http://www.rand.org/pubs/documented_briefings/DB396.html.

37. Ferraiolo DF, Sandhu R, Gavrila S, Kuhn DR: Proposed NIST standard for role-based access control, *ACM Transactions on Information and System Security* 4(3):224–274, 2001.

38. Apache Software Foundation: SSL/TLS strong encryption: an introduction: Error! Hyperlink reference not valid: http://httpd.apache.org/docs/2.2/ssl/ssl_intro.html. (Accessed September 5, 2013).

39. Visweswaran S, Hanbury P, Saul M, Cooper GF: Detecting adverse drug events in discharge summaries using variations on the simple Bayes model, *Proc Am Med Inform Assoc* 689–693, 2003.

40. Jensen PB, Jensen LJ, Brunak S: Mining electronic health records: towards better research applications and clinical care, *Nat Rev Genet* 13(6):395–405, 2012.

HEALTH INFORMATION SYSTEMS: COLLABORATION, ANALYSIS, DESIGN, IMPLEMENTATION, OPERATION

Mary Alice Hanken • Bonnie S. Cassidy

ⓔ Student Study Guide activities for this chapter are available on the Evolve Learning Resources site for this textbook. Please visit http://evolve.elsevier.com/Abdelhak.

CHAPTER CONTENTS

OBJECTIVES

✓ Define key words.
✓ Develop a strong working relationship with information systems staff.
✓ Recognize the strengths of the health information management professional and the information systems professional in developing, selecting, implementing, and modifying health care information systems.
✓ Understand the difference between project activities and operational activities.
✓ Identify the necessary skills to bring an information systems project to completion.
✓ Describe the principles of collaboration between health information management and information systems that help projects be successful.
✓ Recognize the areas where health information management and information systems do not automatically share the same views, information, or approaches to a project.
✓ Discuss the process stages in Nolan's six-stage theory of information system development.
✓ Apply techniques and tools, including hierarchy charts, data flow diagrams, data dictionaries, and entity-relationship diagrams, to perform information systems analysis and design.

✓ Understand and apply strategies and techniques for gathering information for system design and development.
✓ Evaluate information system interfaces from user satisfaction and efficiency perspectives.
✓ Describe the various techniques that are used to evaluate information systems, including benefits realization, break-even analysis, payback period, and discounted payback period.
✓ Describe the activities that take place during system implementation.
✓ Recognize the value of training in project success.
✓ Differentiate between a training manual and a user manual.
✓ Evaluate the success of systems projects.
✓ Identify both measurable metrics and organizational values addressed by a system.
✓ Recognize that systems projects move into an improvement phase after implementation.
✓ Describe the purpose and content of a request for proposal.
✓ Describe the usual process that is followed in purchasing a vendor system.

KEY WORDS

Benefits realization
Business data
Break-even analysis
Computer-aided software
  engineering
Collaboration
Cost-benefit analysis
Cost-effectiveness analysis

Data dictionary
Data flow diagram
Data mapping
Discounted payback period
Downtime
Entity-relationship diagram
Hierarchy chart
Information governance

Information governance plan
Payback period
Physical system design
Project
Prototype
Request for information
Request for proposal
Scenario

Stakeholder
System development life cycle
System life cycle
System testing
Training manual
Use case
User
User's manual

ABBREVIATIONS

ADT	Admission, Discharge, Transfer	**ERD**	Entity-Relationship Diagram
ASP	Application Service Provider	**HIM**	Health Information Management
CASE	Computer-Aided Systems Engineering	**I/S**	Information Systems
CBA	Cost-Benefit Analysis	**IT**	Information Technology
CEHRT	certified electronic health record technology	**MIS**	Management Information Systems
CPOE	Computerized Provider Order Entry	**REG/ADT**	Registration/Admission, Discharge, Transfer
DFD	Data Flow Diagram	**RFI**	Request for Information
EHR	Electronic Health Record	**RFP**	Request for Proposal
EMR	Electronic Medical Record	**ROI**	Return on Investment

COLLABORATION ESSENTIAL TO HEALTH INFORMATION SYSTEMS

The growth of electronic health information systems across all health care provider settings redefines the way information is used for the delivery of products and services. The health care industry, which has been slower to adopt and embrace information technology in all areas, is now firmly engaged in bringing electronic tools to delivering health services of all kinds. This book presents the evolution of technology from many health care perspectives including legal and regulatory frameworks, business process technological advances, patient care outcomes, more effective use of data and, threaded among all of them, recognition of the value, roles, and essential nature of information systems users. To make change happen effectively, health care leaders must identify, engage, and appreciate the user community and customers of organizational health information systems.

Part of the health information manager's responsibility is to help analyze, design, select, and implement health information systems for patient-related and clinical data management use at departmental and enterprise-wide levels. The health information manager's oversight for or responsibilities related to health information, privacy and security for their organization, an enterprise core data dictionary, regulatory requirements, and accreditation standards makes their role essential in the information systems cycle. This chapter outlines a structured approach for accomplishing information systems tasks and provides tools to assist the health information manager to be successful in this process.

The scope of health information systems in a hospital and in an enterprise system are outlined in Chapter 8: Technology, Applications and Security.

CRITICAL THINKING

The manager of the clinical laboratory wants to replace the department's outdated information system to better manage information related to collecting specimens, tracking completion of laboratory tests, and reporting clinical test results. The radiology department director wants to install a voice-recognition information system to replace the current radiology dictation/transcription system as part of a new information system that will help manage patient flow, track the completion of radiology tests, store completed radiology reports, and automatically retrieve patient demographic data from the hospital information system. The vice president for hospital human resources wants to purchase an automated system that will help manage information related to employee demographics, employment status, employee benefits, and salary administration. The director of health information management (HIM) plans to request the purchase or development of a release of information system that will track requests for patient information disclosure, track patient requests for amendments, create structured letters, and provide report generation capability.

The goal of the managers is to use automation as an adjunct in helping them better manage information considering the investment to be made, how can these managers be reasonably confident that the systems selected will meet the needs of their organizations and their various departments? If a stand-alone or special purpose system is considered, how will it be interfaced with existing and planned systems? Is it better to identify a vendor who can offer an integrated system versus using many different vendors whose products each require an interface? How many vendors are using national standards to address interoperability questions? One strategy to help select appropriate systems is to follow a structured approach for analyzing user needs, identifying functional requirements that meet the user needs, choosing a system that has the required functionality, and implementing the system in an organized, well-thought-out manner.

VALUE OF USER PERSPECTIVE

The **user** perspective of health information systems and technologyy projects can help users and respective customers identify and initiate executive project sponsors and stakeholders as well as address fundamental roles for users at multiple levels. Appreciating user roles enables executive sponsors to: (1) understand the dependencies and the work effort involved in systems implementations, (2) hold realistic expectations of process and outcome, and (3) become much more sophisticated buyers of the technology.

An example of the potential users of an electronic health record system includes the users listed in Table 9-1.

TABLE 9-1	Users of the Electronic Health Record
Physicians	Pharmacists
Nurses	Pharmacy technicians
Nurse's aides	Laboratory technicians
Physical therapists	Radiologists
Occupational therapists	Radiology technicians
Speech therapists	Data analysts
Health information staff	Quality improvement analysts
Medical records staff	Utilization review coordinators
Care/case coordinators	Business office personnel
Dieticians	Social workers
Decision support analysts	Mental health specialists
AND THE LIST GOES ON AND ON...	

TABLE 9-2	Projects versus Operations	
Projects	**Operations**	
Peaks and valleys workflow	Steady stream of work
No direct authority, full responsibility	Full authority, full responsibility
Ad hoc teams	Business-aligned teams
Done once	Done repeatedly
Highly time dependent	Function dependent
Defined start and end dates	Not "start date" and "end date" dependent
Product/service driven	Business function/process driven

A Natural Dependence

Collaboration Principle

There is a natural dependence between users of HI systems and the information technology staff in the pursuit of definition, design, development, purchase, implementation, and use of any HI system. Information technology in the workplace includes tools applied to business functions. The tools are the workhorses of business. Computer systems fail to perform if data structure and databases, operating systems, interfaces, and networks are not well planned, robust, and technically compatible. This business community/user and information technology staff dependence should be more than just recognized; it should be embraced.

Environmental basics is a term Ellen Anderson created to define the "human elements" that exist as a natural part of humans composing work teams intended to accomplish specific tasks. The eight environmental basics covered in this chapter include personal commitment, trust, respect, policy setting to manage human behavior, expectations, vocabulary, understanding, and knowledge.[1]

A stakeholder is any individual who has a stake or real interest in the success of the HI systems project, regardless of department, position, or functional role in the organization.

The information technology (IT) division of most organizations has a title that includes the word *information*. This is true in health care organizations as well. A few examples are management of information systems (MIS), information technology (IT), and information services or systems (I/S). The abbreviation I/S is used in this chapter when referring to either the department itself or the staff of individuals in this unit of work activity in any organization. It is not surprising to note that more than one work unit of an organization may use the word *information* in its title. Both the I/S department and the health information department are in the business of managing information for the health care industry.

Webster's New Twentieth Century Dictionary of the English Language defines collaboration as "to labor, especially in literary or scientific pursuits, as the associate of another or others." In this chapter, the term is used to refer to the combined labor of users and I/S staff in the pursuit of HI systems. The important word here is, of course, *together*.

Project, in the context of this chapter, means a unit of work to acquire or build and implement an HI system (software, hardware, and all infrastructure) with a definitive start date, targeted stop date, steps, milestones, and outcome.

Project work is quite different from regular operations in any organization. Table 9-2 illustrates some comparisons. The nuances of projects make collaboration that much more important and that much more challenging.

ENVIRONMENTAL BASICS (REQUIRED FOR TRUE COLLABORATION)

The term system life cycle has been used in describing computer system development for many years. Simply put, the stages of a system can be expressed in simple verbs: *define*, *design/develop* or *buy*, *do/implement*, *operate/support*, and then *obsolescense*. That system life cycle then recycles to *redefine*, *redesign*, *upgrade*, and so forth, in a continuous fashion until the system is no longer used and another takes its place. In many organizations information systems or applications may each be on their own cycle (see Figure 9-1).

Define, *design*, *develop*, *do/implement*, *redesign*, *redevelop*, and *operate/support* are all action verbs that involve groups, and lots of them. Because HI systems happen through groups, environmental basics that are group oriented must be in place before an HI system project is started. All these environmental basics must be intact for project success (see Box 9-1). These same principles apply to a working relationship to improve and expand systems within an organization or in a community setting (see Box 9-2).

Four Shared Environmental Basics

Personal commitment, trust, respect, and policy setting are four mandatory environmental basics shared between HI system users and I/S staff for true collaboration.

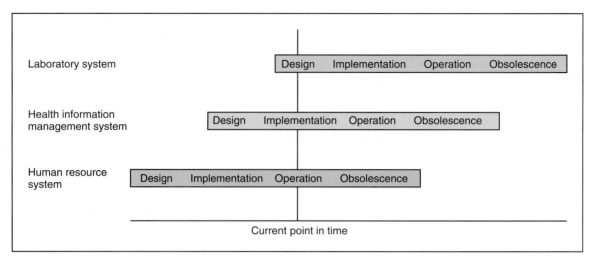

FIGURE 9-1 Comparison of departmental information systems at different life-cycle stages.

BOX 9-1 EHR Implementation Cycle

Change management is the basic foundation underlying all phases of the EHR implementation life cycle that helps achieve EHR meaningful use and practice transformation. The EHR implementation life cycle shown in the following figure illustrates the phases a physician practice or clinic goes through in a successful implementation. Change management strategies and principles must be integrated into all phases of the implementation process.[1,2]

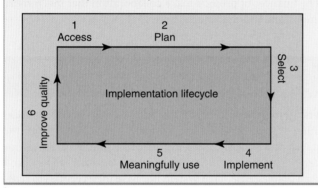

[1]http://www.healthit.gov/sites/default/files/tools/nlc_changemanagementprimer.pdf

Personal Commitment

Collaboration Principle: Personal commitment builds HI system champions.

Commitment is not easy when resources are tight, especially if the capital costs are high, the risks are great, and the resources are limited. Yet personal commitment to a project produces commitment to the success of the implementation of HI systems. Nothing goes further than a user who truly believes. Commitment needs to come, however, from all sides of the collaboration equation—from organizational leaders, system users, and I/S staff. Personal commitment is more than verbalization. It is quite easy to verbalize commitment; it is quite another matter to stand behind that commitment.

If you are starting an HI systems project, use focus groups, surveys, and interviews to assess the level of commitment. Study the positive and negative feedback from all focus groups, surveys, or interviews. Is there a strong personal commitment to this project? What are the major drivers? Is regulatory compliance involved? Are the positive or negative perceptions about the project warranted? Are the perceptions based on correct or incorrect facts? If incorrect, how can you correct them? Will correcting the facts change the degree of personal commitment? If correct facts have created a negative perception, can conditions be altered to raise the level of commitment? If users show strong personal commitment to the project, are they grounded in reality?

Grounded Champions

User leaders and managers make the best HI system project champions. Physicians, nurses, and other clinicians are often part of the leadership for the development of clinical information systems. Sometimes, however, leaders and managers need accurate resource information to be truly grounded in their commitment and genuine excitement. User managers can be very serious about the project but also blind to the resource commitment of their operational people and budget to ensure success. Test their commitment before beginning the project. They will usually underestimate resources in terms of both people and money—it is human nature to wish it done quickly and at a cost less than realistic.

I/S managers and leaders also must be personally committed to the project. They are faced with an overwhelming number of requests to automate or update existing automation from all business units within the organization. Setting a high I/S priority to a project is usually propelled by a combination of (1) a compelling business reason and (2) the right technology fit and direction. For example, it makes no sense to automate a business function when the desired technology is not ready for general usage.

If I/S leaders and managers declare a project a high priority, you are halfway there. Are there true capital dollars behind it? Is it assigned a budget? Is it a shared budget among a number of departments, including I/S? Is the budget "assigned" realistic? Does I/S appear to sign initial project documents if you move forward immediately?

BOX 9-2 Change Management: EHR in Physician or Clinic Practice

A Summary of Must Do's to Be Successful Implementing an EHR in a physician or clinic practice setting involves more than the application of technology. When successful, it results in the transformation of systems, processes, and workflows of a practice. The following list summarizes the change management principles that HIM professionals must implement for change initiatives to be successful.

- Develop a clear vision for what you want the practice to look like in the future. Clearly state what your practice will look like for patients, you, and your staff after a successful EHR implementation.
- Ensure that staff understand they own the practice's future state. Let staff know that each of them will have a role and will be responsible for achieving success.
- Establish urgency. Communicate to staff WHY change is occurring, the implications for NOT changing, and WHY change needs to happen as quickly as possible.
- Build a credible guiding team. Identify practice staff who have credibility with their peers and other staff and can engage staff, build and maintain staff commitment, and sustain momentum.
- Educate all practice staff. Staff must have full knowledge of the CEHRT and understand how using the technology will affect them, their work, and the entire practice. Accurate, timely information will help you control the rumor mill inherent in any change initiative. Remember that education and training will be required throughout your change initiative journey.
- If you are the practice leader, recognize your role in persuading others to adopt a change initiative. Practice leaders must communicate and educate other practice staff on the vision for the future state and how the practice will achieve that vision through the use of technology and other practice transformation strategies.
- Help practice staff reach a positive decision to adopt and maintain the change. Promote the use of the guiding team to help staff with day-to-day problems and to provide timely technical assistance. As the practice leader, establish a culture where it's okay for staff to identify problems and concerns while encouraging them to help find practical solutions.
- Promote confidence and confirmation to sustain the change. Practice leadership must continue to assess, communicate, and intervene, as needed, to promote continued acceptance of the EHR system and other practice transformation initiatives.
- Create short-term wins. Although goals and objectives are generally considered long-term, acknowledging short-term success is necessary to maintain momentum.
- Create a culture of continuous quality improvement by evaluating, adjusting, and rewarding staff. Practice leaders must constantly listen to staff, respond to staff needs, evaluate progress, and intervene to help fix things that aren't going as planned. This support helps shape both the practice and its evolution toward the future state.[3]

Trust

Collaboration Principle: The worst of projects can succeed within a basis of trust, and the best of projects will likely fail without it.

It has been said that the worst of projects were successful because, even during the down-and-out periods, project members and business communities trusted each other. Together they pulled a project through the battles to victory. It has also been said that the best of projects and systems failed because no trust existed.[4] When no trust exists, each source of irritation or project component failure brings the project closer to its knees. A baseline level of trust must be in place as a project begins. Trust develops more completely as a project's work groups or teams grow comfortable in the natural dependencies between them. There are various levels of trust in any collective group of people; HI systems are no exception. All levels within an organization must trust, and be trusted, for maximum use of group synergy.

Those who hold the corporate purse strings, or control the organizational finances, must trust the rest of the organization to be good stewards of the millions of dollars often required to get a system into production. The executive sponsors play an important role in establishing trust and voicing the benefits of the HI system project. They must also trust that the proposed budget reflects the true costs or costs as commonly computed within the organization. If they take the fiscal stewardship of the organization seriously, they will ask for a cost-benefit analysis or strong reasoning for the value to help in their prioritization of this capital expenditure relative to other capital expenditure requests.

Project management is a set of methodologies used to deliver projects on time, on budget, and to meet expectations. Part of project management is the use of a project steering committee. Project steering committee members need to trust that their fight for the capital dollars will result in correctly and appropriately implemented information technology. They also must trust that the people who will be empowered to select or create and implement the system have the talents and the will to do so. They may also trust that the potential system users have or will acquire the computer skills and aptitudes needed to use the system. Do they have these trusts?

User managers are the most trusting of all, especially if they are true champions of a potential system. They trust that the people above them will act on their commitment of resources. They trust that the users they supervise will embrace the system, or at least accept it and make it work. They trust that I/S staff know how to implement and support the desired system, have budgeted appropriately, and will supply resources when needed.

If a system will be purchased, the organization must trust vendor representatives who provide sales information about the product, help to configure the system for use, and support implementation at time of going live and during the operations stage. Do they trust that the vendor will deliver the promised system? Will the vendor work to fit their product to the client's environment or build only what sells in the marketplace? Will the vendor support and upgrade the system?

The I/S staff must trust the user community to know what it wants and needs in system functionality. They must also believe that the users will deliver the human resources necessary to participate actively in the project that the user community will ultimately own. They must also trust that the business community stands ready to basically own and functionally support the system after implementation.

Users, then, must trust all of the above. Do users see these groups as trustworthy? Do they perceive that these groups will deliver? Is this particular project a "wise" use of the organization's dollars in their minds? Will the various departments really support users through initial training, implementation, institutionalized training and retraining, and system support?

Through the focus groups, interviews, and surveys, distrust may appear. Has I/S "let down" the user community in the past on the basis of technical promises not kept or a cost that is three times the estimate? Has the business community ill-defined a system and "wasted lots of I/S dollars" trying to define it while in the middle of system development? These are two very common distrust statements. Neither contributes to future project success.

The potential list of double-sided "done me wrongs" could go on and on. This is truly only project background garbage and needs to be cleaned up before a good working relationship can develop in the dynamics of working groups and team efforts. Distrust does not contribute to positive group synergy.

Respect

Collaboration Principle: Mutual respect breeds collaboration. Disrespect destroys it.

In health information systems projects, the caste system that exists in most health care organizations can quickly disappear. The appointment clerk can be as important or more important than the physician in an appointment scheduling system implementation. This creates some interesting team membership. A baseline level of respect between project players can hasten the comfort level of multidiscipline, multi–business unit project teams who have seldom worked side by side. Individuals need to feel respect, regardless of what role they play in the organization or in a health information system project.

Equally critical factors in system implementation are two common problems with systems work: (1) resource tug-of-war and (2) timeline tag. Because there are so many components included with systems, planned people resources will likely get "shuffled" a lot, and unplanned resources will continually knock on managers' doors for staffing. For example, a user manager may have planned to have two of the staff "free" in May for 2 weeks for user testing, but the user testing will be delayed 3 weeks because of a delay in receipt of equipment. The staff is now needed in June, possibly not a good time from the business unit's perspective.

Using the delayed equipment example, the project timeline has now leaped forward by at least 3 weeks. Project teams will be trying to play timeline tag to catch up or move the "go-live" date forward. If the "go-live" date is a "hard date" (which means it cannot be changed—perhaps it is a regulatory compliance date, for example), the pressure to play the tag intensifies.

Project teams and managers must be sensitive to user frustration resulting from this resource shuffling and the timeline movement, and the user community must be sensitive to what components of the project work are truly under the control of the project manager and teams.

It is also important to understand that the user community can cause the delays as well. Turning the tide, the user community can cause a delay because an operations activity suddenly "takes priority" or a consensus activity within the user community cannot be scheduled for when it was originally planned.

Gauge what mutual respect exists between the business units to be involved with the information systems project and between the collective business units and the I/S staff. Does each appreciate the role and work effort of the other? Does each appreciate the time it takes to accomplish the designated work effort that contributes to the whole of the organization?

Policy Setting

Collaboration Principle: In the absence of clear policies and principles of information management, there will be internal conflict and civil war.[3]

It has been appropriately said that policies and principles manage human behavior. These directives for human behavior guide both system development and the project teams developing them. The establishment of an infrastructure of policies and procedures for information management is information governance. Information governance is the high-level, corporate, or enterprise policies or strategies that define the purpose for collecting data, ownership of data, and intended use of data. Accountability and responsibility flow from governance. The information governance plan is the framework for the overall organizational approach to data governance.

In large measure, data access, data use, data content, data standards, authentication, electronic signature, data exchange standards, data release, and data security are focused subjects for information governance policies and principles directly guiding EHR systems. For example, patient confidentiality will remain a major concern until appropriate policies are in place that address patient identifying interoperable data, secure messaging software, data exchange systems, the Intranet and Internet, and today's rapidly developing wireless mobile technology, and any other technology that develops in the future. The same concern appears as a data warehouse or clinical data repository project emerges or radically changes because data are suddenly pulled from a transaction processing system where individuals have an easily established "need to know" and moved into the organizational hands of an entire enterprise or external vendor. The warehouse or repository will create a need for different policies and procedures related to data access, use, and retention.

As the rate of technology advancement intensifies, policies and principles quickly become outdated and ineffective guides to human behavior amid exciting new automation. Project teams can become foes as one pushes ahead with no clear organizational directive while the other refuses to move without it. The users and I/S staff can quickly become antagonistic. Before this happens, the organization

BOX 9-3 HIM Role in Health Information Governance and Data Stewardship

In choosing a career in health information management, HIM professionals make a commitment to continuously developing new skills and expertise to ensure that they will have a pivotal role in providing quality health care through quality information. HIM professionals are in the midst of the greatest transformation in the history of the U.S. health care system. HIM leadership is imperative to the success of this transformation, as is the ability to develop and excel in providing oversight in information governance.

Current and future HIM professionals should aim to lead the health care industry into the next generation of health informatics and data analytics which require information governance.

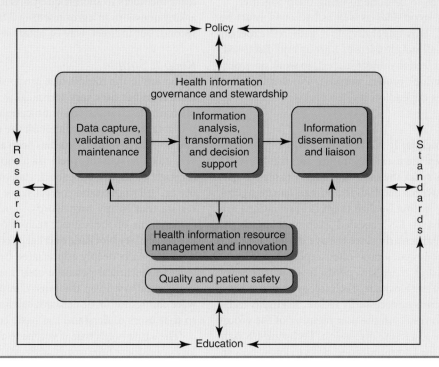

must create the appropriate behavioral framework for use in that organizational culture. Collaboration, then, is not hindered by lack of organizational directives for human behavior.

It takes real courage to develop information governance policies. Those who are pushing hard for the system can label policy makers a hindrance to automation because they anticipate that policy setting will result in a more complex system or a time delay. You cannot implement a health information system without a playbook or user's guide with policies and procedures (see Box 9-3). It is best to establish a culture for information governance through an enterprise-wide group that (1) takes the stewardship of data, especially patient-identifiable data, to heart and (2) takes on the scope of "setting confidentiality criteria that would provide a basis for new applications and for new delivery system models."[5]

SELF-ASSESSMENT QUIZ

1. What are the four Shared Environmental Basics?

Five Unshared Environmental Basics

Collaboration Principle: Expectations, vocabulary, understanding, process, and knowledge are five environmental basics not common between the user community and I/S.

So far, we have presented four shared environmental basics. There are five other environmental basics that are not initially or automatically shared between I/S and the user community. Work on these environmental basics because they will make or break a project.

Expectations

Collaboration Principle: Perception is an individual's reality built on expectations. Individuals in the user community and individuals in I/S will have different initial project expectations.

Everyone has expectations. It's human nature. Users often "expect that the system would do" this or that. I/S developers often "expect that the user would use the system" this way or that way. Positive expectations are important because they have tremendous motivating power. User perception has a powerful influence on the success of EHR and other health information systems. In one very controlled man–machine study, "the most striking finding was that perceived useful-ness was 50% more influential than ease of use in determin-ing usage"[5] of new information systems. When the user community and I/S have shared expectations, projects can embrace common goals and objectives built from those expectations. This builds the ultimate group synergy. If they do not share expectations (and it is human nature that they will not), work needs to be done to bring them together.

All expectations, good ones as well as bad ones, must be "held in common." It is imperative that gathered expecta-tions be brought to all stakeholders as a group and discussed. Shared expectations lead to project success, so work on group consensus. This defines project purpose. Powerful project goals and objectives depend on it.

Vocabulary

Collaboration Principle: It is likely that no common lan-guage exists between the user community and the I/S staff.

We don't always speak the same language. Business buzz-words and I/S buzzwords abound. It's human nature to cre-ate them and then institutionalize them. Abbreviations are the mental shorthand for repeated communications of often-used words. Particularly since the age of the computer and data automation, codes now often replace words and abbreviations. I/S staff especially needs to be consciously aware of the vocabulary blockade. Technology does not have to be discussed in terms unnecessarily technical. Highly tech-nical language often results in the user member of the group sitting quietly, quite lost in the discussion. Technical I/S staff members may lack the communication skills to know how to simplify their terminology. They often face several big stum-bling blocks. The first is their technical terminology anchor-age. Once a new and important term is learned, it can be difficult for them to find another, more relevant term from a business function perspective that would be more success-ful in discussion. The second is detail. Once buried in detail, it can be tough to bring yourself to a higher, conceptual explanation of that detail. Yet the project team members often need and want only the concept. A good conceptual explanation is sufficient. Ask the I/S member to explain and use analogies until the language is clear.

The user member, on the other hand, may use business jargon or abbreviations. The I/S individuals lose concentra-tion and understanding in the midst of this jargon. If the terms are misunderstood, the I/S members can assume that they know the definition of business buzzwords, abbrevia-tions, or codes and make faulty programming errors as a result. This can be very costly to the project and a real waste of organizational resources. Again, it is okay to ask questions and get clarification.

Vocabulary Blockade

Be proactive about vocabulary blockade. Before a group con-venes, grasp the level of jargon a technical person intends to use in group settings. If you know that he or she will "lose the users" and will have difficulty in simplifying the terminology, suggest less technical terms that will get the message across without frustrating the group. After all, the listener usually will need only a conceptual understanding of the term used.

Encourage clarification through establishing and monitor-ing ground rules about vocabulary. "Don't interpret. Ask." should be a ground rule for all project groups. The project leaders should encourage a "no stupid questions" policy and then create a discreet procedure for stakeholders and project team members to submit questions if they are uncomfortable asking questions in a group setting. This gives team members a second, but indirect, way of obtaining clarification.

Keep It Simple

If you are in the middle of a group setting and the technical team member uses very technical words, again suggest sim-ple terms to clear the communication early in the discussion. If that task seems too difficult for the technical team member, and no data definition role has been assigned to a team mem-ber, take a stab at your own nontechnical explanation through a simplified feedback statement. It can start as sim-ply as, "If I understand correctly," or "I'd like to see if I could restate that in my own words," and end with a simplified explanation of the subject technology. This process clears the vocabulary blockade and keeps communications flowing. This is usually deeply appreciated by the user members and gives the technical person a clear message to simplify his or her vocabulary. Even the most complicated computer hard-ware configuration or network can be simplified dramatically so that users understand the basic concept.

The same holds true if you have a user member who uses lots of business buzzwords, abbreviations, or business codes. This often happens with front-line day-to-day operations personnel. Their world is very focused, and those shortened communication aids are second nature to them in their daily work. Ask what an abbreviation stands for or for a descriptive phrase or a word to help others in work groups understand. Sometimes even the manager of the department doesn't know the newest buzzwords or abbreviations. Clarification helps everyone on the team, not just the I/S members. The day-to-day operations personnel may not even know what an abbreviation or code means because they use it only in its shortened form. If so, record the term in question and get clarification after the session; then share it with the team.

Never lose the "business balance" in dealing with vocabu-lary (see Box 9-4). Ultimately, the system exists for business reasons, will use business data, and will be documented pri-marily in business terms. In a health care organization, this includes all aspects of the business, clinical as well as financial.

Understanding

Collaboration Principle: Much of understanding revolves around how people think. I/S people think in systems; users think in business tasks.

Have you ever heard the expression, "I never thought of it that way"? Understanding is dramatically affected by how we think. I/S people tend to think in systems. The business com-munity tends to think in business tasks. For example, a phy-sician may be describing the step-by-step process she uses to

BOX 9-4 | **Certified EHR Systems**

The "business balance" today also requires an understanding of "certified EHRs technology."

To get an incentive payment, you must use an EHR that is certified specifically for the EHR incentive programs. Certified EHR technology gives assurance to purchasers and other users that an EHR system or module offers the necessary technological capability, functionality, and security to help them meet the meaningful use criteria. Certification also helps providers and patients be confident that the electronic health IT products and systems they use are secure, can maintain data confidentially, and can work with other systems to share information.[2] For example, a certified electronic health record system should be capable of electronically receiving and storing discrete lab data using national standards for the format and content of the data (LOINC/HL7).

[2]http://www.cms.gov/Regulations-and-Guidance/Legislation/EHRIncentivePrograms/Certification.html

review critical laboratory test results and radiology results, order additional laboratory work and pharmaceuticals, and finally refer the patient to home-based hospice care. The I/S person is interpreting her words in terms of systems—that laboratory system that feeds results to the clinical results reporting system that provides physicians with data to update orders entered using an order-entry system, and so on. This different way of processing information allows varying views of the same material. Both brains need to work in their own thought process to maximize their skill sets in a successful implementation. The two styles should be encouraged. Problems can occur, however, if either type of thinking misinterprets the facts as presented by the other.

The team may be communicating through a mutually understood vocabulary but in very vague terms. Vagueness blocks understanding. Each team member can then interpret vague language to fit his or her own expectations and knowledge base. This hinders collaboration.

This is a good time to discuss the differences between vagueness and concept and appropriate detail. We looked at concept versus detail in the previous discussion of vocabulary. Concept is most appropriate in "mixed" groups—those encounters where both user team members and various I/S technical team members are present. An example would be identifying the specific physical server placement in the network architecture that will support the new system. (Because the user community may not recognize the term *server*, the technical team needs to make sure that the user community understands the term in this context.) Specific detail, rather than concept, is most appropriate in sessions where everyone in the room not only wants to but needs to understand even the smallest detail. Vagueness is the lack of enough fact to communicate your message clearly.

A clarification feedback exercise is also a helpful activity in team meetings when not all user community representatives are always present at every meeting. For example, one user member describes the desired process one way at a meeting on Monday and is absent at Friday's meeting. Her counterpart describes it another way on Friday. By listening carefully on Friday, you catch the different description. If you have a

user facilitator in the meeting, he or she should catch this. Use the notes from the meeting on Monday, maybe even a model or flowchart or diagram or some visual way to show Monday's description, to verify the discrepancy. Ask that the group stop the discussion and clarify the discrepancy. Validate that clarification with the user member who was absent from the meeting. If there is a true inconsistency of belief between users, allow the whole team to understand that the inconsistency exists and that it needs resolution before moving on with project tasks. This can also work with user understanding of computer hardware layout for the office space or navigational demands on the user through network connectivity. Get the user members to explain their understanding of the configuration or navigational steps in simple language to the I/S people responsible for the placement. An amazing amount of understanding can result through this simple feedback and clarification technique.

Process

Collaboration Principle: Team members must understand not only the content of the project and product but also, equally important, the process by which the team is obtaining the outcome.

How many times in a work effort have you heard the phrase, "I don't have a clue what I'm doing"? If that statement is indeed true, that individual does not understand the process. Often project team members clearly understand what they are working toward. They "don't have a clue," however, about how they are getting there. If the process is clearly known; clearly communicate it for understanding. The effect on team members enables them to truly perform at their very best. If the process is not known, say so. At least give guidance about continuous work effort without a well-defined process. Do not leave project teams in process limbo. As process limbo increases, project team(s) morale decreases.

A word about the unknown is critical here. Many aspects of a project can be "unknown": unknown from an operations side (for example, a new procedure around a system that has never been in place for some new business functionality) and unknown from a technical perspective (for example, new sites are involved in the project or the volume estimated in the operational work expected on the system is much greater than volumes in other systems). The unknowns are constant and predictably there. To have true understanding from all team members, including the user members, project leaders must give members of the team the courtesy of knowing what aspects of the project are "unknowns." A project phenomenon then occurs. It can build incredible team unity, a "we are all on the same, uncharted waters together" camaraderie. It also identifies vulnerabilities that the team as a whole must embrace and work to minimize or mitigate. For example, if there is real concern on the part of I/S staff related to the volume of traffic over their lines with this "additional system," team members will want to take that into consideration in planning business procedures. Understanding the vulnerability allows the team members to do this planning and act. Lacking this knowledge and understanding leaves them in the dark, possibly unknowingly planning a use or activity that will have a negative impact on the system. This sets the project teams up for unnecessary conflict and possible collaboration failure.

CRITICAL THINKING

Value of Certified EHR Systems: In February 2009, Congress acknowledged the value of certification in the language of the American Recovery and Reinvestment Act (ARRA) aimed at stimulating the nation's economy. The law offers a multi-year series of incentive payments to providers and hospitals for the meaningful use of certified EHR technology.[3]

Do certified EHR systems reduce the risk for purchasers? Are certified systems more likely to meet the clinical providers needs? Do certified systems reduce the unknowns of system selection?

Knowledge

Collaboration Principle: I/S and the user community each initially have a knowledge base *not* well known to the other.

Another ground rule for projects should be "Never assume. Know." When a project starts, the user community has a knowledge base not well known to the I/S people. The I/S people have a knowledge base not well known to the user community. The knowledge that each member needs to support the project "rubs off" from other members as a natural part of communicating and understanding throughout the project's life. Each team member evolves into a teacher to the others. Each member also learns to absorb or filter out knowledge on the basis of their perceived need to know that information to function in their role.

Users should be aware of the knowledge base of today's I/S staff. It is never as good as it could be or should be because the speed and volume of today's knowledge in information technology is beyond the mental capacity of any I/S department or individual staff member. I/S staff members tend to specialize to address the amount of information and its ever-changing complexity. The I/S staffers will never know all that they could know about the desired database, operating system, network, workstations, and other components of the system's infrastructure. The question is, do they know enough to make solid technical decisions? Probe the rationale for their potential choices to get clues about the supporting knowledge base.

It is frustrating for user communities when the I/S staff and users disagree over a new system or system component. The disagreement may be based on different I/S staffers gaining different bases of knowledge that lead to differing conclusions. It might be based on the same knowledge base interpreted differently. Try to understand how much knowledge plays into the I/S decision making rather than, for example, a preference toward a vendor or operating system, a likable sales representative, or price, or some other criteria in question. One of the legitimate questions that project teams often tackle is whether to go with a well-known system or component or strike out for the new, better, but untested

technology or perhaps an untested company. This dilemma gets more complex as information technology leaps forward, rapidly outdating the known technology. This issue comes into play when decisions are being made about what health information or electronic health record system vendor is the safest choice.

With all that said, users must still rely on I/S's knowledge for the physical infrastructure of the system through the design, development, selection, implementation, and support stages of the project. That does not preclude, however, users self-educating about these components through their own professional journals or other educational endeavors. As users read and explore this knowledge base, it is helpful for them to use I/S people as a sounding board to discuss their learning outside of the group sessions to clarify their understanding.

I/S units have another kind of knowledge that will be used during the development of a built system or the configuration of a purchased product and as problems are found in testing the system before implementation. This same knowledge spills over to support usage after the product is put into production. The I/S staff has a ready body of knowledge to draw on to "problem solve." When it could be "one of 10 possibilities," they will need to work their way through their problem-solving triage and knowledge bank to find the problem and then resolve it.

The user community has no need to share this knowledge bank in detail. However, if a user is involved in experiencing the problem, he or she should provide specific information to the I/S staff. Users will want to understand the general cause of the problem so that they can learn how to avoid the problem in the future, particularly if is it a "user error" problem. Users will also want to know the solution and have clear directions for what they should do if it occurs again. If triaging the problem and reaching solution involves **downtime** (time when the computer system is not available to the user community), that community also has a need and a right to know whether the resolution process could take an hour or a day. "Stretching" users from a promise of an hour to a day destroys trust.

THE TIDE TURNS

What becomes an interesting twist is the knowledge advantage the user community gains over the I/S people as the system is implemented and then used over time. No one will know that system better than the user. Although I/S people will initially know the system better than the users do, they will become hard pressed to keep up with the learning curve of users who have incorporated the system into their daily lives.

Users can get frustrated by the tendency of the I/S staff members to initially label reported bugs or problems found by the users as "user error" before true knowledge of the problem is unraveled. This is a dangerous practice because it can often be wrong—perhaps it is a programming error, network connectivity error, software error, a client–server communications error, and so on. It also destroys mutual respect because the users feel they are branded as incompetent in the eyes of I/S.

If you have a shared and well-defined proposal, built on relevant policies and principles, that has been validated and driven by users and I/S staff who have a personal commitment to the project and its people on the basis of solid trust and respect that has solidified expectations through the beginnings of a common vocabulary and understanding of departmental knowledge bases, jump on this project. We now have the environmental basics for moving ahead with collaborating on projects successfully.

SELF-ASSESSMENT QUIZ

2. What are the unshared environmental basics?

CRITICAL THINKING

What is your incentive for implementing an EHR system or another health information system? How can you establish ground rules to work together as a team of users and I/S staff members to move through the process of designing or selecting a health information system, implementing the system, and making it operational?

INFORMATION SYSTEMS ANALYSIS PHASES

Faced with the challenge of analysis, design, selection, or development and implementation of an automated system, the health information manager's primary goal is to help design or select a system that meets user, department or enterprise needs, The system should also supports the strategic objectives of the enterprise including current and emerging privacy and security concerns. The basic **system development life cycle** is used to identify, investigate, design, select, and implement information systems. To assist in accomplishing the goal of choosing and maintaining the best systems, the information system process usually consists of six principal phases:

- Initiation phase
- Analysis phase
- Design phase
- Implementation phase
- Operations/maturity phase
- Evaluation phase

Taken as a whole, these phases make up what is typically called the information system life cycle.

Initiation Phase

System initiation is the method through which organizations make decisions to invest in particular information systems. This leading effort is necessary to understand what is involved in replacing existing information systems and in selecting new ones. Often performed in the context of the overall information technology strategic plan for the organization, the purpose of working through an initiation process supports an integrated approach to acquiring new products and ensures a clear identification of the project scope as a starting point. Goals, a budget, a schedule, identification of system integration requirements, and a statement of the problem as understood at this point are outlined. If the organization is working with one or more vendors, then the vendors' future system plans should be included in the process. For example, if an ambulatory care organization is using a software prescribing package that is interfaced to its electronic health record (EHR) package and the vendor selling the prescribing package decides that it will no longer support this package, then the organization will need to research and find alternatives. Alternatives may be available through the EHR vendor or other sources. It is important to consider a vendor's financial viability. In the health care sector, a number of vendors have merged or acquired other companies. In selecting a vendor, the organization may be balancing many variables, including product support, over time. When the problem and the expectations are stated with an initial understanding, a baseline benchmark can be established against which the adjustments that always follow can be measured. The adjustments are tracked as the project progresses. Once agreement on the "problem" or the business opportunity to be addressed has been reached, then work can begin more definitively on the analysis phase. This phase affords early agreements with key users who will be valuable as the work progresses.

Analysis Phase

To provide an information system that meets user requirements, the health information manager must identify how an automated system can support the performance of user tasks. In fact, understanding the environment in which user tasks are performed is an essential part of the analysis phase and provides the context to identify user needs formally. Here, the business process and associated information are documented. The analysis phase lays the foundation and provides the map for system design and implementation. This is a detailed activity that includes the review of current practices, planned processes, and the associated functional requirements so that appropriate decisions can be made. This phase is applicable for existing systems as well. Perhaps an EHR system is in place but some aspects of the system need to be improved. Perhaps the workflow of the clinicians in performing a clinical assessment does not match the flow for data capture in the electronic system or the electronic record system was initially designed on the basis of paper forms and does not take advantage of the capability of an electronic system to move recommendations or plans from the assessment to actions. For example, at the end of the history and physical or initial assessment, there are recommendations for follow-up. The recommendations might be "Obtain an orthopedic consult for left knee" or "Schedule a chemical dependency assessment." If these items are narrative, the system typically does not act on them. If these recommendations are data, they could easily be converted into an action that is pushed forward to begin the scheduling process.

Consideration should be given to any necessary interfaces with other systems as well. This side-by-side planning will ease the transition of system implementation. As was described in the chapter on the EHR, an organization may decide to purchase "best of breed" components. This may result in a lab system designed by one vendor, a radiology system designed by another vendor, and the core EHR designed by a third vendor. All of these components must work together and "talk" to each other.

Several tools and approaches are available to help in the analysis process. Note that some of these tools may be used in a variety of management activities beyond a systems life-cycle development process. Some of these are structured. Examples of structured development tools are graphic flow-charts, decomposition charts, matrix tables, and data flow diagrams. These tools are useful in describing current practices, identifying problem areas, and mapping anticipated new processes and are discussed in more detail later in the chapter.

Although the analysis process remains the underlying activity in developing and acquiring new applications, there are alternative approaches available. One of those approaches, a less-structured approach to identifying user needs, is the use of prototype systems. In this approach, a model or "draft" system is quickly developed to provide a preliminary model or early version application. Called a *prototype*, the system is presented to users and refined after initial use. Before the final product is achieved using this method, there may be several iterations of the prototype. On occasion, an off-the-shelf database program may offer sufficient capability to put a prototype quickly into place. Prototyping is discussed again later in this chapter. Some organizations may use predesigned software that can be modified by in-house information technology (IT) staff. Others may contract with IT services. Another option is leasing packaged software from an application service provider (ASP). Health care organizations are making use of a variety of alternatives to keep pace with the demand for responsive information systems. Other approaches to rapid system or phased development processes are also used.

 SELF-ASSESSMENT QUIZ

3. Understanding the environment in which user tasks are performed is an essential part of which phase of the information system life cycle.

Design Phase

On the basis of the findings or requirements identified in the analysis phase and on a decision to proceed, system design encompasses activities related to specifying the details of a new system or upgrades and additions to an existing system.

Typically, this includes making decisions about the logical and physical design of the system. Through the use of structured design tools such as computer-aided software engineering (CASE) programs, a systems blueprint is developed. This blueprint is analogous to an architect's blueprint and provides the basis for the physical system design. The physical design stage converts the system blueprint into specific detail so that computer code can be developed. In a health care setting, the traditional description of system design applies when the automated system is developed by staff within the organization. However, in today's environment, health care organizations frequently purchase predesigned systems from outside vendors. In these cases, the meaning of system design takes on a different perspective. It usually refers to the assessment of various characteristics of the design of the system rather than the development of the system itself. The vendor system(s) must be able to produce the desired outcomes. Benchmarking with similar organizations that have the vendor's products for similar purposes is an oft-used process.

The design component of any EHR system must include the ability to interface with other systems. Many vendors attempt to offer a complete system, but most hospitals find themselves adding components from other vendors. The costs of these interfaces should be added into project costs.

Implementation Phase

System implementation involves making the system operational in the organization. Implementation characteristically covers a wide range of tasks, including the following:

- System testing
- User training and retraining
- Site preparation
- Managing organization change and system impact

To achieve the primary goal of meeting user needs, the system must function efficiently and effectively. To minimize potential system defects and operational flaws, test data are constructed and entered into the system. The results of system testing are used to correct operational weaknesses and to make programming changes. It is important to stress the system to be sure that it will perform as expected under the load of normal business operating conditions.

User training is an essential component for successful system implementation. If users are not proficient in system use, its effectiveness is reduced. The element of user training is not always sufficiently emphasized, and plans for user training are often ill-conceived and incomplete. Consideration needs to be given to how to organize the training effort, identifying and selecting the most appropriate training strategies for the task and users, and developing the training materials or systems. In major implementations such as EHR systems, user training is supported through available coaches who can serve as resource trainers around the clock as clinicians learn to work with new electronic tools. Also, "just-in-time" computer skills may be needed for clinicians and other staff.

Operations/Maturity Phase

As the use of information systems increases in health care facilities, personnel (clinical and administrative) who use these systems grow dependent on them to do their jobs. These systems need to be reliable and available, often 24/7. Resources are often recognized and planned carefully for a new system acquisition, but it is equally important to plan resources for the operational or ongoing phase of an information system.

Although health care systems may be reliable and "down" for only short periods of time, the downtime can be extremely disruptive after all staff members have moved from paper to the electronic systems. Planning for alternative hot site data storage and restoration is vital. Tom Payne, MD, noted that causes for systems outages at the University of Washington clinical areas have been highly variable, including construction mishaps severing cables, air-conditioning system failures, users mistakenly plugging two ends of a network cable into adjacent wall ports, and denial of service attacks.[8] Once in place, the information systems need to function at an optimal level. If the systems become overloaded and the response time deteriorates, it is not acceptable. Users should report slowdowns and problems with the systems through a central reporting area. This area will then be able to spot trends and help determine what is needed to improve overall system performance.

Evaluation Phase

The evaluation phase is important in any system development effort. Frequently, systems are developed and implemented but never evaluated to determine whether the original goals for implementation are met. Forgoing the evaluation stage may mean that potential system benefits are not realized. Therefore, to achieve maximum benefits realization, all systems should be evaluated against predeveloped criteria and needs requirements. After a system is in place, needs may change, users may become more sophisticated, or technology may change, so reevaluation may also start the life-cycle process over again.

SELF-ASSESSMENT QUIZ

4. Testing by users helps to identify _____ and _____ during the implementation phase of the system life cycle.

THE PLAYERS

To proceed with substantial information system projects, a number of people need to get involved. Everyone in an organization from those who are in upper-level positions who support the overall idea to those whose job may be substantially changed as the result of an implementation and, of course, those who will have a direct role in the project itself will be a player. Even projects that might initially be viewed as discrete and only involving one area of the health care organization may need to interface with other systems, so the right players need to be involved in the process.

A project typically will have individuals who have an interest in the planned information system or perhaps in the existing information system. These individuals are called *stakeholders*. A little closer to the project are those whose budgets fund the project and who must maintain it. These individuals or departments set priorities and policies and may also use the system and are called *owners*. Individuals in upper-level positions who support the overall idea of the project are called *sponsors*.

The project will have a project manager who oversees the project. The project manager's role is to use his or her knowledge and skills and the appropriate tools and people resources to bring the pieces together in a cohesive manner to meet the goals of the project. In an information system project, the desired result is a functioning system that improves (more efficient, more effective) what it replaces and is completed within budget in a timely manner. There are excellent resources on project management and the typical responsibilities of a project manager.

The project is likely to have the following additional team roles assigned to individuals during the project phases:

- **Subject matter or domain expert:** Provides information on what is actually happening or what should happen and the information needed in the process or product under development
- **Functional or business analyst:** Captures the information from the subject matter experts, organizes it, and communicates it to the rest of the project team; lists requirements
- **Solutions architect:** Converts the requirements into an architecture and design for the system being created
- **Development lead:** Puts together the overall architecture on the basis of the work of the solutions architect and the developers
- **Developer:** Translates technical specifications and algorithms into executable code
- **Quality assurance coordinator:** Helps to develop cases and other means to test the system and verify that it will meet the needs of the customers (The entry-level role is running test cases and scripts written by another quality assurance professional.)
- **Deployment coordinator:** Creates a program that can live in and work within a systems environment (i.e., configure changes, identify conflicting software, manipulate other components as needed); tests all the components to make the software work in an environment
- **Trainer:** Creates the training materials for the users. Some of this training material may also be converted into help files and specific user instructions.[9]

The descriptions of these team roles are brief, but they provide a clue to the skills and related tasks involved in each role. These roles may be carried out by a combination of staff within the organization and external contractors or consultants.

Role of the HIM Professional

Within a health care enterprise, the health information manager should be an advocate for use of appropriate strategies and tools that help ensure the development or selection of information systems that meet organizational needs. The health information manager usually chairs or serves on several information-related organization and department committees, such as:

- Committees charged with enterprise-wide information management
- Information privacy
- Information security
- EHR systems
- Templates and forms
- Decision support systems
- Strategic planning for IT
- Departmental IT

As an advocate for effective system development or selection, the health information manager and key HIM specialists should assume a prominent role in the system development life cycle. Tasks assumed may vary from individual to individual, depending on specific job functions. For example, the director of an HIM department may assume overall responsibility for the analysis, design, and implementation of a departmental system. On the other hand, an HIM professional who has oversight for enterprise-wide clinical information systems may have responsibility for assisting clinical areas in carrying out the processes of the system development life cycle. The HIM manager may assume a more technical role and be responsible for direction and day-to-day operations of individual phases of the system development life cycle for a specific project. It is not unusual to see HIM managers leading project development and implementation teams for a variety of clinical and patient-related information systems. As noted in the list of project roles, the HIM professional could serve as a subject-matter expert, a functional analyst, a quality assurance analyst, or a trainer. Once again, the interests and specific background of the HIM professional will determine roles in any given project.

PROJECT MANAGEMENT

One of the crucial factors for ensuring the success of any project is the degree to which it is effectively managed. The information systems life cycle is no different from any other project's life cycle. Success requires good planning, appropriate allocation of resources, and effective monitoring and control. Information system project managers may have a technical background or a management background.

The first step in project management is development of the project plan. One of the most crucial elements of the plan is the definition of the scope of the project. Project scope definition identifies the boundaries of the project. For example, the scope of development and implementation of an order entry system would include considerations of interfacing with the clinical record, laboratory, radiology, and pharmacy systems but would not include concerns with interfacing with a release

of information tracking system. In the case of implementing a computerized provider order entry (CPOE) module for the clinical record system, the team would include physicians, nurses, and other care providers who would be users of the system as well as those individuals representing the systems and functional areas needed to bring the project to successful completion. If the project scope includes developing structured text for progress notes in either the inpatient or outpatient arenas, then the team would include physicians, nurses, other care providers, and the health information manager or health information specialist.

A second crucial component of the planning phase is identification of project deliverables and activities. A *deliverable* is a tangible work product such as a computer code, documents, system specifications, a database design, and so on.

After deliverables have been delineated, activities to support deliverable development must be identified. Good project management relies on breaking down the project into smaller and smaller activities. Frequently, a tool called the *work breakdown structure* is used to break the project into smaller and smaller activities. An example of a work breakdown structure appears in (Table 9-3).

When activities have been identified, resources must be allocated to the project. Resources include budget, personnel,

TABLE 9-3	Sample Work Breakdown Table for Database Deliverable	
Deliverable	Activity 1	Activity 2
Relational database	1.1. Data definition	1.1.1. Define data types
		1.1.2. Provide support for null types
		1.1.3. Provide support for primary keys
		1.1.4. Provide support for foreign keys
		1.1.5. Provide unique indexes
		1.1.6. Provide for multiple views
	1.2. Data model	1.2.1. Identify entity relationships
		1.2.2. Develop entity relationship diagrams
		1.2.3. Develop screen designs
		1.2.4. Develop extended entity relationship diagram
		1.2.5. Develop normal form relations
		1.2.6. Develop files
	1.3. Data dictionary	1.3.1. Define entities
		1.3.2. Define relations
		1.3.3. Define processes
		1.3.4. Define data stores
		1.3.5. Define data structures
	1.4. Backup and recovery services	1.4.1. Provide backup facilities
		1.4.2. Provide journaling facilities
		1.4.3. Provide recovery facilities
		1.4.4. Provide rollback of individual transactions
	1.5. Provide for security services	1.5.1. Password access
		1.5.2. Encryption
		1.5.3. View access

equipment, and materials. Part of resource allocation is identification of the project team and each team member's role and responsibilities. As is evident in the activities outlined in the database work breakdown structure in Table 9-3, many skill sets are needed to ensure that the project is efficiently completed. Individuals included as part of the team in this project would be systems analysts, database administrators, system managers, technical writers, users, domain experts, and managers.

In addition to personnel, project resources include equipment, facilities, and materials. In the database project in Table 9-3, equipment would include computers, case tools, and printers. Facilities could include telephones and office and meeting space. Materials could include such things as office supplies and reference materials. Thus, a significant part of project planning includes identification of project deliverables, activities, and resources necessary for efficient project completion. These elements directly contribute to the development of the project budget.

After deliverables, activities, resources, and budget are established for the program, a project schedule must be developed. The schedule incorporates project activities and personnel, identifying who will perform the activity and when the activity will be completed. Several project management software programs are available. Most of these programs include project scheduling tools such as Gantt charts and other tools such as flowcharts and visuals to help track the deliverables and progress of the project. These methods are described in another chapter of this text.

When a project schedule has been completed, with deadlines, milestones, and personnel identified, the project manager can allocate resources to the project. This includes allocation of money, space, facilities, equipment, and people to the project. The project manager must ensure that there is appropriate resource leveling. This means that resources are appropriated only at the point in the project at which they are actually needed. Projects frequently exceed budget projections because personnel, equipment, materials, or facilities are allocated too far in advance of their need. On the other hand, project budgets can be exceeded when resources are allocated too late, thus holding up vital project activities.

Monitoring and control of the project are crucial components of the project manager's job. If the project is not adequately monitored and controlled, disastrous results may occur. Monitoring and control include tracking the schedule of the project and also include active intervention should the project either fall behind or exceed schedule. The project manager must be able to foresee problems and then readjust and allocate resources appropriately to ensure that deliverables are on time and within budget.

SYSTEM LIFE CYCLES

To appreciate fully the development of a system and its place within the organization, knowledge of the life cycle of systems is necessary. Like human beings, all systems go through a life cycle. Systems originate, develop, and, finally, decline. Several models have been developed that illustrate the concept of a system life cycle.

General System Life Cycle

Information systems are similar to biological, social, and political systems. All systems go through a system life cycle. All systems have a birth or development period, a period of growth, a period of maturity, and a period of decline or deterioration.[10] The following example demonstrates the four phases of the general system life cycle.

Information System Life Cycle

Information systems have a life cycle that is analogous to the general system life cycle. To be more definitive in describing what occurs at each phase in the information system life cycle, more descriptive labels are attached to each phase:[10]
- Design
- Implementation
- Operation and maintenance
- Obsolescence

For example, in the information system life cycle, the development phase of the general system life cycle is usually referred to as the design phase. This is the phase in which analysis of the requirements and design of the information system occurs. The general system life cycle growth phase is normally called the implementation phase. In this phase, development, testing, and implementation take place. The operation/maintenance activity of the information system life cycle is similar to the maturity phase of the general system life cycle. This is the functioning phase of the system in which activities to maintain, update, and operate the system occur. The fourth phase of deterioration or decline is identified in the information system life cycle as system obsolescence.

Information System Life Cycles in the Organization

An organization is composed of hundreds and perhaps thousands of interacting and interfacing information systems. For example, in a health care facility, there are information systems that support clinical functions, such as those that provide order entry, clinical monitoring, nursing care, dietary requirements, rehabilitation needs, and

---

⚙ CRITICAL THINKING

Your hospital has an electronic health record that has been in operation for several years. The oversight team has identified a project to assess the overall system of templates used for data capture across the services; services include Pediatrics, Primary Care, Orthopedics, Gastroenterology, Ophthalmology, ENT (Ear/Nose/Throat), Obstetrics/Gynecology, Cardiology, and Sports Medicine. You have been identified as a subject matter expert and asked to manage this project. Prepare a 2-page preliminary project plan that reflects how you will apply the information just explained.

diagnostic testing. There are also information systems that support administrative functions, such as patient registration, billing, marketing, and human resources. All these systems use some type of IT to assist them in carrying out their functions. Given the number of information systems in any organization, it is easy to recognize that at any one time, multiple information systems are in different phases of an information system life cycle. For example, the clinical laboratory system may be in the maintenance phase of the information system life cycle, whereas the radiology information system is in the design phase of the information system life cycle. On the other hand, the HIM department tracking system for release of information may be in the implementation phase, whereas the marketing information system is in the obsolescence phase. Thus, information systems throughout an enterprise are in a constant state of fluctuation (Figure 9-1).

It is unlikely that at any given time, all organization information systems would be in a state of maturity. It is more likely that there will consistently be variability in information system life cycles. Even when an organization purchases an integrated clinical and administrative system, the system will have a number of modules, and within the modules there may be basic and more advanced functionality or the organization may decide to implement three of the modules initially and then add other modules later. Therefore, the components of an integrated system may still be in different phases of the systems life cycle. Figure 9-1 shows the concept of information system fluctuation. It is important for the health information manager to recognize this variability because this phenomenon of discontinuity causes stress within the organization. This stress can be manifested in multiple ways. One aspect of stress is the competition for resources. There is competition for similar resources, including technical assistance (people) during approximately the same period (time) and use of the same hardware (equipment) resources. There is also competition for financial allocation (budget). The HIM department needs technical assistance and training during the implementation stage of the release of information tracking system. The HIM department will then train other users in the organization. The clinical laboratory needs technical assistance in identifying system design. The human resources system requires technical expertise to perform the upgrade and may require a greater portion of the equipment resource. As in the illustration in Figure 9-1 the systems, although in various stages of their cycles, are all bearing some cost in regard to financial expenditures of the organization. Prioritization of needs and suitable allocation of resources are exceedingly important to meet organizational needs. It is, however, a significant challenge for the organization to balance the allocation of resources appropriately so that maximum benefit is realized. Resource balancing includes competing clinical needs to support improved patient care. It may be that some of these needs converge and can be supported through improved information systems. Once in the maintenance phase the systems need ongoing support and upgrades. Upgrades also include costs for testing, training, and implementation of changes.

Aggregate Information Life Cycle of the Organization

A logical question that might arise after the discussion of information system life cycle is whether the organization as a whole has a life cycle of its own. In other words, can a composite picture of an organization-wide information system life cycle be visualized if all information system life cycles are aggregated into a whole? This is an appropriate question because an organization's level of experience and sophistication with IT has an impact on how it manages the technology. For example, an organization that is just starting to automate its information functions would have a different emphasis in management of its technology than an organization in which most of the information functions were already automated.

Nolan first described the concept of organizations that have information system life cycles.[11] The view postulated by Nolan is that an organization at any given point in time is at a certain maturity or level of sophistication in deployment of IT. Nolan postulated the following stages in his organization-wide information system process:

- Initiation, where the organization begins to automate information functions
- Expansion or growth of information automation, which is usually unplanned
- Control, where the organization tries to manage IT growth and control resources, primarily budget growth
- Integration, where the organization attempts to integrate distributed systems through organization-wide standards, policies, and procedures
- Data administration, where integrated databases are developed and information is considered a critical organizational resource
- Maturity, where growth of applications is focused on their strategic importance to the organization

At each of these stages, the organization usually takes a different approach to management of IT. For example, in the early stages of initiation and expansion, the organization is likely to assume a laissez-faire attitude, allowing expansion of the technology with little or no organization-wide control. For example, a clinician in a particular clinic may develop a small system that works well within that clinic. In the meantime, the organization is looking for an electronic record system that will meet the needs of its ambulatory services. After the organization makes a decision to move forward with an organizational approach, the clinic with its own system will be expected to participate in the organization-wide system. Resources will be redirected to the organizational system.

The organization grows to realize the need for integration of technology and information management. In the stages of integration and data administration, the organization treats information and its associated technologies and management as critical to the survival of the organization. The main focus in these stages is to distribute functions but also to centralize standards for both technology and information management. In the maturity stage the organization views information as a strategic resource and emphasizes development of applications that further the strategic advantage of the enterprise.

At this point in development, the organization's IT planning will align with the business strategic plans.

Expectations of EHR systems include the integration of EHRs and clinical decision support tools. For example, as medications are ordered the clinical decision support tools cross-check interactions with other medications already prescribed for a patient, check patient allergies, and flag potential orders for review. These decision support systems need to be updated regularly on the basis of determinations of quality-of-care profiles, new information on medication interactions, and new medications.

Sometimes information systems become obsolete because of a change in user expectations. For example, a hospital-wide information system may provide the necessary functionality for nursing care, but users expect the functionality to be enhanced in some way. The users might expect to be able to take their computer device with them, perhaps in their pocket rather than having to enter data at a central nursing station/terminal. An EHR system may not take advantage of all the interactive mobile devices. Perhaps follow-up and patient reminders were not built into the system or the system does not have a feature that notes that for patients of a given age or sex, certain exams are due.

As organizations work to advance health information exchange, new requirements for wide area networks require a technology infrastructure that allows access from multiple external locations. Even a single user wants to be able to work from home or use wireless technology to check on information. Many organizations have multiple work sites, and even if this is not the case, health care providers are distributed. Care providers may be visiting a patient at home or simply working from an off-site location. All of this capability must be provided within the bounds of confidentiality and security of protected health information.

At the level of the user interface, another system improvement might use color on the display screen to alert clinical providers to out-of-range laboratory values. Or because clinicians who copy and paste within an EHR's electronic progress notes do not always provide appropriate attribution to the original author, automatically adding color to copied text is a way to alert the reader that the original text can be found elsewhere in this patient's record. Or because certain information may be pulled forward into a note by design, the information added to this visit or progress notes is highlighted in a different color. As users become more sophisticated about how information systems can help them perform their daily tasks more optimally and experience new ways to view data on workstations or on their handheld devices, they are likely to expect system enhancements.

PRINCIPLES OF SYSTEMS DEVELOPMENT

Everyone who undertakes a system development project wants to succeed. Therefore, discussions with colleagues and thorough research of existing systems—both highly successful and those that struggled or failed—provide information for the planning and assessment process. Whitten et al. suggest eight principles to use with the systems approach and technologies:[5]

1. Get the owners and users involved.
2. Use a problem-solving approach.
3. Establish phases and activities.
4. Establish standards (documentation, quality, automated tools, IT).
5. Justify systems as capital expenses (and plan for ongoing costs).
6. Do not be afraid to cancel or revise scope (reevaluate cost-effectiveness, feasibility, scope).
7. Divide and conquer (subsystems can be built into larger systems).
8. Design systems for growth and change.

As a system project emerges, it is recommended that the first phase, the initiation phase, not be skipped or taken lightly. This phase is the opportunity not only to reaffirm that the project should go forward but also to examine carefully the problems, any significant reasons for proceeding, and opportunities that occur as a result of having the system in place.[12] This is the time to set out project scope and objectives accompanied by a narrative to give context. Prepare a preliminary plan with an initial timetable to be presented and negotiated. Assess the value of the project; the value may be monetary, or it may be stated in other terms. This work should lead to a consensus related to the project, everything from "proceed to the next phase" to the "priority problems are . . . ."

SELF-ASSESSMENT QUIZ

5. When organizations view information as a strategic resource the information systems processes are likely to align with the organization's _____ plans.

BUSINESS PROCESS REDESIGN

Individuals may intuitively know that automating a problem will not fix it; therefore, business process redesign should be applied to address and resolve problems first, wherever possible, and then identify where the application of automation makes sense. Many of the quality improvement principles and tools can be used to make improvements to the processes in an organization before the formal systems design process. Doing the process improvement work first will help focus more clearly on how and where to apply automation to the problem.

After the initial phase, the work proceeds to the next phase. Although there may be variation among authors about the names of these steps, the process usually encompasses the areas of analysis, design, implementation, and evaluation. Although the steps in the development cycle are primarily concerned with new development efforts, they are equally appropriate with some modification for selection of already developed products from the vendor market. Because this chapter is concerned with the HIM professional's role in systems development, there is an emphasis on tasks associated

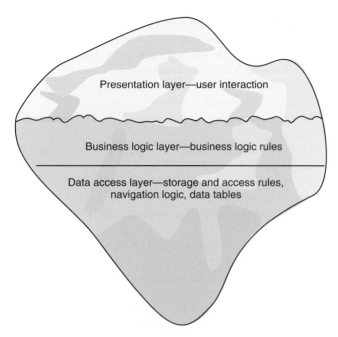

FIGURE 9-2 "Iceberg" diagram showing architectural layers of software.

with analysis, selection, implementation, operations, and evaluation. Users tend to interact with the presentation layer of a software application, but in addition to the presentation layer, there is a business logic layer and a data access layer. It might be helpful to think of the application as an iceberg and the presentation layer as the part of the iceberg that is visible above water. It may be the smallest portion of the iceberg because the business logic layer contains the programmed business rules and the data access layer contains the rules related to the storage and access of information along with the logic to navigate the database. The data access layer also contains the definitions of the data tables (see Figure 9-2).

ANALYSIS

The development or selection of an information system can be an arduous and complex process. In the face of the challenge of information system development, a logical question that arises is, "Where should we begin?" The beginning of any development project effort usually starts with a perceived need or an effort to solve a problem. For example, a supervisor in the HIM department may recognize that a new application for case mix analysis may provide improved decision support capabilities. The launching of the development process may also be initiated by users who believe that new technology is required to support their daily tasks. Whatever the reason for initiation, the goal of the analysis step is to build on the initial work and determine the feasibility of a new system and confirm the scope of the developmental or selection effort. In this context, the analysis will confirm or determine the following:

- Whether there is a need for a new system (or application)
- Whether the organization can afford a new system

- Whether the organization has sufficient technical expertise to develop or operate the new system
- What general functionality is expected
- What benefits are expected from system implementation

Many organizations have invested considerable resources into a system or into modules in a large system. The organization may be working with one or more vendors to support an organization-wide system such as an EHR system. Vendors typically want to keep their customers and want to know whether their system or a module within it is not meeting customer needs. Some fixes may be fairly easy, and the vendor is happy to incorporate the changes into its next system upgrade. Other fixes may require substantial redesign. An organization that is clear about its needs and expectations and has used a systems analysis approach should be able to communicate with vendor development staff. If a vendor is not able to meet the organization's needs, then the organization may explore alternatives.

Tools and Aids for System Analysis

Health information professionals have many tools at their disposal to assist in determining the feasibility and scope of any new information system development effort. These tools are appropriate to use whether the system is being developed internally by the organization or will be purchased from a vendor. Several tools[1,13,14] are used in systems analysis, including the following:

- Action diagrams
- Context diagrams (communication)
- Data analysis diagrams
- Data dictionaries
- Data flow diagrams/process models
- Data mapping
- Data models
- Data navigation diagrams
- Data structure diagrams
- Decision trees and tables
- Decomposition diagrams
- Dialogue design diagrams
- Entity-relationship diagrams
- Fishbone (Ishikawa) diagrams
- State transition diagrams
- Use case–scenarios

The use of each of these tools depends on the desired output from the analysis and analyst preference. In this chapter, only selected tools are discussed. Table 9-4 lists selected tools and gives a brief description of their purpose.

Process Modeling

Remember that the four components we must integrate in system design are technology, people, data, and business process. Events in a business environment trigger various kinds of transaction processing. Process has hierarchy too, much like data, to systems-thinking people. Process hierarchy has been identified as function, process, subprocess, and

TABLE 9-4 Structured Analysis Tools

Development Tool	Purpose
Data dictionary	Data modeling technique that is a repository for all primitive-level data structures and data elements within a system
Data flow diagram/process	Graphical representation of modeling flow of data through a system Can be a logical or physical data flow
Decomposition diagram	Used to break down problems into smaller levels of detail Usually depicted in a hierarchy chart similar to an organizational chart
Entity-relationship	Data modeling technique that depicts the logical design of a database schema

procedure. In an EHR system and in other systems, several challenges will need attention in modeling the current process. First, workflow inconsistencies are possible if two or more persons perform the same subprocess. These inconsistencies may be unknown to the user manager. Second, there may be multiple versions of the same subprocess within the business unit or whole organization, all sanctioned by multiple user managers. Documentation of "variance," sanctioned or unsanctioned, is important for understanding the old way of doing things and in planning and implementing new systems.

Although we are documenting the current work activity, this is a critical step in new system design. Some argue that focus on the "old" fosters a "stuck in a box" approach when they want a "new" visionary path. This visualization of current activity is detailed "baseline data," which becomes invaluable for (1) doing "what if" exercises to analyze the business impact of the new system in system design and implementation planning, (2) a powerful aid in discussions with vendors when buying a new EHR system that will be "retrofitted" to the business environment, and (3) a true measuring stick for "benefits" of the new system once implemented. These models should be sanctioned by the business community before becoming working tools for new system design, development, and implementation. User team members are responsible for this. The finalized model should be documented in writing, possibly by using project method tools including visuals.

Analysis Document

When brought together, results from the various investigative strategies and details outlined in analysis tools depict what is required for the new information system or for an upgrade to an existing one. All pertinent information is synthesized and documented in a systems analysis document. The systems analysis report presents a logical description of what was done during the analysis phase, how it was done, and what results were obtained. In addition to describing the analysis process, strengths and weaknesses of the existing system are documented. Any resource constraints that might preclude the acquisition or development of the new system or upgrading of an existing system should be identified and noted in the report. These constraints may include such things as time, budget, insufficient in-house technological expertise, lack of state-of-the-art technology, and external factors. Seldom does an organization possess all the resources necessary to build or acquire the ideal system. Comparing constraints with the proposed ideal system helps the facility judge what is an affordable or appropriate system, given the current situation.

The content of the systems report varies, depending on the analysis team style and scope of analysis. Martin[3] suggests that the analysis report contain four major sections:

1. Analysis method
   - List of end users contacted
   - Description of analysis methods used
   - Procedures or processes observed or reviewed
   - Records, forms, reports analyzed
   - Strengths and weaknesses of method
2. Statement of user requirements
   - System objectives
   - Output and report requirements
   - User training needs
   - Impact of system on end users
3. Statement of system constraints
   - Description of resource constraints
   - Impact of constraints
   - Description of realistic system, given constraints
4. Documentation
   - Data collection instruments
   - Analysis data (synopsis of interviews, tabulation of surveys)
   - Hierarchy charts, DFDs, data dictionaries, ERDs

Whitten et al.[12] suggest an alternative report approach for those who want to read more from a results perspective and then stop reading when the report exceeds their level of interest in the detail. This administrative format would be organized as follows:

- Introduction
- Conclusions and recommendations
- Summary and discussion of facts and details
- Methods and procedures
- Final conclusions
- Appendixes with facts and details

A group might find that the information that has been gathered needs to be organized and presented in more than one way depending on the audience for the information. Key information and documents may also need to be prepared to be presented in meetings.

Investigative Strategies for Analysis of Requirements

In this chapter, information life cycles and the analysis of system requirements have been discussed. The importance of developing structured tools such as hierarchy charts, DFDs, and data dictionaries when describing a system has been addressed. However, these tools require the gathering of information before they can be constructed. A legitimate question to ask is, "How is the information needed for input to these tools gathered?"

Various investigative strategies can be used to gather information during the analysis phase of system development. Among them are interviews with users, questionnaires, focus groups, observation of tasks, and review of documents, forms, and procedures. This phase of the project is essential to successful systems design.[12] Because HIM professionals often serve as liaisons between system developers and the end-user community, it is important that they understand and become skilled in the techniques for gathering information.

Ways of Gathering Information

Interviews

Interviews are a common method for gathering information about system requirements. The use of the interview strategy has several advantages. First, it provides an opportunity for end users to participate and contribute to the design and development or upgrade of a system. All too frequently, information systems are designed, selected, and changed without appropriate user input. The interview process helps to break down barriers of user resistance by allowing the user to assume a vested interest in the process. If users are involved in the development, design, selection, and upgrade of an information system, they are less likely to resist using the system, and the system will more likely meet users' needs.

The type of questions asked during an interview process, the length of time that an interview takes, and the number of people to be interviewed depend on the system under development and the desired outcomes from the interview process (see Box 9-5).

Target Audience

To be successful, the interview process must adequately identify the target audience—that is, which people are most familiar with system requirements on operational and strategic levels. For example, in the release of information tracking system presented earlier, several groups of people should be interviewed. Naturally, the HIM department staff members responsible for day-to-day release of information activities should be interviewed because they are direct users of the system. The interview process should also be expanded beyond direct system users and include those who are or might be remote users or secondary beneficiaries of the system. Secondary beneficiaries of the system often provide a different perspective and significant insights into system needs; in this case, these beneficiaries include employees and managers in inpatient and outpatient clinical areas and those responsible for oversight of the privacy and compliance areas. The interview process might also include physicians, nurses, and other caregivers working the outpatient areas because certain disclosure of information is most likely occurring in these areas as well. If the organization engages in research, then a research representative should also be included. If the organization offers specialty services such as long-term care, behavioral health, or home health, then representatives from those areas are candidates for the interview process. In this fact-finding process, it will be important to identify any secondary record systems within the organization that contain patient-identifiable data, especially if those areas tend to release information outside the organization. It will also be important to identify events and people in the organization who might also be called on from time to time to respond to a request for patient-identifiable information and to document how they typically respond to those requests. It will also be required to check on mandatory reporting by the organization and to identify the current process. It is also important to identify the people in the organization who are political power brokers and whose support is essential for the system under development. For example, the director of the HIM department, who is knowledgeable about the federal and state regulations and current professional practices, would definitely be an important power broker in the successful development of a release of information tracking system and would be included in the roster of interviewees. Often overlooked in the interview process are the people who have knowledge of the strategic uses of information in the organization.

Too often, information systems are developed from only a day-to-day operational perspective. For example, a point-of-care nursing system might be selected by nurse users because of the system's interface and support of daily tasks. This system, however, may not support the organization's strategic objective of providing accessible data for continuous quality improvement. In this case, the system would support day-to-day operational tasks well but would be inadequate in supporting strategic information needs. Therefore, managers concerned with strategic information needs should also be included in the roster of interviewees when appropriate.

The potential number of people to be interviewed can grow to be quite large. Because the interview process can be time-consuming (between 30 and 60 minutes), the interview audience should be selected carefully. All power brokers significant to the project should be interviewed. The managers who are knowledgeable about the strategic use of

---

BOX 9-5   Factors That Contribute to a Successful Interview Process

- Defining the target audience
- Identifying the objectives of the interview
- Developing appropriate interview questions and format
- Adequately analyzing and documenting responses

depends on what kinds of tabulation and measurement are desired outcomes of the survey.

It is important that the meaning of questions be clear to the survey respondent. A question should ask only one thing. Double-barreled questions that contain two or more concepts should be avoided. An example of a double-barreled question is "Are the daily discharge data you receive complete and accurate?" This question includes two concepts: completeness and accuracy. The data may be complete (include all data elements) but may not be accurate (the information associated with the data elements may be incorrect). It is also important that survey questions be nonbiased. Questions that lead the end user to a conclusion have no place on a questionnaire. An example of a leading question is, "Don't you agree that the health information management department has poor customer service?" A better way to handle this question would be to ask, "How would you rate the degree of customer service of the health information management department—excellent, good, average, poor, or very poor?"

The meaning of questions should be clear to the end user. Many times, surveys include questions that are difficult to understand. The following is an example of an ambiguous question: "Do you favor or oppose health care legislation?" In this example, health care legislation can mean just about anything. Is it referring to a plan for national health insurance, legislation related to security of patient data, Medicare legislation, or some other type of legislation? The answer to this question cannot be interpreted without the analyst making assumptions about what the end user is thinking.

Questionnaire Construction
Having a set of good questions is the foundation for building a questionnaire. However, certain basic principles should be followed in the construction of the questionnaire if the survey is to be successful. A poorly constructed questionnaire, even if it contains good questions, can yield a poor response rate for a variety of reasons. A questionnaire should have a pleasing appearance to the end user, directions should be easy to understand, and the document should be easy to complete. If the survey is unattractive or too difficult or time-consuming to complete, a low response rate is likely.

The following steps are guidelines for beginning questionnaire construction:
Choose a concise, suitable title for the survey document.
Clearly state the purpose of the survey in a brief paragraph at the beginning of the survey instrument, followed by simple, easy-to-follow directions.
Order the questions in a logical sequence.

Survey instruments usually begin with relatively easy-to-answer questions that help get the end user into the questionnaire. The questionnaire should flow easily. It is best to put questions referring to similar concepts together. This provides for easier survey completion and data tabulation. For example, in the customer satisfaction questionnaire, all questions related to troubleshooting might be placed together. Thought-provoking or sensitive questions are usually left to the end of the survey.

A consistent, clear, and attractive format should be decided on for the survey instrument. A practical step is to divide the survey into logical sections and assign titles and numerics or characters to each. For example, the section of a survey that collects data about the end user may be titled "A. Demographics," and all questions in that section are preceded by the character A—for example, A1, A2, A3.

The length of the survey varies, depending on its purpose and objectives. No questionnaire should take more than 30 minutes to complete. Therefore, it is important to select questions carefully, including only those that are directly related to purpose and desired measurements. Like the personal interview protocol, a survey document should be pretested. The pretest should be conducted on a small sample of people. Time estimates of survey completion should be gathered, and problems with question clarity, survey directions, format, and spelling errors should be identified in the pretest and corrected before general survey distribution.

Questionnaire Administration
After the survey instrument has been developed and pretested, it is ready for general administration. A cover letter to the end user should accompany the questionnaire. The cover letter should be a vehicle for getting the end user excited about the survey. It should state the purpose of the questionnaire, what value the results will have to the end user, and how the results will be used. End users should be assured that their responses will be kept confidential. To facilitate follow-up, each questionnaire can be assigned a number. A master log of numbers with associated end-user names should be maintained. As surveys are returned, their numbers can be compared with the master list and the end users' names crossed out. If initial response is low, the master log can be consulted, and users who have not returned their surveys can be sent a reminder notice or another questionnaire. To obtain a good survey response, reminders usually have to be sent once or twice. The initial response rate to a survey is usually about 30%. Reminders significantly increase the response rate. Analysts should strive for a response rate of 60% or more to justify conclusions made from questionnaire results. Another option is to use an online questionnaire, which can be distributed to those individuals who are the target of the survey. Their response to the survey can be tracked by the system. Reminders can easily be sent to nonresponders. The survey can be structured to send responses to a database to assist in the analysis process.

Observation
Observation is an appropriate technique for collection of information about system requirements or identifying tasks performed by end users. Observation is usually used as an adjunct to interview and questionnaire techniques. The results of observation can be used to confirm or expand on information collected from interviews and questionnaires. Observation should not be distracting to the end users.

Conducting an observation takes a high degree of skill. It usually requires a structured technique for recording observations, the details of a system, or how users perform their tasks. When an observation is conducted, the subject of the review should be narrowed down. For example, in determining order processing needs for a hospital information system, the tasks of unit secretaries might be studied. Rather than observing all the tasks performed by a hospital unit support staff member, only one or a few tasks may be observed at a time. Because observation is tedious work, the analyst should not attempt to perform observations over extended periods. Observations can also be distracting to the end user and disruptive to regular workflow, so analysts should be unobtrusive. The maximum period for a single observation should be no more than 60 minutes.

Observation can also be used to confirm whether work tasks and workflow conform to written procedures. Procedure manuals are frequently a point of reference for information-gathering about system needs. However, they are often inaccurate or out of date. Therefore, observation of how a procedure is performed may be essential if incorrect assumptions about the process are to be avoided.

As with other information-gathering techniques, the purpose of the observation should be well defined. A structured observation protocol should be developed to facilitate easy note taking. For example, an analyst may observe how unit secretaries enter laboratory orders in the hospital information system. The purpose of the review may be to reduce duplication of work effort, ascertain whether procedure is being followed, or determine whether data entry flow is optimal. In this case, a list of tasks that make up the function could be compiled. As each task is observed, the analyst can note how many times the task was performed, who performed it, and how long it took to complete. Figure 9-3 is an example of an observation protocol for laboratory order entry by a unit support staff member. This example would change if the provider is creating the order at the time of the interaction with the system as in the CPOE process. One of the reasons for CPOE is to eliminate some of the steps—potential error opportunities—by having the care provider directly interact with the system. The care provider is also able to respond immediately to any alerts and decision questions presented during the order-entry process.

Document and Forms Review

One useful method for gathering data about information needs is to conduct a document or forms review. Review of forms can identify which data elements a facility routinely collects. Paper forms can also help identify those parts of an electronic system that are missing. The forms review can also help to determine information flow by identifying form origination, distribution, and archival locations. Health care facilities are notorious for the number of forms they use to

---

Laboratory Order-Entry Protocol

Unit secretary name: _____   Date: _____   Shift _____

Task performed	Case #/Time	Case #/Time	Case #/Time
Review MD handwritten orders			
Check date and time of orders			
Log on to HIS system			
Select patient name			
Select MD name			
Select lab function			
Review current lab orders against new orders to determine duplicate orders			
Select lab order entry			
Select test			
Select schedule			
Select frequency of test			

FIGURE 9-3 Observation protocol for laboratory order entry.

collect data. Even in an EHR environment, forms continue to develop. If an organization is scanning documents instead of filing paper forms, it is still a paper environment in many ways. Forms review frequently helps to uncover duplication in work effort, variation in data meanings and use, rogue forms, and problems with data integrity.

Ways of Presenting Information

Once the data is gathered it can be organized into several visual presentations to examine tasks and data flow.

Decomposition Diagram/Hierarchy Chart

The hierarchy chart is a type of decomposition diagram. Its purpose is to break down problems into smaller and smaller detail. The hierarchy chart does this by identifying all the tasks in a process and grouping them into various hierarchical levels. The hierarchy chart is organized in a treelike manner. Each task in the chart is called a node. Each node, except for the uppermost one, has a single parent node. Each parent node may have none, one, or multiple children nodes. Sibling nodes are nodes that are all on the same level of the chart. The lowest nodes on each level of the chart (i.e., nodes that have no children) are called functional primitives. The functional primitive nodes are eventually translated into program modules that perform the work of the system.

To construct a hierarchy chart, the first step is to list all the tasks in the order in which they occur.

To develop a tree structure, it is necessary to assemble the processes together in functionally similar groups. Why would an HIM professional want to develop a hierarchy chart? Whether the information system under consideration

is to be developed in house or purchased from a vendor, a hierarchy chart of the system should be developed for the following reasons:

- The process of developing the chart forces a review of the current process. Redundancies in work patterns can be identified and inefficiencies can be corrected.
- The hierarchy chart can provide the foundation for building data flow diagrams (see Figure 9-4).

The chart provides a means to communicate with developers and can also be used to assess whether a vendor product will meet user needs.

Data Flow Diagram/Process Modeling

After tasks within a system are identified, it is necessary to expand this information into a data flow diagram (DFD). DFDs are used to track the flow of data through an entire system. The DFD answers the question, "Now that the basic processes are defined, what data are needed for the processes to be carried out?" DFDs identify the data flow within a system, in essence providing a data map of which data go from an area, which data are received by an area, and which data are either temporarily or permanently stored in an area. In addition to tracking data flow, a DFD identifies transformations on data (processes) and data repositories (data stores).

There are four essential concepts related to DFDs: external entities, processes, data stores, and data flows. An external entity includes people or groups of people who interact with the system but are not internal to it. For example, a patient would be considered an external entity to a system of health care delivery. Processes are actions performed on

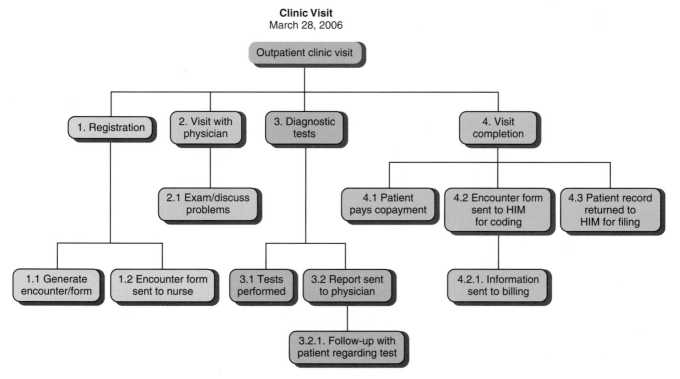

FIGURE 9-4 Hierarchy chart for an outpatient visit.

data. Data stores are repositories for data. They may be either temporary or permanent storage areas. Data flows represent the movement of data through a system. Data move out of entities, to entities, between processes, and into and out of data stores.

Specific symbols are used to identify each DFD component. The external entity is represented by a square. Table 9-5 displays DFD symbols with examples of each. Like the hierarchy chart, DFDs are constructed by moving from the complex to the simple. In other words, the system as a whole is first represented, and successive levels represent more and more system detail. The method and construction rules for developing DFDs vary, depending on whose recommended process is followed. The description and construction of DFDs in this chapter follow general development rules. For readers with an additional interest in developing a greater depth of tool usage, appropriate references are provided.[1,13,14]

The context level of the DFD provides a relatively simple picture of the system under study. The context level identifies the major external entities, data transformation, data flows, and data stores of the system (see Figure 9-5). This

TABLE 9-5 Data Flow Diagram Symbols

Data Flow Name	Data Flow Symbol	Example
External entity: department, person, or group receiving or sending data		Admitting department
Process: changes inputs to outputs		Complete outguide
Data store: location of data storage		Deficiency record file
Data flow		Patient record

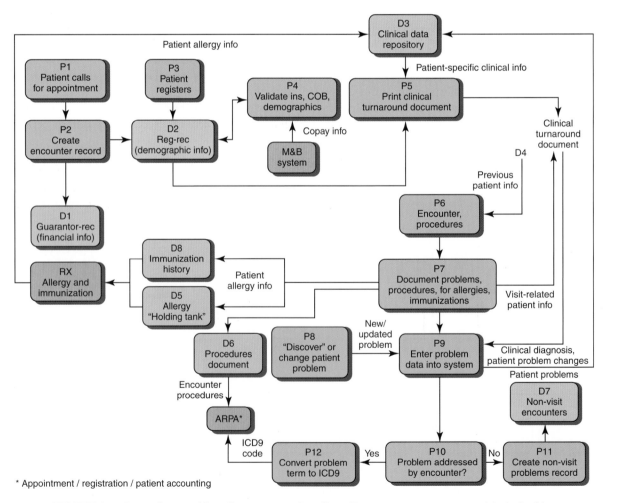

FIGURE 9-5 Outpatient problem list process: data flow. Process components are labeled with a "P" and numbered. Data components are labeled with a "D" and numbered. The purpose of the diagram is to show the relationship between process and data.

diagram shows the relationship between the patient activities and the data that are part of the clinical activity of a visit. The data components are coded with a "D," and the process components are coded with a "P." Each major data and process component is numbered. This process begins with the patient making an appointment and follows the process through registration, clinical service provision, collection and processing of the data needed to bill for service, the review and analysis of patient information, and updating of the patient's problems, allergies, and immunizations. To understand the system fully, it is necessary to break down the process successively into more detailed parts. This is accomplished through explosion diagrams. Information contained in the hierarchy chart can be used to help construct the successive DFD explosions. Why should an HIM professional possess the skills to construct DFDs? Like the hierarchy chart, DFDs should be developed whether the system is to be developed in house or purchased from a vendor. An important aspect of HIM is the design of information systems to support organizational functions and strategic objectives. To design or redesign systems, processes must be systematically described at the level of detail provided by tools such as the DFD. The construction of DFDs provides an avenue to describe the following:

- Where data originate
- How data are transformed
- How data flow
- Where data are deposited

Without this level of detail, an information system cannot be adequately designed or redesigned.

HIM professionals must be able to interact with users and assist them in systematically breaking down complex systems into smaller and smaller components. They frequently serve as intermediaries between users and system developers. The processes represented in DFDs are much easier for users and developers to understand than if the processes were described in narrative or prose form. DFDs often help to resolve discrepancies in perceptions of how something is done or should be performed. Using DFDs helps to avoid confusion, which is a critical element in any system design process.

SELF-ASSESSMENT QUIZ

6. What is a recognized way to answer the following question: "Now that the basic processes are defined what data are needed for processes to be carried out?"

Data Dictionary

The data dictionary describes all the primitive-level data structures and data elements within a system. It is the central repository for all information about the database and functions as a catalog for identifying the nature of all the data in a system. It provides the central resource for ensuring that standard definitions for data elements and data structures are used throughout the system. If you are blending data systems developed over time or by different organizations or vendors,

the process of harmonizing the data dictionary is critical. For example, the terminology used for data elements may vary. The same data element may be called something different in each vendor system (i.e., patient number, billing number, medical record number, sequence number). The typical data dictionary includes information about processes, data flows, data stores, and data elements in a system. For example, in a data dictionary, the data element "gender" used in a master patient index would contain information about the data element's data type, its length, its range, allowed values, and meanings. In this case, the data element "gender" has a data type of alphanumerical, its length would be one character, and allowed values would be "F," "M," "O," and "U." The meaning would be included as a notation indicating that "gender" referred to the patient's gender and that "M" meant male and "F" female, "O" meant other. It would also be possible to add the category of Unknown, "U," if this information is not always available. Work has also been done to expand gender categories, and if your organization needs to track a larger set of values, those can be found in standard tables (see Figure 9-6). Additional discussion on data dictionaries can be found in other chapters.

How is the data dictionary compiled? There are several ways in which a data dictionary can be notated.[3,8] The style used depends largely on the procedures established and the preference of individual information system departments. There is usually a unique notation for data structures, data processes, data flows, data stores, and data elements (see Figure 9-7). The label is daily discharge list. The entry type is data flow. The description gives a more complete explanation of the data flow. There is no alias. Note that in this data dictionary entry, there is no "values/meaning" section. In its place is an area for noting the composition of the flow. In this case, the daily discharge list is composed of current date, medical record number, patient last and first names and middle initial, patient's date of birth, admission date, and discharge date. The location of the data flow is indicated in the last entry of this notation. This list can be generated from the hospital's Reg/ADT system and stored as a report or printed as needed. A primary user of this report is the HIM department.

Project:	Master patient index
Label:	Sex
Entry type:	Data element
Description:	Patient gender
Alias:	None
Values/meaning:	Length: 1 character Type: alphanumeric Value: M = male; F = female

FIGURE 9-6 Data dictionary element: patient gender.

FIGURE 9-7 Data dictionary discharge list.

Project:	Record completion review system
Label:	Daily discharge list
Entry type:	Data flow
Description:	Daily list of patients discharged from the hospital
Alias:	None
Composition:	Daily discharge list 5 currentdate + medrecno + ptlname + ptfname + ptmidinital + ptdob + admitdate + dischgdate
Locations:	Context- and first-level explosions; second-level explosion of process 1, record catalog Data flow → Daily discharge list

For a data element, the length, type, and values that the element can take on would be notated. For a data structure, such as patient account, all the data elements that compose the patient account data structure would be noted. Additional categories such as Source or Location may also be part of a data dictionary.

Another data dictionary example is a data element used both for internal program evaluation and external reporting. A behavioral health organization contracts with managed care organizations to provide a variety of programs from residential services to outpatient counseling. One of the outcome measures used to review the attainment of objectives is the client's "residential arrangement" or where the client lives. This piece of data is collected when the client is admitted or registered for care, at review periods, and at discharge. For example, if a client is homeless at the time of registering for services and 6 months later is living independently in a stable housing setting, then this is a positive outcome. Obviously this measure is combined with other measures such as a problem severity scale to determine whether the client has a reduction in symptoms from registration, to review points, and at discharge. See Figure 9-8 for the residential arrangement data dictionary reporting component and Figure 9-9 for a list of values associated with this data element.

Why is the development of a data dictionary important? One reason is that the data dictionary provides a central repository of standard terminology and the description of data used in all the information systems in the organization. The data dictionary helps to reduce data redundancy and increase the integrity of enterprise-wide data. Without this standardization, it is unlikely that efficient and effective information systems can be created. When used with hierarchy charts and DFDs, the data dictionary helps to document an information

FIGURE 9-8 Data dictionary element: residential arrangement.

Data dictionary

Residential arrangement - used to report behavioral health care outcome

Project:	Outcome reporting to managed care provider
Label:	Residential arrangement
Entry type:	Data element
Description:	An outcome measure that describes the residential arrangement of the client
Alias:	None
Values/meaning:	Valid codes: 10, 20, 22, 25, 26, 30, 41, 47, 50, 61, 62, 82, 83 (See figure 9-9 for code definitions)
Process description:	Collect and report data element after initial assessment and on change of residential arrangement and at discharge
Note:	Combine with action code of: Add = A, Change = C, Delete = D Combine with date: MMDDYYYY

Data Dictionary

Values for Residential Arrangement

Definition: This code describes the housing arrangement of the client on the date of the report.

Procedure: Reports are created after the initial assessment, at a change in residential arrangement and at discharge. For a change in residential arrangement report the date the client actually changed to a new residential arrangement.

Purpose: This is an outcome measure.

Type: Text (2 digits)

Valid codes	Definitions
	Type of Housing
10	Independent housing, alone or with others. Independent housing is defined as housing where no supervision is provided.
20	Supported housing alone or with others. Supervision by mental health staff is provided.
22	Adult family home—licensed as such by the State
25	Residential Drug/Alcohol treatment-treatment for 90 days or more. If the client is in treatment for less than 90 days, use the code for the living arrangements just prior to treatment.
26	Foster Care (for children)
30	Long-term Adaptive Services means a facility-based residential program with 24-hour nursing care and medical supervision, and mental health services which include: (a) Program and case consultation from a mental health professional (b) Individualized treatment, as appropriate (c) Staff training Types of facility include: Skilled Nursing/IntermediateCare Facility, Institute of Mental Disease (IMD), DD facility
41	Congregate Care Facility (CCF)
47	Group Care (children)

50	Long term rehabilitative services (LTR)
61	Jail/Juvenile Correctional Facility—Incarceration for 90 days or more. If the client is incarcerated for less than 90 days, use the code for the living arrangement just prior to incarceration.
62	Psychiatric Inpatient Facility—Voluntary or involuntary hospitalization for 90 days or more. Types of facilities include inpatient Psychiatric Hospital, Psychiatric Health Facility, Veterans Affairs Hospital, or State Hospital. If the client is hospitalized for less than 90 days, use the code for the living arrangement just prior to hospitalization.
82	Homeless—Those persons of all ages who lack a fixed, regular and adequate nighttime residence including persons whose primary nighttime residence is one of the following: Emergency shelter (e.g., missions, churches) where residence is on a "night by night basis"; Living on the streets, in a vehicle, or abandoned building; Being discharged/ discharged from an institution (e.g., jail, medical or psychiatric hospital) with no arranged residence; Temporary living accommodations by a voucher system (e.g., motel vouchers); Living in a public or private place not designated for, or not ordinarily used as, a regular sleeping accommodation for human beings; Children living in transitional housing
83	Temporary housing Temporarily or inadequately housed in a residence which is not their own (e.g., transitional housing, living with family or friends); Living in a temporary non-subsidized living arrangement (e.g., welfare hotel or motel)

FIGURE 9-9 Data dictionary element values for residential arrangement.

system fully. This type of documentation can speed up the process of developing system programs. It also provides information that makes modification of programs and data easier. Without this type of documentation, system maintenance would be extremely difficult if not impossible. Like the development of DFDs, the development of a data dictionary helps to decrease confusion among users and analysts about the purpose and functions of a system.

DESIGN

In the analysis phase, the needs and requirements of a system are specified. During the system design phase, these requirements are translated into specifications needed to build the system. During this stage, decisions about the logical and physical designs of the system are made.

In today's health care environment, major systems or integrated systems (i.e., laboratory, radiology, clinical record, order entry) are usually purchased from a vendor rather than developed by in-house systems personnel. Therefore, the following processes are usually performed within the vendor domain, particularly the physical design phase. It is still important for the HIM professional to know about these processes and what the desired output alternatives are. Knowing both processes and preferred outputs helps the HIM professional better assess a vendor product.

Logical and Physical Design

A specific sequence of events is used in the system design phase. This sequence usually consists of the logical system design and the physical system design. The logical design describes the functionality of the system and is sometimes called the functional specifications of a system. This is where the vision of system performance and its features are presented. In this section, the system conceptualization is stated in general rather than technical terms.

The format of the logical design section varies, depending on individual preferences of the design team and the scope of the project. Stair[8] provides a traditional list of logical design outputs, as follows.

Output Design

Output design covers specifications, including format, content, and frequency, for all output such as forms, screens, and reports. An example of output is the display on the computer monitor of all current laboratory values with outlier values highlighted.

Input Design

Input design covers specifications, including format, content, and frequency, for all input data. An example of input design for an order-entry system is an automatic capability that flags drug contraindications whenever a pharmaceutical is ordered.

Processing Design

Types of data manipulations required, such as calculations, comparisons, and text manipulations are covered in processing design. An example of a processing design feature is the automatic calculation of the net fluid input and output for a patient with an intravenous line in place.

File and Database Design

Specifications of file and database capabilities are the fourth element of logical and physical design. An example of a database capability is the real-time update of a patient file or record.

Controls and Security Design

Controls and security design cover specifications for data access and backup. An example of security is that all users must use a log-on identification and password for entry to the system.

Another method of describing system functionality is to use a scenario-based format. This format was presented earlier in the discussion of investigative techniques. In that context, a scenario or use case was presented to an end user, and questions were posed about how an information system could alleviate the problems presented. The same format is also a good mechanism for describing system functional requirements. The following is an example of the use case/scenario format used for a nursing point-of-care system.

 CRITICAL THINKING

Nursing Point-of-Care System Use Case/Scenario Format: The patient pushes the call button. The nurse goes to the patient's room. The patient requests pain medication and a beverage. The nurse logs on to the patient information system from a terminal at the patient's bedside. The nurse accesses the patient record and checks to see what medication can be administered and what beverages the patient is allowed to have.

A list of general goals and features usually accompanies the scenario-based format. In the preceding case, for example, the general goals might include the following:
- Present data at the bedside.
- Provide for data to be entered in one place and distributed appropriately.
- Provide different formats or views of the same data to accommodate a multidisciplinary team approach.

The physical system design section specifies all the characteristics necessary to implement the logical design. The physical design includes details about the design of hardware, software, databases, communications, and procedures and controls.

Design Principles

Both technical and functional characteristics must be considered during system design. In the technical arena, programmers and designers are interested in the degree of modularity a program has, its cohesion within a single module, and how independent each program module is. Included among other physical design characteristics are program accuracy, augmentability, completeness, consistency, efficiency, maintainability, reliability, and reusability. The HIM professional is commonly not involved in assessing these technical design characteristics. On the other hand, the professional is frequently called on to assess the functional qualities of a system and how they comply with good design principles.

What are basic design principles for system functionality? From an end user's perspective, system functionality usually involves three things: input, output, and system performance. The basic criterion that should be used to measure all three functionalities is "How well is each integrated into the daily work task of the end user?"

Input and Output

The goals of the input process are as follows:

- To make entry of data into an information system easy so that transactions can be quickly and accurately completed.
- To integrate the process to such a degree in the employee workflow that it is transparent to the end user; in other words, the input mechanism is unobtrusive. If nursing personnel must wait in line to access a computer terminal, then the input process is not satisfactory.
- To reduce duplication in work effort while ensuring a better quality product. If one individual has to complete a source document and another individual enters the same data, for example, physician's orders, into the computer system, the input mechanism is duplicative and not satisfactory. On the other hand, if a physician can input directly, there is no duplication. Even if a unit support staff member inputs data directly and the physician performs a quality input check, the input approach reduces duplication of data input.

The goals of the output process include the following:

- To assist the end user in retrieving appropriate data at the appropriate time in the appropriate format. As with the input mechanism, the end user should be able to retrieve data unobtrusively in the regular workflow pattern. Care providers will avoid accessing data from a computer terminal if it does not conveniently fit into their regular workflow process.
- To provide information that is accurate, timely, complete, and specific to the query. If a care provider queries a patient care system for all abnormal electrolyte results during the past 48 hours but the system returns results of all laboratory tests, the output function is not satisfactory.

Screen Design

An important part of input and output is the data display screen and its ease of use. Many options are available to navigate and display elements of a complex software package such as an EHR.

Windows can either be used as views to a document or provide utilities such as tools or commands for the user. For example, document windows contain user data and provide mechanisms for the user to interact with the data. Utility windows are usually smaller, accessory windows that provide additional tools to the user.

Dialogue boxes are a special application of a window. The purpose of a dialogue box is to elicit a response from the user. A common example of a dialogue box is a print options box that asks the user to specify which printer is to be used, how many pages to print, and how many copies of each page to print.

Icons are graphic representations of real-world objects that help convey to the user the purpose of a command executed through the icon. In other words, the icon presents a type of picture that graphically portrays the kind of function that is executed if the icon is selected. For example, a graphic display of a file cabinet may indicate that selection of that icon will open up a directory of files; a graphic display of an open book may indicate that the selection of that icon will initiate a thesaurus look-up function. A common representation in EHR systems is the use of "tabs" on the display that may be clicked to access specific locations within the electronic record. Examples are "tabs" for medications, progress notes, and discharge summary. Other icons may be used to represent pharmacy or laboratory. As data entry devices become smaller with handheld devices, the use of icons helps streamline the visual identification and access to content in the patient record. Icons are useful devices in interface design because many end users recognize and understand pictures of things more easily than verbal commands of the same thing.

General Design

Several general guidelines should be followed regardless of the type of screen or interface developed. A primary virtue of an interface is its degree of simplicity. Simple interfaces are easy to learn, easy to remember, and easy to use by a large target audience. A satisfying interface makes end users think that they are in control of the system. The system should be able to perform the following functions:

- Respond quickly to user commands
- Provide useful and simple messages
- Offer good navigation tools
- Provide adequate power to perform necessary tasks

Whitten et al., Dennis et al., and Kulak and Guiney have described several human–machine interface characteristics.[12,15,16] Input and output interfaces should provide direction and learning. An end user should be able to interact with a system without extensive training. If the interface is designed to fit the normal work pattern of the end user, extensive directions are superfluous. Screens should be layered or windowed and good navigational tools provided. Users should be able to move within the system without getting lost in a maze of screens or commands.

Interfaces should provide the end user with a choice of style. As an example, a physician may want to review the 5-day trend in a patient's white blood cell count and compare it with the count after the administration of a chemotherapeutic agent over the same period. In this case, the system should be flexible enough to present the user with choices of a graphic, tabular, or other format for display.

Interfaces should be forgiving. This means that users should be able to recover easily from input or query errors. Error messages should be polite, meaningful, and informative. A flashing message "Error," for example, does not explain to the user what caused the error or how to recover from it. All interfaces should contain an escape feature. This allows the end user to interrupt a session at will or to recover from an error.

Another important part of an interface is the input device. Among input mechanisms are keyboard, mouse, light pen, touch-sensitive screen, voice recognition, pen-based system, handheld device, bar code reader, smart phone, and laser scanning. The measure of utility of these mechanisms is the degree to which each comfortably augments the normal workflow of the end user. No matter how attractive a technology is, its benefit is diminished if it disrupts rather than assists employees in their normal work. For example, the choice of voice recognition may seem like an attractive alternative to using a keyboard for input. However, the system should be easy to use and contain a medical vocabulary with spell check. The system should also be easy to train to one's voice and take a minimum of training time; otherwise, use of voice recognition would defeat the purpose of a robust interface.

System Performance

Besides input and output considerations, system performance issues must be considered. From an end-user perspective, functional system performance indicators may include such criteria as degree of data accuracy, system response rates, system efficiency, system security, and ease of system use.

Criteria and thresholds for system performance vary depending on the application. For example, the response time in a clinical application may be more critical than in a billing application, or security issues may be more critical in situations that involve patient-identifiable information than in applications that deal with aggregate data. Because of this variability, system performance criteria should be developed with the application in mind. An example of functional system performance criteria for an order-entry system for a unit staff member is presented in Table 9-6. **These criteria would change with an order-entry system for direct provider input.** In this example, three performance issues are identified: accuracy, response rate, and efficiency. For each issue, subissues are

identified. For example, under "accuracy," issues related to input, transaction, and database accuracy have been noted. For each subissue, the criteria and methods for evaluation have been enumerated. In this order-entry example, accuracy has been identified as a major performance issue and is divided into three components: input accuracy, transaction accuracy, and database accuracy. The evaluation of all three of these components is essential to determine the performance accuracy of the system. For example, orders may be correctly entered by unit support staff members, but there may be a transaction error (system error) in processing the order. In other words, the order could be correctly entered, but the order is not received by the recipient department, such as the pharmacy or laboratory. Although this type of error could occur for any number of reasons, it is nonetheless important to document the rate of such errors.

In the order-entry example in Table 9-6 the criterion for measuring input accuracy is entry error rate, and the method for evaluating this error rate is to compare the physician-written orders with the orders entered into the system by the unit support staff members. For transaction accuracy, the criterion for measurement is errors per time period, and the method of evaluation is comparison of orders entered with orders received by the appropriate clinical department. In regard to database accuracy, the criterion for measurement is error rate per record, and the method for evaluation is comparison of orders entered with the patient database.

As this example illustrates, the development of system performance criteria is a nontrivial activity. It is important that every criterion important for system performance and specific to the application is identified and that appropriate methods for evaluation are established. One of the reasons for the emergence of CPOE is the recognition that removing steps in the order-entry process and allowing the individual who created the order to interact with the system's alerts and guidelines should reduce errors.

Auditing current system performance is also helpful in reviewing current performance issues when upgrading software or selecting replacement software.

After the current system is documented, the workflow for the new system is designed. User members should be visionary people, and the team must have the new data defined for the new system to guide new process definition. This will be a conceptual model of process that will change as constraints and opportunities present themselves down the development path as teams take the system design documents and breathe life into them. In fact, using scenarios to describe the basic business processes brings concrete analysis to evaluating vendor products. Health care enterprise decision makers need to provide enough clear descriptions for developers or vendors to fully explain just how their product will be able to perform the processes in question. Investing in the "what if" approach through scenarios is worth the time and effort required.

New, unique system-oriented processes may be handled by the user community as the system is implemented and used. These might include system backup, system table maintenance, data purges and archiving, and so on. Today

TABLE 9-6   Order Entry System Performance Criteria
(If orders are not entered by ordering clinician)

Indicators	Criteria	Evaluation Method
Accuracy		
Input accuracy	Entry error rate	Compare physician orders with orders entered
Transaction accuracy	Errors per time period	Compare orders entered with orders received by department
Database accuracy	Error rate/record	Compare orders entered with patient database
Response Rate		
Input responses	Number of transactions per time period	Measure transactions per time period
Output response	Amount of time for one transaction	Transaction response rate
Downtime	Downtime minutes per time period	Downtime rate
Efficiency		
Input efficiency	Errorless transactions per time period	Transaction error rate
System efficiency	Errors corrected per time period	Error correction rate

as computer systems become "friendlier," more and more system maintenance/support is being designed to be handled by the users—those who have the most stake in system reliability and integrity. Traditionally, these processes have been completed by computer operations/support staff.

Again, user members need to obtain user community acceptance of the conceptual workflow for the new system. The approval should be documented in writing, possibly through some project method document including visuals. Expect multiple queries from front-end users at this time. Suddenly, they begin to understand the system plan and start assessing the personal impact because the proposed workflow directly includes them. They start seeing a living system rather than just plans. It is important for user members to work with user managers to address and honestly answer these queries now. Be honest about the unknowns: there are many of them in this design or conceptual stage of projects.

Database Design

We now move to development activities. The first of these is often the database design. Database designers and administrators take the conceptual model of data turned into a logical model for the new system and plan the physical database.

Entity-Relationship Diagrams

System hierarchy charts, DFDs, and data dictionaries are all important tools in the analysis and design process. Another tool frequently used to help describe the relations among data in an information system is the entity-relationship diagram (ERD). The ERD is used principally to illustrate the logical design of information system databases. This is accomplished by describing diagrammatically the relation between entities and by identifying entity attributes. ERDs are composed of three categories of items:

Entities

Relations

Attributes

Entities are objects such as people, places, things, or events that make up the data of a database. In the manual record completeness review system, entities include physicians (people), patient records (things), deficiency cards (things), and patient care areas (places). In an ERD, an entity is represented by a rectangle.

Relations are links or ties that exist between or among entities. In an ERD, a relation is represented by a diamond. An example of a relation in the record completeness review system is the relation between a patient record (an entity) and a deficiency (an entity). In this relation, a patient record can have many deficiencies (i.e., there may be several clinicians, each having a deficiency, or the record may have several content or signature deficiencies). Another example is the relation between a clinician (entity) and a record content/signature deficiency (entity). In this relation, a clinician can have many content/signature deficiencies in a number of patient records (i.e., have deficiencies for more than one record).

Attributes describe both entities and relations. Attributes may be thought of as the data elements that need to be captured to describe an entity fully. As an example, the attributes of the deficiency card in the manual record completeness review system include patient number, clinician name, clinician number, and list of deficiencies. The attributes of the entity "clinician" would include clinician number and clinician name.

In an ERD, entity and relation symbols are connected by straight lines. In addition to indicating a relation among entities, it is important to indicate how frequently the occurrence can exist at any given point in time. In the preceding example, the relation between a patient record and deficiency cards can occur many times (i.e., a patient record can have more than one deficiency card at any given point in time). This relation is referred to as a one-to-many relation. Other examples of relations include many-to-many (m to m) and one-to-one (1 to 1).

Figure 9-10 shows the use of a simple ERD—in this case, the relationship between a patient record and a data deficiency. Note that both the entities (patient record and data deficiency) are represented by a rectangle. The relation "has" is represented by a diamond. The type of relationship (1 to many) is represented by the characters "1" and "m" on either side of the relationship symbol. This ERD is read in the following way: Each patient record can have more than one (or many) data deficiencies. The reverse of this is that each data deficiency can relate to only one patient record.

Note: In an EHR system, the record deficiency data are posted as a "to do" list for the clinician and tracked by the HIM professional. The HIM professional also uses a related reporting function to aggregate individuals into clinical departments (or programs) and identify the length of time involved in various deficiencies. Depending on the organization's rules, a clinician who does not respond to messages to remove deficiencies of documentation content or signatures may lose the privilege of admitting patients, or other organizational sanctions.

Another example of an ERD is shown in Figure 9-11. This figure shows the conceptual data model for an outpatient problem list. Starting on the left side, the diagram says that a panel of patients/consumers receives services/care events and that certain clinicians are responsible to manage the care for the patients/consumers in their panel. After a consumer/patient receives a service, the patient/consumer's diagnosis or problem is placed on that individual consumer/patient's problem list. The problem list has a vocabulary table to help control and standardize the vocabulary used on problem lists. The problem vocabulary table is also used to categorize the

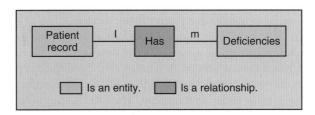

FIGURE 9-10 Entity-relationship diagram for deficiencies.

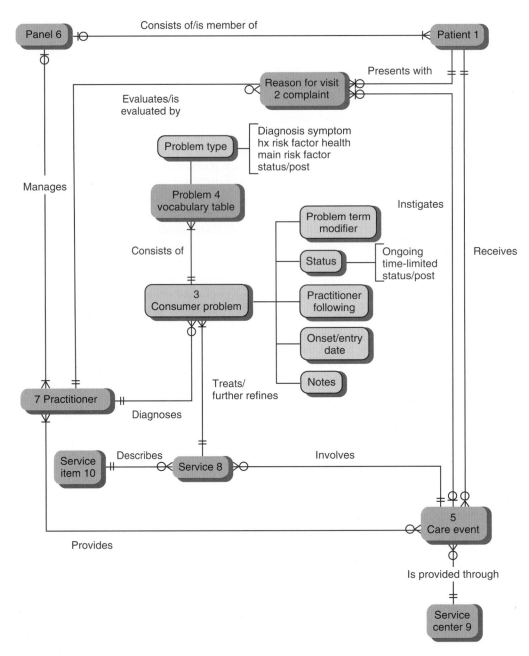

FIGURE 9-11 Conceptual data model for outpatient problem list.

types of problems and the risk factors associated with the consumers/patients in this managed care system. Each problem has the potential attributes of problem term modifier, status, clinician after the problem, onset or entry date, and notes. This diagram also portrays other messages—for example, that a panel consists of many consumers/patients or that a consumer/patient can have many health concerns or complaints and many problems and receive many services.

Why is the ERD important? Development of ERDs should be done whether the system is to be developed in house or purchased from a vendor. In most system development projects, there are hundreds of complex ERDs that describe the entire system under development. The ERD is an important tool for the development of a logical data model of the system. The logical data model reflects a high-level, global view

of information within the organization and forms the basis for the physical design of the database. As such, it prescribes physical database requirements such as number of files, primary keys, and attributes. If the logical structure is badly designed, the databases are likely to be inefficient and ineffective. Therefore, a great deal of attention must be paid to the accuracy and completeness of the logical data model.

The database administrator will likely plan the physical database somehow isolated from the user members, participating periodically to clarify or possibly to determine whether he or she might structure the database one way or the other, depending on the user's response to the database administrator's question about operations impact. This "plan" is usually a textual listing of database tables with "keys" (unique identifiers for each of the subject tables) and component data and identified physical storage mode and location. This is not for user community usage. However, the user members of the teams that identified the desired data should understand and indeed formally accept the proposed physical structure of the new database. This requires a clear understanding of the proposed database presented by I/S staff.

Computer-Aided Systems Engineering Tools (CASE)

A logical question that should arise after studying the various structured analysis tools is, "How are the products derived from each of these tools integrated?" In other words, how are the charts, diagrams, dictionaries, and tables tied together to derive a coherent picture of system design? These development tools are computerized to improve the efficiency, accuracy, and completeness of the system development process. These tools are called computer-aided software engineering (also referred to as computer-aided systems engineering), or CASE, tools.

CASE tools provide a mechanism for the electronic development of systems analysis aids such as structure charts, DFDs, ERDs, and data dictionaries. Instead of developing charts and diagrams manually, the analyst can use a computer program with a graphic interface to assist in development. CASE tools do not automatically develop the various charts and diagrams. Rather, the designer interacts with the CASE program to select the appropriate symbols, connectors, and labels and electronically draw the proper diagram. All diagrams, graphs, tables, and dictionaries that are developed are stored electronically.

CASE tools help designers relate their work electronically by organizing information about a system in a central repository. The central repository may contain data models, logic definitions, and functional models, and may screen and report definitions. After it is developed, designers can query the repository for information about the system. The physical design of databases and program code also can be generated from the repository by system developers. If new processes are added or current ones extended, previously developed models, graphs, tables, and dictionaries can be reused or easily updated.

After the database plan is finalized, the database administrator builds it as a foundation for system features and functionality. The programmers can dig in with actual screen planning and design, menu development, report planning and creation, and so forth.

The user team members usually enjoy this task. This is where all their prior work starts to congeal. They will have defined their data and business rules, anticipated and flow-charted proposed new processes. If the "mock screen" technique was used in any of these earlier tasks, the users and the designers probably have a "gut feeling" for how many screens may work, how the screens would flow through the system, how much of the data would be chosen from "pop-up tables" versus entered as "free-form text," and so on. Find creative but patient people for the job—often a dichotomy. This task can be time-consuming.

Reach consensus on "seed" screens to be used in screen design sessions; there is no limit on number or versions. Screen ideas can be dropped quickly in these sessions, so multiple versions are actually a good idea. If the automated EHR has a data entry staff, plan some design sessions for data entry personnel only. If the system has a large number of data viewers from many departments or units, include them in design sessions. If the system has a lot of report functionality, do report design sessions that include supervisors and managers who request and read them.

Iterative design is the name of the game here. Avoid long time spans between sessions that allow (1) the programmers to get too far into a full-screen design and (2) the users too long to forget their prior creativity.

SYSTEM IMPLEMENTATION

System implementation usually refers to all the tasks associated with getting the information system installed and operating. Planning for implementation should occur as soon as feasible after the initial decision is made to go forward on the design or selection of a system. System implementation can be an enormous undertaking. The key to a smooth implementation process is planning and well-executed management. Many systems fail or encounter significant problems during installation because of inadequate planning or poor execution of plans. The steps in implementing a system may vary, given the project and the scope of installation, but the following activities are usually present to some degree:

- User preparation and training
- Site preparation
- System or module testing
- System conversion or module addition
- System or module startup

It is important to remember that the steps in system implementation are not necessarily linear. Rather, activities associated with two or more of the preceding categories may be occurring concurrently. For example, system testing and user preparation activities may take place in parallel. In fact, some of the implementation processes may also be occurring during the system design phase. For example, preparations for the site may be taking place at the same time as final system design.

User Preparation

The implementation of a system or the addition of a new module should come as no surprise to end users if they have been appropriately included in the analysis and design phases.[9] Early in the implementation process, the system purpose, its general functionality, and its anticipated benefits should be reemphasized to end users, managers, and appropriate others. This can be accomplished through formal or informal presentations given by an implementation team member or through brochures, newsletters, seminars, and workshops. Users should be presented with a realistic view of the system. Although the system may have many benefits, these should not be exploited so that unrealistic user expectations are developed.

Site Preparation

The location of the system and its associated components need to be planned well in advance of installation. If the system is small, management of site preparation is minimal. With larger systems, however, installation site preparation is a major activity. For example, installation of a laboratory or total hospital information system may require special wiring or special wireless configuration planning, special room accommodations, special cables or boxes, and sufficient room for all components. If the system involves a wide area or a local area network, site preparation is likely to require facility-wide planning. For example, plans need to be developed for network backbone wiring, locations for wiring closets and hubs, and conduit for wiring.

Analysis of end-user space requirements should not be forgotten in the site preparation process. Too often, when system installation occurs, it is discovered that the allotted space for end-user terminals or computers is not adequate. Space may be too small, ill-configured, inconvenient to wiring, subject to wireless interference, or not in an appropriate place to allow adequate access. This oversight can turn any installation process into a nightmare.

System Testing and Conversion

All systems must be tested to ensure that they perform in the way intended. It would be a disaster to install a system on an organization-wide basis and then have it fail in one or more transactions. Good system testing is a precursor to successful installation as well as upgrades to a system. The development of test scripts can be a tedious process. Therefore, development of tests will probably begin long before system installation. The adequacy of both the hardware and the software of a system must be assessed. Many manufacturers provide diagnostic routines to test major system components. These routines should be supplemented by organization-developed tests.

Test Phases

Several phases are used to test systematically the performance of software. First, each program is tested (unit testing) by providing test data or audit scripts that force the execution of all program statements. Total system testing is done to determine how well programs interact and execute in an integrated environment. Many times, a system may work well during a test situation in which limited amounts of data are used. Most production systems, however, operate in a data-intensive environment. Therefore, it is important to determine how well the system works during actual production. This is accomplished through volume testing, in which large amounts of data are put through the system. Processing and response times can be more adequately assessed when volume testing occurs. Systems usually do not stand alone but are expected to interact with other systems. For example, the laboratory information system would be expected to interact with the admission and order-entry systems. To determine how well interaction occurs, the new system is tested with other information system components. This is usually referred to as integration testing.

System Conversion

Before a new system is implemented, files from the old system often need to be converted from one medium to another. In some systems, paper is converted into digital images and placed into the electronic health record (e.g., a digital image of a signed patient consent form). This digital image will serve a purpose to verify consent, but it is not data. Conversion can take many forms. For example, it may involve converting from one computer medium to another, from one file structure to another, or from one operating system to another. The technical issues to be addressed during any conversion can be complex. When the transfer occurs, it is extremely important to have quality control procedures in place that ensure the integrity of data and transactions. The HIM professional should be part of the team that determines the criteria and methods for quality control during the conversion process.

Startup

System startup occurs when all activities leading up to installation have been completed. This includes activities related to user training, site preparation, hardware installation, testing, and conversion. The following approaches to the startup phase can be used:

- Abrupt changeover
- Gradual phase-in of applications in selected organizational units
- Gradual phase-in of applications organization wide

Abrupt Changeover

Abrupt changeover refers to the total rollout of a system across all organizational units at the same time. This approach requires preparation, training, and buy-in from the entire organization. Everything and everyone must be ready to begin at the same time.

Gradual Phase-In

Gradual phase-in of applications usually refers to bringing up one application at a time in selected units over a period of time. For example, three units in a hospital might initially bring up an application. After a few weeks, the application would be rolled out in several more units. Once the entire system was successfully operating in the selected units, organization-wide implementation would occur. This approach is lower risk. If problems occur during the installation, the impact on end users and the organization is minimized. Debugging any problems that occur is also easier because the application is tested and debugged as it is implemented. Thus, at any one time, there are fewer sources to search for problem origin.

Systems can also be phased in application by application over the total organization. For example, the order-entry application could be brought up at the same time in all patient care units throughout the facility. When the application is proved to be stable, the next application module is brought online. This approach is not quite as low risk as the previous method. It does, however, provide more insurance than abrupt changeover does. Allowing all organizational units to be at the same point in system installation also has its benefits from both operational and training aspects, provided all system applications are problem free.

Implementation Readiness

System development will never go quite as project managers and teams expect. "Challenges" will surface as the teams attempt to "put it all together." A detail-oriented problem solver from the user community is the best choice to work through "challenges." This task can also be time-consuming and may require the user member or manager to muster resources quickly and without fanfare (see Box 9-8).

Users may need to get creative now. Sometimes solutions lay in choosing among a technical fix, a software fix, or a people fix. For every system created or purchased, there are likely multiple "constraints" involved in implementation that will have a business impact. If environmental basics are solid, project teams and departments can work through constraints to a solution.

User Plans for Updated Processes and Procedures

Users have plans for what operational workflow will likely change with the introduction of the new system. It is now time to review these plans and identify any changes to the plans (see Box 9-9). I/S staff will have little to do with this task. A user or group of users will take on the sole responsibility of "process owner." It should be done in concert with the systems team members configuring the system and defining the database load. Include here direct business activities and also any system support activities that have been delegated to users' responsibility. This is a huge job,

---

BOX 9-8 Project Champion or Advocate for Physician Practice or Clinic

The first step in establishing good leadership for a physician practice or clinic EHR project is to identify a physician champion within the practice. This physician advocate plays a critical role of transformational leadership and should be respected for his/her comfort with and knowledge of IT as well as his/her knowledge and understanding of practice culture. That said, choosing an early adopter of EHR technology may not be the best choice in a physician champion. It is often best to focus on enlisting a medical leader who is well respected, has a good understanding of practice culture, works collaboratively with top-level leadership, can influence broad groups of peers, and demonstrates good IT understanding and use. The physician champion should also be viewed as an advocate by his/her associates. This respected proponent should view the role of technology in health care not as a panacea that will solve all problems, but, rather, as a tool that can improve the efficiency, effectiveness and safety of patient care.[4,17]

Why is the physician leader important to this clinic or practice's implementation of an EHR system?

[4]Daigrepont, J., McGrath, D., Complete Guide and Toolkit to Successful HER Adoption, Chicago, 2012, page 15

BOX 9-9 Discussion Scenario: Outpatient Behavioral Health Clinic

An outpatient behavioral health clinic requires clients/patients to sign a consent for medication for each new prescription medication. Signing the consent form demonstrates the client's participation in the decision and is a reminder trigger to share current information about the medication, its positive effects and potential side effects. Signing the consent is a paper and pen process. Medical team members who prescribe medications (physicians, advanced registered nurse practitioners, and physician's assistants) keep paper consent forms in their offices and use them as needed. Typically, the client is able to sign the consent form during the clinic visit. Clients who are children or who have an appointed guardian typically must have a parent or guardian sign the consent form. The consent form is scanned into the clinical record. Because the organization has an electronic health record and wants to reduce the number of scanned documents, the HIM staff has suggested that the organization use digital signature pads. The digital signature pad can be used for several applications, but beginning with the medication consent form allows a small group to try this technology before it is used for a variety of other applications in the organization.

Discuss the current and future workflows involved. How do before and after flowcharts differ? What are the potential benefits and potential costs?

---

but it is dramatically foreshortened with good planning. Poor process planning is generally one weak area for the user community, who do not comprehend the impact on implementation without carefully defined and orchestrated new workflow. User members should understand that the first go-round will not necessarily be totally functional. Thus, part of implementation is the iterative refinement of the workflow. It is also a helpful message to the user community who may be nervous about the impending implementation.

Transition Plan

Teams should know what the business unit is doing now and what is expected when the new system is in place, but the spatial move between systems can be wrought with bumps. The conversion from one system to another should be planned for a time least disruptive to the business operations. It may be a time, however, when other unautomated but important system rollouts are occurring. It may involve temporary staffing and their logistics or automated work activity to greatly foreshorten the task. Seasoned veterans of implementations are great resources for planning this work. User members need to work closely with the planning staff and the user managers to smooth the conversion path.

Users not only define the implementation process, they completely drive it. Do you want to implement the system throughout the organization, department, or unit, or "phase it in"? If it is phased in, who will go first and why? Do others agree with that rationale? If the system is to be used by many disciplines, do you start with one, or a handful of many, and then spread out the implementation on the basis of your ability to train the users? When is the best time to implement? What other activities are occurring that might interfere with the implementation? Will you implement one module or the whole system at once? Is there space for more hardware in work areas? When can training be scheduled? How will you get appropriate security access for the system to the users? Users must drive these decisions to ensure workflow continuity.

Users will get lots of feedback from existing client interviews and site visits about these decisions, often including conflicting styles of implementation and conflicting opinions about their success or failure. For example, one client will have used only "champions" to begin implementation. Another may have used a mix of users who are computer proficient and computer illiterate or initially trained. The user member must be comfortable with decision making amid conflicting information from the past implementation experiences of others.

Training

The critical task of training is usually underfunded, understaffed, underscheduled, and often only concentrates on system functionality, forgetting process: Users are not interested, nor should they be asked, to separate learning the new system from learning the operational processes in place to support the new system. This combination approach (new system supported by new processes) to training takes more energy if you buy a system because vendor manuals will be geared only to the system's features and functionality. When flexibility is part of the system's design, the flexibility will be discussed at length in the vendor's training materials. The chosen way the organization specifically configured the system to best meet the business needs of that particular organization will not be included. This leads to unnecessary system functionality information directed at the trainees, and the trainee may be lost or confused about how he or she is expected to take the new system and apply it to daily work activities. In other words, the training materials sold by the vendor must be applied to each client's environment and may be rewritten for use by the organization.

Often user members on design and development teams make good trainers. The training plan may call for "train the trainer," in which case system developers or vendor trainers may train the user trainer who will go forth and train the rest of the user community. This is tiring, repetitive work that can be frustrating if users are not grasping the important concepts or seem resistant to change. Sometimes trainers train the user community directly.

Lots of questions will need to be answered in planning training. How much is enough? Who needs it when? How will you backfill your staff with other employees who can do the work during the staff's training time? What prerequisites does the user community need? Do you need to survey their skills and knowledge? If the system is purchased, did you "buy" training? If so, what training did you buy—train the trainer, train the users, and so forth? Does the vendor

have a trainer? Do vendor's training materials—training agenda, training manual, goals, objectives, and evaluations—exist? Are they appropriate for users' needs? Who is going to put documented processes and procedures that support the new system into the training materials and curriculum? If vendor training materials do not exist (often the vendor offers only one manual, which may not be suitable for training), then how do you get these materials? If you built the system, who will produce the training manual and training curriculum? Where can you do training and when? Is a training room temporary, or can it serve continuing training needs? How can you "institutionalize" training and system trainers after implementation? How can you get a practice time and place for users between training and implementation and long after? How do you use an organization's intranet for training and reference materials?

The presentation method for the curriculum must match the knowledge, skills, and availability of the end users. Among presentation options are demonstration, simulation, one-on-one training, online topic-based demonstrations, online interactive learning sessions, exercises, workbooks, and lecture and discussion sessions. Each of these methods has its benefits and drawbacks. The usage of each depends on the degree of skill to be developed, the scope of the system, the skill of the end users, and the need to provide just-in-time learning. For example, a demonstration might be used when the system is simple to operate and the end user does not have to possess a great deal of skill. On the other hand, a more complex system might require demonstration and simulation integrated with exercises and lecture and discussion sessions.

The development of self-paced training modules is an alternative to holding large classroom-style classes. Self-paced modules can be developed so that end users can use them with minimal assistance and they can be placed online. These modules can incorporate methods of lecture, exercise, simulation, and competence testing. They can be especially attractive in the health care environment, where employees work around-the-clock shifts and may not be available to attend training sessions scheduled during the usual daytime work period.

A word here about a training manual versus a user's manual. They are different, and they have different goals, as depicted in Table 9-7. A training manual is intended to train: to teach concepts that serve as background to hands-on exercises that teach system functionality and outcomes. A user's manual should be a complete textual documentation of the system that includes all system features and functionality, complete rationale behind use of particular features, complete picture of system usage within the organization or user environment, solutions to potential problems with usage, sources of help for users, and so forth. One does not replace the other. Part of the plans for training entail securing (or creating) a useful training manual.

Try orienting a few users to the new system and then let them determine what would most help others in learning the system. Test any newly created materials on a few other users

TABLE 9-7 Training versus User (Reference) Manual

Training Manual	User (Reference) Manual
Training is objective	System knowledge reference is objective
Focuses on select, critical system functions	Encompasses documentation of entire system
Exposes trainees to select system features critical to usage of this unique application	Defines and describes all system features, which are available in the system design
Limits explanation of system logic to subject area being taught	Explanation of full system logic incorporated into format and text
Incorporates the adult learning principles of discuss, demonstrate, do, and evaluate	Lacks "exercises" and evaluation components in manual format
Outcome is satisfactory work performance	Outcome is self help in problem solving while accomplishing work tasks

to gain valuable feedback. "Cheat sheets" are helpful in the initial training and in the first month or two of system implementation. They come in many flavors and forms.

CRITICAL THINKING

With the increasing complexity of clinical system implementations, the need for well trained, skilled project managers continues to increase. All projects need not be managed by formally trained project management. However, an experienced project manager can be a valuable resource as organizations commence implementation of complex technologies. If organizations are interested in providing staff with project management training, they can consider certification programs available through a number of colleges and universities or other organizations. There are also a variety of different project management certification credentials that one can pursue.[5,18]

What value do you see in having a skilled project manager?

[5]http://www.hrsa.gov/healthit/toolbox/RuralHealthITtoolbox/Project/skillsehr.html

CRITICAL THINKING

You have been selected as a trainer to assist the medical staff on implementing a new computerized provider order entry system (CPOE). Review the discussion on training in the chapter and a minimum of 2 additional articles on successful implementation of CPOE applications. Identify effective training strategies for CPOE.

Preparation of User Manuals

If you build the system, you are automatically forced to develop a user's manual that serves as a reference to system functionality, navigation, and workflow to support the system. The user member may be asked to document the designed front-end user features and functionality of the

system, whereas other members of the team write other appropriate chapters of the documentation. This will become the bible for the system, so this work must be done to reflect the user's view accurately. It then needs to be updated when system changes occur.

If you buy the system, you will need to review carefully the user's manual that is sold with the system for accuracy, completeness, and ease of use. It will only describe the features and functions of the system. It will not describe any of the processes the user community has put in place to support the new system. This will need to be added before training so that workflow can be learned along with the new system. Include new workflow documentation in the user's manual, which will serve as a reference guide to the system after it is implemented.

An important consideration for training is to tailor it to the specific user community and the criticality of the application. Major EHR implementations may deploy trainers as "coaches" who are readily available at the clinic sites so that the care process documentation can occur safely.

Data Migration

If the decision has been made that data from an old automated system will migrate to the new system, programs must be written to accommodate this. Business units decide the need for such action and the structure of the data through migration, and they influence the timing of the migration. They then need to test for data availability and integrity. This data mapping activity forces users to assess the value of data in legacy systems.

As health care organizations move to new systems, they often have data in legacy systems. The legacy system is usually an older existing system that either may need to be interfaced into the new system and continue its unique function or may be shut down in favor of a newer system. In either event, some or all of the data in the legacy system may need to be mapped to a new system. As decisions are made about purchasing a new system, it will be important to identify legacy systems data that will be needed in the new system environment. Data mapping and the data dictionary have relevance to one another in that the data dictionary may carry alias terms that help systems recognize that a term has several synonyms. For example, one system may call an individual who is receiving care a patient, another may call the individual a client, and another system may use the term resident. There are more complex mapping activities as well; for example, as health care organizations move from ICD-9 coding to ICD-10 coding, those terms must be mapped. If an individual is pulling a research study, the authors of the study may have been using data from legacy systems. Older code books and references tend to disappear, so being able to use a map will help to identify the same diagnoses or procedure in both coding systems. Sometimes a health care facility is required to report to an external organization. The external organization might have fewer values for a data element than the health care facility. In this instance, the larger set of values is mapped to the smaller set of values. For example, a health care facility may track the discharge to location for patients, residents, or clients discharged alive. The health care organization may keep a detailed list, but the external organization only wants to know whether the individual was discharged to his or her home/residence or other location.

User Acceptance Testing

System testing is a BIG DEAL. It is often called the "user acceptance test," and it means just that. If this is an EHR application, I/S staff will set up a "test database" that consists of the full system features and functions complete with dummy patients supplied by users. This test database is isolated from the "production" database and made available to selected users who add fake data and then test the system's features and functionality. Performance is measured against test plan criteria established earlier. Does it work like you expected? Are you getting "strange messages"? What does it not do that you thought it would? System testing will also occur when a system is being upgraded. Users should actively participate in the testing process for initial and ongoing implementations. Just as business process scenarios add strength to vendor evaluation earlier in the process, the careful provision of test scenarios strengthens the testing experience.

"Go Live"

"Go live" implementation is a time to be highly organized because things happen quickly. A response plan aids in focusing on the immediate tasks at hand. Identify what roles team members will play at "go live." Clearly and completely communicate to the user community the series of events that are about to occur. Implementation teams can expect to do lots of hand holding on the initial days of "go live." There is a natural learning curve to every system, every user, and every I/S staff member involved in implementation. Everyone is learning: the user community, all of the I/S staff, the vendor representatives (if the system was purchased), everyone.

This is the time when the "unknowns" strike as problems and test the teams that designed, developed, and implemented the system for their patience and endurance. If you are supporting the system in any way during this time, you will be "going the extra mile"—probably putting in long hours in problem solving, helping users navigate through difficulties, supporting the user community through technical "snags," and so forth. It is an exciting and tiring time, and tempers can fly. Draw heavily on the environmental basics to sustain the teams and add humor whenever possible. Keep track of problems and issues that arise by using a formal log; these could need immediate attention or could be fodder for system improvement or phase II work.

The implementation will not happen perfectly. The odds are against perfection with so many new variables in the pot. Be prepared to document and problem solve for at least the first several months of system usage. Keep a log that serves to track the problem, triage, and solution status because the volume identified soon overwhelms the human brain (see Box 9-10). Problem solving after "go live" is a continuation of major testing of the environmental basics in systems work.

SYSTEM AND PROJECT EVALUATION

Although system evaluation in this chapter is discussed at the end of the system development life cycle, this should not be construed to mean that the evaluation process begins only after system installation. In fact, planning for system evaluation and realization of benefits should start in parallel with the system design effort. What is system evaluation, and why is it important to begin the process early in the system life cycle?

The purpose of system evaluation is to determine whether the system functions in the way intended. All too often, systems are installed, but the degree of benefit derived from them is never measured. Organizations that fail to measure system benefits cannot systematically determine whether expenditures on system development or purchase were justified. As a result, such organizations have no method to determine what impact the time, effort, and expense of a system development or selection process has had on the organization. In today's environment of competition, continuous quality improvement, and cost justification, no organization can afford not to justify information system expenditures.

In all the efforts that led up to system implementation, you should have accumulated some real figures to measure change or new business impact. Use these as a baseline to determine system implementation success or failure. Ask whether the system implementation is the only factor that has caused the change. Users will likely be asked to measure against these baselines because much of the data will be coming directly from their units. Once the changes to baselines are measured, it is time to review the implementation. Was it a success or failure? What made it so? If problems exist, can and should they be corrected now? Can some things wait until an identified phase II or upgrade?

For example, an EHR system evaluation should evaluate how the system performs against both strategic values of the organization and value benchmarks.[6] See Tables 9-8 and 9-9. Once electronic systems are in place, the sharing of episodes of care enhance the quality and continuity of care. The benefit may be stronger in ambulatory settings because of the longitudinal nature of care; however, all care settings should benefit. A number of opportunities to measure improvements are listed in Box 9-11.

Use of a value-based approach will help an organization assess both the financial and more intangible values associated with a major system, such as the EHR system.

Use of value benchmarks will give an organization a broader view of measuring the potential value of an EHR system. If the system is realizing a value benefit that translates into cost reduction, the most operationally valid benchmark

BOX 9-10   Go Live Checklist for Physician Practice or Clinic

The following is a Day of Go-Live EHR Checklist for a physician practice or clinic.

Staff

- Staff has been trained on any new EHR policies and procedures and has signed off, indicating that they understand the new policies and procedures.
- Staff has completed EHR application training (education session sign-in logs have been verified).
- All morning staff has been instructed to arrive to work 30 minutes early to prepare for the first patients.
- Staff has performed a "system walk through" of a patient visit from beginning to end, allowing questions to be answered and minor glitches to be corrected.

The Practice

- Appointment times/schedules have been modified to allow for the EHR learning curve.
- Signs have been placed around the practice to let patients know that an EHR is being implemented and requesting patience with delays.
- Phone tree message has been updated with an informative message stating that the practice is implementing a new EHR and requesting patience with delays.
- Go-live day "break area" has been established with snacks and drinks for the staff.
- Expectations have been set that the go live day might not be perfect, but that all will get through it if everyone does the best job they can.

Application

- All users have signed on to the EHR system with their user names/passwords.
- Everyone can log on and has the correct privileges.
- The EHR build is complete and has been signed-off on.
- The EHR has been tested and has been signed-off on.
- Paper reports/forms that will be generated out of the EHR have been tested

Support

- Support escalation procedures (procedures that define what actions will be taken in the event there is a problem, who will manage the problem internally, and if necessary, who will report the problem to the vendor) have been completed and are in place. The escalation plan has been communicated to all staff and to the vendor.
- The practice support team has been trained and is aware of their roles/functions for go live.
- Morning, noon and evening support team "huddles" have been established to check in and review issues.
- A point person has been identified and will be available to make critical system changes on the fly.
- Your EHR vendor has been notified of your live event and is on site or on standby for support.

Backups and Downtime

- System backups have been tested and validated. Offsite storage of backups has been arranged.
- Downtime procedures have been established and are ready to go, if necessary.
- Paper copies of all patient forms, templates, etc., have been made available in the event of a system failure.

Connectivity

- All PCs have been checked and the EHR application can be accessed.
- Wireless PCs/connections have been checked and areas without connection or "dead spots" have been identified.
- If you are using an ASP connection, redundant lines have been checked.
- EHR system faxes have been tested and are working.
- EHR system interfaces have been tested and are working.
- All PC's/wireless devices can connect to a printer and print from the EHR.[6,19]

[6]Electronic Health Record (EHR) Implementation Go-Live Planning Checklist, Checklist Provided By: The National Learning Consortium (NLC), Developed By: Health Information Technology Research Center (HITRC) Doctor's Office Quality Information Technology (DOQ-IT)

TABLE 9-8   Electronic Health Record: Strategic and Operational Values

Strategic Value	Operational Value
Improved patient satisfaction	Faster registration
Improved clinician satisfaction	Improved work flow
Improved data resources	Elimination of data entry
Better and safer patient care	Elimination of duplicate data storage
Enhanced decision support capabilities	Reduction of identification and billing errors
Improved ability to integrate into community care systems	Greater access to complete and accurate information
Improved standardization of information resource	Direct entry of orders by responsible clinician
	Clinical reminders and alerts
	Access to new sources of medical information
	Enhanced development and use of multidisciplinary clinical pathways/protocols
	Activity-based costing
	Standardization of quality of care measures
	Outcomes measurement

Integral components: Master Patient Index (MPI), Electronic Health/Patient Record (EHR), Clinical Data Repository (CDR).

TABLE 9-9 Sample Value Benchmarks

Opportunity	Basis	Benchmark
Pharmacy		
FTE reduction	Improved efficiency	FTE/thousand pharmacy orders
Error reduction	Bar-coded inventory	Dispensing errors/per thousand orders
Improved drug utilization	Limited formulary Decrease in drug costs	% Reduction in formulary Drug cost/patient day Drug cost/thousand covered lives
Enterprise Master Patient Index		
Reduction in denied claims	Improved eligibility verification	% Claims denied FTE/claim
Dollars saved	Improved cash flow	Days in AR
Increased revenue	Income growth from improved service	% Increase in net income
Enterprise Scheduling		
FTE reduction	Improved efficiency	Transactions/FTE
Increased revenue	Reduced no-shows and cancellations, improved service	% Increase in net income
Clinical documentation		
Overtime reduction	Decreased shift overlap	% Nursing overtime hours
Full-time equivalent reduction	Improved efficiency	Nursing FTEs/AOB Nursing FTEs/thousand covered lives
Health information management		
FTE reduction	Reduced manual chart processing Reduced storage costs	HIM FTEs/AOB Total paper charts stored Health information management FTEs/thousand covered lives
Order/Results Management With Decision Support		
Reduced test volume	Guided ordering/protocols	Tests/unit of service
Reduced morbidity	Clinical rules	Adverse medical events
Reduction in length of stay	Results flags/alerts	Average length of stay
Enterprise-wide benchmarks		
Improved efficiency	Integrated systems	Cost/unit of service Cost/diagnosis-related group Cost/pathway

Adapted from Murphy G, Hanken MA, Waters K: *The electronic health record: changing the vision*, Philadelphia, 1999, Saunders/Elsevier.
FTE, full-time equivalent; AR, accounts receivable; AOB, adjusted occupied bed.

BOX 9-11 EHR System Evaluation

- Improved access to medical history, allergies, and medications should reduce the number of adverse reactions from treatment.
- Improved access should reduce the amount of time spent in obtaining and reviewing patient history before ordering diagnostics or treatment, which should shorten the time it takes to provide care and should reduce the cost of care.
- Improved access should allow caregivers to place orders that are legible, timely, and screened for possible errors, which should result in fewer errors in the treatment process.
- Improved access to patient information should reduce the need to delay seeing drop-in or emergency care patients until a record is obtained from current or remote storage, which should reduce the amount of time patients spend waiting for this information to be available to the treating clinician.
- System prompts and reminders should reduce the possibility of adverse reactions to care.
- Use of electronic and embedded disease protocols should result in consistent comparison to an agreed on standard of care.

- Use of online formularies should save time for the ordering caregiver and result in lower medication costs.
- Use of electronic clinical decision support systems should improve the efficiency and effectiveness of care.
- Use of electronic systems should result in standardization of terms and data, which should allow comparison of both the quality and cost of care.
- Legibility is improved, which should reduce medication errors.
- Laboratory technicians can check and see when a medication was ordered/administered, which should allow better timing of specimen collections.
- Caregivers can complete their documentation without obtaining access to a paper record, which should allow more timely completion of documentation.
- Administrative access to clinical records for billing, coding, and release of information can be completed without access to a paper record, which should allow more timely completion of these functions.

BOX 9-12 Physician Practice/Clinic System Improvement

There is also a quality improvement process post–go live which will continue indefinitely. This is when you will develop a strategy to move beyond just using the features and functions of the EHR and start focusing on the data in the system to maximize the benefits that the system can provide.

To maximize the benefits of having an EHR in your practice, you need to be able to utilize it to its fullest extent. Once the EHR is up and running, you can immediately and easily refer back to your goals developed in the assessment phase to measure the overall success of the EHR deployment to date. This method will give you a good general indication of what the affects of the EHR have been since go live.[7,20]

[7]http://www.ddcmultimedia.com/doqit/EHR_Adoption/Evaluate_Improve/L1P6.html

is the "average cost per case."[4] Value benchmarks can help measure the achievement of objectives and expectations for an EHR system.

It is safe to say the quest for new and better ways to conduct business is an eternal one that continually requires collaboration between the user community and the I/S staff. Out of implementation and usage will come new desires for improving the system (see Box 9-12). This starts the project cycle all over again in search of new and better information systems.

Evaluation Methods

The following methods are used to evaluate systems:
- Benefits realization
- Cost-benefit analysis
- Cost-effectiveness analysis
- Other evaluation approaches

Benefits Realization

In benefits realization, the criteria used for system evaluation evolve from the analysis and design sections of the systems life cycle. Take, for example, a computerized release of information system. Suppose that in the systems analysis document some of the goals of this system were as follows:
- Decrease response time to requests for information
- Assist in/improve gathering of standard data and standard data sets
- Assist in/improve preparation of standard documents and standard document sets
- Accurately report metrics related to requests for information and their release
- Accurately report pending release and reasons, if any, that may delay release
- Accurately measure the productivity of each staff member responsible for release of information
- Accurately document what is being released, when, why, how, and to whom
- Identify those releases made with patient or guardian consent
- Identify those releases required by law and not requiring patient consent
- Identify and track performance on those releases for which local law may require notification of the patient to allow the patient to object to a mandatory release (subpoena) and the outcome
- Identify discretionary releases (where the laws are permissive)
- Identify the requests for information that were denied or not answered and the reason
- Reduce errors in the release of information to external entities
- Reduce employee time in documenting the release of information data elements
- Provide for reporting capability (i.e., releases of information made without the patient's consent)
- Calculate daily, weekly, and monthly work volumes
- Provide for retention of the database for a period of at least 6 years

In the evaluation of the release of information tracking system, these goals would be used as the basic criteria for determining the benefits of system installation. Using this method for evaluation of a system is usually referred to as benefits realization. In other words, has the system delivered the benefits that were anticipated? To determine the exact benefits derived from the system, good measurements must be established for each criterion. For example, the response time for responding to requests for information must be known before system implementation. If these and other data are not known, post-implementation benefits cannot be calculated. This points out the need for understanding and applying the necessary tracking of metrics.

The work of planning and accomplishing effective evaluation begins with a clear idea of what is to be improved by the new application. The case for purchasing or developing systems is made early on in project initiation and analysis phases, and the foundation for future evaluation must be established and data collected for future evaluation collected before implementation. The examples given are related to processes; however, the organization could add other expected outcomes directly related to patient care improvement and patient safety, establish baseline data before implementation, and then reassess. The reassessment findings might prove useful, although attributing changes solely to the implementation of a new system may not be possible.

Cost-Benefit Analysis

The benefits realization method is not usually economics based, although the potential costs in inappropriate release of information could be discussed. In other words, system benefits are not necessarily compared with an economic outcome. Cost-benefit analysis (CBA), on the other hand, attempts to measure benefits compared with system costs. Basically, the goal of CBA is to determine whether the information system decreases or increases benefits and whether it decreases or increases cost for the organization. Cost-benefit methods are frequently used before system development or selection of system alternatives. These methods are applied in an attempt to justify the selection of one alternative over another. For example, CBA would be used to justify selection of one vendor's product over another or to justify the purchase of a proposed information system.

The term *cost-benefit analysis* is used somewhat loosely in the information systems field as opposed to its use by economists. Basically, CBA uses microeconomic models to assist in making good decisions. In CBA, dollar values are assigned to the cost and benefits of a proposed information system. These dollar values are then compared to help make a decision between alternative systems. Several techniques are used to evaluate alternative solutions. Among them are break-even analysis, payback period, discounted payback period, return on investment, and internal rate of return. (These techniques are also discussed in the financial management chapter of this book.)

Break-Even Analysis

Break-even analysis is probably the simplest CBA technique. In break-even analysis, costs to operate the current system are compared with those to operate the proposed system. The point at which old system costs equal new system costs is called the break-even point. After the break-even point, the proposed system should begin to generate a positive monetary return compared with the old system. With this analysis, a set period is usually targeted ahead of time for monetary return (e.g., 2 to 5 years).

Payback Period

Calculation of the payback period is often done to determine whether a new system will fully recover its investment (development) costs before the end of its life cycle. To determine the payback period, a comparison between total old system costs and total new system costs (including investment) is made. The difference between new system and old system costs is calculated on a year-by-year (cumulative) basis. When the difference between old system and new system costs reaches zero, the payback period has been reached.

Discounted Payback Period

Another CBA technique uses the discounted payback period. In this method, an organization determines how much a system costs in future dollars. The basic concept underlying this approach is that today's dollars are worth more than future dollars. This is because an organization can usually invest today's dollars at a certain interest rate and receive a return on investment (ROI). Therefore, future dollars that are anticipated to be made by installing an information system are discounted in calculations used to determine the discounted payback period. For example, say a health care facility can invest $1 today at 8% interest. The value of that dollar next year will be $1.08. To determine the present value of today's dollar at any time in the future, the following formula is used:

$$1/(1 + ROI)^n,$$

where ROI is the facility's expected return on investment and n is the number of years into the future.

Cost-Effectiveness Analysis

As opposed to CBA, cost-effectiveness analysis attempts to evaluate certain beneficial consequences in nonmonetary terms. Therefore, in cost-effectiveness analysis, desirable benefits are not valued in monetary terms but are measured in some other unit. For example, what price could be placed on saving one life or making a patient's record available to a patient care unit more quickly? Or, can the investment in a new information system decrease medication errors or increase timelier drug administration? The determination of how much it is worth to decrease one medication error is a social question, not a technical or economic one. How much a nonmonetary item is worth is left for the specific facility to determine given current situations and constraints. There are and will be a number of organization-wide systems that do not meet monetary criteria but will still be necessary to build infrastructure and as business investments. Health care has been slow to recognize that investing in information systems is a continuing process and a regular budget item once a system is in place. As health care attempts to raise the level of consistency in the use of known quality performance in health care, it will be easier to quantify and attach dollars to the difference between high-quality and mediocre care. The information systems such as the EHR will help in this endeavor.

To evaluate the costs and benefits of a system objectively, a variety of analytic techniques should be used, including CBA and benefits realization. As noted, other dimensions could be added to these examples to prove the cost effectiveness and return on investment.

Other Evaluation Approaches and Methods

In addition to the three previously discussed evaluation methods (benefits realization, cost-benefit analysis, and cost-effectiveness analysis), many other evaluation techniques can be used to assess the functional, technical, and economic outcomes of system implementation. Evaluation of computer systems should be approached in the same manner as any evaluation study. As a first step, the evaluation question(s) should be framed. For example, an evaluation question may be, "Does the system work as it was intended to work?" In other words, does the system perform well technically? For an ADT system, can the admitting clerk retrieve a patient's previous admission and discharge dates? Does the system provide the patient's medical record number and demographics? Can the admitting clerk update the demographic information? Can the system easily identify possible duplicate medical record numbers for the same patient?

Another type of evaluation question might be to assess whether the system is being used as it was intended. For example, who uses the system? What functions of the systems are being used most often? Which functions are being rarely or never used? Still another question for evaluation might be

"What impact has the system had in the delivery of patient care?" For example, have medication errors been reduced since system implementation? Are laboratory results being reported faster? Are laboratory tests being processed faster? Is the waiting time in the emergency department or clinics significantly reduced? It is apparent that an infinite number of evaluation questions can be developed. The important point is that the evaluation questions must be narrowed to those that are deemed most important and critical to the enterprise.

After the evaluation questions have been chosen, the next step in the evaluation process is to choose a research method. The types of research methods that can be used include qualitative, survey, and experimental methods, as well as mathematical and computer simulations and methods that use a combination of these approaches. Each of these methods has its own strengths and weaknesses. The choice of any method is directly dependent on the evaluation question(s) to be answered.

Qualitative research attempts to answer questions about how and why specific outcomes occur. This type of research frequently uses structured observation, focused interview of participants, and analysis of formal and informal notes and reports. A principal objective of qualitative research is to study a system in its natural environment or setting. Words, rather than numbers, are used to describe the results of the analysis. This type of research is particularly useful in studying the design, use, and implementation of health care information systems. For example, observing how clinicians actually use a system may provide better information about how the system facilitates ease of use than conducting a survey because it allows the evaluator to study the dynamics of a process. A drawback of the qualitative research technique is that it relies on the observation and interpretation of one or a few evaluators. This method may introduce bias into the evaluation results unless countermeasures are built into the evaluation process. The role of qualitative research is increasing in significance to answer questions that quantitative measurement does not answer. Freidman and Wyatt[21] note that the motivation of qualitative studies is to address what people really want to know, such as, "Is the information resource working as intended? How can it be improved? Does it make any difference? Are the differences beneficial? Are the observed effects those envisioned by the developers or are they different?" Like quantitative analysis, quantitative evaluation relies on a method to guide the process.

Survey methods are frequently used to study the outcomes of health care information systems. The type of survey conducted is dependent on the evaluation question selected for study. Survey evaluation can be used to assess the level of user satisfaction with a system and the level of user compliance. Survey data are also collected to describe the demographics of groups of system users or nonusers, identify the status of implementation or use of a system, measure attitudes toward computer use, and measure the degree of adaptation to computer usage. Survey evaluation is conducted by using a structured or standardized survey instrument or questionnaire applied to a population or sample of a population. Using a survey approach is usually an easier evaluation method then using a qualitative approach. A strength of survey research is that it is usually nonintrusive, easy to administer, and easy to compile data. A major drawback of survey research is that it cannot assess adequately the dynamics of how change occurs or assess the relationships between information systems and their external environment.

Experimental research methods can also be used to evaluate various aspects of information system implementation and use. However, these methods demand a much more rigorous environment and require the use of control groups. For these reasons, much of the experimental research conducted on health information systems has been performed in laboratory settings. Key requirements for an experimental research approach are random assignment of subjects to experimental and control groups and the manipulation of one or more independent variables. In addition, the evaluator must be able to control other independent and intervening variables that may affect the dependent variable under study and ultimately the outcome of the evaluation.

For the reasons cited, applying true experimental research design on health information systems is difficult. Therefore, a modification of the experimental design is often used. This is called a quasi-experimental or field design. In these situations, the evaluator frequently uses intact groups as opposed to randomly assigned groups. In addition, the evaluator does not have as much control over independent and extraneous variables. Although not as rigorous as the experimental design, the field evaluation does allow the study of an information system in its natural environment. As long as potential biases are recognized, the field design can be an important evaluation tool.

Mathematical and computer simulations are good strategies for studying the operational effectiveness of a computer system. For example, a computer simulation may be able to predict how an information system may affect the wait time of a patient being admitted to the hospital. Or it may be able to predict the throughput of laboratory tests and results given a certain volume of patients and laboratory tests. In one study, a computer simulation model of the order-entry process was developed and used to perform computer simulation experiments to estimate the effects of two methods of order entry on several outcome measures.[2] The results indicated that the personal order sets for order entry could result in significant reduction of personnel and errors.

After the evaluation question and method have been chosen, the evaluation project must be managed in the same way as any other project. Resources must be allocated, including staff, equipment, money, and facilities, to carry out the evaluation. A project manager should be assigned to oversee the total evaluation process. Steps in the process must be identified. Responsibilities must be assigned and a timeline developed. Monitoring of the project by the project manager must be a constant process to ensure that the project stays on time, has adequate resources, and is appropriately managed.

There is no one right question to ask, nor is there one right way to conduct an evaluation. The evaluation questions that are chosen and the methods used are highly dependent on the enterprise, its specific needs, and its individual context. What is important to one organization may not be important to another. Therefore, there is no "cookie-cutter" or "one quick fix" approach to evaluation of information systems. It should be apparent, however, that evaluation of information systems should go beyond the technical aspects of the system. Because there is strong evidence that computer systems "affect the structure and functioning of operations, the quality of work life of employees within them, and ultimately the cost and quality of the goods and services they provide,"[11] each enterprise should have a rigorous program of evaluation. The program of evaluation should include study of how information systems affect the organization and functioning of the enterprise, the quality of work life of the employees, and the delivery and outcome of patient care. In health care, some of the questions to be studied cross over into quality improvement projects. For example, evaluation can be designed to look at both the information system and the quality of care or the efficiency of the service.

PURCHASING PROCESS: REQUEST FOR PROPOSAL

Information system development for most health care applications is an enormous undertaking. Few health care facilities have the budget, expertise, or other resources necessary to develop most health care applications. Although every health care facility is unique, there are enough similarities across many functions to make the development of "vanilla" systems by vendors practical. These systems usually have general functionalities that can be modified to meet the needs of many health care facilities. For example, a health care facility would not usually develop a laboratory information system because this type of system is complex and the facility would probably not be able to justify the cost of development for benefit received. This type of system, however, is an ideal candidate for vendor development. Because most laboratories have similar functions, a general information system can be developed to meet the needs of many clinical laboratories. The cost of development, which is initially assumed by the vendor, can then be spread across many purchasers, making the individual cost to any one client less than if the client developed the system in house.

When a decision is made to purchase a system from a vendor rather than develop the product in house, a request for proposal (RFP) process is usually undertaken. An RFP is a document that details all required system functionality, including functional, technical, training, and implementation requirements. The document is distributed to a selected number of vendors, who are invited to respond to the proposal. The vendor response to the proposal indicates to what degree the vendor's product meets the proposed system requirements.

Request for Information

During the system specification process, the committee may issue a request for information (RFI) to vendors. Enough is generally known at this point about system capabilities so that an intelligent decision can be made about which vendor products are most likely to be competitive in a response to an RFP. The RFI basically solicits general information from vendors about their products. The RFI may state in general terms what the facility is looking for in system functionality. Vendors respond with information about their product lines and their experience in the marketplace and provide copies of their annual reports. The RFI is a good way for health care facilities to narrow down the field of vendors to whom an RFP will be sent.

Before an RFP is prepared, functional specifications for the new system must be generated. To produce the specifications, the same techniques used in the system life cycle should be used. This includes development of hierarchy charts, DFDs, preliminary data dictionaries, and ERDs. Many health care facilities fail to do a thorough systems analysis when developing an RFP. This results in poorly drafted system specifications. When this occurs, the facility places itself in a vulnerable position. No RFP should be generated without a thorough analysis of user needs and projected system capabilities.

Planning Steps Before Request for Proposal Preparation

When the purchase of an information system is being considered, a steering committee is usually appointed to oversee the process. Membership of the committee is commonly multidisciplinary, including users, managers, and representatives from administration and information systems. The primary responsibility of the committee is to provide overall management of the system selection and implementation process. It is the committee's responsibility to develop a work plan and timetable and ensure that the process is completed. Specific tasks of the committee vary from institution to institution but broadly encompass the following:
- Development of project work plan and timetable
- Oversight of systems analysis
- Development of system specifications
- Determination of costs and benefits
- Compilation and distribution of the RFP
- Evaluation of responses to the RFP
- Selection of the system
- Conducting vendor negotiations
- Oversight of system implementation

Analysis of System Requirements

Although the decision has been made to purchase a system rather than develop a system, this does not obviate the need for an analysis effort. This process of identifying user requirements and determining system capabilities is essentially the same as in the system life cycle. The steering committee may assign members of the committee analysis responsibilities, delegate these to in-house information system professionals, or contract with consultants to perform the function. No matter who is chosen to perform the function, the steering committee still has the final responsibility for the analysis process.

A detailed analysis document should be prepared. A benefits realization process should be identified and developed at this point, as well as the feasibility of the proposed system together with estimates of cost and benefits.

The results of analysis provide the foundation from which system functionality is determined. They also provide the basis for developing the function specifications of the RFP and the criteria by which vendor products are evaluated. Because of its importance, the analysis document should be complete and accurately reflect user requirements.

Development of System Specifications

System specifications include both the functional and the technical specifications of the system—the logical and physical descriptions of the system. Among logical system specifications are those related to output, input, processing, database, and security design. Physical specifications include details of hardware, database, communication, and control needs. Training needs and implementation requirements are initially identified at this time. The details of system specification are later translated into the functional requirements section of the RFP document. Therefore, it is important that specifications be appropriate, complete, and accurate.

Development and Distribution of the Request for Proposal

After the analysis has been performed and system specifications identified, the RFP is prepared. The RFP is usually a lengthy document. Depending on the complexity of the system, an RFP can be several hundred pages long. Although format varies, an RFP usually includes the following sections:

- Proposal information and format
- Enterprise profile
- Conditions of response
- Functional requirements
- Technical requirements
- Training requirements
- Implementation requirements
- Vendor profile
- System costs

An RFP is a professionally prepared document. It is important that it be correct in all areas because sometimes it also functions as a legal document. Many times, the RFP and the response of the vendor who wins the bid are included in the final contract. Therefore, the importance of the accuracy of the RFP cannot be overemphasized.

Table of Contents

I. General information
  A. Proposal information
  B. Proposal format
II. Enterprise information
  A. Description of the enterprise
  B. Hardware and software environment
  C. Departmental operations
III. Vendor responses
  A. Specific instructions
  B. Functional requirements
  C. Technical requirements
    1. Interface requirements
    2. Processing environment requirements
    3. Support and maintenance requirements
    4. Installation requirements and approach
    5. Training requirements
  D. Vendor background
  E. System costs and financing arrangements
  F. Contractual arrangements

FIGURE 9-12 Typical request for proposal table of contents.

Disclaimer and Table of Contents

An RFP usually begins with a disclaimer that the information contained in the document is considered proprietary and is to be considered in strict confidence and that no information contained in it can be disclosed without written permission from the organization issuing the RFP. A table of contents that functions as an index to the RFP is usually included. Figure 9-12 shows the table of contents of a typical RFP.

Proposal Overview

After the table of contents, an overview of the proposal is usually presented. Here the proposal format, timetable, and requirements for proposal submission are detailed. One of the most important parts of this section is the proposal timetable. Here, milestones of the process are listed with associated time frames. The time frames in each proposal vary, depending on the complexity of the system being considered and on organizational constraints.

Enterprise Profile

The next section of the RFP usually contains a profile of the enterprise. This consists of a brief description of the organization and its demographic data. Statistics such as bed size, occupancy rate, and number of admissions, discharges, procedures, and outpatient visits are frequently provided. These data provide the vendor with a perspective of the facility's volume of data and transactions. General information about the facility services and organization department operations is included. The current hardware and software environments are detailed in this section as well. This includes specifics about what type of hardware is in place, what applications are running, and who the developers of each application are. This provides vendors with important information to determine whether their products can easily interface with current applications or operate under the current hardware environment.

This section also includes a description of activities of all departments that are planning to use the proposed information system. These descriptions provide an overview of current departmental operations and usually include appropriate statistics related to work volumes that may affect system performance requirements.

Conditions of Response

In this section, guidelines to the vendors for response to the proposal are provided. This typically contains information about what format should be used, the date and time the response is to be submitted, detailed instructions for completing each section of the proposal, and the name and telephone number of the person to contact if questions arise.

Functional Specifications

The functional specifications together with the technical requirements section are the heart of the RFP. In this section, all system functionality is listed. Various formats are used to allow vendors to indicate whether their product has the desired functionality. The format of the response usually allows the vendor to indicate whether the feature is currently developed and operational, can be custom developed, is planned to be developed, or is not available. The length of and areas covered in the functional specification section depend on the system under consideration. For example, if a total hospital information system is being considered, there will be a listing of hospital-wide systems such as the EHR and a subsection for almost every hospital department—for example, subsections for clinical laboratory, radiology, admission, HIM, and nursing. Functional specifications for a decision support system intended to support managerial personnel specifications would be limited to such areas as cost accounting, case mix, and budgeting. Functional specifications for a clinical decision support system would link strongly to the clinical components of the system and add features to support clinical decision making. Figure 9-13 provides a use case for electronic signatures as part of an EHR system, and Figure 9-14 provides an example of the business rules associated with the electronic signature of a particular document (Consult) with the EHR system. Figure 9-15 provides sample functional specifications for a pharmacy module, and Figure 9-16 shows sample specifications for an executive decision support system.

A trend for describing functional specifications is to state requirements in a use case or scenario-based format. This format was discussed earlier in this chapter. One format of the use case/scenario-based description is to present the goal of the ideal system, followed by a scenario of current problems. Vendors are asked to explain how their systems will support the general goal and how each will address the problems presented. The following is a brief example of such a format of a point-of-care RFP.

Example of a Point-of-Care Request for Proposal

Following are the goals and problems for our system. Please respond to each by indicating how your system would meet each goal and how it would address each problem.

Goal: Deliver information to nurse caregivers at the patient's bedside.

Problem: Vital signs are taken at the bedside and then written down on a scratch pad by the nurse. The nurse then takes the data to the nursing station and rewrites the data onto the vital signs sheet. The data are then retranscribed and placed in the patient health record. These notes may not be entered into the clinical record until the nurse finishes rounds.

Technical Requirements

The technical requirements section of the RFP contains information about specifications for hardware, software, interfaces, processing environment, and communications. The following is an example of the technical interface requirements needed for a managerial decision support system.

Example of Technical Interface Requirements

1. Explain how your system accommodates the following interfaces:
   - Accept payroll information from a personnel/payroll system
   - Accept cost information from a general ledger system
   - Update general ledger system with budget information
   - Accept detail charge, payment, and patient information from patient billing, receivables, and registration systems
2. For those interfaces provided by you, describe the following:
   - Who writes the interface
   - Who maintains the interface
   - Language used for the interface

In this section, vendors are expected to provide information about the performance of their systems. They may also be asked to submit samples of their system documentation, such as technical system, user, installation, and operations manuals. Support and maintenance details are also requested. For example, the RFP may ask the vendor to supply the following information:

- Indicate the location of personnel who would be assigned to the maintenance function.
- Describe the type of support the company is capable of providing on a continuing basis.
- Describe the means of support, such as hotlines, dial-up services, e-mail, and direct interactive support.
- Describe the procedure for requesting application software changes.

Installation and Training Requirements

In this section, vendors are requested to submit their installation work plans. Vendor responsibility, length of installation, customer responsibility, and skill level of installation

Organization: Community Behavioral Health Center

Use case name: Electronically sign documents and entries in the EHRS
Date:
Use case #:
Version #:

Iteration: Focused

Summary: Only individuals authorized to create entries/documents in clinical records or authorized to review entries/documents in clinical records may sign the entries/documents. Each authorized signer must also be an authenticated user in the system. Signatures will be designated as required on certain clinical entries/documents. Certain individuals will require a cosigner on their clinical entries/documents. Certain individuals will have the authority to cosign. Certain individuals will be able to sign independently.
This organization has a number of interns in their professional fields who will require cosignatures to demonstrate supervision of their work.
The organization will use the signature(s) as a means of finalizing and locking the entry/document so that it cannot be changed without invoking an amendment process.

Basic course of events:

1. Authenticated user who is also authorized to document in the clinical record enters the electronic health record system.
2. User finds correct client/patient, one that he/she is associated with as a caregiver or administrative contact.
3. User identifies correct category for documentation of entry/document.
4. User completes the entry/document the client/patient.
5. User electronically signs and locks the entry/document.
6. Entry document is made available in the system to all legitimate users.

Alternative paths:

1. User clinician dictates the entry/document into the organization's dictation system.
2. Another user, designated as a transcriber, transcribes the document.
3. The transcribed document is placed in a queue or electronic "to do" list for the user clinician to review and sign. If the clinician is satisfied with the document, the path goes back to #5 in the basic path. If the clinician is not satisfied with the document, it is routed back to the transcriber for revision and then the document is again listed on the "to do" list for review and signature.
4. If the entry or document needs a cosignature (and a cosignature may be for a variety of reasons), then at step #5 in the Basic Course the entry/document would be placed on the cosigner's "to do" list for review and signature.
5. The cosigner reviewer may change the entry/document and sign it or may send it back to the original author of the entry/document for revision, Once it is revised it would again go the "to do" list of the cosigner reviewer for review and signature. Once signed by the reviewer the document is "locked" and the document is made available to all legitimate users.

Exception paths: If entry remains unsigned for a period of time clinician is renotified through "to do" list. If entry remains unsigned for more than 2 weeks the clinician's manager is notified. If clinician is no longer available to sign (resigned, etc.) then the manager reviews entry, determines its appropriateness and may sign as the reviewer which allows the entry/document to be accessible to other legitimate users.

Extension points:

Trigger: The user attempts to document in the EHRS and sign the entry/document.

Assumptions: The act of signing electronically signing the document "locks" the document when the authorized individual can sign independently or when a required reviewer signs.

Precondition: The EHRS is operational and the user has authorized access.

Postconditions: The signed entries are available to all authorized EHRS users.

Related business rules: Designation of who is authorized to document in the clinical record. Identification of which users or users types require cosignatue. Amendments/corrections to locked documents.

Author:

Date:

FIGURE 9-13 Use case for electronic signatures.

Sample Business Rules for Electronic Consult Documents
1. An unsigned consult may be deleted by a provider who is also an author/dictator.
2. An unsigned consult may be deleted by a clinical student who is also an author/dictator.
3. An uncosigned consult may be viewed by a provider who is also an expected signer/cosigner.
4. An uncosigned consult may be printed by a clinical student who is also an author/dictator.
5. An uncosigned consult may be printed by a provider who is also an expected cosigner.
6. An uncosigned consult may be edited by a provider who is also an expected signer/cosigner.
7. An unsigned consult may be viewed by a provider who is also an author/dictator.
8. An unsigned consult may be viewed by a clinical coordinator.
9. A completed consult may be viewed by an authorized user.
10. A completed consult may be viewed by a provider.
11. A completed consult may be viewed by a clinical student who is also an author/dictator.
12. An unsigned consult may be printed by a manager HIM.
13. An uncosigned consult may be amended by a provider who is also an expected cosigner,
14. An unsigned consult may be deleted by a manager HIM.
15. An unsigned consult may be viewed by designated HIM staff.
16. A completed consult may have its title changed by a manager HIM.

FIGURE 9-14 Business rules for consultation.

Application	Function currently available	Custom available	Planned	Not available
Order may be entered on any terminal by MD, nurse, unit clerk, or pharmacist.				
System automatically notifies individual entering order if drug is not available in hospital formulary.				
All new drug orders are automatically screened against patient's drug profile for possible interactions.				

FIGURE 9-15 Sample functional specifications: pharmacy system.

Application	Function currently available	Custom available	Planned	Not available
System allows for user-defined product lines.				
System stores a standard treatment profile for a product.				
System allows for online review and modification of standard treatment profiles.				

FIGURE 9-16 Sample functional specifications: executive decision support system.

personnel are described. Training requirements are also outlined in this section. Vendors are asked to describe the training they provide in areas of application usage, system operations, and continuing training. A description of training techniques and samples of training materials may also be requested. Vendors may be asked to describe what resources are needed for training (e.g., type of site), the number of people they will train, and the training time. All costs associated with training should be requested.

Vendor Profile

In any selection process, it is extremely important to ascertain the stability of the vendor. Too often facilities purchase systems only to have the vendor go out of business, leave the marketplace for some reason, or be acquired by another company. To minimize risk to the client, a thorough background analysis of the vendor should be done.

Information requested in the vendor profile includes demographic data, such as number of employees, number of support personnel, number of employees with installation experience, years the system has been available, and the number of systems installed. Vendor annual reports should be requested, including total revenues for several years, research and development expenditures, and systems contracted within the past few years. The facility may also want to ask whether a user group exists and, if so, how frequently it meets and how many members it has.

System Costs and Financing Arrangements

A system cost schedule should be prepared for both lease and purchase options. For each item in the schedule, the vendor should be requested to indicate the one-time cost, annual maintenance, and total cost over a certain period (e.g., 5 years). Among the categories in the cost schedule are hardware, software, software installation, software maintenance, custom development and interfaces, training, and consulting fees.

Contractual Information, References, and Other Materials

A sample copy of all contracts and addenda that are required for the facility to contract for the proposed system should be requested. It should be noted in the RFP that the facility reserves the right to negotiate the final terms and conditions of any resulting agreements. References for facilities that are using the vendor's product should be requested. The vendor should be asked to supply a list of all installations of their product, the contact person at each of these sites, and whether the site can be available for a visit. Any other manuals or references that the vendor may want to provide can be added in this section.

Distribution of the Request for Proposal

After the RFP has been developed, it is ready for distribution to the vendors. Before distribution, a short list of vendors who probably have systems that will meet functionality specifications is identified. The short list is usually compiled from information received during the RFI process. Remember that for every RFP that is sent, a potential response is possible. Because responses tend to be longer than the RFP itself, review of these can be costly and time-consuming. The facility will want to send out an RFP only to vendor candidates who are truly viable. The number of RFPs distributed depends on the vendor market. Once distributed, the RFP timetable is invoked, and the process follows the time line prescribed in the RFP document.

Evaluation Criteria

Before distribution of the RFP, the steering committee develops evaluation criteria for analyzing and comparing vendor responses. Many methods are used for evaluation, and the type used depends on the system scope and individual preference of the facility. The following general categories of evaluation are usually considered:

Hardware/software configuration
• Processing options • Ease of use • Potential to handle projected volume increases • Proven system • Quality of sample documentation
Functions and features
• Number or percentage or required functions/features currently accommodated • Number or percentage of required functions/features that can be custom developed • Quality of sample documentation
Economic considerations
• One-time installation cost • Recurring costs • Consulting charges • Conversion costs • Other costs
Technical considerations
• Reliability and performance • Security • Architecture • Interface capabilities
Vendor considerations
• Support and training • Contract flexibility • Financial stability • Management strength

FIGURE 9-17 Evaluation criteria.

- Hardware and software configuration
- Application functions and features
- Economic considerations
- Technical considerations
- Vendor considerations (Figure 9-17)

Some type of weighting scheme or priority measurement is assigned to each item within a category. One method of evaluation is to develop a weighting scale. The scale may range in value from 1 to 5. Each characteristic is then assigned a weight in relation to its importance. For instance, a hospital may consider security an extremely important item for its system. In this case, on a scale of 1 to 5, security may be assigned the weight of 5, which is the highest weight on the scale. On the other hand, management strength under vendor considerations may not be a highly valued characteristic, and this item may be assigned a lower weight of 2.

In addition to weighting each characteristic, each vendor's response can be evaluated by use of a Likert scale. This is usually referred to as scoring. For example, a scale of 1 to 3 might be used. If the vendor responded that the system currently had a required feature, then 3 points would be assigned for that option. If the vendor could custom configure the feature, then 2 points would be assigned. If the vendor has plans for the feature to be developed in the future, then 1 point would be assigned. If the system does not include the feature, then 0 points would be assigned. The weighted value of each characteristic is usually multiplied by the vendor's score for that feature, resulting in a weighted score for each characteristic. The weighted score is then added across all features to arrive at a final weighted score for each vendor. Table 9-10 shows

TABLE 9-10 Weighted Scores for Pharmacy Information System Vendors

FUNCTIONS	SCORE*			WEIGHTED SCORE	
	Weight†	Vendor A	Vendor B	Vendor A	Vendor B
Order may be entered on any terminal by physician, nurse, unit support staff member, or pharmacist.	5	3	3	15	15
System automatically notifies person entering order if drug is not available in hospital formulary.	3	2	3	6	9
All new drug orders are automatically screened against patient's drug profile for possible interactions.	4	2	3	8	12
Total weighted scores				29	36

*Score: 3, currently has; 2, can customize; 1, plans to have.
†Weight: 5, essential; 4, very important; 3, important; 2, somewhat important; 1, nice to have.

how a weighted score would be calculated for the set of sample functional characteristics for a pharmacy system. Table 9-10 compares the products of Vendor A with those of Vendor B. The calculations indicate that, overall, Vendor B's product appears to offer more functionality than Vendor A's product, given the preestablished weights.

There is no specific checklist of evaluation criteria that can be applied to every vendor product. Therefore, the categories listed in Figure 9-17 must be expanded or contracted depending on the system that is being evaluated. For example, if the product being evaluated were a laboratory information system, the specific functional requirements would include those listed in Table 9-11. However, if the system being evaluated were a different product, the vendor evaluation criteria would be different.

There is not total agreement that the use of a weighting scheme such as that just described provides the best comparison method. For example, one vendor may score higher than all other contenders, but the product may in fact be mediocre in most categories. It is important, therefore, to look at the scores of each criterion individually as well as the overall weighted scores. In reality, such a weighting method is only one input into the total decision process. The weighting process can also be helpful if individuals score the systems independently and then compare and discuss their reasons for the scoring. This should lead to more clarity and an opportunity to identify those vendors that are front runners in the selection process.

Use of a checklist of features and requirements against which vendors measure their own products has several drawbacks. One drawback of the checklist method is that frequently the scoring method of criterion evaluation does not ensure that the best product receives the highest score. Another drawback of the checklist method is that only the vendor's viewpoint is represented. Although this viewpoint is necessary, it may be biased.

Another shortcoming of the checklist method is that it is a static technique. This means that the features or

TABLE 9-11 Sample Functional Specifications for Laboratory Information System

Functional Specification	Currently Available	Custom Available	Planned	Not Available
1.1. Order processing				
1.1. Test request with automatic accessioning				
1.2. Duplicate order checking				
2.1. Specimen collection				
2.1. Automatic generation of label				
2.2. Generation of specimen bar code labels at collection point				
2.3. Specimen location printed on label				
3.1. Result reporting				
3.2 Electronically transmit results using national standards (HL7, LOINC)				
3.3 Interface with electronic health record system to report results				
3.4 Electronically transmit FAX results when needed				
3.5 Print reports remotely for different locations as needed				
3.6 Result inquiry by patient name				
3.7 Result inquiry by patient medical record number				
3.8 Remote verification of test status.				
3.9 Remote transmission of results via phone				

requirements listed on the checklist might exist in the product, but there is no way to evaluate how these features work together. Therefore, demonstration use cases or scenarios are included in many RFPs to try to minimize the static nature of the checklist method. Demonstration use cases or scenarios are "stories" or simulations of processes that the system is expected to accommodate. For example, in a laboratory information system a demonstration use case/scenario might describe processes for ordering test procedures, reporting test results, or printing work lists and reports. For example, an electronic signature scenario in a university hospital would illustrate that documents such as the history and physical may require two signatures to reflect the author clinician and the supervising physician.

Demonstrations and Site Visits

Demonstrations

After responses to the RFP have been reviewed, the steering committee culls the list of vendors. The vendors that come out highest in the evaluation process are invited to present demonstrations of their products. The demonstrations usually take place at the facility and, depending on system complexity, may last several hours to 1 to 2 days. Before the demonstration, the steering committee should have established a demonstration schedule. This schedule should include a list of all functions to be demonstrated and a schedule of end users who are to witness the demonstration. A set of evaluation criteria (e.g., apparent ease of use, interface flexibility, evaluation of inputs and outputs) should be developed by the steering committee. These criteria are then applied by the end users to evaluate the demonstration. Other methods, such as focus groups, can be used to debrief end users and gather their opinions about system functionality. All opinions and evaluations should be documented and evaluated by the steering committee. This evaluation will probably result in some vendors being eliminated from consideration.

Site Visits

After demonstrations have taken place, the steering committee usually schedules site visits to observe the vendor product in production mode. Site visits take place at facilities where the vendor product is installed. Usually 1 to 2 days are arranged for each site visit. The site visit team should have a visit protocol prepared in advance. The protocol should allow formal and informal observations of the system and discussion with end users at the selected site. This may be the only opportunity the team has to view the system in production mode. Therefore, it is extremely important that the site protocol is complete and affords the best possible opportunity for overview of the system and its management. After each site visit, the steering committee should be debriefed. Evaluations should be compiled. Discrepancies between what was reported in the vendor response to proposal and what

was observed in production mode should be noted and investigated. A site visit may illustrate how a facility is using the vendor system and the fit may closely follow and be a good fit for the workflow processes of that organization; however, the workflow processes of the organization shopping for a vendor may be very different or the site visit facility may not be using all modules of the vendor software. These differences should be discussed in the context of workflow and fit.

System Selection and Contract Negotiation

After all data have been gathered, demonstrations held, and site visits completed, the steering committee should be ready to select a vendor product. When a product has been selected, contract negotiations begin. The contractual process is extremely important because it lays down the rules through which the client and vendor are to operate. In complex installations, the vendor and health care facility are partners for months or even years. Therefore, it is important that the contract minimizes risk to both parties. Commonly, a special team is formed to carry out contract negotiation. Members of the team should have negotiation experience. Representatives from administration, information systems, legal counsel, and significant others are usually included in the facility negotiation team. It is important that the leaders of both the vendor and the facility teams be authorized to make decisions for their respective businesses.

The negotiation of a good contract is one of the most important elements in ensuring a successful system installation. The following items are usually part of any software contract:

- Identification of products and services: This should include detailed specifications for the software and support materials to be licensed.
- License grant: This includes the scope of rights to be transferred, the number of sites, and intellectual property rights.
- Delivery terms: This includes such things as time and date of delivery, method of delivery, schedule of delivery, and recourse for damages or slippage.
- Installation: This includes such items as site preparation, timing of installation, and training.
- Warranties: This includes such items as express and implied warranties, scope and term of warranties, and conditions on warranties.
- Remedies and liability: This includes such items as limitations on liability and types of liability.
- Acceptance and testing: This includes such items as how the system will be tested, timing of testing, and specifications for testing.
- Price and payments: This includes method of payment, such as lump sum or spaced payments, conditional payments, royalties, taxes, and prices for updates or modifications, service, or maintenance.

- Term and termination: This includes such items as effective date of agreement; notice of breach, insolvency, or bankruptcy; and termination for cause.
- Support and maintenance: This may include such items as training, documentation, maintenance, emergency and preventive maintenance, and access to source code.

It is important to remember that a contract is a binding document. Therefore, software contracts should be negotiated by a team of people who have expertise in both legal and technological arenas. No matter how small the contract in monetary terms, the health care facility should always seek legal advice before signing any software contract. Entering into an initial contract with a vendor may lead to a long working relationship.

OPERATION/MATURITY PHASE

Investing in software for an EHR or other major components of health care systems is a major commitment. The organization must fund the ongoing operation and upgrades to health care systems and the people to support and use the systems. Systems will need to be redesigned and upgraded on a regular basis. Use of the systems will change the delivery of care. Users must continue to be involved in the systems process. As users become more sophisticated they will expect more of an information system. New technology emerges. Maintenance and system upgrades will require analysis, planning, testing, implementation, and evaluation. And so the cycle continues.

CHAPTER REVIEW

1. Give examples of activities in the life-cycle phases of design, implementation, and operation.

2. Why does the discontinuity of life-cycle phases cause stress in an organization? Give examples of how the stress might manifest itself.

3. System implementation relies heavily on good planning. List several examples of plans that need to be developed to ensure a smooth system implementation.

4. Why is system evaluation after implementation important?

5. Describe and give an example of benefits realization as a component of the systems process.

6. What is the purpose of a request for proposal (RFP)? What information should it contain?

REFERENCES

1. Murphy G, Hanken MA, Waters K: *The electronic health record: changing the vision,* Philadelphia, 1999, Saunders/Elsevier.
2. http://www.healthit.gov/sites/default/files/tools/nlc_change management-primer.pdf.
3. ibid.
4. Kloss L: The politics of information system integration, *JAHIMA* 68:18, 1997.
5. Murphy G, Anderson E: An organizational model for data access and management—work in progress, *JAHIMA* 65:52, 1994.
6. http://www.cms.gov/Regulations-and-Guidance/Legislation/EHRIncentivePrograms/Certification.html.
7. https://www.cchit.org/about.
8. Payne TH: *Practical guide to clinical computing systems: design, operations and infrastructure,* Amsterdam, 2008, Elsevier, p. 5.
9. Bogue R: *Anatomy of a software development role:* http://www.developer.com/img/articles. (Accessed 01.01.06.).
10. Martin MP: *Analysis and design of business information systems,* New York, 1991, Macmillan.
11. Nolan RL: Managing the crisis in data processing, *Harv Business Rev,* 1979, March-April.
12. Whitten J, Bentley L, Dittman K: *Systems analysis and design methods,* ed 6, Boston, 2007, McGraw-Hill.
13. Davis F: User acceptance of information technology: system characteristics, user perception and behavioral impacts, *Int J Man Machine Stud* 38:475–487, 1993.
14. Ciotti V: Applying TQM/CQI principles to information system selection, *Healthcare Fin Man* 49:56, 1995.
15. Dennis A, Wixon BH, Tegarden D: Systems analysis and design with UML, *version 2.0,* Hoboken, 2005, Wiley & Sons.
16. Kulak D, Guiney E: *Use cases: requirements in context,* Boston, 2000, Addison Wesley.
17. Daigrepont J, McGrath D: *Complete Guide and Toolkit to Successful EHR Adoption,* Chicago, 2012, HIMSS, p. 15.
18. http://www.hrsa.gov/healthit/toolbox/RuralHealthITtoolbox/Project/skillsehr.html.
19. Electronic Health Record (EHR) Implementation Go-Live Planning Checklist, Checklist Provided By:The National Learning Consortium (NLC), Developed By: Health Information Technology Research Center (HITRC), Doctor's Office Quality Information Technology (DOQ-IT).
20. http://www.ddcmultimedia.com/doqit/EHR_Adoption/Evaluate_Improve/L1P6.html.
21. Freidman CP, Wyatt JC: *Evaluation methods in biomedical informatics,* New York, 2006, Springer.

STATISTICS AND DATA PRESENTATION

Valerie J.M. Watzlaf

ⓔ Student Study Guide activities for this chapter are available on the Evolve Learning Resources site for this textbook. Please visit http://evolve.elsevier.com/Abdelhak.

CHAPTER CONTENTS

OBJECTIVES

After reading this chapter, the reader will be able to do the following:

✓ Compute health care statistics, including mortality and morbidity rates, autopsy rates, measures of central tendency, and dispersion, and determine the most appropriate use of these health care statistics in health information management.

✓ Organize data generated from health care statistics into appropriate categories, including nominal, ordinal, discrete, and continuous.

✓ Display data generated from health care statistics using the most appropriate tables, graphs, and figures, including frequency tables, bar graphs, histograms, Pareto diagrams, pie charts, and frequency polygons.

✓ Determine which tests of significance should be used to test specific hypotheses and which are most appropriate for certain types of data.

KEY WORDS

Alternative hypothesis	Fetal death rate	Morbidity rates	Proportion
Anesthesia death rate	Frequency distribution	Mortality rates	Random sample
Autopsy rate	Frequency polygon	Neonatal death rate	Range
Average daily inpatient census	Gross death rate	Net death rate	Rate
Average length of stay	Histogram	Nominal data	Ratio
Bar graph	Hypothesis	Nosocomial infection rate	Ratio data
Bed turnover rate	Incidence	Null hypothesis	Regression analysis
Census statistics	Incidence rate	Ordinal data	Sampling error
Coefficient of variation	Infant death rate	p value	Standard deviation
Community-acquired infection	Inpatient bed occupancy rate	Pearson correlation coefficient	Standardized mortality ratio
Comorbidity	Interval data	Percentage	Stratified random sample
Confidence interval	Length of stay	Percentage of occupancy	Systematic sampling
Contingency table	Level of significance	Pie chart	Test statistic
Continuous data	Maternal death rate	Postoperative death rate	Tests of significance
Direct method of age adjustment	Mean	Postoperative infection rate	Variance
Discrete data	Median	Prevalence	Vital statistics
Dispersion	Mode	Prevalence rate	Weighted mean

ABBREVIATIONS

AIDS Acquired Immunodeficiency Syndrome
ALOS Average Length of Stay
ANOVA Analysis of Variance
CV Coefficient of Variation
dfb Degrees of Freedom, Between Groups
dfw Degrees of Freedom, Within Groups
DRG Diagnosis-Related Group
HIM Health Information Management

ICD *International Classification of Diseases*
MSB Mean Square Between Groups
MSW Mean Square Within Groups
NCHS National Center for Health Statistics
SMR Standardized Mortality Ratio
SSB Sum of Squares Between Groups
SSW Sum of Squares Within Groups

OVERVIEW OF STATISTICS AND DATA PRESENTATION

Health care organizations continuously generate health care data. These data are used internally by patients, medical staff, nursing staff, and physical, occupational, and speech therapists and externally by state and federal regulatory agencies, The Joint Commission, and insurance companies, to name just a few. No matter whom the user may be, statistics and data presentation focus on answering the user's questions while complying with the standards of the health care facility. To accomplish this goal, various methods are used to calculate specific types of statistics. Different rates, ratios, proportions, and percentages are used to evaluate mortality, autopsy, and morbidity rates and census and vital statistics.

Organizing and displaying health care data are necessary. To choose appropriate methods of displaying and analyzing data, the health information management (HIM) professional must identify the level of measurement (nominal, ordinal, interval, or ratio) for variables and determine whether data are continuous or discrete. Measures of central tendency (mean, median, and mode) and dispersion (variance and standard deviation) and tests of significance are used to describe and analyze data. It is also important for the HIM professional to understand basic principles of sample size determination and to be familiar with commonly used statistical tests such as analysis of variance (ANOVA), correlation, and regression.

This chapter explains basic and advanced health care statistics that are used in the health care field. Each statistic is defined and the formula for calculating each statistic is provided along with examples of how each statistic is used. Various methods of displaying data are described and illustrated.

Role of the Health Information Management Professional

Now more than ever, health care data are being collected to serve many purposes. One primary purpose is to establish health care statistics to compare trends in incidence of disease, quality and outcomes of care, and management of health information departments; another primary purpose is to conduct epidemiologic research. The HIM professional's goal is to collect, organize, display, and interpret health care data properly to meet the needs of the users. Data can be manipulated in many ways to demonstrate one result or another. HIM professionals need a broad base of knowledge to determine which data elements should be used and when data are being analyzed appropriately or inappropriately. To do this, an understanding of health care and vital and public health statistics is necessary. Furthermore, knowledge of statistical analysis is necessary so that HIM professionals can be the forerunners in data analysis. Because

HIM professionals oversee a vast array of health data, it is imperative that the interpretation of the analysis and results of health care data start with them.

The HIM professional should assume the lead in recommending and using statistical tests that promote improvement in the analysis, use, and dissemination of health care data. The HIM professional fills many diversified roles and responsibilities, such as clinical vocabulary manager, data miner, or clinical trials manager.

In each of these roles, understanding and applying the methods used to collect, analyze, display, interpret, and disseminate data are essential. Responsibilities undertaken in these roles may vary from person to person. For example, the clinical trials manager may play a clearly visible role in cancer research study analysis and interpretation of the data, the clinical vocabulary manager may play a key role in developing vocabularies and standards that can be effectively used in the design of the electronic health record, and the data miner may determine the appropriate databases to use when analyzing clinical and financial data.

The HIM professional may assume other managerial roles in which statistics are used to assess productivity in coding, transcription, correspondence, and record analysis. The HIM professional should have sufficient knowledge and skills to do the following:

- Collect quality health data
- Organize the data into databases
- Statistically analyze the data collected
- Develop, generate, and interpret health care statistical reports

HEALTH CARE STATISTICS

Vital Statistics

Vital statistics include data collected for vital events in our lives, such as births and adoptions, marriages and divorces, and deaths, including fetal deaths. Birth, death, and fetal death certificates are familiar reports to HIM professionals. Birth, death and fetal death information is collected on every birth, death, and fetal death that occurs throughout the United States. Birth certificate information includes demographic data on the child, mother, and father as well as medical and health information regarding the pregnancy and the newborn. Death certificate information includes demographic information on the decedent as well as the place and cause of death. A fetal death is the spontaneous intrauterine death of a fetus at any time during a pregnancy. The fetal death certificate information includes demographic information on the mother and father as well as the cause of the fetal death and any contributing medical and health information on the mother. Although each state can determine the format and content of its certificates, the National Center for Health Statistics (NCHS) recommends standard forms that most states have adopted. The purpose of the NCHS standard forms is to have a national uniform reporting system of vital statistics. These standard forms are revised periodically. The attending physician is responsible for the completion of birth, death, and fetal death certificates. The accurate completion of these certificates is supervised by the HIM department, and a copy of the birth or death certificate is kept in the medical record. A copy of the fetal death certificate is kept in the mother's medical record.

When the certificate is complete, the original is sent to the local registrar, who keeps a copy and forwards the original to the state registrar. At each of these stages, the certificate is checked by the registrar to make sure it is complete. Individuals can obtain from the state registrar certified copies of birth, death, and fetal death certificates. Each state sends electronic files of birth and death statistics to the NCHS. The death statistics are then compiled in the National Death Index. The Death Index is a central computerized index of death record information used for research purposes by epidemiologists and other workers involved in health care research.[1] The natality, or birth, statistics are compiled in the monthly vital statistics reports, and the data files are also available for purposes of research.

Refer to your state health data center or division of vital statistics to receive state-specific information on preparing and registering vital records.

Rates, Ratios, Proportions, and Percentages

A rate is defined as the number of individuals with a specific characteristic divided by the total number of individuals or, alternatively, as the number of times an event did occur compared with the number of times it could have occurred.

A rate contains two major elements: a numerator and a denominator. The numerator is the number of times an event did occur. The number of events under study, or the numerator alone, conveys little information. However, when the numerator is compared with the denominator or the population of people in which the event could have occurred, a rate is determined. The results of a quality improvement study showed that 20 patients with diabetes had a stroke while taking a certain medication. What does this tell you? Should this medication be discontinued in this population? The data provided here include only the numerator. To compute a rate, the denominator is needed—for this example, total number of patients with diabetes who are taking the medication. This particular example included a sample size of 1000 patients. The rate is 20 in 1000 or 2 in 100. A rate is normally expressed in the following manner: 20 in 1000, 2 in 100, 1 in 100,000, 10 in 1,000,000, and so on.

However, rates are also commonly expressed as percentages by converting the rate into a decimal and then multiplying the decimal by 100. A percentage is based on a whole divided into 100 parts. In the preceding example, the rate could also be expressed as a percentage by taking $20/1000 = 0.02 \times 100 = 2\%$ or by taking $2/100 = 0.02 \times 100 = 2\%$. This tells us that 2% of the patients with diabetes (in the study) had a stroke while taking a certain medication. To express a fraction, such as $1/5$, as a percentage, the first step is converting the fraction into a decimal by dividing the numerator, 1, by the denominator, 5, to obtain 0.20. The decimal is then converted into a percentage by multiplying the decimal by 100, which can be accomplished by moving the decimal point two places to the right. The result of this process is 20%.

A **proportion** and a **ratio** are similar to a rate. A proportion, which is a part considered in relation to the whole, is normally expressed as a fraction—$^{20}/_{1000}, ^{2}/_{100}, ^{1}/_{100,000}, ^{10}/_{1000,000}$, and so on. A ratio is a comparison of one thing to another, such as births to deaths or marriages to divorces. A ratio is expressed as 20:1000, 2:100, 1:100,000, 10:1,000,000, and so on. The number of physicians relative to patients or teachers relative to students is normally expressed as a ratio. For example, if a physician group practice has 10 physicians and 1000 patients, the ratio is 10:1000, which reduces to 1:100.

Table 10-1 summarizes examples of rates, proportions, ratios, and percentages.[2,3]

Once percentages are calculated, they can be compared across different subgroups, as seen in Table 10-2. This table

TABLE 10-1	Examples of Ratios, Proportions, Percentages, and Rates		
Ratio	Proportion	Percentage	Rate (per 100,000)
1:100	1/100 = 0.01	1.0	1000 in 100,000
3:10,000	3/10,000 = 0.0003	0.03	30 in 100,000
250:100,000	250/100,000 = 0.0025	0.25	250 in 100,000

TABLE 10-2	Percentage of Elderly by Age (Years): 1990–2025			
Region	Year	Age 65 and Over	Age 75 and Over	Age 80 and Over
Europe*	1990	13.7	6.1	3.2
	2010	17.5	8.4	4.9
	2025	22.4	10.8	6.4
North America	1990	12.6	5.3	2.8
	2010	14.0	6.5	4.0
	2025	20.1	8.5	4.6
Oceania	1990	9.3	3.6	1.8
	2010	11.0	4.8	2.8
	2025	15.0	6.6	3.6
Asia	1990	4.8	1.5	0.6
	2010	6.8	2.5	1.2
	2025	10.0	3.6	1.8
Latin America, Caribbean	1990	4.6	1.6	0.8
	2010	6.4	2.6	1.2
	2025	9.4	3.6	1.8
Near East, North Africa	1990	3.8	1.2	0.5
	2010	4.6	1.6	0.8
	2025	6.4	2.2	1.1
Sub-Saharan Africa	1990	2.7	0.7	0.3
	2010	2.9	0.8	0.3
	2025	3.4	1.0	0.4

*Data exclude the former Soviet Union.
Source: U.S. Bureau of the Census: Center for International Research, International Data Base on Aging.

concisely shows differences among geographic areas in the percentage of elderly people by age categories. It even allows a glance toward the future by projecting percentages from 2010 and 2025. Comparing percentages among areas shows that Europe has the highest percentage of population aged 65 years or older (13.7% in 1990) and that it should remain the world leader for at least the next 3 decades. North America and Oceania also have relatively high percentages of elderly people, which are projected to increase substantially from 1990 to 2025.[4]

DID YOU KNOW?

Did you know statistics are kept on the number of Facebook users, the percent that use Facebook daily, and its yearly revenue increases?

Mortality Rates

Mortality rates are computed because they demonstrate an outcome that may be related to the quality of the health care provided. There are many types of mortality rates. Table 10-3 provides definitions and formulas for the most commonly used mortality rates.[2,3]

Gross Death Rate

The **gross death rate** is a crude death rate for hospital inpatients because it does not consider such factors as age, gender, race, and severity of illness, which also play an important part in death rates. The use of the gross death rate as a measure of quality in health care has been questioned because it does not take these factors into account. As long as the HIM professional is aware that other factors influence this rate and that they have not been taken into account in the calculation, the gross death rate can be a quick, useful means of analyzing mortality in hospital inpatients (see the following example of gross death rate).

Example of Gross Death Rate

The discharge analysis report of Anywhere Health Care Facility shows 752 discharges (including deaths) for October 200X. Twelve deaths were also shown in the report.

Gross death rate:

$$= \frac{12 \text{ inpatient deaths}}{752 \text{ discharges (including deaths)}} \times 100$$

$$= 1.60\%$$

This means that 1.60% of total discharges from Anywhere Health Care Facility during October 200X ended in death or that the gross percentage of deaths, or the hospital death rate, for October was 1.60%.

TABLE 10-3 Mortality Rates	
Rate	Formula
Gross death rate (hospital death rate)	$\dfrac{\text{Total number of inpatient deaths}}{\text{Total number of discharges (including deaths)}} \times 100$
Net death rate	$\dfrac{\text{Total number of inpatient deaths} - \text{Inpatient deaths} < 48\,\text{hours}}{\text{Total discharges (including deaths)} - \text{Deaths} < 48\,\text{hours}} \times 100$
Anesthesia death rate	$\dfrac{\text{Total number of anesthetic deaths}}{\text{Total number of anesthetics administered}} \times 100$
Postoperative death rate	$\dfrac{\text{Total number of deaths (within 10 days of surgery)}}{\text{Total number of patients who received surgery}} \times 100$
Maternal mortality rate	$\dfrac{\text{Total number of direct maternal deaths}}{\text{Total number of obstetrical discharges (including deaths)}} \times 100$
Neonatal mortality rate	$\dfrac{\text{Total number of neonatal deaths}}{\text{Total number of neonatal discharges (including deaths)}} \times 100$
Infant mortality rate	$\dfrac{\text{Total number of infant deaths}}{\text{Total number of infant discharges (including deaths)}} \times 100$
Fetal Death Rates	
Early fetal death (abortion) rate	$\dfrac{\text{Total number of early fetal deaths}}{\text{Total number of births (including early fetal deaths)}} \times 100$
Intermediate fetal deaths	$\dfrac{\text{Total number of intermediate fetal deaths}}{\text{Total number of births (including intermediate fetal deaths)}} \times 100$
Late fetal (stillborn) deaths	$\dfrac{\text{Total number of late fetal deaths}}{\text{Total number of births (including late fetal deaths)}} \times 100$

Note: The numerator and denominator in each formula must be for the same time period.

Net Death Rate

The net death rate is different from the gross death rate because it does not include deaths that occurred less than 48 hours after admission to the health care facility. The net death rate is useful because it provides a more realistic account of patient deaths related to patient care provided by a specific health care facility. For example, a 90-year-old patient arrives at the emergency department with shortness of breath, chest pain, and arrhythmia. After being evaluated, the patient is admitted, and it is determined that he has had a severe myocardial infarction (see the example of net death rate).

Approximately 24 hours later, the patient has cardiac arrest and dies. This particular death would be included in the gross death rate but not the net death rate because it occurred less than 48 hours after admission. Reporting agencies sometimes request net death rates because they may provide a more realistic reflection of patient care provided than gross death rates do. However, net death rates still do not take into consideration other risk factors that may also affect death, such as age, gender, race, and so forth. Therefore, an important note is that health care facilities are not necessarily responsible for deaths that occur more than 48 hours after patients are admitted; on the other hand, health care facilities are not necessarily free of responsibility for deaths that occur within 48 hours of admission. For this reason, some health care facilities do not make use of or report the net death rate.

Another consideration when computing any mortality rate is a health care facility must decide whether newborn inpatients will be included in these calculations. This decision is up to the health care facility; however, if a facility decides that newborn inpatient deaths will be included in the numerator, all newborn discharges must also be included in the denominator.

Example of Net Death Rate

Inpatient deaths at Anywhere Health Care Facility for 200X totaled 50. Inpatient deaths that occurred less than 48 hours after admission to the facility totaled 15. Total discharges (including deaths) were 15,546.

Net death rate:

$$= \dfrac{\begin{array}{c}50\ \text{inpatient deaths}\\ -15\ \text{inpatient deaths} < 48\ \text{hours}\end{array}}{15,546\ \text{discharges (including deaths)}} \times 100$$
$$\quad -15\ \text{inpatient deaths} < 48\ \text{hours}$$

$$= 0.23\%$$

This means that 0.23% (fewer than 1%) of the deaths of discharges for 200X occurred more than 48 hours after admission to the health care facility, or that the net percentage of deaths or net death rate for 200X was 0.23%.

Anesthesia Death Rate

The anesthesia death rate can also be referred to as a cause-specific death rate because the death is determined by a physician or medical examiner to be due to a specific cause (e.g., an anesthetic agent). This rate indicates the number of deaths that are due to the administration of anesthetics for a specified period of time. If the recent anesthetic death rate is higher than the rate in previous periods, a focused evaluation may be necessary to determine why this is so (see the example of anesthesia death rate).

Example of Anesthesia Death Rate

Anywhere Health Care Facility performed 492 surgical procedures during November and administered 452 anesthetics. Deaths resulting from the administration of an anesthetic totaled two for the month.

Anesthesia death rate:

$$= \frac{2 \text{ anesthetic deaths}}{452 \text{ anesthetics administered}} \times 100$$

$$= 0.44\%$$

This means that 0.44% (fewer than 1%) of anesthetics administered resulted in a patient's death, or that the anesthesia death rate for November was 0.44%.

Postoperative Death Rate

The postoperative death rate may be considered a cause-specific death rate as well. This death rate indicates the number of patients who die within 10 days of surgery divided by the number of patients who underwent surgery for the period; therefore, it expresses the number of deaths that may have resulted from surgical complications. In both the anesthesia and the postoperative death rates, other risk factors, such as age, gender, race, and severity of illness, are not considered. Therefore, if it is found that these rates are higher in certain periods than in others, specific evaluations are necessary to determine whether the increase is truly due to the anesthesia or surgery or to other risk factors (see the example of postoperative death rate).

Example of Postoperative Death Rate

Surgery was performed on 492 patients in the Anywhere Health Care Facility during November, and 27 of those patients died within 10 days of surgery.

Postoperative death rate:

$$= \frac{27 \text{ postoperative deaths}}{492 \text{ patients having surgical procedures}} \times 100$$

$$= 5.49\% \text{ or } 5.5\%$$

This means that 5.5% of the patients who underwent surgery died within 10 days of the procedure or that the postoperative death rate for November was 5.5%.

Maternal Death Rate

Death rates are further categorized according to the type of service or department, such as the maternal mortality or death rate. A maternal death results from causes associated with pregnancy or its management but not from accidental or incidental causes unrelated to the pregnancy. The maternal death rate is the number of maternal deaths divided by the number of obstetric discharges. Again, like all the rates described previously, the maternal death rate does not take into account any other risk factors. The maternal death rate is useful because maternal deaths are rare. Therefore, if there is even one maternal death in a period, it is necessary to examine the cause of death in more detail (see the example of maternal death rate).

Example of Maternal Death Rate

Anywhere Health Care Facility had a total of 752 discharges for October, including 120 obstetrical discharges (including deaths) and 1 maternal death.

Maternal death rate:

$$= \frac{1 \text{ maternal death}}{120 \text{ obstetrical discharges (including deaths)}} \times 100$$

$$= 0.83\% \text{ or } 0.8\%$$

This means that 0.8% (fewer than 1%) of obstetrical patients discharged during October died, or that the maternal death rate for October was 0.8%.

Neonatal, Infant, and Fetal Death Rates

The formulas for these rates are given in Table 10-3. Neonatal and infant death rates are computed to examine deaths of the neonate and infant at different stages. A neonatal death is the death of an infant within the first 27 days, 23 hours, and 59 minutes of life. An infant death is death of an infant at any time from the moment of birth through the first year of life. Both of these figures are compared with the number of neonates and infants, respectively, who were discharged and died during the same period.

Fetal death rates are computed to examine differences in the rates of early, intermediate, and late fetal deaths. The definition of early, intermediate, and late fetal deaths may vary from state to state. These deaths are distinguished by the length of gestation or the weight of the fetus.

- Early fetal death (abortion) = less than 20 weeks of gestation or weight 500 grams or less
- Intermediate fetal death = 20 completed weeks of gestation but less than 28 weeks of gestation or weight 501 to 1000 grams
- Late fetal death (stillborn) = 28 weeks of completed gestation and weight more than 1001 grams

See the example of neonatal, infant, and fetal death rates.

Example of Neonatal, Infant, and Fetal Death Rates

Anywhere Health Care Facility developed the following discharge analysis report for 200X. A segment of the report shows the following:

Live births 127
Neonatal discharges 115
Neonatal deaths (before 28 days) 2
Infant discharges 50
Infant deaths (before 1 year and at or after 28 days) 5
Intermediate fetal deaths 13

Neonatal mortality rate:

$$= \frac{2\,\text{neonatal deaths}}{115\,\text{neonatal discharges} + 2\,\text{neonatal deaths}} \times 100$$

$$= 1.71\% \text{ or } 1.7\%$$

This means that 1.7% of the neonates discharged/died or that the neonatal mortality rate for 200X was 1.7%.

Note: Because the intermediate fetal death rate is most commonly used, an example of that rate is given.

Intermediate fetal death rate:

$$= \frac{13\,\text{intermediate fetal deaths}}{127\,\text{live births} + 13\,\text{intermediate fetal deaths}} \times 100$$

$$= 9.29\% \text{ or } 9.3\%$$

This means that intermediate fetal deaths made up 9.3% of live births (excluding the live births at or before 20 weeks' gestation), or that the intermediate fetal death rate for 200X was 9.3%.

Infant mortality rate:

$$= \frac{5\,\text{infant deaths}}{50\,\text{infant discharges} + 5\,\text{infant deaths}} \times 100$$

$$= 0.09\% \text{ or } 9.1\%$$

This means that 9.1% of infants discharged died, or that the infant mortality rate for 200X was 9.1%.

Using and Examining Mortality Rates

Mortality statistics and trends are analyzed and used in many ways. When trends in mortality are examined, the possible reasons for differences in mortality rates should be considered. The influences can be grouped into three variables: time, place, and person. Changes over time include the following:
- Revisions in the rules for *International Classification of Diseases* (ICD) coding of death certificates
- Improvements in medical technology
- Earlier detection and diagnosis of disease

In relation to place, the following factors influence mortality trends:
- Changes in the environment
- International and regional differences in medical technology
- Diagnostic and treatment practices of physicians

Finally, the following characteristics of groups of people can also influence mortality:
- Age
- Gender
- Race
- Ethnicity
- Social habits (diet, smoking, alcohol intake)
- Genetic background
- Emotional and behavioral health characteristics

All these factors must be taken into consideration when mortality trends are examined within the health care facility or across health care facilities in relation to the quality of care provided.[5]

When examining mortality rates within a specific population, as in the gross and net death rates, it is important to show age-specific rates or to adjust for age. Mortality rates are routinely adjusted for age because it is the most important influence in relation to death. As a person ages, the likelihood that the person will die increases. Age-specific rates can be used, but it becomes difficult to make comparisons of data with four or more age levels or categories. Therefore, age adjustment is performed. Statistically, age adjustment removes the difference in composition with respect to age.[1]

Two methods can be used to perform age adjustment. One is the **direct method of age adjustment**, and the other is the indirect method of age adjustment or **standardized mortality ratio** (SMR). The calculations for these two methods are shown in Table 10-4.

The direct method uses a standard population and applies the age-specific rates available for each population. The expected number of deaths in the standard population is then determined. To use the direct method of age adjustment, age-specific rates must be available for both populations and the number of deaths per age category should be at least five. The indirect method, or SMR, is used more often and can be used without age-specific rates and when the number of deaths per age category is small or fewer than five. Standard rates are then applied to the populations being compared to calculate the expected number of deaths, which is compared with the observed number of deaths.[6]

Because the SMR is used in most national and statewide mortality reports, it is explained in more detail here. For example, in Table 10-5, hypothetical data for hospitals are examined for death rates associated with heart failure and shock.

The actual or observed number of deaths in the hospital is compared with the expected number of deaths. The expected number of deaths is taken from a comparative national database adjusted for age and patient severity for each diagnosis. Table 10-5 shows a sample of the hospitals that treated patients included in the diagnosis, heart failure and shock, and the actual and expected number of deaths. An SMR of 1 means that the number of observed deaths and the number of expected deaths are equal, and therefore the mortality rate

TABLE 10-4   Age Adjustment Methods

Direct Method	Formula
Age-adjusted death rate (A)	$\dfrac{\text{Total expected number of deaths at population A rates}}{\text{Total standard population}} \times \text{Constant}$
Age-adjusted death rate (B)	$\dfrac{\text{Total expected number of deaths at population B rates}}{\text{Total standard population}} \times \text{Constant}$
Compare ages = adjusted death rates for populations A and B	

Indirect Method	Formula
SMR for population A	$\dfrac{\text{Observed deaths in population A}}{\text{Expected deaths in population A at standard rates}}$
SMR for population B	$\dfrac{\text{Observed deaths in population B}}{\text{Expected deaths in population B at standard rates}}$
Compare the two SMRs for populations A and B.	

SMR, Standardized mortality ratio.

TABLE 10-5   Heart Failure and Shock

Hospital	Number of Patients	Actual # of Deaths	Expected Number of Deaths
1	268	23	21.03
2	312	25	33.08
3	155	10	12.16
4	208	8	16.56
5	567	25	40.31
6	199	13	9.56
7	347	36	21.65
8	291	20	18.15
9	455	11	13.45
10	677	32	32.43

is equal to what is expected from national norms. An SMR less than 1 means that the observed deaths are lower than the expected deaths, and therefore the mortality rate is lower than expected from national norms. An SMR of greater than 1 means that the observed deaths are greater than the expected deaths, and therefore the mortality rate is higher than expected from national norms (see the examples of use of SMR).

Example Use of Standardized Mortality Ratio (SMR)

For hospital 1, an SMR of 1.09 means that the hospital had a 9% higher mortality rate for heart failure and shock than is expected from national norms. This is calculated as follows:

$$SMR = \frac{23\,\text{actual deaths}}{21.03\,\text{expected deaths}} = 1.09$$
$$(1.09 - 1) \times 100 = 0.09 \times 100 = 9\%$$

Example Use of Standardized Mortality Ratio

For hospital 4, an SMR of 0.48 means that the hospital had a 52% lower mortality rate for heart failure and shock than is expected from national norms. This is calculated as follows:

$$SMR = \frac{8\,\text{actual deaths}}{16.56\,\text{expected deaths}} = 0.48$$
$$(1 - 0.48) \times 100 = 0.52 \times 100 = 52\%$$

SELF-ASSESSMENT QUIZ

1. Statistics relating to vital events in our lives, such as births and adoptions, marriages, divorces, and deaths, including fetal deaths are called:
   a. Vital statistics
   b. Census statistics
   c. Mortality statistics
   d. Morbidity statistics
2. 50/1000; 50/100; 4/100,000 are all examples of a:
   a. Ratio
   b. Proportion
   c. Percentage
   d. Measures of central tendency
3. An early fetal death occurs at less than 20 weeks gestation or when fetal weight is 500 grams or less. This may also be referred to as a(n):
   a. Abortion
   b. Infant death
   c. Neonatal death
   d. Infant mortality ratio

Autopsy Rates

Autopsy rates are computed so that the health care facility can determine the proportion of deaths in which an autopsy was performed. This enables the facility to examine why a higher or lower autopsy rate may be seen from one month to another. Autopsies are performed to determine the cause of death, to better understand the disease process, or to collect tissue samples, as in patients with Alzheimer's disease. Autopsy rates can be further broken down to show the gross autopsy rate, or the rate of autopsies performed for total inpatient deaths; the net autopsy rate, or the rate of autopsies performed for inpatient deaths, excluding unautopsied coroner cases; and the adjusted hospital autopsy rate or the autopsy rate performed for all deaths of hospital patients whose bodies are available or brought to the hospital for autopsy (those not removed by coroners, medical examiners, and so on). Autopsies may be performed after the deaths of inpatients, outpatients, home care patients, skilled nursing care residents, patients who died at home, previous patients, and so on (see example of hospital autopsy rates). Table 10-6 presents the most commonly used autopsy rates.[3]

Example of Hospital Autopsy Rates

Anywhere Health Care Facility developed the following report regarding discharges, deaths, and autopsies during January 200X.

Hospital Statistics
Discharges (including deaths) 1000
Total deaths 56
    Inpatient (including two coroner cases) 52
    Outpatient 2
    Home care 2
Autopsies 13
    Inpatient 10
    Outpatient 1
    Home care 2

Gross autopsy rate:

$$= \frac{10 \text{ autopsies on inpatients}}{52 \text{ inpatient deaths}} \times 100$$

$$= 19.23\% \text{ or } 19.2\%$$

This means that 19.2% of the hospital inpatients who died during January received an autopsy, or that the gross autopsy rate was 19.2%.

Net autopsy rate:

$$= \frac{10 \text{ autopsies on inpatients}}{52 \text{ inpatient deaths} - 2 \text{ unautopsied coroner's cases}} \times 100$$

$$= 20\%$$

This means that 20% of the hospital inpatients who died during January received an autopsy within the hospital, or that the net autopsy rate was 20%.

Hospital autopsy rate (adjusted):

$$= \frac{13 \text{ total hospital autopsies}}{\substack{52 \text{ inpatient deaths} - 2 \text{ coroner cases} \\ + 2 \text{ outpatients} \\ + 2 \text{ home health care patients} = 54}} \times 100$$

$$= 24.07\% \text{ or } 24.1\%$$

This means that 24.1% of all health care facility patients who died in January (inpatients, outpatients, and home care patients) received an autopsy within the hospital, or that the adjusted hospital autopsy rate was 24.1%.

Morbidity Rates

Morbidity rates can include complication rates, such as community-acquired, hospital-acquired or nosocomial, and postoperative infection rates. They can also include comorbidity rates and the prevalence and incidence rates of disease.

Hospitals use each of these rates to study the types of disease or conditions that are present within the health care facility and to examine the quality of care provided by the facility. These rates can aid health care facilities in planning specific health care services and programs. Table 10-7 provides a summary of the more common morbidity rates and the formulas used to compute them.[3]

Complications include infections, allergic reactions to medications, transfusion reactions, decubitus ulcers, falls, burns, and errors of medication administration. The complication rates for any of these complications can also be computed by using the formula for complication rates listed in Table 10-7.

One of the most common complications is infections. Infection rates are computed so that the health care facility can determine when infections developed and, therefore, how they may be prevented. A nosocomial, or facility-acquired, infection rate includes infections that occur more than 72 hours after admission.[7] Health care facilities may be more interested in this rate because it may show infections that occur as a result of the care that is provided in the facility. Further analysis of the nosocomial infection rate may

---

TABLE 10-6   Autopsy Rates

Autopsy Rate	Formula
Gross autopsy rate (ratio of inpatient autopsies to inpatient deaths)	$\dfrac{\text{Total inpatient autopsies}}{\text{Total inpatient deaths}} \times 100$
Net autopsy rate	$\dfrac{\text{Total inpatient autopsies}}{\text{Total inpatient deaths} - \text{unautopsied coroner's cases}} \times 100$
Hospital autopsy rate (adjusted) Total hospital autopsies 100	$\dfrac{\text{Total hospital autopsies}}{\substack{\text{Number of deaths of hospital patients whose bodies} \\ \text{are available for hospital autopsy}}} \times 100$

Note: Numerators and denominators in each formula must be for the same time period.

TABLE 10-7 Morbidity Rates

Definition	Formula
Complication (condition that occurs during hospital stay that extends length of stay by at least 1 day in 75% of cases)*	$\dfrac{\text{Total number of complications}}{\text{Total number of discharges}} \times 100$
Nosocomial infection rate (infection that occurs >72 hours after admission to hospital)*	$\dfrac{\text{Total number of infections that occur} > 72 \text{ hours after admission}}{\text{Total discharges}} \times 100$
Postoperative infection rate*	$\dfrac{\text{Total number of postoperative infections}}{\text{Total number of discharges}} \times 100$
Community-acquired infection rate (infection that occurs in community or <72 hours of admission)*	$\dfrac{\text{Total number of community-acquired infections that occur} < 72 \text{ after admission}}{\text{Total number of discharges}} \times 100$
Total infection rate (includes both nosocomial and community-acquired infections)*	$\dfrac{\text{Total number of community-acquired and nosocomial infections}}{\text{Total number of discharges}} \times 100$
Comorbidity (preexisting condition that will, because of its presence with principal diagnosis, increase the length of stay by at least 1 day in 75% of cases)*	$\dfrac{\text{Total number of comorbidities}}{\text{Total number of discharges for a given period}} \times 100$
Prevalence (number of people with specific disease at specified period of time; number of existing cases of disease)	$\dfrac{\text{Number of cases of disease present in a population at specified time period}}{\text{Number of people in population at specified time period}} \times 100$
Incidence (number of people with disease during specified time period; number of new cases of disease)	$\dfrac{\text{Number of new cases of a disease occurring in population during a specified time period}}{\text{Number of people in population at specified time period}} \times 100$

*Numerators and denominators in each formula must be for the same time period.

show that other risk factors, such as age, compromising conditions such as cancer, the use of chemotherapy treatment, and the overall severity of the disease, may make an individual patient more susceptible to infection. Therefore, as with several of the mortality rates, other factors play a part in the development of the nosocomial infection. The postoperative infection rate is normally calculated to pinpoint how the infection may have developed. Postoperative infection rates are important to examine because the health care facility can determine which infections occur after surgery and are probably a result of the surgical procedure.

Distinguishing between nosocomial and community-acquired infections is important because community-acquired infections are typically present less than 72 hours before admission to the health care facility. Health care facilities may be interested in this rate because it demonstrates the infections that patients probably had before admission to the facility. If the facility finds that their community-acquired infection rate is high, they may need to develop community-wide prevention programs, such as administering a vaccine for pneumonia. Health care facilities can benefit from analysis of their total infection rate (both nosocomial and community-acquired infections) to determine the additional cost, length of stay, and overall effect the infections have on the quality of care provided to the patient.

Comorbidities are preexisting conditions, such as diabetes, hypertension, and osteoporosis. Analysis of the comorbidity rate is important because comorbidities can increase the length of stay and affect the outcome of care provided.

Comorbidities include some of the other risk factors that affect mortality and morbidity rates.

Morbidity Data for Anywhere Health Care Facility During March 200X

Discharges (including deaths) 2000
  Surgical operations 1543
  Number of comorbidities 238
  Number of complications 120
  Nosocomial infections (includes postoperative infections) 22
  Postoperative infections 8
  Community-acquired infections 30

  Complication rate:
  $$= \dfrac{120 \text{ total complications}}{2000 \text{ discharges (including deaths)}} \times 100$$
  $$= 6.0\%$$

This means that 6.0% of all discharges for March had at least one complication, or that the complication rate for March was 6.0%.

  Nosocomial infection rate:
  $$= \dfrac{22 \text{ nosocomial infections}}{2000 \text{ discharges (including deaths)}} \times 100$$
  $$= 1.1\%$$

This means that 1.1% of all discharges for March had a nosocomial or hospital-acquired infection, or that the nosocomial or hospital-acquired infection rate for March was 1.1%.

Postoperative infection rate:

$$= \frac{8\,\text{postoperative infections}}{1543\,\text{surgical operations}} \times 100$$

$$= 0.52\%$$

This means that 0.5% of all those with surgical operations performed during March developed a postoperative infection, or that the postoperative infection rate for March was 0.5%.

Community-acquired infection rate:

$$= \frac{30\,\text{community-acquired infections}}{2000\,\text{discharges (including deaths)}} \times 100$$

$$= 1.5\%$$

This means that 1.5% of all discharges for March had a community-acquired infection, or that the community-acquired infection rate for March was 1.5%.

Total infection rate:

$$= \frac{52\,\text{total infections}}{2000\,\text{discharges (including deaths)}} \times 100$$

$$= 2.6\%$$

This means that 2.6% of all discharges for March had an infection, or that the total infection rate for March was 2.6%.

Comorbidity rate:

$$= \frac{238\,\text{total comorbidities}}{2000\,\text{discharges (including deaths)}} \times 100$$

$$= 11.9\%$$

This means that 11.9% of all discharges for March had at least one comorbidity, or that the comorbidity rate for March was 11.9%.

Prevalence and incidence rates are determined to examine the frequency of specific types of disease, such as cancer, acquired immunodeficiency syndrome (AIDS), and heart disease. Prevalence means the number of existing cases of disease, whereas incidence refers to the number of new cases of disease (see the examples of prevalence and incidence rate determinants).

The prevalence rate is the number of existing cases of a disease in a specified time period divided by the population at that time. The quotient is then multiplied by a constant, such as 1000 or 100,000.

Example of Prevalence Rate

In a community of elderly people, the number of women alive with osteoporosis in the year 200X is 3593. The population of women in this community is 100,000.

Prevalence rate:
$$= \frac{3593\,\text{women with osteoporosis}}{100,000\,\text{women in population}} \times 1000$$
$$= 35.93, \text{or 36 osteoporosis cases per 100,000 women in this community}$$

The incidence rate is the number of newly reported cases of a disease in a specified time period divided by the population at that time. The quotient is then multiplied by a constant such as 1000 or 100,000.

Example of Incidence Rate

In the same elderly community, the number of new cases of osteoporosis reported in 200X is 1113, and the population of women in the community at that time is 100,000.

Incidence rate:
$$= \frac{1113\,\text{new cases of osteoporosis}}{100,000\,\text{women in this community}} \times 1000$$
$$= 11.13, \text{or 11 new osteoporosis cases per 100,000 women in population}$$

To manage health care services effectively, the HIM professional should analyze prevalence and incidence rates of specific diseases that are prominent within a particular region or state. National sources of morbidity data include the National Health Care Survey. Originated in 1956, this survey is performed annually on a representative sample of 40,000 persons. Many subprograms are part of the National Health Care Survey, such as the National Hospital Discharge Survey, National Hospital Ambulatory and Medical Care Survey, and National Nursing Home Survey. Results of these surveys include incidence and prevalence rates of disease for specific geographic areas, length of hospital stays, cause of hospitalizations, and use of ambulatory care services.[1] The HIM professional should be aware that this information exists and can be used in conjunction with other morbidity rates to analyze further the distribution and effectiveness of health care services.

Characteristics similar to those that influence trends in mortality also influence trends in morbidity—time, place, person. For example, infectious diseases tend to occur more often at specific times of the year. The place of employment or geographic location can also increase susceptibility to disease. Age can influence the occurrence of infectious diseases; for example, diseases such as measles and chickenpox are more common in the young. Gender can influence morbidity trends, with differences in coronary artery disease for men and women. Race also influences morbidity trends, with hypertension being more prevalent in African Americans.[5]

Census Statistics

Ratios, percentages, and averages related to the length of stay, occupancy, bed turnover, and total number of patients present at a specified time within the institution can be useful both to health care administrators and HIM professionals. Such data can be used for the following purposes:
- To evaluate the current status of the health care facility
- To plan for future health care events
- To compare utilization of various units within a health care organization

The census statistics are extremely useful in the overall analysis of how much, how long, and by whom the health care facility is being used. Table 10-8 provides the formulas for the common census statistics[3] (see the example of census statistics).

Example of Census Statistics

A 500-bed health care facility, during the month of June (30 days), had a total of 3600 discharges (including deaths), a total of 14,647 inpatient service days, and a total of 15,567 discharge days.

Inpatient bed occupancy rate (percentage of occupancy)

$$= \frac{14,647 \text{ inpatient services days}}{500 \text{ (beds)} \times 30 \text{ (Number of days in June)}} \times 100$$

$$= 97.6\%$$

This means that 97.6% of the available beds were occupied, or that the inpatient bed occupancy ratio was about 14,647:15,000, or that the percentage of occupancy was 97.6%.

Average daily inpatient census:

$$= \frac{14,647 \text{ inpatient services days}}{30 \text{ (Number of days in June)}} = 488$$

This means that the average number of inpatients during June was 488 or that the average daily inpatient census for June was 488.

Average length of stay:

$$= \frac{15,567 \text{ discharge days}}{3600 \text{ discharges (including deaths)}} = 4.3 \text{ days}$$

This means that patients stayed in the health care facility an average of 4.3 days during June, or that the average length of stay (ALOS) for June was 4.3.

TABLE 10-8   Census Statistics

Definition	Formula
Daily inpatient census (no. of inpatients present at census-taking time plus any inpatients who are both admitted and discharged after census-taking time the previous day).	Formula is presented as the definition.
Inpatient service day (unit of measure including services received by one inpatient in one 24-hour period). Synonyms: patient day, inpatient day, census day, bed occupancy day.	Formula is presented as the definition.
Inpatient bed count (no. of available inpatient beds [occupied and vacant] on any given day. Note: Not all beds are included in the inpatient bed count. These include beds in examination rooms, therapy, labor rooms, and recovery rooms as well as bassinets. (Beds set up for temporary use are not included.)	Formula is presented as the definition.
Average daily inpatient census (average number of inpatients in a facility for a given period of time).	$\dfrac{\text{Total number of service days for a period}}{\text{Total number of days in that period}}$
Length of stay (for an inpatient, number of calendar days from admission to discharge). Synonyms: discharge days, duration of inpatient hospitalization, days of stay. Total length of stay (for all inpatients: total days in facility of any group of inpatients discharged during specified period). Synonyms: discharge days, total inpatients days of stay.	Duration of hospitalization for one inpatient. Day of admission is not counted unless it is the day of discharge or the day of discharge is not counted unless it is the day of admission. Either method is correct if done consistently.
Average length of stay (average length of stay of inpatients discharged during specified period).	$\dfrac{\text{Total length of stay (discharge days)}}{\text{Total number of discharges (including deaths)}}$
Inpatient bed occupancy rates (proportion of inpatient beds occupied, defined as ratio of inpatient service days to inpatient bed count days in specified period). Synonyms: percentage of occupancy, occupancy percentage, occupancy rate.	$\dfrac{\text{Total service days for a period}}{\substack{\text{Total bed count days in the period}\\ \text{(Bed count} \times \text{number of days in period)}}} \times 100$
Bed turnover rate (number of times a bed, on average, changes occupants during a given period of time).	Direct formula: $\dfrac{\text{Number of discharges (including deaths) for a period}}{\text{Average bed count during the period}}$ Indirect formula: $\dfrac{\text{Occupancy rate} \times \text{number of days in period}}{\text{Average length of stay}}$

Example of Census Statistics for Oncology Department

Discharges (including deaths)	1322
Hospital days for discharged patients	10,576
Patient A	admitted June 18 and died the same day
Patient B	admitted June 18 and discharged on June 19
Patient C	admitted on June 19 and discharged June 25
Patient D	admitted June 25 and discharged on August 8

Average length of stay for Oncology Department:

$$= \frac{10,576 \text{ discharge days for oncology patients}}{1322 \text{ discharges from oncology department}} = 8.0 \text{ days}$$

Patients in the Oncology Department stayed an average of 8.0 days during June, or the average length of stay for the Oncology Department for June was 8 days. The Oncology Department average length of stay (8 days) can then be compared with the overall facility length of stay (4 days) and determine why the Oncology Department length of stay is double that of the facility length of stay.

Length of Stay for individual patients

Patient A = 1 day because the patient was admitted and died on the same day

Patient B = 1 day because the patient was admitted one day and discharged the next

Patient C = 6 days by subtracting the date of admission from the date of discharge because the patient was admitted and discharged within the same month

Patient D = 44 days = 5 days in June + 31 days in July + 8 days in August

The individual patient lengths of stay can be compared with one another, especially if the patients received the same services or were from the same department.

Bed Turnover Rate:

Direct method:

$$= \frac{3600 \text{ discharges (including deaths)}}{500 \text{ beds}} = 7.2$$

Indirect method:

$$= \frac{97.6\% \text{ (percentage of occupancy)} \times 30 \text{ days in June}}{4.3 \text{ (average length of stay for June)}}$$

$$= \frac{0.976 \times 30}{4.3} = 6.8$$

This means that during June each of the hospital's 500 beds changed patients about 7.2 times according to the direct method and 6.8 times according to the indirect method—a small difference between the two methods.

SELF-ASSESSMENT QUIZ

4. Fifty-five lymphedema newly diagnosed cases per 1000 women with breast cancer in San Diego is an example of what type of rate:
   a. Prevalence rate
   b. Incidence rate
   c. Mortality rate
   d. Morbidity rate
5. Two-hundred Alzheimer's disease cases per 1000 men under age 50 in Minneapolis is an example of what type of rate:
   a. Prevalence rate
   b. Incidence rate
   c. Nosocomial infection rate
   d. Community-acquired infection rate
6. Ratios, percentages, and averages related to the length of stay, occupancy, bed turnover, and total number of patients present at a specified time within the institution are statistics referred to as:
   a. Infection rates
   b. Mortality rates
   c. Census statistics
   d. Morbidity statistics

ORGANIZING AND DISPLAYING THE DATA[8]

Types of Data

Before deciding how to display data, it is important to recognize that different methods of display are appropriate for different types of data. Variables or data can be grouped into the following four categories on the basis of what kind of information or meaning the numbers convey:

- Nominal
- Ordinal
- Interval
- Ratio

Variables can also be classified as discrete or continuous based on how many possible values the variable can assume.

Nominal Data

The term nominal data is used to describe data collected on variables for which qualitative (what kind) rather than quantitative (how much or how many) differences exist between individuals. Nominal data are also called categorical, qualitative, or named data. Examples of nominal variables include the gender and race of subjects in a research study. To facilitate tabulating and analyzing data, numerical values are often assigned to the categories of nominal variables. Using the variable "gender" as an example, the female category could be coded as "0" and the male category could be coded as "1." The variable employment status could be coded "10" for employed and "9" for unemployed, and so on. It is important to realize the numerical values used to represent nominal data only serve as labels for categories. The values or codes convey no quantitative (how much or how many) information. Therefore, the choice of numerical values is arbitrary; gender could also be coded as 1 for female and 2 for male, and so forth. Table 10-9 shows nominal data for types of treatments for patients with Alzheimer's disease by gender.

Ordinal or Ranked Data

Ordinal data are data expressing rankings from lowest to highest according to some criterion. An example of the use of ordinal data is found in severity of illness scores used in assessing quality of care outcomes. Atlas, a severity of illness system, uses the following ordinal data to describe the severity of illness:

0 = no or minimal risk of vital organ failure
1 = low risk of vital organ failure
2 = moderate risk of vital organ failure
3 = high risk of vital organ failure
4 = presence of vital organ failure

Ordinal data can also include responses to questionnaires or interviews:

1 = strongly disagree
2 = disagree
3 = neutral
4 = agree
5 = strongly agree

Commonplace examples of ordinal data include class rank of graduating high school seniors and the ranking of sports teams within a league. A key feature of ordinal data is that the equal distances between ranks do not necessarily correspond to equal distances on the underlying criterion. For example, the distance between class ranks of 1 and 2 is equal to the distance between class ranks of 3 and 4. However, when we consider the underlying criterion of grade point average, those of the students ranked as 1 and 2 may be closer to each other than are those of the students ranked and 3 and 4. See Table 10-10 for an example of ordinal data

TABLE 10-10 Frequency Table—Ranked Ordinal Data: *Ranked Score Used to Compare the Ability of ICD-10-CM to Capture the Diagnosis

Ordinal Scale	Number of Cases %
5 = Diagnosis is fully captured by code	120 (60.0)
4 = Diagnosis is almost fully captured	40 (20.0)
3 = Diagnosis is partially captured by code	10 (5.0)
2 = Diagnosis is less than partially captured by code	10 (5.0)
1 = Diagnosis is not captured by code	20 (10.0)
Total	200 (100)

*Ranking was determined by examining the number of codes, the level of specificity, and the ability of the code description to fully capture the diagnostic term.

used in a frequency table explaining the use of a ranked score to determine the ability of ICD-10-CM to capture the diagnostic term.

Interval Data

Interval data convey more precise quantitative information than do ordinal data because it is assumed that equal differences between numbers correspond to equal differences in the trait or characteristic being measured. Examples of interval data include scores on college examinations and scores on nationally administered tests such as the SAT (Scholastic Aptitude Test). If Student A received a score of 400 on the verbal section of the SAT, Student B received a score of 450, Student C received a score of 500, and Student D received a score of 550, it is assumed that the difference in verbal aptitude between Student A and Student B is equal to the difference in verbal aptitude between Student C and Student D.

Ratio Data

Ratio data share the property of equal differences with interval data. What is unique about ratio data is that the value of 0 represents the total absence of the trait or characteristic being measured. For example, if the speed of a car when it is stopped at a red light is 0, the value of 0 can be interpreted as the absence of speed; the car is not moving. Other examples of ratio data include height and weight of patients and length of stay at a hospital.

Discrete Data

Discrete data are data on quantitative variables that can only take on a limited number of values, typically only whole numbers. Examples of discrete data include the number of medications a person is taking, the number of children in a family, or the number of records that are coded. See Table 10-11 for an example of discrete

TABLE 10-9 Frequency Table—Nominal Data: Type of Treatment by Gender for Alzheimer's Patients

Treatment	Male (n=200) Number (%)	Female (n=200) Number (%)	Total Number (%)
Cognitive Therapy	26 (13.0)	20 (10.0)	46 (11.5)
Exercise	54 (27.0)	25 (12.5)	79 (19.75)
Medication	50 (25.0)	75 (37.5)	125 (31.25)
Combination of Treatments	68 (34.0)	70 (35.0)	138 (34.5)
Diet Modifications	2 (1.0)	10 (5.0)	12 (3.0)
Total	200 (100)	200 (100)	400 (100)

TABLE 10-11   Example of a Frequency Table—Discrete Data: Records Coded Using Computer-Assisted Coding Software by Type of Admission

Type of Admission	Number of Records Coded Number (%)
Inpatient	50 (50)
Outpatient	10 (10)
Emergency	20 (20)
Skilled Care	20 (20)
Total	100 (100)

BOX 10-1   Guidelines for Displaying Data

Ask yourself what is the main message you wish to convey to the reader and then choose the type of graph that is most appropriate for the information you want to communicate.

Be careful to choose a type of graph that is consistent with the type of data shown in the graph. For example, do not choose a histogram for nominal data.

Create an effective graph that is visually attractive and numerically accurate.

Aim for simplicity; unnecessary detail in a graph can be distracting to the reader.

When applicable, give careful consideration to the scaling of the vertical axis (the minimum and maximum values displayed, and the number of units between consecutive labeled values).

data used in a frequency table on number of records coded using computer assisted coding software by type of admission.

Continuous Data

Continuous data are data on quantitative variables that can assume an infinite number of possible values. Examples include height, weight, temperature, and costs or charges. See Table 10-12 for an example of continuous data for the total cost of hospitalizations at an acute care hospital.

Types of Data Display

Many methods are used to display data effectively (Box 10-1). Some methods of particular value to the HIM professional are frequency distribution tables, bar graphs, pie charts, histograms, frequency polygons, and Pareto diagrams.

Frequency Distribution

A frequency distribution table presents the number of times that each category of a qualitative variable or value of a quantitative variable is observed within a sample. When continuous variables that have a large number of possible values are represented, it is common for the frequencies to be reported in ranges or intervals of values, rather than the frequencies of individual values. For example, a frequency table

representing the age of patients could show the number of patients whose ages are between 20 and 29 years, 30 and 39 years, 40 and 49 years, and so forth. To allow comparisons to be made across samples of varying size, percentages that represent relative frequency are usually reported along with the frequency count. To compute these percentages, the number of observations within a category is divided by the total sample size, and the result is multiplied by 100. The frequency table should be self-explanatory and not show so much data that the table becomes uninterpretable. The table should be clearly labeled, the total sample size displayed, and units of measurement included. When intervals are used, the number of intervals should be not less than 5 and no more than 20, of equal width, with end points of the intervals that are mutually exclusive and do not overlap. Tables 10-9 through 10-12 are examples of frequency distribution tables for nominal, ordinal, discrete and continuous data, respectively.

Bar Graph

Bar graphs are normally used to illustrate nominal, ordinal, and discrete data. The discrete categories are shown on the horizontal, or x, axis and the frequency is shown on the vertical, or y, axis. The purpose of the bar graph is to show the frequency for each interval or category. The scale of the vertical axis must begin at zero so that the heights of the

TABLE 10-12   Frequency Table—Continuous Data: Cost of Hospitalizations at Acute Care Hospital

Cost of Hospitalization ($)	Absolute Frequency	Relative Frequency (%)	Cumulative Frequency	Cumulative Relative Frequency (%)
0-2999	55	33.3	55	33.3
3000-5999	61	37.0	116	70.3
6000-8999	20	12.1	136	82.4
9000-11,999	13	7.9	149	90.3
12,000-14,999	4	2.4	153	92.7
15,000-17,999	3	1.8	156	94.5
18,000-20,999	4	2.4	160	97.0
>21,000	5	3.0	165	100.0

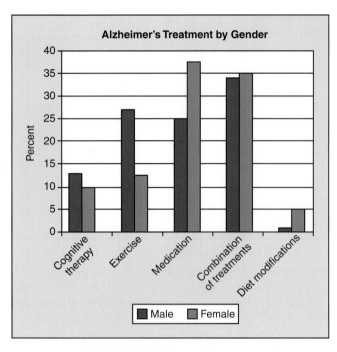

FIGURE 10-1 Bar graph.

bars are proportional to the frequencies. By using different colors or patterns of bars to represent different samples, bar graphs can be used to compare the frequency of categories or intervals in two or more samples. Figure 10-1 is an example of a bar graph using the data in Table 10-9. Other types of bar graphs are shown in Figures 10-2 and

10-3. These graphs are still considered bar graphs but incorporate a line over the bars to show the total number of admissions and number of infections (see Figure 10-2). Also, Figure 10-3 shows the number of Stage IV cases of disease compared to the total cases of disease over time with use of a stacked bar graph.

Pie Chart

A **pie chart** is effective for representing the relative frequency of categories or intervals within a sample. It is constructed by drawing a circle, 360 degrees, and dividing that circle into sections that correspond to the relative frequency in each category. For example, if the relative frequency is 15%, then the slice of pie should span (0.15) × (360 degrees), or 54 degrees. Figure 10-4 is an example of a pie chart based on the data in Table 10-11.

Histogram

Did you know that histograms are usually used for larger data sets or "big data" and are also used to see if a data set is approximately normally distributed.

The **histogram** is usually used to present a frequency distribution for continuous data. It is similar to a bar graph, but the horizontal axis of the histogram usually represents intervals of a continuous variable rather than a discrete variable. Because theoretically there is no separation between the end point of one interval and the starting point of another, the bars of a histogram touch. The heights of the bars correspond to the frequency within each interval. Because intervals are

FIGURE 10-2 Example of bar graph and line graph.

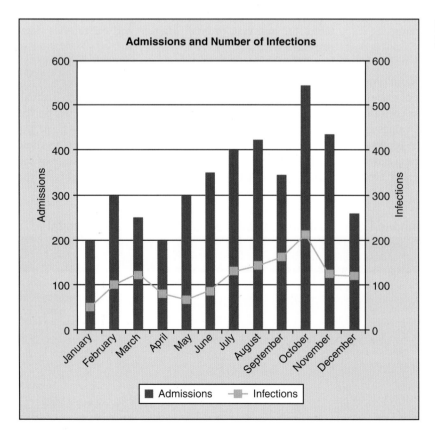

FIGURE 10-3 Example of stacked bar graph.

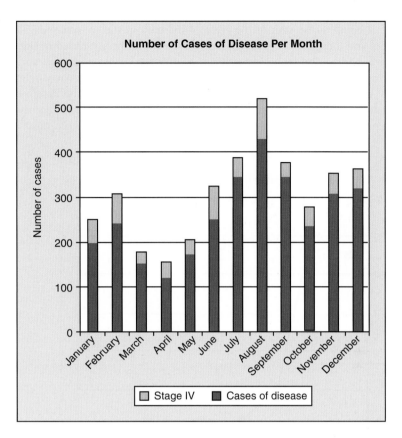

Number of Cases of Disease Per Month

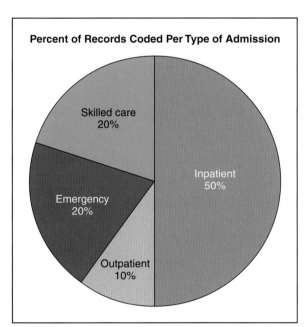

Percent of Records Coded Per Type of Admission

FIGURE 10-4 Pie chart.

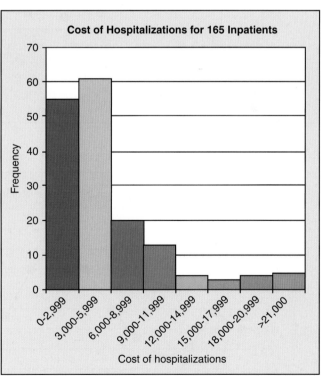

Cost of Hospitalizations for 165 Inpatients

FIGURE 10-5 Histogram.

usually of equal width, the width of all bars of a histogram is usually the same. If the areas (interval width × interval frequency) of all the bars are summed, the result should be equal to the total sample size multiplied by the common interval width. Figure 10-5 is an example of a histogram using absolute frequency data from Table 10-12.

Frequency Polygon

The frequency polygon is another method used to present a frequency distribution with continuous data. It is constructed by joining the midpoints of the tops of the bars of a histogram with a straight line. The total area under the polygon is equal to the sum of the areas of the bars in the histogram and therefore equal to total sample size multiplied by interval width. The frequency polygon is effective when comparing the distribution of a variable in two or more data samples. Figure 10-6 is an example of a frequency polygon using data from Table 10-12. Figure 10-7 is an example of a frequency polygon comparing two data sets.

The reader may find variations of these data presentation methods. For example, statistical process control, which is used in the quality improvement process, uses many of the graphs and figures displayed previously but may change them slightly or call them different things. For example, the Pareto diagram (Figure 10-8) is similar to the bar graph and the histogram and is used to order causes or problems from most to least significant.

FIGURE 10-6 Frequency polygon/line graph.

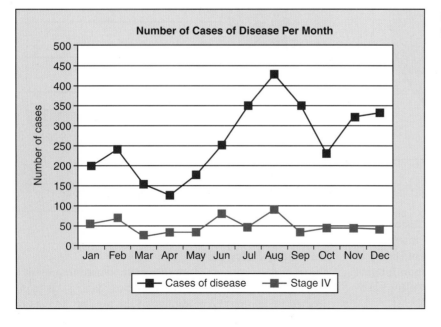

FIGURE 10-7 Frequency polygon comparing two types of data.

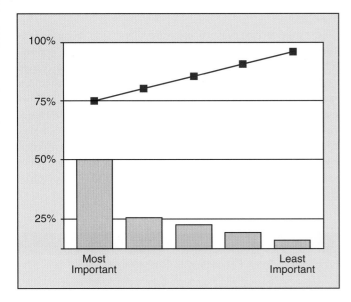

FIGURE 10-8 Pareto diagram.

Measures of Central Tendency

The common measures of central tendency are the following:

- Mean
- Median
- Mode

These measures are used to locate the middle, average, or typical value in a data set. The selection of which one of these measures is most suitable in a given situation depends on the type of data and the purpose for which the measure is being reported.

Mean

The **mean** is the most common measure of central tendency because it is easily understood by audiences and also because determining the mean is a step toward deriving other statistics discussed later, such as the variance and standard deviation. The purpose of the mean is to summarize an entire set of data by means of a single representative value. The mean or average is calculated by adding up the values of all the observations and dividing the total by the number of observations. Sometimes it is necessary to calculate an overall mean for a total sample when separate means are reported for different subdivisions of the sample. In this situation, a **weighted mean** can be calculated, as illustrated in the example that follows.

Example of Mean and Weighted Mean

The lengths of stay in the hospital for eight patients in a pediatric department are 6, 4, 2, 5, 20, 25, 18, and 4 days. The mean, or average, length of stay is calculated as follows:

$$\text{Average length of stay (mean)}:$$
$$= \frac{6+4+2+5+20+25+18+4}{\text{(lengths of stays of each patient)}}$$
$$= \frac{\text{(lengths of stays of each patient)}}{8 \text{ patients}}$$
$$= \frac{84}{8}$$
$$= 10.5 \text{ days}$$

Weighted Mean:

Department	Number of Patients	Average Length of Stay (days)
Internal medicine	40	6
General surgery	20	4
Pediatrics	5	2

If the average lengths of stay are 6, 4, and 2 days for three departments that have seen 40, 20, and 5 patients, respectively, the weighted mean, or average, length of stay is as follows:

$$= \frac{(40 \times 6) + (20 \times 4) + (5 \times 2)}{40 + 20 + 5}$$
$$= \frac{330}{65}$$
$$= 5.1 \text{ days}$$

SELF-ASSESSMENT QUIZ

7. Gender, race, and insurance class are all examples of which type of data?
   a. Nominal
   b. Ordinal
   c. Interval
   d. Ratio
8. Scores on the Registered Health Information Administrator (RHIA) and Registered Health Information Technician (RHIT) examinations are examples of which type of data?
   a. Nominal
   b. Ordinal
   c. Interval
   d. Ratio
9. The major differences between the histogram and the bar graph are:
   a. The bar graph has space between the bars and is normally used for discrete data, whereas the histogram has no space between bars and is normally used for continuous data.
   b. The histogram has space between the bars and is normally used for discrete data, whereas the bar graph has no space between bars and is normally used for continuous data.
   c. There are no differences between these two types of graphs.
   d. The histogram is used for discrete data only, and the bar graph is used for continuous data only.

STATISTICAL MEASURES AND TESTS

Descriptive Statistics

The following measures and methods are often referred to as descriptive statistics because the objective is to summarize and describe significant characteristics of a set of data.

Median

The **median** represents the middle value within a data set. When the values are arranged from lowest to highest, the number of values above the median is equal to the number of values below the median. For an odd number of observations, the median is the middle number in the ordered set of numbers; for an even number of observations, it is the mean of the middle two numbers.

The median is the most appropriate statistic to use for describing ordinal or ranked data because it allows for more meaningful descriptions of the data (e.g., the median response was between "strongly agree" and "agree"). It may also be useful to report the median for interval or ratio data when the data set contains extreme values, in other words, values that are much higher or much lower than the majority of other values. Although the mean can be strongly affected by extreme values, the median is not affected. Therefore, the median may provide a better representation of central tendency than the mean in some situations.

Example of Median (Odd Number)

Data: 1, 8, 6, 4, 2, 5, 9
Data after ordering: 1, 2, 4, 5, 6, 8, 9
Median = 5
Example of Median (Even Number)
Data: 16, 4, 21, 100, 7, 1

Data after ordering: 1, 4, 7, 16, 21, 100 =

$$\frac{7 + 16}{2} \text{(two middle numbers)}$$

Median = 11.5

Mode

The **mode** is the value that occurs most frequently in a given set of values. Some distributions do not have a mode, whereas others may have two modes (bimodal). The mode is the only measure of central tendency that can be used with nominal data. In Table 10-9, the modal health insurance is Medicare because it is the one that occurs most often.

Measures of Dispersion

When interval or ratio data in a sample are summarized, determining the amount of dispersion or variability within the data set is important. **Dispersion** or variability refers to the extent to which scores within a set vary from each other. Measures of dispersion describe the extent to which scores in a set are spread out (or clustered together) around the mean.

Range

The **range** is one way to measure dispersion because it is the difference between the highest and lowest values. The major disadvantage of the range is that it is concerned only with the most extreme values and ignores all other values. When the range is reported, the highest and the lowest values should be included as well as the difference between them. The following statistics show length of stay for patients with pneumonia and how the range is computed by taking the highest length of stay minus the lowest length of stay for both community-acquired and nosocomial pneumonia.

Example of Range

Length of Stay: Patients with Pneumonia

Community-Acquired		Nosocomial	
Medical Record Number	Length of Stay (days)	Medical Record Number	Length of Stay (days)
207658	20	123579	15
214592	10	275816	22
221459	7	254137	18
158645	14	321096	10
129876	8	153992	8
Mean	11.8	Mean	14.6

The range for the length of stay for patients with community-acquired pneumonia was as follows:

20 (highest value) − 7 (lowest value) = 13

The range for the length of stay for patients with nosocomial pneumonia was as follows:

22 (highest value) − 8 (lowest value) = 14

Variance and Standard Deviation

The variance and standard deviation demonstrate how values are spread around the mean. The calculation of these measures is based on deviations (differences) between the value of each score and the value of the mean. The **variance**, or s^2, is computed by squaring each deviation from the mean, summing the deviations, and then dividing their sum by 1 less than n, the sample size.[9] The **standard deviation**, represented by the symbol s, is the square root of the variance. The reason for taking the square root is to express dispersion in terms of the same units as values of the variable. (If height is measured in inches, the variance of height would express dispersion in units of square inches, but the standard deviation would express dispersion in units of inches.) Because of this property, the standard deviation is the most commonly reported measure of dispersion.

Example of Computation of Variance and Standard Deviation of Length of Stay of Patients with Pneumonia

Community-Acquired Pneumonia Variance

$$s^2 = \frac{\begin{array}{c}(20-11.8)^2 + (10-11.8)^2 + (7-11.8)^2 \\ + (14-11.8)^2 + (8-11.8)^2\end{array}}{5-1}$$

$$= \frac{67.24 + 3.24 + 23.04 + 4.84 + 14.44}{4}$$

$$= \frac{112.8}{4} = 28.2$$

Standard Deviation

$$s = \sqrt{28.2} = 5.3$$

Nosocomial Pneumonia Variance

$$s^2 = \frac{\begin{array}{c}(15-14.6)^2 + (22-14.6)^2 + (18-14.6)^2 \\ + (10-14.6)^2 + (8-14.6)^2\end{array}}{5-1}$$

$$= \frac{0.16 + 54.76 + 11.56 + 21.16 + 43.56}{4}$$

$$= \frac{131.2}{4} = 32.8$$

Standard Deviation

$$s = \sqrt{32.8} = 5.7$$

The greater the deviations of the values from the mean, the greater the variance. Therefore compare the variance of the length of stay of the patients with community-acquired pneumonia (28.2) and the variance of the length of stay of the patients with nosocomial pneumonia (32.8). This shows that there is greater deviation from the mean of length of stay values in the nosocomial pneumonia group than in the community-acquired pneumonia group.

The standard deviation for length of stay for patients with community-acquired pneumonia was 5.3. This means that, on average, observed length of stay values fall 5.3 units from the mean. The standard deviation for the nosocomial pneumonia group was 5.7, which means that, on average, observed length of stay values fall 5.7 units from the mean. Therefore, there is greater variation or dispersion in the length of stay for patients with nosocomial pneumonia than in the length of stay for patients with community-acquired pneumonia. The health care facility may want to examine this further to determine whether there are more outliers in the nosocomial group and to examine the outlier cases in more detail.

Coefficient of Variation

When two samples or groups have very different means, the direct comparison of their standard deviations could be misleading. Therefore, when two groups have very different means, it is best to compare their standard deviations expressed as percentages of the mean. The **coefficient of variation** (CV) is used to do

this. The coefficient of variation can also be used to compare dispersion in variables that are measured in different units.

$$CV = \frac{s}{|\bar{x}|} \times 100$$

where
s = standard deviation
$|\bar{x}|$ = absolute value of mean

Examples of Coefficient of Variation for Community-Acquired and Nosocomial Pneumonia

Coefficient of variation for community-acquired pneumonia:

$$= \frac{5.3}{|11.8|} \times 100 = 45\%$$

Coefficient of variation for nosocomial pneumonia:

$$= \frac{5.7}{|14.6|} \times 100 = 39\%$$

The CV was computed because it was important to determine whether the variation of length of stay values in the community-acquired pneumonia group was greater or less than the variation of length of stay values in the nosocomial pneumonia group. By using the CV, the variation can be computed exactly. The CV for the length of stay of the patients with community-acquired pneumonia was 45%, and the CV for the length of stay of the patients with nosocomial pneumonia was 39%. This means that the variation in the length of stay of the patients with community-acquired pneumonia was somewhat greater than that of the patients with nosocomial pneumonia.

SELF-ASSESSMENT QUIZ

10. The most common measure of central tendency is the:
    a. Mean
    b. Median
    c. Mode
    d. Variance
11. The most common measure of dispersion is called:
    a. Variance
    b. Standard deviation
    c. Weighted mean
    d. Range
12. If a coefficient of variation for cholesterol levels is computed to be 42% for males and 56% for females, this means that the variation in cholesterol levels for females is somewhat _____ than that for males.
    a. Greater
    b. Less
    c. Different
    d. The same

Inferential Statistics

In almost all research studies, researchers can collect data from only a sample of the population of the cases about which they are interested in making conclusions. For example, a researcher interested in finding out whether the average salaries of entry-level HIM professionals differ across four geographic regions of the United States could not possibly collect data from every entry-level HIM professional in the country. However, through the use of a family of statistical tools known as inferential statistics, it is possible to make inferences (or generalizations) about a population based on data collected from a sample. With inferential statistics, the generalizations are made that go beyond the particular sample from which data are collected. The domain of inferential statistics can be subdivided into two main areas: tests of significance and estimation of population parameters.

Tests of Significance

The purpose of tests of significance is to determine whether observed differences between groups or relationships between variables in the sample being studied are likely to be due to chance or sampling error or whether they reflect true differences or relationships in the population of interest. The term *sampling error* refers to the principle that the characteristics of a sample are not identical to the characteristics of the population from which the sample is drawn. Even if the average salaries of entry-level HIM professionals were equal across regions in the population, the sample means would still differ.

Although there are a number of tests of significance, all are based on the same underlying logic and all involve a similar series of steps. The first step in carrying out a test of significance is to state the null and alternative hypotheses. A hypothesis is a claim or statement about a property or characteristic of a population. It indicates the nature of the difference or relationship between characteristics. Each hypothesis can be expressed in two forms: as a null hypothesis or as an alternative hypothesis. The null hypothesis states that there is no difference or relationship in the population. If the null hypothesis is true, any differences or relationships that are observed in the sample are purely the result of chance. By contrast, the alternative hypothesis states that there is a true difference or relationship in the population. If the alternative hypothesis is true, the differences or relationships that are observed in the result are the true effect plus chance variation. In the example of the salaries of entry-level HIM professionals, here is how the null and alternative hypotheses could be stated:

> *Null hypothesis:* There is no difference in the mean salaries of entry-level HIM professionals across geographic regions of the United States.
> *Alternative hypothesis:* There is a difference in the mean salaries of entry-level HIM professionals across geographic regions of the United States.

The next step in carrying out a test of significance is computation of a statistic, sometimes referred to as the test statistic, which is based on the relevant data from the sample. The test statistic measures the size of the difference or relationship observed in the sample. In the example of the salaries of entry-level HIM professionals, the test statistic would reflect the size of the difference among sample means from the four geographic regions.

After the test statistic is computed, the probability that the observed value of the test statistic could occur in the event that the null hypothesis is true is determined. This probability is known as a *p* value and can range from 0 to 1. The *p* value provides an answer to the following question: How likely is it that we could observe a difference or relationship of this size in the sample if, in reality, the difference or relationship did not exist in the population? A second way of posing the same question is: How likely is it that the observed difference or relationship is due only to sampling error? A third way of phrasing the question is: What is the probability that the observed difference or relationship could occur through chance alone? The smaller the *p* value, or closer it is to 0, the less likely the null hypothesis is true and the smaller the probability that the observed difference or relationship could be due to chance or sampling error alone.

The availability of models of probability derived by statistical theorists makes it possible to determine the *p* value or probability associated with a given value of a test statistic. These models, known as theoretical sampling distributions, are discussed in greater depth in statistics textbooks. Commonly used theoretical sampling distributions include the normal, *t*, chi-square, and *F* distributions. Software programs that calculate test statistics determine the associated *p* values as well.

As an example of a model of probability that is familiar to you already, think about tossing a coin 10 times. It is well known that if a fair coin, that is, one that has not been tampered with, is tossed an infinite number of times, 50% of the tosses will result in a head and 50% of the tosses will result in a tail. Suppose you tossed a coin 10 times and every toss resulted in a head. You would suspect that the coin had been tampered with based on your knowledge of the model of probability. In fact, it can be shown that the probability of 10 heads when a fair coin is tossed 10 times is .001 or one in a thousand.

The last step in carrying out a test of significance is to decide whether the *p* value is small enough to support making the decision to reject the null hypothesis. How small is small enough? It is up to the researcher to choose the criterion or standard, which is known as the level of significance. The levels of significance that are most commonly chosen are .05 and .01. Setting the level of significance at .05 means that the decision will be made to reject the null hypothesis if the probability is smaller than 5 in 100 that the observed difference or relationship could be due to sampling error; setting it at .01 means the decision to reject will be made if the probability is smaller than 1 in 100. The recommended practice is for the researcher to choose the level of significance *before* carrying out the significance test.

When the *p* value is greater than the level of significance (usually either .05 or .01), the conclusion is stated as either

- ✓ Explain how each epidemiologic research study design can be used in health information management.
- ✓ Demonstrate knowledge of the most applicable computer software to use when applying epidemiologic research study design principles.

- ✓ Recognize outcome measures and discuss how epidemiologic study designs can facilitate executing outcome studies.

KEY WORDS

Analytic study
Bias
Case
Case-control study
Case finding
Case studies
Censored
Clinical trial
Close-ended questions
Cohort study
Community trial
Confounding variables
Control
Correlation coefficient
Cross-sectional study
Dependent variable

Descriptive study
Double blind
Epidemiology
Experimental epidemiology
Exposure characteristics
Focus groups
Generalizability
Historical prospective study
Hypothesis
Incidence rate
Incidence study
Incident case
Independent variable
Institutional review board
Interobserver reliability
Intraobserver reliability

Life-table analysis
Literature review
Methodology
Nosocomial
Odds ratio
Open-ended questions
Outcome measures
Participant observation
Peer-reviewed
Period prevalence rate
Pilot testing
Point prevalence rate
Prevalence rate
Prevalence study
Prospective study
Qualitative research

Relative risk
Reliability
Research question
Response rate
Retrospective study
Risk factors
Sensitivity
Single blind
Specific aims
Specificity
Subject blind
Survey design
Triple blind
Validity
Variables

ABBREVIATIONS

ADL Activities of Daily Living
AHIMA American Health Information Management Association
ALOS Average Length of Stay
ASTM American Society for Testing and Materials
BMI Body Mass Index
CAD Coronary Artery Disease
CAI Community-Acquired Infection
DRG Diagnosis-Related Group
EHR Electronic Health Record
FN False Negatives
FP False Positives
HIM Health Information Management

ICD-9-CM *International Classification of Diseases,* Ninth Edition, Clinical Modification
IRB Institutional Review Board
IR Incidence Rate
K Kappa Statistic
NI Nosocomial Infection
PHR Personal Health Record
r Correlation Coefficient
RR Relative Risk
SPSS Statistical Process for Social Sciences
TJC The Joint Commission
TN True Negatives
TP True Positives

Epidemiology and health information management (HIM) are two fields that complement each other. Validity and reliability of the data managed by HIM professionals are essential to the soundness and integrity of epidemiologic research studies. The epidemiologic research techniques provide a basis for HIM professionals to take part in designing and conducting research studies that examine several clinical, financial, and administrative areas. Epidemiologic techniques aid the HIM professional not only in conducting clinically based research studies but also in the study of specific HIM department functions, such as whether concurrent coding is more beneficial and cost-effective than coding performed at discharge or whether productivity standards developed for HIM employees are effective.

Because HIM professionals oversee a vast array of health data, it is essential that all epidemiologic methods known to examine these data be used. **Epidemiology** is the study of disease and the determinants of disease in populations;

however, it is also the study of clinical and health care trends or patterns and the ability to recognize trends or patterns within large amounts of data. When HIM professionals master the basic epidemiologic techniques, they become premier detectives seeking out the most prominent, logical, and important trends in the data. This is not an easy task and takes a great deal of practice and thought. However, when the epidemiologic techniques are known, used, and understood, the HIM professional becomes more competent.

? DID YOU KNOW?

Did you know that John Snow was the first person to actually conduct an epidemiologic study on the cholera outbreak in Soho, London, in 1854 by using maps to determine that one water pump (the Broad Street Pump) was causing the outbreak? His work was not accepted until much later and after his death. A pub in England is named after him today.

OVERVIEW OF RESEARCH AND EPIDEMIOLOGY

Leadership in the field of HIM begins with knowledge. Research provides knowledge. It enables individuals to learn something valuable about their profession. Research also provides new ideas to be shared, new methods and systems to be tried, and new infrastructure to be constructed. The purpose of research is to discover or learn something new about a specific area that was not known before. It enables researchers to take a question, review the literature related to that question, collect data related to that question, analyze the data collected, and then formulate answers to the question. Research is not formulating answers to your questions from your own opinions or perceptions without the collection of new data.

This chapter introduces the reader to research methods and epidemiology. It also includes the types of statistical tests that are most appropriate to use when certain types of epidemiologic studies are conducted. This chapter discusses the relationship between epidemiology and outcomes studies and provides an example of an epidemiologic study that is also a clinical outcomes study. The actual database, methods of data collection and data analysis, and areas of future research are explained and discussed. HIM professionals who are actively involved in analysis, interpretation, and complex research study design should continuously supplement their knowledge through coursework, seminars, and in-service training in these areas as well as work closely with a statistician and an epidemiologist.

Familiarity with research study protocol (Figure 11-1), including formulating a hypothesis, reviewing and analyzing the literature, developing specific aims, determining the significance of the research, and defining the methodology for collecting and analyzing the data, is necessary for the HIM professional. When the steps of the research design are well formulated and understood, then the data, statistics, and data display are easier to interpret.

Familiarity with the different types of epidemiologic research study designs is necessary to determine whether the health care data generated from a research study are accurate and appropriate. The different epidemiologic research study designs to be examined are the descriptive study (cross-sectional or prevalence), analytic study (case-control or retrospective, cohort or prospective, and historical prospective), and experimental study (clinical and community trials). The selection of the study design depends on the hypothesis or research question.

HIM professionals should recognize that every research study involves some degree of bias or error. This may be due to sampling variability, methods of data collection, or confounding variables.

ROLE OF THE HEALTH INFORMATION MANAGEMENT PROFESSIONAL

Medical language and classification expert and domain manager are two roles that are included in the "Report on the Roles and Functions of the e-Health Information Management by the American Health Information Management Association" (AHIMA).[1] Do you feel capable of taking on these new roles? Becoming a leader in research in the HIM field and using epidemiologic principles to enhance that research could help you get there.

Becoming a leader in research[2] should be a goal of every HIM professional because research leads to advanced knowledge and advanced knowledge leads to advancement of issues that directly affect patient care. The research process can be difficult, and it sometimes takes years before results are established and used. Nevertheless, research enables an individual to test an idea and to determine whether an association between two variables exists. Sometimes this idea has been tossed around for years but, because of priorities given to other aspects of the HIM department, has not been studied. It is important that every HIM professional take the time to perform research on topics that are of interest and relevant to the field.

Healthy People 2020[3] is a prevention agenda for the nation that identifies the most significant preventable issues related to health and focuses public and private sector efforts to address those issues. It is a comprehensive agenda organized into more than 40 topic areas with goals and specific objectives under each area. One of the topic areas, as well as goals and specific objectives most related to HIM are shown in the following example.

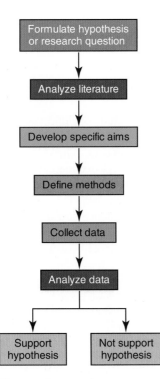

FIGURE 11-1 Nature of research.

Example of *Healthy People 2020: Topic Area, Goal and Objectives Related to Health Information Management*

Topic Area: Health Communication and Health Information Technology

Goal: Use health communication strategies and health information technology (IT) to improve population health outcomes and health care quality, and to achieve health equity.

Objective: HC-HIT 5: Increase the proportion of persons who use electronic personal health management tools.

Sub-Objective: HC-HIT 5.1: Increase the proportion of persons who use the Internet to keep track of personal health information, such as care received, test results, or upcoming medical appointments.

The baseline for this specific aim is 14.3% and the target is 15.7% by 2020.

One factor in eliminating health disparities includes improving data collection methods used to accurately assess the health status for specific populations, especially small ones. One way to reach this goal is through the development and use of the personal health record (PHR) which is on the forefront of the HIM profession and will have a direct impact on public health. The HIM professional can work toward developing effective tools so that accurate health information is received either through the electronic health record (EHR), the Internet, or other clinical databases or registries. In *Healthy People 2020*, goals focus on preventing illnesses on a population basis. The HIM professional, through work with the EHR, PHR, or with other clinical databases and registries, has a direct impact in the prevention of diseases.

These are national priorities that, when examined through research studies, could make a difference that may affect the world. More specific research goals could also be examined and may include determining the prevalence of specific HIM functions across the country through observation and surveys, determining a national coding accuracy rate, or studying the performance (work) satisfaction levels of HIM employees in different health care settings.

All the areas described are examples of potential research projects. However, choose one that is of great interest to you and proceed. The HIM professional is a leader, and as a leader, he or she should strive to advance the profession. Research provides the avenue for that advancement.

DESIGNING THE RESEARCH PROPOSAL

Several steps should be taken when a research or grant proposal is designed that will make the entire process interesting, rewarding, and fulfilling.[4] These steps include the following:

- Identification of a research hypothesis or question
- Review of the literature
- Draft of research methods
- Development of the research plan or study design
  - Specific aims
  - Significance and preliminary research
  - Experimental design and methods
  - Human subjects (when human subjects are involved the researcher must seek approval of the **institutional review board** [IRB])
  - Literature cited
- Development of the research budget
- Design of the appendix

Hypothesis and Research Questions

A **hypothesis** or **research question** identifies the goal of the research. The hypothesis is an educated guess about the outcome of the study. It poses an assertion to be supported and may predict a relationship between two or more variables; a research question asks a question to be answered. A hypothesis is not an opinion or value judgment. For example, the statement that every American has the right to health care is a value judgment that cannot be proved right or wrong. Some statements that seem like an opinion on the surface can become a hypothesis with definition of the concepts. The statement "The poor do not have access to health care" can become a testable hypothesis by defining the concept of poor by income level, adequacy by the average in the United States, and health care by the number of physician office visits within a specified period of time. Research questions are used in a new area when not much is known about the topic. Answers to the question will help determine the relationships.[5]

The concepts in the hypothesis are the **variables**, which are either **independent** or **dependent**. The variable that causes change in the other variables is called an **independent variable**. A variable for which the value is dependent on one or more other variables but that cannot itself affect the other variables is called a **dependent variable**. The hypothesized relationship between the variables of interest determines their category. The dependent variable is the variable we wish to explain, and the independent variable is the factor that we believe may explain it. In a causal relationship, the cause is an independent variable and the effect is a dependent variable. For example, because smoking causes lung cancer, smoking is an independent variable and lung cancer a dependent variable.[5]

Suppose a researcher wanted to test whether the medical record would prove to be a useful collection tool for factors suspected of being associated with ovarian cancer. Previous research has found that at least 20 factors may be associated with this disease[6]. However, few studies used the medical record alone to collect data pertaining to these factors. Ovarian cancer is a devastating disease that defies early detection. If a link could be made to one or more specific factors, then preventive measures could be taken by women with the factors to decrease the risk of developing ovarian cancer. This study has the following research question:

Is the medical record a useful tool for collecting data pertaining to factors suspected of being associated with ovarian cancer?

and the following hypothesis:

An association exists between risk factors suspected of being linked with ovarian cancer. The ovarian cancer is the dependent variable and the risk factors are the independent variables.

How do you propose an effective hypothesis or research question? Often, a researcher proposes a hypothesis or research question on the basis of ideas that are generated by reading the literature. Other times a researcher has an idea that is generated from personal experiences and then through the review and analysis of the literature develops an insightful hypothesis or research question. Either way, an extensive review of the literature is necessary.

Review of Literature

Once the hypothesis or question is established, the second step of a sound research study design is to conduct an extensive literature review (Figure 11-2). A review must be conducted to determine the research that has already been performed in this area. The best way to accomplish this task is to conduct a literature search. Most librarians can conduct a literature search by entering key words and phrases into a computer that then searches through journals, books, and other publications. How far back in time to search must also be specified. A literature search can also be performed independently by searching the Internet or by using other online sources such as MEDLINE. Depending on the type, the search will produce a list that includes the title, author's name, and journal title and an abstract, if one is available, summarizing each article.

The key words and phrases that are used can make or break the literature search, so they should be chosen with

care. If there is uncertainty about which key words to choose, the wording should be discussed with the reference librarian. For example, the key words chosen for the ovarian cancer study included *epithelial ovarian cancer*, *risk factors*, *epidemiology*, and *medical record*. The Internet is also an excellent resource for conducting the literature search; however, care should be taken because some articles that are found through the Internet may not be peer reviewed (as discussed subsequently). Even so, the Internet can link you to many peer-reviewed articles through MEDLINE, OVID, and other excellent online searches. OVID is an international resource of electronic medical, scientific, and academic research information. It supports researchers, students, and others by providing methods on how to search for specific information relevant to a specific research topic.

When the literature search is concluded, it must be carefully examined and any articles of interest should be collected and reviewed. An important step here is to determine whether a particular article is valuable for your research study. For example, the type of journal should be examined. Some journals are peer reviewed, and others are not. **Peer reviewed** means that peers within the specific research area have extensively reviewed the article and provided comments and feedback to the authors to incorporate into their revision of the article before publication. Some journals, editorials, government reports, and so forth may not be peer reviewed, and although the information in the report may still be important and useful, it did not go through the extensive review process just described.

A critical review of a research article through a peer-review process normally focuses on the following areas:

- Content is of value, interest, and importance to the reader
- Hypothesis or research question is clear and appropriate
- Review of the literature supports the study
- Study design chosen is appropriate for the hypothesis/research question
- The methods are appropriate and support the specific aims
- Statistical analysis is appropriate for the study design
- The discussion and conclusions are appropriate on the basis of the results
- Writing, illustrations, tables, and so forth are clear, well organized, and accurate
- Replication of the methods described could be performed by the reader
- Qualitative comments including an overall impression (accept or reject) and any major problems and suggested revisions.

It is also important when collecting information for the literature review to distinguish among the citations, references, and bibliographies that are contained in some research articles. Citations provide information about the source of the written material in the body of the article. The citation, which is usually depicted as a number or author's last name, depending on the style manual used, does not provide much information by itself. You need to go to the reference list or

FIGURE 11-2 Relationship between peer-reviewed journal, research articles, and professional literature.

bibliography to get the exact title, author, journal name, and so forth. The reference list is usually at the end of the article and includes only the articles cited within the body of the article. The bibliography is like a list of references; however, it includes additional articles and books not cited in the text but that were reviewed to prepare to write the article and are included for further reading. Therefore, the bibliography may contain many more articles and books than are cited in the article itself.

The purposes of the literature review are:
- To develop a solid foundation in the particular field through study of that topic
- To become an expert through reviewing past literature to determine how one's hypothesis is different from previous research studies
- To determine what it is about one's idea or hypothesis that makes it worth carrying out
- To find gaps or problems with existing studies and begin thinking about how to design a study to fill those gaps

Another important task to incorporate into the literature review is to organize all the articles selected into a table that includes the following:
- Title of the article and journal, book, or report
- Author(s)
- Publisher, date, and so on
- Summary of the article
- Advantages of the article specific to study design for your research topic
- Disadvantages of the article specific to study design

By developing a table such as this, the researcher will be better able to determine the gaps of previous research studies and will then know where to focus the research study design.

Methodology (Draft)

At this point, the researcher should begin to think about how to design the study so that the hypothesis can be properly tested. The methodology can be the most difficult task and, therefore, should be started as soon as possible. The methodology should include a step-by-step process of what is done in the research study and why this process is necessary to test the hypothesis properly. A rough draft of the methodology should be developed to determine whether the study is feasible. It also allows the researcher to realize how much is known about the subject matter and to think about what the research involves.

Research Plan

When a draft of the method has been written and the feasibility of the study confirmed through the literature review, the research plan should be written. It includes the following:
- Specific aims or objectives
- Significance (review of literature or preliminary research)
- Research design and method

- Population under study-sample selection
- Time frame
- Place of study
- Data collection process
- Application to the IRB
- Analysis of the data
- Human subjects (if applicable)
- Literature cited

Specific Aims

The specific aims should briefly describe the project's goals or objectives. The goals, objectives, aims, or purposes should be enumerated for better clarification. The list should include both short- and long-term goals. For example, the specific aims in the ovarian cancer study are as follows:
- To determine whether the medical record is a useful tool for collecting data pertaining to risk factors and other health history information (short-term goal)
- To narrow the number of factors suspected of being linked to ovarian cancer by providing evidence that a potential risk factor is found more in the cases (women with the disease) than in the controls (women without the disease; short-term goal)
- To identify groups of women who may be at high risk for development of ovarian cancer and work toward designing and implementing preventive measures to control the disease (long-term goal)
- To benefit future researchers who examine chromosomal markers and ovarian cancer so that they begin to incorporate risk factors in the analysis of their data (long-term goal)

Significance (Review of Literature and Preliminary Research)

This section should detail the importance of the research project by including a review of past research studies on the same subject (literature review) and preliminary research or pilot studies (if any) performed by the researcher. It should state why the research study must be performed, how it is different from previous research studies, and who the research will benefit. This section should also demonstrate the researcher's knowledge by including a discussion of existing research that has been performed in the same area and showing the gaps in that research. When these deficiencies are discussed in detail, this part of the plan should reveal how the current research will address these deficiencies.

The key to this section is to be succinct, clear, and organized to convey why the research is important. If the preliminary research is brief, it can be included in the significance section, particularly if it adds to the study's importance. If the preliminary research is extensive, it should be included in a separate section titled "Preliminary Studies" or "Preliminary Research."

An excerpt of the significance section is shown in the following example to demonstrate how the preliminary research is used to show the importance of the proposed study.

Example of a Significance Section of a Research Proposal

Ovarian cancer is the most lethal of all gynecologic cancers. It is an almost-silent disease in a deep-seated organ that defies early detection. In fact, the appearance of vague, non-specific symptoms (pelvic pain, low backache, aching legs, bloating, nausea) may be a manifestation of already advanced disease. Epithelial cancers predominate (incidence rate of ovarian cancer is approximately 20,000 cases per year, and epithelial ovarian cancer makes up about 65% of that amount); except for a minority in which torsion or hemorrhage occurs, the majority of patients are asymptomatic. At present, ovarian cancer is responsible for half of the deaths related to female genital malignancy, and although mortality rates for gynecologic cancers are declining, those for ovarian cancer are slowly increasing.[2,3]

A number of risk factors are suspected of being linked to epithelial ovarian cancer. These include nulliparity, infertility, menstrual tension, abnormal breast swelling, marked dysmenorrhea, early menopause (50 years), irradiation of pelvic organs, exposure to talc, high socioeconomic status, smoking, alcohol use, breast cancer, cervical fibroids, endometrial cancer, obesity, oral contraceptive use (inverse relationship), use of fertility drugs, history of colorectal cancer, white ethnicity, age older than 40 years, and family history of ovarian cancer.[4,6–12]

A research study has been performed through a small grant from the School of Health Related Professions' Research and Development Fund in which risk factors in 20 ovarian cancer cases and in 40 randomly selected age-related controls were evaluated. Interpretation of the data has been limited because 30% of the risk factors were not found in the medical record for the cases or controls. These results may be due to the small sample size and collection of data from only one hospital.

The proposed project will be able to analyze effectively the large number of risk factors suspected of being linked to ovarian cancer by evaluating the disease at an earlier stage and by incorporating an improved method of epidemiologic assessment. By examining the risk factors in incident cases and in age-matched control subjects from the medical record and from telephone interviews, we will be able to pinpoint the risk factors cited immediately after diagnosis and follow-up with a telephone interview to add any risk factors not collected from the medical record. This proposed project would enable us to remedy inadequacies of the past study and therefore determine a risk factor truly linked to the development of epithelial ovarian cancer. This identified risk factor will lead to the identification of women at high risk for development of ovarian cancer. Future prospective studies can be designed to follow women with and without the risk factor to determine whether ovarian cancer develops.

(Footnotes/references are not provided because this is an example of the significance section.)

Methodology

The method should include a research design in relation to time, place, and persons. It should consist of the following:

- Time frame. This should state exactly when the study will be conducted and why it is necessary to conduct the study for this specific time period.
- Place of study. This section should explain where the study will be conducted and whether it will include one facility or multiple facilities and why.
- Population under study. This includes which subjects will be in the study, how they will become part of the study, why these specific subjects will be part of the study, whether a representative sample of the population will be used and why, and how sample size will be determined.

The method should also include a step-by-step plan of how the study is to be performed. This is called the "Procedures" and can include the following:

- Data collection process. This section should reveal how the data will be collected (by questionnaire, interview, abstracting techniques); what data will be categorized and why; how the data will be categorized and why; who will collect the data; whether training techniques will be needed and, if so, what the training will consist of; where the data will be stored; whether the data will include patient identifiers and why; and how the data will be accessed. A separate paragraph or statement regarding how the confidentiality of the subjects will be protected should be included.
- Application to the IRB. The methodology section should state that the study will be submitted for approval to an IRB. An IRB, or research and human rights committee, is part of most health care facilities and meets at least quarterly. Some boards may meet more often, depending on the number of applications they receive. The aim of any IRB is to protect human subjects or patients from research risks and invasion of privacy. The IRB reviews all research studies that involve subjects or patients, including experiments, interviews, and questionnaires and any study that collects data from a patient's medical record. The scientific merits of a proposal are considered in the context of assessing the risks and benefits of the proposed research.
- Analysis of the data. This section should describe how the data will be analyzed and the types of statistical tests that will be performed (e.g., frequency distribution, chi-square, confidence intervals, and assessment of validity and reliability, to be addressed later in this chapter). The researcher must be sure to describe why this type of statistical analysis will be used.

An excerpt from an actual methodology section is described in the following example.

Example of a Methodology Section of a Research Proposal

Objective/Time Frame: The current research will evaluate the relationship between epithelial ovarian cancer and characteristics suspected of being linked to the disease in a population of individuals newly diagnosed with epithelial ovarian cancer over a 1-year period.

Place of Study: New or **incident cases** of a particular disease will be ascertained from several hospital-based cancer registries. Incident cases will be used because the medical record provides a more complete past history of medical information when a patient is newly diagnosed with a condition. Also, if the patients are well enough and willing, telephone interviews will be performed. Telephone interviews can be performed with family members, physicians, and so on, if the patient is unable to provide information.

Population Under Study: The controls will be randomly selected from a population of women undergoing surgery or hospitalization for reasons unrelated to cancer. Each control will be matched with the case on age (within 5 years), admission date (within 1 week), and hospital. The number of cases with epithelial ovarian cancer will be 150. The number of controls will be 300.

Procedures—Data Collection Process: The 150 cancer cases will be categorized by stage, histologic grade, metastases, demographic data, and risk factors as listed in the significance section. The 300 controls will be categorized by risk factors and demographic data.

Application to Institutional Review Board: The hospitals will be notified and the study will be explained and submitted for approval by their IRBs. Consent to participate in the study will be obtained from the cases and controls by mail 1 week after discharge.

Data Collection Process: The hospital will notify the research team whenever a patient with ovarian cancer is admitted. The research team will match the case with the control and after discharge will abstract data from the medical record using a pretested data collection instrument (see the sample questionnaire in Figure 11-3). The abstractors will be trained so that each one is certain about where to find specific information in the record when a risk factor or characteristic is not applicable, not documented, or not present in the case or control.

After the data are collected, a telephone interview will be performed using the pretested data collection instrument to collect any data not found in the medical record and to assess the validity of the data in the medical record.

Analysis of the Data: The data will be entered into a personal computer, and statistical analysis will include frequency distribution, chi-square, and odds ratios. Because the examination of risk factors from medical records may vary from one abstractor to another, various members of the research team will repeat the abstracting of another member, levels of agreement will be determined, and a kappa (κ) statistic will be computed.

Human Subjects

The human subjects section is necessary only if human subjects are used in the research or if there are any risks to a human subject. The following should be included in this section:

- Demographic description of the subject population, including age, percentage of males and females, race
- How informed consent will be obtained
- If necessary, how confidentiality (risk of privacy) will be safeguarded
- Potential risks and benefits of the study to the people enrolled

---

Sample of Ovarian Cancer Questionnaire (Abstracted from 119 Total Elements)

1. Do you know of any blood relatives in your family who have or have had any type of cancer?

   ☐ Yes   ☐ No   ☐ Not documented

   If yes, what relation?

   ☐ Mother   ☐ Niece   ☐ Grandmother
   ☐ Father   ☐ Sister   ☐ Nephew
   ☐ Aunt   ☐ Brother
   ☐ Uncle   ☐ Grandfather

   ☐ Other _____

   If yes, what type:

   ☐ Lung   ☐ Liver   ☐ Lymphomas
   ☐ Brain   ☐ Breast   ☐ Colon
   ☐ Skin   ☐ Pancreas   ☐ Blood-related (leukemia)

   ☐ Other: _____

2. Do you smoke cigarettes?

   ☐ Yes   ☐ No   ☐ Not documented

   If yes, how many cigarettes do you smoke each day?

   ☐ 1/2 pack or less   ☐ 1 pack
   ☐ 1 to 2 packs   ☐ More than 2 packs

FIGURE 11-3 Excerpt of ovarian cancer questionnaire.

Any letters validating IRB approval should be placed in this section to show that the facility where the research will be conducted has approved the study methodology.

Literature Referenced

All literature discussed or reviewed in any section of the research proposal should be numbered or cited in that section and a full reference listed at the end of the proposal. Different formats for references are used depending on the preference of the funding agency. Use the format that the funding agency specifies. The general format for a journal reference includes the author(s), year of publication in parentheses, title, name of journal, volume, and page numbers. For a book, it generally includes the author(s), year of publication in parentheses, title, and place and name of publishing company.

Budget Development

A detailed budget is necessary to determine the actual costs of the research project and is required for most funding agencies. The budget can include the following:

- Salary and fringe benefits for personnel
- Equipment
- Supplies
- Travel
- Patient care costs, if applicable to the research problem
- Contractual costs, such as including another agency or organization to assist with the study
- Consulting costs
- Telephone or fax costs
- Internet access
- Paper
- Computer usage
- Equipment maintenance

Justification is essential in the budget and should include the specific functions of the personnel, consultants, and collaborators. At times, incentives to study subjects may be necessary to encourage them to participate in the research study. If that is done, the amount of dollars or the specific health care benefit should be listed in the budget as well.

An outline of the budget for the ovarian cancer study if it were carried out today is shown in the example.

Example of a Budget of a Research Proposal

Secretarial Salary Total: $1056.00
Duties include typing study protocol for review by IRB at hospitals and universities, copying the study protocol, preparing envelopes for mailing, and typing preliminary and final results of study.
80 hours × $10.00/hour = $800.00
Fringe benefits: $0.32 × $800.00 = $256.00

Research Assistant Salary Total: $5220.00
Abstractors (Each abstractor will review 450 records to determine agreement levels. Total of three abstractors will be used.)
450 records × 0.30 hours/record × 3 = 405.00 hours × $8.00/hour = $3240.00
Abstractor for data entry
450 records × 0.25 hours/record = 112.50 hours × $8.00/hour = $900.00

Telephone interviews
450 interviews × 0.30 hours/interview = 135 hours × $8.00/hour = $1080.00

Travel to Hospitals Total: $2141.40
To decrease the amount of travel, visits can be made to hospitals at the end of the month because more cases will be available. Because 78 cases were available from three hospitals, six hospitals can be used with 33 visits.
33 visits × 3 abstractors × 20 miles × $0.33 per mile = $653.40
Parking = 33 × 3 = 99 × $10.00 = $990.00
Travel will also include visits by a principal investigator to each of the hospitals initially and throughout the study.
5 visits × 6 hospitals = 30 visits × 20 miles × $0.33/mile = $198.00
Parking = 30 × $10.00 = $300.00

Supplies Total: $2100.00
Photocopying, postage, disks, paper, fax, telephone costs

Total Budget $10,517.40
There will be no costs or payments made to or from the subjects.

Appendix Design

The appendix can comprise tables, figures, laboratory tests, data collection forms, and letters of support. It can include anything that is important and relative to the research study or that better clarifies a topic described in the study but that may be too voluminous to include in the body of the proposal. Information such as research articles reviewed or a sample of a database from a preliminary study is not pertinent to the research project and should be excluded. For the ovarian cancer study, the data collection instrument was included in the appendix section of the grant application.

Additional Considerations

Most research proposal guidelines have page-length limitations for each of the sections just discussed. It is important to adhere to any page limitations or any other instructions because failure to do this may make the research application ineligible for review by the funding agency.

SELF-ASSESSMENT QUIZ

1. The study of disease and determinants of disease in populations is called:
   a. A clinical trial
   b. An outcomes study
   c. Epidemiology
   d. Clinical medicine
2. After the hypothesis is established, the second step of a good research study is to conduct a:
   a. Preliminary study
   b. Selection of subjects
   c. Review of IRB rules
   d. Literature review
3. The research plan is an important part of the entire research proposal development. List the components of the research proposal that make up the research plan.

VALIDITY AND RELIABILITY

Validity

Validity assesses relevance, completeness, accuracy, and correctness. It measures how well a data collection instrument, laboratory test, medical record abstract, or other data source measures what it should measure. Validity can assess, for example, whether a thermometer truly measures temperature or whether an IQ test really measures intelligence.

It is crucial that the HIM professional be aware of validity problems in specific types of studies. The data collection instrument and the method of data collection have a great impact on the validity of data. To determine whether the validity of a research study is upheld, specific methods should be used. One such method includes gaining confirmatory information from different sources to determine whether the information collected for the study is correct. For example, information recorded in the medical record regarding the patient's method of payment or insurance carrier can be validated by further examining financial records, physicians' office records, and pharmacy records. Brief interviews with family members can further confirm or validate the accuracy of correctness of the insurance type.

Sensitivity and Specificity

Validity also refers to correct measurement or correct labeling. Assessments of methods used to test whether a person has a disease are considered tests of validity regarding the correctness of measurement or labeling. Two measures of this are sensitivity and specificity. To use sensitivity and specificity, one must know the following definitions:

- True positives (TP) correctly categorize true cases as cases—valid labeling.
- False negatives (FN) incorrectly label true cases as noncases—not valid.
- True negatives (TN) correctly label noncases as noncases—valid.
- False positives (FP) incorrectly label noncases as cases—not valid.

Sensitivity is the percentage of all true cases correctly identified—TP/(TP + FN) or TP/Total positives (or total cases).

Specificity is the percentage of all true noncases correctly identified—TN/(TN + FP) or TN/Total negatives (or total noncases).[7,8]

Analysis and Discussion

Table 11-1 shows the accuracy of a specific blood test in detecting prostate cancer. The specificity rate of 91% suggests that this blood test correctly labels noncases 91% of the time and misses the noncases 9% of the time. The sensitivity rate of only 83% suggests that the blood test misses 17% of the true cases, or patients with prostate cancer. This blood test could pose serious health problems when true cases may

TABLE 11-1	Sensitivity and Specificity: Accuracy of Blood Test to Detect Prostate Cancer	
Test	Prostate Cancer	No Prostate Cancer
1	TP (100)	FP (20)
—	FN (20)	TN (200)
Totals	TP + FN (120)	FP + TN (220)
Sensitivity = TP/TP + FN = 100/100 + 20 = 100/120 = 83.3%		
Specificity = TN/TN + FP = 200/200 + 20 = 200/220 = 90.9%		

TP, True positives; FP, false positives; FN, false negatives; TN, true negatives.

be missed, and therefore diagnosis and treatment may be delayed or missed. Each researcher must determine when the sensitivity and specificity levels are accurate enough to use the test.

Coding validity is a major area of research in the field of HIM. However, there is a paucity of literature in the area of coding accuracy or validity of HIM professionals. Often it is difficult to assess the validity of a principal diagnosis, ICD-9-CM (*International Classification of Diseases*, Ninth Revision, Clinical Modification) code, or diagnosis-related group (DRG) because the basis of the categorization may be subjective. However, the accuracy or validity of coding can be established when a "gold standard" is determined. The gold standard is used as the correct code when conducting research studies. However, one must be aware of the limitations in using such a standard and must strive to lessen the error. The correct diagnosis, code, or DRG can be determined on the basis of coding standards and agreement by expert coders. For example, the validity of coding quality can be determined by having the coding supervisor recode a random sample of records of patients with a principal diagnostic code of coronary artery disease (CAD; Figure 11-4). Two coders—coder A and coder B—did the coding. The recoding performed by the coding supervisor can be considered the gold standard. The validity (sensitivity and specificity) could then be recorded as shown in Figure 11-4. Coder B's coding is more accurate than coder A's in coding true cases of CAD (100% vs. 60%) and in accurately coding noncases as noncases (80% vs. 73%).

Specific factors cause incorrect or inaccurate labeling. In the coding example, these factors can include inexperience and lack of knowledge regarding the disease (CAD), ICD-9-CM coding principles, and proper review and analysis of the medical record. Other factors may be related to the equipment, such as outdated coding books. Also, it is obvious that validity is influenced by the gold standard that is selected. When results of such studies are assessed, it is important to consider the subjectivity of the standard.

Reliability

Reliability refers to consistency between users of a given instrument or method. In many research studies, more than

CODING SUPERVISOR/VALIDATOR		
Coding Status	True Case CAD	True Noncase No CAD
Coder A		
CAD (+)	9 (TP)	4 (FP)
No CAD (-)	6 (FN)	11 (TN)
Totals	15	15
Coder B		
CAD (+)	15 (TP)	3 (FP)
No CAD (-)	0 (FN)	12 (TN)
Totals	15	15

	Coder A	Coder B
Sensitivity = True positives (TP)/All true cases (Total)	9/15 = 60%	15/15 = 100%
Specificity = True negatives (TN)/All non cases (Total)	11/15 = 73%	12/15 = 80%

FIGURE 11-4 Recoding of a random sample of patient records with a principal diagnostic code of coronary artery disease (CAD).

one research assistant collects the data. For example, in the ovarian cancer study, an abstract was used to collect the information from the medical records for both cases and controls. Because different research assistants were used to abstract the medical records to collect the data, the classification of the results might differ from one assistant to another. Reproducibility or reliability between more than one research assistant or observer is called interobserver reliability. However, even one individual observer's responses may vary over time. Reliability within one research assistant or observer is called intraobserver reliability.

To test for the reliability of risk factors that were collected from the medical record between research assistants in the ovarian cancer study (described in more detail later in the chapter), each medical record was abstracted three times to determine levels of agreement. Levels of agreement ranged from 71% to 100% for all the characteristics or risk factors collected for the study. A kappa statistic (κ) was also calculated. This statistic enables the researcher to determine whether the agreement levels that are seen are real or are due to the result of chance. A statistic can range from 0.00 to 1.00. A kappa statistic greater than 0.75 equals excellent agreement or reproducibility; $0.4 = \kappa = 0.75$ denotes good

agreement; and $0 = \kappa < 0.4$ denotes marginal agreement. After deliberation with our statistician and review of the literature, a statistic of 0.60 was chosen as the standard level for this study; anything below 0.60 was determined not to be real and caused by chance or sampling variability. Therefore, the usefulness of the agreement levels for those risk factors could be limited.

Another method of testing interobserver reliability when interviewing is to use different research assistants on the first and second interviews of the same subject. One can then measure consistency of recall and variations of response to different research assistants. To measure intraobserver reliability, the same research assistant can be used at different times while measuring consistency of the subject's response.

Sometimes reliability is measured and reported in the form of a correlation coefficient (r) rather than a proportion or percentage. A correlation coefficient is a statistic that shows the strength of a relationship between two variables. A correlation coefficient, when used to measure degrees of reliability, can range from −1 to +1. The closer r approaches −1 or +1, the stronger the reliability or the relationship between two variables. The closer r approaches zero, the weaker the relationship or reliability.[9] For example, if an

HIM professional was interested in the correlation between the number of health care providers attending medical record documentation seminars and the number of complete medical records received in the HIM department on discharge of the patient 1 week after the seminar was conducted, a correlation coefficient can be used. A high positive score, such as 0.91, means that as the number of health care providers attending the seminar increased, the number of completed medical records at discharge increased. A high negative score, such as −0.91, means that as the number of health care providers attending the seminar increased, the number of completed medical records decreased.

✓ SELF-ASSESSMENT QUIZ

4. The ability of a test instrument to measure what it is supposed to measure is called:
   a. Validity
   b. Reliability
   c. Agreement
   d. Kappa statistic
5. What is the reproducibility (or reliability) between more than one research assistant or observer called?
   a. Intraobserver reliability
   b. Interobserver reliability
   c. Bias
   d. Consistency
6. Describe the kappa statistic.
   a. What is a kappa statistic and when should it be used?
   b. What is a good standard value for this statistic?
   c. What is the conclusion for a kappa statistic of 0.40?

BIASES

No research study is perfect. No matter how well designed a research study is, there is always some type of error or **bias**. Therefore, it is imperative that researchers be aware of the types of bias that can occur and the methods used to decrease the amount of bias. The following are examples of common types of error or bias.[10]

Confounding Variables

If other characteristics such as age or sex are known to be associated with both the independent (risk factor or exposure characteristic) and the dependent (disease) variables, these confounding variables should be controlled so that they are not the reason an association is seen. Methods to control for age, for example, include matching (discussed later in this chapter) cases and controls on age or performing age adjustment when analyzing the data.

Sampling Variability

The results of a study may be false because of improper sample size and selection. It is important to obtain an effective sample so that the results of the research study can be generalized to the population under study. Sometimes this is difficult but very necessary because when the sample is large enough, random, and truly represents the population under study, the results can be generalized or extrapolated to the entire population under study. This is discussed in more detail in Chapter 10.

Ascertainment or Selection Bias

When selecting subjects, researchers are more likely to choose people who are frequently under medical care. If a disease or condition is asymptomatic or mild, it may escape routine medical attention and may have an impact on the condition under study.

In addition, volunteers and paid subjects may be very different from the general population. Volunteers may volunteer to be in a study because they are very healthy or because they have a special interest in the study.

Diagnosis Bias

Certain diseases are not easy to diagnose, and different health professionals may offer different opinions. For example, when the stage and grade of certain types of cancers are determined, a standard review of slides by one or more pathologists who are unaware of the specimens' origin can be used. This method may provide more clarity in assessing an accurate diagnosis, which can be extremely important when obtaining cases and controls for a study.

Nonresponse Bias

Subjects who refuse to participate in a study may be different from the subjects who do participate. The solution is to collect basic demographic characteristics on participants and nonparticipants to see whether the characteristics are similar. In this way, the researcher can determine whether the study participants represent the general population and are not different in relation to health or risk characteristics.

Survival Bias

Survival bias occurs with cross-sectional studies because only those who have lived long enough to be in the study are examined. The solution is to use incident or new cases to relieve this bias.

Recall Bias

Recall bias can be attributed to faulty memory or to subjects who tend to remember certain types of information because of the exposure or disease. Before the study begins, list possible biases and ways to reduce them. For example, mothers of children with anomalies or complications tend to remember more about their deliveries than do mothers of healthy children. Mothers of children with anomalies are the cases, whereas controls can be mothers of children with a different type of anomaly or adverse pregnancy outcome. Mothers with healthy children could be yet another comparison group. In this way, recall bias should be reduced because cases and controls would be similar in recalling specific events relevant to their children given that both groups would have children with anomalies.

> **? DID YOU KNOW?**
>
> Did you know that some of the most difficult items to remember are related to the amount and type of foods we eat as well as exercise habits? Smartphone apps are being used to make it easier for people to collect and record their diet and exercise habits and then send the data directly to the researcher for analysis.

Interviewer Bias

Interviewers tend to ask questions differently or may probe more if they know which subjects have the characteristic of interest. To reduce interviewer bias, the solution is to standardize the interview form and to provide intensive training for the interviewers, stressing that they must be consistent when performing the interview.

Prevarication Bias

Prevarication bias occurs when an individual tends to exaggerate a response in an interview or questionnaire. A worker who receives disability compensation might exaggerate his or her exposure. The solution is to use several independent raters and several sources of data to validate the information collected.

> **✓ SELF-ASSESSMENT QUIZ**
>
> **7.** When selecting subjects for a research study, researchers are more likely to choose people who are frequently under medical care. What type of bias is this called?
>   **a.** Survival bias
>   **b.** Diagnosis bias
>   **c.** Selection bias
>   **d.** Recall bias
> **8.** Subjects with faulty memory, or who tend to remember certain types of information because of their exposure or the disease under study, lead to what type of bias?
>   **a.** Nonresponse bias
>   **b.** Recall bias
>   **c.** Prevarication bias
>   **d.** Sampling variability
> **9.** What two methods may reduce interviewer bias?

EPIDEMIOLOGIC/RESEARCH STUDY DESIGNS

An important step in designing a research study is to choose the most appropriate study design to test the hypothesis. The HIM professional can appropriately choose the study design

TABLE 11-2	Types of Epidemiologic Research Study Designs
Study Design	**Description**
Descriptive studies—cross-sectional or prevalence study	Examine the distribution of disease or health characteristics in populations at one point in time. Used to generate hypotheses.
Analytic studies Case-control or retrospective Cohort or prospectives Historical prospective	Examine a disease to determine whether certain health characteristics are causing the disease.
Experimental studies Clinical trials Community trials	Modify the health characteristics that are found to cause the disease by using health care interventions that control progression of the disease or prevent the disease from occurring.

to use if he or she is aware of the many designs that exist. Because epidemiology is so closely related to the HIM field, the study designs described in this chapter include epidemiologic research study designs. Epidemiology is the study of the distribution and determinants of disease or events in populations. The results of the study are used to prevent and control public health problems. The most common types of study designs are described in detail here and summarized in Table 11-2. Examples of each design are provided, and common statistics that are generated from these studies are described.

Descriptive Study

The descriptive study describes the frequency and distribution of diseases in populations. It is usually the first study design chosen when little is known about the disease or health characteristics. Qualitative studies or exploratory studies also describe or explore a new area of study and will be explained later in this section. First, let us look at a cross-sectional design.

Cross-Sectional or Prevalence Study

The cross-sectional or prevalence study is one type of descriptive study; it concurrently describes characteristics and health outcomes at one specific point or period in time. The cross-sectional or prevalence study cannot answer questions regarding cause and effect or whether the health characteristic came before the disease. This study design is used to generate hypotheses, not to test them. For example, a health care facility may be interested in examining the prevalence of community-acquired pneumonia in elderly people. Pneumonia is debilitating and increases the cost and length of stay when pneumonia develops in an elderly person who is hospitalized for another condition.

The cross-sectional or prevalence study can be used to determine the prevalence of pneumonia in the region within the elderly population. To do this, the condition under study (i.e., pneumonia) needs to be defined.

Specific criteria related to the type of pneumonia are necessary, along with any other criteria necessary to define the condition further. Positive results of culture and sensitivity and chest x-ray studies and clinical symptoms such as fever and malaise can be used as criteria to define pneumonia. This can be further validated by the DRG and ICD-9-CM codes for pneumonia and a review of the medical record by an infectious disease physician or epidemiologist. Further clarification of the pneumonia should specify that it is community acquired and not **nosocomial** (developing 72 hours after hospitalization).

Then the **prevalence rate** is determined as shown in the following example.

> ## Example of Prevalence Rate
>
> Prevalence rate = Number of people aged 65 years or older with community-acquired pneumonia in a specific region during 200X × 1000
> Number of people aged 65 years or older in a specific region during 200X

After the prevalence rates are determined, they can be compared across certain groups. For example, further defined prevalence rates for pneumonia may be calculated for people younger than 65 years and a comparison of the two groups can be made. One cannot determine from this study design that being elderly (age 65 years or older) causes an increase in pneumonia incidence. However, one can make statements of associations; that is, older age has a greater association with the development of community-acquired pneumonia. One can then develop a hypothesis such as that community-acquired pneumonia is more prevalent in individuals aged 65 years and older than in those younger than 65 years and conduct further studies to determine whether the hypothesis is true or false.

Prevalence rates can facilitate **case finding**, assist health care administrators in planning for diversified health care facilities and special care units, aid health planners in developing appropriate health programs, and assist HIM professionals in further describing morbidity rates within the health care facility. Case finding includes targeting individual cases that have a particular disease or exposure so that health care services can be provided for them.

Prevalence rates can be categorized into two types: **point prevalence rates** and **period prevalence rates**. Point prevalence refers to evaluating a health condition at a specific point in time. Therefore, each study participant is assessed only once at one point in time, although the actual point prevalence study may take months or years to conduct. Period prevalence refers to evaluating a health condition over a period of time, such as 1 year. Study participants are counted for period prevalence even if they die, migrate, or have a recurrence of the disease during the period.[6] Figure 11-5 demonstrates the difference between point and period prevalence when examining specific cases within a study.

FIGURE 11-5 Chronology of cases in a community to measure prevalence.

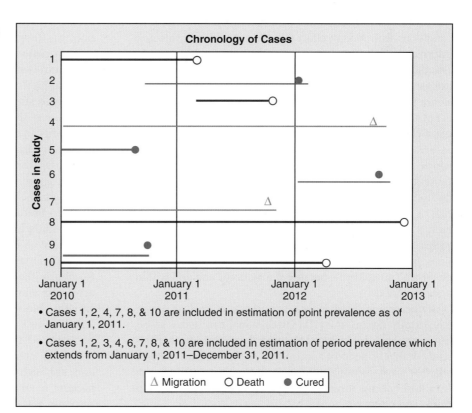

TABLE 11-3	Advantages and Disadvantages of Cross-Sectional or Prevalence Study Design	
Advantages	**Disadvantages**	
Takes less time than other studies before results are seen	Describes only what exists at the time of the prevalence study; does not answer whether the health characteristic or the disease came first	
Inexpensive	Examines only survivors and those alive to be found as cases	
Helpful in case finding, program planning, planning of health care facilities or special units, and sample size determination	Not good for rare conditions or diseases	
Stimulates new ideas or hypotheses	Given a health characteristic, fails to identify future likelihood of developing the disease	

Advantages and Disadvantages

Table 11-3 indicates the advantages and disadvantages of the cross-sectional or prevalence study design. It is a useful study design when time and resources are limited. Using the cross-sectional design is appropriate when little is known about the health characteristics or disease under study. This study can provide new or beginning information on a multitude of conditions with modest effort and time. Analysis of this new information will stimulate the researcher to develop hypotheses that would motivate further testing and the use of more extensive study designs. Because the cross-sectional or prevalence study may be considered a descriptive study, its intent is not to show cause-and-effect relations between, for example, a characteristic such as alcohol intake and a disease such as breast cancer. Analytic and experimental study designs, which are discussed later in this chapter, can assess the cause-and-effect relation. Unlike the analytic and experimental study designs, the cross-sectional design cannot assess the risk or likelihood for development of a disease. Other limitations of the cross-sectional design include dealing only with survivors, not being effective in studying rare conditions because a large sample is necessary to obtain cases, or missing an epidemic because it may occur and end within a short period.[7]

By becoming familiar with the cross-sectional or prevalence study design, the HIM professional can better assess how prevalence rates are determined, determine whether this study design is the most appropriate one to use, and evaluate whether cross-sectional studies performed within the health care facility have formed appropriate conclusions (i.e., not cause-and-effect relations).

Survey Research

Other types of descriptive study designs include the survey design. Here, the research focuses on collecting data with a survey instrument such as a questionnaire or interview guide. When surveys are constructed, there are certain elements to pay particular attention to. These elements include the following:

- Framing of questions—Include questions that collect data to answer the research question or address the study's specific aims.
- Wording—When constructing the survey instrument, think about your audience or recipients and write so that it is clear to them. Also, work with an expert in survey design, who can help formulate effective questions that are clear and appropriate for the particular audience.
- Cover letter—The cover letter that will accompany the survey is very important. It should briefly describe the study, identify the research sponsor and the researcher's qualifications, ask for the recipient's participation, stress that responses will be kept confidential, list the date when the survey should be returned, and state that a copy of the results will be provided after the study is completed. Incentives related to completion of the survey can also be included to increase the response rate. (See example of cover letter later in this section.)
- Mail, fax, e-mail, Web—Choose the medium to present the survey. With the wide distribution of the Internet and its related technologies, online questionnaires have become a rational carrier of survey investigation compared with traditional methods such as mail, fax, or phone surveys.[11] The commonly cited advantages include easy access, instant distribution, and reduced costs. In addition, the Internet allows questionnaires and surveys to reach a nationwide or even worldwide population with minimum cost and time. Other reported benefits include the graphical and interactive design on the Web. The automated storage of data from the Web server into the database at the back end, after the responder submits the form, can save the time of tedious data entry and create fewer data-entry errors. Also, it can prevent the responder from sending inappropriate data by using certain programming restrictions. Additional features that may help the respondents complete the survey include the help button, as in the example that follows this list. In the study by Schleyer and Forrest,[11] the authors state that the Web-based survey will be more economical than the mail survey when the sample size is more than 275. Recognize the bias in using the Internet: those without access are eliminated from participating.
- Length—Most surveys should be limited to a maximum length of two to three pages so that they will most likely be answered. In the electronic health record (EHR) study described later, the Web-based survey totaled 13 pages and, although the authors thought this would still work because it was Web based, it was too long for effective response and data collection.

- Question ordering—It is important to think about the order of specific questions. Normally, the demographic questions are listed first, then the more content-related questions, and then the open-ended questions.
- Open versus closed questions—Open-ended or unstructured format questions are those that ask a question and do not provide a list of responses to choose from, similar to an essay question. They enable the recipient to write out his or her thoughts in free form. Close-ended or structured format questions are those that ask a question and provide a list of responses to choose from, similar to multiple-choice questions, dichotomous or yes/no questions, or questions based on level or measurement or ranking. In the EHR study, both close-ended and open-ended questions were used. We decided to add the open-ended or unstructured questions so that richer data could be obtained.
- Pilot testing—Every survey should be pilot tested with a small sample of the potential recipients. The recipients should go through the survey as if they are going to answer the questions and provide feedback on any changes or additions to the survey. After the feedback is received by the research team, the survey should be changed to meet the feedback received, where applicable.
- Sample size (one can choose to use the following available lists)
  - Faculty/student lists
  - Insurance lists
  - Clinic/hospital list
  - Organization list
  - Society list
- After deciding who will be surveyed, it is easy to choose a systematic sample from an existing list. For example, after the sample size of 100 is decided on and your recipients are members of AHIMA who joined in the past year, a list of the recipients can be obtained, and then a systematic random sample can be taken from this list.
- Response rate—Researchers always strive for a very high response rate. Wyatt states that to have valid results from survey studies, a response rate of at least 80% should be obtained.[12] However, this can be difficult to achieve, and extensive follow-up techniques are needed. After 2 weeks, if facilities/respondents do not respond, a follow-up e-mail or phone call (or both) should be made to the facility asking them to complete the survey, reiterating the importance of the study and its results, and asking if they have any questions regarding the survey. Including different types of survey media and follow-up e-mails or phone calls are essential in obtaining a high response rate.
- Low response—Do not be that alarmed if the intended response rate is not reached. If it is found that the recipients who did respond are similar in demographics to all the intended recipients, then this allows the researcher to state that the responses received, although lower than expected, are similar to what can be expected from the entire sample. Because the list of intended recipients is available, the demographic information can be obtained from the list provided and compared with the recipients who did respond.
- Coding survey and data entry—After all data are received from the survey, they should be coded and then entered into an appropriate statistical software package for analysis. If a Web-based survey is used, then the coding and data entry do not have to be performed because this is completed when the survey is designed. Data entry is automatic because as the recipient responds, the data are automatically downloaded to a database management system for data quality checks and statistical analysis. See Figure 11-6, which outlines how the survey is built on the Web and sent to the respondent through the Internet, where it can be automatically reviewed by the researcher as it is being stored on the database server.

Following is an example of a descriptive/prevalence study with a Web-based survey focus. The purpose of the study was to measure the awareness of individuals of the American Society for Testing and Materials (ASTM) standards for content and structure of the EHR.[13] The examples include the cover letter and part of the Web-based survey (Figure 11-7) used to collect data.

Example of Cover Letter

Dear _____:

IRB #

Thank you for agreeing to participate in the research study titled "Standards for the Content of Electronic Health Records" sponsored by the American Health Information Management Association (AHIMA).

As we described to you previously, your participation in this study is extremely important because your responses could lead to the uniform data standards for the electronic health record (EHR), which HIPAA is recommending.

As we described to you previously, the focus of this research is the American Society for Testing and Materials (ASTM) E1384 Standard Guide on Content and Structure of Electronic Health Records and the corresponding ASTM E1633 Coded Values for Electronic Health Records. We are investigating the level of awareness and measuring the extent of usage of the standards for the content of the EHR. We are also attempting to collect feedback on how the standards for EHR content meet users' needs.

Your prompt participation is extremely important and will aid in the next revision of the standards. For your efforts in completing the survey, we are offering an opportunity for your name to be entered into a drawing to win $200! There will be two $200 prizes awarded from the pool of people completing the survey!

In addition, you will receive the overall results of the study and a complimentary copy of the most recent edition of the *Journal of the American Health Information Management Association* (JAHIMA) or, if you already receive that journal, another comparable AHIMA journal of your choice.

Your responses will be kept completely confidential and will only be reported in aggregate form. Completion of the survey will take approximately 20 minutes. Please click here to access the survey.

Once you access the Web site, please follow the directions included in the survey. Please provide your responses to us not later than _____ to be eligible for the drawing.

Your responses will be kept completely confidential.

If you have any questions or concerns regarding completion of the survey, please contact Valerie Watzlaf or Patti Firouzan at _____.

Thank you very much.
Sincerely,
Valerie J. M. Watzlaf
Patti Firouzan

Qualitative Research

Qualitative research is another type of descriptive study design that is used when little is known about a specific topic. It is quite effective and popular in HIM research because much of what is studied within the HIM context has not been examined before. Qualitative research designs provide a foundation for larger quantitative studies. It also provides richer information than can be obtained from quantitative-based studies alone. It is most appropriate to use in examining attitudes, feelings, perceptions, or relationships, but it can also be used to obtain more extensive information than what can be collected with quantitative methods. For example, in the obesity and breast cancer recurrence study by Katoh et al.,[14] quantitative methods were used to collect the data. Thus, when data were examined in relation to survival, for example, the length of survival was collected but not the

quality of life. This is one variable that could have been collected through a qualitative design by asking the study participants about their quality of life through focus groups or interviews. Sometimes, a mixed-methodology design can be used in which quantitative methods and qualitative methods are used together to collect the data.

There are three main types of qualitative research: participant observation, focus groups, and case studies.

The first, participant observation, is when the researcher is immersed into the subject's environment to learn what the subject experiences firsthand. The researcher pays special attention to the physical, social, and human environment, as well as formal and informal interactions and unplanned activities. The researcher can choose to be disguised or undisguised and is basically there to describe a problem to outsiders on the basis of the understanding of the insider's perspective.[5] For example, participant observation in HIM may include observing employees' perceptions and interactions after an EHR system is implemented in their health care facility. The researchers should focus their observations on activities surrounding the use of the EHR and how well the activities are carried out when using the EHR: who is in command or control of using the EHR for HIM functions, the channels of communication when the EHR is in use, and how effective the communication is. The participant observation experience should help to address the whys and hows of the research questions.

Focus groups or focus group interviews include a small group of people (usually experts in the field or people whose opinion on the topic is being sought—for example, a study in Nebraska of the uninsured and underinsured involved focus

INFRASTRUCTURE

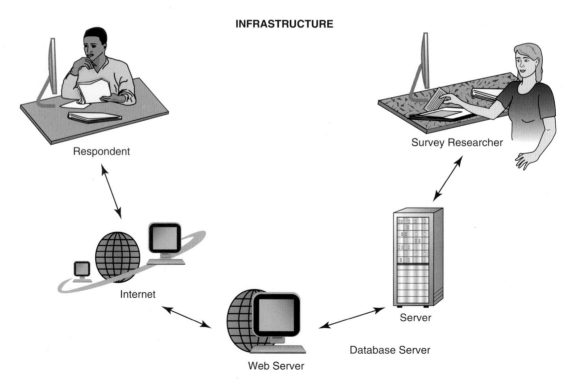

FIGURE 11-6 Web-based survey process.

EHR and Data Elements Survey

1. What is the current stage of your EHR system?

☐ **Planning** (Initial stage of EHR implementation and involves identification of the purpose and features of the proposed system.)

☐ **Development** (Involves design of the EHR system and includes both the conceptual design and the physical design.)

☐ **Modular Installation** (Implementation of the EHR system that can include portions of the entire system and adding components over time or implementing the entire system at once.)

☐ **Fully In-Place** (The EHR system collects data from multiple sources throughout the organization, provides decision support, and is used by all caregivers at the point of care as the primary source of information.)

☐ **Other** (Please specify in text.)_____

Below is a list of data elements related to the **TREATMENT PLAN** for the EHR. This includes data entries that direct a patient's treatment and detailed data on deliverance of orders and compliance with any diagnostic or therapeutic treatment plans, whether written, oral, or standing.

2. Please indicate which of those elements you collect (will collect) in your existing system.

Elements of Treatment Plan*	Already included/will include in EHR?		
	Yes	No	Not applicable
Treatment Plan	☐	☐	☐
Treatment Plan ID	☐	☐	☐
Date-time	☐	☐	☐
Care/treatment plan (text)	☐	☐	☐
Clinical order(s) (full text)	☐	☐	☐
Date-time of order	☐	☐	☐

3. What other data elements related to the TREATMENT PLAN do you believe are needed to be included in the EHR? _____

_____

_____

4. What data elements related to the TREATMENT PLAN do you believe should be removed from the standard data set? _____

_____

_____

5. Do you have additional comments on the listed data elements related to the ORDER-CARE/TREATMENT PLAN? _____

_____

_____

*Respondents were able to click on a term and the definition of the term was provided in a pop-up box.

FIGURE 11-7 Excerpts of a Web-based survey used to examine the use of the EHR and data elements included.

groups of those individuals who fit the category—and what living without insurance was like) who are brought together to answer and discuss specific questions. Here, the study participants can discuss issues, hear one another's viewpoint, and comment on those views. It enables the researcher to learn more about the topic because a group of experts is brainstorming. It also provides the researcher with the ability to examine interactions among members of the group. There is usually a moderator and a recorder, and sometimes the focus group is videotaped. Also, more than one focus group can frame a particular study. For example, in a study examining the effectiveness and efficiency of public health reporting with ICD-10-CM and ICD-10-PCS, a group of experts in ICD-10 and public health would be solicited to form a focus group to answer questions related to information accumulated from the first three study parts and to make recommendations on where changes need to be made. Some questions may include the following:

- After review of the public health diagnoses and procedures reportable list, are there any diagnoses or procedures that you believe should be added, deleted, or changed? If so, please explain.
- Based on the information provided to you, what recommendations do you have to improve the ICD-10-CM and ICD-10-PCS coding systems for public health reporting?

Notice how the questions are framed to elicit discussion. The focus group interview is flexible and is usually of low cost because in just one setting, data from 6 to 12 individuals can be gathered. The focus group data can be difficult to analyze and control and can sometimes be difficult; however, a good moderator can diminish the negative effects.

Case studies seek to provide a richly detailed portrait of an individual, program, event, department, time period, culture, or community.[5] For example, case studies can be conducted on health care facilities by use of report cards on their clinicians to determine their effects on the quality of patient care and outcomes. Extensive interviews can be carried out with physicians and other health care providers, patients, administrators, and other staff to determine their perceptions of the use of the report cards and their thoughts on how it has affected patient care. Then, additional sources can be used to substantiate and complement what was found, such as medical records, report card databases, and observations of relevant quality management committee meetings.

One of the most difficult parts of conducting qualitative research is making sense of the data that have been collected. Sometimes the data are extremely voluminous, leading to hours of organization and analysis. However, the researcher can examine qualitative data quite effectively if the following questions are examined:

- What patterns and common themes emerge from the data collected?
- Can these patterns or themes be narrowed to three or four basic themes in which data can be categorized?
- Can data matrices be developed to answer the research questions?

Based on the study described earlier on report cards and quality, one example of a matrix describing common themes may look like this:

Report Cards	Quality	Cost	LOS	Outcomes
Clinicians				
Management				
Staff				

LOS, Length of stay.

One of the major weaknesses of qualitative research is its lack of generalizability or extrapolation of the results. This is because the sample size is usually small and cannot be taken as representative of the population under study. Also, the reliability of the results is another problem because the collection and analysis of the data can be quite different across researchers. However, when one wants to obtain more comprehensive information in an inexpensive and less time-consuming way, and when one is exploring new areas, it is an excellent design to use.

> ### ✔ SELF-ASSESSMENT QUIZ
>
> 10. Which type of study design is normally used to generate hypotheses?
>   a. Analytic study
>   b. Experimental study
>   c. Descriptive study
>   d. Quasi-experimental study
> 11. One disadvantage of this type of epidemiologic study design is that it only examines survivors and those living as cases. It is called a:
>   a. Clinical trial
>   b. Community trial
>   c. Prospective study
>   d. Cross-sectional prevalence study
> 12. When is it best to use a qualitative study design?
> 13. What is a mixed-methodology design?

Analytic Study Design

Case-Control or Retrospective Study Design

In an analytic study, a disease or health condition is examined to determine possible causes. Intensive research related to the disease is necessary to determine characteristics that may cause the specific disease. These characteristics are also referred to as exposure characteristics or risk factors because they may increase the risk for development of the disease. The exposure characteristic or risk factor may also be referred to as the independent variable and the disease under study as the dependent variable. The case-control or retrospective study is one type of analytic study design. The researcher collects data on the cases (those who have the disease that is under study) and controls (those who are similar to the cases but do not have the disease that is under study) by looking back in time. For example, in the ovarian cancer study described earlier in this chapter, the cases included patients with epithelial ovarian cancer and the controls included patients with other diagnoses who were admitted to the same hospital during the same time period as the cases. The cases and controls were also similar in age. Specific exposure characteristics (possible risk factors) were collected for both groups by retrieving the data from medical records and through personal interviews.

When conducting a case-control or retrospective study, the following design issues must be considered:

Randomly select cases by using incidence or prevalence rates, and obtain information on the patients' past history of exposures or risk factors. Specify criteria for the cases (i.e., epithelial ovarian cancer, ICD-9-CM code of 183.0, pathology reports, and slides indicating that the case truly is a case and does have the disease under study).

Randomly select controls similar to the cases in characteristics such as age and sex but without the disease and obtain a past history of their exposures. Select controls from populations such as hospitals and other health care facilities and residents of a community and neighbors, friends, or siblings of the cases. Cases and controls should come from similar populations to demonstrate that those who have the disease under study are similar to other people in the community except for the disease of interest. For example, if the cases are hospital patients, controls should also be hospital patients but with a different disease or illness from the one under study.

Determine whether matching will be used. Some studies match on variables such as age and sex because these variables affect both the independent variables (exposure characteristic or risk factor) and the dependent variables (disease). When variables affect the dependent and independent variables, they are referred to as confounding variables. In the ovarian cancer study, cases and controls were matched on age within 5 years because age is related to several of the risk factors, such as use of birth control pills and nulliparity and incidence of ovarian cancer.

Design the research instrument. To collect the data, the research instrument should be developed. The following are the different types of research instruments that may be used in a case-control study:
- Interviewer-administered questionnaire (in person or by phone)
- Self-administered questionnaire through the mail or on the Internet
- Worksheet to collect data abstracted from medical records
- Data collection worksheets for recording data from slides, laboratory tests, observations from physical examinations, and so on

The following list provides steps used in the design and development of the research instrument:

List all variables to be measured.

Develop the data collection instrument. Precode each variable on the data collection form with a number. When the data are entered into the computer for analysis, each variable will be recognized. Use closed-ended questions because they are easier to code. Use of pictures and lists will improve the subject's recall.

Pilot test the data collection instrument to verify collection of the variables.

Select the data sources so that comparable details for cases and controls are provided.

An example of some sections of the research instrument used in the ovarian cancer study is presented in Figure 11-3, sample of ovarian cancer questionnaire.

Hypothetical Example of How Subjects Are Selected into a Case-Control Study

Figure 11-8 is a hypothetical example of how subjects are selected from a health care population into a case-control study. In this example, the independent variable (exposure characteristic or risk factor) is alcohol use and the dependent variable (disease) is breast cancer. The cases are subjects with breast cancer separated into alcohol users and nonusers. The controls are subjects with other diseases, such as heart disease, separated into alcohol users and nonusers. In most research studies, a larger number of controls than cases are chosen to better determine differences between the cases and controls.

Determining the Odds Ratio

The **odds ratio** is an estimate of the relative risk a person has if he or she is exposed to a certain characteristic. One should

FIGURE 11-8 Example of case-control study population.

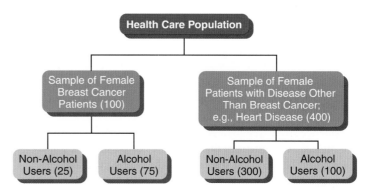

use the odds ratio only with case-control studies, when the disease is rare, and when cases are true representatives of all cases and controls are true representatives of all controls.[6]

Example of the Odds Ratio

	Breast Cancer	Control	Total
Alcohol	75 (a)	100 (b)	175 (a + b)
None	25 (c)	300 (d)	325 (c + d)
	100 (a + c)	400 (b + d)	500 (a + b + c + d)

a = Subjects with the independent variable (alcohol) who have the disease (breast cancer)

b = Subjects with the independent variable (alcohol) who did not have the disease (breast cancer)

c = Subjects without the independent variable (alcohol) who have the disease (breast cancer)

d = Subjects without the independent variable (alcohol) who did not have the disease (breast cancer)

If a disease is rare, then a/(a + b) is about equal to a/b because a is small relative to b. Also, c/(c + d) is about equal to c/d. Therefore, by assuming that a + b is about equal to b and that c + d is about equal to d, the formula for the odds ratio is as follows:

$$\frac{(a/b)}{(c/d)} = \frac{ad}{bc}$$

Therefore, in the hypothetical case shown before:

$$\frac{(ad)}{(bc)} = \frac{(75)(300)}{(100)(25)} = \frac{22,500}{2500} = 9$$

This means that a person who drinks alcohol is nine times more likely to get breast cancer than a person who does not drink alcohol. Further refinement of this odds ratio could include defining alcohol levels to the actual amount a person drinks. Then 2 × 2 tables (such as the table used in the preceding example) could be constructed to examine levels of alcohol intake, and odds ratios could be developed and compared. Other confounders for the development of breast cancer, such as age, are not addressed here. More advanced statistical analysis beyond the scope of this chapter would be necessary to examine the risk of alcohol intake and breast cancer while controlling for confounding variables.

Advantages and Disadvantages

Table 11-4 summarizes the advantages and disadvantages of the case-control study design. Like the cross-sectional or prevalence study design, it is useful when time and resources are limited. The intent of the researcher is to establish some association between the disease and the exposure characteristic. This study design does have drawbacks because it relies on recall or past information from the subjects, making

validation of that information somewhat difficult. Also, obtaining an appropriate control group for the case-control study to be valid is difficult. It is recommended that four controls be obtained for each case. Finding that large a control group while matching for specific characteristics such as age and sex can be difficult. Another major limitation of the case-control study is that the true relative risk cannot be determined; it can only be estimated by using the odds ratio. However, when one wants to determine quickly and inexpensively whether an association exists between a health condition and a characteristic, the case-control method is an appropriate route to take.[7]

The HIM professional can perform research with the case-control study design when directing a disease registry, such as a cancer or trauma registry, and when performing departmental and facility-wide performance improvement studies. Also, performing and aiding researchers in carrying out this study design are important roles of the HIM professional.

Prospective, Cohort, or Incidence Study Design

The prospective study design does something that neither the cross-sectional nor the case-control method can do. It determines whether the characteristic or suspected risk factor truly preceded the disease or health condition. The prospective study design is the best method for determining the magnitude of risk in the population with the characteristic or

---

TABLE 11-4 Advantages and Disadvantages of the Case-Control Design

Advantages	Disadvantages
Well suited for rare diseases or those with a long latency period, such as cancer and heart disease	Relies on recall or records for information on past exposures of certain factors; accuracy may be difficult to obtain
Takes less time before results are seen than the prospective or cohort study but more time than a cross-sectional or prevalence study	Validation of information collected difficult to obtain
Inexpensive	Occurrence of exposure obtained from selected cases and controls
Requires comparatively few subjects	Selection of an appropriate control group may be difficult
Uses existing records	Rates of disease in the exposed and unexposed subjects cannot be determined because the subjects are not being followed over time
Minimal risk to subjects	Probability of bias may be greater than in the cohort study
Allows a study of multiple potential causes of disease	Supports causal hypothesis by establishing an association but does not prove it

suspected risk factor. A prospective study typically includes the following steps:

Identify subjects with the characteristic under study who are free from the disease.

Identify subjects without the characteristic under study who are free from the disease. These subjects are considered the comparison group.

Follow both groups forward in time to determine if and when they develop the disease or health condition under study.

The initial assessment to determine who should be included in the prospective study is the same as that for a cross-sectional or prevalence study. In both designs, the researcher must identify cases and noncases and determine whether they have the characteristic under study. However, when the disease under study begins to develop in subjects in the prospective study, incident cases or new cases are collected. Prospective study participants are usually volunteers. They are examined to make sure they do not have the disease at the beginning of the study. To do this, the researcher collects data related to their occupations, medical histories, and social status. Physical examinations and laboratory tests may also be needed to ensure that the subjects do not have the disease.

Some prospective or cohort studies begin in a community or an industrial setting or within a hospital. The subjects are separated into two groups on the basis of their exposures or health characteristic and then are followed forward to determine whether the disease develops. A hypothetical example would be subjects who are asked to participate in a prospective study to determine whether at any time after delivery they have postpartum depression. The hypothesis for this study is that women with babies who spend some time in the neonatal intensive care unit may have a higher incidence of postpartum depression than women whose babies do not spend time in the neonatal intensive care unit. Data on prenatal care, history of depression, family history of depression, and family life after delivery of the baby are collected from both groups. The women in both groups are then followed forward in time to see whether postpartum depression develops.

Another common example is comparing a group of people in the community who have certain social habits, such as comparing a group of people who exercise with a group of sedentary people. In this example, both groups receive physical examinations and laboratory tests to be certain that they are not hypertensive. Interviews to collect data on family and personal histories are also conducted. Both groups are then followed to determine whether they become hypertensive. The hypothesis for this study is that people who exercise have a decreased incidence of hypertension compared with those who do not exercise. Data on specific types, amounts, and levels of exercise also need to be collected and analyzed.

To determine whether one group does have an increased risk for development of a disease as a result of health habits or characteristics, incidence rates must be determined. As stated previously, an incidence rate (IR) is as follows:

$$\frac{\text{Number of new cases over a time period}}{\text{Population at risk (those free of disease at start of study)}} \times 1000$$

For the preceding examples, the IRs would be as follows:

$$\frac{\text{Number of postpartum depression cases during a time period}}{\text{Women who delivered babies in hospital during a given time period}} \times 1000$$

$$\frac{\text{Number of new cases of hypertension during a time period in a specific community}}{\text{Population (both sedentary and those who exercise) in the specific community during a given time period}} \times 1000$$

To determine which groups have a greater risk for development of the disease under study, the relative risk (RR) is determined according to the following formula:

$$RR = \frac{\text{Incidence rate exposed (IRe)}}{\text{Incidence rate unexposed (IRo)}}$$

By using the data displayed in Table 11-5, one can calculate the RR. The IR of the group who does not exercise is 145 and the IR of the group who does exercise is 50. The RR for this study is $145/50 = 2.9$. Therefore, the people who do not exercise are about three times more likely to have hypertension develop than are the people who do exercise.

Although there are more advantages than disadvantages to using the prospective study (Table 11-6), a major benefit of this design is that it accurately determines whether the characteristic was present before the disease developed.[6] Because the IRs and RRs can be calculated, the researcher can determine the number of cases that can be prevented if a specific characteristic or exposure is controlled. This is a major advantage over the study designs discussed earlier.

Historical Prospective Study Design

In the historical prospective study design, past records are used to collect information regarding the exposure characteristic or risk factor under study. Then, over the next 10, 15, or 20 years, medical records, death certificates, and so on are monitored to determine the number of cases of a particular disease that have developed. The time of the actual study and the end of the follow-up period happen some time in the future. IRs and RRs are then calculated for the exposed and unexposed groups.

TABLE 11-5	Determining the Relative Risk: Incidence Rate per 1000 of Hypertension by Levels of Exercise		
	Population	Cases	Incidence Rate
Exercise	1000	50	50
No exercise	1000	145	145
Total	2000	195	97.5

TABLE 11-6 Advantages and Disadvantages of Prospective, Cohort, or Incidence Study

Advantages	Disadvantages
Describes which came first—the characteristic or the disease	Not good with rare diseases because it takes so long to follow them
Relative risk is determined, not established	Subjects are lost during follow-up because of death, withdrawal, migration.
Analytically tests the hypothesis of cause and effect	Long time to see results
Decreases the amount of bias caused by recall or memory	Expensive Unexpected changes in environment or social habits may influence the health outcome. Subjects tend to participate less because of the amount of time they must spend in the study.

The purpose of the study illustrated in Figure 11-9 was to examine the association between obesity using body mass index (BMI) levels and recurrence and mortality in breast cancer. The risk factor or independent variable is obesity and the dependent variable is recurrence of breast cancer or mortality with breast cancer as the primary cause of death. Both the obese and nonobese cohorts were identified some time in the past (before 2000) from medical records, an existing database from the oncology department, and cancer registry data. The study required all subjects to be free of a breast cancer recurrence from 1977 to 2000. The groups were stratified on the basis of their BMI levels. They were followed by use of both the cancer registry and medical record to determine their rates of breast cancer recurrence and mortality caused by the breast cancer.

Advantages and Disadvantages

The major advantages of this study design compared with the prospective study design are that less time and effort are expended and the cost is lower. All other advantages and disadvantages listed in Table 11-5 for the prospective design hold true for the historical prospective design, except that the RR is really an estimate of risk similar to an odds ratio.

✅ SELF-ASSESSMENT QUIZ

14. Which statistic is an estimate of the relative risk and is used in case-control studies when the disease under study is rare and when cases are true representatives of all cases and controls?
    a. Odds ratio
    b. Life analysis
    c. Correlation
    d. Regression

15. Which study design is well suited for rare diseases or those with a long latency period, such as cancer and heart disease?
    a. Prospective study
    b. Clinical trial
    c. Descriptive study
    d. Case-control study

16. Compare the prospective study design with the historical prospective study design.
    a. What is the major difference between the prospective study design and the historical prospective study design?
    b. What is the major advantage of the historical prospective study design compared with the prospective study design?

Examined medical records and tumor registry data to determine those women who were diagnosed with breast cancer. Data on height and weight at diagnosis were also determined to evaluate obesity levels.	Monitored both obese and non-obese groups to determine their health outcome: 1) Breast cancer recurrence 2) Death due to breast cancer 3) Alive and free of disease	Study period ends. Incidence rates of breast cancer recurrence are determined as well as mortality rates for both obese and non-obese groups.
From 2000	2001-2008	2013

FIGURE 11-9 Historical prospective study design.

Experimental Epidemiology

Clinical and Community Trials

Two types of studies are referred to in experimental epidemiology. They are the clinical trial and the community trial.

The clinical trial and the community trial are similar to the prospective study in that they comprise two groups that have different exposures and that are followed to determine their outcomes. In this design, a certain medication or treatment is given to a group, and their outcomes are compared with those of a control or comparison group (subjects who do not have the intervention). In the clinical or community trial, the researcher provides the "exposure" in a controlled environment by providing some intervention procedure (e.g., medicine, education, surgical procedure). The researcher decides what the intervention will be and which subjects will receive it and which will not.

Before beginning the trial, the researcher must obtain informed consent from subjects and IRB approval to conduct the study and select the methods that will be used to randomize subjects into specific groups.

The researcher must also consider the following when conducting a clinical or community trial:
- How will adverse reactions and other complications be recorded and addressed?
- What criteria will be used to exclude and include subjects?
- Will the study be single blind (subject blind as to which group he or she is in), double blind (subject and observer blind), or triple blind (subject, observer, and statistician blind)?
- Ethical considerations: If the treatment group responds favorably to treatment, should the study be stopped and the treatment offered to both groups?

The difference between a clinical trial and a community trial is that the clinical trial usually begins in a clinical setting, and the intervention medication, treatment, or procedure is tested on selected subjects. In a community trial, the intervention medication, treatment, or procedure is tested on a group of subjects as a whole within a particular community, outside a clinical setting.[7]

Life-Table Analysis

Life-table analysis is most appropriate for prospective studies or experimental studies when the researcher has a loss of subjects as a result of follow-up or the study ends before recurrence or death has occurred in some subjects. Life-table analysis examines survival times of individual subjects. Survival time includes the time subjects are free of disease after diagnosis or the time to recovery or improvement after the start of a specific intervention medication, treatment, or procedure. Subjects tend to enter a study sample at different times as they enter for treatment. Each subject is followed until death, and during that time, a subject may be lost to follow-up because the researcher is not able to locate the subject and therefore cannot determine whether death has occurred. Also, some subjects may withdraw from the study because they do not want to participate in it or because it has ended. When a survival time is censored, this means that the

subject is alive at the time of analysis or was alive when last seen. Survival times are flagged with a plus sign (+) to indicate that they are censored.[15]

Life-table analysis operates on a premise called the person-time denominator. This is a special denominator that must be used in calculating rates for small study groups when subjects in the study are not all observed for the entire study period because of withdrawal, death, or loss to follow-up.

Assumptions for use of the life-table analysis are as follow:
- The risk of the outcome event (death) should not be different if a patient enters the study during the first year of the study versus the second or third year.
- The rate of the outcome event should not be higher at the end of 2 years of observation than at the end of 1 year.
- The rate of the outcome event is similar among subjects lost to follow-up and among subjects who remain under observation.

One type of life-table analysis is the Kaplan-Meier product limit method, which is appropriate for both small and large sample sizes. The result of the Kaplan-Meier product limit method is a survival curve.

The following is a hypothetical example of subjects in a clinical trial and how the Kaplan-Meier product limit method is calculated.

Example of Kaplan-Meier Product Limit Method

Subject Number	Survival Time (months)
1	47
2	40+
3	37
4	34
5	48+
6	41
7	41
8	45
9	23
10	43

+, censored observations, withdrawn alive or lost to follow-up.

Survival Time (1)	Rank (2)	Uncensored Rank (3)	Cumulative Proportion Surviving (4)	Proportion Surviving (5)
23	1	1	9/10 = 0.90	0.900
34	2	2	8/9 = 0.889	0.800
37	3	3	7/8 = 0.875	0.700
40+	4	—	—	—
41	5	5	5/6 = 0.833	0.583
41	6	6	4/5 = 0.80	0.466
43	7	7	3/4 = 0.75	0.350
45	8	8	2/3 = 0.667	0.233
47	9	9	1/2 = 0.50	0.117
48+	10	—	—	—

(1) Survival time (t_i) months; (2) rank; (3) uncensored ranks (r_i); (4) proportion surviving ($n - r$)/[($n - r$) + 1]; (5) cumulative proportion surviving $s(t)$.

Column 1 lists all survival times, both censored and uncensored, in order from smallest to largest. (Uncensored observations are listed first if censored and uncensored observations have the same survival times.)

Column 2 lists the rank of each observation shown in column 1.

Column 3 lists the rank of uncensored observations only, where $t(r) = t$.

Column 4 shows the estimated proportion of subjects in the sample who survive longer than t. To calculate the proportion of subjects surviving through each time interval, n is sample size (10) and r is the uncensored rank, compute $(n - r)/(n - r) + 1$. Therefore, $9/10 = 0.90$ means that 90% of the subjects in the sample have survived longer than 23 months.

In *Column 5*, all values in column 4 up to and including t are multiplied for each survival time. For example, $9/10 = 0.900$; $9/10 \times 8/9 = 0.800$; $9/10 \times 8/9 \times 7/8 = 0.700$, and so on.[16]

An example of the Kaplan-Meier curve for obesity and breast cancer survival is shown in Figure 11-10. This figure shows that approximately 80% of both groups survived about 58 months, or 4.8 years. At about 110 months, or 9.2 years, approximately 68% of the nonobese group had survived, whereas only 54% of the obese group had survived.

SELF-ASSESSMENT QUIZ

17. Which type of study design modifies the health characteristics that are found to cause the disease by using health care interventions that control the disease from progressing or prevent the disease from occurring?
    a. Analytic study
    b. Descriptive study
    c. Outcomes study
    d. Experimental study
18. Which type of life analysis is appropriate for both large and small sample sizes and provides a survival curve as a method to examine survival between two groups?
    a. Rank and survival method
    b. Kaplan-Meier product limit method
    c. Standardized mortality method
    d. Censorship and survival method
19. Describe life-table analysis.
    a. What is a person-time denominator and when is it used?
    b. What are the assumptions that must be met before life-table analysis is used?
    c. For which study designs is life-table analysis most appropriate?

Comparison

Selection of the study design will greatly affect the results of the research. Table 11-7 compares the various research designs discussed in this chapter.

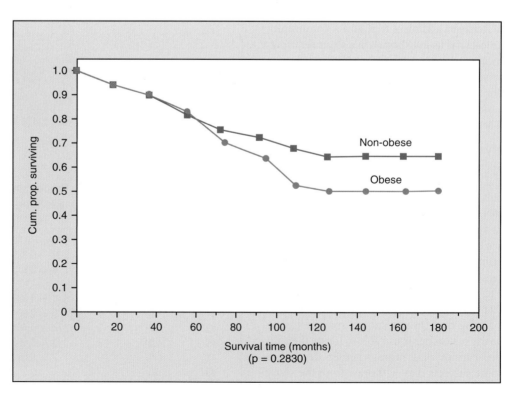

FIGURE 11-10 Kaplan-Meier estimation of survival.

TABLE 11-7 Epidemiologic Research

ANALYTIC STUDIES

Type	Descriptive Cross-Sectional Prevalence Study	Case-Control Retrospective	Cohort Prospective, Incidence	Historical Prospective	Experimental Studies: Clinical and Community Trials
Description	Examines the distribution of disease or health characteristics in populations at one point in time Useful when little is known about the disease or characteristics under study	Examines a disease to determine whether certain health (risk factor) characteristics are causing the disease			Modifies the health characteristics that are found to cause the disease by using health care interventions that control progression of the disease or prevent the disease from occurring
Outcomes	• Hypotheses • Further research • Case finding • Program planning • Planning of health care facilities or special units • Determining sample size • Morbidity rates within a health care facility	• Studies of multiple potential causes of diseases • Supports causal hypothesis by establishing an association but does not prove it • Odds ratio	• Describes which came first, the characteristics or the disease • Determines relative risk (not estimates) • Analytically tests the hypothesis of cause and effect	Outcomes are the same as in the cohort study except that the relative risk is really an estimate of risk that is similar to an odds ratio	• Compares changes in a disease over time in a treatment and control group • Life-table analysis is used to compare survival times in the two groups • Determines whether an experimental intervention is effective
Time	Takes less time than other types of studies	Takes less time before results are seen than the prospective or cohort studies but more time than the cross-sectional or prevalence studies	Requires a great amount of time on part of subject (subjects may participate less because of it) because they must be monitored to determine whether they develop the disease	Takes less time than the full prospective study but somewhat more time than the cross-sectional or case-control study	Time varies depending on the type of trial being performed; most experimental studies take longer than the cross-sectional, case-control, and historical prospective.
Financial resources	Uses modest effort and financial resources	Inexpensive; uses existing records	Expensive because of the time needed to follow the subjects	Less expensive than the full prospective study but more than the case-control or cross-sectional studies	Expenses vary depending on type of intervention and length of time of the trial but can be very high.
Sample size	Large sample size is necessary, so does not work well with rare conditions	Requires comparatively few subjects Well suited for rare diseases or those with a long latency period, such as cancer and heart disease	Large random sample is always better to truly represent the population under study	Same as prospective	Sample sizes vary and may be small depending on the type of intervention and the appropriateness of the subjects who receive it.

Continued

TABLE 11-7   Epidemiologic Research—cont'd

ANALYTIC STUDIES

Limitations					

• Fails to identify future likelihood of developing the disease
• Does not answer the question of whether the health characteristic or the disease came first
• Does not assess risk or likelihood of developing the disease
• Examines only survivors and those alive found as cases
• Misses an epidemic that may only be present for a short period
	• Because of reliance on subjects' recall or records for information of past exposures to risk factors:
	  ○ Accuracy may be difficult to obtain
	  ○ Difficult to validate information
	• Selection of appropriate control group may be difficult
	• Rates of disease in the exposed and unexposed subjects cannot be determined because the subjects are not being followed over time
		• Subjects are lost during the study period from death, withdrawal, and migration
		• Not good with rare diseases because of the length of time needed for following the cases
		• Unexpected changes in the environment may influence the health outcome
			Same as prospective study except that subjects lost to follow-up may be fewer because of the shorter time period to follow them	• Adverse reactions
				• Ethical considerations
				• Loss of subjects through death, withdrawal
				• Compliance of subjects	

USE OF COMPUTER SOFTWARE IN RESEARCH

Because most research studies generate large amounts of data, a variety of computer software are used to sort and analyze the data, depending on the type of statistics that are generated. An initial database can be constructed with any spreadsheet or database software or statistical software such as SPSS (Statistical Process for the Social Sciences; SPSS, Inc., Chicago, IL). Then further statistical analysis can be performed using software to perform frequency distributions, tests of significance, or life-table analysis.

For example, the HIM professional in conjunction with risk management personnel has been collecting data on the number of falls by both patients and employees that have occurred within the health care facility. Data collected include where and how the fall occurred; the type of injury that was sustained; the cause of the fall; and the age, sex, and race of the patients and employees who fell. The data have been coded and entered into an electronic spreadsheet. Further analysis is necessary to determine a frequency distribution on the total number of falls and the number of falls per nursing unit. Spreadsheet software can determine these distributions and can generate graphics to display the data. However, using spreadsheet software to determine more extensive statistical analysis may not be the most efficient route to take. To determine whether there is a significant association between a specific nursing unit and the number of falls, correlation coefficients and tests of significance may be necessary. These types of statistics may be more easily generated with statistical software. Further analysis to examine health outcomes 1 month, 6 months, or 1 year after the fall may include life-table analysis with SPSS software.

The HIM professional should know the types of software that are available to perform certain statistical tests. Statisticians should be consulted to aid in this process and in the interpretation and explanation of the data. Remember that the computer software or statistical analysis performed is only as good as the data that are collected and entered into the computer. It is up to the researcher to determine whether the results make sense and, therefore, how they should be applied and interpreted.

Other types of statistical software can aid in the collection of the data for a research study by assisting in the development of the questionnaire or data collection instrument. One example of such software is Epi Info™ (Centers for Disease Control and Prevention, Atlanta, GA). This software, which can be obtained at a low cost, not only aids in constructing the data collection instrument but also includes features such as SPSS to perform basic and advanced statistical analysis of the data.

Many types of computer software and statistical analysis applications are available. It is beyond the scope of this chapter to discuss all of them. However, the HIM professional should be aware of the computer software available to assist in database development and analysis of data. This may be the most important step the HIM professional takes when conducting research studies in the health care environment.

OUTCOME STUDIES AND EPIDEMIOLOGY

Today more than ever before, health care facilities, managed care organizations, federal and state governments, and the like are focusing on the outcomes of care and designing and carrying out outcomes studies. The HIM professional will be able to conduct unique, thorough, and sound outcomes research with a thorough understanding of epidemiologic research methods and the specific outcome measures that are being studied. In the beginning of this chapter, the epidemiologic study designs were explained and discussed, and the design of a research proposal or plan was explained. Now, the outcomes measures are briefly explained, and an outcomes study that was performed by the author and colleagues is discussed in relation to how it applies to outcomes research.

Outcomes research can focus on several measures. In the past, its main focus was on mortality rates. Now, because health care facilities are interested in knowing many other things about the end results of care, and The Joint Commission and the ORYX initiative require health care facilities to provide clinical outcome measures, the HIM professional must think of many different ways to study outcomes. The outcomes may focus on causation, efficiency (cost), treatment impact, or more generic measures such as morbidity, mortality, satisfaction, physical function, pain, emotional function, social function, cognitive function, vitality, and overall quality of life. Disease-specific measures are also common and require intense design and analysis to find accurate results.

The outcomes study that was performed by the author and colleagues[17] is a descriptive epidemiologic study that used a cross-sectional study design. Past research demonstrated that the medical record alone is not always an effective epidemiologic research tool when data are collected on specific risk factors associated with ovarian cancer.[18,19] However, when the medical record, as well as financial data and physician input, was used to study the cost of infections in an elderly population, an effective database emerged. This pilot study was designed to analyze noninstitutionalized elderly patient hospitalizations for type of diagnosis and procedures, DRGs, and infections. The hypothesis tested was that the elderly patient hospitalized with an infection has an increased length of stay and cost compared with those hospitalized without infections.

Study Procedures

All Medicare patients who were participating in the Good Health Study and admitted to a hospital in Pittsburgh, Pennsylvania, from July 1, 1986, through December 31, 1987, were studied.

The Good Health Study[20] examined noninstitutionalized elderly individuals for incidence rates of clinical infections, organisms responsible for infection, patterns of transmission, and the outcome of the infections measured by mortality, morbidity, and the adverse effects of treatment. This free-living elderly population is representative of the elderly in general. Comparisons of the Good Health Study population for health habits, living arrangements, medical conditions, and activities of daily living (ADLs) were consistently similar across three other studies of elderly persons in Boston, Massachusetts; New Haven, Connecticut; and Iowa.[21]

Medicare patient hospitalizations ($n = 165$) were analyzed by abstracting the medical records to determine the principal and secondary diagnoses and procedures. Diagnoses and procedures were recorded if they appeared anywhere in the medical record, including the discharge summary, progress notes, operative reports, and data on laboratory and clinical findings. The criteria for infections used in the Good Health Study were used to determine whether the symptoms, signs, and laboratory findings documented in the medical record reflect an infectious disease.[22] Any infections recorded that differed from what was recorded by the hospital were reviewed by an infectious disease physician to determine whether the differences seen were accurate. An infection was considered to be nosocomial if it developed after 72 hours of hospitalization and community acquired if it developed before 72 hours of admission.

The diagnoses and procedures were coded according to ICD-9-CM. The age, sex, disposition, admission and discharge dates, diagnosis, and procedure codes were entered into a DRG grouper system (same software used by the hospital for past DRG groupings). This step enabled computation of a final DRG and relative weight. Data such as total charges, cost, DRG payment, total payment, and whether there was a gain or loss for the hospital were obtained from the financial department at the hospital. With this information, the total payment for the abstracted hospitalizations could be calculated.

An example of sections of the database used to analyze some of the study data can be found on the Evolve Web site. Patient hospitalizations without infections are listed first, followed by those with infections. The format of the database works well with Access and Excel software for performing data analysis.

Data Analysis

Because this was a descriptive, pilot outcome study, basic statistical analysis was used. To determine whether there were differences in cost, length of stay, and reimbursement for hospitalizations with and without infections, the average length of stay (ALOS), average DRG payment, average total payment, and the difference between the average total payment and average cost by specific weight categories were analyzed. This was done in the following ways:

ALOS, cost, DRG, and total payment by relative weight for patients with and without infections (Table 11-8)

ALOS, cost, DRG, and total payment by relative weight for patients with community-acquired infections (CAIs) and patients without infections (Table 11-9)

ALOS, cost, DRG, and total payment by relative weight for patients with nosocomial infections (NIs) and patients without infections (Table 11-10)

The weight of the DRG must be controlled to determine whether the differences seen in Tables 11-8 through 11-10 are due to the infection. This was analyzed in the following ways:

- Average cost and total payment per weight for patients with and without infections by low and high relative weights (Table 11-11)
- Average cost and total payment per weight for patient hospitalizations with CAI and patient hospitalizations without infections by low and high relative weights (Table 11-12)
- Average cost and total payment per weight for patient hospitalizations with NI and hospitalizations without infections by low and high relative weights (Table 11-13) Length of stay also had to be controlled. This was done in the following way:
- Average cost and total payment by length of stay (= 1 week and >1 week) for hospitalizations with and without infections (Table 11-14)

- Average cost and total payment per day (<1 and >1) per weight for hospitalizations with and without infections (Table 11-15)

The results are described as follows:
- The average cost and ALOS were higher in hospitalizations with infections than in hospitalizations without infections.
- When the DRG and length of stay were controlled simultaneously, however, lower average costs per day per weight were seen for hospitalizations with infections.
- Similar results (lower average costs per day per weight) were found when comparisons were done to separate infection types NI and CAI.
- Sixty-eight percent of all NIs developed on or after day 5, and the risk of infection increased in hospitalizations with longer lengths of stay.

TABLE 11-8 Average Length of Stay, Cost, DRG, and Total Payment by Relative Weight for Hospitalizations with or Without Infections

| DRG Weight | Total Hosp. | INFECTION | | | | | | NO INFECTION | | | | | |
		n	ALOS	Acost	Adrg	Atot	Diff.	n	ALOS	Acost	Adrg	Atot	Diff.
<0.70	39	12	6.8	4260	2263	3629	−631	27	5.5	3487	2388	3632	145
0.7–0.89	42	20	8.9	5032	3191	4548	−484	22	6.1	4258	2788	4300	42
0.9–1.19	36	12	5.5	3298	3483	4607	1309	24	5.7	3588	3677	4986	1398
1.2–1.9	22	10	10.8	6635	5599	7907	1272	12	9.1	5875	5032	7187	1312
2.0–2.9	21	11	29.4	40,819	9344	26,483	14,336	10	22.3	15,937	9277	13,088	2869
Without outlier	19	10	20.5	18,448	9216	15,546	−2902	9	13.8	10,815	9240	12,838	2023
≥3	5	1	13.0	7669	12,167	14,918	7249	4	14.7	16,733	15,465	20,940	4207

Hosp., Hospitalization; Acost, average cost; Adrg, average DRG payment; ALOS, average length of stay; Atot, average total payment; Diff., average total payment — average cost; DRG, diagnosis-related group.

TABLE 11-9 ALOS, Cost, DRG, and Total Payment by Relative Weight for Hospitalizations with Community-Acquired Infections and Hospitalizations Without Infections

| DRG Weight | Total Hosp. | COMMUNITY-ACQUIRED INFECTION | | | | | | NO INFECTION | | | | | |
		n	ALOS	Acost	Adrg	Atot	Diff.	n	ALOS	Acost	Adrg	Atot	Diff.
<0.70	38	11	6.3	3728	2065	3270	−458	27	5.5	3487	2388	3632	145
0.7–0.89	40	18	8.4	4659	3242	4481	−178	22	6.1	4258	2788	4300	42
0.9–1.19	32	8	5.9	3493	3965	5259	1766	24	5.7	3588	3677	4986	1398
1.2–1.9	22	10	10.8	6635	5599	7907	1272	12	9.1	5875	5032	7187	1312
2.0–2.9	17	7	31.1	53,363	9780	33,257	20,106	10	22.3	15,937	9277	13,088	2869
Without outlier	16	6	16.6	18,170	9640	16,158	−2012	9	13.8	10,815	9240	12,838	2023
≥3	4	0	—	—	—	—	—	4	14.7	16,733	15,465	20,940	4207

Hosp., Hospitalization; Acost, average cost; Adrg, average DRG payment; ALOS, average length of stay; Atot, average total payment; Diff., average total payment — average cost; DRG, diagnosis-related group.

TABLE 11-10 ALOS, Cost, DRG, and Total Payment by Relative Weight for Hospitalizations with Nosocomial Infections and Hospitalizations Without Infections

DRG Weight	Total Hosp.	NOSOCOMIAL INFECTION						NO INFECTION					
		n	ALOS	Acost	Adrg	Atot	Diff.	n	ALOS	Acost	Adrg	Atot	Diff.
<0.70	29	2	9.5	6081	2360	4443	−1638	27	5.5	3487	2388	3632	145
0.7–0.89	24	2	13.5	8390	2742	5151	−3239	22	6.1	4258	2788	4300	42
0.9–1.19	29	5	9.4	5136	3672	5402	266	24	5.7	3588	3677	4986	1398
1.2–1.9	13	1	12.0	7564	6987	9741	2177	12	9.1	5875	5032	7187	1312
2.0–2.9	17	7	39.0	57,904	9222	33,981	23,923	10	22.3	15,937	9277	13,088	2869
Without outlier	15	6	25.8	23,467	8989	17,002	−6465	9	13.8	10,815	9240	12,838	2023
≥3	5	1	13.0	7669	12,167	14,918	7249	4	14.7	16,733	15,465	20,940	4207

Hosp., Hospitalization; *Acost,* average cost; *Adrg,* average DRG payment; *ALOS,* average length of stay; *Atot,* average total payment; *Diff.,* average total payment − average cost; *DRG,* diagnosis-related group.

TABLE 11-11 Average Cost and Total Payment per Weight for Hospitalizations with and Without Infections by Low and High Relative Weights

DRG Weight	Total Hosp.	INFECTION				NO INFECTION			
		n	Cost/wt	Tpay/wt	Diff.	n	Cost/wt	Diff.	n
<1	90	34	6073	5546	−527	56	5368	5587	219
>1	75	32	7629	6574	−1055	43	4263	4969	706
Without outlier	73	31	4972	5296	324	42	3800	4948	1148

Hosp., Hospitalization; *Cost/wt,* average (cost/weight); *Tpay/wt,* average (total payment/weight); *Diff.,* average (total payment/weight) − average (cost/weight).

TABLE 11-12 Average Cost and Total Payment per Weight for Hospitalizations with Community-Acquired Infections and Hospitalizations Without Infections by Low and High Relative Weights

DRG Weight	Total Hosp.	COMMUNITY-ACQUIRED INFECTION				NO INFECTION			
		n	Cost/wt	Tpay/wt	Diff.	n	Cost/wt	Diff.	n
<1	86	30	5791	5452	−339	56	5368	5587	219
>1	67	24	8102	6899	−1203	43	4263	4969	706
Without outlier	65	23	4542	5190	648	42	3800	4948	1148

Hosp., Hospitalization; *Cost/wt,* average (cost/weight); *Tpay/wt,* average (total payment/weight); *Diff.,* average (total payment/weight) − average (cost/weight).

TABLE 11-13 Average Cost and Total Payment per Weight for Hospitalizations with Nosocomial Infections and Hospitalizations Without Infections by Low and High Relative Weights

DRG Weight	Total Hosp.	NOSOCOMIAL INFECTION				NO INFECTION			
		n	Cost/wt	Tpay/wt	Diff.	n	Cost/wt	Diff.	n
<1	61	5	8954	6454	−2500	56	5368	5587	219
>1	56	13	13168	8981	−4187	43	4263	4969	706
Without outlier	54	12	6768	5879	−889	42	3800	4948	1148

Hosp., Hospitalization; *Cost/wt,* average (cost/weight); *Tpay/wt,* average (total payment/weight); *Diff.,* average (total payment/weight) − average (cost/weight).

| TABLE 11-14 | Average Cost and Total Payment by Length of Stay for Hospitalizations with and Without Infections |

	INFECTION					NO INFECTION			
Length of Stay	Total Hosp.	n	Cost/wt	Tpay/wt	Diff.	n	Cost/wt	Diff.	n
<1 week	81	26	731	1533	802	55	771	1294	523
>1 week	84	40	667	625	−42	44	697	712	15
Without outlier	82	39	627	611	−16	43	698	725	27

Hosp., Hospitalization; *Cost/wt*, average (cost/weight); *Tpay/wt*, average (total payment/weight); *Diff.*, average (total payment/weight) − average (cost/weight).

| TABLE 11-15 | Average Cost and Total Payment per Day per Weight for Hospitalizations with and Without Infections |

	INFECTION					NO INFECTION			
DRG Weight	Total Hosp.	n	Cost/wt	Tpay/wt	Diff.	n	Cost/wt	Diff.	n
<1	90	34	883	1328	445	56	1031	1344	313
>1	75	32	424	563	139	43	474	769	295
Without outlier	73	31	413	568	155	42	479	785	306

Hosp., Hospitalization; *Cost/wt*, average [(cost/day)/weight]; *Tpay/wt*, average [(total payment/day)/weight]; *Diff.*, average [(total payment/day)weight] − average [(cost/day)weight].

Two models were developed to explain the results. In the first model, individuals have an increased length of stay, leading to the development of the NI, which then further increases length of stay with attendant increased costs. In the second model, there may be sicker individuals who have an increased risk of infection, which leads to a longer length of stay and therefore higher cost.

This outcome study demonstrates what can be accomplished when the medical record and financial data are used. By using the medical record as well as financial data and input from the infectious disease department, a detailed analysis of infections in an elderly population in relation to cost and length of stay (two important efficiency outcome measures) was completed. This outcome study also enabled the hospital to determine the types of studies that should be done in the future. Performance improvement studies that examine the effectiveness of infection control procedures over time, the importance of examining both CAIs and NIs, and the differences that severity of illness may have on cost and length of stay are all areas that have been identified as needing further study. Future outcome studies in this area and other areas will continue to use the medical record. However, the data obtained from the medical record should not be examined alone. The data should be analyzed along with data from other sources, such as severity of illness data, financial data, quality improvement data, infection control data, and risk management and patient safety data to examine epidemiologic trends over time. Only when several data sources are used together to investigate a particular aspect of care can that aspect of care be thoroughly and completely examined. The EHR may be the key to bringing all of these data sources together. As research in these areas moves forward, it will inevitably promote the advancement of the EHR. What a major breakthrough research can provide for HIM and health care in general.

❓DID YOU KNOW?

Did you know that the Centers for Medicare and Medicaid (CMS) and the Agency for Healthcare Research and Quality (AHRQ) now require health care organizations to report outcome measures related to hospital-acquired infections such as pneumonia, pressure ulcers, and catheter-associated urinary tract infections?

SUMMARY

The HIM professional has a strong voice in health information and informatics research. Much of the research that has been completed in the field of HIM was done by HIM professionals. Knowing the types of study designs and methodologies to use when conducting HIM-related research is important and should be examined and used carefully. Research study protocol is important for all types of study designs, as demonstrated when conducting clinical trials. No study is perfect, but it is important to conduct HIM-related research so that results are obtained and move the field of HIM one step further.[23]

CHAPTER REVIEW

1. The specific aims should include the project's,
   _____ and should be both _____ and _____.
   a. goals or objectives; short and long term
   b. end results or conclusions; succinct and clear
   c. hypothesis; explicit and concise
   d. budget; salaries and equipment

2. Which section of the research proposal should include
   the importance of the research project supported by a
   review of past research studies (literature review) and
   preliminary research performed by the author?
   a. methodology
   b. significance
   c. specific aims
   d. hypothesis

3. Which section of the research proposal includes such
   things as data collection process, IRB application,
   statistical analysis of the data, time frame, sample
   size, and place of study?
   a. procedures
   b. process
   c. significance
   d. methodology

4. Informed consent, confidentiality, risks and benefits
   of people enrolled in the study, and the demographic
   description of the subjects are all included in which
   section of the research proposal?
   a. human subjects
   b. appendix
   c. literature cited
   d. specific aims

5. In a case-control study, why are the cases and controls
   often matched on variables such as age and sex?
   a. so that cases and controls are similar except for the
      disease and health characteristic under study
   b. so that cases and controls are similar for all aspects of
      the study
   c. so that cases and controls are similar except for the
      disease under study only
   d. so that cases and controls are similar except for the
      health characteristic only

6. What is a tentative assertion called that is assumed by
   the researcher but not positively known until it is
   tested?
   a. significance
   b. hypothesis
   c. method
   d. specific aims

7. The incidence rate of the exposed group divided by
   the incidence rate of the unexposed group is the
   formula used to determine:
   a. relative risk
   b. odds ratio
   c. incidence
   d. prevalence

8. The outcome study that examined infections and cost
   in an elderly population demonstrates what can be
   accomplished when what two data sources are used?
   a. incident reports and medical record
   b. infection control reports and medical record
   c. financial data and medical record
   d. GEMs and medical record

9. This study design must deal with possible adverse
   reactions of interventions, ethical considerations, loss
   of subjects through death, withdrawal, and
   compliance of subjects. It is called:
   a. experimental studies
   b. descriptive studies
   c. prospective studies
   d. retrospective (case-control) studies

10. In this study design, subjects may be lost during the
    study period from death, withdrawal, and migration,
    and it is not good with rare diseases because of the
    length of time needed for following the subjects over
    time, as well as unexpected changes in the environment
    that may influence the health outcome. It is called:
    a. retrospective (case-control) study
    b. experimental study
    c. prospective study
    d. prevalence study

REFERENCES

1. e-Health Task Force of the AHIMA: *Report on the roles and functions of e-health information management,* April 2002.
2. Watzlaf VJM: The leadership role of the health information management professional in research, *Top Health Inform Manage* 15:47–58, 1995.
3. U.S. Department of Health and Human Services: *Healthy People 2020,* 2013. Washington, DC, http://www.healthypeople.gov/2020/topicsobjectives 2020/overview.aspx?topicid=18.
4. Watzlaf VJM: The development of the grant proposal, *J Am Med Rec Assoc* 60:37–41, 1989.
5. Shi L: *Health services research methods,* Albany, NY, 1997, Delmar.
6. Hunn J, Rodriguez GC: Ovarian Cancer: Etiology Risk Factors and Epidemiology, *Clin Obstet Gynecol* 55(1):3–23, 2012, Type: Journal Article, Review. http://dx.doi.org/10.1097/GRF.0b013e31824b4611.
7. Slome C, Brogan D, Eyres S, et al: *Basic epidemiological methods and biostatistics: a workbook,* Belmont, CA, 1986, Jones & Bartlett.
8. Lilienfeld A, Lilienfeld D: *Foundations of epidemiology,* ed 2, New York, 1980, Oxford University Press.
9. Kuzma J: *Basic statistics for the health sciences,* Mountain View, CA, 1998, Mayfield.
10. Schlesselman JJ: *Case-control studies—design, conduct, analysis,* New York, 1982, Oxford University Press.
11. Schleyer TKL, Forrest JL: Web-based survey design and administration, *J Am Med Inform Assoc* (7), 2000.
12. Wyatt JC: When to use Web-based surveys [editorial comment], *J Am Med Inform Assoc* (7), 2000.
13. Watzlaf VJM, Zeng X, Jarymowycz C, et al: Standards for the content of the electronic health record, *Perspect Health Inform Manage* 1(1)2004. http://www.ahima.org/perspectives.
14. Katoh A, Watzlaf VJM, D'Amico F: An examination of obesity and breast cancer survival in post-menopausal women, *Br J Cancer* 70:928–933, 1994.

15. American College of Surgeons: *Module 14-Statistics fundamental tumor registry operations,* Chicago, 1991, Commission on Cancer.

16. Kramer S, Jarrett P: *Biostatistics and epidemiology for the tumor registry professionals,* Harrisburg, PA, 1984, Pennsylvania Department of Health and Pennsylvania Tumor Registrars Association.

17. Watzlaf VJM, Kuller LH, Ruben FL: The use of the medical record and financial data to examine the cost of infections in the elderly, *Top Health Rec Manage* 13:65–76, 1992.

18. Watzlaf VJM: Is the medical record an effective epidemiological data source? *Proceedings of the National Center for Health Statistics Public Health Conference on Records and Statistics,* July 1989, Washington, DC.

19. Watzlaf VJM: The medical record as an epidemiological database, *Top Health Rec Manage* 7:61–67, 1987.

20. Ruben FL, Dearwater SR, Norden CW, et al: Clinical infections in the noninstitutionalized geriatric age group: methods utilized and incidence of infections. The Pittsburgh Good Health Study, *Am J Epidemiol* 141:145–157, 1995.

21. National Institute of Aging: Established population for epidemiologic studies of the elderly: *Resource data book,* Bethesda, MD, 1986, National Institutes of Health Publication No. 86, 2443.

22. Mandell GL, Douglas RG, Bennett JE, editors: *Principles and practice of infectious disease,* New York, 1979, Wiley.

23. Layman E, Watzlaf V: *Health informatics research methods: principles and practice,* Chicago, 2009, American Health Information Association.

CHAPTER 12

PERFORMANCE MANAGEMENT AND PATIENT SAFETY

Patrice L. Spath • Donna J. Slovensky

Student Study Guide activities for this chapter are available on the Evolve Learning Resources site for this textbook. Please visit http://evolve.elsevier.com/Abdelhak.

CHAPTER CONTENTS

OBJECTIVES

After reading this chapter, the reader will be able to do the following:

✓ Define key quality management and patient safety terminology.
✓ Identify major societal and regulatory drivers for quality and safety initiatives in health care organizations.

✓ Identify regulatory and accreditation requirements for performance management activities in health care organizations.
✓ Describe the primary stakeholders in health care quality and patient safety.

✓ Differentiate among structure, process, and outcome measures of performance.

✓ Identify sources of data for calculating performance measures.

✓ Discuss various approaches used by health care organizations to improve quality and patient safety.

✓ Describe and apply improvement tools frequently used in problem analysis and performance management.

✓ Describe the process of conducting a root cause analysis.

✓ Describe the process of conducting a proactive risk assessment.

✓ Identify key risk management and utilization management activities in health care organizations.

✓ Describe the hospital process for ensuring competence of physicians and licensed independent practitioners.

KEY TERMS

Accreditation
Accountable care organizations
Adverse event
Affinity diagram
Aggregate data
Baldrige National Quality Award
Bar graph
Benchmarking
Brainstorming
Case management
Cause-and-effect diagram
Checksheet
Claims management
Clinical practice guidelines
Concurrent review
Conditions of Participation
Control chart
Correlation analysis
Credentialing
Credentials verification organization
Data sheet

Decision matrix
Discharge planning
Electronic health record
E-measures
Evidenced-based medicine
External benchmarking
Failure mode and effect analysis
Federal Register
Fishbone diagram
Flowchart
Force field analysis
Healthcare Effectiveness Data and Information Set
Histogram
Incident report
Indicator
Intensity of service/severity of illness
Internal benchmarking
Lean thinking
Leapfrog Group
Licensed independent practitioners

Line graph
Loss reduction
National Committee for Quality Assurance
National Practitioner Data Bank
National Quality Forum
Never events
Nominal group technique
Outcome measures
Pareto chart
Patient advocacy
Patient safety improvement
Patient safety indicators
Patient safety organizations
Pay for performance
Peer review
Performance assessment
Performance measure
Performance target
Physician advisor
Plan-Do-Check-Act (PDCA)
Potentially compensable event

Privilege delineation
Proactive risk assessments.
Prospective review process
Process measures
Retrospective review
Quality improvement
Quality improvement organizations
Rapid cycle improvement
Reliable measure
Risk
Risk management
Root cause analysis
Run chart
Sentinel event
Simulation
Six Sigma
Structure measures
Surgical Care Improvement Project
The Joint Commission
Threshold
Utilization management

ABBREVIATIONS

ACO   Accountable Care Organization
AHRQ   Agency for Healthcare Research and Quality
CMS   Centers for Medicare and Medicaid Services
COP   Conditions of Participation
DMAIC   Definition, Measurement, Analysis, Improvement, and Control
EBM   Evidence-Based Medicine
EHR   Electronic Health Record
FMEA   Failure Mode and Effect Analysis
HCO   Health Care Organization
HEDIS   Healthcare Effectiveness Data and Information Set
HIM   Health Information Management
IOM   Institute of Medicine
IS/SI   Intensity of Service/Severity of Illness
LIP   Licensed Independent Practitioner
NCQA   National Committee for Quality Assurance
NICU   Neonatal Intensive Care Unit

NPDB   National Practitioner Data Bank
NQF   National Quality Forum
P4P   Pay for Performance
PCE   Potentially Compensable Event
PDCA   Plan, Do, Check, Act
PDSA   Plan, Do, Study, Act
PSI   Patient Safety Indicator
PSO   Patient Safety Organization
QI   Quality Improvement
QIO   Quality Improvement Organization
RCI   Rapid Cycle Improvement
SCIP   Surgical Care Improvement Project
SOW   Statement of Work
TJC   The Joint Commission
UM   Utilization Management

Most people expect quality in the delivery of health care services, although the definition of quality is often unique to the individual. Consumers expect to receive the right medical interventions, achieve good physical outcomes, and to be satisfied with personal interactions with caregivers. Additionally, consumers expect the physical facilities where care is provided to be clean and pleasant and to have the "best" (i.e., most current) technology available. Each of these characteristics is a part of quality; none is the whole. The way a health care consumer defines quality quite often differs from what providers or purchasers view as important quality attributes in the delivery of health services.

Without question, "quality" should be an integral component of all health care services. Despite this universally accepted belief, how to measure performance and what constitutes an acceptable level of quality continue to be greatly debated. Scholars and researchers, health care providers and payers, and individual consumers of health care all bring different perspectives into the debate.

There is ongoing concern worldwide regarding the safety of health care services. Media reports about errors made in the delivery of patient care have raised consumer awareness of the potential for medical mishaps. In November 1999, the Institute of Medicine (IOM) released the report, *To Err Is Human: Building a Safer Health System.*[1] The report purported to show, for the first time, the extent to which medical errors may cause preventable deaths in the United States. It was estimated at that time that between 44,000 and 98,000 deaths occurred each year in hospitals as a result of medical errors by physicians, pharmacists, and other health care providers. More recent estimates suggest the true number of premature deaths associated with preventable harm to hospital patients is more than 400,000 per year.[2]

The IOM report suggested that most medical errors are a result of the complexity of health care services, not incompetent individuals.

DID YOU KNOW?

The number one cause of death in the United States, and worldwide, is heart disease.

In the 2001 IOM report *Crossing the Quality Chasm: A New Health System for the 21st Century,*[3] the Committee on Quality of Health Care in America identified six key dimensions of health care quality. Although the report was published at the very beginning of the 21st century, its references continue to be relevant to quality management activities. The six key dimensions include:

Safe—avoiding injuries to patients from the care that is intended to help them.

Effective—providing services based on scientific knowledge to all who could benefit and refraining from providing services to those not likely to benefit (avoiding underuse and overuse, respectively).

Patient centered—providing care that is respectful of and responsive to individual patient preferences, needs, and values and ensuring that patient values guide all clinical decisions.

Timely—reducing waits and sometimes harmful delays for both those who receive and those who give care.

Efficient—avoiding waste, including waste of equipment, supplies, ideas, and energy.

Equitable—providing care that does not vary in quality because of personal characteristics such as gender, ethnicity, geographic location, and socioeconomic status.

The 2010 Affordable Care Act required the Secretary of the Department of Health and Human Services (HHS) to establish a national strategy for health care quality improvement that sets priorities and includes a strategic plan for how

to achieve these priorities. The three broad aims of this strategy are:

- Better Care: Improve the overall quality, by making health care more patient-centered, reliable, accessible, and safe.
- Healthy People/Health Communities: Improve the health of the U.S. population by supporting proven interventions to address the behavioral, social, and environmental determinants of health in addition to delivering higher-quality care.
- Affordable Care: Reduce the cost of quality health care for individuals, families, employers, and government.

More information about the national health care quality strategy can be found online at the AHRQ sponsored Web site, Working for Quality: http://www.ahrq.gov/workingforquality/index.html.

DID YOU KNOW

An easy way to distinguish between efficiency and effectiveness: efficiency = doing things right; effectiveness = doing the right things.

SELF-ASSESSMENT QUIZ

1. List the six dimensions of quality as identified in the Institute of Medicine report.
2. List the three broad aims of the National Quality Strategy.

THE BIG PICTURE AND KEY PLAYERS

Although health care providers have numerous internal incentives for improving the quality and safety of services, the details for accomplishing these activities are often influenced by external mandates. Some requirements are grounded in law; others are stipulated by agencies with which a health care organization (HCO) interacts on a voluntary basis. Purchasers and consumers also play a role in influencing performance management in health services. This section focuses on the key players and how these groups affect health care quality and patient safety.

Federal Oversight Agencies

Because most HCOs provide services to Medicare or Medicaid beneficiaries, the regulations of the Centers for Medicare and Medicaid Services (CMS) have significant impact on the "what" and "how" of performance improvement activities at the provider level. Regulations governing providers of services to Medicare beneficiaries are detailed in the Conditions of Participation (COP). These regulations require that providers develop, implement, and maintain an effective organization-wide, data-driven quality assessment and performance improvement program. The regulation specifics vary according to the provider setting. For instance, hospices must monitor the effectiveness and safety of services and quality of care to identify opportunities for improvement, take actions aimed at performance improvement, and measure the success of improvement actions.[4]

DID YOU KNOW

The Conditions of Participation are published in the Federal Register, which is available online at http://www.gpo.gov/fdsys/.

CMS also conducts nationwide health care performance measurement, with providers required to submit measurement data to CMS. Current measures and measurement results can be found on the Medicare Web site. CMS contracts at the state level with quality improvement organizations (QIOs) to direct and oversee improvement initiatives. Requirements for QIOs that contract with CMS are outlined in comprehensive triennial documents, the QIO Statement of Work (SOW), numbered consecutively beginning in 1983. The Tenth SOW, encompassing August 1, 2011, through July 31, 2014, includes initiatives related to reducing hospital-acquired infections, improving care for nursing home residents, advancing implementation of electronic health records in physician offices, and improving patient transitions between health care settings. The current SOW is available on the CMS Web site (http://www.cms.gov/Medicare/Quality-Initiatives-Patient-Assessment-Instruments/QualityImprovementOrgs/index.html).

SELF-ASSESSMENT QUIZ

3. What does the acronym SOW stand for?
4. What is the current SOW number?
5. What is the SOW cycle?

Accrediting Bodies

Many health care organizations voluntarily participate in national accreditation programs. Accreditation is a credential given to an organization that meets defined standards, some of which relate to performance management. Only organizations seeking accreditation must comply with these mandates. All health care accreditation programs include some requirements related to performance management. The two main accrediting bodies in the United States are The Joint Commission and the National Committee for Quality Assurance. The requirements of these two groups are summarized in the following section.

The Joint Commission

The Joint Commission (TJC) is a not-for-profit, nongovernmental entity that offers voluntary accreditation programs for all types of health care facilities. It provides education, leadership, and objective evaluation and feedback to health care organizations in the quest for health care quality and patient safety. TJC standards require accredited organizations to collect data to monitor performance, compile and analyze performance data, and improve performance.

DID YOU KNOW

The Joint Commission, which has been accrediting HCOs since 1951, accredits or certifies more than 20,000 health care organizations and programs in the United States.

Since 2002, TJC has sponsored a comparative performance measurement project that involves collection and analysis of data received from accredited hospitals. The initial core measure data focused on hospital performance in four areas: acute myocardial infarction, heart failure, community-acquired pneumonia, and pregnancy and related conditions. A hospital's actual performance in these areas is one of the elements taken into consideration by TJC when accrediting the organization. As with all regulations in health care, TJC standards are subject to change. Current performance measurement and improvement initiatives, accreditation issues, and other information are available on TJC's Web site (www.jointcommission.org).

National Committee for Quality Assurance

The National Committee for Quality Assurance (NCQA) is a private, not-for-profit organization established in 1990. NCQA accredits a variety of organizations from health maintenance organizations to accountable care organizations to managed behavioral health care organizations, and each accreditation program has distinct performance management requirements. More than 110 million Americans (70.5% of all health plan members) are covered by an NCQA-Accredited health plan.[5] NCQA also sponsors the Healthcare Effectiveness Data and Information Set (HEDIS), a comparative performance measurement project that evaluates a health plan's clinical and administrative systems. These data are made available to purchasers and consumers to assist them in making choices about health care providers.

SELF-ASSESSMENT QUIZ

6. What is the purpose of HEDIS?
7. Which accrediting body sponsors HEDIS?

NCQA accreditation and participation in HEDIS is voluntary, but many large employers require or request accreditation or HEDIS reporting for the health plans they make available to their employees. Additional information about the NCQA's programs and activities is available on their Web site (www.ncqa.org).

National Quality Awards

Some health care leaders seek to advance performance improvement by voluntarily participating in quality award programs at the state and national levels. An example of such a program is the Malcolm Baldrige National Quality Award, established by Congress in 1987 to recognize organizations for their achievements in quality and business performance and to raise awareness about the importance of quality and performance excellence as a competitive edge. The Baldrige Healthcare Criteria for Performance Excellence, first published in 1998, are intended to help organizations use an integrated approach to organizational performance management that results in[6]:

- delivery of ever-improving value to patients and other customers, contributing to improved health care quality;
- improvement of overall organizational effectiveness and capabilities as a health care provider; and
- organizational and personal learning.

 DID YOU KNOW

The first HCO winner of the Baldrige award was SMS Health Care, a Franciscan Sisters of Mary organization in St. Louis, Missouri, in 2002. Since that early award, an additional 15 HCOs have been recognized with the Baldrige Quality Award.

The Baldrige Healthcare Criteria are designed as an interrelated system of items that address major areas of performance excellence. The 2013 criteria are organized into seven categories or management disciplines that cover[6]:

- leadership
- strategic planning
- focus on customers
- measurement, analysis, and knowledge management
- staff focus
- operations focus
- organizational results

The Baldrige Criteria help HCOs stay focused on improvement goals and align all activities to achieve these goals. The criteria are the basis for many national quality award programs sponsored by professional organizations. An example is the American Health Care Association's Quality Award that addresses the key requirements of performance excellence in long-term care facilities. The criteria for the American Hospital Association Quest for Quality prize cover many of the concepts found in the Baldrige Criteria.[7] Information about the Baldrige Award and the criteria underpinning it is available on the National Institute of Standards and Technology Web site (http://www.nist.gov/Baldrige).

Purchasers

Federal and state governments are by far the largest purchasers of health care services. The quality of these services is regulated by the COP and by state health department regulations. There are also many private health insurance companies, as well as employers that purchase health insurance for their employees, which have a vested interest in health care quality. Like federal and state governments, these purchasers want to receive good value for the dollars they expend on health care services. In response to the rising cost of health care, nongovernment health care purchasers are taking a more assertive role in advancing quality and patient safety.

The Leapfrog Group, a collaboration of large employers, came together in 1998 to determine how purchasers could influence the quality and affordability of health care. Annually this group conducts a survey to evaluate hospitals' adherence to evidence-based, high-quality, and safe practices. Purchasers use the survey responses to recognize providers that have met Leapfrog's safety, quality, and resource standards and to educate health plan enrollees about quality and patient safety. More information about the Leapfrog Group initiatives can be found on its Web site (http://www.leapfroggroup.org).

Some health plans have initiated payment systems that financially reward providers that achieve specific quality or patient safety goals. These initiatives are commonly called Pay for Performance (P4P). The fundamental principles of P4P are (1) common performance measures for providers (usually represent a balance of patient satisfaction, prevention, and long-term care management) and (2) significant health plan financial payments on the basis of that performance, with each plan independently deciding the source, amount, and payment method for its incentive program.

In 2008, the CMS announced that Medicare will no longer pay most hospitals a higher rate for an inpatient stay if the reason for the enhanced payment is a "never event." Never events are hospital-acquired conditions considered by CMS to be (1) preventable, (2) high cost or high volume (or both), and (3) result in additional costs. Never events include[8]:

- Foreign object retained after surgery
- Air embolism
- Blood incompatibility
- Stages III and IV pressure ulcers
- Injury following falls and other trauma
- Catheter-associated urinary tract infection
- Vascular catheter–associated infection
- Surgical site infections or mediastinitis after coronary artery bypass graft, certain orthopedic procedures, bariatric surgeries, and cardiac implantable electronic device procedures
- Certain manifestations of poor control of blood sugar levels
- Deep vein thrombosis or pulmonary embolism following total knee replacement and hip replacement
- Iatrogenic pneumothorax with venous catheterization

State Medicaid programs and some commercial insurance plans have adopted similar "never event" payment strategies.

Consumers

Consumers do not have the power to mandate specific health service performance management activities; however, they do influence what is required by federal regulations and accreditation standards. This influence occurs in many ways. There are numerous consumer/patient advocacy groups that work in partnership with legislators, providers, and purchasers to promote health care quality and patient safety improvements. Often one or more consumer representatives serve on the governing board or advisory groups of accreditation organizations to provide the "public perspective" when accreditation standards are revised. Individuals and consumer groups have the opportunity to comment on proposed changes in the Medicare COP, which are published in the publicly available Federal Register.

Patient advocacy services may be available in individual HCOs as a proactive approach to ensuring patient satisfaction with the process and outcomes of care episodes. In addition to responding to individual patient complaints, HCOs often monitor overall patient satisfaction with the facility and with staff interactions by use of written questionnaires or telephone surveys. Hospitals that care for Medicare patients are required to participate in the CMS patient satisfaction measurement system.[9] Satisfaction survey results for individual hospitals are publicly available on the Medicare Web site (www.medicare.gov).

 DID YOU KNOW

Press-Ganey is a consulting organization with a special focus on improving patient experience. Their services are used by more than 10,000 HCOs. See more info on their Web site at http://www.pressganey.com.

National Health Care Quality Measurement Priorities

During the 1990s, great emphasis was placed on the need for public accountability of providers and insurers to furnish comprehensive, high-quality health care at an acceptable cost.[10] In support of public accountability, the National Quality Forum (NQF) was created in 1999 to develop and implement a national strategy for health care quality measurement and reporting. The NQF, a not-for-profit membership group, includes representatives from a diverse group of national, state, regional, and local organizations, including purchasers, consumers, health systems, health care practitioners, health plans, accrediting bodies, regulatory agencies, medical suppliers, and information technology companies. The mission of the NQF is to improve American health care through endorsement of consensus-based national standards for measurement and public reporting of health care performance data that provide meaningful information about whether care is safe, timely, beneficial, patient centered, equitable, and efficient. The specific goals of the NQF are as follows[11]:

- Set national priorities and goals for performance improvement
- Endorse national consensus standards for measuring and publicly reporting on performance
- Promote the attainment of national goals through education and outreach programs

At this time, the NQF has endorsed several condition-specific performance measure sets that address the quality of patient care across the continuum. For instance, sets of measures that can be used to evaluate the quality of hospital care cover conditions such as the following:

- Acute coronary artery syndrome
- Cerebrovascular disease

- Heart failure
- Pneumonia
- Pregnancy, childbirth, and neonatal conditions

Many of the condition-specific measures in the NQF-endorsed measure sets are being used by CMS, TJC, NCQA, and other accrediting and regulatory groups to evaluate the performance of HCOs. Information about the work of the NQF and the measure development and dissemination process can be found on the NQF Web site (http://www.qualityforum.org).

Although there are numerous factors influencing health care performance management and differing stakeholder incentives and priorities, the fundamental elements are constant: performance measurement, assessment, and improvement. These are the basic building blocks of performance management. To promote a systematic organization-wide quality management approach, providers may have a written performance management plan. This plan describes the organization's structure and processes for measuring, assessing, and improving performance.

 SELF-ASSESSMENT QUIZ

8. What is the purpose of the NQF?
9. What are the fundamental elements of health care performance management?

As the health care delivery system struggles to achieve a balance between costs and access, performance management and clinical outcomes become increasingly important. HCOs and other players in the industry will inevitably compete in terms of quality. Orme[12] succinctly describes the goals of quality improvement (QI) efforts in health care as "to improve the processes of delivering care and thereby increase customer satisfaction with the quality of care (service outcomes), to improve the functional health of patients (clinical outcomes), and to reduce the costs of providing care."

PERFORMANCE MEASUREMENT

Performance measure is a generic term used to describe a particular value or characteristic designated to quantify input, output, outcome, efficiency, or effectiveness. Input refers to the materials or resources used in a process, such as x-ray film and the radiographer's time. Output is the product or end results of a process, such as a transcribed record document or a completed diagnostic test, or a "complete" health record or a patient's satisfactory physical condition after a surgical procedure. Efficiency refers to "doing things right," or using an acceptable ratio of resources used to output or outcome achieved. Five ruined films before an acceptable diagnostic image is achieved would not be considered efficient! Effectiveness refers to "doing the right thing." For example, using only the appropriate diagnostic tests to establish a treatment plan that returns a patient to a state of wellness is effective.

In recent years, medical professionals have increasingly relied on evidence-based medicine (EBM) to select the "right thing" to do for a patient. EBM involves the use of current best research evidence in making decisions about the care of individual patients. This research is incorporated into clinical practice guidelines—statements of the right things to do for patients with a particular diagnosis or medical condition. Hundreds of examples of evidence-based clinical practice guidelines can be found on the Internet at the National Guideline Clearinghouse sponsored by the Agency for Healthcare Research and Quality.

Performance measures are composed of a number and a unit of measure. The number provides the magnitude (how much), and the unit is what gives the number its meaning (what). For example, "Percent of patients undergoing hip replacement surgery who receive prophylactic antibiotics as specified by the treatment protocol" is an example of a performance measure. Performance measures are often described as "indicators." An indicator is a quantitative measure of an aspect of patient care. It is not a direct measure of quality; rather, it is a screen or flag that indicates areas for more detailed analysis. For instance, a low percentage of patients receiving the correct antibiotic is an indication that antibiotic prescribing practices need to be examined more closely.

Performance measures are typically classified as one of two types: important single events or patterns of events evident in aggregate data. An important single event is an infrequently occurring, undesirable happening of such magnitude that each occurrence warrants further investigation. Examples are obstetrical death, severe transfusion reaction, and surgery on the wrong body part. When an important single event occurs, there is an immediate investigation to determine the cause and to initiate corrective actions to prevent the event from recurring. These events, often referred to as sentinel events, are discussed in greater detail in relation to patient safety.

SELF-ASSESSMENT QUIZ

10. Who sponsors the National Guideline Clearinghouse?
11. What is EBM?
12. How are clinical practice guidelines related to EBM?
13. Are indicators qualitative or quantitative?
14. True or False? an indicator is a direct measure of quality.

The second type of measure (patterns evidenced in aggregate data) reflects performance that is less dramatic or injurious than an important single event and can reasonably be expected to fluctuate. For example, hospital meal trays delivered late or delayed administration of medication are undesirable events but can be expected to occur occasionally in the normal course of operations. Typically, these types of events are monitored until performance levels trigger a predetermined threshold. At that point, a focused review is undertaken to initiate corrective action. For instance, a hospital monitoring compliance with the use of prophylactic antibiotics for patients undergoing hip replacement surgery might

set a performance expectation of 95% or better. When actual performance falls below 95%, a focused review is conducted to determine the cause of less-than-desired results.

To evaluate the quality of health services adequately, the performance of many aspects must be measured.

Structure, Process, and Outcome Measures

Avedis Donabedian, physician and professor of public health at the University of Michigan from 1966 to 1989, was internationally known for his research on health care improvement. His work in the definition and assessment of health care quality resulted in one of the most widely acknowledged models for measuring quality in health care.[13] Donabedian defined a comprehensive approach to assessing quality of care by using measures that examine structures, processes, and outcomes associated with the delivery of health care. Table 12-1 contains examples of structure, process, and outcome measures used for the purpose of evaluating performance in health care organizations.

? DID YOU KNOW
Dr. Donabedian was born in Beirut, Lebanon, in 1919. He died in 2000.

Structure Measures
Structure measures indirectly assess care by looking at certain provider characteristics and the physical and organizational resources available to support the delivery of care. Structure measures look at the capability or potential for providing quality care. By their nature, structure measures are static:

TABLE 12-1	Donabedian's Model of Structure, Process, and Outcome Measures
Structure	Percent of physicians with board certification
	Number of fire safety inspections completed annually
	Computer system able to electronically transmit medication prescriptions to pharmacy
	Nurse–patient ratio in a hospital
Process	Percent of nursing home residents that received an influenza vaccination in the last 12 months
	Percent of patients seen by a physician within 12 hours of hospital admission
	Percent of health records that contain an up-to-date list of the patient's allergies
	Percent of patients suspected of having a heart attack who are given an aspirin upon arrival to the hospital
Outcome	Mortality rate of patients undergoing coronary artery bypass surgery
	Percent of nursing home residents that develop stage 3 or stage 4 pressure ulcers
	Percent of hospitalized patients that report their pain was adequately managed
	Percent of patients with kidney failure that develop hemodialysis-related complications

the organization or individual is evaluated at a unique point in time. The organizational makeup of a facility, operational policies and procedures, technologic capabilities, staffing, compliance with safety regulations, and workforce competence are all examples of structures that can be measured.

Process Measures

Process measures focus on what is done during the delivery of health care services. Some process measures evaluate the quality of health care professionals' decisions as they direct a patient's course of treatment. For instance, are caregivers complying with clinical practice guideline recommendations? Some process measures evaluate staff member compliance with specific procedures or activities. For instance, are hospital admissions employees making input errors when entering patient demographic information into the computer? Health care delivery involves many tasks, both clinical and nonclinical. For this reason, process measures are the most common measurements used to evaluate the quality of health care services.[14]

Outcome Measures

Outcome measures look at the end results of the patient's encounter with the health care system. A commonly used outcome measure in acute health care settings is patient mortality rates. Although the mortality rate is certainly an important measure, other variables may be necessary to examine adequately the quality of care provided to patients. For instance, what if the patient's diagnosis is terminal metastatic carcinoma? Would death suggest poor quality care for this patient? Process measures are often necessary to supplement outcome measures to evaluate whether the "right" things are done, such as provision of adequate pain control and provider adherence to living will requirements. Other examples of outcome measures include patient complication and infection rates, average cost of care, and other results of health services.

Patient experience measures, a type of outcome measure, focus on health services from the patient's perspective. These measures are used to evaluate satisfaction as well as patient-reported outcomes such as level of pain and ability to conduct activities of daily living following surgery. Patient experience measures have an increasing role in research and health policy decision-making although there is controversy as to whether the measures are legitimate indicators of health care quality.[15]

SELF-ASSESSMENT QUIZ

15. Is a structure measure a direct or indirect measure of quality?
16. Is a process measure a direct or indirect measure of quality?
17. Is an outcome measure a direct or indirect measure of quality?
18. Is a patient experience measure a direct or indirect measure of quality?
19. What is the most common type of measure?

Developing Performance Measures

The choice of performance measures is an important consideration for an HCO because it is impossible to measure all aspects of patient care and services. Several factors must be considered when performance measures are selected. These factors include the following[16]:

- External accreditation and regulatory requirements
- National quality measurement priorities
- Clinical importance
- Strategic priorities of the HCO
- Available resources
- Reporting techniques and analytical tools

Often HCOs choose to use measures developed by national groups that sponsor performance databases. For instance, CMS and TJC have several health care measurement projects involving hospitals, home health agencies, skilled nursing facilities, and other providers. One set of measures is focused on compliance with clinical practice guidelines to prevent postoperative infections. Surgical procedures studied for the Surgical Care Improvement Project (SCIP) include coronary artery bypass graft procedures, cardiac procedures, colon procedures, hip and knee arthroplasty, abdominal and vaginal hysterectomy, and selected vascular surgery procedures. Performance measures for this project, as of 2013, are listed in Table 12-2.[17]

SELF-ASSESSMENT QUIZ

20. What was the purpose of the SCIP project?

Details about the performance measures in the CMS and TJC measurement and improvement projects and those sponsored by other regulatory agencies, accreditation bodies, and professional groups can be found on the National Quality Measures Clearinghouse Web site sponsored by the Agency for Healthcare Research and Quality (http://www.qualitymeasures.ahrq.gov). Development of a performance measure involves three basic steps:

- Identify what you want to know.
- Identify the raw data necessary for creating the measure.
- Define a data collection strategy.

TABLE 12-2   Surgical Care Improvement Project Performance Measures

Antibiotic within 1 hour of surgical incision
Prophylactic antibiotic selection
Antibiotic discontinued within 24 hours of anesthesia end time (48 hours for cardiac patients)
Appropriate hair removal
Urinary catheter removed by postoperative day #1 or #2
Perioperative temperature management
Venous thrombo-embolism (VTE) prophylaxis ordered & administered within 24 hours of anesthesia end time
Beta blocker given in the perioperative period if on beta blocker prior to arrival

FIGURE 12-1 Example of measurement development steps.

> **We want to know:** For patients recovering from surgery, is the patient's pain assessed and documented every 2 hours while awake for the first 24 hours following surgery?
>
> **Raw data needed:** The number of patients whose pain was assessed and documented every 2 hours while awake for the first 24 hours following surgery.
>
> **Performance measure:** $\dfrac{\text{\# cases meeting criteria}}{\text{\# surgery cases (total)}} \times 100$
>
> **Data collection strategy:** Records of consecutive surgery patients will be reviewed and results reported monthly.

These steps are illustrated in Figure 12-1 for a measure of postoperative pain management.

Collecting Measurement Data

Two types of paper-based forms are commonly used to gather performance measurement data. A checksheet is a form specially designed so that the results can be readily interpreted from the form itself. This form of data collection is ideal for capturing data concurrently (during actual delivery of patient care or services) because the employee can interpret the results and take corrective actions immediately. A data sheet is a form designed to collect data in a simple tabular or columnar format. Specific bits of data (e.g., numbers, words, or marks) are entered in spaces on the sheet. As a result, additional processing is typically required after the data are collected to construct the performance measure. Illustrated in Figure 12-2 is a data sheet used to capture information about the occurrence of particular events that might take place during a patient's hospitalization.

One form is completed for each patient record reviewed. Although the example shown is a paper form, the data could be captured in an electronic form or simply entered into a spreadsheet or database application. Those tasked with performing the data collection should understand the data definitions (the exact intended meaning of the variables being

FIGURE 12-2 Example of data sheet used for record reviews.

SAMPLE HOSPITAL Unexpected Outcomes Occurrence Screening Report	
INDICATOR	**PRESENT**
1. Unexpected transfer to another acute facility	
2. Unscheduled return to operating room	
3. Unplanned organ removal/repair subsequent to or during surgery	
4. Neurological deficit not present on admission	
5. Patient fall resulting in injury	
6. Nosocomial infection	
7. Hospital-acquired decubitus	
8. Unscheduled admission following outpatient surgery	
9. Patient discharged against medical advice	
10. Post-surgical death	
11. Medication error or adverse drug reaction	
12. Transfusion error or transfusion reaction	
13. Return to intensive care unit within 24 hours of transfer to nursing unit	
14. Abnormal physiological findings documented without further investigation or resolution	
15. Complications attributed to anesthesia	

collected), have the necessary forms at hand, and be trained in the data collection process. This training should include specific guidance about where in the health record or other data source this data item would be located.

E-Measures

With the growth in electronic health records (EHRs), data that were previously gathered manually are increasingly available in electronic format. This will reduce, but not totally eliminate, the need for manual data gathering. Promoting the use of EHRs for quality measure reporting was part of the 2009 Health Information Technology for Economic and Clinical Health (HITECH) Act. Some of the NQF endorsed performance measures have been converted to electronic measures (known as e-measures). The data for calculating e-measures are extracted automatically from EHRs without the need for manual review of records.

As with other complex electronic information, the underlying algorithms for extracting the data needed to construct the measures are created in a structured language using standard data categories and specified data types. The algorithm must account for all possible data configurations. Figure 12-3 shows three common data categories and several types of data that must be acknowledged within each category. When this sample is conceptually expanded to include the full scope of data categories and all likely data types, the magnitude of the system design is evident. The NQF has published a monograph on Automation of Quality Measurement that provides a good overview of quality data sets, available at: http://www.qualityforum.org/Publications/2009/11/Health_Information_Technology_Automation_of_Quality_Measurement__Quality_Data_Set_and_Data_Flow.aspx.

Even when an HCO has a central data repository for information about patients and their health care experiences, it may be necessary to gather information from other sources. Data warehouse systems provide consolidated and consistent historical data about patient care activities; however, careful planning is necessary to ensure that the information supports performance measurement activities.

Other sources of data for performance measures include interviews, surveys, and direct observation. Data for patient experience measures are often collected through face-to-face interviews and with paper or electronic surveys. In some situations the only way to gather performance measure data is by actually witnessing how things are being done. This data gathering technique is commonly used to report the percentage of caregivers that follow proper hand hygiene practices.

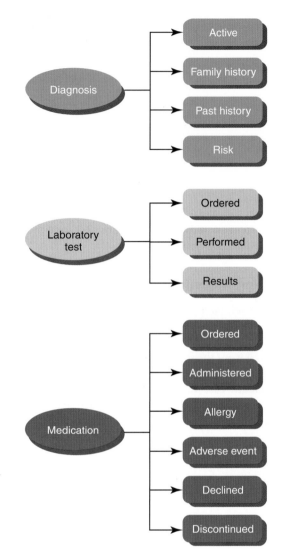

FIGURE 12-3 Sample data categories and data types.

Data Quality

To achieve their potential value, performance measures must be valid and reliable. Validity refers to the following[18]:

- Degree to which all items in the measure relate to the performance being measured
- Extent to which all relevant aspects of performance are covered
- Extent to which the measure appears to measure what it is intended to measure

A reliable measure is stable, showing consistent results over time and among different users of the measure. A reliable measure has low levels of random error. For example, a properly calibrated scale will measure an individual's weight accurately each time he or she steps on the scale no matter who reads the weight value. A coding skills test is valid if it accurately distinguishes between high-performing coders and low-performing coders; it is reliable if the distinction is made each time the test is administered, even if the grader changes.

A vital element of data collection is the need for accuracy. Inaccurate data may give the wrong answer to questions

---

SELF-ASSESSMENT QUIZ

21. A _____ data collection form is designed to interpret data from the form.
22. A _____ data collection form requires further data processing for usability.
23. Data for e-measures are obtained from what source?
24. True or False? The EHR will eliminate all manual data collections in HCOs.

about performance. One of the most troublesome sources of error is called bias. It is important to understand bias and to allow for this during the development and implementation of any data collection system. Well-designed data collection strategies and processes can reduce bias. Some types of bias that may occur include the following:

- Some part of the process or the data has been left out of the data collection process.
- The data collection itself interferes with the process it is measuring.
- The data collector distorts the data.
- The data collection procedures were not followed or were incorrect or ambiguous.
- Some of the data are missing or were not obtained.
- The time period or frequency selected for data collection distorts the data, typically by missing significant events or cyclical occurrences.

SELF-ASSESSMENT QUIZ

25. Distinguish between validity and reliability.
26. Missing or incomplete data can introduce _____ into data analysis.

Health information management (HIM) professionals play a vital role in ensuring valid and reliable data collection. From the front-end capture of data to back-end reporting of measurement results, no nonclinical department has greater influence.[19] As coordinators of data quality, HIM professionals can influence consistent recording and capture of data that later become worthwhile performance measurement information.

PERFORMANCE ASSESSMENT

Performance assessment (sometimes called evaluation, appraisal, or rating) involves a formal periodic review of performance measurement results. If the data collection strategy has been carefully planned, the resulting information should provide a good understanding of performance. After the performance data have been verified for accuracy, it is time for the assessment phase. However, before the results can be analyzed, the information needs to be assembled and presented in a meaningful way. The performance data should help people answer the following questions:

- What is the current performance?
- Is there a trend over time?
- Should we take any action? If yes, what kind of action?
- What contributes the most to undesirable performance (the vital few factors)?
- Are we focusing on the highest priority actions?

Reports for Analysis

To facilitate performance assessment, data must be presented in a format that makes it easier to draw conclusions. This grouping or summarizing may take several forms: tabulation, graphs, or statistical comparisons. Sometimes a single data grouping will suffice for the purposes of performance assessment. Where larger amounts of data must be dealt with, multiple groupings are essential for creating a clear base for analysis. Spreadsheets and databases are useful for organizing and categorizing performance measurement data to show trends. Performance measurement reports may take many forms. Some of the more common graphical presentations are described in greater detail later in this chapter.

At the assessment stage, the objective is to transfer information to the responsible decision makers. Reports will likely consist of sets of tables or charts of performance measurement results, supplemented with basic conclusions. Before actually presenting any performance information, it is beneficial to evaluate and understand a few key factors:

- Who is the audience?
- What is the intended use of the data? Will it be used to support decisions and take actions, or is its purpose simply to monitor performance?
- What is the basic message you want to communicate (for example, here is where we are and how we are doing)?
- What is the best presentation format (report, brochure, oral presentation, etc.)?

The image provided by a well-constructed graph or table is often the most compelling way to communicate performance measurement data. Statistical tools can elaborate on the story told by the graphs or tables and provide validation for the information displayed on the graph or table. Two fundamental concepts are important in statistics: summarizing numbers and distributions. Summarizing numbers condense information from many numbers into one meaningful number (e.g., mean, median). Describing the distribution establishes an association between different observed values of a variable and a summarizing number that quantifies that association (e.g., range, standard deviation).

SELF-ASSESSMENT QUIZ

27. Summarizing numbers include: _____, _____, _____, and _____.
28. Distribution measures include: _____, _____, and _____.

Performance Goals and Targets

In years past, HCOs judged their performance one patient at a time. It wasn't until 1917, when the American College of Surgeons developed minimum hospital standards, that hospitals began to look more closely at performance in the aggregate (e.g., mortality rates, complication rates). In 1953, when TJC took over the Hospital Standardization Program from the College of Surgeons, new performance measurement requirements were gradually added. However, even then performance assessment was still done in a vacuum. A provider evaluated its current data and compared the results with its own past performance, asking questions such as the following: Is our mortality rate going up or down? Have complications decreased over past years' performance? Before the mid-1980s, it was rare for an HCO to assess performance on the basis of what other providers were able to achieve. For the most part, comparative health care performance data were hard to come by. Today, instead of evaluating performance on the basis of past performance alone, HCOs have all kinds of tools at their disposal for assessing the quality and safety of clinical services.

HCOs may use their own historical experience to establish performance expectations (sometimes called **thresholds**). If comparative performance data from other providers are available, these results are often taken into consideration when an HCO sets expectations. For example, the mortality rate for hospitalized patients over the age of 65 with the diagnosis of hip fracture is 2.5% (2009 national average for all hospitals).[20] An individual hospital would want to set mortality rate expectations that are similar to or better than what other providers are able to achieve. If the mortality rate has historically been higher at the individual HCO, then the national rate can be established as a **performance target**. The target is a "stretch goal" that represents a future performance expectation that the HCO will work toward achieving.

Thresholds and targets are used for performance assessment purposes. If current performance does not vary significantly from expected results, performance measurement continues. If current performance does vary significantly from expected results, improvement activities are undertaken.

SELF-ASSESSMENT QUIZ

29. Distinguish between a "threshold" and a "stretch goal."

PERFORMANCE IMPROVEMENT

When an opportunity for improvement is identified, an improvement activity is undertaken. Performance improvement involves an investigation of the cause of undesirable performance and implementation of solutions to prevent recurrence of the undesirable events. There are a variety of problem-solving approaches and a plethora of investigation techniques. Common approaches and techniques are described in the following section.

Performance Improvement Models

An improvement model is a description of the steps required to achieve better performance. Most performance models are variations on the scientific method (i.e., controlled, systematic investigation of empirical evidence). A widely used model of performance improvement is the **Plan-Do-Check-Act** (PDCA) cycle developed in the 1920s by Walter Shewhart, a statistician and quality expert at Western Electric Company in Cicero, Illinois (Figure 12-4).[21]

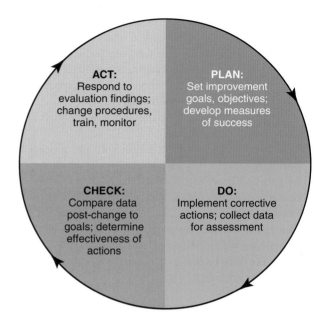

FIGURE 12-4 PDCA (Plan, Do, Check, Act) cycle.

❓ DID YOU KNOW

Did you know that Dr. Shewhart's academic discipline was physics? Review his biography at http://www-history.mcs.st-and.ac.uk/Biographies/Shewhart.html.

The diagram of the PDCA improvement model is depicted as a circular form for a reason. It is intended to be a model that is applied through recurring improvement cycles, as follows:

- Plan for improvements. How is the process performing? What are the constraints to improvement? What are you trying to accomplish? Develop improvement actions on the basis of the evidence. A question to be answered during the plan stage: How will you know if a change is improvement? Select process measures that correlate with expected results and make predictions of how the changes will affect performance.
- Do the improvement actions. On a small scale, perhaps a pilot test in one area, implement the process changes that are expected to achieve better performance. Collect data that can be used to assess the effect of these process changes accurately.
- Check the results of improvement actions. Compare the effects of the process changes with the predicted outcomes. When expectations are realized, the theories about what will work (the plan) have been supported, and the changes are implemented on a wider scale. When expected performance is not realized, the theories about what would work are wrong (not validated).
- Act on the evidence. Make the changes permanent, run new trials, revise improvement actions, or whatever is appropriate to the findings. Share the learning from the project with other people in the organization—the specifics of the process improvements and the general change principles—so that

others may benefit from the lessons learned. Sharing is key to organizational learning and continuous improvement.

Another renowned statistician, W. Edwards Deming, modified Shewhart's original model and renamed it the Plan-Do-Study-Act (PDSA) cycle. The steps of the PDSA model are similar to those in Figure 12-4.[22]

> **? DID YOU KNOW**
>
> A W. Edwards Deming quote: "If you do not know how to ask the right question, you discover nothing."

HCOs are also using other performance improvement models, derived from the PDCA cycle, that originated in business and manufacturing industries. Three approaches gaining popularity in the health care industry are rapid cycle improvement, Six Sigma, and lean.

Rapid Cycle Improvement

Rapid cycle improvement (RCI) has been successfully applied to improving both the operational aspects of health care delivery and clinical patient care processes. RCI is based on the PDSA model, using an accelerated method (usually less than 4 to 6 weeks per improvement cycle) to collect and analyze data and make informed changes based on that analysis.[23] This is then followed by another improvement cycle to evaluate the success of the change. RCI relies on small process changes and immediate, careful measurement of the effect of these changes.

The model entails four steps: set the aim (the goal), define the measures (the expected improvements), make changes (action plan), and test changes (the solution). The process is considered "rapid cycle" because it focuses on small, concrete changes that can be put into action and tested quickly, usually in a "pilot" situation.

Setting the aim involves taking a clear and deliberate look at what is to be accomplished. For example, a hospice unit might set a goal of improving patient satisfaction if patient satisfaction surveys reveal lower scores than is desirable. The aim or goal drives the next step—defining the measure. The measure should describe what the process will accomplish if a solution is successful. It may be necessary to set more than one measure for a goal, and the focus should be on key measures that address the goal as directly as possible. For example, a measure to meet the goal of improving patient satisfaction might be the average time from assessment of a patient's level of pain to administration of appropriate pain medication.

The third step is to select process changes that are expected to achieve the aim. Although many organizations search relevant literature for ideas for process changes, frontline staff and project team members can be invaluable sources. Possible processes to investigate for the example presented might be those related to medication ordering and administration.

The last RCI step is to test the changes using a rapid-cycle PDSA process. Evaluating the solution in a short time is a key factor. If the changes do not work, iterative PDSA

cycles are initiated until a workable solution is found. Repetition of the improvement cycles leads to continuous improvement and facilitates creation of internal performance benchmarks.

Many health care improvement initiatives use the RCI model, including the breakthrough projects sponsored by the Institute for Healthcare Improvement and national improvement projects such as the *Expecting Success: Excellence in Cardiac Care* national collaborative sponsored by the Robert Wood Johnson Foundation (RWJF).[24]

Six Sigma

Like many other quality and performance improvement approaches, Six Sigma has its roots in the manufacturing industry. In the late 1980s, Motorola began an initiative to eliminate defects and improve the efficiency of its operations. The overall goal was to reduce defective work so that the company could deliver its products at a lower cost while offering superior customer service. Motorola's approach came to be known as Six Sigma, derived from the Greek symbol sigma ($\sum$), used by statisticians to denote the measure of standard deviation of a population.

In Six Sigma terminology, results that fail to meet performance standards are called "defects," typically reported as defects per million opportunities. Six Sigma quality is attained when a process yields only 3.4 defects per million opportunities. The goal is to achieve an almost perfect level of quality (defect free). This requires understanding and eliminating defects in a process to move continually closer to the goal of "six sigma."

Six Sigma projects follow a highly structured process of five sequential steps illustrated in Figure 12-5. Taking the first letter from each of these steps creates an acronym, DMAIC (pronounced as dee-MAY-ick), which is typically used to label the method.

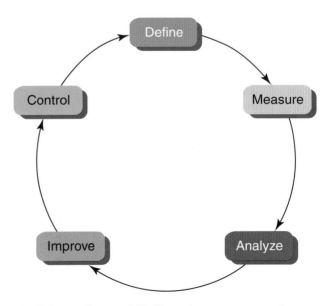

FIGURE 12-5 Steps of Six Sigma improvement project.

Problem definition requires knowing the customers of the process and their requirements (both output and service). Once customer wants are known, it is possible to measure performance against these requirements. Measuring and sampling systems are employed to understand what is actually happening in the processes. The collected data are used to calculate a Sigma score for the current process. Analysis of the information and hard facts obtained through measurement activities leads to prioritizing the potential causes of the problems being investigated. At this time, an initial hypothesis of the cause is formulated. Further information analysis is conducted until the root causes of undesirable performance are identified. Potential solutions are selected based on the probability of the solution actually solving the problem and the ease and cost of implementation. After improvements are implemented, the Sigma score for the process is recalculated to quantify the actual improvements made. Performance measures are established to capture deviations from standards and to predict future problems before they occur and to sustain the improvement.

Lean

In the 1980s, Japanese success in the global marketplace brought QI philosophies and techniques to international attention. Although initially applied in the manufacturing sector, these principles are now gaining popularity in the service sectors, including health care. One example is the Toyota Production System, also called "lean manufacturing" or "lean thinking."[25] Lean thinking principles, listed below, are applicable to a variety of health care processes and work settings.

- Eliminate waste and retain only value-added activities.
- Concentrate on improving value-added activities.
- Respond to the voice of the customer.
- Optimize processes across the organization.

The central tenet of lean thinking is value—providing "perfect" value to the customer by using only value-adding processes and eliminating waste. In health care, this means that every process should add to the value of the services provided to patients, their families, and other customers. Although activities such as diagnostic testing are of obvious value, others are more difficult to "see." For example, clerical services may seem unrelated to patients' view of the care they received. At the structural level, however, clerical inefficiencies may compromise the organization's ability to provide excellent patient care.

Eliminating waste and non-value-adding activities requires a focus on the entire value chain of a process or linked processes. Lean principles encourage health care managers to concentrate on optimizing the flow along the entire value chain and forego manipulation of separate tasks and activities in their efforts to improve performance, which may improve one subprocess to the detriment of another or to the entire process.

The steps of a lean improvement project are similar to other improvement projects; however the objective is always consistent—create a leaner, more efficient process that meets the needs of customers. Although there is some variation in how a lean project is conducted, the following steps are often carried out:

- The performance problem is stated through the eyes of the process customer. For instance, physicians are a customer of the HIM department. If the process of retrieving patient records is selected for a lean project, a performance problem from the physicians' perspective would be: duplicate tests are ordered when patient's previous health records are not available in an emergency.
- Current work procedures are examined, and a diagram of the current process is created. The illustration of the current process is based on what is actually happening. Direct observation is the preferred way to gather this information. The picture of the process helps in understanding the cause of performance problems.
- Specific improvement opportunities are identified and quantified. Data are gathered to determine how often each problem occurs and how it affects the process customers.
- Underlying causes of the specific problems are investigated. A common approach is to ask why this problem occurs five times in series to get to the root of it.
- A better way to do the work is proposed, and this new way is illustrated in a process diagram.
- A plan for implementing process changes is developed. The plan describes the steps needed to make the process changes happen and assigns implementation responsibilities and completion deadlines to specific individuals.
- The performance improvements expected as a result of implementing changes are predicted. How measurement data will be gathered is specified.
- After process changes are made, the actual performance improvement results are measured and compared with what was predicted to occur.

Benchmarking

Benchmarking is the act of comparing one's performance to high-quality performers. The purpose of this comparison is to identify how high-quality performers are able to achieve better performance and incorporate what works best into your way of doing things. As the health care environment becomes increasingly competitive and cost conscious, benchmarking is becoming a commonly used tool to identify ways to improve processes and initiate change at all operational levels. Most benchmarking processes are derived from the model developed by Xerox in the early 1980s. Organizations adapt, modify, and rearrange various steps to fit their goals. A generic model is shown in Figure 12-6.

SELF-ASSESSMENT QUIZ

30. What is the purpose of benchmarking?

Basically, two types of benchmarking are used to stimulate the improvement process: internal and external. Internal benchmarking compares performance between functional areas or departments *within* an organization. The goal is

FIGURE 12-6 Flowchart of benchmarking process.

to decrease or eliminate process errors or to improve process efficiency. For instance, the well-organized patient registration process in one department is studied and adopted by another department with a less efficient registration process. Internal benchmarking can often be done with minimal investment of time and money.

External benchmarking, sometimes called performance benchmarking, is used to close the gap between an organization's performance and that of other organizations. Such efforts often examine patient care practices, as well as vendor or supplier relationships and operational cost controls. For instance, a neonatal intensive care unit (NICU) seeking to reduce its infant mortality rate would contact practitioners at NICUs with very low rates of mortality to discuss practice differences. Through these discussions, a high-mortality NICU can learn new and better ways to care for vulnerable newborns.

External benchmarking may involve examination of processes in industries outside of health care. For example, an HCO might examine the ticket sales and itinerary planning process in the airline industry to improve its patient registration and scheduling processes.

PROCESS IMPROVEMENT TOOLS

During any type of improvement project, various tools and techniques are used to measure and improve performance. These improvement tools are structured analytical and evaluation techniques that help to advance the improvement initiative. Although the list of available performance improvement tools is extensive, it can be collapsed into three general types of techniques:

- Idea-generating techniques
- Information organization methods
- Data presentation and analysis methods

Figure 12-7 lists the steps of an improvement project and common tools that may be used during each step.

Idea Generation

Brainstorming is a structured but flexible process designed to maximize the number of ideas generated by a group of people. It is primarily used in the exploratory phase of problem analysis and solution development.

Brainstorming requires a leader who serves primarily as a facilitator and recorder and a team of six to ten persons brought together to generate ideas about a particular performance issue. The issue is defined, a time limit set for discussion, and ideas recorded for later team member discussion. All ideas should be expressed vocally, and criticism should be avoided. The goal is to produce a large number of ideas. Brainstorming has become an integral part of performance management in response to emphasis on worker empowerment and the need to solicit opinions from all levels of

FIGURE 12-7 Common tools used during an improvement project.

Process Improvement Tools and Techniques	Identify opportunity	Analyze the process	Generate solutions	Implement solutions	Evaluate results
Brainstorming	X	X	X		
Nominal group technique	X	X			
Affinity diagram	X	X			
Flowchart	X	X	X	X	
Decision matrix	X	X	X		
Cause-and-effect diagram	X	X	X		
Force field analysis			X	X	
Histogram	X	X			X
Bar graph	X	X			X
Pareto chart	X	X			X
Line graph	X	X			X
Control chart	X	X			X
Correlation analysis		X			X

workers within an organization. **Nominal group technique** is similar to brainstorming but uses silent generation of ideas and a sequential reporting approach to ensure participation by all group members.

SELF-ASSESSMENT QUIZ

31. What is the key distinction between brainstorming and NGT?

DID YOU KNOW

Brainstorming methods were first introduced in 1953 as a group creativity technique by Alex Faickney Osborn in his book *Applied Imagination.*

Affinity diagrams may be used to bridge the gap between idea generation and organization of the ideas. After the initial brainstorming session, affinity diagrams often are used to organize and prioritize information into clusters or categories (Figure 12-8). In the example, the tool is used to identify causes of a problem. It can also be used for brainstorming and categorizing solutions.

Affinity diagrams are particularly useful when dealing with large amounts of complicated information. This technique reduces what may seem to be an unmanageable amount of information into a smaller number of homogeneous categories. As in the case of brainstorming, discussion time limits should be set to keep the amount of new information generated manageable.

Information Organization

Flowcharts are graphic representations of a sequence of activities or steps in a process. A flowchart can be created to show the current process that needs improving. It can also be used to illustrate how the process will look after improvements are made. A flowchart consists of a series of connected symbols that represent process steps (Figure 12-9).

Flowcharts are used during an improvement project to help people:

- Agree on the steps of a process and the order in which they occur

FIGURE 12-8 Affinity diagram.

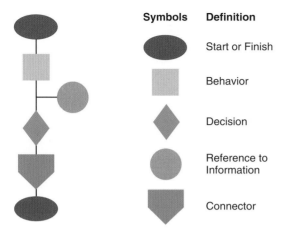

Symbols	Definition
	Start or Finish
	Behavior
	Decision
	Reference to Information
	Connector

FIGURE 12-9 Flowchart.

- See duplicated efforts and other non-value-added steps that might be lurking in a process
- Clarify working relationships between people and organizations
- Target specific process steps that need improving

Creation of a flowchart begins by deciding on the starting and ending points. Tasks are sequentially arranged and decision-making points identified. The goal is to illustrate a real-life situation accurately in an ordered and understandable format.

The **decision matrix** is another information organization tool. This multidimensional tool is used to organize and categorize information into a more usable form for decision-making purposes. Information generated through the use of brainstorming or other idea-generating tools is entered on the matrix and then prioritized according to predefined criteria. The decision matrix will allow a team to analyze the pros and cons of each idea.

To use a decision matrix for selecting the best possible improvements to the existing process, the team would first develop a list of criteria for evaluating all the solutions that have been suggested. The criteria are specific to the solutions offered and the improvement goal. Sample criteria include the following:

- Will the proposed solution make a positive impact?

- Will the people involved in the process and upper management support the proposed solution?
- Can the people involved in the process implement the needed changes?
- What will be the cost of the proposed solution?
- Does the proposed solution fix the performance problem?
- How difficult is the proposed solution to implement?

A matrix is then created, listing solutions down the left side and selection criteria across the top. Next, the team answers the criteria questions for each solution proposed. By comparing the criteria answers against each solution, either a clear winner will appear or the team may be able to reduce the list of possible solutions. From the remaining solutions, either a new decision matrix with other criteria can be developed or further analysis can be done.

Illustrated in Figure 12-10 is a decision matrix used to evaluate solutions to a performance problem in the HIM department. A decision matrix can also be weighted. In place of a yes or no answer, there might be numerical values such as +1 or −1. The relative values might state that one criterion is 5 times more important than another, therefore responses in this column could range from +5 to −5.

> **? DID YOU KNOW**
>
> The cause-and-effect diagram is sometimes referred to as an Ishikawa diagram, in recognition of its creator Kaoru Ishikawa.

Cause-and-effect diagrams are useful tools for solving complicated problems by helping people see the relationship between performance factors and an end result. They are also called **fishbone diagrams** because they look something like fish skeletons (Figure 12-11).

Cause-and-effect diagrams are particularly useful in the plan phase of the PDCA cycle. Constructing a fishbone diagram requires only a few simple steps. First, an effect (an outcome or goal) is placed on the right side of the diagram at the end of the horizontal causal line. Second, major causes are directly linked to the causal line in an ordered sequence. Finally, minor causes are linked to each of the major causes along the time line. Often brainstorming is used to generate the list of major and minor causes. The completed diagram

Solutions	Decision Criteria				
	Positive Impact	Management Support	Can Implement	Low Cost	Easy to Implement
Hire more HIM staff	Yes	No	Yes	No	Yes
Retrain existing HIM staff	Yes	Yes	Yes	Yes	Yes
Automate the process	Yes	No	Yes	No	No
Transfer process to another department	Yes	Yes	Yes	Yes	No

FIGURE 12-10 Decision matrix.

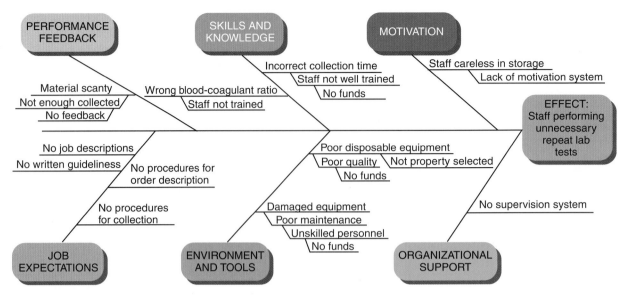

FIGURE 12-11 Fishbone diagram.

organizes all possible causes into categories (somewhat like an affinity diagram). Next, the improvement team must determine which problems should be tackled first. A decision matrix might be used to make this determination.

Force field analysis is a tool that also shows the relationship between performance variables and outcomes. When used during the solution generation step of an improvement project, force field analysis makes it easier to identify the variables that help and variables that hinder reaching the desired outcome. It depicts the situation as a balance between two sets of forces: one that tries to change the status quo and one that tries to maintain it (Figure 12-12).

This tool is particularly useful during the plan stage of the PDCA cycle when it is often important to reduce the impact of process variables hindering improvement plans. Brainstorming is used to identify the positive (driving forces) and the negative (inhibiting forces) to achieve a particular outcome. Expected positive effects (drivers) are placed in the left column, and negative effects (inhibitors) are placed in the right column.

Data Presentation and Analysis

Histograms are graphic representations of frequency distributions. They are useful for identifying whether the variation that exists in the frequency distribution is normal or skewed. To construct a histogram, create a vertical and a horizontal axis. The groupings or classes, which must be continuous data, are shown as contiguous bars placed on the horizontal axis. The frequency of occurrence for each class is plotted on the vertical axis, with the height of the bar representing the count. A bar graph is used to report count values of categorical data, such as the number of outpatient visits for each day of the week. The categories are labeled on the horizontal axis with the frequency count plotted on the y-axis (Figure 12-13). This may seem similar in appearance to a

FIGURE 12-12 Force field diagram.

Acquire New Transcription Equipment	
Driving Forces ⟶	⟵ Restraining Forces
Work completed in half the time	All stakeholders not in agreement
Fewer errors	Existing equipment not that old
Physicians will love it	High capital costs
Lower maintenance costs	Budget
Transcriptionists will love it	Purchasing policy committee

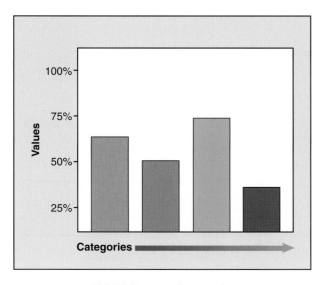

FIGURE 12-13 Bar graph.

histogram; however, the bars are separated as the x-axis is a label, not a continuous variable.

SELF-ASSESSMENT QUIZ

32. Distinguish between a histogram and a bar chart.

Pareto charts are similar to bar graphs. The primary difference is that occurrences plotted on a Pareto chart are ordered from the largest or most frequently occurring category (and presumably most important) to the smallest or least frequently occurring category (Figure 12-14).

To create a Pareto chart, first select the data to be displayed and then determine the standard for comparison (i.e., frequency, cost, or amount). Draw and appropriately label the vertical and horizontal axes. Finally, draw bars that represent the frequency of each factor according to a predetermined rank ordering. Pareto charts are often used to demonstrate the most frequent performance problems that are most in need of fixing. A second y-axis may be used to plot a cumulative frequency line as an additional visual tool to establish the relative magnitude of a category.

? DID YOU KNOW

A cumulative frequency curve, which is sometimes used with a Pareto chart, may also be referred to as an ogive.

SELF-ASSESSMENT QUIZ

33. Distinguish between a bar chart and a Pareto chart.

Line graphs, sometimes known as **run charts**, provide a simple visual method of monitoring performance trends over time. To create a line graph, first decide the time period for which data are to be collected and analyzed (e.g., continual or time restricted). Second, draw a graph with a vertical and a horizontal axis. Here, the horizontal axis indicates increments of time, and the vertical axis indicates increments of measurement. Finally, plot the data points and evaluate any trends evident in the data (Figure 12-15). Multiple data sets can be plotted on a single graph to allow easy comparisons. For example, a line could be added representing performance expectations, and the line graph could visually display the gap between expected and actual performance.

Control charts are a special type of line graph used to monitor performance. They add another dimension to performance analysis—that is, the ability to determine whether a process is statistically in control. In the 1920s, Walter A. Shewhart, a physicist, was charged with improving the

FIGURE 12-14 Pareto chart.

FIGURE 12-15 Line graph.

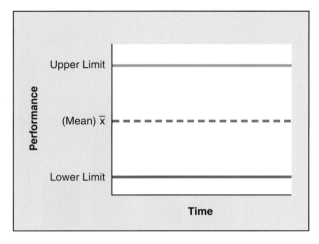

FIGURE 12-16 Control chart.

quality of telephone production in Bell Laboratories. Shewhart developed a theory of process variation that forms the basis of statistical process control.[21] The critical feature of Shewhart's theory of variation is that it categorizes variation according to the action needed to reduce it. To reduce common cause variation, one must change the process. To reduce special cause variation, one must find and eliminate unusual occurrences. Common cause variation occurs in any process, and it results from routine, random events. For example, a clerk assembles 10 records during the first hour. However, the second group of records contains more documents than the first group, and the clerk only assembles eight records in the second hour. The number of records assembled each hour may randomly go up and down, but if this number were to be plotted on a line graph, you would see that it varies in a predictable manner. Special cause variation is not random and is due to an unusual event. For example, a clerk can routinely photocopy documents at an average rate of 50 pages per minute. If a paper jam occurs, the time taken to correct the jam and reset the documents will extend the average rate of production. To help distinguish between these two kinds of process variations, Shewhart devised the control chart (Figure 12-16).

Control charts have three important lines. The central line is the mean or median for the data, and the upper and lower lines are known as control limits. The control limits are established as a specified number of standard deviations (σ) from the mean. Recall that when data are normally distributed, approximately 95% of the data points will fall within +/=2 standard deviations. Data points outside the control limits (or unusual data patterns) indicate a special cause that should be found and eliminated.[26] The simplest control chart is the individual's chart. This chart is used for processes that produce one value in each time frame. An example of this might be daily output from coding staff. To use this kind of chart, the data should have a normal distribution.

To create an individual's control chart (Box 12-1), 20 or more data points are necessary. Fifteen is the absolute minimum.

If all values plotted on a control chart fall between the upper and lower control limit lines and there are no significant trends, the process is considered to be stable or "in control." If a process is in control and no changes are made to how work is done, it is possible to predict what future performance will be. Process performance is predictable only if it is in control—that is, unaffected by extraordinary or special cause variation. The usefulness of the control chart is enhanced when it is integrated with other performance improvement tools such as cause-and-effect diagrams, Pareto charts, and flowcharts.

BOX 12-1   Steps to Create an Individual's Control Chart

List the data points in time order.

Determine the range between each of the consecutive data points. The range is the absolute difference between two consecutive data points. The range is always positive, even if the next data point is lower than the one being compared with. There will be one less range value than there are data points.

Find the mean range. To do this, total the ranges and divide by the number of range values. The symbol for the mean range is $\bar{R}$.

Find the mean or average of the data point values. To do this, total the values of all the data points and divide by the number of data points. The symbol for the mean data value is $\bar{X}$.

Calculate the control limits. $[2.66\bar{R} = 3\sigma.]$ Upper Control Limit $= \bar{X} + (2.66\bar{R})$ Lower Control Limit $= \bar{X} - (2.66\bar{R})$

Draw a solid horizontal line representing the data mean. Label the line and write the actual mean value next to it.

Draw two dotted horizontal lines representing the upper and lower control limits. Label the two control limit lines and write the actual upper and lower limits next to them.

Plot the data points in time sequence. Connect each point to the next point in the sequence with a line.

The symbols for mean range and mean data value are defined in the box text. The only other symbol used in the box is σ (standard deviation).

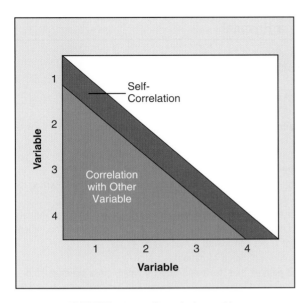

FIGURE 12-17 Correlation table.

Correlation analysis determines the strength, direction, and statistical significance of a relationship between one or more performance variables (Figure 12-17). Correlation coefficients provide an exact interpretation of the relationship noted on the run chart. In correlation analysis, scores range from −1.0, signifying a perfect negative relationship, to 0.0, signifying no relationship, to 1.0, signifying a perfect positive relationship.

To use correlation analysis, first select variables with a relationship of interest. Second, set the acceptance level of significance. Finally, examine the coefficients to determine significance, direction (positive or negative), and strength of association. Correlation analysis provides easily interpretable numbers and a straightforward method of examining relationships between various performance variables.

PATIENT SAFETY

Driven by media attention and growing concerns about medical mistakes, patient safety improvement has become a national imperative. Although some believe that purchasers and consumers are having the greatest influence on patient safety improvement activities, researchers identified TJC as the primary driver of hospital patient safety initiatives.[27] Professional and market initiatives have also facilitated improvement, but hospitals report that these have had less impact to date. The National Patient Safety Goals issued by TJC each year have strongly influenced adoption of safer patient care practices in all provider sites.

Starting in 2003, TJC published National Patient Safety Goals to promote specific changes intended to improve patient safety. Accredited organizations are evaluated for continuous compliance with the requirements associated with these goals. For example, one of the 2013 goals applicable to all accredited organizations is to improve the accuracy of patient identification. Caregivers are expected to use at least two patient identifiers (neither to be the patient's room

number) whenever providing care, treatment, or services to a patient. The current National Patient Safety Goals can be found on the TJC Web site (www.jointcommission.org).

It can sometimes be difficult to differentiate between patient safety improvement and other types of health care performance management activities. In truth, there is no clear-cut distinction. For the purposes of this text, **patient safety improvement** is defined as actions undertaken by individuals and organizations to protect health care recipients from being harmed by the effects of health care services.

Patient safety improvement involves the familiar performance management building blocks: measurement, assessment, and improvement. Many of the same process improvement tools described earlier in this chapter can also be used to improve patient safety. Some concepts that are unique to patient safety improvement are detailed in this section.

Safety Measurement

Information about patient incidents is obtained primarily from **incident reports**. These are paper-based or electronic reports completed by health care professionals when an incident occurs. Common categories of reportable patient incidents are listed in Table 12-3.

Incident reports have been used in health care organizations for many years. Health care facilities require the staff to fill out an incident report when a variance has occurred from the usual process of patient care or when a mishap or injury occurs involving a patient, staff member, or visitor. These reports are meant to be nonjudgmental, factual accounts of the event and its consequences, if there were any. Incident reports are prepared to assist the organizations in identifying and correcting problem-prone areas and in preparation for possible legal action. Incident reports are not incorporated into the health record at any time. They are considered administrative documents prepared to facilitate the organization's quality and patient safety improvement efforts.

Obtaining reliable information about patient incidents is not without its challenges. An individual's willingness to report an incident is strongly linked to the organizational culture and how the information is used. If the involved staff member is blamed for the event and disciplined or dismissed by management because of his or her involvement, it is unlikely people will voluntarily incriminate themselves or their colleagues by completing incident reports. Experience has shown that when caregivers are provided protection from disciplinary actions, they are more willing to report incidents.[28]

The value of collecting patient incident data is in the knowledge that can be gained from analysis of the data. Figure 12-18 illustrates a patient safety report created from incident data.

The bar graph provides information about the type of medication errors that occurred in a hospital during a 6-month period. The largest percentage of errors relate to accidental omission of a medication. The hospital will focus

TABLE 12-3 Examples of Reportable Patient Incidents in a Hospital

Suicide gesture. Suicidal behavior that does not meet the definition for suicide attempt
Suicide attempt. Suicidal behavior that is either medically serious or psychiatrically serious
Suicide. Act of taking one's own life voluntarily and accidentally
Alleged patient abuse. Includes acts of physical, psychological, sexual, or verbal abuse
Rape/attempted rape. Sexual assault with or without penetration
Homicide. Death of a patient or staff caused by a patient or death of patient caused by another individual
Patient-on-staff abuse. Physical injury, intentionally striking staff
Patient-on-patient abuse. Patient injured or assaulted by another patient
Falls. All patient falls whether observed or not observed and whether or not there is injury
Blood transfusion error. Blood or blood products erroneously administered to the wrong patient, therapy not ordered, administered wrong blood product, error in typing or cross-matching, with or without any reaction or evident adverse effect
Medication error. A dose of medication that deviates from the physician's order as written in the patient's chart or as written on an outpatient prescription or from standard medical center procedures (Except for errors of omission, the medication dose must actually reach the patient; a wrong dose that is detected and corrected before administration to the patient is not considered a medication error.)
Medication reaction. Anaphylaxis or other adverse reactions seriously affecting the well-being of patient
Idiosyncratic reaction to blood or blood products. Reaction to blood or blood product that has been properly typed, cross-matched, and administered
Surgery-related death. Includes death in operating room, recovery room, during induction of anesthesia, and death within 48 hours of surgery
Unexpected death. Includes events such as death during or following procedures such as cardiac catheterization, biopsy, radiological procedure, endoscopy; cause of death unknown; death reportable to local medical examiner or coroner; death due to previously unknown problem or diagnosis; death due to misadventure such as respirator malfunction, medication error, failure to diagnose, or failure to treat appropriately
Patient involved in fire. Patient sets the fire, is involved in a fire, is burned, or is exposed in smoke of fire (i.e., smoke inhalation)
Inaccurate counts in surgery. Needle, sponge, or pad counts
Other. Any incidents that result or may result in significant patient disability or disfigurement

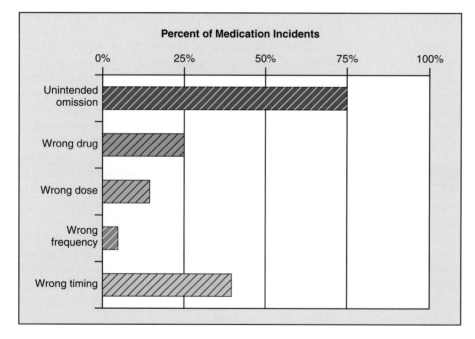

FIGURE 12-18 Type of medication errors.

its medication safety improvement efforts on eliminating this type of error. Collection, analysis, and reporting of patient incident data are often responsibilities assigned to the quality or risk management department.

In March 2003, the Agency for Healthcare Research and Quality (AHRQ) published the first set of patient safety indicators (PSI), which measure potentially preventable complications (adverse events).[29] AHRQ has created software that hospitals can use to screen billing records to provide a perspective on patient safety. Examples of the current indicators are found in Table 12-4.

Specifically, PSIs screen for problems that patients experience as a result of exposure to the health care system and that are likely amenable to prevention by changes at the system or provider level. Although quality assessments based on administrative data cannot be definitive, the measures can be used to flag potential patient safety problems that require further investigation.

TABLE 12-4 Agency for Healthcare Research and Quality Patient Safety Indicators

- Death in low-mortality diagnosis-related groups
- Pressure ulcer
- Death among surgical inpatients with treatable serious complications
- Foreign body left in during procedure
- Iatrogenic pneumothorax
- Central venous catheter–related bloodstream infections
- Postoperative hip fracture
- Postoperative hemorrhage or hematoma
- Postoperative physiologic and metabolic derangements
- Postoperative respiratory failure
- Postoperative pulmonary embolism or deep vein thrombosis
- Postoperative sepsis
- Postoperative wound dehiscence
- Accidental puncture or laceration
- Transfusion reaction
- Birth trauma—injury to neonate
- Obstetric trauma—vaginal delivery with instrument
- Obstetric trauma—vaginal delivery without instrument

Source: AHRQ: Patient safety indicators overview: http://www.qualityindicators. ahrq.gov/Modules/psi_resources.aspx. Accessed September 2013.

Patient Safety Databases

A number of groups are gathering and analyzing information about patient incidents that occur at many facilities to identify the error-producing factors in repeat mishaps. This analysis provides important learning opportunities for health care organizations. Some examples of these patient safety database projects are listed in Table 12-5.

In December 1999, the patient safety panel of the IOM recommended that hospitals and other health care providers be required to report medical errors that lead to a serious patient injury or death to a nationwide reporting system.[1] Data compiled from the reporting system could be used to learn how to prevent future occurrences. The panel also endorsed the development of voluntary reporting systems for less serious errors to detect system weaknesses that may ultimately lead to serious patient harm. Several states already require that health care facilities report certain types of patient incidents to the state health department.[30]

The nationwide reporting system envisioned by the IOM is now in place. The AHRQ has certified a number of entities throughout the United States to function as patient safety organizations (PSOs).[31] These entities serve as independent, external experts that can collect, analyze, and aggregate information about patient safety events to develop insights into the underlying causes. Health care organizations can voluntarily report patient safety events to a PSO. Patient safety events include the following:

- Incident—patient safety events that reached the patient, whether or not there was harm;
- Near miss or close call—patient safety events that did not reach the patient; and

TABLE 12-5 Examples of National Patient Safety Databases

Sponsoring Organization	Description
American Society of Anesthesiologists http://www. asaclosedclaims.org	This database, known as the Closed Claims Project, contains an in-depth investigation of closed anesthesia malpractice claims designed to identify major areas of loss, patterns of injury, and strategies for prevention.
Food and Drug Administration (FDA) http://www.fda.gov	The FDA collects and analyzes data about patient incidents involving medical device failures. Through the FDA's Medical Products Reporting Program, MedWatch, information about product safety problems is rapidly communicated to the medical community, thereby improving patient care. The Vaccine Adverse Event Reporting System is a cooperative program for vaccine safety of the FDA and the Centers for Disease Control. Health care professionals and the public are encouraged to report incidents of adverse events or side effects after vaccine administration.
Institute for Safe Medication Practices (ISMP) http://www. ismp.org	The ISMP provides an independent review of medication errors that have been voluntarily submitted to the Medical Errors Reporting Program sponsored by the U.S. Pharmacopeia. Information about the common factors causing medication errors and how to reduce them is distributed to health care facilities by the ISMP through their biweekly *Medication Safety Alert* newsletter and various other educational offerings.
The Joint Commission http://www. jointcommission.org	The Joint Commission has been collecting data about sentinel events since 1996. The review findings are regularly summarized and shared with the health care community through sentinel event alerts. The alerts also serve as the basis for development of National Patient Safety Goals.

- Unsafe condition—any circumstance that increases the probability of a patient safety event.

AHRQ has developed common definitions and reporting formats that allow health care providers to collect and submit standardized information regarding these events.[32]

SELF-ASSESSMENT QUIZ

34. Who certifies entities as PSOs?
35. What are three categories of patient safety events to be reported to a PSO?

The network of patient safety databases to which PSOs, health care providers, and others voluntarily contribute non-identifiable patient safety event data is used by AHRQ to analyze national and regional statistics, including trends and patterns, regarding these events. Findings are made public and included in AHRQ's annual National Healthcare Quality Report.

Safety Improvement

Ensuring patient safety involves the establishment of operational systems and processes that minimize the likelihood of errors and maximize the likelihood of intercepting them when they occur.[33] Techniques for establishing safer health care systems and processes are similar to any performance improvement initiative. First, the process to be improved is identified and then analyzed to determine where improvements are needed. Then actions intended to achieve desired improvement goals are implemented.

Patient safety improvement projects initiated after a serious patient incident are considered reactive. The impetus for starting the project is an undesirable event that needs to be investigated. These projects are often called "root cause analyses." Some patient safety improvement projects are proactive. These projects are initiated prospectively for the purpose of avoiding an undesirable event. These projects are often called proactive risk assessments.

Root Cause Analysis

Root cause analysis is a systematic investigation process that occurs after a complication or adverse event that resulted in a patient injury caused by medical management rather than by the underlying disease or condition of the patient.[34] The Joint Commission uses the term *sentinel event* to describe serious patient incidents that should have a root cause analysis. Following are examples of sentinel events:

- Any event that results in an unanticipated patient death or major permanent loss of function, not related to the natural course of the patient's illness or underlying condition
- Suicide of a patient in a setting where the patient receives around-the-clock care, treatment, and services (e.g., hospital, residential treatment center, crisis stabilization center)
- Unanticipated death of a term infant
- Infant abduction or infant discharge to the wrong family
- Hemolytic transfusion reaction involving administration of blood or blood products having major blood group incompatibilities
- Surgery on the wrong patient or wrong body part

Simply stated, a root cause analysis is a process designed for investigating what, how, and why something happened and for determining how to prevent the same thing from happening again. Understanding why an event occurred is the key to developing effective improvement recommendations. Imagine you find that one of the people in the HIM department is not documenting release of information requests as required by the procedure. Typically, the manager might conclude that the cause of this mistake is a noncompliant employee. However, stopping here in the investigation only tells the manager what happened and how it happened. If the manager does not probe deeper to understand the reasons for the mistake, then preventing its recurrence will be difficult. Mistakes do not just happen. They can often be traced to some root causes. In this case, the manager might ask, "Why didn't they follow the procedure?" "Is the procedure clear, understandable, easy to follow?" "Am I asking the employee to do something that is beyond the scope of his or her training?" "Are there incentives for not documenting each release of information, such as productivity bonuses?" "Do the employees have someone to answer their questions?" "Are any other employees having the same issues?" Each question leads to more questions. This constant questioning, asking "why," "why," "why," will help determine the root causes so that meaningful corrective actions can be designed.

Root cause analysis is a four-step process. The first step is to collect the data. Generally a team of individuals is brought together to review what happened, when it happened, and how it happened and to begin to explore why it happened. This may include participants or witnesses to the events, individuals who are expert in various aspects of the event (clinicians, human resources, technicians, etc.), and organizational leaders who can clear away barriers that may impede process improvements. The second step is to identify the causal factors. Causal factors are events or conditions that collectively, with other factors, increased the likelihood of an incident. By themselves the causal factors may not have caused the incident, but when they occurred concurrently, the probability of an incident increased.

Step three is to identify the root causes. These are the causes that, if corrected, would prevent recurrence of this and similar incidents. Root causes are fundamental factors that address underlying system issues rather than single problems or factors. Root causes can include system deficiencies, management failures, inadequate competencies, omissions, nonadherence to procedures, and inadequate communication. This step may involve the use of a cause-and-effect diagram. This diagram structures the inquiry process by helping people consider all the reasons why a particular causal factor exists. For example, you may find the HIM department procedure for recording in the release-of-information log is too cumbersome (a causal factor). To discover the root cause of inadequate or missing log entries, you would consider all the reasons the procedure is too cumbersome. Eventually, through this questioning process, you would get to the root cause of the problem.

The final step of a root cause analysis is to generate recommendations for corrective action. Actions can fall into three categories: eliminate the chance for error, make it easier for people to do the right thing, and mitigate the effects of the error after it has occurred. Process changes may be necessary, staff may need some additional training, or any number of actions may be taken. The goal is to reduce or eliminate the root cause of the event so that future similar events do not occur. The completed root cause analysis is documented and shared with appropriate staff, physicians, and leaders in the organization.

Students can review actual serious patient incidents and the investigations of these events on the Morbidity and Mortality Rounds Internet Web site (http://webmm.ahrq.gov) sponsored by the AHRQ. The case studies on this site illustrate the importance of tracking down the causes of sentinel events and significant "near-miss" events so that health care processes can be changed to prevent similar occurrences in the future.

 DID YOU KNOW

The AHRQ WebM&M (http://webmm.ahrq.gov/) site includes expert analysis of medical errors. Each month one case is spotlighted with expanded commentary, readers' polls, and quizzes. Providers can earn continuing education credits by taking the quizzes.

Proactive Risk Assessment

In addition to improving patient safety through use of traditional performance improvement techniques, in July 2001, TJC began to require accredited organizations to conduct proactive risk assessment projects. Many organizations are meeting this requirement by using a method known as **failure mode and effect analysis** (FMEA). FMEA is a risk analysis technique used in manufacturing, aviation, computer software design, and other industries to conduct safety system evaluations. It is now being used in HCOs to analyze existing systems and evaluate new processes before implementation. It is a technique that promotes systematic thinking about the safety of a patient care process in terms of [35]:

- What could go wrong?
- How badly might it go wrong?
- What needs to be done to prevent failures?

During an FMEA, the people involved in the process work together to answer these questions objectively. The fundamental purpose of the FMEA is to take actions that reduce the likelihood of a process failure.

The first step in conducting an FMEA is to define the process to be analyzed. Because these projects can be labor intensive, it is best to select a process that is high risk or known to be problematic. For example, FMEA is a good tool for health care facilities to use in analyzing various medication administration processes because these activities have been shown to be at high risk for errors. [36]

After the process has been selected, a multidisciplinary team is convened consisting of subject matter experts and people representing various viewpoints. The team members include both management and staff-level positions. The team starts out by creating a flowchart of the process. Next, for each process step, the team determines how that step might fail. For example, at the step of ordering medication, the physician may order the wrong medication or the wrong dosage. The physician may write an illegible order or use abbreviations that can be misinterpreted by the pharmacist. The team brainstorms all possible failures that can occur at each step in the process.

For each possible failure, the team defines the effect of the failure by answering several questions [34]:

- What would likely happen if this failure occurred?
- How serious would it be if this failure occurred?
- What are the chances that this failure will actually happen?
- What are the chances that this failure will be detected and corrected before patients are harmed?

Determining the effect of each failure is as important as describing the failure itself. The process improvement actions ultimately recommended by the team will be directed toward the "vital few" failures that will cause the greatest harm to patients should they occur. The next step in the FMEA is to identify the causes for the failures. For each significant failure, a "mini" root cause analysis is done. Although the failure is theoretical, the team tries to identify the factors that could contribute to or cause the failure. Recommendations for improvements and corrective actions are then developed to prevent significant failures. Just as the team would do in any type of performance improvement project, the corrective actions are pilot tested to ensure they are effective and do not introduce new problems into the system. If effective, the corrective actions are fully implemented and monitored to ensure continuing effectiveness. Other than the demand on human resources and time, the main limitation of FMEA is that it deals with process failures one at a time. In most cases, adverse events are typically the result of multiple failures and preexisting hazardous conditions. [37]

 DID YOU KNOW

The concept of identifying the "vital few" failures with FMEA is consistent with the Pareto Principle (sometimes called the 80/20 rule), which separates the "vital few" from the "trivial many."

A variety of other prospective risk assessment tools and techniques are available to HCOs. One technique that is gaining popularity for improving patient safety is simulation. **Simulation** is a technique to replace or amplify real-life experiences with guided experiences that evoke or replicate substantial aspects of the real world in a fully interactive manner. [38] This technique is helpful in preparing people for error-prone, high-risk, or unusual situations. By simulating possible adverse events, people learn to recognize problems and understand the effects of their responses in a safe environment. Simulation forces people to review processes on a detailed level, which can help to improve patient safety. Typical results of simulations include changing the process flow, reducing process times, changing material handling methods, reassigning functions, bringing in new technologies, updating information processing methods, and adding or replacing resources. These changes, when appropriate, can help to improve patient safety.

The fundamental purpose of all proactive risk assessment techniques is to recommend and take actions that reduce the likelihood of a process failure. Any process can be chosen for a risk assessment; it does not have to be a process involving direct patient care. Proactive risk assessment techniques can be applied to the work activities in the HIM department to help reduce mistakes and improve service efficiency.

RISK MANAGEMENT

In the context of an HCO, a risk is any event or situation that could potentially result in an injury to an individual or in financial loss to the HCO. The definition of injury as used in legal terms is more encompassing than its general definition of physical harm. In the legal sense, harm or injury may be defined as any wrong or damage done to a person or to a person's rights or property. As social welfare agents, HCOs hold a public trust. Risk management programs acknowledge accountability to the public for a safe physical environment and adherence to accepted standards of clinical practice. Although malpractice litigation often captures public visibility with large monetary awards for death or personal injury resulting from medical treatment, the organization's administrative and governance bodies must be concerned with potential injury to all people who enter the facility or its grounds for any reason. These potential claimants include patients, employees, visitors, contractual and business affiliates, and members of the medical staff.

Risk management encompasses all policies, procedures, and practices directed at reducing risk and subsequent liability for injuries that occur in the organization's immediate environment. The policies and procedures that constitute a risk management program are developed in collaboration with the HCO's legal counsel because judicial interpretation of statutory law in the court system is a continually evolving process. In general, risk management activities are intended to minimize the potential for injury occurrence, ensure prompt and appropriate response to injured parties, and anticipate and plan for ensuing liability when injuries occur. Activities are directed at preventing or reducing financial loss, allocating funds for compensable events, and diminishing negative public image resulting from injury claims.

Risk management documentation must be created and maintained in strict accordance with legal guidelines to prevent discoverability. Attorney-client privilege cannot be invoked for records maintained in the ordinary course of business or in provision of patient care.[39] Therefore, information about specific incidents or individual patients should be documented only as private communications between the risk manager or HCO leadership and the legal counsel. This communication may serve as the basis for administrative decisions or action plans to respond to an identified risk or potentially compensable event (PCE). A PCE is an adverse occurrence, usually involving a patient, that could result in a financial obligation for the HCO.

Claims resolved through the court system often require defensive legal action over a period of several years. A finding against the HCO that results in a monetary award to the claimant usually is paid out several years after the injury occurred. Substantial costs associated with the defense are incurred whether the courts find for or against the HCO.

Financial planning to ensure adequate resources to meet future legal obligations requires accurate, complete information from the claims management program. Many claims by injured parties are settled without legal action. The insurance carrier or the organization may determine that settlement is preferable to trial for several reasons, including insufficient information for adequate defense, risk of greater financial loss than the settlement amount, and adverse impact on public image.

Loss Prevention and Reduction

The best protective risk management strategy is prevention. Prevention requires identifying and monitoring high-risk and problem-prone processes and physical plant locations. Historical aggregate data on injuries, safety hazards, complaints, and liability claims can provide information about potential risks. Monitoring includes ongoing evaluation of individual behaviors (e.g., correct hand-washing practice), physical safety (e.g., prominently displayed signs to indicate wet floors), personal security (e.g., functional locks on employee lockers), or some other aspect of corporate risk. Action to correct identified problems and follow-up to prevent recurrence are critical to the risk prevention process.

Loss reduction focuses on a single incident or claim and requires immediate response to any adverse occurrence. Injured people should receive prompt medical attention. Investigation of the incident should include examining the site and interviewing witnesses immediately after the occurrence to collect all pertinent facts. If the incident is considered potentially compensable, a claims representative for the liability insurance carrier should be contacted to ensure that all necessary information has been collected and appropriate responsive action taken. In many cases, prompt, sincere efforts to correct the problem can avert a claim for financial damages.

Claims Management

Claims management refers to the administrative and legal procedures initiated following an adverse event. For individual cases, these procedures may include the following:

- An internal audit of the charges billed
- Examination of the health record for completeness
- Sequestration of financial and health records
- Interrogatories
- Settlement negotiations
- Preparation for trial
- Tracking of the status of claims
- Analysis of aggregate claims and losses
- Objective use of resulting information to improve individual and organization performance

Aggregate data generated through facility-wide monitoring and evaluation activities, hazard surveillance, infection control, and other quality review activities are properly integrated into performance and patient safety improvement functions. Information is thus available to achieve the following objectives:

- Improve system processes
- Increase patient and employee satisfaction
- Improve clinical outcomes
- Decrease risk factors

UTILIZATION MANAGEMENT

Utilization management (UM) activities are intended to ensure that facilities and resources (both human and nonhuman) are used appropriately to meet the health care needs of patients. Both underutilization (unmet patient needs) and overutilization (provision of care or services not medically necessary) are undesirable outcomes. HCOs, providers, and health plans are all involved in UM activities.

The goal of UM is to maintain or increase quality of care and to improve access to timely and quality care for those who need it through efficient provision of resources. UM involves the three familiar building blocks of performance management:

- Measurement of how organizations and providers are using resources
- Assessment of how well resources are being used
- Improvement of resource use

UM encompasses the dual objectives of cost containment and quality of care. Although UM activities are often independent in an HCO, these activities are interdependent with performance and patient safety improvement functions.

External Requirements

The Medicare COP includes requirements for utilization management activities. Hospitals must have a process for reviewing services furnished by the institution and by members of the medical staff to patients entitled to benefits under the Medicare and Medicaid programs. These review activities include analyses of the medical necessity of hospital admissions, continued hospital stays, and professional services furnished.[40] Medical necessity means that a patient's clinical condition, as documented by a diagnostic test or physical finding, warrants services that can be provided only as an inpatient. Hospitals are required to have a committee that oversees the UM functions. At least two members of the committee must be doctors of medicine or osteopathy.

For the most part, TJC standards are silent on the topic of UM. The standards include some aspects of UM but are not labeled as such. For instance, the Provision of Care standards for hospitals include performance expectations related to ensuring continuity of care for patients discharged to another care setting or to home. Data collected during UM activities are to be integrated with the organization's overall performance improvement activities.

The UM activities of health plans are governed by CMS regulations (for federally funded beneficiaries) and state insurance commission regulations. Health plans accredited by the NCQA must comply with prescriptive UM standards that are similar to the CMS and state regulations. Organizationally, UM may be a program area within a health plan, or it may be a service provided by a third-party vendor (stand-alone UM outsourcing company). Health plans may delegate UM for various aspects of health care to different organizations. For example, UM for behavioral health, pharmacy services, and medical review may be provided by separate entities. Many health plans and stand-alone UM companies offer purchasers multiple medical management programs and often share staff and data systems among the program areas.

Accountable care organizations (ACOs) are a relatively new model of health care delivery in which providers are economically rewarded for high-quality, cost-efficient patient care. An ACO is a group of hospitals, physicians and other providers that agree to be held collectively accountable for the cost and quality of care delivered to a population of patients.[41] ACOs accredited by the NCQA are required to have an infrastructure for effectively managing its resources. To be financially successful ACO providers must deliver the right amount of care to patients at the right time. To accomplish this goal, UM activities, including ongoing monitoring of services rendered and the cost for those services, are necessary.

Program Components

Review of health care utilization is intended to reduce overuse and underuse of services by examining the appropriateness of care. Appropriate care means that services provided to a patient are consistent with their clinical needs. For example, an elderly patient may require rehabilitation services after hip replacement. The UM function involves four activities: prospective review, concurrent review, discharge planning/case management, and retrospective review.

Prospective Review

The prospective review process is initiated before a patient actually receives health services. If the patient's health plan requires prior approval of high-cost services (such as nuclear imaging studies or elective surgeries), the provider or facility contacts the UM company or health plan to obtain approval on behalf of the patient. UM personnel at the health plan gather clinical information about the patient's condition and use criteria to determine whether the planned health services are medically necessary. These criteria are often supplied by a commercial entity such as Milliman or McKesson. McKesson's InterQual criteria are referred to as IS/SI criteria—intensity of service/severity of illness—because they describe where services should be provided (intensity) on the basis of the level of the patient's physical impairment (severity).

 DID YOU KNOW

InterQual published its first IS/SI criteria in 1978. The criteria were used to evaluate the need for inpatient admission and level of service.

Cases that meet criteria are approved for payment by the health plan. Cases that do not meet criteria undergo additional review. Additional review may include gathering of more detailed clinical information, clinical consultation between physicians, or review by a specialist. The health plan's final determination of medical necessity is communicated to the provider or facility, often in an electronic format. All health plans have some type of appeals process that can be initiated by patients if there is disagreement about the medical necessity of planned services.

Concurrent Review

Hospitals, skilled nursing and rehabilitation facilities, and home health agencies conduct concurrent UM at the time of a patient's admission (usually within 24 hours or one working day) and periodically during provision of services. These UM activities are termed concurrent reviews because need for services is assessed simultaneously with provision of care. InterQual IS/SI criteria are often used for both admission and continued stay reviews. The intent of these reviews is to determine the point at which the patient no longer requires services at the current level of care. For instance, is a hospitalized patient medically able to return home and be adequately managed with home care services? The InterQual IS/SI criteria assist the UM staff, usually nurses or HIM professionals, in making these determinations. As with any criteria or guideline, the recommendations are not considered hard-and-fast rules. The final decision regarding what's best for the patient is left to the patient's physician.

Most providers use a two-stage review process with non-physician personnel conducting the initial and subsequent reviews. The UM staff screen patient health records (or information submitted by the admitting physician for prospective reviews) for documentation to establish compliance with medical necessity criteria. If documentation is sufficient and criteria are met, admission or continued stay is deemed appropriate. If criteria are not met, the patient's physician is asked to provide additional information or the case will be referred to a physician advisor. The facility's physician advisor for UM activities reviews the case and discusses the patient's condition with the attending physician. If the patient does not appear to need the services currently being provided, the facility risks payment denial from the health plan. When a patient's admission or continued stay is not considered medically necessary, the provider notifies the patient of probable noncoverage by their health plan. After receipt of the notice detailing the review process and outcome, the patient is expected to assume personal responsibility for payment of charges incurred beyond the date specified in the letter. In most cases, the patient is discharged promptly. For many reasons, including the loss of community goodwill, HCOs prefer to avoid this type of review outcome.

Health plans and ACOs often conduct concurrent review to determine the need for continued services. This review may be done remotely, with the facility's UM staff providing information about patients by phone or electronically (fax or secure e-mail). Some health plans employ UM staff to go on site in a facility to review records of patients currently receiving care. Figure 12-19 is a flowchart of the concurrent review process used by a health plan to evaluate the medical necessity of care provided to hospitalized beneficiaries.

Discharge Planning/Case Management

Discharge planning is a UM function designed to assist patients in transitioning from one level of care to another. Often UM staff conducts an initial discharge assessment but will refer patients in need of intensive discharge planning to case management services. Case management is patient focused and provides additional care coordination for patients with complex medical needs or in need of post-hospital health care services. Case managers, often registered nurses or social workers, interact with patients and providers to optimize efficient care. Unless postdischarge needs are adequately planned for, a patient's inpatient stay may be unnecessarily prolonged beyond the point of medical necessity. The Medicare COP and TJC standards require that hospitals have a process that identifies patients in need of discharge planning and ensures that appropriate arrangements for posthospital care are made before discharge.[42]

Retrospective Review

Retrospective review occurs after care has been rendered. Examples of cases in which a health plan might conduct a retrospective review include an emergency department visit for a nonemergent condition or after receiving a bill for services that were not preauthorized by the plan. Medical necessity and appropriateness of care also may be investigated by an HCO after services have been rendered to a patient. Although retrospective review offers no opportunity to prevent overuse or underuse of services, the reviews can provide valuable information about patterns of undesirable practices that can be used to improve future performance.

Retrospective review often involves an analysis of resource use to determine where there are opportunities to improve the efficiency of care or decreasing costs. Figure 12-20 is an example of a utilization report that would be useful for retrospective review in a hospital.

The report shows the hospital's average costs in ten revenue centers for patients treated for gastrointestinal hemorrhage compared with the average costs at other hospitals in their market area. In 5 of the 10 revenue centers, the hospital has higher average costs compared with other hospitals (the center line marked 100% represents the average cost). Physicians and other caregivers investigate the cause(s) of these higher costs and initiate improvement actions on the basis of what they find. The data in the figure originated from the Medicare MEDPAR files, and the comparative analysis was provided by Thomson Reuters, a health information vendor.

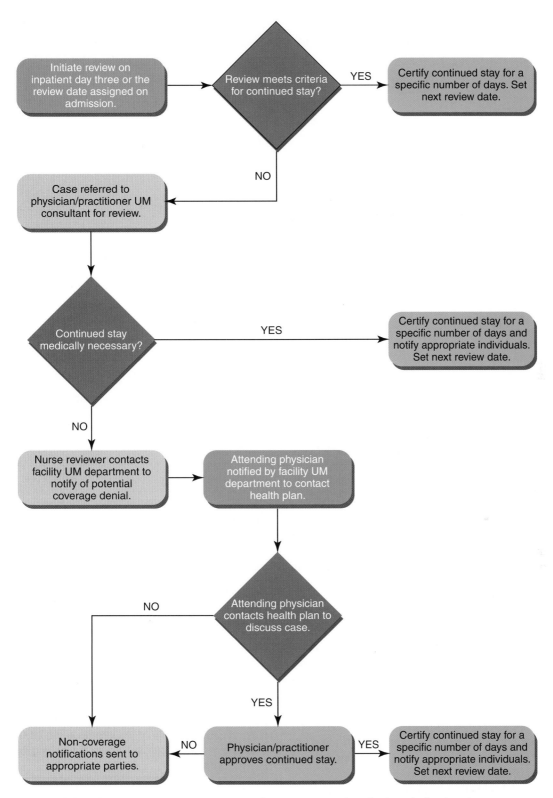

FIGURE 12-19 Health plan process of concurrent review for hospitalized patients.

36. What are some situations where concurrent UM review is appropriate?
37. What are some situations that would trigger a retrospective UM review?
38. How does case management benefit the HCO?

Plan and Program Structure

HCOs, health plans, and ACOs have a utilization management plan that describes the processes that support measurement, assessment, and improvement activities. The plan fixes authority and responsibility for the UM process, accountability and reporting mechanisms, the role of physician advisors,

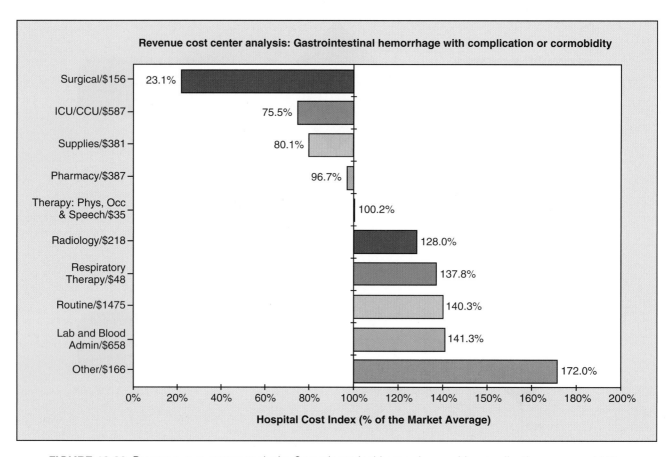

FIGURE 12-20 Revenue cost center analysis: Gastrointestinal hemorrhage with complication or cormobidity.

the review processes, and procedures for handling review decisions and payment denial appeals.

In a hospital, the UM activities are overseen by a distinct UM committee, or the task may be assigned to another medical staff committee. Although UM committee membership may vary according to whether it is a separate group or part of another, the committee is primarily composed of staff physicians representing all clinical departments. This includes representatives from surgery, family practice, internal medicine, psychiatry, pediatrics, obstetrics, and the other specialties. Nonphysician members of the committee may include the director of case management or utilization management, a senior leader from hospital administration or nursing, the performance improvement director, the director of HIM, and a representative from the finance department. The primary responsibility of the UM committee is to review utilization data and recommend changes in patient care practices and health care delivery processes.

Staffing of the UM function in an HCO will vary depending on the size of the facility. In many smaller HCOs the person responsible for UM wears a number of other hats. UM coordinators often have a clinical background. Many UM departments also employ data analysts to assist with concurrent and retrospective review activities.

Physician involvement in the UM process is critical. Health plans and ACOs have a designated medical director to oversee UM activities. Some HCOs have medical directors that oversee UM activities while others may appoint one or more volunteer physician advisors to serve as support to the UR process. Some hospitals have a rotating schedule assigning each physician a time in which he or she functions as physician advisor. Others employ full-time physician advisors. A growing trend is to use the title "medical advisor" rather than "physician advisor," although the responsibilities are essentially the same.

Students may find it helpful to compare and contrast performance improvement, risk management, and utilization management on several dimensions to distinguish elements unique to each. A brief comparison is provided in Table 12-6.

SELF-ASSESSMENT QUIZ

39. What is the role of physicians in the UM process?
40. What is the primary driver for having a robust UM program?

MEDICAL STAFF CREDENTIALING AND PRIVILEGING

Physicians and licensed independent practitioners (LIPs) should perform only those services for which they are qualified through education, training, and experience. The Joint Commission defines an LIP as "any individual permitted by law and by the organization to provide care, treatment, and

TABLE 12-6 Comparison of Performance Improvement, Risk Management, and Utilization Management

	Performance Improvement	Risk Management	Utilization Management
Purpose	Improve quality of care and services	Avoid or manage financial liability	Efficient and effective use of resources
Reference population	Cohorts of similar cases	Individual patients, employees, visitors, and professional staff	Individual patients
Process used	Criterion-referenced documentation review	Review causes of single events or occurrences and patterns of events	Individual patient needs/characteristics compared with criteria to determine need for health care services
Tools/techniques	Statistical analysis	Occurrence screening	Discharge planning case management
Primary question(s)	Can the outcome of care or service be improved?	Could the occurrence have been prevented? Can we minimize the loss?	Can the necessary treatment or service be provided elsewhere more cost-effectively or equally effectively by use of a less-invasive approach?
Actions	Revise policies, procedures, or processes	Revise processes; change environment; allocate financial resources	Approve or deny patient access to or payment for diagnostic services and clinical treatments
Key external driver	Accrediting and regulatory agencies, MCOs, and payers	Liability insurers	MCOs and payers

MCO, Managed care organization.

services, without direction or supervision." In other words, if the practitioner can deliver patient care directly without physician orders or supervision, then he or she is most likely an LIP.

Since the 1960s, the courts consistently have held HCOs accountable for ensuring the competence of physicians and LIPs (whether employed by the HCO or practicing independently). A major cause for the formalization of the process for ensuring physician and LIP competence throughout the health care industry was the *Darling v. Charleston Community Hospital* lawsuit in 1965, which established the principle of corporate negligence and liability for hospitals.[43] Corporate negligence is defined as the failure of the corporation to follow the established standards of conduct in providing accommodations and facilities necessary to carry out the purposes of the corporation. These standards of conduct have been held to include confirming the competence of the members of the medical staff. Over the years since the *Darling* case, courts have held that liability includes cases where the HCO *should* have known about substandard practices of a physician or LIP. In the current age of electronic information, failure to thoroughly investigate a practitioner's background and professional credentials is indefensible. The Medicare COP and TJC accreditation standards require HCOs to have a credentialing and privileging process. This involves three primary activities: credentialing, privilege delineation, and ongoing evaluation.

✓ SELF-ASSESSMENT QUIZ

41. True or False? HCOs are accountable for ensuring competence of both LIPs and physicians.
42. What case established the principle of corporate negligence and liability for hospitals?

Credential Verification

Credentialing is defined as the process of evaluating an individual's knowledge and experience against a standard to determine whether the individual is qualified to perform certain tasks. Credentialing can be done for individuals functioning in any number of professional roles. This section focuses exclusively on the HCO process of credentialing physicians and LIPs.

The credentialing process is an objective mechanism used by the HCO governing body to demonstrate accountability for professional staff practice behaviors and associated clinical outcomes. In the simplest sense, the credentialing process serves as a performance appraisal of medical staff members. Data are used to assess physician and LIP knowledge and skills, behaviors and attitudes, and quality of patient care practices.

The credentialing process starts when a physician or LIP applies for membership to the hospital's organized medical staff. The new applicant is required to complete a questionnaire that includes information about his or her education, professional credentials and licenses, work and health history, and other personal and professional background information. In addition, letters of reference from educators and colleagues familiar with the applicant's work are required. Exact documentation requirements and application procedures for appointment to the medical staff vary among HCOs, but requirements are documented and made known to all applicants. At a minimum, all organizations should require proof of the following:

- Education and training
- Liability insurance coverage
- Current licensure
- Clinical competence

- Satisfactory health status

In addition, the HCO queries the National Practitioner Data Bank (NPDB) to identify any available adverse quality-of-care determinations, civil judgments, criminal convictions, and actions taken by licensing agencies about the applicant.

> **? DID YOU KNOW**
>
> Providers can self-query the NPDB to see what information is maintained about them. There is a nominal fee per request.

Because verifying the validity of documents and statements attesting to professional credentials is a time- and resource-consuming process, many HCOs outsource the document verification process to an external agent. These entities, referred to as credentials verification organizations, make the contacts necessary to verify an applicant's education, training, experience, and professional licenses and certifications through primary source agencies.

Once core credentialing elements have been verified (which include licensure, education and training, current clinical competence, and the ability to perform the requested privileges), the physician members of the medical staff review the applicant's credentials. Depending on facility size, this review might be done by a credentials committee of the medical staff, by a subcommittee of the relevant medical staff department, or by the medical executive committee. Following are "red flags" that might cause the medical staff to request additional information from the applicant or recommend the applicant be denied medical staff membership.

- A high-mobility practitioner who has moved from state to state or from hospital to hospital every couple of years, who is licensed in several states, or who is a member of the medical staffs of several hospitals in several geographic locations.
- A practitioner with a high number of professional liability suits or who has had disciplinary actions taken by another hospital or licensing board.
- A practitioner whose application reveals an unexplained time gap (anything over 30 days) in training or professional practice.

- An incomplete application, especially when the incomplete sections relate to questions about licensure, hospital disciplinary actions, liability claims history, and health status.

Finally, the HCO governing board receives the medical staff recommendations regarding the new applicant and grants or denies membership. At least every 2 years, each physician and LIP undergoes credentialing (known as reappointment). The same documentation and review process is followed.

Privilege Delineation

Privilege delineation refers to the process of determining the procedures and services a physician or LIP is permitted to perform under the jurisdiction of the HCO. At the time of initial credentialing and reappointment, the applicant also formally requests privileges. Listed in Figure 12-21 are examples of privileges that a hospital pathologist might request. A pathologist with no specialty training would be limited to Category 1 privileges. A pathologist with more extensive training could request Category 1 privileges and one or more Category 2 privileges.

Any award of privileges must be supported with documentation of the practitioner's training, education, and other evidence of qualification or competence. For example, a physician requesting cytopathology privileges would need to submit evidence of training and experience in procedures such as retrieval of cytologic material (generally fine-needle aspiration biopsies). The medical staff reviews privilege requests to determine the applicant's ability to perform competently. Privilege recommendations for physicians and LIPs are presented to the HCO governing board, the group ultimately responsible for making final determinations regarding the privileges granted to practitioners.

Ongoing Evaluation

The HCO must evaluate the credentials and performance of physicians and LIPs when initially appointed to the medical staff and at the time of reappointment. In addition, the organization must conduct ongoing measurement of various

---

Category 1 Basic Privileges: Patient management, including diagnostic procedures and interventions encompassing the areas described below and similiar activities

Basic privileges in anatomic pathology includes examination and diagnostic analysis of routine and special stains and frozen sections of surgical specimens; cytology specimens; diagnostic electron microscopy; and autopsy pathology; diseases of the skin, nervous and hematoproliferative systems.

Category 2 Subspecialty Privileges
1. Forensic pathology
2. Hematology
3. Neuropathology
4. Dermatopathology
5. Cytopathology

FIGURE 12-21 List of available privileges for hospital pathologist.

aspects of performance. Performance data for each physician and LIP is collected through observation, record review, and monitoring of diagnostic and treatment techniques. Additional information may be obtained through discussion with other professional staff involved in care, consulting with physician assistants involved in surgery, and interviewing nursing and administrative staff. The goal of ongoing evaluation, sometimes called peer review or professional practice evaluation, is to assure the continued competence of physicians and LIPs. It is not sufficient to only evaluate performance during initial credentialing and once every two years during the reappointment process.[43]

Joint Commission standards specify some particular aspects of performance that must be routinely evaluated. These include medication usage, blood usage, and appropriateness of operative procedures (see TJC standards for specific requirements). Many hospitals monitor physician and LIP performance in patient care practices selected for measurement by CMS or TJC (see the earlier section in this chapter on national health care quality measurement priorities). In Figure 12-22 is a report used at one hospital to monitor physician compliance with SCIP measurements. The physician is identified by number, and his or her performance is reported for each quarterly time period.

Review of patients' records is another way the medical staff evaluates performance of physicians and LIPs. This is often called peer review because the individual whose practice is being reviewed is evaluated by individuals who have similar training, work in similar environments, and have similar proficiency in a clinical practice area or specialty. If the case being examined is about general medical care, then any unbiased physician may be able to function as a peer reviewer. However, if the issue requires specialist knowledge, the peer physician must be competent in that specialty and similarly licensed and trained.[44]

Patient records are also reviewed by peers to evaluate various aspects of the care provided to the patient. This may include evaluations of the following:
- Medical assessments and treatments
- Medication use

- Use of blood and blood components
- Appropriateness of operative and other procedures
- Appropriateness of care, including significant departures from generally accepted standards of practice

Peer review committees comprise physicians and LIPs who meet the qualifications established by the medical staff. Some hospitals establish one independent multidisciplinary peer review committee. Others choose to create multidisciplinary peer review subcommittees within medical staff departments. A third approach is to delegate peer review to the medical executive committee.

Performance expectations or targets are established by the medical staff. When physicians fail to comply with expectations, the medical staff is expected to take action. These actions often involve peer pressure to improve performance. However, the actions could be as serious as recommending a physician's privileges be taken away if performance does not improve. The range of improvement actions available to the medical staff and how these actions must be carried out is detailed in the medical staff bylaws and procedures. TJC standards require the organized medical staff in a hospital to have defined processes for credentialing, privileging, and ongoing professional practice evaluation.

At the time a physician or LIP is reappointed to the medical staff, a summary of his or her professional practice evaluation results from the previous 2 years is created and shared with the credentials committee. This summary, often called a physician profile, is used to evaluate the practitioner's continued competence for credentialing and privileging purposes. A sample reappointment profile for a radiologist is shown in Figure 12-23. Often HIM professionals are involved in identifying patient records for peer review purposes and gathering data for physician profiles.

ROLE OF MANAGERS IN QUALITY AND PATIENT SAFETY

Performance management and patient safety improvement cannot simply be delegated to staff. To create and sustain an environment that promotes continual improvement, it

FIGURE 12-22 Physician performance report: Surgical Care Improvement Project measures.

Physician #127	Calendar Quarter			
Measure	1st	2nd	3rd	4th
Prophylactic antibiotic received within 1 hour prior to surgical incision	56.0%	78.0%	72.6%	95.5%
Appropriate prophylactic antibiotic ordered	93.7%	95.0%	95.0%	90.7%
Prophylactic antibiotic discontinued within 24 hours after surgery end-time	33.6%	73.0%	73.0%	82.5%
Cardiac surgery patients with controlled 6 A.M. post-operative serum glucose	45.0%	66.0%	84.0%	100%
Surgery patients with appropriate hair removal	80.3%	76.0%	78.0%	73.0%
Colorectal surgery patients with immediate post-operative normothermia	100%	94.0%	90.3%	95.5%

Practitioner: Dr. Xavier Ray	Time Period:	
	Year one	Year two
Number of interpretation discrepancies	3	<15
Number of cases referred for peer review	22	n/a
Number of peer review concerns identified	0	<3
Complication rate	.05%	<2.0%
Percent of patients undergoing outpatient radiology procedure that have an unplanned admission to the hospital post-procedure	2.5%	<5.0%
Number of adverse events while patient is receiving moderate sedation	0	0
Number of sentinel events	0	0
Number of patient praises	2	n/a
Number of patient complaints	1	n/a
Number of reported incidents of use of an unapproved abbreviation	3	<10
Number of reported incidents of an illegible order	6	<10
Number of reported incidents of noncompliance with universal protocol	0	0
Number of reported incidents of noncompliance with policy regarding communication of critical test results	2	0
Average dictation turnaround	28 hours	<24 hours
Number of reported behavior-related incidents	0	n/a
Number of validated behavior concerns	0	0
Number of suspensions for delinquent patient records	2	0
Percent of department meetings attended	75%	>50%

FIGURE 12-23 Performance profile for a hospital radiologist.

is necessary for senior leaders and managers to set the tenor, provide support, and clear away barriers. Improving performance takes investments. People must receive training in problem solving, process improvement tools, and team building. Although training can be a substantial expenditure in terms of financial and human resources, it is one of the better investments that can be made.

Performance management and patient safety improvement also require patience and discipline. Experience demonstrates that positive changes do not come as quickly as one would like. There are some false starts. People may be threatened by process changes or increased employee involvement in decision-making. A temptation is to accept quick-fix process "tweaks" rather than commit resources to sustainable process redesign and system enhancements. It is no coincidence that W. Edwards Deming's first principle of total quality management is "Practice Constancy of Purpose."[45] Deming, one of the early leaders in performance improvement in manufacturing, had a profound impact on quality management in all industries through the application of statistical principles.

Financial and human resources are expended on improvement projects, and processes are undergoing almost constant redesign. Yet familiar problems seem to creep back into the system to disrupt the performance of key processes. Some suggestions for achieving lasting performance improvements include the following:

- Change things and behaviors. Often performance improvement efforts focus on standardizing or streamlining work steps, and unfortunately the human part of the process is overlooked. Modifying attitudes and behaviors is important. Otherwise people will lapse into the old way of doing things without giving the new process a chance to become a habit. Empowerment, delegating responsibility to permit employees to make decisions and institute needed changes in their work processes, requires the employees to be adequately trained and competent to make those decisions.
- Train people. Educating people in the use of the performance improvement skills they need to get the job done is critical. Everyone should know how to apply the organization's fundamental improvement model and, at a minimum, how to use basic improvement tools.

- Test redesigned processes. An important way to ensure that improvements are sustainable is to test possible process changes with a small subset of activities. Quantitative and qualitative data should be collected during the pilot phase for the purpose of learning what effect changes in a process will have on related processes and systems.
- Do not order change and ignore support. For health care services to get better every day requires knowledge, diligence, effort, focus, and resources. You can't give employees training about performance improvement, tell them which processes to improve, and then turn and walk away. Managers must take an active role in steering the improvement efforts of the department.
- Process management is a dynamic activity. Regulations and incentives that guide performance measurement, assessment, and improvement activities in health care organizations are constantly changing. HIM professionals must keep abreast of the latest changes to be ready to meet the current information needs of health care leaders.
- Focus on results and creating value. Performance measurements of health care activities need to focus on key results. The results are used to create value for the key stakeholders: patients and their families, employees, payers, and the community at large. By creating value for key stakeholders, the organization builds loyalty and contributes to public good.
- Manage information assets. The contemporary operating environment in health care organizations is challenging. To survive, everyone needs to be well informed. Health care organizations must continually measure and analyze performance. Many types of data and information are needed for performance management to support organizational decision-making and operational improvement. HIM professionals have an important role in providing physician leaders and the senior executive team with information on the organization's current performance and the direction it is heading.
- HIM involvement is crucial. Collection and analysis of performance data are expensive in terms of monetary and human resources. Inadequate planning can result in misdirected endeavors, causing wasted efforts or, worse yet, incorrect patient care decisions. The HIM professional's advice, support, and expertise are crucial to the success of health care performance management. Regardless of how often regulations change or accreditation standards are revised, there is always one certainty: valid, reliable, and timely information about organizational performance will always be needed by managers and caregivers.

✓ CHAPTER REVIEW

1. Which of the following IS NOT one of the aims of the national strategy for health care improvement established by the Secretary of the Department of Health and Human Services (HHS)?
   a. deliver patient-centered, reliable, accessible, and safe health care.
   b. support proven interventions to address the determinants of health.
   c. decrease regional variations in timely access to health care services.
   d. reduce the cost of quality health care services.

2. Which group sponsors the Healthcare Effectiveness Data and Information Set (HEDIS).
   a. National Committee on Quality Assurance
   b. The Joint Commission
   c. National Quality Forum
   d. American Hospital Association

3. An example of a hospital "never event," considered by the Centers for Medicare and Medicaid Services to be preventable is:
   a. extended hospital stay representing an outlier.
   b. discharge against medical advice.
   c. nosocomial pneumonia.
   d. vascular catheter–associated infection.

4. An example of an outcome measure that could be used in a nursing home to evaluate performance is:
   a. percent of residents with an up-to-date plan of care.
   b. number of fire safety inspections conducted each year.
   c. percent of residents that develop a urinary tract infection.
   d. average daily census in the Alzheimer Unit.

5. Which of the following is an example of a process measure that could be used in an outpatient surgery center to evaluate performance?
   a. percent of records with documentation of patient allergies
   b. number of patients with postoperative complications
   c. percent of patients that report their pain was well controlled
   d. average number of surgeries performed each week

6. Data for calculating which of these performance measures are extracted automatically from EHRs without the need for manual review of records?
   a. patient experience measures
   b. e-measures
   c. pay-for-performance measures
   d. structure measures

7. Which of the following is an activity of the hospital's organized medical staff that involves the evaluation of physician practices by other physicians with similar training and experience?
   a. case management

b. credentialing
c. peer review
d. due process

8. An example of an AHRQ patient safety indicator is:
   a. average patient wait time in the emergency department.
   b. percent of Medicare patients referred to hospice services.
   c. percent of patients that develop postoperative respiratory failure.
   d. average number of deficiencies found during health inspections.

9. The goal of this type of improvement project is to create a less wasteful, more efficient process that meets the needs of customers.
   a. lean
   b. six Sigma
   c. rapid cycle improvement
   d. root cause analysis

10. This improvement tool is used to illustrate the steps of a process.
    a. brainstorming
    b. cause and effect diagram
    c. decision matrix
    d. flowchart

REFERENCES

1. Kohn LT, Corrigan JM, Donaldson MS, editors: *To err is human: building a safer health system*, Washington, DC, 2000, National Academy Press.
2. James JT: A new, evidence-based estimate of patient harms associated with hospital care, *J Patient Saf* 9:122–128, 2013.
3. Committee on Quality of Health Care in America, Institute of Medicine: *Crossing the quality chasm: a new health system for the 21st century*, Washington, DC, 2001, National Academy Press.
4. Department of Health and Human Services, Centers for Medicare and Medicaid Services: 42 CFR Part 481 Medicare and Medicaid Programs: Hospice Conditions of Participation: quality Assessment and Performance Improvement (effective on December 2, 2008), Sec. 418.58. In *Conditions of participation: quality assessment and performance improvement*, Washington, DC, 2008, Department of Health and Human Services.
5. Accreditation programs: http://www.ncqa.org. Accessed September 2009.
6. National Institute of Standards and Technology: *2013-2014 Baldrige Health Care Criteria for Performance Excellence*, Washington, DC, 2012.
7. Spath PL: *Leading your healthcare organization to excellence: a guide to using the Baldrige criteria*, Chicago, IL, 2005, ACHE Management Series/Health Administration Press.
8. Centers for Medicare and Medicaid Services: Hospital-acquired conditions: http://www.cms.gov/Medicare/Medicare-Fee-for-Service-Payment/HospitalAcqCond/Hospital-Acquired_Conditions.html. Accessed September 2013.
9. Centers for Medicare and Medicaid Services: Hospital quality initiatives. HCAHPS: patients' perspectives of care survey: http://www.cms.gov/Medicare/Quality-Initiatives-Patient-Assessment-Instruments/HospitalQualityInits/HospitalHCAHPS.html. Accessed September 2013.
10. Spath PL, editor: *Provider report cards: a guide for promoting health care quality to the public*, Chicago, 1999, American Hospital Association Press.
11. National Quality Forum: Mission: http://www.qualityforum.org/About_NQF/Mission_and_Vision.aspx. Accessed September 2013.
12. Orme CN: Customer information and the quality improvement process: developing a customer information system, *Hosp Health Serv Adm* 37:197–212, 1992.
13. Donabedian A: *Explorations in quality assessment and monitoring, volume 1: the definitions of quality and approaches in assessment*, Chicago, IL, 1980, Health Administration Press, 1980.
14. Spath PL: *Introduction to healthcare quality management*, ed 2, Chicago, IL, 2013, ACHE Health Administration Press.
15. Manary M, Boulding W, Staelin R, et al: The patient experience and health outcomes, *N Engl J Med* 368:201–203, 2013.
16. Spath PL: Taming the measurement monster, *Front Health Serv Manag* 23:3–14, 2007.
17. Joint Commission, The. Surgical care improvement project. http://www.jointcommission.org/surgical_care_improvement_project. Accessed September 2013.
18. Agency for Health Care Policy and Research: *Using clinical practice guidelines to evaluate quality of care, vol. 1, Issues*, Washington, DC, 1995, U.S. Department of Health and Human Services, AHCPR Pub. No. 95-0045.
19. AHIMA Task Force on Healthcare Quality and Patient Safety: HIM functions in healthcare quality and patient safety, *JAHIMA* 82:42–45, 2011.
20. Norton Healthcare: Other indicators. http://www.nortonhealthcare.com/OtherIndicators. Accessed September 2013.
21. Best M, Newhauser D: Walter A Shewhart, 1924, and the Hawthorne factory, *Qual Saf Health Care* 15:142–143, 2006.
22. Best M, Newhauser D: W Edwards Deming: father of quality management, patient and composer, *Qual Saf Health Care* 14:137–145, 2005.
23. West B: Rapid cycle improvement: avoid the pitfalls, *Nurs Manage* 43:50–53, 2012.
24. Siegel B, et al: A quality improvement framework for equity in cardiovascular care: results of a national collaborative, *J Healthc Qual* 34:32–43, 2012.
25. Zidel T: *A lean guide to transforming healthcare*, Milwaukee, WI, 2006, American Society for Quality, Quality Press.
26. Provost LP, Murray SK: *The health care data guide: learning from data for improvement*, San Francisco, CA, 2011, Jossey-Bass.
27. Devers KJ, Pham HH, Liu G: What is driving hospitals' patient-safety efforts? *Health Aff* 23:103–115, 2004.
28. Snijders C, Kollen BJ, van Lingen R, Fetter WP, Molendijk H: Which aspects of safety culture predict incident reporting behavior in neonatal intensive care units? A multilevel analysis, *Crit Care Med* 37:61–67, 2009.
29. *AHRQ quality indicators—guide to patient safety indicators*, Rockville, MD, 2003, Agency for Healthcare Research and Quality: AHRQ publication No. 03-R203: http://www.qualityindicators.ahrq.gov.
30. Hurtado MP, Swift EK, Corrigan JM, editors: *Envisioning the national health care quality report*, Washington, DC, 2001, National Academy Press.
31. Agency for Healthcare Research and Quality: patient safety organizations: http://www.pso.ahrq.gov. Accessed September 2013.
32. Agency for Healthcare Research and Quality: Patient safety organization privacy protection center: https://www.psoppc.org/web/patientsafety. Accessed September 2013.
33. Aspden P, Corrigan JM, Wolcott J, et al., editors: *Patient safety: achieving a new standard for care*, Washington, DC, 2004, National Academy Press.
34. Croteau RJ, editor: *Root cause analysis in health care: tools and techniques*, Oakbrook Terrace, IL, 2010, Joint Commission on Accreditation of Healthcare Organizations.
35. Spath PL: Using failure mode and effects analysis to improve patient safety, *AORN J* 78:16–37, 2003.
36. Dlugacz YD: Medication safety improvement. In Spath P, editor: *Error reduction in health care: a systems approach to improving patient safety*, 2 ed, San Francisco, CA, 2011, Jossey-Bass.
37. Woolf SH, Kuzel AJ, Dovey SM, Phillips RL: A string of mistakes: the importance of cascade analysis in describing, counting, and preventing medical errors, *Ann Fam Med* 2:317–326, 2004.
38. Gaba DM: The future vision of simulation in health care, *Qual Saf Health Care* 13:12–110, 2004.

39. Pozgar GD: *Legal aspects of health care administration,* ed 11, New York, NY, 2011, Jones & Bartlett Learning.

40. Department of Health and Human Services, Centers for Medicare and Medicare Services: Part 482—Conditions of Participation for Hospitals, Sec. 482.30, Condition of participation: Utilization review, October 1, 2011.

41. Blumen H, Lenderman T: *How using care management guidelines can help accountable care organizations achieve success, 2011:* http://publications.milliman.com/publications/healthreform/pdfs/how-using-care-management.pdf. Accessed September 2013.

42. Department of Health and Human Services, Centers for Medicare and Medicare Services: Part 482—Conditions of Participation for Hospitals, Sec. 482.43, Conditions of participation: Discharge planning, October 1, 2011.

43. *Darling v. Charleston Community Hospital,* 33 Ill. 2d 325, 211 N.E.2d 253 (1965), cert. denied, 383 U.S. 946 (1966)

44. AllMed Healthcare Management: *How to apply the 2007 joint commission standards to hospital peer review: a practical guide, 2007.* http://allmedmd.com//landing-pages/ppc-downloads/copy_of_Allmed-JCAHO-Standards.pdf. Accessed September 2013.

45. Deming W: *Out of the crisis,* Cambridge, MA, 1986, Massachusetts Institute of Technology, Center for Advanced Engineering Study.

DATA ANALYTICS: REPORTING, INTERPRETATION, AND USE

Kay Clements • Shannon Houser

ⓔ Student Study Guide activities for this chapter are available on the Evolve Learning Resources site for this textbook. Please visit http://evolve.elsevier.com/Abdelhak.

CHAPTER CONTENTS

OBJECTIVES

After reading this chapter, the reader will be able to do the following:
✓ Define key words.
✓ Describe various registries and their purposes and/or uses.
✓ Distinguish between primary and secondary data.
✓ Describe how public and private agencies and organizations use health care data to assess costs, quality, and patient outcomes of health care services.

✓ Discuss why data collection methods have changed since the implementation of electronic health records.
✓ Discuss how health care data can be used for performance management, research purposes, administrative and clinical decision-making, and consumer education.
✓ Discuss the importance and methods of formulating a data dictionary for a health information system.
✓ Discuss the concept of data governance and the benefits to the health care organization.

KEY WORDS

Abstracting
Active case ascertainment
  surveillance systems
Applied research
Attribute
Basic research
Benchmarking
Big data
Business intelligence
Case
Case eligibility
Case finding
Clinical case definition

Clinical decision support
Comorbidity
Core measure
Data
Data analysis
Data analytics
Data dictionary
Data element
Data warehouse
Domain
Entities
Epidemiologic case definitions
External users

Field
Follow-up
Grading
Health care data users
Hospital cancer data system
Incidence
Internal users
Logical data model
Major birth defects
Metadata
Morphology
Outcome
Population-based cancer registries

Primary data
Public health
Public health informatics
Record
Reference date
Registry
Research
Secondary data
Stage
Surveillance system
Topography
Value/coding

ABBREVIATIONS

AAFP American Academy of Family Physicians
ACG Adjusted Clinical Group
ACIP Advisory Committee on Immunization Practices
ACS American College of Surgeons
ACSCOT American College of Surgeons Committee on Trauma
AHRQ Agency for Healthcare Research and Quality
AIS Abbreviated Injury Scale
AJCC American Joint Committee on Cancer
ANSI American National Standards Institute
APACHE Acute Physiology, Age, and Chronic Health Evaluation
APR-DRG All Patient Refined Diagnosis Related Groups
ASTM American Society for Testing and Materials
CCS Clinical Classification Software
CDC Centers for Disease Control and Prevention
CHCA Child Health Corporation of America
CHDA Certified Health Data Analyst
CMS Centers for Medicare and Medicaid Services
CoC Commission on Cancer
CPT Current Procedural Terminology
CTR Certified Tumor Registrar
DCE Distributed Computing Environment
DCG Diagnosis Cost Group

DHHS Department of Health and Human Services
EHR Electronic Health Record
EMS Emergency Medical System
FIGO International Federation of Gynecology and Obstetrics
HCUP Healthcare Cost and Utilization Project
HEDIS Health Plan Employer Data and Information Set
HIM Health Information Management
HISPP Healthcare Informatics Standards Planning Panel
HITSP Healthcare Information Technology Standards Panel
HL7 Health Level 7
HOI Health Outcomes Institute
ICCS International Classification of Clinical Services
ICD-10-CM *International Classification of Diseases*, Tenth Revision, Clinical Modification
ICD-9-CM *International Classification of Diseases*, Ninth Revision, Clinical Modification
ICD-O-3 *International Classification of Diseases for Oncology*, Third Edition
IDDM Insulin-Dependent Diabetes Mellitus
IWG Informatics Working Group
MACDP Metropolitan Atlanta Congenital Defects Program
MHCA Mental Health Council of America

NAACCR	North American Association of Central Cancer Registries
NCDB	National Cancer Data Base
NCI	National Cancer Institute
NCQA	National Committee for Quality Assurance
NCRA	National Cancer Registrars Association
NIDDM	Non-Insulin-Dependent Diabetes Mellitus
NIH	National Institute of Health
NOTA	National Organ Transplant Act
NTDB	National Trauma Data Bank
NVAC	National Vaccine Advisory Committee
OPTN	Organ Procurement and Transplantation Network
OSF	Open Systems Foundation
PEPPER	Program for Evaluating Payment Patterns Electronic Reports
ROADS	Registry Operations and Data Standards
SEER	Surveillance, Epidemiology, and End Results
SQL	Standard Structured Query Language
TJC	The Joint Commission
TNM	Tumor, Lymph Node, and Metastases
UHC	University HealthSystem Consortium
UNOS	United Network for Organ Sharing
WHO	World Health Organization
XML	Extensible Markup Language

Significant portions of Chapter 13 related to data dictionaries and decision support were adapted from chapters by Maida Herbst and Kathleen Aller in *Electronic Health Records: Changing the Vision.*

DATA

While data can refer to a collection of elements, it can also be defined simply as "factual information, especially information organized for analysis."[1] Data analysis is the process of evaluating data using analytic and logical reasoning to examine each component of the data. Data analytics refers to the field of data analysis and often involves studying past historical data to research potential trends for decision-making.

The term big data is used to distinguish data sets that are very large. In the McKinsey report, "Big Data: The Next Frontier for Innovation, Competition, and Productivity," "big data refers to datasets of a size that is beyond the ability of typical database software tools to capture, store, manage, and analyze; the speed at which the data is acquired and used; and the variety of different types of data that are available to collect and analyze."[2] As organizations accumulate large amounts of data, they strive to use it meaningfully and make decisions in real time. Business intelligence is the general term used for the identification, extraction, and analysis of data.[2] When business decisions are based on data, the integrity of the data is accessed. Data integrity is defined by one source as "the accuracy and consistency of stored data, indicated by an absence of any alteration in data between two updates of a data record."[3] According to the Data Management Association, the management of data incorporates governance over architecture, analysis, design, security and quality management as well as data management warehousing.[2] In Chapter 4, Health Data Concepts and Information Governance, integrity is also described as "the property of data that indicates the data are true to the source and have not been altered or destroyed in an unauthorized manner or by unauthorized users, the extent to which data are complete, accurate, consistent, and timely."

This chapter identifies the various sources of health care data, the internal and external users, the need to assess the quality and provide accurate data, and the reporting of health care data to a variety of agencies and organizations to assess costs, access, and quality of health care services provided. An example of big data being used in health care is studying a specific respiratory condition (asthma, flu, etc.) to predict where a disease outbreak will occur geographically or to identify the demographic characteristics for the patient population being affected.

Another example of using big data is trending readmission rates within 30 days for patients with specific diseases such as congestive heart failure. To reduce not only the morbidity for the patient but also the costs associated with the readmissions for the hospital, both administrative data and clinical data are utilized to identify protocols to educate and follow-up the patient population to reduce the chance that they will be readmitted.

For health care professionals some of the data from a data warehouse are pushed to managers' dashboards so they can track how services are provided, verify staff compliance with documentation standards, check client service volumes, and trend financial performance indicators.

SELF-ASSESSMENT QUIZ

1. Discuss "big data" and its impact on health care data by identifying the characteristics associated with big data.

HEALTH CARE DATA

Health care data are created from a patient's health-related event as depicted in Figure 13-1. This figure illustrates a patient receiving services in the health care environment in the form of prescribed medications, diagnostic testing, treatment, and/or medical care. From these encounters, health care data are recorded in the patient's health record, and pertinent information is abstracted and coded for reimbursement. The patient's health record is considered a source of primary data on health. Data generated from these individual health care encounters can be stored in databases, aggregated, and used by various health care individuals, organizations, and agencies for multiple purposes. These databases represent sources of secondary data on health.

Traditionally, a patient's health care data were documented in a paper-based medical record. Recently health care organizations have transitioned to electronic health records or are in the process of transitioning and maintain a hybrid medical record. However, simply because clinical information is now available in electronic formats does not necessarily imply that it is quality data. Having the data available in

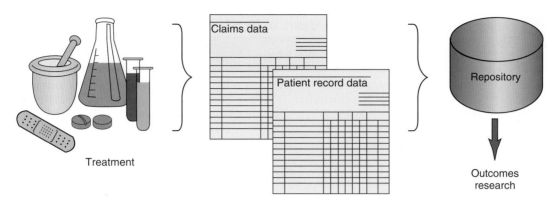

FIGURE 13-1 Outcomes research. (From Murphy GF, Hanken MA, Waters KA: *Electronic health records: changing the vision*, Philadelphia, 1999, Elsevier.)

electronic format is the first step in rendering data into legible, transferable, exchangeable elements that can be shared with internal and external users.

Health Care Data Users

Health care data users range from individual patients, health care providers, and organizations to epidemiologists, researchers, health care payers, grants funding organizations, politicians, and public agencies. Data users can be divided into two groups, internal users and external users. Individuals who are affiliated with the organization are referred to as internal users. Users from outside the organization are considered external users. Table 13-1 gives examples of the public and private organizations that collect and disseminate data for a variety of purposes.

HEALTH CARE DATA QUALITY, REPORTING, AND USES

Many electronic health records systems provide an enterprise-wide data warehouse built with individual data elements entered by providers as they care for their patients. However, before data are collected and reported internally or externally, the quality of data should be evaluated. The HIM professional is in a unique position to develop internal processes in the HIM Department to evaluate the quality of the data in the electronic health record. With input from care providers, the definition of a complete electronic record needs to be defined based on the documentation standards in place in the organization. Next, what constitutes an error(s) should be defined. Examples may include copying and pasting the same progress note for several days without adding new data elements, entering data for one patient into another patient's record, or associating a note in a wrong encounter for a patient. Electronic health record deficiencies and/or errors need to be defined in order for the quality of the data to be assessed. Deficiencies that were identified for the paper-based record are not applicable in many instances in the electronic health record (e.g., signatures along with a data/time stamp may be captured at the time of entry of the progress note). Repetitive types of errors should be identified with feedback

in the form of education provided to the individual care providers.

The uses vary as much as the users. The primary purpose of health care data is to document the care and treatment provided to the patient. Secondary uses include validation of medical services for reimbursement by health care payers, evaluation and planning related to health care services, surveillance and prevention of disability and disease, health policy analysis, measurement and tracking outcomes of treatment, and assisting individuals and communities in achieving better health.

Health care data are often used in the form of coded data that translate narrative prose into numeric or alphanumeric codes (numbers and letters). This information can be recoded or translated into other coding schemes beyond the original through a mapping process. Coded data are discussed in depth in Chapter 7.

Given the importance of these coded data, attention to the quality of coding process is paramount. The accuracy of coded data is based on how well the codes match the clinical information they represent. The quality of the coded data can be affected by several factors, including how it is generated, the training of the individuals who are assigning the codes, and the supporting documentation that is available for review. Coded data are compiled from individual health encounters into large databases. Within databases, it is possible to generate a variety of descriptive reports from the aggregate data, including the number of each type of diagnosis patients have during a given time period, the number and type of procedures, and provider statistics and demographics. These summary reports are indices of the types of diagnoses treated, procedures performed, and providers who treated the patients in a given setting during a given time period.

As previously mentioned, information contained in the actual patient record is considered primary data, whereas the information that is generated from the record is considered secondary data. Both primary and secondary data are stored in databases. This chapter highlights important uses of health data to include an overview of selected registries currently tracking patient information and defines public and private users of health data. The development of data dictionaries and standards is also discussed.

TABLE 13-1 Examples of Public and Private Users of Health Care Data

Organization	Available Data	Purpose(s)	Publicly Reported	Description of Organization	Web Site
University HealthSystem Consortium (UHC)	UHC's Key Indicator Report, Quality and Safety Management Report, Clinical Outcomes Report, Hospital Quality Measures Reports	Administrative Benchmaking Quality assessment	No	The UHC was formed in 1984 and is an alliance of 107 academic medical centers and 220 of their affiliated hospitals representing approximately 90% of the nation's nonprofit academic medical centers.	http://www.uhc.edu/12443.htm
Child Health Corporation of America (CHCA)	Various reports to member organizations using pediatric-specific data	Administrative Benchmaking Performance improvement Quality assessment	No	CHCA is a network of 43 leading children's hospitals in North America providing programs and services to improve performance: reducing hospital costs, increasing revenue, and improving the quality of care for children.	http://www.chca.com/company_profile/index.html
Health Grades	America's 50 Best Hospitals Report	Superior quality Clinical excellence	Yes	Health Grades is a leading independent health ratings company that uses a five-star rating system for hospitals, nursing homes, and physicians.	http://www.healthgrades.com
Centers for Medicare and Medicaid Services (CMS)	Reporting Hospital Quality Data for Annual Payment (RHQDAPU)	Quality assessment	Yes	RHQDAPU reports data on quality measures, the Surgical Care Improvement Project (SCIP), mortality measures, patient survey, Agency for Healthcare Research and Quality, and safety indicators.	http://www.cms.hhs.gov/apps/media/press/factsheet.asp?Counter=3225
CMS	Hospital-Acquired Infections and Present on Admission Indicator	Value-based purchasing	Yes	SCIP is a national quality improvement project designed to improve surgical care in hospitals.	http://www.cms.hhs.gov/apps/media/press/factsheet.asp?Counter=3043
CMS	Hospital Compare	Quality assessment	Yes	Hospital Compare was created through the efforts of the CMS, the Department of Health and Human Services, and other members of the Hospital Quality Alliance: Improving Care Through Information (HQA). Participating hospitals have agreed to submit quality information for Hospital Compare to make available for public reporting.	http://www.cms.gov/Medicare/Quality-Initiatives-Patient-Assessment-Instruments/HospitalQualityInits/HospitalCompare.html
Texas Medical Foundation (TMF) Health Quality Institute for CMS	Program for evaluating payment patterns electronic (PEPPER) Report	Benchmarking	Yes	An electronic report that provides hospital-specific data for Medicare severity diagnosis-related groups (MS-DRGs) and discharges at high risk for payment errors.	http://texasqio.tmf.org/ResourceCenter.aspx

TABLE 13-1 Examples of Public and Private Users of Health Care Data—cont'd

Organization	Available Data	Purpose(s)	Publicly Reported	Description of Organization	Web Site
The Joint Commission (TJC)	Strategic Surveillance System (S3TM)	Quality assessment	No	A tool that generates reports that allow accredited hospitals to assess and compare their performance with national and state benchmarks for the purpose of identifying areas needing improvement. Data from past survey findings, ORYX core measure data, data from the Office of Quality Monitoring, data from the organization's electronic application, and Medicare Provider Analysis and Review (MedPAR) data are used in compiling reports for facility use.	http://www.jointcommission.org/performance_measurement.aspx
The Leapfrog Group	The Leapfrog Hospital Survey	Quality services Cost-effectiveness	Yes	The Leapfrog Group is a voluntary program aimed at mobilizing employer purchasing power to alert America's health industry that big leaps in health care safety, quality, and customer value will be recognized and rewarded. The survey is the gold standard for comparing hospitals' performance on the national standards of safety, quality, and efficiency.	https://leapfroghospitalsurvey.org/
Agency for Healthcare Research and Quality (AHRQ)	Healthcare Cost and Utilization (H-CUP) Project State Inpatient Database Healthcare Cost and Utilization Project (H-CUP) State Emergency Department Database	Performance improvement Health care utilization, access, quality service Patient outcomes	Yes	The AHRQ is the lead federal agency charged with improving quality, safety, efficiency, and effectiveness by collecting data on published Patient Quality (PQI) and Patient Safety (PSI) Indicators.	http://www.ahrq.gov/professionals/systems/hospital/qitoolkit/index.html

Health care organizations generate so much health care data (administrative, clinical, and financial) that without tools for analysis and interpretation, the data in its raw form cannot be used in decision-making or performance improvement. The health information management (HIM) practitioner is responsible for monitoring and auditing HIM operations to ensure that accurate data are abstracted, coded, and entered by HIM personnel. In addition to the HIM department, other areas in the health care facility (quality, performance improvement, etc.) abstract and enter data into various databases for the organization to submit data to organizations externally for the purposes of analysis, interpretation, benchmarking, and reporting. Reports that are generated from such efforts can be categorized by organization and purpose.

See Table 13-1 for examples of the private and public organizations for which data analysis, interpretation, and reporting requirements need to be well known by HIM practitioners.

✓ SELF-ASSESSMENT QUIZ

2. Distinguish between primary data and secondary data and provide examples of each.

Benchmarking

Health care organizations benchmark or compare their organizations against peer organizations that are known for their excellence. In today's competitive environment with the focus on quality and patient safety and the required reporting of patient safety and quality indicators, benchmarking has become a common tool in health care organizations. Benchmarking is discussed in more detail in Chapter 12.

Clinical Decision Support

Clinical decision support is typically presented as a system that brings knowledge to caregivers to assist them in making decisions about patient care. The system may generate an alert for an abnormally high laboratory test result or for a patient taking two medications that may interact negatively. The caregiver is then given the opportunity to review the situation and determine the appropriate course of care. The system can also automatically provide time-based reminders (i.e., this patient is due to have a routine bone density screening). Clinical decision support systems may provide links to the caregiver to other resources. These resources may be clinical guidelines or reference materials that can be accessed online. The overall objective is to bring knowledge resources to the caregiver in real time during the delivery of care process. A clinical decision support system includes a controlled vocabulary, a central data repository with appropriately structured clinical data, a knowledge representation scheme, an inference engine, and output mechanisms such as the electronic health record (EHR).

Consumer Education

Through the efforts of the Centers for Medicare and Medicaid Services (CMS), the Department of Health and Human Resources, and members of the Hospital Quality Alliance (HQA), data on the quality of health care services have been made available to the public with the purpose of making the public a better informed consumer of health care services. This quality tool was developed for Medicare beneficiaries to locate information for specific medical conditions or undergoing specific procedures and is available publicly for use.[4] Please refer to Table 13-1, Examples of Public and Private Users of Healthcare Data and find Hospital Compare to review the purpose and description.

 DID YOU KNOW?

Definition of Core Measure
Standardized performance measures developed to improve patient safety and the quality of health care such as the ones published by The Joint Commission (TJC) and the Centers for Medicare and Medicaid Services.[4] In 2003, TJC and CMS cooperated in an effort to adopt the same measurements for reporting by hospitals.

Performance Management

The Joint Commission uses data from core measures to evaluate the quality improvement process addressing patient safety and quality of care. The data are transmitted to The Joint Commission from the accredited health care organizations. After transmission and evaluation, the quality data are provided to the public. It is also used to assess The Joint Commission accreditation and by health care organizations to internally analyze areas that can be improved.[5] Performance measurement is used by health care organizations to evaluate and support performance. It is also used externally, to show accountability to consumers, payers, and accreditation organizations. It provides statistically valid, data-driven information. This enables a health care organization to evaluate itself. This type of information is particularly beneficial to consumers, enabling them to make critical decisions about where to seek quality health care.

For example, a section of The Joint Commission Web site discusses the derivation and reporting of core measures. *The Specifications Manual for National Hospital Inpatient Quality Measures* provides information about how the care provided for patients with acute myocardial infarction, heart failure, pneumonia, pregnancy and related conditions, and surgical infection prevention are measured. Information about these areas are continuously monitored and reported to The Joint Commission. The statistics derived from these data is one area of focus that The Joint Commission uses to prepare for an accreditation visit. The CMS is also using core measures to monitor the quality of care for its Medicare beneficiaries.

The Joint Commission's Web site has a section called "Quality Checks" where anyone can locate the accreditation status of accredited organizations. Consumers can search for accredited organizations to find information about the services provided and the organization's performance on the basis of various measures, including the core measures.[6]

 SELF-ASSESSMENT QUIZ

3. Describe the purpose of core measurements and provide an historical overview of how The Joint Commission and Centers for Medicare and Medicaid Services aligned their core measurements.

Planning and Assessment

As discussed earlier in the chapter, information from the various disease registries can be used by organizations to assess services and quality of care as well as to assist in planning. For example, American College of Surgeons (ACS)–approved cancer programs publish an annual report that provides summary information about the treatment provided to cancer patients and how that care compares with the care in other ACS-approved programs throughout the country. The data from the annual analysis can also help determine future patient needs for expansion of facilities and services.

Similarly, hospital discharge data can be used for strategic planning and outcome analysis. For example, the Intermountain Heath Care System, a nonprofit integrated health system in Salt Lake City, uses statewide data to compare itself with other organizations. Further, the New Hampshire Hospital Association develops an annual market share report. This allows hospitals to evaluate their market position and to determine how to position themselves and reallocate resources in a way that is beneficial to both the institution and the patient population it serves.[7]

Regulatory Reporting

The health care industry is highly regulated, and health care organizations are required to report data to federal, state, and county agencies, as well as voluntarily reporting to accrediting bodies, such as The Joint Commission. As Chapter 12 mentions, the data reported by health care facilities are focused on access, quality, utilization management, patient outcomes, and cost of care. With the federal government's emphasis on educating the public and making people informed consumers of health care services, it is in the health care facility's best interest to report accurate data. Public reporting of data from public and private Web sites such as Hospital Compare[8] and Health Grades[9] allows consumers to identify facilities with lowest average length of stay, the lowest cost for performing specified services, and the mortality rate of medical and surgical services in the health care facility. Health care organizations also join consortia and share data for benchmarking within their peer groups. This information is not publicly available but is accessible to members only.

DID YOU KNOW?

Hospital Compare

Hospital Compare is a Centers for Medicare and Medicaid Services tool that offers information on quality of services. This tool is used to locate information on how well hospitals care for patients with certain medical conditions or surgical procedures and provides results from surveys of patients about the quality of care they received during a recent hospital stay.[8]

SELF-ASSESSMENT QUIZ

4. Discuss five ways in which health care data are used by the health care organization.

DID YOU KNOW?

Health Grades

Health grades is an independent rating system for public use health grades. This independent health care ratings organization uses a five-star system to rate physicians, hospitals, and nursing homes.[9]

SELF-ASSESSMENT QUIZ

5. Name three organizations that use health care data to assess the quality of care provided by health care providers/organizations.

REGISTRIES OVERVIEW

A **registry** is a systematic collection of data specific to a type of disease (e.g., cancer, acquired immune deficiency syndrome), exposure to hazardous substances or events (such as Agent Orange), or trauma and treatment (such as implanted medical devices). The data collected, methods of data collection, reports generated, and the uses vary with the kind of registry. Registries provide surveillance (collection, collation, analysis, and dissemination of data) mechanisms and, for some, **incidence** (occurrence) measures. A registry can be established for any disease; an overview of the characteristics of well-known registries will be provided in this chapter. Registries can also vary by location or type of agency. Some are specific to an organization such as a hospital.[10] Others are operated by a governmental agency and collect data for a geographic area such as a city, county, or state.

Case Definition and Eligibility

A **case** is defined as a person with a given disease or condition that will be included in the registry. Criteria for the disease or condition are established to determine who should be included. The decision to enter the person into the registry is based on the established set of criteria. Some definitions are defined as reportable conditions by the Centers for Disease Control and Prevention (CDC) as **epidemiologic case definitions**. These are diseases that must be reported to a public health agency. Epidemiologic analysis is then undertaken on the basis of the specific issues of interest regarding the disease being studied.

A **clinical case definition** may be established as well. A clinical definition is a list of signs and symptoms that establishes a clinical diagnosis. A clinical case may be reported as a reportable disease if it meets the epidemiologic case criteria. In addition to the clinical diagnoses, other criteria may need to be met for the condition to meet the epidemiologic definition. A patient may have the clinical signs and symptoms requiring treatment and yet may not meet the strict definition for reporting designated by the CDC.[11]

Case definitions are provided for all reportable diseases, and the case definitions for specific types of registries are discussed later in applicable sections of the chapter.

Case Finding

Case finding is the method through which all the eligible cases to be included in the registry are identified, accessioned into the registry, and abstracted. Case finding mechanisms should be redundant and include multiple methods to identify all the cases. This may result in the same patient being identified more than once; care should be taken to include a patient only once in the database. For example, receiving information from multiple data sources such as the pathology department or laboratory, the HIM department, the radiology department, the operating suite, and outpatient departments that may interact with the patients who are served by the registry will likely result in identifying several episodes of care for the patient. Electronic case finding has been implemented in registries where specific diagnostic/procedural codes identify potential patients that need to be included in the registry database.

Electronic Abstracting

With the rapid implementation of electronic health records, many data elements can be found in the patient's record. The data are collected primarily from the electronic health record since the elements are stored in a data warehouse. These data items are collected because of their relevance to the disease or condition addressed in the registry. Data items constitute the information included in the database for the registry. Software applications may be available that allow for transfer of specific data elements into the registry software. Depending on the type of registry, the follow-up information can be obtained electronically. Abstracting this information provides a succinct summary characterizing various issues, including demographic information about the patient, diagnostic information, treatment data, outcome of treatment, and follow-up information.

Follow-Up

An important function in the cancer registry is the annual follow-up conducted on patients after they are accessioned and entered into the database. Registries that perform follow-up require a tracking system to generate a list of patients on a monthly basis. Information is requested from various facilities regarding a patient's readmission, outpatient encounters, and clinic visits. The patient's primary physician may be contacted requesting the date of the patient's most recent office visit. Tracking the continued well-being of the patient and determining patient status at specified intervals is a major focus for Certified Tumor Registrars (CTRs). The American College of Surgeons (ACS) Commission on

Cancer (CoC) also requires a minimum of 90% of follow-up for the cancer registry to maintain approved status.

Registry Data Quality Integrity

Visual and computerized edits on data entered into the database should be performed by the registry staff responsible for data entry into the database of the registry. This may be required by the organization external to the registry or simply to ensure that the database has consistent, complete, accurate data. Accuracy and completeness of data are essential to ensure data integrity. The value of registry data is directly related to the validity of the data collected. Generally, to ensure data validity, a systematic quality control sampling of a minimum of 10% of the annual analytic caseload and a maximum of 300 cases annually in the registry should be reviewed for data quality.[12] The linkage of computerized information may allow cross-referencing of data to ensure that all cases have been included and that the data elements in the records match other records.

Confidentiality and Release of Registry Information

Registries contain patient-identifiable information that is derived from primary patient record information. All information in the registry must be kept confidential. Confidentiality policies and procedures are required in all phases of registry operations and should address protection of the privacy of individual patients, facility information, and the privacy of the physicians and health care providers who report the cases. They should also provide public assurance that the data will not be abused and that all confidentiality-protecting legislation or administrative rule(s) will be enforced. As a result of the Health Insurance Portability and Accountability Act of 1996, health care organizations are required to track patient registry information that is reported externally to state agencies to provide an accounting of disclosures to a patient, if requested.[13] Penalties can be imposed if disclosures are made without the proper authorizations.

CANCER REGISTRIES

Cancer registries collect, store, analyze, and manage cancer data.[14] Cancer registries are important to physicians, epidemiologists, and researchers concerned with assessing cancer incidence, treatment, and end results. There are three types of cancer registries: hospital registries, state registries, and special cancer registries.[14]

The National Cancer Act of 1971 mandated the collection, analysis, and dissemination of data for use in the prevention, diagnosis, and treatment of cancer. This mandate led to the establishment of the Surveillance, Epidemiology, and End Results (SEER) Program, a continuing project of the National Cancer Institute (NCI). The SEER Program operates population-based cancer registries in various geographic areas of the country covering about 28% of the U.S. population. The selection of demographic areas is based primarily on the areas' epidemiologically significant subgroups to provide a sampling of the U.S. population. Trends in cancer incidence, mortality rates, and patient survival in the United States are derived from this database.[15]

With the passage of the Cancer Registries Amendment Act (Public Law 102-515) in 1992, a national program of population-based cancer registries was created. Funding of $16.83 million was allocated by Congress for 1994 to set up statewide registries in states where none existed and to enhance existing registries. Today, there are more than 2000 hospital-based cancer registries, and all states have population-based registries. The categories of cancer registries are based on the type of facility or organization sponsoring the cancer registry.[12]

Some patient types, such as patients admitted to hospice care, may be ineligible for inclusion in the hospital-based cancer registry.

Hospital Cancer Registries

A hospital cancer registry is one of the components of a cancer program approved by the ACS Commission on Cancer (CoC). The latest edition of the Cancer Program Standards, available on the CoC's Web site, delineates the total program requirements. Hospitals that are accredited through the ACS CoC also follow the ACoS/CoC abstracting rules and standards. Cancer registries transmit abstract data to their state's cancer registry and, if the facility is AcoS/CoC-accredited, to the National Cancer Data Base (NCDB).[14]

> **? DID YOU KNOW?**
>
> The National Cancer Data Base (NCDB), established in 1989, is a joint program of hospital registries of the Commission on Cancer (CoC) and the American Cancer Society. Its purpose is to ensure quality cancer care by providing data to:
> - Evaluate patient management within hospitals and other treatment centers
> - Make comparisons of cancer care and outcomes between institutions
> - Set standards to help improve quality of cancer care[14]

View the latest edition of the Cancer Program Standards available from the ACS Commission on Cancer at www.facs.org.

The case eligibility for most cancer registries is defined as all the organization's patients diagnosed (clinically or histologically) or treated for active diseases on or after the reference date or at the beginning of the registry, and are eligible for inclusion. The registry's policy and procedure manual will define specifically the types of cases to be included.

Accessioning

The primary case finding sources are the pathology department, HIM department information, and outpatient services areas. As a key resource, cancer registry personnel examine the reports from the pathology department for all pathologic diagnoses of cancer and today many registries use electronic systems to screen for these cases. The types of reports that can be screened include surgical specimen, autopsy, bone marrow, hematology, and cytology reports. The second most common source is the organization's database of diagnosis codes.

Population-Based/State Cancer Registries

There are three types of population-based cancer registries: incidence only, cancer control, and research. Most incidence-only registries are operated by a government health agency and are designed to determine cancer rates and trends in a defined population. Monitoring cancer incidence is legislatively mandated in most states.[16]

Cancer Registry Abstracting

The cancer registry abstract contains information about each patient from the time of diagnosis and continuing throughout the patient's life. Cancer registrars must follow abstracting rules set by their individual state central registries. Registrars accredited through the American College of Surgeons Commission on Cancer must also follow their abstracting rules and standards. Cancer registries submit data to their state's cancer registry and, if they have an ACoS/CoC-accredited registry, to the National Cancer Data Base.

You may search the Internet and find additional information at:
- The North American Association of Central Cancer Registries Data (NAACCR) Standards and Data Dictionary for Abstracting: www.naaccr.org/StandardsandRegistry Operations/VolumeII.aspx
- The National Program of Cancer Registries (NPCR) Standards for Abstracting: www.cdc.gov/cancer/npcr/ standards.htm

Cancer Registry Coding

Cancer registries use different coding applications from the Health Information Management Department. The case definition for cancer registries consists of neoplasms that are to be reported to the registry. The best classification system for developing a reportable list for a cancer registry is based on the *International Classification of Diseases for Oncology*, Third Edition (ICD-O-3)[15] and is used to code the histology, behavior, and grade of the patient's tumor. The American Joint Committee on Cancer (AJCC) Staging Manual is used to derive a correct staging of the tumor, nodes, and distant metastasis. The Collaborative Staging Manual is used to derive a stage after completing multiple questions about how the tumor has spread and how the information was collected.[14]

Cancer Registry Staging

The extent of the spread of cancer, or stage, at the time of initial diagnosis and treatment is recorded for every case included in the registry.[17] Historically, the staging system most commonly used was developed in 1977 by the SEER Program of the NCI, *Self Instructional Manual for Tumor Registrars,* Book 6, or the Summary Staging Guide. This system is used to stage cases as in situ, localized, regional spread to lymph nodes or adjacent tissue, or distant spread to lymph nodes in other areas of the body or distant sites. Although the TNM system was designed for use by physicians, in some hospitals, staging is performed by the registry staff.[18,19] A working knowledge of both the SEER and the AJCC staging systems is necessary.

Collaborative Staging (CS) is a group of data items set up by a joint task force including representatives from the American Joint Committee on Cancer (AJCC), CoC, NAACCR, NCRA, NPCR, and SEER, designed to provide a single uniform set of codes and rules for collecting extent of disease and stage information to meet the needs of all of the participating organizations. The CS schema incorporates all of the fields from SEER 10-digit EOD, in a modified form, and adds several additional fields. When CS data items are coded, a computer algorithm allows generation of AJCC 7th Edition Tumor, Nodes, and Metastasis (TNM) stage, SEER Summary Stage 1988, and SEER Summary Stage 2000.[20] CS was implemented in the year 2003. However, an announcement was made on August 23, 2013, by the American Joint Committee on Cancer (AJCC), the Centers for Disease Control and Prevention (CDC), the Commission on Cancer (CoC), and the National Cancer Institute (NCI) that it is not feasible to continue support of Collaborative Staging beyond diagnosis year 2015. Beginning with cases diagnosed in 2016 support of Collaborative Stage will cease and CDC, CoC, and NCI will transition to the direct coding of the AJCC TMN staging.[21]

Quality Management of the Cancer Program and Registry Data

To be effective, the quality management program must be multidisciplinary and must include four components: quality planning, measurement, evaluation, and improvement. The cancer committee is responsible for establishing the quality improvement priorities of the cancer program and for monitoring the effectiveness of quality improvement activities.[10] The usefulness of the data collected by a registry depends on the quality of the data. Quality control procedures are important to ensure the completeness, accuracy, and timeliness of the data collected.

The Cancer Registrar Profession

Certified Tumor Registrars enjoy career opportunities in many settings, from hospitals and state registries to national cancer programs, and even consulting firms.[22] The Council on Certification of the NCRA approved the definition of the cancer registry field.

The NCRA is a nonprofit, professional organization representing the cancer registrars. It promotes education, credentialing, and advocacy for cancer registry professionals.

The Council on Certification of the NCRA certifies the professionals who meet the eligibility requirements and are successful on the national examination as Certified Tumor Registrars (CTR). To learn more about the NCRA, go to: www.lncra-usa.org/i4a/pages/index.cfm?pageid=3299.

BIRTH DEFECTS REGISTRIES

Birth defects are the leading cause of infant mortality in the United States. According to the CDC, a baby is born with a birth defect every 4.5 minutes.[23,24] In addition, birth defects are the leading cause of years of potential life lost and contribute to childhood morbidity and long-term disability. Major birth defects account for more than 1 of every 5 infant deaths.[25] Population-based birth registries have operated since the 1920s, with the earliest being in the state of New Jersey. In the early years, birth registries strictly used vital records to identify malformations. The Birth Defects Prevention Act of 1998 requires that data are collected and analyzed, epidemiologic research is undertaken, and information and education efforts with the aim of preventing birth defects are facilitated. In 2002, there were 35 operational programs and 10 planning programs that were collecting data on birth defects.

A variety of data collection methods are used, including printed abstracts or reports that are completed by the program's staff or reports completed by the health care facility's staff. Today, information can be obtained using electronic devices such as laptops, Web-based data entry, or electronically submitted reports.[26]

Birth defects surveillance systems are characterized as either active or passive case reporting systems (see Table 13-2).

Active case ascertainment surveillance systems identify cases in all hospitals, clinics, or other medical facilities through systematic review of patient records, surgery records, disease indexes, pathology reports, vital records, and hospital logs (obstetric, newborn nursery, neonatal intensive care unit, postmortem) or by interviewing health professionals who may be knowledgeable about diagnosed cases.

Passive case ascertainment surveillance systems rely on reports submitted to the registry by hospitals, clinics, or other facilities, supplemented with data from vital statistics. In some states, staff members submit reports voluntarily, but, in general, reporting requirements are established by state legislation. One example of a passive surveillance system is the national Birth Defects Monitoring Program. Newborn hospital discharge summaries are obtained from electronic health information systems, and investigators have no opportunity to review the rest of the patient record.

Many state and regional birth defect registries are modeled after the Metropolitan Atlanta Congenital Defects Program (MACDP), which is the first active case ascertainment system in the United States. The MACDP criteria include cases in which the infant has a serious or major structural defect that can adversely affect health and development and cases of live-born infants and stillbirths, 20 weeks of gestation or more, weighing 500 grams or more. Pregnancies with birth defects prenatally diagnosed and terminated

TABLE 13-2 Legislation Mandating Registries		
Name of Legislation	Purpose	Reference Source
Birth Defects Prevention Act of 1998[25,27]	(1) Collect, analyze, and make available data on birth defects in a manner that facilitates compliance with this act, including data on the causes of such defects and on the incidence and prevalence of such defects; (2) operate regional centers for the conduct of applied epidemiologic research on the prevention of such defects; and (3) provide information and education to the public on the prevention of such defects.	http://www.cchconline.org/privacy/bdact.php3#sum
Safe Medical Devices Act of 1990[28,29]	Medical device reporting is one of the U.S. Food and Drug Administration's (FDA's) means of obtaining information on medical device problems. (1) Congress passed the Safe Medical Devices Act of 1990 (SMDA) to strengthen the Medical Device Amendment of 1976 and to broaden the reporting criteria for device-related adverse events (60 Fed Reg 63579 [1995]). In December 1995, the FDA issued its final rule on medical device reporting, which clarified and expanded existing reporting requirements for medical device manufacturers and health care facilities. (2) These new FDA regulations went into effect July 31, 1996, and provide guidance to people required to report incidents under the SMDA.	http://thomas.loc.gov/cgi-bin/bdquery/z?d101:H.R.3095:
National Organ Transplant Act (NOTA) 1984[30]	The National Organ Transplant Act (1984 Public Law 98-507), approved October 19, 1984, and amended in 1988 and 1990, provided for the establishment of the Task Force on Organ Transplantation; authorized the secretary of Health and Human Services to make grants for the planning, establishment, and initial operation of qualified Organ Procurement Organizations (OPOs); and established the formation of the Organ Procurement and Transplantation Network (OPTN) and Scientific Registry of Transplant Recipients (SRTR).	http://history.nih.gov/research/downloads/PL98-507.pdf

before 20 weeks of gestation are ascertained whenever possible, but because of incomplete ascertainment, the records are kept as separate data.[27]

Birth Defects Case Definition and Coding

In all birth defects registries the goal is to capture data about specific types of congenital anomalies and conditions. However, the goals vary by the type of case surveillance system (active vs. passive) used. These anomalies are identified and coded with *International Classification of Diseases, Ninth Revision, Clinical Modification* (ICD-9-CM) codes that fall within the range 740.0 to 759.9. However, in October of 2015 the coding classification system may move to ICD-10-CM.

In approximately 70% of cases, birth defects occur as isolated defects.[23] Attempts are being made to classify infants with multiple birth defects according to biologically meaningful categories to assist in identifying etiologic and pathogenetic mechanisms. Birth defects can also be classified as major or minor; major birth defects are those that affect survival, require substantial medical care, or result in marked physiologic or psychological impairment.

The CDC has defined a set of core data items to be included in a birth defects registry. Some of the items include syndrome identification, demographic data, pregnancy history, birth-related data, cytogenetic and laboratory data, family history, and etiologic information.

Quality Control of Birth Defects Registry Data

To evaluate the completeness and accuracy of data collection, reabstracting procedures similar to those used by cancer registries are often followed. The linkage of computerized discharge summary indexes with prenatal records is another quality control procedure that is used. The abstracts are reviewed by clinical geneticists, who evaluate them for accuracy and completeness of the diagnosis as well as for defect coding.[31]

Use of Birth Defects Registry Data

The analysis of birth defects surveillance data allows health care planners and epidemiologists to monitor the birth defect rates in different areas as well as changes in the rates. The data are monitored by statistically evaluating the difference between observed and expected numbers of specific defects or defect combinations for a specified time in a defined area. Comparisons may lead to the identification of clusters of birth defects. Investigation of such clusters may yield useful etiologic information. The goal of many birth defect registries is to provide health care providers and policy makers with information necessary to plan, develop, and implement strategies for the treatment and prevention of serious congenital malformations.[27]

Because individual birth defects are rare, researchers have difficulty obtaining enough cases for etiologic studies. Data for population-based state systems are an important source of information to improve knowledge and understanding of birth defects and to further prevention and intervention. The CDC funds some state and regional birth defects registries.

Other examples of the uses of registry data are illustrated by reports provided by the Illinois Department of Public Health at their Web site. Issued by the Illinois Department of Public Health's Adverse Pregnancy Outcomes Reporting System, the reports include information on the prevalence of birth defects in Illinois. For example, the prevalence of birth defects among Illinois and Chicago neonates from 1999 to 2001 is presented with graphs reporting quarterly data since 1989. Some of the other reports address neural tube defects, birth defects resulting from maternal diabetes, and prenatal exposure to controlled substances.[32]

DEATH REGISTRIES

Mortality statistics are considered part of the vital statistics kept by the National Center for Health Statistics. These statistics are used to develop reports that are available to the public and to researchers. Examples of reports are tables of life expectancy, fetal death rates, and causes of death.

Electronic filing of death certificates with the state departments of health is now possible with the use of information technology. The Electronic Death Registration System (EDRS) allows for multiple users to contribute information needed to complete the death certificate, such as the funeral home director, the family, and the health care provider at the time of death. These electronic systems are accessed using the Internet and allow for individual users to enter data in real time with edits to assist in obtaining the correct elements.

Early efforts for the development of the EDRS by the Social Security Administration date back to the late 1990s. At that time, EDRS Standards & Guidelines were developed. In the early 2000s funding became available through SSA and NCHS, and a national model was developed in 2002. Although there are still challenges in implementation, there are many benefits to be derived from electronic filing of death certificates such as improved timeliness, higher-quality mortality data, increased security, and mortality data that is readily available for surveillance of medical conditions and outbreaks of diseases.[33]

The causes of death from the death certificate are translated into medical codes through use of the classification contained in the applicable revision of the ICD, published by the WHO. These coding rules make statistics useful by giving preference to certain categories by consolidating conditions and by systematically selecting a single cause of death from a reported sequence of conditions. The single tabulation requires that the underlying cause of death be reported.[34]

DIABETES REGISTRIES

The detection and management of diabetes can result in significant improvement in health outcomes and reduce morbidity and mortality. Diabetes was identified as the seventh most common cause of death in the United States in 2011.[35] Diabetes registries' surveillance data are used to identify high-risk groups, target intervention programs, evaluate disease prevention and control activities, and establish an infrastructure for community-sponsored disease prevention programs.[36] Population-based registries provide an excellent foundation for family studies of autoimmune disease.[36] Monitoring diabetes at a regional, state, or national level is crucial to identifying where diabetes is the greatest problem so that resources can be allocated for primary and secondary prevention. Moreover, registries are useful for evaluating the effectiveness of prevention programs.

The types of diabetes that are monitored include the following:
- Insulin-dependent diabetes mellitus (IDDM), or Type 1
- Non-insulin-dependent diabetes mellitus (NIDDM), or Type 2
- Gestational diabetes
- Maternal diabetes

The rates of complications and the methods by which they develop are important aspects of diabetes. Complications of diabetes include severe eye disease (e.g., blindness), amputations of the lower extremities, and end-stage renal disease. Diabetes also places the patient at an increased risk for cardiovascular disease. Type 1 diabetes is an autoimmune disease that represents about 5% of diabetes cases; 90 to 95% of diabetes cases are Type 2. Other factors associated with Type 2 diabetes include older age, obesity, physical inactivity, and a family or gestational history of Type 2 diabetes.[37]

Diabetes Registry Case Finding

Because the treatment and follow-up of this patient population involves tracking of specific data elements, a registry is an excellent tool to use for disease management. Case finding has been a manual process in the past, but now with the implementation of electronic health records, patients can be identified electronically.[38] For example, a large registry operated by the Kaiser Foundation in Northern California identifies new cases by using a passive surveillance system. The sources of information include pharmacies (prescriptions for diabetic medications), laboratories (HbA1c = 7.0%), and outpatient, emergency department, and hospitalization records listing a diagnosis of diabetes.[39]

Medical and demographic data are obtained by reviewing hospital patient records and data reporting forms submitted by physicians and pharmacies or by populating the registry from other databases. For example, a registry maintained by a health care insurer can populate a registry with information from all relevant encounters. Data variables include patient demographics, diagnoses, reasons for admission, treatments, medications, diabetic education, attending physicians, complications, and lengths of stay.

No uniform software system is used by all diabetes registries. Software is usually designed by and for the registry and is tailored to meet its needs. The Indian Health Service, an agency of the U.S. Public Health Service, encourages each of its clinics and hospitals to maintain a diabetes registry. (American Indians and Inuits have one of the highest known prevalence rates of Type 2 diabetes.) Although the registries may be maintained in manual or electronic format, integration of the diabetes registry with the hospital clinical information system is recommended.[28]

Diabetes registries can be utilized in academic health centers to identify and follow patients, by third-party payers to monitor quality of care and patient outcomes, and by the Veterans Affairs Health System, which uses the data to trend outcomes and affect the quality of care provided to their patients.[38]

IMPLANT REGISTRIES

In 1986 the General Accounting Office completed a study that indicated that problems with medical devices were underreported, even though the FDA had required the reporting of deaths related to medical devices since 1984. Congress passed the Safe Medical Devices Act (SMDA) in 1990 to increase the reporting of significant problems with medical devices from hospitals, physicians, and manufacturers. The main objectives of the reporting requirements are to track patients so that their whereabouts are known and to facilitate timely, accurate communication among manufacturers, health care providers, and patients.[29,40]

Millions of patients have medical devices implanted in or on their bodies. These devices include pacemakers, heart valves, artificial joints, ocular lenses, defibrillators, breast implants, insulin pumps, and other devices. Although these medical devices have improved the quality of life for many people and have saved the lives of countless others, numerous safety alerts and voluntary manufacturer recalls have been issued for them. These safety alerts and recalls have raised procedural questions with life-threatening implications: Who is responsible for notifying the patients? Through the International Implant Registry, physicians are notified when important safety information needs to be communicated. If the physician cannot be contacted, patients are notified directly and told to contact their physicians or the manufacturers of their devices.

The SMDA of 1990 requires manufacturers to register and track certain implantable medical devices and to notify recipients regarding important safety information. It also requires hospitals, ambulatory surgical facilities, nursing facilities, and outpatient diagnostic or treatment facilities other than physicians' offices to file reports with the Food and Drug Administration or device manufacturers when there is a probability that a device caused or contributed to a death, serious illness, or serious injury.[29,40] Hospitals may choose to keep internal implant registries to identify patients and answer manufacturer recall or other research questions. Maintaining this information in a retrievable mode facilitates current and future requests for data on these patients.

IMMUNIZATION REGISTRIES

Immunization registries collect vaccination information about children within a geographic area. Registries provide a central location to collect vaccination records of children from multiple providers and to generate reminders and recall vaccination notices. They also can provide official vaccination forms and vaccination coverage assessments.

Immunization registries are a useful tool in achieving one of the national health objectives for *Healthy People 2020* discussed in Chapter 1. This objective sets the goal to increase immunization rates and reduce preventable infectious diseases. A "fully operational" registry is defined as one that includes 95% enrollment of all area children younger than 6 years of age with two or more immunization encounters administered within the geographic area. This definition is described in a 2002 report from the Advisory Committee on Immunization Practices (ACIP) and the American Academy of Family Physicians (AAFP) that provides recommendations regarding the provision of immunizations.[41]

Children are entered into the registry through a variety of mechanisms including linkage with electronic birth records and by a health care provider at the time of a child's first immunization. Immunization registries also can be used to enhance adult immunization services and coverage.

Immunization Registry Case Finding and Data Use

The registry stores data electronically on the basis of all National Vaccine Advisory Committee (NVAC)–approved core data elements. These data elements are used to establish a registry record within 6 weeks of birth for each child born in the geographic area. This enables access to and retrieval of immunization information in the registry at the time of the patient encounter. The registry should receive and process immunization information within 1 month of vaccine administration and must have safeguards and policies to protect the confidentiality and security of medical information. The software must exchange immunization records according to Health Level 7 (HL7) standards and automatically determine the routine childhood immunization(s) needed, in compliance with current recommendations of the ACIP, when an individual is seen for a scheduled immunization. The registry also should automatically identify individuals who are due or late for immunization(s). This requires enabling the production of reminder/recall notifications. By virtue of the registry data, immunization coverage reports can be automatically produced according to providers, age groups, and geographic areas. The registry is also required to be able to produce official immunization records as needed. The CDC National Immunization Program provides useful information about national and statewide registry systems.[41]

Healthy People 2020 has developed new objectives that include states, local public health departments, and nongovernmental agencies working together by calling attention to specific vaccine-preventable diseases in the United States that result in morbidity and mortality. Vaccine administration is appropriate at various stages in a person's lifetime. Some immunizations are recommended based on a previous medical condition, because of travel to a foreign country, or simply because an individual has reached an age when contracting a medical condition such as pneumonia or a type of flu could be life-threatening. Examples of vaccines for the older population include pneumonia, flu, and shingles vaccines.[42]

ORGAN TRANSPLANT REGISTRIES

The first successful organ transplantation operations were performed in 1954. Thanks to medical advances, today's technology makes transplantation a recognized and accepted mode of treatment for patients with organ failure. The success of transplantation and the scarcity of organs have raised many ethical, legal, and economic issues.[30]

The National Organ Transplant Act (NOTA, Public Law 98-507) was passed by Congress in 1984. The NOTA called for a national task force on organ transplantation that was charged with conducting an in-depth study of transplantation and making recommendations about medical, ethical, legal, economic, and social issues pertaining to human transplantation. In 1986, the task force recommended the establishment and operation of a national scientific registry. In October 1986, the United Network for Organ Sharing (UNOS) was established. It is a nonprofit, scientific, educational organization that administers the nation's only Organ Procurement and Transplantation Network (OPTN). Through the OPTN, UNOS does the following:

- Collects and manages data about every transplant event occurring in the United States
- Facilitates the organ matching and placement process with use of UNOS-developed data technology and the UNOS Organ Center
- Brings together medical professionals, transplant recipients, and donor families to develop organ transplantation policy[43]

UNOS members include transplant centers, independent procurement organizations, tissue-typing laboratories, consortia, public members, and voluntary health and professional associations.

Transplant Case Registration and Data Use

All UNOS member institutions and organizations involved in organ procurement, tissue typing, and organ transplantation are required to submit comprehensive data concerning transplant activities. To place a patient on the waiting list, the transplant center submits information that contains such patient information as address, race, ethnicity, education level, cause of organ failure, number of previous transplants, and whether the patient's name appears on any other lists.

The registry collects data through the whole transplant process from before transplant until graft failure or death. Transplant centers and organ procurement organizations enter data into the OPTN database through the Internet by using the secure Web-based application UNet.

The online database system UNet is used for the collection, storage, analysis, and publication of all data pertaining to the patient waiting list, organ matching, and transplants. Launched on October 25, 1999, this system contains data regarding every organ donation and transplant event occurring in the United States since 1986. UNet enables the nation's organ transplant institutions to register patients for transplants, match donated organs to waiting patients, and manage the time-sensitive, life-critical data of all patients before and after their transplants.

Data regarding transplants can be used by the government, the scientific community, and the public. Uses include the development of health care policy regarding reimbursement, performance standards, and public health research, and patients and their families can also assess their treatment options. Data from the UNOS database are currently used to monitor the efficacy of the organ allocation process. Data recorded on the potential recipient form are especially useful for this purpose. These data, combined with waiting list information, can be used to determine retrospectively the patient with highest priority to receive each organ.[44]

The quality assurance department at UNOS provides training for data coordinators and related personnel on data collection and offers assistance to members when they have questions or concerns about reporting requirements.

TRAUMA REGISTRIES

The CDC identified traumatic injury caused by accidental or unintentional injuries as the fifth leading cause of death for 2011. Intentional injury was listed as the tenth leading cause of death.[35] Trauma typically involves young adults and results in the loss of a great number of productive work years. Traumatic injury kills more people between ages 1 and 34 years than all other causes combined. The loss of productivity and the spending for health care costs the general public billions of dollars a year.[45]

Regional or statewide trauma systems of emergency trauma centers and emergency medical systems (EMS) have been shown to reduce mortality and morbidity rates and the loss of productivity from traumatic injuries. The evidence to support this claim has been based on data from hospital-based trauma registries. The data in these independent registries vary in their content and structure, thus impeding comparisons.[45]

In response to this concern the ACS Committee on Trauma (ACSCOT), with funding from the federal government, developed the National Trauma Data Bank (NTDB) and the associated data dictionary. The data dictionary spells out inclusion criteria and uniform registry variables to be used in all trauma registries. Annually, local, regional, or state registries are encouraged to report a subset of these variables to become the National Trauma Registry.[45]

Trauma registries gather data about patients who are injured. These registries can be hospital based or population based. The registry contains demographic information, data collected by EMS personnel before hospitalization, and medical information based on the patient hospital record. The medical information will be used to determine injury severity measurement. Injury measurements can be based on ICD codes (ICDMAP) or anatomic descriptors of tissue damage caused by the injury (Abbreviated Injury Scale [AIS]). The injury severity measurement is also included in the trauma registry.[46,47]

Trauma Registry Case Finding and Data Use

Case finding is performed by reviewing emergency department logs, admitting department face sheets, patient records, and the disease indices—injury codes 800 to 959.9 and E codes listed in the ICD-9-CM. After appropriate cases are identified, information is abstracted from the record. Data elements that are important in trauma registry include patient-specific and demographic information, place of accident, cause of injury (E code), site of injury, condition of patient at the scene of the accident, transport modality, prehospital interventions, vital signs on admission, consciousness status, blood transfusions, procedures and treatment, total days in the intensive care unit, complications, discharge recommendations, and other information.[48]

Both the AIS scores and the Injury Severity Scale scores are routinely documented. The Glasgow Coma Scale is required by the ACS Trauma Registry on admission to the emergency department.[49]

TRAUMATIC BRAIN INJURY REGISTRY

Traumatic brain injury (TBI) registries collect data about patients who have experienced a traumatic central nervous system injury to the brain or the spinal cord. The injury is termed a TBI or traumatic spinal cord injury (SCI). The TBI Registry can be a stand-alone registry or included in the Trauma Registry.

Traumatic Brain Injury Case Finding and Data Use Case Definition and Coding

Case definition is based on codes that identify all traumatic brain injuries and spinal cord injuries using the ICD-9-CM. States may further define the population that is included (e.g., whether to include only residents of the state versus all patients incurring injuries).

Traumatic Brain Injury Registry Abstracting

Legislation at the state level has mandated the reporting of TBI by hospitals in 17 states. The collection of data on brain injuries began as early as 1984.[50] Basic demographic information is abstracted in addition to the reporting of ICD-9 or ICD-10 codes. A state may use several resources such as a surveillance system, a trauma registry, or a TBI registry or use hospital discharge information to collect patient information such as Glasgow Coma Scale scores, the cost of care, cause of the TBI, and contributing factors (such as the use of alcohol or safety belts, level of disability upon discharge, and disposition). At the state level, information may be collected under the supervision of the state's public health department or the department of rehabilitation services.

Data Use—National Level (Reporting)

The Traumatic Brain Injury Model Systems National Data and Statistical Center (TBINDSC) is a central resource for data collected on traumatic brain injuries for the Traumatic Brain Injury Model Systems (TBIMS) Program. The data collected at the TBINDSC is used by researchers to advance the knowledge of rehabilitative measures to enhance the quality of life for TBI patients.[51]

Data Use—State Level (Reporting)

The CDC has provided funding that has allowed some states to conduct injury surveillance and collect injury data that examines causes of injury rather than the nature of the injury. At the state level, annual or biannual reports of aggregate data are compiled and published.[52]

> **? DID YOU KNOW?**
>
> **Difference Between Surveillance Systems and Registries.**
> Jean Langlois of the Centers for Disease Control and Prevention has identified the difference between a surveillance system and a registry:
> A **surveillance system** is systematic and ongoing data collection using methods that are practical, uniform, and often focus on rapid data collection rather than complete accuracy; it may or may not be population-based (includes all cases of traumatic brain injury in a defined population, e.g., a state).
> A **registry** is a method of systematic and ongoing data collection that is population-based (includes all cases of traumatic brain injury [TBI] in a defined population, e.g., a state), includes personal identifying and contact information for each case, and may be used for follow-up of TBI cases over time and/or linking TBI cases to services.[50]

> **✓ SELF-ASSESSMENT QUIZ**
>
> 6. Distinguish between a registry and a surveillance system and provide an example of each.

RESEARCH AND USE OF DATA

The roles and responsibilities of HIM professionals have expanded with the increased use of patient data reported from the HIM-related information-gathering processes. In addition, these data contribute to and are used in research efforts in public health studies. According to 45 CFR 56, research is "a systematic investigation, including research development, testing and evaluation, designed to develop or contribute to generalizable knowledge."[53] Research can be categorized into two types, basic and applied.[54] Basic research focuses on theoretical concepts and fundamental principles, whereas applied research uses accumulated theories, knowledge, methods, and techniques to solve the practical problems identified in a clinical setting.

HIM professionals have access to a vast amount of information that can be used in research. This research can evaluate clinical services provided or affect government policy. It can also provide data for clinical studies or be used to analyze HIM practice. Data from registries can be used at the organizational or the population level to prevent disease or mitigate disability. Further, the data can provide the basis to support the need for new health care programs or to substantiate funding a research project. In addition to the use of registry data, the coded data that are generated for reimbursement are also used for health services, medical, and public health research.

HIM plays an important role in research as providers of health care data from primary and secondary resources. Data that have been reviewed and "cleaned" are much more valuable for researchers. Data can be combined in a variety of ways depending on the request from the researchers. The key issue for the HIM professional is to identify errors and correct the data before it is needed by the researchers who will validate the research question posed by the study.

PUBLIC HEALTH RESEARCH

Public health is "the science and art of preventing disease, prolonging life, and promoting health through the organized efforts and informed choices of society, organizations, public and private, communities and individuals."[55]

Data from the surveillance of disease and health status support three core public health functions:[56]

- The assessment and monitoring of the health of communities and populations at risk to identify health problems and priorities
- The formulation of public policies designed to solve identified local and national health problems and priorities
- The assurance that all populations have access to appropriate and cost-effective care, including health promotion and disease prevention services, and evaluation of the effectiveness of that care

The knowledge of the HIM professional is strategic to the work of each core public health function. HIM professionals participate in a variety of roles, acting as data collectors, data

analysts, data reporters, and project managers on public health research studies. The traditional HIM professional roles associated with paper-based health records have expanded into roles that assist with the transition to electronic health records using data standards (e.g., ICD-10, Systemized Nomenclature of Medicine [SNOMED], HL7, etc.) to assist public health research.

PUBLIC HEALTH INFORMATICS

Public health informatics is the systematic application of information from public health practice and research, using computer science and technology.[57] The majority of the work in public health informatics in the United States occurs at the local and state level, in the state, county, or parish departments of public health.

The core activities for state public health departments include:[58]

- Receiving, collecting, and maintaining vital statistics (birth and death records)
- Receiving reports of communicable disease cases from physicians, health care facilities, and laboratories used for infectious disease surveillance
- Reporting infectious disease statistics and trends
- Collecting child immunization and lead screening information
- Collecting and analyzing emergency room data daily to detect early evidence of biological threats
- Collecting hospital capacity information to allow for planning of responses in case of emergencies

To promote interoperability, the CDC has encouraged the adoption in public health data exchange of several standard vocabularies and messaging formats from the health care arena: HL7, which are standards for health care messaging; the LOINC system for encoding laboratory test and result information; and the SNOMED, which is a vocabulary of health care concepts.[58] Several organizations support the collaboration among public health agencies, including the following:

- Public Health Informatics Institute (see Chapter 3, Table 3-4): Through a collaborative approach, the institute brings public health professionals together to define the requirements for health information systems and discuss the current and emerging issues facing public health.
- Public Health Information Network

USE OF POPULATION-BASED DATA

Coded data can be used in many applications as described earlier, but to compare populations the data must be risk adjusted. Several methods have been used to accomplish this, including the Elixhauser Comorbidity Measurement,[59] the All Patient Refined Diagnosis Related Groups (APR-DRGs),[60] Diagnostic Cost Groups (DCGs), and Adjusted Clinical Groups (ACGs),[61] to name a few. These methods use coded data to derive a way to risk adjust groups.

According to Petersen et al.,[61] health-based risk adjustment is the means by which the disease risk is evaluated when determining payment rates, assessing outcomes, researching variation in the use of health services, and performing other comparisons of patient populations. The variables that constitute the method of risk adjustment can also be used to predict outcomes in some cases. For example, the Elixhauser Comorbidity Measurement[59] uses approximately 30 ICD codes to predict increased length of stay, inpatient mortality rates, and charges. Another recent development is the creation of Clinical Classification Software (CCS),[62] which can be used in lieu of ICD codes to predict outcomes. These means of risk adjustment are readily derived from the coded data that HIM professionals generate.

Table 13-3 shows examples of database and data collection systems in federal, state, and international levels.

HEALTH SERVICES RESEARCH

Health services research is an applied field that encompasses many disciplines. The focus of research is generation of knowledge through scientific inquiry about how resources, organization, financing, and policies relate to the provision of health services. There are two main areas of research; the first focuses on the organizational level and the second on the policy level. Major areas of interest include social and economic determinants, organizational design of health services at the population level, and the consequences of health policy.[63]

HIM practice is intertwined with the research interest areas of health service researchers. This is primarily due to the impact the HIM department has on the reimbursement

TABLE 13-3 Database and Data Collection Systems, Databases, and Repositories

Level	Database	Agency	Description
Federal	CDC Wonder	Centers for Disease Control and Prevention (CDC)	A query system that allows access to a variety of online databases of statistical public health data published by CDC. Databases include AIDS public use data, births, cancer statistics, infant deaths, mortality, tuberculosis information system, population data from the census, sexually transmitted disease morbidity, and vaccine adverse event reporting.
	CMS Chart Series	Centers for Medicare and Medicaid Services (CMS)	Chart Series with data on spending, operations, and quality of care. It includes CMS facts and figures (agency programs and operations); Health Care System facts and figures (charts on the entire U.S. health care system); Medicaid facts and figures (Medicaid program).
	CMS: Data and Systems	CMS	Link to CMS information technology; computer data & systems; monitoring programs; research; statistics, trends, & reports; and files for order.
	Healthcare Cost and Utilization Project (HCUP)	Agency for Healthcare Research and Quality (AHRQ)	This AHRQ project has collected data since 1988 and has become the largest longitudinal collection of hospital data in the United States. The data include all-payer, encounter-level information and can be used for trending and monitoring the utilization of health services, as well as quality of care, access, and outcomes of treatment at the national, regional, and state level.
	Hospital Compare	CMS Department of Health and Human Services (DHHS) U.S. Hospital Quality Alliance: Improving Care Through Information	Survey data collected from patients who have been treated during a recent hospital stay. This quality tool allows consumers to search and find comparative information evaluating the quality of care provided by hospitals in a geographic area for specific medical conditions or surgical procedures.
	National Center for Health Statistics (NCHS)	CDC	The CDC, the nation's principal health statistics agency, provides health statistics including diseases, pregnancies, births, aging, and mortality.
	SEER-Medicare Linked Database	National Cancer Institute (NCI), National Institutes of Health	Population-based sources on elderly with cancer for epidemiologic and health services research.
State	State Cancer Profiles	NCI	Descriptive statistics that contains comparison tables, graphs, and maps and support data focused on cancer sites that have known preventable risk factors or screening tests for early detection, and effective treatment options.

Continued

TABLE 13-3 Database and Data Collection Systems, Databases, and Repositories—cont'd

Level	Database	Agency	Description
	State Inpatient Databases (SID)	AHRQ	A database that contains discharge abstracts information across all payers, including Medicare, Medicaid, private insurance, and the uninsured. This database allows for multistate analyses and comparison of discharge data.
International	WHO Statistical Information System (WHOSIS)	World Health Organization (WHO)	This statistical information system (SIS) is an interactive database comprising more than 100 indicators. The database can be accessed by a quick search, by major categories (mortality and burden of disease, health service coverage, risk factors, health systems resources, inequities, and demographic and socioeconomic statistics), or through user-defined tables. Data are published annually.
	Global Health Atlas	WHO	Standardized data and statistics collected for analysis and comparison at country, regional, and global levels for the major infectious diseases of poverty, such as malaria, HIV/AIDS, tuberculosis, and others. The database is updated on an ongoing basis.

process. Further, HIM professionals have intimate knowledge of the structure and organization of health care. Because of this, HIM professionals may be especially well suited to work in health services research and to contribute to the data needs of researchers in this area. An example of research is health care financing and health outcomes. A summary of research using discharge databases can be found in the report titled *The Value of Hospital Discharge Databases*. Studies cited involve evaluating the effect of market competition on hospital costs, studying the effect of insurance status and intensive care unit resources, and the relationship between nurses' education level and surgical outcomes, among others.[7]

MEDICAL RESEARCH

Comorbidity is a condition that is in addition to a primary condition and that affects the course or treatment of a condition. Comorbid conditions can be used in health services research to adjust for the effect of secondary conditions. Typically they can be used in clinical research related to inpatient care, but as research continues, outpatient comorbid conditions could also be developed. The outcomes of interest can vary but usually involve one or more of the following: mortality, cost of health care, and length of stay.

To assist in determining the impact of comorbid disease, a variety of tools have been developed. For example, Anne Elixhauser developed one that uses ICD codes.[59] In a study that predicted mortality in the intensive care unit, comorbid disease measured by the 30 Elixhauser conditions was more predictive than was the Acute Physiology, Age, and Chronic Health Evaluation (APACHE) method.[64]

CERTIFIED HEALTH DATA ANALYST

The Certified Health Data Analyst (CHDA) is a credential offered by the American Health Information Management Association (AHIMA).[65] The credential is designed to

recognize the HIM professional who specializes in data analysis in the health care industry. The analysis of health data has become a critical element in day-to-day operations and health care facilities management. More and more health information management professionals are involved in managing and analyzing health data in various job settings. Following the current changes in the health care industry such as health reform and EHRs, a demand for HIM professionals with CHDA credentials will increase in coming years. According to AHIMA, CHDA skills focus on data management, data analytics, and data reporting. See the following Did You Know box for sample job responsibilities and qualifications of the CHDA.

 DID YOU KNOW?

Sample Job Responsibilities of the Certified Health Data Analyst (CHDA)

Job Summary

This position is responsible for collecting, ongoing analysis, interpreting, and reporting of health care data obtained from a variety of sources, including patient care, financial, and demographic data. A practitioner with CHDA credentials assists with planning, designing, analyzing, and reporting health data to provide accurate information to organizational health care leaders.

Required Knowledge and Skills

- Manage data elements, data sets, and databases (such as UB-04, OASIS, relational).
- Select, design, and implement electronic health records systems.
- Manage health care data (such as financial, clinical, administrative, and research).
- Comply with external data standards (such as HL7).
- Manage standard industry coding and classification systems (such as CPT, ICD-9-CM) and groupers (such as MS-DRGs, APR-DRGs, APCs).

- Plan for the implementation of industry coding and classifications (such as ICD-10-CM, ICD-10-PCS, SNOMED).
- Analyze, interpret, and present data for organizational needs (such as quality, utilization management, benchmarking, external reporting).
- Employ statistical methodologies in design, analysis, and reporting for research.
- Utilize statistical software (such as SAS, SPSS, Excel, Access).
- Interpret and apply HIPAA related standards for privacy and security of protected health information.
- Apply project management techniques and tools.
- Possess strong analytical and problem-solving abilities.

Potential Job Responsibilities

I. Data Management

Assist in the management of clinical, financial, and demographic data for collection, analysis, review, clarification, and reporting to the health care management team.

Maintain patient data in a HIPAA compliant manner.

Interact with health care professionals to organize, analyze, and preserve medical information used to evaluate patient care and validate reimbursement.

Implement data management procedures that are compliant with federal regulations, state licensing rules, and voluntary accrediting standards such as The Joint Commission.

Ensure consistent implementation of data standards.

Coordinate internal and external data users to effectively manage information flow, data collection, review, and analysis, as well as reporting to appropriate regulatory or benchmarking organizations.

Demonstrate the ability to describe how information is used and exchanged in various health care settings.

Select and utilize standard vocabularies, terminologies, and classifications to facilitate the flow of information.

II. Data Analysis

Interact with end-user personnel to develop application data access requirements, transaction rates, volume analysis, and other pertinent data required to develop and maintain integrated databases.

Interact with the health care management team to establish benchmarks, identify deviations, analyze data, and prioritize goals and objectives for performance improvement.

Assist in the development of new approaches and techniques of data analysis.

Provide statistical analysis to the health care management team.

Assess analytical requirements for fellow team members.

Use statistical analytical tools to identify deviations within specialty areas of health care management.

Collaborate with internal and external resources to ensure consistency of methods, interpretation, and approach to analysis of health care data.

Collaborate with other health care team members to review and evaluate process improvements based on improved process methods.

III. Data Reporting

Generate routine, recurring, and ad hoc reports from statistical analysis of health care data.

Develop and/or present data in an appropriate format for targeted audience.

Interpret and report results from statistical analysis to the health care team to provide data for decision support, identifying opportunities for performance improvement, reporting data for benchmarking purposes, complying with government requirements for quality reporting, core measures, etc.

Provide health care management and providers' results from outcomes data analysis.

Facilitate meetings and communicate outcomes to a diverse set of stakeholders.

Qualifications

- Bachelor's degree in health information management required
- Master's degree in health informatics or health information management preferred
- 3+ years of working experience in health care data management
- Registered Health Information Administrator (RHIA) credential with CDHA credential preferred

DATA DICTIONARY

The quality of the data abstracted and entered into various health care applications is essential to providing accurate data to external users such as The Joint Commission for accreditation, Agency for Health Care Research and Quality (AHRQ) for reporting on quality indicators, and for CMS's core measures. In addition, data quality is also necessary for internal users from departments such as utilization management, quality and performance improvement, business office, and the health care organization's administration. One important tool used in controlling the quality of data entered into administrative and clinical applications is the data dictionary.

An understanding of data dictionaries is useful to better understand all types of data, to enhance the ability to analyze data, and to use the data appropriately to assess outcomes and support clinical decision-making.

The data dictionary is as critical to the EHR as the English dictionary is to other forms of communication. The data dictionary conceptually is no different from any other dictionary except that it must be more precise and complete in its definitions.

Data Dictionary Definitions

Metadata—The term metadata is defined as "data about data."[66] It defines the structure that will be used to define all of the characteristics about data so that different individuals looking at characteristics of a data element would arrive at the same conclusion as to what the data mean and how they are to be used. Properly created, the metastructure of data allows for a clearer understanding of the meaning and greater reliability of the quality of information that is part of any electronic record.[67]

Data element—The data element is the atomic level of information.[68] It is best described as a single question that demands a singular defined response. For example, the data element "gender" implies a question about the gender of a person. It demands a defined response that may include "male," "female," or "unknown." The data dictionary describes the nature of the data element sufficiently so that any user of the system will understand what the question and the response means, what it does not mean, and the limits of what it can express.

Field—A field is a physical term that refers to the place in a computer system in which a data element might reside. It is best described as the container for the data. The field container may accommodate the data element in terms of data size or data type, or it may impose limits on how the data element can be defined because of the limits of the system. In many instances, the terms "field" and "data element" have been used interchangeably.[68]

Entities—An entity (or subject) represents a higher level than the data element.[69] It refers to a subject of information that may be a thing, a concept, or a process. The entity may contain many data elements that act as attributes, or descriptors of the entity, and are used to identify the nature of an instance of the entity. For example, the entity "physician" might have many data elements that define the gender, age, address, license number, and so forth, of the instance of a physician.

Table—A table is the physical representation of the entity. Like the field, it is the container that has the data elements that will describe many instances of the entity in the manner established by the logical data model (see Table 13-4).

Record—A record is a row within the table. It contains the data elements within fields that will provide sufficient data to identify a unique instance of the entity. For example, a record in the table that represents the entity "physician" would contain an identifier number and the age, gender, address, and other information about an individual physician to record him or her in the table as a unique instance of the entity "physician."

Attributes—An attribute is a data element that describes the entity. It is generally represented as a column in a table (e.g., city).[70]

Domain—The domain represents the type of value that is allowable for a specific element.[69] For example, an alphabetic character cannot be included in the domain of the data element "date of birth." The domain might specify that 01/01/1997 is acceptable, but Jan. 1, 1997, is not.

Value/coding—The value or coding for a data element represents a more specified way that values may be returned to the data element question. In general, it represents a tighter leash on the domain of the element by specifying more specifically what the answer to the data element question can be. For example, the definition for data element "gender" might specify that only the characters "M," "F," or "U" are acceptable values and that "M" equals "male," "F" equals "female," and "U" equals "unknown."

Logical data model—The logical data model represents the structure of the relationship of data elements and entities within an information system. The logical model is crucial to the proper functioning of any system within an enterprise.[70] The logical model allows for elegance in system design so that the system is adaptable to the changing information needs of the enterprise. The data dictionary is important to complete a good logical data model, but the dictionary should not be dependent on the logical model. By use of the data dictionary to define elements independent of the model, different systems with different logical models will be able to share data that are defined precisely and independently of the manner in which the data elements are structured in different logical models.

Purpose of the Data Dictionary

The data dictionary is a critical part of any information system design. To understand this significance, it is important to first understand the context in which the data dictionary should operate. An information system is not computer hardware, software, or even paper forms. It is a consensus among individuals to share information in a specified way so that all participants derive the same meaning from the content and all participants contribute content in a manner that expresses the intended meaning of the contributor.[71] The data dictionary is a point of consensus that institutionalizes the structure and meaning of the individual elements of the information system. EHRs are tools that support this consensus and allow for a more efficient sharing of the information. Because most computerized information systems are less tolerant than nonelectronic information systems, they help enforce the rules and definitions that have been established. The more effort put into the establishment of the data dictionary, the greater the quality of the information product of the system.

TABLE 13-4 Comparison of Core Health Data Elements

PhyID	Lst_nm	Fst_nm	Addr	City	State	ZIP
239879	SMITH	TOM	234 GREEN ST	SEATTLE	WA	98104
234098	WHITE	MARY	234 LINCOLN AVE	TACOMA	WA	98234
239487	BROWN	JAMES	256 TENDAL PL	PUYALLUP	WA	98398

From Murphy GF, Hanken MA, Waters KA: *Electronic health records: changing the vision*, Philadelphia, 1999, Elsevier.

The development of the data dictionary does not occur by default. A great deal of effort and forethought is required to create a data dictionary that will consistently provide for a meaningful information system. Many institutions have failed to see the value of a formal effort to establish a common enterprise-wide data dictionary and have paid the price in systems that will not integrate and reports and analysis that are worse than meaningless. It is surprising how many sophisticated institutions are relying on invalid or inconsistently defined data that lead to decisions based on misinformation. Many simply assume they understand the meaning of their data or the calculations associated with those data.

Scope of the Data Dictionary

The data dictionary should include all the elements that are required for a person or institution to make key business decisions. In building toward an EHR, institutions will need to map out the foundation data and agree on a strategy to address it. A great deal of effort is necessary to define the functional requirements of an information system that supports decision-making. Further effort is necessary to define the structure or logical data model that will support those requirements. After this is understood, then the logical model will dictate which data elements are necessary to support these functional requirements. These elements will form the scope of the dictionary. The scope of the information systems frequently expands beyond their intended boundaries. The process of building the data dictionary and defining the logical data model can bring criteria and discipline to help control this "scope creep."

Meta-Content of the Data Dictionary

The data dictionary must have a meta-content that defines the attributes that will be included in the data dictionary for each element.[68] We recommend the following attributes be included for each data element:

- Logical name—A long name given to the element on the basis of a naming convention. For example, a name that proceeds left to right from the broadest (largest granularity) to most specific (smallest granularity) term, such as [hospital_department_admit_phone_ number].
- Physical name—A short name given to the element limited by the size of the physical database system. This name will be the name that is identified by the computer as the data element in the physical database, for example, [adm_ph_no].
- Category—The dictionary should attempt to categorize the element in a broad category such as demographic, health history, symptom, physical sign, and so forth.
- Definition—The definition of the data element.
- Type—The data type (character, numeric, date, logical, calculated, free text/memo, etc.).
- Length—The size of the field required to hold values for the data element.
- Decimal—A description of the number of decimal places that might be required in a numeric field.

- Domain—The description of the allowed values for the data element, including the rule for exclusion of invalid data.
- Coding—A description of coded values if they are required for the data element.
- Reference—A reference for the source that was used to define the data element in the dictionary, if applicable. This might be a standard such as American National Standards Institute (ANSI) X12, American Society for Testing and Materials (ASTM), or HL7.

Building the Data Dictionary

Most information systems do not begin as brand-new systems in health care environments. In most instances, health care institutions have had multiple systems for recording a great deal of information. Each application uses a set of definitions appropriate to the application or department. Thus radiology systems would have items such as "gender," "date of birth," "height," "weight," and so forth, whereas the laboratory or admission department might have similar elements that are defined differently in "their" systems. The problem is intensified when different institutions wish to compare their data.[72] As institutions try to integrate new systems or automate paper systems, they begin to grapple with the decision support functions they require. Many of these institutions simply layer on new data elements and structures rather than reassess or overhaul their existing systems. Although some institutions make a valiant effort to integrate and upgrade their information environment, they quickly identify the cost and complexities involved in replacing old systems and cultures. The process of building a fully integrated information structure appears so daunting at times that many institutions just give up or delay developing the system's integration capabilities.

There is a solution to the dilemma, however, if the process of building a new data model and data dictionary is done intellectually, systematically, and with an eye to the future. This process cannot be driven by vendors but rather should be used to drive vendors' response to the institutional needs.[73]

Step 1: Inventory of an Existing Enterprise

The first step in building the data dictionary for any information system is to inventory the content of the existing system. To do this appropriately, all aspects of the enterprise-wide data collection process must be analyzed. Every form and every computer input screen must be reviewed so that data elements that are collected by the institution are cataloged. Similar elements need to be grouped, and the source and purpose of each needs to be recorded. After all data elements are assembled and grouped, a meticulous and time-consuming effort must be undertaken to analyze each element and to identify those elements that are synonymous.

Step 2: Identifying New Data Content Needs

The process of identifying new data content is complex and requires a great deal of planning and discipline to accomplish appropriately. This process falls into the realm of logical data modeling, which is outside the scope of this chapter. The processes for logical data modeling and data dictionary development are intimately linked and must occur together. The data dictionary provides the structured container for the product of this process and represents one piece of the overall data design of any enterprise.

Step 3: Consensus Development

As described previously, information systems are totally dependent on a consensus of the users about the definition and management of all the atomic (cannot be further divided) bits of information within an enterprise. Without a solid consensus, the information system is severely compromised. The ability to build an EHR requires that users of the system understand and buy into the definitions of elements that will be used in the system. Otherwise, the data will lack validity and integrity. Box 13-1 shows an example of a process for developing that consensus through the use of an informatics work group that is given a specific work plan to accomplish its goal.

BOX 13-1   Developing a Data Dictionary Through Consensus by Using an Informatics Work Group

Phase 1: Data Gathering

1. The Informatics Working Group (IWG) meets to present the members with the goals and background of the data dictionary structure. Each member receives the following:
   - A process consensus document
   - Guidelines and procedures
   - An example of data dictionary elements
   - A copy of the data element worksheet
   - A review of the database program used to store and retrieve the elements
2. The IWG accepts its work charge that specifies the content area selected to be addressed. This content area might have a number of specific elements already listed to include as part of the charge, or it might be left fairly open to the IWG to identify elements within that content area. Examples of content areas are demographic data, plan and coverage data, and encounter data.
3. IWG members provide comment on existing elements and begin reviewing other data elements to consider for further discussion.
4. All proposed data elements are evaluated to see whether they are appropriate for inclusion on the basis of a defined set of criteria.
5. The IWG confirms the initial set of elements for data dictionary development.
6. Data element general descriptions are compiled by project staff.
7. IWG members submit additional elements, with preliminary coding and definition recommendations from respected sources, to the staff for investigation as additions to the set under development. Elements with defined definitions and coding should be referenced by individual group members supplying the data elements. The governing board appoints a task force to serve as a resource to the content area and connect to the IWG to assist in content, definition, and coding in specialty areas.
8. All work is documented in the data dictionary software and appropriate documentation is prepared.

Phase 2: Organization and Task Completion

1. Staff compiles the list supplied by the task force and begins research through as many sources as possible (including members of the task force) to complete specific definitions and coding of the elements. Each element is also assessed to see that it meets basic criteria for inclusion. Each element is evaluated to see whether it could be used in a logical data modeling process.
2. Staff prepares documentation on each data element that notes the following:
   - Data element definition
   - Data element source (where the element came from; e.g., form, person, contract requirement)
   - Data element priority (significance to users for billing, clinical needs)
   - Data element references (who requires the element for what purposes)
   - Data element code references where appropriate
   - Data element inclusion within a data model
   - Category (content area) in which the data element most commonly resides
3. The first iteration of the data element definitions and coding is delivered to the IWG. When the task force reconvenes, its members review the current product; critique the elements' definitions and coding; suggest changes, additions, or deletions; and specify any additional follow-up required.
4. Staff perform follow-up tasks and return the product to the IWG for final review.
5. The IWG reviews one more iteration of the definition content product to that point and makes additional changes. Final recommendations are secured by consensus.

Phase 3: Validation

1. The reconciled product of the IWG is submitted for a 30-day review and comment process by stakeholders or any interested party. All comments are summarized from a questionnaire tool. Both objective ratings and written comments are requested.
2. Comments are returned to the staff and organized for an initial review by the IWG.
3. The IWG provides preliminary recommendations for action to the governing body when specific changes are recommended.
4. The governing body reviews recommendations from the IWG along with the feedback from the questionnaire and makes a final determination on data element changes.
5. Revisions on content are added to the existing data dictionary and disseminated to stakeholders and interested parties through the established dissemination process carried out by the staff.

Phase 4: Maintenance

1. The value of the dictionary will grow over time. Changes that need to be made will be considered for compelling clinical/business reasons.
2. All modifications to the dictionary will follow a prescribed protocol that includes the following steps:
   - Any health care entity can submit a request for modification of existing elements or addition of new elements to existing elements within the data dictionary as new standards are developed or modified nationally and the need for new content areas develops.
   - Indicators will be maintained to reference archive data and original documentation where changes occur. This will support continuity and accuracy of data over time.
   - The governing body reviews requests, determines when changes should be considered, and refers proposed changes to the IWG to be considered using the standard process identified in this work plan.

Criteria for Data Element Inclusion

Each data element to be included in the data dictionary should be evaluated to see whether it is appropriate for inclusion on the basis of a set of criteria. The following are our recommendations for criteria to apply to proposed data elements.

- The element should belong to the enterprise under development.
- The element should be a variable used to make decisions important to the enterprise.
- The element should be obtainable as a normal part of the transactions that occur within the enterprise.
- The element must be unique and clearly definable.
- Each element must have only one defined value response that may include a prescribed set of coded values (e.g., acceptable gender options) or any other single response type allowed by the database management system.
- Collection of the data element should not produce an undue burden on the data reporter.
- In general, the value returned for a data element should not contain more than one meaning. For example, an alphanumerical member number might have buried within the string a number of attribute values such as member date of birth, plan type, risk type, program type, or any other variables about the member, any or all of which might change over time, which might be less than desirable.

Cataloging Standards

Standards are nothing new to most health care practitioners. Their relevance and importance in many areas of health delivery are well understood and appreciated. Few organizations are not subject to measurement against standards established by The Joint Commission, the National Committee for Quality Assurance (NCQA), and other accrediting bodies. Manufacturers of medical devices, particularly those companies that produce patient-monitoring and life-sustaining equipment, must comply with very specific standards set forth by government regulatory agencies.

In many disciplines, standards of practice are international and universally recognized. For example, the notations and intonations associated with the standard musical scale are used by musicians throughout the world. Thus, listeners to Beethoven's Fifth Symphony as performed by the Vienna Philharmonic orchestra should be capable of identifying the same piece when it is delivered by a local high school orchestra (although the quality of its delivery might vary). Likewise, agencies within the European Economic Council have decreed that the dimensions of door hinges produced by hinge manufacturers in any member country must adhere to mutually agreed standards. This enables a French housing contractor to purchase door hinges from a low-cost supplier in Belgium for use in constructing homes in Portugal.

The standards of music and European door hinges are well documented and cataloged. The highly variable and complex nature of health care information renders it much more difficult to standardize. However, as noted previously, this variability is often the source of confusion when clinical data recorded by one practitioner are later interpreted by another practitioner. Similarly, if the content and attributes of a broadly used patient identifier (i.e., the enterprise medical record number) are not uniform within various department-based systems, the ability to merge these data for various analyses is thwarted.

After standards of data capture and retention are instituted and incorporated into the enterprise data dictionary, they must be cataloged and distributed to all users of the dictionary. The source of these standards can vary. Whenever possible, standards ordained by broadly acknowledged agencies and parties should be adopted. Thus, ICD-9-CM or ICD-10 would be referenced as the approved means of recording diagnoses in light of its general acceptance as a disease classification scheme.

Intraorganizational standards should also be acknowledged and referenced by the data dictionary. If a "customized" approach to calculating patient acuity has been developed within an acute-care hospital, only those scores resultant from its use should be cataloged. It would be futile to reference the format and content of a commercially available severity scoring system if it is not used in nursing practice.

Ideally, the format and content of a corporate-wide data dictionary are defined before the design and development of automated systems. However, most organizations, particularly health care entities, do not have the luxury of "scrapping" extant applications and rebuilding them from scratch. Hence, data dictionaries are often implemented after many organizational systems have been implemented and are in broad use.

Even if a start-up health care facility possessed the opportunity to construct its data dictionary, there are no national or international standards that dictate and direct its complete design. The complexity of our health care delivery system has produced a more fragmented approach to the design and standards. These have typically arisen from specialty organizations or cooperatives that are associated with a particular specialty (the American College of Radiology's standards for image archiving) or function (the use of the American Medical Association's Current Procedural Terminology (CPT)-4 for the coding of various types of procedures).

Lacking any nationally recognized composite data model, health care organizations should strive to pursue and implement standards for specific types of information (such as those mentioned above) wherever possible. With the increased demand for the exchange of clinical information among providers, government agencies, payers, and other parties, the need to adhere to recognized standards is obvious. Use of established taxonomies and guidelines greatly enhances the "exchangeability" of medical data and reduced administrative costs.

DATA INTERPRETATION AND OUTCOMES

Patients, purchasers, payers, and providers are clamoring for objective data about what really works in health care. The term outcome refers to an indicator of the results of a process. Although that process may be of almost any type, typically it is related to the content and delivery of health care.

Those whose primary concern is with quality of life may look for different outcomes from those interested in years of life or others more concerned with costs. Although there are certainly instances in which all indicators point to the same conclusion, often it is necessary to balance quality, cost, or other considerations to some degree.

Many lists of outcomes variables have been assembled. For those looking to develop outcomes information systems, a more straightforward approach to the data issue may be to recognize that nearly all health care information can be considered some component of outcomes data, segmented along the dimensions of:

- Administrative: Demographics, billing events, cost and payment models, and so on
- Patient perceptions: Physical health status, mental health status, access, satisfaction, and so on
- Clinical: Interventions, observations, conditions, results, and so on
- Life domains: Employment, housing, community supports, and so on

Researchers obtain access to large sets of claims data, sometimes supplemented with paper medical records. Claims data include data from insurers, the CMS, and regional data sets. Claims data contain some limited number of coded data elements representing clinical condition, procedures or treatments, discharge disposition, and possibly some other indicator of how the case was resolved. This information source represents a large, fairly uniform set of data that is readily available in coded form, online, and theoretically ready for use. It can be combined into a longitudinal record and analyzed for specific conditions and patient populations, as depicted in Figure 13-1.

Unfortunately, claims data tend to provide a limited clinical picture, are often fragmented, and usually contain inaccuracies such as mismatched patient identifiers. They may also have been distorted as a result of coding practices that are driven more by reimbursement requirements than by a concern for clinical accuracy. One study found that claims data failed to identify as many as half the prognostically important clinical conditions found in a clinical information system.[74]

Outcomes Data and Information Systems

Those with some right to the data from a large number of organizations include insurers or benefits managers, regulatory or watchdog groups, and private health care database developers. Like the academic researchers, this group must confine itself to the set of coded data submitted, so the scope of its work is limited. However, it is often in a position to specify the content of the data submitted to it, so it is able to focus on specific areas of interest, usually through the periodic submission of defined indicators. For example, the NCQA has defined a set of indicators for the Health Plan Employer Data and Information Set (HEDIS). This set is limited, but it permits comparison of health plans across a large, consistent data sample. Performance measurement is intended to lead to quality improvement within participating provider organizations by highlighting trends and offering comparisons to similar organizations. Likewise, most insurers have available large case samples with common data elements from a diverse group of providers that help them to identify organizations and practices they wish to encourage.

Outcomes Data Use

Outcomes may also be presented in terms of life domains and being able to return to the activities of living. Some managed care systems include information on life domains. This information is usually important when care spans a period of time. For example, on entry into the care process, the individual was not able to work or live independently because of his or her condition. After completion of the treatment process, the individual is able to return to work and to an independent living situation.

Intraorganizational outcomes teams use their own data and are more likely to focus on local processes. Their goal tends to be outcomes management through profiling, guidelines, performance improvement, and the like. These teams have access to a wider range of data elements and information systems, which may provide a more comprehensive clinical picture. They may also be able to make modifications to the data collection systems to allow them to expand their data sets to reflect specific interests and to address data quality issues. Intraorganizational outcomes teams generally have cleaner, more comprehensive data sets available to them, but the sample size is often too small to be significant. Further, few provider organizations have personnel with the time and training to analyze and interpret outcomes data effectively.

Outcomes and the Electronic Health Record

In the absence of both a comprehensive EHR and true outcomes information systems, all these groups have had to make do with the information systems available to them. General health care information systems (HIS) are operational systems that work with the transactional data on a single patient at a time. Although they may have a comprehensive information set, it is usually not readily accessible across patients or time. Patient survey data management and analysis products aggregate data across time and patients but tend to lack core operational data necessary to the analysis. Health care decision support packages are also strong in the aggregation and analysis components but have historically lacked the comprehensive data set desired. Generic databases and statistical packages are excellent tools but lack health care domain knowledge and require the users to build their own data model.

It is imperative that EHRs explicitly support these requirements. In simplified form, they may be diagrammed

FIGURE 13-2 Outcomes information systems requirements. (From Murphy GF, Hanken MA, Waters KA: *Electronic health records: changing the vision*, Philadelphia, 1999, Elsevier.)

as seen in Figure 13-2. That is, comprehensive data drawn from clinical and operational management systems must be warehoused in a format that allows necessary indicator data to be transmitted to those who need the data. The data must be supplemented with other relevant information such as benchmarks or standards of care. Health care–specific applications need to operate over the combined data to support analysis and reporting needs for outcomes research and management.

This ideal record is a complete, longitudinal picture of all health-related activities from birth to death, including occupational, physical fitness, nutritional, and other relevant lifestyle data. With it, the researcher can look for correlations between treatments, prior conditions, lifestyle, and long-term outcomes. Further, it allows groups of related health care events to be grouped together into episodes of care. This ideal record is a logical whole, not necessarily a single physical record. It might be stored on many computers but is entirely online, and the components can be easily linked together when needed.

Figure 13-3 shows the reality of an encounter-based record, distributed across multiple providers. Actual health care records are often discontinuous and impossible to integrate. The patient is identified differently in each piece, and there is little or no health-related information apart from formal encounters. Large portions of the record are not online at all. There are many reasons for this. Some are inherent in the structure of the health care industry, others in the history of

health care information systems, and still others in the nature of the data itself.

The health care industry is still characterized by large numbers of autonomous or semiautonomous business entities involved in the provision of, administration of, or payment for care. These organizations are linked in an intricate network of relationships, but each has its own data set. The standard concerns of any business regarding proprietary data apply to health care organizations and are compounded by the uniquely confidential nature of health care data.

Providers involved with many managed care organizations cannot possibly use all these information systems and may not have the resources and expertise necessary to generate each of the data sets requested by the organizations. Even if they can, differing data definitions, and the encounter-based orientation of most provider data, may seriously limit analysis at the level of the managed care organization. There may be gaps where systems are entirely absent or where key types of information, such as clinical data or critical specialty information, are not available. Finally, it must be acknowledged that no matter what the structure of the health care system, there is no current way to capture routinely complete data about such issues as patient participation in or compliance with a treatment regimen.

Within a given health care enterprise, there is no guarantee that the computerized data that does exist can be linked into a coherent longitudinal record of care. Many large

FIGURE 13-3 Longitudinal data. (From Murphy GF, Hanken MA, Waters KA: *Electronic health records: changing the vision*, Philadelphia, 1999, Elsevier.)

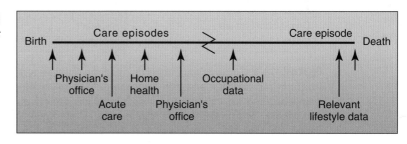

providers, such as hospitals, have a number of information systems. These often come under the ownership of individual departments, each with differing priorities and data definitions. The systems may or may not communicate with each other effectively, making it difficult to link the records of a single patient across systems (see Figure 13-4).

Outcome Indicators

Outcome measures are still in the early development stage. Most outcomes are condition- or process-specific, making it difficult to identify a single, simple set of outcomes data. Various groups have developed indicators such as blood transfusion or maternal deaths to monitor outcomes of specific events. Others have relied on diagnosis and procedure codes, discharge status, length of stay, and proxy measures such as cost. Within a health care organization, researchers can collect data such as unplanned returns to surgery, but they are often limited to data from a single encounter and cannot track long-term outcomes if the patient receives future care outside the organization.

One major area of research and development within this field has been in the development of survey instruments to measure health status, access to care, and satisfaction, as reported by the patient. Much of the effort has gone into the development of standard, easy-to-complete instruments that can be readily incorporated into the patient care process and that provide a comparable set of data across health care providers. Some of the best-known health status measures are the SF-36 and SF-12 from the Medical Outcomes Trust, and the HSQ and HSQ-12 from the Health Outcomes Institute. Mental health has standard client satisfaction surveys as well, notably one from the Mental Health Council of America (MHCA) and Telesage.

Survey data have not traditionally been incorporated into the clinical information system as a part of the patient care process but are a critical component of the complete outcomes data set. The need for better and more comparable outcome indicators has spawned myriad indicator development, cataloging, and standardization efforts. For example, the Health Outcomes Institute (HOI), which was spun off from Ellwood's initial outcomes work, promotes the development, dissemination, and use of public domain outcomes measures. In 1996, it worked with the American Medical Group Association on a software package known as the Outcomes Data Conversion Utilities. The utilities provide access to a database of standardized survey questions for developing survey instruments and also translate existing indicators into standard equivalents for comparative purposes.[75] Good indicators reflect outcomes over which caregivers have some degree of control. They are also readily collected, thoroughly tested, and widely accepted so that they can be used for comparative purposes.

Outcomes and Coding Issues

There has been considerable incentive for payers to standardize medical coding and for providers to code medical activities. A number of researchers have developed coding systems for nursing diagnoses and care, but there is to date no one standard model. (Coding and vocabulary issues are discussed in more depth in Chapter 7.) From an outcomes research standpoint, this is disastrous because a significant component of care is lost to handwritten textual notes or organization- and vendor-specific coding schemes. A similar, even more pronounced situation holds for other allied health professions.

Coding schemes may also differ by setting. Thus, if one wishes to compare inpatient and outpatient surgery outcomes, it has been necessary to look at both CPT-4 and ICD-9-CM codes to identify all similar procedures. These coding systems may not be useful when looking at outcomes

Actual Health Care Record

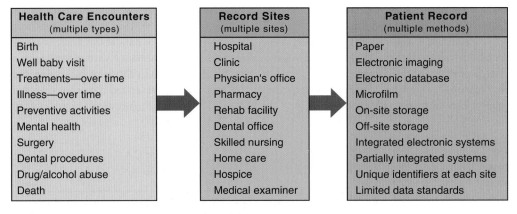

Health Care Encounters (multiple types)	Record Sites (multiple sites)	Patient Record (multiple methods)
Birth	Hospital	Paper
Well baby visit	Clinic	Electronic imaging
Treatments—over time	Physician's office	Electronic database
Illness—over time	Pharmacy	Microfilm
Preventive activities	Rehab facility	On-site storage
Mental health	Dental office	Off-site storage
Surgery	Skilled nursing	Integrated electronic systems
Dental procedures	Home care	Partially integrated systems
Drug/alcohol abuse	Hospice	Unique identifiers at each site
Death	Medical examiner	Limited data standards

FIGURE 13-4 Current health records describe multiple types of treatment and preventive activities from birth to death in an often fragmented delivery system. The records themselves are also in transition, and an individual's records may be stored at multiple sites in a variety of formats and media. (From Murphy GF, Hanken MA, Waters KA: *Electronic health records: changing the vision*, Philadelphia, 1999, Elsevier.)

for specialty care such as mental health or drug treatment. Different settings typically capture differing levels of detail within the record as well. For example, in the inpatient hospital setting, it is common for information systems to store 15 or more diagnosis codes, whereas in a physician-office setting, there are generally only four. Again, the reasons may be traced to billing and payment issues. Furthermore, these are U.S. standards. Comparisons across national boundaries may require that other coding schemes such OPCS4 (United Kingdom) for procedures or ICD-10 for diagnoses be incorporated in the analysis.

The coding issue is important and extends beyond coding data to identify diagnoses and procedures because uncoded textual data are difficult to analyze in any comprehensive, automated fashion given today's information systems technology. Although there are limitations inherent in all coding systems, they do provide a structured approach to storing comparable data. Data that are coded according to organization-specific coding schemes such as billing or service codes can be analyzed locally, but, unless it is mapped to some universal scheme or crosswalk, it cannot be compared across organizations. Given that a typical acute care hospital has thousands of service codes, this is a formidable task. An example of a universal coding scheme is the International Classification of Clinical Services (ICCS), originally developed by Stan Mendenhall at the Commission on Professional and Hospital Activities in an attempt to standardize descriptions of treatments and to provide more clinical data within codes.

Further, health care payers are using financial incentives to improve practice. The primary mechanism is through initiatives that reward good-quality care with financial reward. One of these programs is called pay for performance and may be referred to as P4P or PFP. The main goal is to improve quality of care and patient safety by linking patient outcomes to reimbursement and payment incentives. Pay for performance systems are often associated with the private sector, while in the public sector, the same programs or systems are known as value-based purchasing (VBP). VBP is used in the federal health care reimbursement systems.[76] Included in this program is the incentive to stimulate implementation of the electronic health record (EHR) in physician offices.

Finally, it must be acknowledged that some of the most important elements of care can never be coded. The intangibles of a sunny room, a cheerful smile, or an empathetic listener may affect outcomes but cannot be quantified or captured within the clinical record. It should be noted that mental health systems do include items that are often not included in other aspects of health care. For example, the client has and uses his or her natural support system (family or friends) to help address the problem.

Desirable Outcome Systems

It is desirable that data collection systems be available wherever care is rendered—whether in an office, at a bedside, in a home, or at a remote location—and that the data be entered by the person first acquiring it.[77] This is important, too, in that we want not only to gather information but to provide it back to the caregiver in such a manner as to influence care in a positive way.

Ideally, the outcomes data warehouse will be structured around persons, not the patient—that is, it will include information on a population of people who have either received care in the past or who may receive care at some time in the future. This larger population is helpful for indicator denominators, for example, "x% of women of childbearing age within our sample received regular Papanicolaou smears." It is also important for modeling future patient populations, and it can help us to understand why some people become patients and others do not. If there are nonpatients for whom we have some responsibility (e.g., as a capitated provider or as a payer) and about whom we have specific demographic or survey data, these should be included. Information about the larger community may not be as detailed but can still be descriptive of demographics, use rates, risk factors, and so forth. It is also beneficial to include comparative or benchmark data on treatment approaches, resource allocation, and outcomes of particular interest. In recent years, there have been many public and private regional and national data pools created. These should provide ready access to comparative data. They may also provide large enough data samples for statistically valid studies.

It should be noted that the need for a master identifier is just as critical for caregiver records as it is for patients because we cannot hope to do effective provider profiling unless we can accurately identify the care rendered in many different locations by the same individuals. The national provider identifier will help in this regard.

To understand what contributed to an outcome, it is beneficial to know the entire course of care, from the onset of symptoms to full recovery, which implies the presence of a mechanism to identify all the components of an episode of care. On the surface, this seems straightforward, but automating the process for huge numbers of patient records poses both theoretical and processing challenges. For example, where does one episode end and another begin? What do we do if services rendered during a single encounter apply to more than one condition? How do we categorize similar episodes for comparative purposes? This process is complex enough for relatively straightforward disease processes. Where there are chronic or comorbid conditions, it becomes far more so. Further, we should also be able to identify preventive care as an episode in and of itself. The whole concept of episodes of care, in the context of data management, is still in its infancy. A few providers have begun tagging encounter records with an episode at the outset of care for administrative purposes. This is problematic because a visit that initially appears to be for one condition may ultimately be seen to be the result of some other condition entirely or a part of more than one concurrent episode of care.

Episodic groupers are a fairly recent development in health care information processing. These have been developed by companies that process millions of health care claims a year for benefits management firms, payers, and managed care plans. Although each episodic grouper uses proprietary logic to assign claims events to a condition and an episode, the groupers all have certain points in common:

- Clinical groupings—Each episodic grouper begins by categorizing individual claims by medical condition, usually on the basis of proprietary groupings of ICD-9-CM diagnosis codes that represent some level of clinical or treatment homogeneity. There are usually several hundred conditions within a given model.
- Assigning events to episodes—Where services are clearly linked to a single diagnosis on the claim, the grouper is able to assign them to an episode fairly easily. Other services can only be assigned with use of clinically based logic that takes into account expected time frames, concurrent episodes, and sophisticated data reconciliation processes.
- Determining the end of an episode—Groupers use either discrete time periods or a window of time during which there are no services for a condition to decide when an episode is at end. Each approach has some drawbacks. Under the discrete time period approach, all appropriate services during the expected duration of the episode are included. If actual care exceeds this time period, the grouper may end up counting too many episodes for the same condition because a new episode would start when the time period expires. Under the clear window approach, the end of the episode is determined by the absence of treatment for defined periods of time. This may result in counting too few episodes when a new instance begins during the expected window and is assumed to be part of the previous episode.

Early generations of episodic groupers were limited to claims data and focused on ambulatory and physician billing data. As they begin to move into the provider and acute care arena, we can expect to see increasing sophistication in the modeling process. Over time, these systems should prove invaluable to the outcomes movement.

The data warehouse relies on internal codes to provide comprehensive analytic functionality. Whether these codes are user defined or standard, data from multiple source systems will need to be interpreted and mapped to the codes. There are now powerful, commercially available mapping engines that can assign codes, compute event durations, fill in gaps within records, and generally scrub and reconcile data as they are fed into a warehouse. More experimental are processors to read and interpret text so that it can be stored in a format useful for analysis. At the same time, clinical information systems are becoming better at guiding the user through structured text entry in a way that allows data to be stored behind the scenes in code but presented to the user as text.

The data warehouse must be complemented by a robust set of tools designed and built with an understanding of health care and outcomes information requirements. These allow information to be derived from the outcomes warehouse and interpreted. At a minimum, this tool set needs to include functionality for the following:

- Data sampling—Identifying the characteristics and volume of records to be included in a given analysis. Some data sampling tools allow records to be selected by number or value (e.g., include all records in DRG 50 or exclude abnormal white blood cell counts). Others look across records to allow such samples as the physician who treated the fewest cases during the month of July or the diagnosis with the highest variable cost per case.
- Grouping—Continuing analysis requires that data be segmented into meaningful subsets. Grouping functions allow the creation of subsets based on flexible criteria that may be as simple as age or gender cohorts or complex combinations of diagnoses, interventions, and outcomes.
- Tabular and graphical reporting—Reporting functionality runs the gamut from rigid, standardized reports in flat, tabular formats to flexible ad hoc reports that allow the user to drill through increasing layers of detail, shift perspectives, resort, and present the information in a variety of graphical formats. Reporting functionality also varies widely in its usability and its efficiency. Some "user-friendly" report writers may be simple to use but offer limited functionality or they may be downright unfriendly. Standard Structured Query Language (SQL)–based reporting functions have no "knowledge" of health care and so require considerable expertise to perform such functions as properly counting cases in which each uses multiple services. Even well-designed, health care–oriented reporting tools require that the user have knowledge of the data model to use them effectively, so a strategy of offering tiered reporting tools for power users versus the occasional or casual user is perhaps most realistic.
- Modeling—Changes in treatment patterns, resource mix, staffing, and so forth are all of interest.
- Indicator reporting functions—Performance measurement requires the collection and dissemination of indicators both internally and to third parties such as the NCQA and The Joint Commission. These should be automatically gathered from within the warehouse and formatted for the necessary review and transmission.
- Benchmarking and comparative reporting capabilities—All these tools should be able to operate over both detailed internal data and external comparative data.

For outcomes management, it is also beneficial to have specific functionality for process improvement studies and for the development and use of standards of care such as pathways and guidelines. One other function that deserves mention is data mining. This is another term with a range of connotations, depending on the source. The idea is to extract gems of information from mountains of data. Data mining software is intended to facilitate the review of large volumes of data for insights, trends, patterns, and hypotheses. This can be done by using a basic set of sampling and reporting tools. It can also be pursued with more experimental software designed to identify patterns and relationships in raw data. The latter have not yet achieved broad acceptance for general health care applications but show promise for outcomes research purposes.

Information dissemination requirements are dependent on the audience and the purpose. Audiences with an interest in outcomes information include the following:

- Caregivers and provider organizations
- Patients and consumer groups
- Health care purchasers
- Regulators and accrediting bodies
- Researchers

Each of these audiences has its own perspective on what may be the same information. Although a patient may want outcomes data to assist in deciding on a provider and a course of treatment, he or she will probably want that information highly processed in an explanatory format. The researcher, on the other hand, is likely to want data in their raw form. The information dissemination approach will also be affected by the purpose of the data; for example, purposes may include the following:

- Education
- Behavior modification
- Quality optimization
- Resource management
- Evaluation
- Research

From an information systems development standpoint, this means that no single information dissemination module will be designed, coded, and implemented. Instead, information dissemination must be a function of the entire system. Table 13-1 gives examples of strategies that may be effective for selected audiences and purposes.

The results of outcomes research should be available to caregivers in a variety of forms: through online bibliographic tools, guideline lookups, and the clinical decision support functions provided within the workstation. This last feature will include reminders, alerts, order sets reflecting the results of outcomes research, and detailed analytical tools for the caregiver who is also a researcher.

Some of the most significant trends of benefit to the outcomes movement include the following:

- Standard data definitions and interchange mechanisms for health care data. The work of standards developers and promoters such as HL7, ASTM, and the ANSI's Healthcare Informatics Standards Planning Panel (HISPP) and ANSI Healthcare Information Technology Standards Panel (ANSI HITSP). This work is intended to break down barriers between information systems caused by differing data definitions. This allows not only the information systems from various newly affiliated health care organizations to exchange data, but also often-incompatible systems within single organizations to exchange data.
- Open systems, including communications and database standards. These remove the technical barriers to systems integration, just as standard data definitions remove the data barriers. Common database access formats such as SQL mean that data can be retrieved easily from a number of sources and combined to build up a complete picture of conditions, interventions, and outcomes. This approach should allow the merging of local organizational data with state,

regional, and national public databases and with proprietary data sets from specialty companies. Common methods of identifying data between systems, such as that used by extensible markup language (XML), are also helpful.

- Security. Network-based security standards such as the Open Systems Foundation's (OSF) Distributed Computing Environment (DCE) provide vehicles for controlling system and data access, whereas field definitions within databases guard specific data elements from inappropriate usage. Data security and confidentiality is a major concern of health care consumers. The ability to ensure it is critical to the public's acceptance of outcomes data sharing.
- Local and wide area networking, with and without wires. Not only do networks enhance communication, they also make it possible for everyone to "work off the same page." That is, caregivers in many locations can have access to the same applications and information at the same time, thus increasing the uniformity and integrity of the data set. Without networks, each caregiver accesses and enters data on a separate, local computer system, duplicating some, misspelling others, and leaving some out entirely, making it difficult to build a single, comprehensive record of care. Wireless networks provide the additional benefit of allowing the computer to move with the caregiver.
- Graphical user interfaces. These make information systems more approachable and easier to use, thereby helping to expand the user community to caregivers and even patients. This in turn should enable the capture of a richer, far more complete information set for outcomes analysis. It should also improve the accuracy of the data by moving health care data capture to the point of care.
- High-powered, commodity hardware. Inexpensive and interchangeable hardware makes it feasible to collect data at the point of care, wherever that may be. Powerful hardware makes it feasible to work with distributed data, enormous databases, and huge transaction volumes. This supports not only the data collection effort but the manipulation of large data sets for analysis purposes.
- The Web, the Internet, and Intranets. These are significant information dissemination vehicles. They also provide a platform for the rapid and relatively low-cost development and deployment of distributed applications.

Most acute care hospitals have some type of case mix analysis capability. Even a fairly simple system should permit a general analysis of such proxy outcome measures as length of stay and discharge status by type of case. This information can be used to develop guidelines, critical pathways, or other process improvement approaches. For example, you might look at reducing the length of stay for total hip replacement cases. Using the case mix system, you can examine the characteristics of cases with differing outcomes—in this example, length of stay—and develop a plan to adopt a similar pattern of care on the basis of the characteristics of the cases with the lower length of stay. This plan can be loaded into existing clinical systems, to the extent that those systems can support it. For example, if you have nursing care plans online, the new plan can be incorporated in those. If you have an order entry system with standard order sets, the new plan can be set up as a standard order. As you begin to collect data on patients treated under the new plan, you will be going back to your case mix system to assess the impact of the change and possibly to fine-tune it.

Simultaneous with the change in clinical process, you will want to consider how to enhance your existing systems to further support this change. You might want to add additional data elements to measure outcomes more effectively within your case mix system. You might want to implement system modules you have purchased but not yet installed. You may want to purchase additional modules for systems you already have, such as advanced nursing functions. Or it may be time to begin moving forward with major new components of your long-term information systems strategy and architecture. Both sides of the process, the analysis and systems implementation and the modification of clinical processes and ways of thinking, are iterative. The goal is to discover how much outcomes data are already available to you and how best to use the data while moving forward with your long-term plan. As new system components and data elements are put in place, the outcomes information and functionality available will expand, enabling you to reap the benefits of the outcomes movement. This will help support clinical decision-making as well.

CHAPTER REVIEW

1. Which one of the following is NOT a step in building a data dictionary?
   a. perform an inventory of the current system
   b. identify new data content needs of the current system
   c. mandate the adoption of your preferred definitions of data elements
   d. develop a consensus between all users of the system

2. The AIS scores would be found in which of the following registries?
   a. Trauma Registry
   b. Cancer Registry
   c. Birth Registry
   d. Diabetes Registry

3. Health care organizations and providers are required to report data on specific core measures. This is an example of which use of health care data reporting?
   a. benchmarking
   b. clinical decision support
   c. consumer education
   d. performance management

4. CMS attempts to make the Medicare beneficiary a better-informed public consumer of health care for inpatient services by providing which of the following:
   a. Health Grades
   b. Hospital Compare
   c. Texas Medical Foundation Health Quality Institute
   d. Agency for Healthcare Research and Quality

5. Which of the following registries would report information on the national health objectives set for *Healthy People 2020*?
   a. cancer registries
   b. trauma registries
   c. immunization registries
   d. diabetes registries

6. Identify which one of the following is NOT a core public health function.
   a. assessment and monitoring of the health of communities and populations at risk
   b. formulation of public policies designed to solve identified local and national health problems and priorities
   c. assurance that all populations have access to appropriate and cost-effective care, including health promotion and disease prevention services
   d. oversight of transplant, death, cancer, trauma, and immunization national registries

7. The selection of a data element should meet all of the following criteria EXCEPT for:
   a. can be reused in a different system if it has a different definition
   b. should be obtainable in the normal work process
   c. must be unique and clearly definable
   d. should be used to make decisions important to the organization

8. Which of the following lead agencies has the primary responsibility to improve quality, safety, efficiency, and effectiveness by collecting data on published patient quality and patient safety indicators?
   a. The Leapfrog Group
   b. Agency for Health Care Research and Quality
   c. Texas Medical Foundation Health Quality Institute
   d. Health Grades

9. Identify the function that is NOT common to all registries.
   a. case definition and eligibility criteria
   b. abstracting and entering specified data elements into a database
   c. staging of the disease process and periodic follow-up for ACS approval
   d. data reporting for use by agencies, the scientific community, and the public

10. When health care organizations compare their organization's patient safety and quality indicators against peer organizations that are known for their excellence, they are using which of the following tools?
    a. benchmarking
    b. decision support
    c. administrative analysis
    d. Consumer Assessment of Health Providers and Systems Survey (CAHPS)

REFERENCES

1. The Free Dictionary by Farlex. http://www.thefreedictionary.com/data. Accessed August 27, 2013.
2. DataInformed: *Big data and analytics in the enterprise: data and analytics glossary.* http://data-informed.com/glossary-of-big-data-terms/.
3. Business Dictionary.com. http://www.businessdictionary.com/definition/data-integrity.html.
4. Joint Commission Core Measure definition. http://www.jointcommission.org/core_measure_sets.aspx. Accessed August 27, 2013.
5. Quality Net. https://www.qualitynet.org/dcs/ContentServer?pagename=QnetPublic/Page/QnetHomepage. Accessed August 27, 2013.
6. Joint Commission on Accreditation of Healthcare Organizations. http://www.jointcommission.org. Accessed August 27, 2013.
7. Schoenman J, Sutton J, Kintala S, et al.: *The value of hospital discharge databases,* Salt Lake City, UT, 2005, National Association of Health Data Organizations.
8. U.S. Department of Health and Human Services: *Hospital quality compare—a quality tool provided by Medicare.* http://www.medicare.gov/hospitalcompare/About/What-Is-HOS.html. Accessed August 27, 2013.
9. HealthGrades, The leading independent healthcare ratings organization. http://www.healthgrades.com. Accessed August 27, 2013.
10. *Standards of the Commission on Cancer, cancer program standards,* Chicago, 2004, American College of Surgeons.
11. *Case definitions for infectious conditions under public health surveillance,* Atlanta, Centers for Disease Control and Prevention. http://www.cdc.gov/mmwr/preview/mmwrhtml/00047449.htm. Accessed August 27, 2013.
12. Cancer Program Standards 2012: *Ensuring patient-centered care, version 1.1, page 50,* National Cancer Registrars Association, Chicago, 2012, Commission on Cancer, American College of Surgeons.
13. Code of Federal Regulations, Title 45, 164.501—Privacy of individually identifiable health information. http://www.law.cornell.edu/cfr/text/45/164.501. Accessed August 27, 2013.
14. National Cancer Registrars Association Education Foundation: *An introduction to the cancer registry instructor's guide.* www.ncra-usa.org. Accessed September 14, 2013.
15. Cancer Program Standards 2012: *Ensuring patient-centered care, version 1.1, page 19,* National Cancer Registrars Association, Chicago, 2012, Commission on Cancer, American College of Surgeons.
16. Menck HR, Smart CR, editors: *Central cancer registries: design, management and use,* Bethesda, MD, 1994, American Association of Central Cancer Registries.
17. National Cancer Institute: *Staging: questions and answers.* http://www.cancer.gov/cancertopics/factsheet/Detection/staging. August 27, 2013.
18. American Cancer Society: *Learn about cancer, The Surveillance, Epidemiology and End Results Program (SEER).* http://www.cancer.org/cancer/cancerbasics/cancer-surveillance-programs-and-registries-in-the-united-states. Accessed January 21, 2014.
19. National Tumor Registrars Association, Council on Certification. http://www.ctrexam.org/eligibility/index.htm#status. Accessed August 27, 2013.
20. Collaborative Staging: http://www.facs.org/cancer/coc/naaccr2004.pdf.
21. Email announcement: Info@ncra-usa.org. August 23, 2013.
22. NCRA's Formal Education Program Review Committee. www.ncra-usa.org/i4a/pages/index.cfm?pageid-3299.
23. Pregnancy and Newborn Health Education Center: *Fact sheet.* http://www.marchofdimes.com/professionals/14332_1206.asp. Accessed August 27, 2013.
24. Center for Disease Control and Prevention: *Facts about birth defects.* http://www.cdc.gov/ncbddd/birthdefects/facts.html. Accessed January 21, 2014.
25. Centers for Disease Control and Prevention: *State-based tracking systems.* http://www.cdc.gov/ncbddd/birthdefects/states/index.html. Accessed January 21, 2014.
26. Edmonds L: *State birth defects surveillance,* Centers for Disease Control and Prevention. National Center on Birth Defects and Developmental Disabilities. http://ncvhs.hhs.gov/030422p5.pdf.
27. Centers for Disease Control and Prevention: *Metropolitan Atlanta Congenital Defects Program (MACDP).* http://www.cdc.gov/ncbddd/birthdefects/MACDP.html. Accessed January 21, 2014.
28. Indian Health service, Division of Diabetes Treatment and Prevention: *The HIS diabetes care and outcomes audit.* http://www.ihs.gov/MedicalPrograms/Diabetes/index.cfm?module=resourcesAudit. Accessed January 21, 2014.
29. U.S. Food and Drug Administration: *Medical devices, FDS safety and innovation act.* http://www.fda.gov/MedicalDevices/DeviceRegulationandGuidance/Overview/ucm310927.htm. Accessed January 21, 2014.
30. New York Organ Donor Network, Transplantation. http://www.donatelifeny.org/all-about-transplantation/organ-transplant-history/. Accessed January 24, 2014.
31. Texas Department of State Health Services, Birth Defects Epidemiology & Surveillance Branch: *Texas birth defects registry fact sheet.* http://www.dshs.state.tx.us/birthdefects/. Accessed January 21, 2014.
32. Illinois Department of Public Health, Adverse Pregnancy Outcomes Reporting System. http://www.idph.state.il.us/about/epi/aporsrpt.htm. Accessed August 27, 2013.
33. Heim RT: Electronic death registration. In *National conference on health statistics August, 2010,* National Association for Public Health Statistics and Information Systems. http://www.cdc.gov/nchs/ppt/nchs2010/26_Trasatti.pdf.
34. Centers for Disease Control and Prevention: *Mortality data from National Vital Statistics System.* http://www.cdc.gov/nchs/nvss.htm. Accessed August 27, 2013.
35. Leading Causes of Death. FastStats Homepage. Centers for Disease Control and Prevention. http://www.cdc.gov/nchs/fastats/lcod.htm.
36. Centers for Disease Control and Prevention: *National diabetes prevention program, registry of recognized programs.* http://www.cdc.gov/diabetes/prevention/recognition/registry.htm. Accessed January 21, 2014.
37. Centers for Disease Control and Prevention: *Chronic disease prevention and health promotion, diabetes.* http://www.cdc.gov/chronicdisease/resources/publications/AAG/ddt.htm. Accessed January 21, 2014.
38. Khan L, Mincemoyer S, Gabbay R: Diabetes registries: where we are and where are we headed? *Diabetes Technol Ther* 11(4), 2009.
39. Kaiser Permanente, Division of Research, Diabetes Registry: http://www.dor.kaiser.org/external/DORExternal/research/distance.aspx. Accessed August 27, 2013.
40. U.S. Food and Drug Administration: *Medical device reporting for user facilities.* http://www.fda.gov/downloads/MedicalDevices/DeviceRegulatinsandGuidance/GuidanceDocuments/UCM095266.pdf. Accessed January 21, 2014.
41. National Immunization Program, Centers for Disease Control and Prevention. http://www.cdc.gov/vaccines/programs/iis/index.html. Accessed August 27, 2013.
42. Immunizations and Infectious Diseases: *Healthy people 2020—improving the health of Americans.* http://www.healthypeople.gov/2020/default.aspx.
43. United Network for Organ Sharing: *Who we are.* http://www.unos.org/about/. Accessed August 27, 2013.
44. United Network for Organ Sharing. http://www.unos.org/. Accessed August 27, 2013.
45. American College of Surgeons: *Trauma programs.* http://www.facs.org/trauma. Accessed August 27, 2013.
46. Centers for Disease Control and Prevention, 2005. http://www.cdc.gov/nchs/data/injury/DicussionDocu.pdf. Accessed August 27, 2013.
47. Trauma. Org: *Abbreviated Injury Scale (AIS) score.* http://www.trauma.org/index.php/main/article/510/. Accessed January 24, 2014.
48. Washington State Department of Health, Office of Community Health Systems: *Washington state trauma registry users guide, September 2011.* http://www.doh.wa.gov/Portals/1/Documents/Pubs/346043.pdf. Accessed January 24, 2014.
49. Department of Health and Human Services, Centers for Disease Control and Prevention Chicago Glasgow Coma Scale, http://www.bt.cdc.gov/masscasualties/pdf/glasgow-coma-scale.pdf. Accessed January 14, 2014.
50. National Association of State Head Injury Administrators: *Data collection.* http://www.biausa.org/About-Us/about-brain-injury-association.htm. Accessed August 27, 2013.

51. National Data and Statistical Center for Brain Injury Model. http://www.tbindsc.org.

52. National Center for Injury Prevention and Control: *CDC TBI registry abstracting.* http://www.cdc.gov/ncipc/profiles/tbi/al/default.htm.

53. *Code of federal regulations: title 45, public welfare.* http://www.hhs.gov/ohrp/humansubjects/guidance/45cfr46.html. Accessed September 3, 2013.

54. Layman EJ: Research and health informatics. In Layman EJ, Watzlaf VJ, editors: *Health informatics research,* Chicago, 2008, American Health Information Association, pp 3–21.

55. American Public Health Association: *Advocacy & policy, overview.* http://www.apha.org/advocacy/. Accessed January 14, 2014.

56. Institute of Medicine of the National Academies: *The future of the public's health in the 21st century, November 11, 2002:* http://www.nap.edu/openbook.php?isbn=030908704X. Accessed September 3, 2013.

57. American Health Informatics Association: *Informatics areas, public health informatics.* http://www.amia.org/applications-informatics/public-health-informatics. Accessed January 24, 2014.

58. Public Health Informatics: Core state department activities. http://en.wikipedia.org/wiki/Public_health_informatics.

59. Chu YT, Ng YY, Wu SC: Comparison of different comorbidity measures for use with administrative data in predicting short- and long-term mortality, *BMC Health Serv Res* 10:140, 2010. http://www.ncbi.nlm.nih.gov/pmc/articles/PMC2897792/pdf/1472-6963-10-140.pdf. Accessed on January 24, 2014.

60. CMS Premier Hospital Quality Incentive Demonstration Project: *What are APR-DRGs? An introduction to severity of illness and risk of mortality adjustment methodology, 2003.* https://www.premierinc.com/p4p/hqi/downloads/premier-hqid-final-white-paper-28nov2012.pdf. Accessed September 3, 2013.

61. Petersen L, Pietz K, Woodard L, et al.: Comparison of the predictive validity of diagnosis-based risk adjusters for clinical outcomes, *Med Care* 43:61–67, 2005.

62. Agency for Healthcare Research and Quality: *CCS software.* http://www.hcup-us.ahrq.gov/toolssoftware/ccs/ccs.jsp.

63. Williams S, Torrens P: *Introduction to health services,* ed 7, Albany, NY, 2008, Cengage Learning, Inc.

64. Johnston J, Wagner D, Timmons S, et al.: Impact of difference measure of comorbid disease on predicted mortality of intensive care unit patients, *Med Care* 40:929–940, 2002.

65. AHIMA Certified Health Data Analyst. http://www.ahima.org/certification/chda/default.aspx. Accessed January 18, 2010.

66. Bargmeyer BE, Gillman DW: *Metadata standards and metadata registries: an overview.* Bureau of Labor Statistics, Washington D.C. http://www.bls.gov/ore/pdf/st000010.pdf. Accessed January 14, 2014.

67. Government HealthIT: *On healthcare metadata and Dublin Core, May 16, 2012.* http://www.govhealthit.com/blog/healthcare-metadata-and-dublin-core. Accessed January 14, 2014.

68. Kendall KE, Kendall JE: *Systems analysis and design,* ed 8, Camdens, NJ, 2011, Prentice Hall.

69. Brackett M: *Data sharing, using a common data architecture,* New York, 1994, Wiley.

70. Simsion G, Witt GC: *Data modeling essentials,* ed 3, San Francisco, 2005, Morgan Kaufmann Publishers, Elsevier, Inc.

71. Batini C, DiBattista G, Santucci G, et al.: *Design of data dictionaries,* Amsterdam, 1992, IOS Press.

72. Clayton C, Genton S: Health information managers and clinical data repositories: a natural fit, *J AHIMA* 67:48–51, 1996.

73. Institute of Medicine: *The computer-based patient record,* Washington, DC, 1991, National Academy Press.

74. Jollis JG, Ancukiewicz M, DeLong ER, et al.: Discordance of databases designed for claims payment versus clinical information systems, *Ann Intern Med* 119:844–850, 1993.

75. Association jumps into outcomes software game, *Health Data Network News* 5:4, 1996.

76. Casto AB, Layman E: *Principles of healthcare reimbursement,* ed 3, Chicago, 2011, AHIMA.

77. American Health Information Management Association: *Automated coding software: development and use to enhance anti-fraud,* Chicago, 2005, American Health Information Management Association.

CHAPTER 14

PUBLIC HEALTH INFORMATICS

Bryant Thomas Karras, MD • Mary Alice Hanken, Ph.D., RHIA, CHPS

(e) Student Study Guide activities for this chapter are available on the Evolve Learning Resources site for this textbook. Please visit http://evolve.elsevier.com/Abdelhak.

CHAPTER CONTENTS

OBJECTIVES

✓ Identify how public health and medical care activities and interests converge.

✓ Explain the purpose of the Healthy People 2020 goals and objectives.

✓ Compare progress on Healthy People 2020 objectives with targets.

✓ Identify major achievements in the United States' use of vaccines to control infectious diseases.

✓ List at least 5 immediately reportable communicable disease conditions.

✓ Discuss vaccine targets in Healthy People 2020 that are not being met.

✓ List the meaningful use objectives in stage one and stage two related to public health.

✓ Explain the potential information system gains possible for public health by using health information exchange tools.

✓ Explain why population-based health data is useful to a community and to the United States.

✓ List the services provided by public health agencies and the value of each service to the community.

✓ Describe the public health system's efforts to establish information systems to support its services.

✓ Identify at least three significant events prior to 2010 that shaped the current U.S. public health system.

✓ Provide current examples of how the public health system contributes to the health of U.S. citizens.

✓ Identify at least 3 of the agencies under the umbrella of the Public Health Service.

KEY WORDS:

Health Information Exchange
Meaningful use
Public health
Syndromic Surveillance

ABBREVIATIONS

ADT   Admission, Discharge, Transfer (also RegADT: Registration, Admission, Discharge, Transfer)

ARRA   American Recovery and Reinvestment Act; Stimulus Bill

CDC   Centers for Disease Control

CMS   Centers for Medicaid and Medicare Services

EH   Eligible Hospital

EHR   Electronic Health Record (sometimes abbreviated EMR or cEHRT)

EP   Eligible Professional

HEDIS   Healthcare Effectiveness Data and Information Set

HITECH   Health Information Technology for Economic and Clinical Health; HIT Stimulus Bill

HIE   Health Information Exchange

HL7   Health Level 7

IOM   Institute of Medicine

LOINC   Logical Observation Identifers Names and Codes

MU   Meaningful Use

NBS   NEDSS Base System

NCQA   National Committee for Quality Assurance

NEDSS   National Electronic Disease Surveillance System

nwHIN   Nationwide Health Information Network

ONC   Office of the National Coordinator for Health IT

PHIN   Public Health Information Network

SNOMED   Systematized Nomenclature of Medicine

PUBLIC HEALTH AND MEDICAL CARE

As we take a more overall view of health, we recognize the value of lifestyles, safe and clean communities, and the myriad things we can do to prevent injuries at home, at work, and in our communities. As organizations prepare to manage individuals' health care, they realize that the power and payoff are not in treating individuals for expensive diseases and conditions but in preventing disease and in educating consumers to take care of themselves. This shift is the impetus needed to bring the public health sector and the medical care sectors together. The long-range goals of both groups are similar, but to many observers it appears that the two sectors are not strongly connected.

Public health provides both direct clinical services and community services. It addresses both the individual and the population being served in a community or wider region. Public health goals for the year 2020 are expressed in terms of the entire population in the United States and is called Healthy People 2020. These goals are developed with broad input from many sources in the United States. The goals and specific objectives are published, updated, and measured by the Centers for Disease Control (CDC). Periodic updates are published by the CDC.

HEALTHY PEOPLE 2020

Healthy People 2020 covers 42 topic areas and 1200 objectives. It is a source of reliable public health measures that are supported by data.[1] Over time, the number of objectives have increased and the overall goals have changed. (See Figure 14-1.)

Immunizations and Infectious Diseases

One of the Healthy People 2020 topics is immunization and infectious diseases. There are a number of goals and

Target Year	1990 HEALTHY PEOPLE 1990	2000 HEALTHY PEOPLE 2000	2010 HEALTHY PEOPLE 2010	2020 HEALTHY PEOPLE 2020
Overarching Goals	• Decrease mortality: infants-adults • Increase independence among older adults	• Increase span of healthy life • Reduce health disparities • Achieve access to preventive services for all	• Increase quality and years of healthy life • Eliminate health disparities	• Attain high-quality, longer lives free of preventable disease • Achieve health equity; eliminate disparities • Create social and physical environments that promote good health • Promote quality of life, healthy development, healthy behaviors across life stages
# Topic Areas	15	22	28	42
# Objectives/ Measures	226 / NA	312 / NA	467 / 1,000	1,200 / 1200

FIGURE 14-1 Evolution of Health People. (Source: Healthy People 2020 Progress Review (Power Point), April 18, 2013, Violence Across the Lifespan, Office of Disease Prevention and Health Promotion, CDC.)

objectives in this section, including the following goal and objectives related to adolescents:

- Immunization and Infectious Diseases: Increase routine vaccination coverage levels for adolescents. (IID-11)

There are four more specific objectives under that goal. They are:

- IID-11-1 Increase vaccination coverage level of 1 dose of tetanus-diptheria-acellular pertussis (Tdap) booster vaccine for adolescents aged 13 to 15 years. Baseline: 46.7% of adolescents aged 13 to 15 had received at least 1 dose of a Tdap booster in 2008. Target: 80.0%.
- IID-11-2 Increase the vaccination coverage level of 2 doses of varicella vaccine for adolescents by aged 13 to 15 (excluding chidren who have had varicella) in 2008. Baseline: 36.7% of adolescents aged 13 to 15 had received at least 2 doses of varicella vaccine (excluding adolescents who have had varicella) in 2008. Target: 90.0%.
- IID-11-3 Increase the vaccination coverage level of 1 dose meningococcal conjugate vaccine for adolescents aged 13 to 15. Baseline: 43.9% of adolescents aged 13 to 15 years had received at least 1 dose of meningococcal conjugate vaccine in 2008. Target: 80.0%.
- IID-11-4 Increase the vaccination coverage level of 3 doses of human papillomavirus (HPV) vaccine for females aged 13 to 15. Baseline: 16.6% of females aged 13 to 15 had received at least 3 doses of human papillomavirus (HPV) in 2008. Target: 80.0%.[2]
- Figure 14-2 shows vaccination coverage of adolescents aged 13 to 15 for 2009 through 2011.[3]

The health and longevity of people in the United States is due to many factors, one of which is the decrease in infectious disease. Prevention through vaccines is a major contributor to this success. There are now 17 recommended vaccines to prevent various diseases throughout a person's lifespan. We are all familiar with the push to vaccinate infants and young children, and efforts in this area are close to their

targets. However, adolescent health is emerging as an area where the United States can do better. Vaccine use is one component of improving adolescent health.

? DID YOU KNOW?

Vaccines in the United States reduce direct health care costs by $14 billion dollars and prevent 20 million cases of disease.[4]

(Source: CDC. Ten Great Public Health Achievements – United States 2001-2010. *MMWR*, May 20, 2011.)

In the United States in 1900 infectious diseases were the top three leading causes of death (pneumonia/influenza, tuberculosis, and diarrhea/enteritis). By 1950 pneumonia/influenza had dropped to sixth place as a cause of death and tuberculosis to seventh place. (The top three causes of death were heart disease, cancer, and stroke.) In 2010 only pneumonia/influenza remained in the top ten at ninth place. (The top three causes were heart disease, cancer, and chronic lung disease.)[5]

? DID YOU KNOW?

Tuberculosis is still present in the United States. and Mexico. In 2010 Mexico had 18,848 cases and the United States had 11,171 cases. Data collected about prevalence in the U.S. border states in 2010 showed that California had 2,324 cases, Texas had 1,385 cases, and Arizona had 282 cases. The rate per 100,000 people in the United States was 3.6 cases; the rate per 100,000 people was 6.2 cases in California, 5.5 cases in Texas, 4.4 cases in Arizona, all exceeding the national rate 3.6 per 100,000 cases.

Mexico's border states also had high rates: Baja 54.1, Tamaulipas 35.9, and Sonora 31.2. Mexico's overall rate was 16.8 per 100,000.[6]

Public health carries out surveillance of infectious diseases through its infrastructure at the local, state, and federal levels

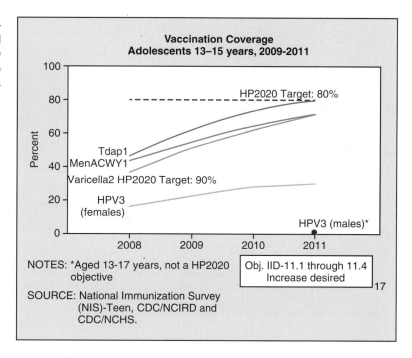

FIGURE 14-2 Vaccination coverage of adolescents 13–15 for 2009–2011. (Source: National Immunization Survey (NIS) Teen, CDC/NCIRD and CDC/NCHS. Published in the Healthy People 2020 Progress Review: The Burden of Tuberculosis and Infectious Diseases in the U.S. and Abroad, July 30, 2013.)

and encourages communities to take advantage of vaccines and current treatment. Prevention is the goal and vaccines are a cost-effective method of prevention. Achieving recommended levels of vaccination and tracking immunization data require the coordination of the medical and public communities. The use of vaccines saves lives, reduces disease, and reduces the costs of health care.

Infections such as pneumonia and influenza are among the top 10 causes of death each year. In 2009 H1N1 influenza caused an estimated 270,000 hospitalizations and 12,270 deaths (1,270 of which were people under age 18).[7] Tuberculosis and hepatitis can be prevented, but more emphasis is needed on using TB and hepatitis prevention approaches. Because people travel around the world today, infections also travel easily (see Box 14-1).

Some of the public health challenges related to infectious disease are international travel, migration into the United States, food and agricultural practices, inappropriate use of antibiotics, and threats of bioterrorism.

BOX 14-1 Middle East Respiratory Virus: Tracking Health Issues

Middle East Respiratory Syndrome (MERS) is caused by a coronavirus. Most people with this confirmed diagnosis develop severe acute respiratory illness including fever, cough, and shortness of breath. About 30% of people confirmed to have MERS infection die. On May 2, 2014 the first U.S. case of MERS was confirmed in a recent traveler from Saudi Arabia. A second case was confirmed a few days later from another traveler from Saudi Arabia. The third U.S. case is a U.S. resident who was in close contact with the first case, the traveler from Saudi Arabia. The CDC has provided guidance to travelers and healthcare providers with the goal of preventing the spread of MERS in the U.S. Individuals with acute respiratory illness and any history of connection to an individual who recently visited the Middle East can be tested for the MERS virus. What is the status of MERS in the U.S. now?[8]

Injury and Violence: Public Health Impact

Another topic area in Healthy People 2020 is injury and violence in the United States. Injuries and violence are the leading cause of death for individuals ages 1 through 44. Injury and violence affects all age groups. There were 181,000 deaths in 2010—one every 3 minutes attributed to injury/violence. There were 33,700 motor vehicle deaths for all ages. Poisoning deaths for people ages 25 through 64 totaled 36,600. There were 22,000 deaths attributed to falls for individuals 65 and older. Homicide deaths for ages birth through 24 totaled 5,600, including 1,500 deaths from child abuse/neglect.[9,10]

In 2010 2.9 million workers were injured on the job; approximately 110,000 were hospitalized and 4,690 died. The United States also had 137,400 work related assaults seen in emergency departments in 2009. Each year these work related injuries, deaths, and illnesses cost $250 billion dollars. (See Figure 14-3.)

The CDC's National Center for Health Statistics (NCHS) is the principal health statistics agency in the U.S. NCHS compiles statistical information to help guide public health and health policy decisions. The goal of NCHS is to collect accurate and timely data on injuries and other health issues. Injury data rely on NCHS's data from multiple sources (see Figure 14-4). Sources for injury data include:

National Vital Statistics System collects mortality data from death certificates in all 50 states and the District of Columbia, including characteristics of the decedent and underlying and contributing causes of death. Injury deaths are annual counts of persons who died for whom the death certificate lists an external cause as the underlying cause of death.[11]

National Health Care Surveys collects data about the facilities that supply health care, the services rendered, and the characteristics of the patients served. Data are obtained from hospitals, office-based physician practices, emergency and outpatient departments,

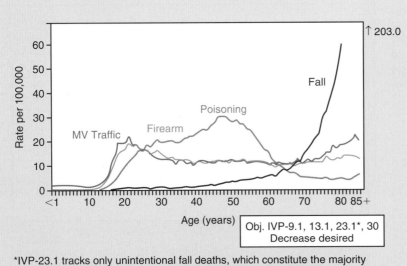

FIGURE 14-3 Injury deaths by cause and age, 2009–2010. (Source: National Vital Statistics System—Mortality (NVSS-M), CDC/NCHS)

*IVP-23.1 tracks only unintentional fall deaths, which constitute the majority of fall deaths. IVP-23.1 does not include fall deaths that are of intentional or of undetermined intent. Data for all fall deaths are shown here.

SOURCE: National Vital Statistics System–Mortality (NVSS-M), CDC/NCHS.

FIGURE 14-4 Injuries in the United States. (Source: National Vital Statistics System 2009, National Hospital Discharge Survey, National Hospital Ambulatory Medical Care Survey, National Health Interview Survey.)

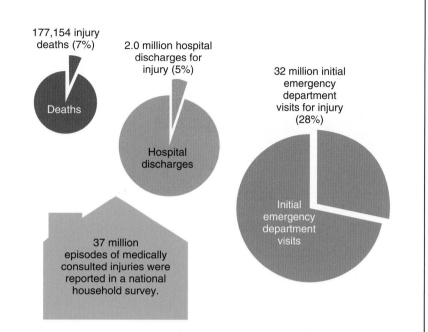

177,154 injury deaths (7%)

Deaths

2.0 million hospital discharges for injury (5%)

Hospital discharges

32 million initial emergency department visits for injury (28%)

Initial emergency department visits

37 million episodes of medically consulted injuries were reported in a national household survey.

More striking that the number of injury deaths is the number of injuries seen in hospitals and emergency departments.

- In 2009, for each death by injury, there were about 11 times as many hospitalizations and 182 times as many emergency department (ED) visits.
- In 2009, the average length of hospital stay for treatment of an injury was 4.8 days.

Data on the nature of the injury and the part of the body involved provide important information on health care utilization and assist in targeting prevention strategies. Mortality data and hospital survey data from 2009 show:

- Fractures accounted for 54 percent of hospitalized injuries. Among adults ages 65 and over, hip fractures accounted for 30 percent of hospitalizations and were mentioned in 16 percent of injury deaths.
- Traumatic brain injury resulted in 51,000 deaths, 245,000 hospitalizations, and 507,000 initial ED visits.

ambulatory surgery centers, nursing homes, and home health and hospice agencies.[12]

National Health Interview Survey collects data on all medically consulted injuries and poisonings occurring to any family member during the 3-month period prior to the interview. Information is available about the external cause and nature of the injury or poisoning episode, the activity the individual was engaged in at the time of the injury or poisoning episode, and the place of occurrence. Information is also obtained from the individual describing how the person was injured or poisoned.[13,14]

The CDC would like to see improved external cause of injury coding in all hospitals and emergency departments. In 2010 the hospital discharge data system was reporting external cause of injury codes for 64% of hospital discharges. The target for 2020 is 85% and the goal is 90%. Emergency departments in 2010 were reporting external injury codes for 78% of visits. The 2020 target is 85% and the goal is 90%. Another improvement in data reporting would be to select a main injury diagnosis among all injury diagnoses

contributing to an injury death. The CDC also encourages full use of the death certificate to include the circumstances of injury. The improved data will help in the development of injury prevention efforts.

Injuries take a toll on the population of the U.S., including social and economic costs. Injuries are still among the leading causes of death in the U.S. If we understand more about the causes of injuries, more can be done to prevent them (see Figure 14-5, Injury Death by Mechanism). In 2009 drug poisoning became the leading cause of injury death in the U.S. During the last three decades, the number of drug poisoning deaths increased sixfold from about 6,100 in 1980 to 37,000 in 2009.

Data on the nature of the injury and the part of the body involved provide important information on health care utilization and help in targeting prevention strategies. Mortality data and hospital survey data from 2009 show that fractures accounted for 54% of hospitalized injuries. Among adults ages 65 and over, hip fractures accounted for 30% of hospitalizations and were mentioned in 16% of injury deaths. It is

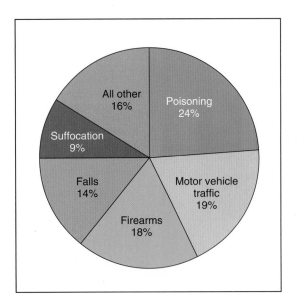

FIGURE 14-5 Injury deaths by mechanism: United States, 2009. (Source National Vital Statistics System, 2009.)

also helpful to know what an injured person was doing and where his or her injury occurred. Many nonfatal injuries occur at home.

The use of the health care system is demonstrated by 2009 data showing that for each death by injury there were about 11 times as many hospitalizations and 182 times as many emergency department visits. The average length of hospital inpatient stay for an injury in 2009 was 4.8 days. See Figure 14-6 to compare injury deaths with other categories of cause of death.

One of the Healthy People 2020 goals is to reduce the number of emergency department visits for nonfatal traumatic brain injuries; the real goal is to reduce the number of traumatic brain injuries. The baseline data for 2007 is 407.2 emergency department visits per 100,000 population for initial emergency department visits for nonfatal traumatic brain injuries (see Figures 14-7 and 14-8). However, instead of decreasing the rate has increased, and in 2010 the rate was 681.0 emergency department visits per 100,000 population. The most dramatic increase is in the age group 0 to 4 years of age. In 2009 persons age 0 to 4 had a rate of 2,272.2 visits per 100,000 population.

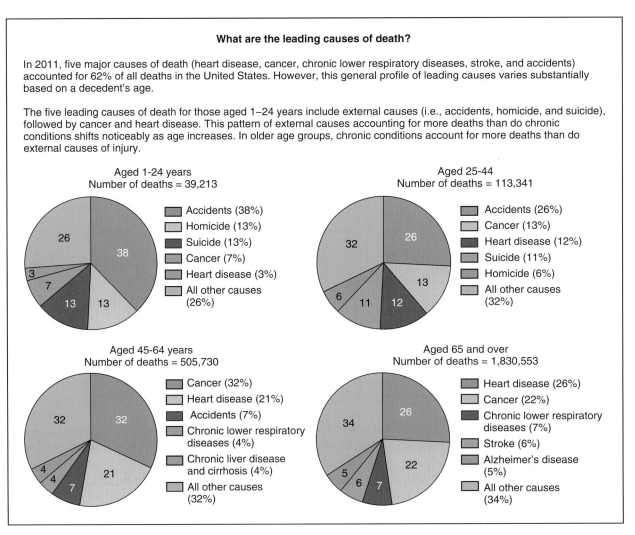

FIGURE 14-6 Leading cause of death by age group. (Source: National Vital Statistics Data Brief, No. 115, March 2013.)

To examine the data in more detail the CDC also breaks the data into groupings by sex, race/ethnicity, age group, geographic location, and health insurance status (see Box 14-2). This breakdown is provided to help examine goal IVP-2.3, Reduce emergency department visits for nonfatal traumatic brain injuries (see Table 14-1).

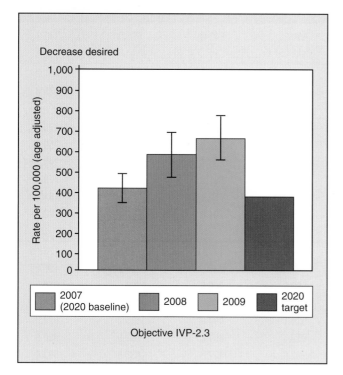

FIGURE 14-7 Initial emergency department visits for nonfatal traumatic brain injuries 2007-2009.

BOX 14-2 How Can You Use the Population Data on ED Visits in Your Community?

After review of figures related to ED initial visits for nonfatal traumatic brain injuries, how could you use this data in your community?

In 2009 traumatic brain injury resulted in 51,000 deaths, 245,000 hospitalizations, and 507,000 initial emergency department visits.

Tobacco use has been a target of public health campaigns for many years. Adults have reduced their use of tobacco significantly to about 12% of the U.S. adult population. Many organizations have made significant changes about smoking in the workplace, in restaurants, and on airplanes. However, the CDC is finding in its youth risk behavior surveys that 26% of adolescents in grades 9 through 12 have used tobacco in the last 30 days. The 2020 target for youth is to reduce this risk behavior to 21%.

Insurance companies also recognize that a number of health problems are related to use of tobacco and are beginning to provide tobacco cessation programs. Public health organizations are also working to establish laws related to smoke-free indoor air in worksites, restaurants, bars, daycare centers, public transportation, multiunit housing, prisons, correctional facilities, vehicles transporting children, school/college/university campuses, and all health care sites. The use of e-cigarettes has not yet made the list of 2020 goals and targets related to improved health, although the substances being used in most e-cigarettes are recognized as addictive. If you are collecting data about smoking and tobacco use for meaningful use and other public health purposes you may want to consider including the use of e-cigarettes.

Healthy People 2020 provides a combination of goals and targets as well as data that can easily be accessed and combined with programs to improve the quality of individual and community health.

FIGURE 14-8 Initial emergency department visits for nonfatal traumatic brain injuries by Age groups 2007–2009. (Source: CDC Healthy People 2020.)

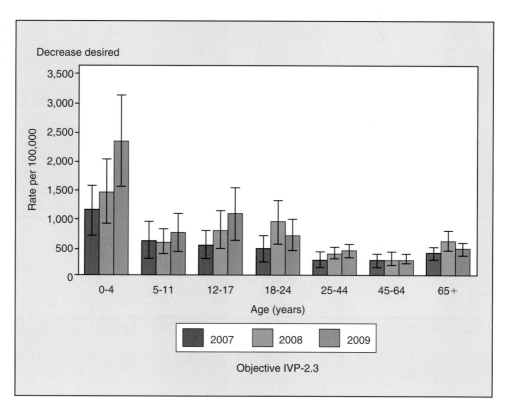

TABLE 14-1

Injury and Violence Prevention
IVP-2.3 Reduce emergency department (ED) visits for nonfatal traumatic brain injuries
Emergency department visits for nonfatal traumatic brain injuries (age adjusted, per 100,000 population)
2020 Baseline (year): 407.2 (2007) **2020 Target:** 365.3 **Desired Direction:** Decrease desired

Populations	2007	2008	2009	2010	2011
Total	407.2	569.6	645.9	681.0	770.3
Sex					
Male	436.1	652.7	810.2	747.7	901.2
Female	367.6	482.5	472.0	609.1	625.6
Race/Ethnicity					
Black or African American only	658.1	711.2	761.1	930.9	993.7
White only	389.7	563.6	638.0	677.5	750.1
Hispanic or Latino	458.8	392.7	435.9	—	740.2
Not Hispanic or Latino	416.9	613.3	691.2	—	778.4
Black or African American only, not Hispanic or Latino	684.1	721.3	750.1	—	1016.4
White only, not Hispanic or Latino	400.6	625.6	704.8	—	773.8
Age Group[†§]					
<18 years	714.0	881.9	1282.0	1207.5	1268.9
0–4 years	1103.1	1416.0	2272.2	1913.8	1957.9
5–11 years	603.5	560.6	748.5	888.2	618.5
12–17 years	517.4	791.9	1044.1	969.5	1458.1
18–44 years	305.7	524.1	497.8	585.2	627.3
18–24 years	446.6	923.5	691.8	989.9	906.9
25–44 years	256.5	382.6	427.3	435.6	522.4
45–64 years	250.9	282.8	279.8	280.5	413.9
45–54 years	205.9	340.4	266.3	292.4	492.7
55–64 years	311.3	DSU	297.0	265.8	321.4
65 years and over	385.8	612.6	471.5	653.0	850.9
65–74	DSU	328.4	276.5	412.6	622.8
75–84 years	DSU	566.5	578.6	777.4	1127.5
85 years and over	DSU	1717.5	DSU	DSU	1109.4
Geographic Location (of provider)					
Metropolitan	439.2	603.2	667.4	710.7	808.0
Non-metropolitan	277.8	467.1	609.8	583.4	647.6
Health Insurance Status (<65 Years)					
Insured	322.7	448.5	523.5	584.4	601.9
Private	277.3	450.5	510.4	569.1	511.4
Public	536.5	538.6	647.9	713.6	937.9
Uninsured	351.0	628.1	604.0	489.0	641.3

[†]Target is not applicable for this population group.
[§]This population group is not age adjusted.
DSU: Data do not meet the criteria for statistical reliability, data quality, or confidentiality.
—: Data are not available.
Data are subject to revision and may have changed since a previous release.
Unless noted otherwise, any age-adjusted data are adjusted using the year 2000 standard population.
Data are not available or not collected for populations not shown.

Data Source: National Hospital Ambulatory Medical Care Survey (NHAMCS), CDC/NCHS; Population Estimates, Census

MEANINGFUL USE AND PUBLIC HEALTH REPORTING

Meaningful use is an incentive program established by the Centers for Medicare and Medicaid (CMS) using the American Recovery and Reinvestment Act (ARRA).[16] The program provides funds to encourage eligible professionals (EP) and eligible hospitals (EH) to adopt and use certified electronic health record systems. To receive the incentive funding providers and hospitals must meet various public health and operational objectives. The long-range plan is to improve patient care. Qualified electronic health record systems must be certified to assure that they have the functionalities that can be used to improve care and health (both individual and population). The incentives are largest for early adopters who can reap the benefits of the incentives of this time-limited program over a period of years. Once the certified electronic record systems are in place, the providers and hospitals must meet both core and menu objectives to quality for continued incentive funding. Professionals and hospitals must meet all core objectives as determined by Medicare or Medicaid. Stage one and Stage Two meaningful use objectives linked to public health practice are listed in Table 14-2. Providers and hospitals must meet all core objectives.

- Providers and hospitals must meet 5 of the menu objectives, one of which must be a public health objective.

Further, the Stimulus bill of 2009 (ARRA: American Recovery and Reinvestment Act; HITECH: Health Information Technology for Economic and Clinical Health) requires state-of-the-art health information technology system EHRs to automatically report certain types of data to public health, thus bringing closer together clinical and public health practice. The initial requirement (Stage One) was to pick one of the public health objectives and test that data could actually be submitted. Stage Two requires actual submission of data. Public health agencies will be expected to be able to receive HL7 messages for registry and reportable conditions, receive de-identified data based on syndromic surveillance rules and send alerts to health care providers about public health events.

HEALTH INFORMATION EXCHANGE AND PUBLIC HEALTH

With the increased use of EHR systems and health information exchanges (HIEs), clinical care information and public health information systems can leverage the interest in data exchange to more actively prevent, detect, and manage disease. Both clinical providers and public health providers will have access to reliable information that is available at the right time, delivered to the right people, and in a format that is useful for all parties. The plan is to inform decision-making at the patient and community level.

Public health is actively using the policies and guidelines developed by the Nationwide Health Information Network (nwHIN) and supported by the ONC. The Public Health Information Network (PHIN) sees itself as the Population and Public Health component of the nwHIN, joining with the components of Care Cordination; Patients and Families; Quality, Safety, and Efficiency; and Privacy and Security.

In Washington State the health information exchange is called One Health Port. One Health Port is designed to be low cost, accessible, and secure.[17] The HIE offers a number of services and has a growing list of subscribers. Initially the most popular tool was eligibility verifications. Several standard message transactions include:

Standard Testing Process: Designed to allow trading partners to test trading sample data before a "go-live"

Continuity of Care Document: Standard mapping for the continuity of care document

Prescription Monitoring Program: Standard mapping for medication history request from the Washington State Department of Health Prescription Monitoring Program database. The database contains all controlled substance prescriptions filled in Washington State in the last year.

Electronic Laboratory Reporting: Electronic transmission from laboratories to public health (Washington State Department of Health) of laboratory reportsthat identify reportable conditions

---

TABLE 14-2 Meaningful Use and Public Health Objectives

	Public Health Objectives	Hospitals (EH)	Clinics (EP)	Requirement
Stage 1	Electronic Laboratory Reporting (ELR)	Must pick 1 of 3	N/A	1 test submission of data
	Immunization Information Systems		Must pick 1 of 2	
	Syndromic Surveillance			
Stage 2	Electronic Laboratory Reporting (ELR)	Required	N/A	Ongoing Submission
	Immunization Information Systems	Required	Required	
	Syndromic Surveillance	Required	Menu Option	
	Cancer Registry Reporting	N/A	Menu Option	
	Specialized Registry (e.g. Prescription Monitoring Program, newborn/hearing screening)	N/A	Menu Option	

(Source Department of Health, WA State http://www.doh.wa.gov/ForPublicHealthandHealthcareProviders/Healthcare Professional 3/5/2014.)

BOX 14-3   What Is Syndromic Surveillance?

Syndromic surveillance is a process that regularly and systematically uses health and health-related data in near "real-time" to make information available on the health of a community. This information includes statistics on disease trends and community health seeking behaviors that support essential public health surveillance functions by public health agencies. Syndromic surveillance is particularly useful to local, state, and federal public health agencies for supporting public health situational awareness, emergency response management, and outbreak recognition and characterization. Patient encounter data, including de-identified data, are a critical input for syndromic surveillance.[19]

Syndromic Surveillance: Electronic transmission of patient encounter information from providers to public health (Washington State Department of Health) for disease trends and public health surveillance functions

HL7 Canonical Guide (Lab, Radiology, ADT): The more routine components are available for results reporting with the ADT transaction.

Immunization Registry: HIE intends to support the statewide immunization registry.

Community Referral and Consult Report: The referral and consult report can be sent and received by participants in the HIE (see Box 14-3).[18]

The Washington State One Health Port is using the CDC format for transmitting syndromic surveillance data. The CDC Public Health Information Network (PHIN) Guide includes case studies. One case study is for an urgent care or emergency department visit (see Figure 14-9). The patient's chief complaint or reason for visit is captured as text. The plan is to pull data elements as appropriate from the registration data (ADT system) of the electronic health record system at the urgent care site and transmit them to the local public health department system. In the sample messages the urgent care center is identified as "MidTwnUrgentC" and the reason for visit is "Fever, chills, smelly urine with burning during urination." The second sample message after diagnosis and treatment adds an ICD9CM diagnosis of "Urinary tract infection, site not specified."

One Health Port also hosts non-standard community forms and transactions between trading partners (see Box 14-4). This allows two or more trading partners to agree to exchange certain information important to their health care process. For example providers are interested in using One Health Port as a secure means of exchanging referral information. As a result the HIE has developed a sample referral form (see Table 14-3).

POPULATION-BASED DATA

Managed care organizations that take on a group of enrollees are now asked to express their data in terms of the population they serve. The Healthcare Effectiveness Data and Information Set (formerly the Health Plan Employer Data and Information Set) (HEDIS) report card system looks at data using much the same approach as the Healthy People approach by the Centers for Disease Control (CDC). The HEDIS program is sponsored by NCQA to measure performance of America's health plans. HEDIS uses 80 measures across 5 domains of care. Some of the health issues addressed are similar to the Healthy People 2020 goals/objectives (see Box 14-5).

As the data is aggregated across health plans it provides information on the status of meeting a quality of care goal for a given population. NCQA produces a report titled the "State of Health Care Quality".

Employers and consumers who purchase health care need feedback regarding the quality of care purchased for the dollar spent. While weighted toward measures based on data available on billing claims, data extracted from clinical records is also used to evaluate these measures. For example, use of appropriate medications for people with asthma. Many health care visits, hospitalizations, missed work and school days could be avoided if individuals have appropriate medications and disease management.

When data for all HEDIS health plans are combined it covers a significant share of the U.S. population. The HEDIS reporting combines reference data from the CDC with HEDIS data. For example, the 2013 State of Health Care Quality Report by NCQA includes a section on influenza. HEDIS tracks the number of adults who receive the annual flu vaccination. The goal is to prevent the flu through vaccination because of the health risk but also because of the economic burden it creates. The overall goal for adult annual flu vaccination is 90%. The adult levels of vaccination (ages 50 and older) show some gains during the most recent reporting but much work is needed to achieve the 90% goal (see Tables 14-4 and 14-5).

As communities discuss and implement regional data systems, they expand the base of population data available. While most care providers hope that these systems will also support individual direct care through coordinating and reduction of duplication, most policymakers and researchers see the benefit in gaining access to more population-based data. As HEDIS and regional and national systems demonstrate, data are valuable only if they are accurate and reliable. This requires appropriate definitions for data, standards for the content, collection, and quality of the data—all skills of the health information manager.

INFORMATION NEEDS AND CORE PUBLIC HEALTH FUNCTIONS

The public health and managed care/medical care systems have similar information needs. The following discussion focuses primarily on public health. Public health is not simply medical care funded or provided through public means. The goal of public health is prevention of disease, injury, disability, and premature death (see Box 14-6). Some services of public health are less visible and may be more difficult to understand than medical services. We may not think of clean water as contributing to our health, but

Syndromic Surveillance Messaging Example
Brief Urgent Care or Emergency Department Visit

Case Study 1 provides an example of a brief patient visit that could take place in either urgent care or emergency department clinical settings. The patient's chief complaint is captured as an unstructured, free-text value using the patient's own words. ADT A04 and A03 messages are generated and sent to the PHA about this visit.

Step 1: Registration Trigger - ADT A04

A 35 year old female walks into Midtown Urgent Care on August 17, 2012 at 12:00 PM. The patient is registered by a clerical assistant who records the patient's name, date of birth, residence information, race, ethnicity, and records that the patient's reason for visit is, "Fever, chills, smelly urine with burning during urination."

At 12:30 PM on August 17, 2012, the facilities electronic health record module for syndromic surveillance data assembles and transmits a Registration message to Big City Health Department about this visit.

Example Message - Step1, Case 1:

```
MSH|^~\&|| DownTownProcessing^2231237890^NPI|||201208171230||ADT^A04^ADT_A01|NIST-SS-001.12|P|2.5.1|||||||||PH_SS-NoAck^SS Sender^2.16.840.1.114222.4.10.3^ISO

EVN||201208171230|||||MidTwnUrgentC^2231231234^NPI
PID|1||2222^^^^MR||^^^^^~^^^^^S|||F||2106-3^^CDCREC|^^^^30303^^^^13121|||||||||||2135-2^^CDCREC
PV1|1||||||||||||||||||||2222_001^^^^VN|||||||||||||||||||||||201208171200
OBX|1|CWE|SS003^^PHINQUESTION||261QU0200X^Urgent Care^HCPTNUCC||||||F
OBX|2|NM|21612-7^^LN||35|a^^UCUM||||||F
OBX|3|CWE|8661-1^^LN||^Fever, chills, smelly urine with burning during urination||||||F
```

Step 2: Discharge Trigger: ADT A03

At 12:35 PM a nurse practitioner examines the patient and diagnoses the patient with urinary tract infection. The nurse assigns an ICD-9-CM diagnosis code of 599.0 within the EHR, and orders a course of antibiotics for the patient. The patient is discharged from the Urgent Care Center at 12:45 PM.

At 2:30 PM on August 17, 2012 the facility's electronic health record module for syndromic surveillance data assembles and transmits a Discharge message to Big City Health Department about this visit.

Example Message - Step 2, Case 1:

```
MSH|^~\&|| DownTownProcessing^2231237890^NPI|||201208171430||ADT^A03^ADT_A03|NIST-SS-001.22|P|2.5.1|||||||||PH_SS-NoAck^SS Sender^2.16.840.1.114222.4.10.3^ISO
EVN||201208171430|||||MidTwnUrgentC^2231231234^NPI
PID|1||2222^^^^MR||^^^^^~^^^^^S|||F||2106-3^^CDCREC|^^^^30303^^^^13121|||||||||||2135-2^^CDCREC
PV1|1||||||||||||||||||||2222_001^^^^VN|||||||||||||||||01||||||||201208171200
DG1|1||599^Urinary tract infection, site not specified^I9CDX|||F
OBX|1|CWE|SS003^^PHINQUESTION||261QU0200X^Urgent Care^HCPTNUCC||||||F
OBX|2|NM|21612-7^^LN||35|a^^UCUM||||||F
OBX|3|CWE|8661-1^^LN||^Fever, chills, smelly urine with burning during urination||||||F
```

FIGURE 14-9 Syndromic surveillance messaging example.

BOX 14-4   Use Cases Available on Washington State Health Information Exchange

Eligibility verifications
Lab and radiology results
Continuity of care document
Immunization reporting and checking
Electronic prescribing
ADT discharge summaries/patient demographics (see Table 14-2)

BOX 14-6   Public Health Obligations

The fundamental obligation of agencies responsible for population-based health is to:
- Prevent epidemics and the spread of disease
- Protect against environmental hazards
- Prevent injuries
- Promote and encourage healthy behaviors and mental health
- Respond to disasters and assist communities in recovery
- Assure the quality and accessibility of health services

BOX 14-5   Health Issues Tracked in HEDIS

Breast Cancer Screening
Childhood and Adolescent Immunization Status
Asthma Medication Use
Childhood and Adult Weight/BMI Assessment

contamination of drinking water results in sickness. Even today, when floods or earthquakes hit areas of the United States, water supplies may be disrupted or contaminated. Leaching of chemicals from farmland fertilizers and pesticides or industrial plants is another source of contamination.

TABLE 14-3   Sample Use Cases HIE One Health Port

The following sample use cases are provided to give examples of how the data exchange works.

Character	Systems	Wants to Send	Wants to Receive
Dr. Kant	Does not have an EMR	Transcription, forms	Lab reports and CCD via web browser
Dr. Able	Has a qualified EMR & practice system (PMS)	eRx, CCD, forms, immunizations	CCD, eRx, immunizations, ADT, eligibility
My Neighborhood Pharmacy	Has a real-time pharmacy system	eRx, Med history, immunizations	eRx, CCD, lab results, immunizations
Northwest Lab	Several	Lab results	Lab orders, ADT, eligibility
Images Anywhere	Several	Rad results, images	CCD, orders, eligibility
General Hospital	Several	ADT, Lab, Rad	CCD, eligibility
My Health Plan	Several	Eligibility, med history	ADT, CCD
Public Health Agency	Several	Immunizations, reportable labs	Immunizations, ADT, CCD, Labs

TABLE 14-4   Flu Shots for Adults Ages 50 to 64

| Year | COMMERCIAL | | MEDICAID | MEDICARE | |
	HMO	PPO	HMO	HMO	PPO
2011	53.3	51.4	-	-	-
2010	52.5	51.6	-	-	-
2009	51.3	50.5	-	-	-
2008	49.8	49.2	-	-	-
2007	48.6	48.1	-	-	-

TABLE 14-5   Flu Shots for Older Adults

| Year | COMMERCIAL | | MEDICAID | MEDICARE | |
	HMO	PPO	HMO	HMO	PPO
2011	-	-	-	68.8	69.5
2010	-	-	-	68.8	69.4
2009	-	-	-	64.5	65.1
2008	-	-	-	65.8	66.7
2007	-	-	-	68.6	68.9

BOX 14-7   Public Health Essential Services

Assessment

Monitor health status to identify community health problems.

Diagnose and investigate health problems and health hazards in the community.

Policy Development

Inform, educate, and empower people about health issues.

Mobilize community partnerships to identify and solve health problems.

Develop policies and plans that support individual and community health efforts.

Assurance

Enforce laws and regulations that protect health and ensure safety.

Link people to needed personal health services and assure the provision of health care when otherwise unavailable.

Assure a competent public health and personal health care workforce.

Evaluate effectiveness, accessibility, and quality of personal and populations-based health services.

Serving All Functions

Research for new insights and innovative solutions to health problems.

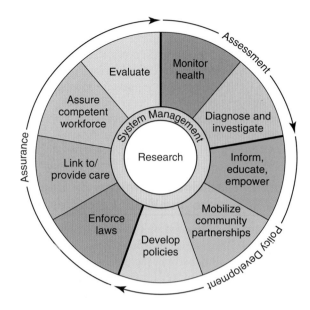

FIGURE 14-10 Public health functions. (Source: Public Health Functions Steering Committee, 1994, http://www.health.gov/phfunctions/images/pubh_wh2.gif)

Public health prevention measures are designed to protect entire communities or populations from such threats as communicable diseases, epidemics, and environmental contaminants.

Public health functions are organized around several core activities, which include:

- Assessment: collecting, analyzing, and disseminating information on health status, personal health problems, population groups at greatest risk, availability and quality of services, resource availability, and concerns of individuals
- Policy development: using the assessment data to consider alternatives and determine which actions and policies to pursue
- Assurance: monitoring actions and policy decisions of public health and other community partners to attain the goals of public health [20] (see Box 14-7 & Figure 14-10).

PUBLIC HEALTH INFORMATION NETWORK

As with paper clinical records, the collection of public health data began as a paper-based system. As data moved to computer-based systems and storage, the data were stored in a variety of formats and databases, such as a database for tuberculosis, another for sexually transmitted disease, and another for investigation of epidemiology reports. Although some data are still collected and transmitted to local and state systems on paper or through a unique system, web-based collection of public health data is increasing. CDC is promoting the use of standard vocabularies and messaging formats to encourage interoperability, such as HL7, LOINC, SNOMED. These are the same standards being adopted and used in healthcare.

National Electronic Disease Surveillance System and NEDSS Base System

The National Electronic Disease Surveillance System (NEDSS) is a conduit for exchanging information that supports the national disease surveillance system. This electronic system is using data standards to facilitate timely, secure reporting of data.

Use of the Public Health Information Network supports the transmission of data from health care sources to local public health agencies, then to state agencies, and finally on to the CDC. At each level the agencies are expected to receive the data, store it, aggregate it properly, and transmit it to the next level.

? DID YOU KNOW?

The CDC level publishes a weekly online newsletter, the *Morbidity and Mortality Weekly Report* (MMWR), that includes data reported by each state. One example of this data is infectious disease reporting, specifically the increase in measles cases in 2014. The resulting data are then published in the *Morbidity and Mortality Weekly Report*. Subsequently, the general news media pick up the articles and the data are disseminated widely through general news channels.

Do you know why there was an increase in measles in 2014? Do you know which state had the largest number of measles cases in 2014? Do you know why the public health departments are concerned about this increase?

In order to make this system work it must work on all levels. If resources, awareness, or technical system expertise are missing the system breaks down.

The NEDSS Base System (NBS) is provided by CDC to help public health agencies report disease data to the CDC using the Public Health Information Network standards. This system helps to transfer data efficiently and securely over the Internet. The NBS also provides support for managing disease outbreaks and prepares data for geographic analysis.

As the health information exchanges mature it will be easier to collect needed data and transmit it horizontally and vertically (i.e. within the community and to the national centers).

Institute of Medicine Committee on Health Threats Resilience and Work Force Resilience

This committee is sponsored by the Department of Homeland Security's Office of Health Affairs. Its purpose is to plan for and provide studies pertinent to emergency response and recovery activities related to catastrophic health events and integrated biosurveillance, including public health capabilities to respond to actionable events. (See Box 14-8.) The goal is to help prepare communities and regions to respond effectively to emergencies. Each time a major natural or manmade disaster occurs that disrupts the lives of a large group of people and affects their ability to maintain their health, the public health system is tested.[21]

Public health threats are always present. Being prepared to prevent, respond to, and rapidly recover is critical for protecting and securing public health. States and local entities are working together on emergency preparedness. Emergency exercises and real incidents give the community an opportunity to test and improve its planning (see Box 14-9). State and local public health departments are often first responders for

---

BOX 14-8 Public Health Preparedness Capabilities

CDC identified the following 15 public health preparedness capabilities as the basis for state and local public health preparedness:

- Biosurveillance
  - Public Health Laboratory Testing
  - Public Health Surveillance and Epidemiological Investigation
- Community Resilience
  - Community Preparedness
  - Community Recovery
- Countermeasures and Mitigation
  - Medical Countermeasure Dispensing
  - Medical Material Management and Distribution
  - Nonpharmaceutical Interventions
  - Responder Health and Safety
- Incident Management
  - Emergency Operations Coordination
- Information Management
  - Emergency Public Information and Warning
  - Information Sharing
- Surge Management
  - Fatality Management
  - Mass Care
  - Medical Surge
  - Volunteer Management

BOX 14-9 Example of a Performance Measure for Emergency Preparedness

Community Recovery

Definition: Community recovery is the ability to collaborate with community partners (e.g., health care organizations, behavioral health care organizations, business, education, and emergency management) to plan and advocate for the rebuilding of public health, medical, mental/behavioral health systems to at least a level of functioning comparable to pre-incident levels, and improved levels where possible.

This capability supports National Health Security Strategy Objective 8: Incorporate Post-Incident Recovery into Planning and Response. Post-incident recovery of the public health, medical, and mental/behavioral health services and systems with a jurisdiction is critical for health security and requires collaboration and advocacy by the public health agency for the restoration of services, providers, facilities, and infrastructure within the public health, medical, and human services sectors. Monitoring the public health, medical, and mental/behavioral health infrastructure is an essential public health service.

Functions and Associated Performance Measures: This capability consists of the ability to perform the functions listed:
  Function 1: Identify and monitor public health, medical, and mental/behavioral health system recovery needs.
  Function 2: Coordinate community public health, medical, and mental/behavioral health system recovery operations.
  Function 3: Implement corrective actions to mitigate damages from future incidents.

(Source: Centers for Disease Control and Prevention, Office of Public Health Preparedness and Response, Public Health Preparedness Capabilities: National Standards for State and Local Planning, March 2011.)

---

public health incidents. The planning and testing of these preparedness plans includes local health care groups, behavioral health organizations, community partners, volunteers, and emergency management groups.

PUBLIC HEALTH PROGRAMS

Proven cost-effective public health measures include water fluoridation to prevent tooth decay, smoking cessation among pregnant women to prevent low birth weight, immunizations to prevent measles and mumps, and health education of consumers to reduce their need for medical services. Many Americans take public health programs for granted. However, much like the health care system, there is a cadre of trained professionals with a system in place to prevent public health problems and to respond when an epidemic breaks out or a toxic chemical is spilled. When young children were being admitted to the hospital for treatment of *Escherichia coli* infection, it was the public health department that tracked down the source of the problem as contaminated hamburger meat and undercooking of the hamburger. All states have health departments with county and city coverage. Most public health departments work with the medical community on some aspects of care. For example, the *E. coli* outbreak was both a clinical treatment problem and a public health problem. Pediatricians and family practitioners usually work closely with the public health department in immunizing children against many childhood diseases. Both the medical care system and the public health system take an interest in prevention of injury, illness, and disease. The most intense development of those interests may be the catalyst that brings the community together.

For much of the last 40 years, public health has been defined by a series of categorical programs and problems such as AIDS, tuberculosis, sewage treatment, immunizations, food-borne illnesses, and primary care for the underserved. When a problem was identified and brought into public view, legislators enacted laws and appropriated funds to address that specific problem. Public health agencies responded by organizing themselves to carry out disease-specific or problem-specific programs.

The result of these disease- and program-specific efforts and their reporting requirements was a disconnected, dysfunctional information system—the components each intended to meet a specific program need. In many states this resulted in program-specific data systems. This is commonly referred to as stove piping. In analyzing its data collection forms for all programs, one state found that it was asking for the individual's address more than 300 times. A coordinated system that allows "registration" once would be a tremendous step forward in reducing the administrative paperwork burden. The next step in the transition would be to build a coordinated database and eliminate program-specific, free-standing information systems.

National Initiatives

Public Health Information Network

The Centers for Disease Control is working to help public health agencies to electronically exchange data across organizations and jurisdictions, between clinical care and public health and federal reporting systems. The goal is efficient and effective exchange and use of information to improve population health and well-being.

National Vaccine Program

At the national level the vaccine program is responsible for coordinating federal agencies involved in vaccine and immunization activities. The national program provides leadership, goals, objectives, and strategies to prevent infectious diseases through immunizations.

State Initiatives

Birth Defects Registry

Washington State has a registry and surveillance system in which any child up to age one year diagnosed or treated with a reportable birth defect who was a Washington State resident at the time of birth or treated in a Washington facility is reportable. The data reported include: child's name, medical record number, date of birth, sex, admission date, Zip code, discharge date, ICD-CM code for diagnosis, the diagnosis, ICD code for procedure, and the procedure. The causes of about 70% of all birth defects are unknown. However, there are concerns about environmental pollutants, occupational

hazards, dietary factors, medication, infections, personal behaviors or genome factors. Some of the reportable birth defects are spina bifida, cleft palate, Down syndrome, and fetal alcohol syndrome.

Immunization Information

The Washington State Immunization Information System was previously called the Child Profile Immunization Registry. The previous system title implied that it was only for children. The new name reflects a change to a lifetime registry of immunizations from birth to death. The new system recognizes that there are significant immunization events during adolescence and adulthood. This system is a secure Web-based tool that helps health care providers keep track of the immunizations they give to patients of all ages in their practice. The immunization records remain available when families move or change providers within the state.

The goal is to help ensure that people get the right vaccines at the right time. The information system is important to the physicians, nurses, public health staff, health educators, and others. The database will serve as a resource during outbreaks of vaccine-preventable disease. Also, schools can verify records of vaccine status for students. Providers can also order vaccine through this system.

There are also information resources on the Washington State site to inform individuals about vaccines. For example, Adolescent Immunizations Frequently Asked Questions discusses why immunizations are important for teens and the recommended immunizations for teens. There are several vaccines on this list, including hepatitis B, human papillomavirus (HPV), influenza, measles-mumps-rubella, polio, meningococcus, tetanus-diphtheria-pertussis, and varicella.

 SELF-ASSESSMENT QUIZ

1. Why was the name of the Washington State Vaccine Registry changed?

Focused Health Problem: Asthma in Washington State

Asthma is a complex, common, chronic respiratory condition that in Washington State affects more women than men. Approximately 18% of women in Washington State have lifetime asthma compared to 11% of women in the United States. More women than men died of asthma between 2010 and 2012 in Washington State: 148 deaths of women and 84 deaths of men.[22]

In 2010 more than 780,000 adults were estimated to have lifetime asthma in Washington State. Hospitals reported that they charged about $73 million for asthma-related hospitalizations in 2010, and another $4.8 million was charged to patients for self-payment. The proportion of adult-onset asthma that can be attributed to workplace exposures has been estimated at 20%. Many individuals have "triggers" in their homes that make their asthma worse (carpet, pets, mold, secondhand smoke). Outdoor air quality may also affect asthma (vehicle exhaust, outdoor burning, industrial emissions). In 2010, 22% of Washington adults with asthma missed work or could not do normal activities, for a total of 4.3 million person-days of lost productivity. [23] This is an area of concern for both public health and the medical care community. It is also clearly an issue that involves education of the individual with asthma and those who may affect the health of individuals with asthma.

Environmental Public Health Data

The environmental component of public health responsibilities in Washington State uses the Washington Tracking Network to gather and analyze data about environmental health hazards, exposure to hazards, and health outcomes based on exposure. Areas under this umbrella include safe drinking water, food safety, shellfish protection, radiation safety, wastewater management, pesticide exposures, vector-borne disease, and general environmental health and safety issues. The Office of Environmental Health, Safety, and Toxicology provides support and expertise on retail food protection, indoor and outdoor air quality, illegal drug lab cleanup, pesticide-related illnesses, school environment safety, recreational water safety, and a variety of toxicological assessments.

The Washington State Department of Health Strategic Plan 2009-2013 contains several recommendations related to information technology, including data integration, development of a data warehouse, collaboration and agreement on standard data definitions, increasing the accuracy of the data, development of business rules for data, and online systems for vital statistics documents. Each of these topics and objectives is tracked from baseline to target during the stated timeframe. Reports are prepared and submitted to the Department of Health to assess performance. [24]

HEALTH PROBLEMS AND COSTS

Public health takes a long look at the real causes of health problems in the United States. It is estimated that about half of all deaths are caused by tobacco use, improper diet, lack of physical activity, alcohol misuse, microbial and toxic agents, firearm use, unsafe sexual behavior, motor vehicle crashes, and illicit use of drugs. The element of personal and community responsibility in these causes of health problems is inescapable. With the possible exception of some microbes and toxic agents, all the causes listed are primarily a result of human behavior.

In 2010, nearly 7,500 Washingtonians died from tobacco-related illnesses. Tobacco-related illnesses are the leading cause of preventable death in Washington State. More than 800,000 people in Washington State smoke, but there are 295,000 fewer adult smokers than there were at the beginning of the smoking-reduction program in Washington State. This reduction in the number of adult smokers is estimated to save $2.8 billion. One of the current targets in Washington State is to reduce smoking rates among low-income individuals (income below $25,000) since this group has been less likely to quit or engage in smoking cessation programs. [24]

Since the introduction of electronic cigarettes the questions for data collection need to be adjusted. Many individuals do not see the connection between electronic cigarette smoking and nicotine/tobacco use. Also there is a concern that tobacco users who chew tobacco do not see themselves as at risk.

The burning cigarette, the moving car, the raw hamburger, and the failed on-site sewage system are all carriers of health threats that are best dealt with early.

IMPROVING HEALTH

Public health can be a powerful tool. Its population-based focus helps to accomplish changes and evaluate the magnitude of the problem. Public health professionals also actively participate in public education efforts.

The connection between public health and better health is well established. Since 1900 the average life expectancy of United States citizens has gone up from 45 to 75 years of age. Public health improvement in sanitation, the control of diseases through immunizations, and other activities are responsible for 25 of the 30 additional years that Americans can now expect to live. In addition, population-based public health of the 1970s contributed greatly to recent improvement in reduced tobacco use, blood pressure control, diet, use of seat belts, and injury control, which in turn have contributed to declines of more than 50% in deaths due to stroke, 40% in deaths due to heart disease, and 25% in overall death rates for children.

Public health uses a variety of approaches to improving health, including an evidence-based approach. "Evidence-based public health is defined as the development, implementation, and evaluation of effective programs and policies in public health through application of principles of scientific reasoning, including systematic uses of data and information systems, and appropriate use of behavioral science theory and program planning models." [25]

Public health research and practice is aimed at whole communities. Evidence-based approaches to public health require an understanding of the complexities of organizational structures, interactions, and myriad other dynamics that shape and influence decision making at local, state, and national levels. Technology has markedly improved access to public health and health care statistics. Technology also makes it easier to find related examples of successes and failures. The Agency for Healthcare Research and Quality is continually funding and publishing work that can be used in the pursuit of evidence-based practices.

Public health has its own datasets which typically fall into two categories: the first is related to services provided and events, and the second describes populations through the use of sampling techniques.

Health statistics and data are important because they measure a wide range of health indicators for a community. A community could be the entire United States, a region, a state, a county or a city. Data on vital statistics and national expenditures cover the entire population. Most data on morbidity and utilization of health resources cover portions of the population. Some information is collected using surveys and estimates of the same statistic may vary among surveys. For example, a number of surveys may ask about cigarette smoking or tobacco use and the results of their data may vary due to sampling frames, various methodologies, definitions, or questionnaires.

Public health uses a wide variety of data and data sources to shape and evaluate its programs and policies, including data from service provision and health events and population-based data.

INTEGRATING THE INFORMATION SYSTEM

Initial public health datasets were not integrated. Because of the amount of data and the complexity of questions to be addressed, more sophisted systems are being developed. As commonality in data standards emerges between facets of the public health system and the health care system, data will be easier to exchange in a timely manner and interoperability between systems will be easier to achieve.

To achieve goals and to demonstrate that goals are met, public health needs an integrated information system. While some basic systems are in place, improvements are still needed. Public health systems still need:

- Redesign of program-specific, free-standing data systems into integrated systems
- An integrated, centrally managed, electronic network that provides access to federal, state, and local information systems
- Data systems that facilitate the provision of services to consumers
- Data management systems that meet the local needs to systematically collect, analyze, and monitor standardized baseline data
- Data systems that contain decision support modules to help identify potential outbreaks of certain infectious diseases and alert communities to contamination of food or water or intentional introduction of harmful bacteria

- Linkage between local and statewide databases in both the private and public sectors
- Data use and dissemination standards
- Technical assistance to ensure a high standard of data analysis, dissemination, and risk communication
- A fully integrated, secure computer network
- Evaluation and dissemination of new health information technologies
- Tracking of clinical and environmental laboratory information

Public health professionals need good data systems to be able to provide accurate, understandable information for policymakers, community leaders, health plans, and health care providers. Outcome measures need to be tracked. Policy outcomes need datafor evaluation. The main concern running through all of this data collection, analysis, and dissemination is the need for balancing the privacy and confidentiality of the individual with the protection of the public good. Most health care providers are aware of regulations that require reporting of communicable diseases. This reporting to the public health department allows the department to take further action, if necessary, to prevent spread of the illness. In most instances, the reporting does not endanger the privacy of the individual.

The reports of identified individuals related to public health concerns such as venereal disease are not published as public information; however, some diseases do require follow-up with others who may have had contact with the infected individual.

Efforts to ensure access and quality of care require partnerships among many affected parties. The sharing of data and the tracking of measurements, programs, and changes over time are essential to obtain community and client perspectives on quality of care and services.

All states have plans and target goals for public health as well as a broad array of services. Tracking services and goals, and assessing progress requires data. (See Table 14-6.)

Health information management professionals have the knowledge and skills to support the data and information systems of the public health system and can contribute to the overall health and well-being of the entire population.

TABLE 14-6 List of Core Public Health Activities

Assuring a Safe and Healthy Environment

- Food safety (inspections, education, permitting, data management including local responsibilities for shellfish monitoring)
- Water recreational facility safety (inspections, education, permitting, data management)
- Hazardous materials management (drug lab inspection, testing oversight, cleanup oversight)
- Solid waste management (permitting, inspection, enforcement, education)
- Water quality control: sewage (permitting, inspection, enforcement, education, and operations and management), groundwater, drinking water (permitting, inspection, enforcement, education, drinking water data), surface water (drinking water permitting, inspection, enforcement, education, and environmental monitoring)
- Vector/rodent control/zoonotic disease (inspection, enforcement, education, and sampling)
- Air quality monitoring (indoor investigations)
- Environmental laboratory services

Continued

TABLE 14-6 List of Core Public Health Activities—cont'd

- School safety (inspection, education, and consultation)
- Environmental health community involvement
- Environmental sampling
- Review of land use decisions

Protecting People from Disease

- Detection/case investigation: screening (specimen collection and analysis), testing, lab (identification and diagnosis), diagnosis (clinical and lab identification)
- Surveillance, reporting (transmission of information), data analysis (monitor and interpret), data gathering (collecting information and collection systems), epidemiologic investigations, case finding (identifying cases and location), contact tracing (identifying potential exposure)
- Regional epidemiology
- Laboratory (identification and diagnosis)
- System intervention: immunizations (preventive pre- or post-exposure), treatment and prophylactic treatment (dispensing, shots, application, and observation), counseling (one-on-one education and therapy), tuberculosis program
- Public and provider education (informing general public and outbreak specific)
- Surveillance of chronic disease trends and behavioral changes, identifying clusters, special studies to identify risk factors and focus prevention efforts, prevention activities focused on behavioral and environmental/policy interventions, and evaluation
- Outreach and prevention with high-risk populations
- Plans and surge capacity for response to emergency situations that threaten the health of people

Understanding Health Issues

- Epidemiology (infectious and noninfectious disease trends; monitoring, collection, and analysis of data on health risk behaviors, health status, and critical health services)
- Dissemination of assessment information in the community to support decision-making
- Technical assistance, education and leadership for community-level data utilization

Evaluation of Public Health Program Results

- Prevention is best: promoting healthy living
- Capacity for health education and systems work related to the following activities: engaging community agencies, organizations and constituencies to address and develop locally designed programs driven by locally identified health issues, strategic planning based on community needs, local data gathering and analysis, and coalition and stakeholder-building
- Resource assessments (develop assessment of resources based on specific needs), generate resources (design materials, find funding, write grants), designing and providing promotional materials and/or social marketing campaigns evaluating results of efforts, and collecting and disseminating research-based best practices
- Assure and support healthy pregnancies, healthy birth outcomes, early brain development; includes maternal and child health programs, early intervention, health and safety promotion in child care centers, children with special health care needs, family planning, First Steps/MCM/MSS community outreach and WIC
- Evaluating results of efforts, collecting and disseminating research-based, replicable best practices (including about chronic illnesses and health behaviors), provider and public education

Helping People Get the Services They Need

- System assurance role: bring people together and provide leadership and support, system infrastructure, support for local community SWOT assessment
- Provide information and education about critical public health services; create conditions that make action possible.
- Information and referral activities (maintain inventory of services, referral, resource broker)
- Create conditions that make action possible (standards, policy, quality assurance, materials and supplies, information, and education)
- Safety net services (direct services as identified through local assessment, Menu of Critical Health Services)

Administration

- Leadership, planning, policy development, and administration
- Financial and management services (accounting, budget, contracts, procurement, grants, and asset management)
- Leadership and governance (communication, public relations, relationship building, program planning, and fundraising)
- Legal authority (policies, procedures, and regulations)
- Human resources (personnel, employee development and recognition, compensation and benefits management, and employee policies)
- Information systems (hardware/software systems, networking, data sharing, policies)

Source: Public Health Improvement Plan 2004, Washington State Department of Health.

LEGAL CONTEXT

Federal Laws

The Public Health Services Act of 1944 structured the current public health service. The original agency was founded in 1798 and reorganized and renamed several times.

DID YOU KNOW?

Did You Know that Agencies within the Public Health Service include:
- Agency for Healthcare Research and Quality (AHRQ)
- Agency for Toxic Substances and Disease Registry (ATSDR)
- Centers for Disease Control and Prevention (CDC)
- Food and Drug Administration (FDA)
- Health Resources and Services Administration (HRSA)
- Indian Health Services (IHS)
- National Institutes of Health (NIH)
- Substance Abuse and Mental Health Services Administration (SMHHSA)

The Public Health Service also includes a commission corps that employs more than 6,000 public health professionals.

Public Law 78-410, codified as 42 U.S.C. Health and Social Welfare, was signed July 1, 1944. It has been amended several times to include the following:
- National Cancer Act of 1971
- Health Insurance Portability and Accountability Act of 1996
- Muscular Dystrophy Community Assistance Research and Education Amendments of 2001
- Hematological Cancer Research Investment and Education Act of 2001
- Newborn Screening Saves Lives Act of 2007
- Patient Protection and Affordable Care Act of 2010
- Pandemic and All-Hazards Preparedness Reauthorization Act of 2013

State Laws

The Washington State Department of Health has a broad range of responsibilities and significant regulatory authority. For example, the Revised Code of Washington (RCW) Title 43 states that its primary responsibilities include the preservation of public health, the maintenance of minimal standards for quality in health care delivery, and the general oversight and planning for all the state's activities as they relate to the health of its citizenry. It is also the intent to improve illness and injury prevention, and support health promotion. Title 70 contains the specific work of state and local public health agencies. Title 69 covers activities related to control of pharmaceuticals, food, and shellfish safety. Title 26 addresses the public health department role as keeper of vital records: birth, marriage, divorce, adoption, death.

Public health services in Washington State are defined in RCW 43.70.514 as services that address: "Communicable disease prevention and response; preparation for, and response to, public health emergencies caused by pandemic disease, earthquake, flood, or terrorism; prevention and management of chronic diseases and disabilities; promotion of healthy families and the development of children; assessment of local health conditions, risks, and trends, and evaluation of the effectiveness of intervention efforts; and environmental health concerns."

All states have a set of diagnoses that are referred to as notifiable conditions. These are largely highly contagious communicable diseases that require the health department to intervene to prevent the further spread of disease in the community. Table 14-7 contains the set of diseases for

TABLE 14-7 Immediately Reportable Communicable Disease Conditions (Wa)

Animal bites
Botulism
Cholera
Diphtheria
Diseases of suspected bioterrorism
Domoic acid poisoning
E. coli
Emerging condition with outbreak potential
Haemophilus influenza, invasive disease, children under age 5
Influenza, novel, of unsubtypable strain
Measles (rubeola)
Meningococcal disease (invasive)
Monkeypox
Outbreaks of suspected food-borne origin
Outbreaks of suspected water-borne origin
Paralytic shellfish poisoning
Plague
Poliomyelitis
Rabies (confirmed human or animal)
Rabies, suspected human exposure (suspected human rabies exposures due to a bite from or other exposure to an animal that is suspected of being infected with rabies)
Rubella, including congenital rubella syndrome (acute disease only)
SARS
Shiga toxin producing E. coli infections including but not limited to E. coli 0157:H7
Smallpox
Tuberculosis
Tularemia
Typhus
Vaccinia transmission
Viral hemorrhagic fever
Yellow fever

Effective 2/4/11 (Source: WAC 246-101-101 Notifiable Conditions)
Note: A number of other conditions must be reported within 24 hours, or 3 business days. Check the WAC for the full list of reportable conditions.

Washington State that require immediate notification of the public health department.

Several states, including Washington, have laws that permit the reporting of clusters of cases that could be an indication of an epidemic from a variety of causes including bioterrorism. To enable this analysis, a limited data set including the chief complaints and preliminary diagnosis is permitted to be reported to public health. Although the exact value of syndromic surveillance is not yet known, this methodology in one form or another represents the future of modern disease surveillance.

Despite all the media attention that public health has gotten in the wake of anthrax and SARS scares, the budget to support the task of public health to monitor and detect disease is woefully underfunded.

Hospitals, clinics, and other health providers have no direct financial gain from providing required information to their local health jurisdiction. However, the effect on the community could be devastating if this data were not shared with public health officials in a timely manner. As the sophistication of health departments increase, the methods for transmitting these reports securely will become commonplace. Electronic transmission of these reports will save time and resources of all health care provider and facility staff members. Timely sharing of data plus improved information systems in public health settings will help improve the health of the community and wider populations.

WHAT PUBLIC HEALTH DOES WITH DATA

Figure 14-11 shows a simplified view of the existing Public Health infrastructure. This figure shows a simplified view of the existing public health infrastructure. This describes the structure of the public health IT environment. Federal agencies include the Centers for Disease Control and Prevention, the Region X health director of the Department of Health and Human Services. State Department of Health and the County and Local Health Districts are shown and the flow of information is represented. The granularity of the data depends on the authority of the agency.

ANALYSIS AND USE OF DATA AND INFORMATION

Public health touches many aspects of the health of individuals and communities. It is clear that public health agencies often are collecting and using the data to change people's behaviors or to change policies or laws to improve aspects of our health. Once the data is collected they often are published and then used to influence change.

For example, the CDC's Injury Center works at putting science into action. It is the leading authority on violence and

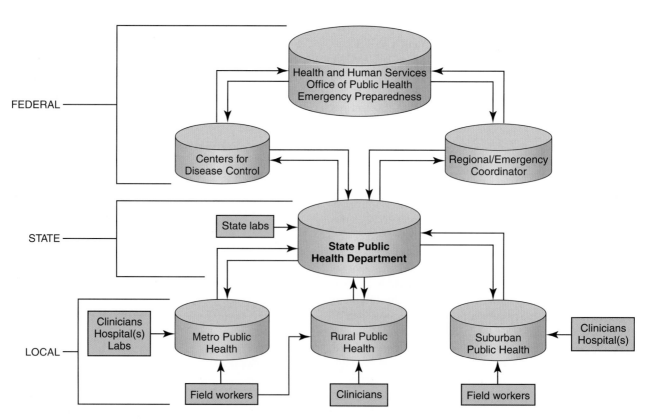

FIGURE 14-11 Simplified view of the existing public health infrastructure.

injury. The CDC Center studies violence and injury and researches the best way to prevent violence and injury with the goal of finding real-world solutions to keeping people safe, healthy, and productive. Action areas include the following:

Identifying and monitoring injuries by studying patterns in data and working on prevention initiatives.

Conducting research to find vital knowledge to influence policy decisions. For example, research shows that state laws that use the 0.08% blood alcohol concentration have effectively reduced alcohol-related traffic deaths.

Building Effective Partnerships for Prevention. which works with a variety of partners to make people safer. For example, a partnership with the National Collegiate Athletic Association helps raise awareness of concussions and improve prevention and treatment of traumatic brain injuries.[26]

Another example is the creation of a one-page Prescription Drug Overdose Fact Sheet (see Box 14-10) that outlines the problem, the most common drugs involved in overdoses, the costs, and the risk factors for drug overdose.[27]

In a third example, collection of data related to child pedestrian safety indicated that children ages 15 to 19 years have the most pedestrian injuries. Factors that increased the risk of injury included living in a dense, low-income urban residential area, being male, being on the street between 3 pm and 7 pm, and texting while walking. To call attention to this concern a safety poster was created and made available through the Children's Safety Network[28] (see Figure 14-12).

Public health has a wide range of activities that touch many aspects of our lives and our communities. Almost all of these activities use and rely on data. As public health and health care become more integrated in their approach to improving the health of individuals and the communities they serve we will support more integrated data and information systems.

BOX 14-10 Prescription Drug Overdose in the United States: Fact Sheet

Overview

Definitions

Drug: Any chemical compound used for the diagnosis or treatment of disease or injury, for the relief of pain, or for the feeling it causes. A drug is either a pharmaceutical (including both prescription and over-the-counter products) or illicit.

Overdose: When a drug is eaten, inhaled, injected, or absorbed through the skin in excessive amounts and injures the body. Overdoses are either intentional or unintentional. If the person taking or giving a substance did not mean to cause harm, then it is unintentional.

Misuse or abuse: The use of illicit or prescription or over-the-counter drugs in a manner other than as directed.[2]

Deaths from drug overdose have been rising steadily over the past two decades and have become the leading cause of injury death in the United States.[1] Every day in the United States, 114 people die as a result of drug overdose[1], and another 6,748 are treated in emergency departments (ED) for the misuse or abuse of drugs.[2] Nearly 9 out of 10 poisoning deaths are caused by drugs.[3]

The Problem

- Drug overdose was the leading cause of injury death in 2012. Among people 25 to 64 years old, drug overdose caused more deaths than motor vehicle traffic crashes.[1]
- Drug overdose death rates have been rising steadily since 1992 with a 117% increase from 1999 to 2012 alone.[1]
- In 2012, 33,175 (79.9%) of the 41,502 drug overdose deaths in the United States were unintentional, 5,465 (13.2%) were of suicidal intent, 80 (0.2%) were homicides, and 2,782 (6.7%) were of undetermined intent.[1]
- In 2011, drug misuse and abuse caused about 2.5 million emergency department (ED) visits. Of these, more than 1.4 million ED visits were related to pharmaceuticals.[2]
- Between 2004 and 2005, an estimated 71,000 children (18 or younger) were seen in EDs each year because of medication overdose (excluding self-harm, abuse and recreational drug use).[4]
- Among children under age 6, pharmaceuticals account for about 40% of all exposures reported to poison centers.[5]

Most Common Drugs Involved in Overdoses

- In 2012, of the 41,502 drug overdose deaths in the United States, 22,114 (53%) were related to pharmaceuticals.[6]
- Of the 22,114 deaths relating to pharmaceutical overdose in 2012, 16,007 (72%) involved opioid analgesics (also called opioid pain relievers or prescription painkillers), and 6,524 (30%) involved benzodiazepines.[6] (Some deaths include more than one type of drug.)
- In 2011, about 1.4 million ED visits involved the nonmedical use of pharmaceuticals. Among those ED visits, 501,207 visits were related to anti-anxiety and insomnia medications, and 420,040 visits were related to opioid analgesics.[2]
- Benzodiazepines are frequently found among people treated in EDs for misusing or abusing drugs.[2] People who died of drug overdoses often had a combination of benzodiazepines and opioid analgesics in their bodies.[6]
- In the United States, prescription opioid abuse costs were about $55.7 billion in 2007.[7] Of this amount, 46% was attributable to workplace costs (e.g., lost productivity), 45% to healthcare costs (e.g., abuse treatment), and 9% to criminal justice costs.[7]

Risk Factors for Drug Overdose

Among those who died from drug overdose in 2012:

- Men were 59% more likely than women to die;
- Whites had the highest death rate, followed by American Indians/Alaska Natives and then blacks;
- The highest death rate was among people 45–49 years of age; and
- The lowest death rates were among children less than 15 years old because they do not abuse drugs as frequently as older people.[1]

Among people who misused or abused drugs and received treatment in emergency departments in 2011:

- 56% were males;
- 82% were people 21 or older.[2]

References

1. Centers for Disease Control and Prevention: *Web-based Injury Statistics Query and Reporting System (WISQARS)* [online], 2014. Available from http://www.cdc.gov/injury/wisqars/fatal.html.
2. Substance Abuse and Mental Health Services Administration: *Highlights of the 2011 Drug Abuse Warning Network (DAWN) findings on*

drug-related emergency department visits. *The DAWN Report*, Rockville, MD, 2013, US Department of Health and Human Services, Substance Abuse and Mental Health Services Administration. Available from http://www.samhsa.gov/data/2k13/DAWN127/sr127-DAWN-highlights.html (http://www.cdc.gov/Other/disclaimer.html).

3. Paulozzi LJ: Prescription drug overdoses: a review. *J Safety Res* 2012. http://dx.doi.org/10.1016/j.jsr.2012.08.009 (http://www.cdc.gov/Other/disclaimer.html).

4. Schillie SF, Shehab N, Thomas KE, Budnitz DS: Medication overdoses leading to emergency department visits among children. *Am J Prev Med* 37:181–187, 2009.

5. Mowry JB, Spyker DA, Cantilena LR, Bailey JE, Ford M: 2012 Annual report of the American Association of Poison Control Centers' National Poison Data System (NPDS): 30th annual report. *Clin Tox* 51:949–1229, 2013.

6. Centers for Disease Control and Prevention: *National Vital Statistics System mortality data*, 2012. Available from http://www.cdc.gov/nchs/deaths.html.

7. Birnbaum HG, White AG, Schiller M, Waldman T, Cleveland JM, Roland CL: Societal costs of prescription opioid abuse, dependence, and misuse in the United States. *Pain Med* 12:657–667, 2011.

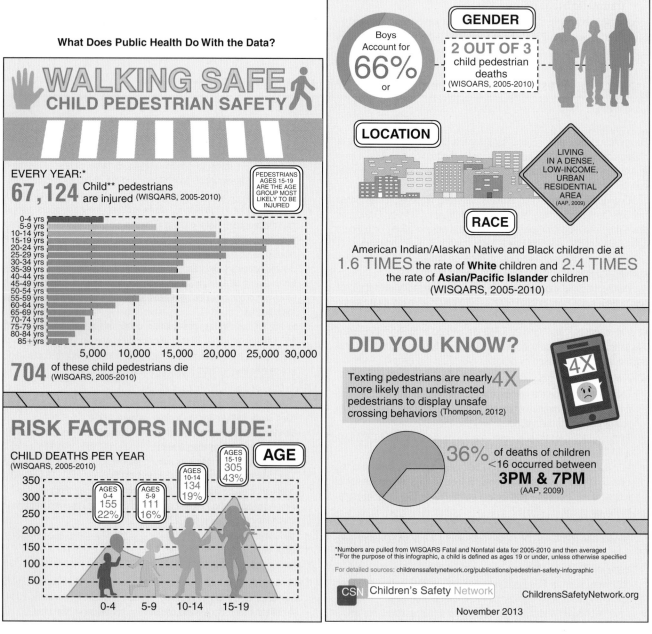

FIGURE 14-12 Walking Safe—Pedestrian Safety. (Source: childrenssafetynetwork.org/publications/pedestrian-safety-infographic.)

✓ CHAPTER REVIEW

1. Which age group is least likely to die from accidents in the United States?
   a. 1-24 years of age
   b. 25-44 years of age
   c. 45-64 years of age
   d. 65 and older

2. Children and young adults (age 1-20) who die of an injury in the United States are most likely to die from:
   a. motor vehicle/traffic accident.
   b. firearm.
   c. poisoning.
   d. fall.

3. True or False: Healthy People 2020 is a relatively new program started by the CDC in 2012.

4. The leading cause of injury death in the United States in 2010 was
   a. auto accidents.
   b. drug overdose.
   c. gunshot wounds.
   d. traumatic head injury.

5. True or False: The CDC recommends that adults over 60 years of age receive the shingles vaccine.

6. List at least three Public Health Obligations.

7. Environmental hazards included in public health responsibilities include:
   a. food safety
   b. pesticide exposures
   c. vaccines
   d. a. and b.

8. Agencies within the U.S. Public Health Service include:
   a. Food and Drug Administration.
   b. Agency for Healthcare Research and Quality.
   c. National Institutes of Health.
   d. All of the above.

9. List at least three infectious diseases/events that are immediately reportable to public health.

10. True or False: Meaningful Use objectives include syndromic surveillance reporting to public health agencies.

REFERENCES

1. Healthy People 2020 Progress Review (Power Point) April 18, 2013, Violence Across the Lifespan, Office of Disease Prevention and Health Promotion, CDC. http://www.cdc.gov/nchs/ppt/hp2020_IVP_OSH_progress_review.pdf. Accessed 7/5/14.
2. http://www.healthypeople.gov/2020/topicsobjectives2020–2/8/2014.
3. National Immunization Survey (NIS) Teen, CDC/NCIRD and CDC/NCHS.
4. CDC: Ten great public health achievements—United States 2001–2010, *MMWR,* May 20, 2011.
5. National Vital Statistics System—Mortality (NVSS-M), CDC/NCHS.
6. Healthy People 2020 Progress Review: The Burden of Tuberculosis and Infectious Diseases in the U.S. and Abroad, CDC, July 30, 2013.
7. http://www.healthypeople.gov/2020/topicsobjectives2020/overview, accessed 2/8/2014.
8. http://www.cdc/coronavirus/mers, accessed 2/8/14.
9. Healthy People 2020 Progress Review (Power Point) April 18, 2013, Violence Across the Lifespan, Office of Disease Prevention and Health Promotion, CDC, http://www.cdc.gov/nchs/ppt/hp2020_IVP_OSH_progress_review.pdf. Accessed 7/5/14.
10. National Vital Statistics System—Mortality (NVSS-M), CDC/NCHS.
11. http://www.cdc.gov/nchs/nvss.htm.
12. http://www.cdc.gov/nchs/nchs.htm.
13. http://www.cdc.gov/nchs/nhis.html.
14. National Vital Statistics System 2009, National Hospital Discharge Survey, National Hospital Ambulatory Medical Care Survey, National Health Interview Survey.
15. *National Vital Statistics Data Brief,* No. 115, March 2013.
16. http://www.cms.gov/Regulations-and-Guidance/Lesgilation/EHRIncentivesProgram, accessed 7/5/14.
17. http://www.onehealthport.com/HIE.
18. www.onehealthport.com/content/hie-transactions.
19. PHIN Messaging Guide of Syndromic Surveillance: Emergency Department, Urgent Care and Inpatient Settings, CDC. April 2013.
20. Public Health Functions Steering Committee: 1994. http://www.health.gov/phfunctions/images/pubh_wh2.gif.
21. Centers for Disease Control and Prevention, Office of Public Health Preparedness and Response, Public Health Preparedness Capabilities: *National Standards for State and Local Planning March 2011.*
22. Washington State Department of Health, Healthy Communities Report February 2014; also WWW.doh.wa.gov/healthycommunities.
23. Washington State Department of Health: *The burden of asthma in Washington State,* 2013 Update, DOH 345–2013, February 2013. http://www.doh.wa.gov/Portals/1/Documents/Pubs?345–240-AsthmaBurdentRep13.
24. http://doh.wa.gov-. DOH Strategic Plan 2009–2013. Accessed 3/8/14.
25. Brownson RC, Baker EA, Leet TL, Gillespie K, editors: *Evidence-based public health,* New York, 2003, Oxford University Press.
26. CDC Injury Center. http://www.cdc.gov/injury/overview/index.html 5/26/14.
27. http://www.cdc.gov/homeandrecreationalsafety/overdose/facts.html 5/26/14.
28. childrenssafetynetwork.org/publications/pedestrian-safety-infographic.

CHAPTER

PRIVACY AND HEALTH LAW

Jill Callahan Klaver

ⓔ Student Study Guide activities for this chapter are available on the Evolve Learning Resources site for this textbook. Please visit http://evolve.elsevier.com/Abdelhak.

CHAPTER CONTENTS

*Health Information Management Department Security
    Measures to Prevent Unauthorized Access*
Duty to Provide Care That Meets Professional Standards
Duty to Obtain Informed Consent to Treatment
Duty to Provide a Safe Environment for Patients and Visitors
Duty to Supervise the Actions of Employees and the
    Professional Staff
    Medical Staff Credentialing Process

*Accessibility of Credentials Files and Quality Profiles
    Legal Risks*
Contract Liability Issues and the Health Information
    Management Department
Legal Resources for Health Information Management
    Professionals
Chapter Review
References

OBJECTIVES

After reading this chapter, the reader will be able to do the following:
✓ Define key words.
✓ Explain why health information management professionals must be knowledgeable about medicolegal issues.
✓ Distinguish between confidential and nonconfidential information within a health information system.
✓ Describe general legal principles governing access to confidential health information in a variety of circumstances.
✓ Distinguish proper or valid requests for access to health information from improper or invalid requests.

✓ Have a basic understanding of the federal and state court systems.
✓ Describe the four components of negligence.
✓ Distinguish between properly executed consents and authorizations and incomplete or improper consents and authorizations.
✓ Identify major resources for locating information on laws, rules, regulations, and standards related to health information.

KEY WORDS

Advance directive
Alternative dispute resolution
Antitrust
Arbitration
Assault
Authentication
Authorization
Bailiff
Battery
Best evidence rule
Breach of contract
Burden of proof
Business associate agreement
Case law
Charitable immunity
Clerk of the court
Common law
Complaint
Confidential communications
Consent
Contemporaneous documentation
Contract

Corporate negligence
Court order
Court reporter
Covered entity
Credentialing
Defamation
Defendant
Deidentified
Deposition
Designated record set
Discovery
Due process
Durable power of attorney for
    health care
Emancipated minor
Evidence
False imprisonment
Fraud
Health care operations
Hearsay rule
Incident report
Informed consent

Institutional review board
Intentional tort
Interrogatory
Invasion of privacy
Jurisdiction
Legal medical record
Libel
Living will
Malpractice
Minimum necessary
Motion to quash
Negligence
Occurrence report
Plaintiff
Pleading
Power of attorney
Precedent
Preempt, preemption
Preponderance of evidence
Privacy
Privileged communication
Protected health information

Proximate cause
Qui tam
"Reasonable man" standard
Regulation
Res ipsa loquitur
Respondeat superior
Restraint of trade
Right of privacy
Satisfactory assurance
Security of health information
Slander
Standard of care
Stare decisis
Statute
Statute of limitations
Subpoena
Subpoena duces tecum
Tort
Whistleblower
Workforce

ABBREVIATIONS

AHA   American Hospital Association
AHIMA   American Health Information Management Association
ARRA   The American Recovery and Reinvestment Act of 2009
CFR   Code of Federal Regulations
CMS   Center for Medicare and Medicaid Services
DHHS   Department of Health and Human Services
DRS   Designated Record Set
EMTALA   Emergency Treatment and Active Labor Act
FOIA   Freedom of Information Act
HIM   Health Information Management

HIPAA   Health Insurance Portability and Accountability Act
HIV   Human Immunodeficiency Virus
IIHI   Individually Identifiable Health Information
IRB   Institutional Review Board
TJC   The Joint Commission
MIB   Medical Information Bureau
NPDB   National Practitioner Data Bank
OIG   Office of the Inspector General
PHI   Protected Health Information

WHY ARE LEGAL ISSUES IMPORTANT TO HEALTH INFORMATION MANAGEMENT PROFESSIONALS?

At this moment, personal information about the health care or health status of millions of people is being collected, recorded, reviewed, analyzed, transmitted, used, and even misused. For every person who goes to a physician, clinic, hospital, or other treatment provider, somewhere there is a data set related to that visit or treatment. There is a record of all births, every operation, every treatment episode, every test result.

Health information management (HIM) professionals design and manage the information systems that hold these vital records. Earlier chapters have discussed some of the reasons these records are kept. Scores of people and organizations want and need health information. As a result, health care providers are required by law to maintain these records. HIM professionals must ensure that the information systems they manage, run, or design meet these obligations. This chapter discusses some of those obligations.

Some requests for health information are legitimate. Others are not. How do HIM professionals decide which requests are valid and which are not? For the requests that are granted, how do HIM professionals decide what can be disclosed and what cannot? HIM professionals are called on to make these decisions every day. In a health care facility, the HIM professional is often the resident expert on these questions. Legal counsel is not always readily available. To make wise decisions—decisions that appropriately protect the confidentiality of health information—HIM professionals must be aware of the rules, regulations, and laws that govern access to health information. A large part of this chapter is devoted to access issues. The rules that govern access to and disclosure of health information are fluid and often thorny. For many HIM professionals, these issues are among the most interesting they encounter in their career.

Why are legal issues so important to HIM professionals? It is because HIM professionals are relied on to understand these issues by the following people and entities:

- Patients or clients whose health information they manage
- Health care organizations in which they are employed
- All users of health information, such as public health officials, who track communicable and other disease patterns, and government agencies responsible for setting health policy

HIM professionals must take this trust seriously. By gaining a good understanding of legal issues, HIM students and professionals can be worthy of that trust.

Fundamentals of the Legal System

In civilized societies, laws guide actions. These laws set forth principles and processes for our actions and for handling disputes over those actions. Laws govern both our private relationships (the relationships between private parties) and our public relationships (the relationships between private parties and the government).

Private law consists of two types of actions: tort actions and contract actions. In a tort action, one party alleges that another party's wrongful conduct has caused him or her harm. The party bringing the action to court seeks compensation for that harm. In a contract action, one party alleges that a contract exists between himself or herself and another party and that the other party has breached the contract by failing to fulfill an obligation that is part of that contract. The party bringing the contract action seeks either compensation for the breach or a court order to force the breaching party to fulfill that obligation.

Public law is composed of rules, regulations, and criminal law. Congress has charged various governmental agencies with the responsibility of overseeing various aspects of many of our nation's most important industries, including health care. These agencies, acting under the authority of state and federal statutes, issue rules and regulations that touch every department of every health care organization. They cover diverse subjects, such as laboratory safety, incineration of medical waste, employment policies, confidentiality of health records and peer review records, and mandatory reporting of medical device failures or problems. Failure to follow these rules can involve monetary penalties as well as criminal penalties. In addition to these rules and regulations, public laws include a body of criminal law—laws that bar conduct considered harmful to society—and set forth a system for punishing "bad acts."

SELF-ASSESSMENT QUIZ

1. Lawsuits based on private law (relationships between two private parties) can be classified as: (choose best answer below)
   a. Tort or contract actions
   b. Criminal or contract actions
   c. Tort or regulatory actions
   d. All of the above

Sources of Law

Laws that affect the health care system come from four main areas:

- Federal and state constitutions—the supreme law of the nation and state, respectively
- Federal and state statutes—laws enacted by Congress and state legislatures, respectively
- Rules and regulations of administrative agencies—acting under powers delegated to them by the legislature
- Court decisions—decisions that interpret statutes, regulations, and the Constitution and, where no such statutes or regulations are applicable, that apply common law (the large body of principles that have evolved from prior court decisions)

Constitutional Law

The U.S. Constitution grants certain powers to the three branches of the federal government: executive, legislative, and judicial. It also grants certain powers to the individual states. Powers granted by the Constitution may be either express or implied. Express powers are those specifically stated in the Constitution, such as the power to tax and the power to declare war. Implied powers are not specifically listed in the Constitution. They are the actions considered "necessary and proper" to permit the express powers to be accomplished.

The Constitution also limits what federal and state governments can do. For example, the first 10 amendments to the Constitution—the Bill of Rights—protect the rights of citizens to, among other things, free speech, freedom of religion, and due process before deprivation of life, liberty, or property. In a public health care facility (which is considered a governmental unit, as opposed to a private nongovernmental facility), a physician's appointment to the medical staff is considered a property right. Therefore, before that appointment could be terminated or rejected, the hospital would be obliged to provide due process to that physician, such as by a full hearing.

Another constitutional right important to the health care industry is the right of privacy, although that right is not an express one. What is the right to privacy? Generally, it is considered to be a constitutionally recognized right to be left alone, to make decisions about one's own body, and to control one's own information. In the 1965 court decision of *Griswold v. Connecticut*, the U.S. Supreme Court recognized a constitutional right of privacy.[1] This right limits the government's power to regulate abortion, contraception, and other reproductive issues. The constitutional right to privacy has also been interpreted as permitting the terminally ill (or their legal guardians) to make decisions regarding the termination or withholding of medical treatment to prolong life.

It is important to note that the Constitution is the overriding, or highest, law in the United States. If lower laws (e.g., state or federal laws) conflict with principles in the Constitution, the Constitution overrides the conflicting law. When a law has been struck down because it is "unconstitutional," that means that the lower law conflicts with the Constitution and is thus invalid.

> **DID YOU KNOW?**
>
> Since the *Griswold v. Connecticut* ruling regarding contraception use for married couples, the Supreme Court has cited the right to privacy in several other rulings, including *Roe v. Wade*, (1973) regarding abortions, *Eisenstadt v. Baird* (1972) regarding contraception use for unmarried couples, and *Lawrence v. Texas* (2003) regarding homosexual activities.

Federal and State Statutes

Laws enacted by legislatures, be they Congress, state legislatures, or local city councils, are another important source of laws that affect health care facilities. One federal law that dramatically affects health care facilities as well as other businesses is the Americans with Disabilities Act (1990).[2] This law not only affects the hiring and employment practices of businesses but also forces public facilities to remove or modify physical plant characteristics that may serve as access barriers for the disabled. The Safe Medical Devices Act (1990) is another federal statute that affects all health care facilities.[3] It requires that certain incidents that involve medical devices and equipment be reported to a national data bank.

> **DID YOU KNOW?**
>
> According to the ADA, an individual with a disability is a person who:
> - Has a physical or mental impairment that substantially limits one or more major life activities;
> - Has a record of such an impairment; or
> - Is regarded as having such an impairment.

Another very important federal law that affects U.S. health care facilities is The American Recovery and Reinvestment Act of 2009 (Public Law 111-5), specifically, the provisions found in the Health Information Technology for Economic & Clinical Health provisions. This law not only put into place certain incentives for adoption and meaningful use of electronic records, it also substantially affected health information privacy- and security-related practices. It continues to affect health information privacy- and security-related practices through periodically issued regulations.

When federal and state laws conflict, valid federal laws supersede the state laws. When state laws and local laws conflict, the valid state law supersedes the local laws.

Rules and Regulations of Administrative Agencies

Among the powers delegated to administrative agencies and departments of the executive branch by legislatures is the power to adopt rules and regulations to implement various laws. These rules and regulations provide instruction in how to comply with the law. Some of the most important agencies and departments at the federal level that affect health care are the Department of Health and Human Services (DHHS) and its Centers for Medicare and Medicaid Services (CMS), the Food and Drug Administration, the Internal Revenue Service on tax matters, the Department of Justice and the Federal Trade Commission on antitrust issues, and the Department of Labor and the National Labor Relations Board on labor and employment issues.

The rules and regulations of these bodies are valid only if they are within the limits of authority granted to them in their charter. Congress, in passing legislation creating these bodies, decides the broad areas in which these federal agencies may regulate, just as state legislatures do for state agencies. In promulgating their rules and regulations, federal agencies and many state agencies must follow administrative procedure acts passed by the legislature. These acts set forth the steps that administrative agencies must follow in issuing new rules and regulations and deciding disputes about those regulations. The Federal Administrative Procedure Act and most of the states' acts provide for advance notice of proposed rules and opportunity for public comment. Many federal agencies must publish both proposed and final rules in the daily *Federal Register* (https://www.federalregister.gov/). An HIM professional should be familiar with the *Federal Register* and with how to scan it for notices of proposed rule making. By doing so, a facility can have early warning of upcoming changes that may affect facility operations. By commenting on proposed rules, the facility can also influence the language of the final rule.

Court Decisions (Case Law)

When cases are brought before them, federal and state courts interpret statutes and regulations, decide their validity, and follow or create common law (also referred to as case law) when no statutes or regulations apply. In deciding cases, courts generally adhere to the principle of *stare decisis* (let the decision stand). This can be described as following precedent. By referring to similar cases that have been decided in the past and by applying the same principles, courts generally arrive at the same ruling in the current case as in similar previous cases. Sometimes, however, even slight factual differences can result in departures from precedent. Sometimes courts decide that the precedent no longer adequately serves society's needs. One of the most important examples of this from a health care standpoint was the elimination of the doctrine of charitable immunity, which had until the early to mid-1960s protected nonprofit hospitals from liability for harm to patients. Courts now permit harmed patients to sue hospitals for their wrongful acts. The landmark case on this point is *Darling v. Charleston Community Memorial Hospital* (1965) (Box 15-1).[4]

BOX 15-1 Facts of the *Darling* Case Guidelines

In the *Darling* case, a college football player fractured his leg during a game. He was taken to the emergency department of a community hospital, where the physician on emergency department duty was a general practitioner who had not treated a major leg fracture for several years. The physician ordered a radiograph, which revealed a fracture of the tibia and the fibula. The physician reduced the fracture and applied a cast that extended from the patient's toes to just below his groin. Shortly after the cast was applied, the patient began to complain of pain, and he was admitted. The physician split the cast and visited the patient frequently while he was an inpatient. Complaints of pain continued. No specialist consultation was called.

After 2 weeks, the patient was transferred to a larger hospital and placed under the care of an orthopedic surgeon. The surgeon found much dead tissue in the fractured leg and over the next 2 months removed increasing amounts of tissue in an effort to save the leg. Finally, it became necessary to amputate the leg eight inches below the knee.

The patient's father filed suit against the physician and the first hospital, alleging negligence. The physician settled out of court, but the hospital chose to go to court. Darling alleged that the hospital was negligent in its failure to provide enough trained nurses for bedside care of all patients at all times. In this case, Darling claimed that the nurses should have been capable of recognizing the progressive gangrene in the leg and should have called it to the attention of the medical staff and hospital administration so that adequate consultation could have been obtained. The hospital argued that its liability as a charitable corporation—if there was liability at all—was limited to the amount of its liability insurance.

Judgment was eventually returned against the hospital in the amount of $100,000. The court decided that the doctrine of charitable immunity should no longer apply. On appeal, the Illinois Supreme Court agreed, stating: "We agree that the doctrine of charitable immunity can no longer stand . . . [A] doctrine which limits the liability of charitable corporations to the amount of liability insurance that they see fit to carry permits them to determine whether or not they will be liable for their torts and the amount of liability, if any."[4]

As a result, hospitals are held liable for the negligent acts of their employees and, in some circumstances, their physicians. Health care organizations' liability is discussed in more detail later in the chapter.

DID YOU KNOW?

Currently, 36 states have implemented "apology laws," which offer a form of legal protection for physicians who apologize to patients after an unforeseen circumstance. Although some states only prohibit expressions of empathy or sympathy from being admissible in court, others prohibit admissions of fault.

Not all disputes are resolved by courts, however. In health care, for example, health care facilities sometimes avoid the need to resort to the courts by participating in mediation or arbitration, also described as alternative dispute resolution, in which a neutral party or panel hears both sides of a dispute and renders a decision, or by settling claims against them by negotiating a direct payment to the parties bringing the claim in exchange for the claimants' dropping the claim.

SELF-ASSESSMENT QUIZ

2. Which of the following are sources of legal obligations for health care organizations? (choose best answer below)
   a. Federal and state constitutions
   b. Federal and state laws
   c. Administrative rules and regulations
   d. Court decisions that apply common law principles from prior court decisions
   e. All of the above

THE LEGAL SYSTEM

The Court System

Federal Courts

The federal court system and many state systems have three levels of courts: trial courts, intermediate courts of appeals, and a supreme court. The federal trial courts are called U.S. district courts. They cannot hear just any case. To be eligible to hear a case, a court must have jurisdiction. To be heard in a federal court, a case must involve either a federal question or diversity of jurisdiction. Federal question cases involve questions of federal law, such as possible violations of federal law or violations of a party's federal constitutional rights. Diversity cases, which involve citizens of different states, are heard in federal courts, but rather than use federal law, federal judges apply the laws of the applicable states in deciding these cases. In many of these diversity cases, a minimum of $10,000 must also be involved.

Appeals from federal trial courts (U.S. district courts) go to a U.S. court of appeals. The United States is divided into 12 circuits. These courts are typically referred to as the U.S. Court of Appeals for the First (Second, Third, Eleventh, or D.C.) Circuit.

The U.S. Supreme Court is the nation's highest court. It decides appeals from any of the U.S. courts of appeals. It may also hear appeals from the highest state courts if those cases involve federal laws or the U.S. Constitution. In some instances, if a U.S. court of appeals or the highest state court refuses to hear an appeal, the case may be appealed directly to the U.S. Supreme Court. The U.S. Supreme Court need not and could not possibly hear all cases. Because the Court's time is limited and the volume of cases is large, the Supreme Court picks and chooses most of the cases it hears. There are no cut-and-dried criteria for which cases are chosen, but the Court attempts to hear the cases involving the most important questions of law or having the greatest potential impact on society. With a few exceptions, the Supreme Court may decide not to review an appealed case. This does not mean that the Supreme Court necessarily approves of the lower court's decision; it merely means that it chooses not to review the decision.

State and Territory Courts

In some states, trial courts are divided into special branches that hear certain types of cases. Probate court, traffic court, juvenile court, and family and divorce courts are examples. In addition to these special branches, there are trial courts with general jurisdiction—the power to hear all disputes not otherwise assigned to one of these special branches or not otherwise barred from state courts by law.

The job of the trial court is to hear the facts, review the applicable law, and decide the outcome. Sometimes there are no factual disagreements, but the parties to the lawsuit simply disagree over what the law provides. At other times, there may be no disagreement over the law, but the facts are in dispute. Often a case involves questions of law and facts.

Most states also have an intermediate appellate court that hears appeals from state trial court decisions. These appellate courts do not hold a new trial and hear new evidence; they generally limit their review to the trial court record to determine whether proper procedures were followed and whether the law was correctly interpreted.

Every state has a single high court, usually called the supreme court.* A state supreme court hears appeals from the intermediate appellate court or, if no intermediate court exists, the state trial courts. The high court often has other duties as well, such as formulating procedural rules for the lower state courts to follow.

Roles of the Key Players: Court Procedures

The plaintiff is the party who initiates the lawsuit. Plaintiffs initiate suits by filing a complaint, petition, or bill with the clerk of the court. This complaint is a written statement by the plaintiff that states his or her claims and commences the action. Plaintiffs sue one or more defendants, the party or

parties from whom relief or compensation is sought. The defendant then files an answer to the complaint, which may also be called a responsive pleading. In this answer, the defendant denies or otherwise responds to the plaintiff's claims. If the case is not immediately settled, it proceeds into a process of discovery. Sometimes HIM directors are involved in the discovery phase of lawsuits by providing certain information used in the discovery devices described next.

During discovery, each party seeks to discover important information about the case through a pretrial investigation. It includes obtaining pertinent testimony (through depositions, sworn verbal testimony, and through interrogatories, sworn written answers to questions) and documents that may be under the control of the opposing party. For example, a patient who is suing a clinic for negligent care of an infected cut needs to obtain copies of the clinic's patient records that describe the care that was provided to the patient.

The purpose of the discovery phase is to encourage early out-of-court resolution of cases by acquainting all parties with all pertinent facts. If the case cannot be settled out of court, it proceeds to trial. Evidence properly uncovered during the discovery phase is available in court. The judge is in charge of deciding which laws are applicable and also uses the state or federal rules of evidence (as applicable to the setting) in deciding whether certain pieces of evidence are admissible at trial. Not all evidence produced during the discovery phase is admissible. Often, certain evidence is judged to be unfairly prejudicial to one side or the other or is subject to certain protective laws (such as the laws that protect peer review information in health care organizations). The judge examines the evidence, hears arguments on both sides of the question, and then uses the applicable rules of evidence to decide whether the information can be fairly used at trial.

The judge also keeps order and makes decisions necessary to facilitate a fair, impartial trial. If the case involves a jury, the jury's job is to determine the facts as presented in court, at least in part by deciding which witnesses and which evidence to believe, and to apply the law as instructed by the judge.

Even when a jury is present, the judge has substantial influence over the trial result. If he or she finds that insufficient evidence has been presented to establish an issue for the jury to resolve, the judge may in various circumstances refuse to send the case to the jury, dismiss the case, or direct the jury to decide the case one way or another. In civil cases, even if the jury has already rendered a verdict, the judge may decide in favor of the other side, setting aside the jury's verdict. This is called a judgment n.o.v.—judgment *non obstante verdicto* (notwithstanding the verdict).

Some of the other players involved in trial proceedings are the clerk of the court, court reporter, and bailiff. The clerk of the court is the administrative manager of the court and handles the paperwork associated with lawsuits. Complaints are filed with the clerk, as are other pleadings and documents. The court reporter is responsible for

---

*In some states, the terminology is quite different. In New York, the highest court is the New York Court of Appeals, and the trial courts are called supreme courts.

creating a verbatim transcript of court proceedings. Bailiffs are courtroom personnel who are present to assist in keeping order, administering oaths, guarding and the assisting the jury, and performing other duties at the direction of the judge.

SELF-ASSESSMENT QUIZ

3. The federal court system has how many levels of courts? (choose best answer below)
   a. 2 levels: appellate courts and the Supreme Court
   b. 1 level: trial courts
   c. 3 levels: trial courts, intermediate courts of appeals, and the Supreme Court

Cases That Involve Health Care Facilities and Providers

Malpractice and Negligence

Among the most frequent types of claims made against health care facilities and individual providers are claims of negligence or malpractice (professional negligence). Negligence is conduct that society considers unreasonably dangerous because "first, the [individual or party] did foresee or should have foreseen that it would subject another or others to an appreciable risk of harm, and second, only the magnitude of the perceivable risk was such that the [individual or party] should have acted in a safer manner."[5]

At this point, some readers may ask, "How can hospitals be held accountable for actions when they are simply the bricks and mortar within which people work?" Two theories of negligence are used to hold hospitals and other health care organizations accountable for their conduct. Under the first theory, *respondeat superior* (meaning "let the master answer" for the actions of the servant—the doctrine of "agency"), the legal system imputes the negligent actions of the organization's employees or agents over whom it has control to the health care organization itself. Using this theory, courts hold employers responsible for the acts of their employees or agents that are performed within the scope of employment. For example, a hospital can be held responsible for the actions of its nurses while they are acting within the scope of their employment (e.g., when they are performing some aspect of their job assignment), but a hospital would not be held responsible for the actions of a nurse in its employ while the nurse is grocery shopping after work.

Under the second, more current theory of corporate negligence, courts can hold health care organizations liable for their own independent acts of negligence. This theory holds organizations responsible for monitoring the activities of the people who function within their facilities, whether those people are employees or independent contractors, such as physicians, and for complying with appropriate industry standards, such as accreditation (The Joint Commission) standards, licensing regulations, and Conditions of Participation issued by Medicare. Health care organizations are no longer considered to be merely physicians' "workshops." They retain some responsibility for all who are authorized to function within their facilities (see examples of situations that can lead to malpractice claims against health care organizations and providers).

Examples of Situations Leading to Malpractice Claims

- Failure to properly diagnose a condition, such as cancer
- Failure to properly treat a condition—for example, not cleaning a wound before stitching it
- Failure to monitor or supervise a patient's condition and take appropriate action—for example, in the *Darling* case described earlier in the chapter, the nurses failed to note and report the leg's worsening condition
- Failure to credential medical staff members properly (e.g., granting a physician privileges to perform some types of surgery for which he or she is not qualified)

Malpractice claims are not the only kind of claims against health care organizations and providers. The following are some of the other types of claims that HIM professionals may encounter in their professional careers.

DID YOU KNOW?

In 2004 The Joint Commission introduced the Universal Protocol for Preventing Wrong Site, Wrong Procedure and Wrong Person Surgery™ for all accredited hospitals, ambulatory care, and office-based surgery facilities. These requirements seek to address and prevent sentinel events (unexpected occurrences involving death or serious physical or psychological injury) related to medical professionals performing the wrong procedure on a patient, on the wrong site or location on the body, or on the wrong patient.

Intentional Torts

Intentional tort claims that may be brought against health care facilities include assault and battery, false imprisonment, defamation of character, invasion of privacy, fraud or misrepresentation, and intentional infliction of emotional distress.

When one thinks of assault and battery, one often thinks of a mugging or an attack of some sort. However, an assault is simply a deliberate threat, coupled with the apparent ability, to do physical harm to another person without that person's consent. No contact is required. For example, if a nurse stood over a patient with a syringe, stating that he or she was going to inject the patient with a strong sedative regardless of whether the patient agreed to it, that would constitute an assault if the patient was aware of the threat. If the nurse proceeded to inject the patient against the patient's will, that would constitute a battery. A battery is nonconsensual, intentional touching of another person in a socially impermissible manner. Awareness of the victim is irrelevant. An unconscious patient who has surgery performed without express (actual) or implied consent (such as when a patient is brought to the facility for life-saving treatment) is the victim of a battery.

Could assault and battery ever really happen in a health care facility? In *Peete v. Blackwell* (1986), a nurse was awarded damages after a physician with whom she was working struck her and cursed at her while ordering her to turn on suctioning equipment.[5] Although there were no lasting injuries, the jury awarded $1 in compensation and $10,000 in punitive damages.

The laws concerning battery are one of the prime reasons behind the requirement to obtain the patient's written consent to treatment. Allegations of battery against health care facilities most often involve situations in which improper or no patient consent was obtained before a surgical procedure. Regardless of whether the procedure helps or harms the patient, invasions of the patient's person without consent entitle the patient to at least nominal damages.**

False imprisonment is unlawful restraint of a person's personal liberty or the unlawful restraining or confining of a person. Physical force is not required; all that is required is a reasonable fear that force will be used to detain or intimidate the person into following orders. How could this apply to a health care facility? If a facility tried to prevent a patient's departure from the facility until the patient's bill was paid, this could qualify as false imprisonment. The use of physical restraints to keep a patient in bed for no other reason than inadequate staffing available to monitor patients could also qualify.

False imprisonment issues can be complex. For example, if an intoxicated driver involved in a motor vehicle accident is treated for minor cuts in an emergency department and then wants to be discharged to drive home but is still extremely intoxicated, must the facility release that patient, or may he or she be restrained until capable of driving safely? Statutes in some states permit intoxicated or mentally ill people to be detained by a hospital if they are dangerous to themselves or others. This is one example of why it is so important for the staff in health care organizations to be familiar with state laws. In judging reasonableness of a health care provider's actions in detaining a patient, documentation in the patient record is often vital.

Defamation of character is oral (slander) or written (libel) communication to a person (other than the person defamed) that tends to damage the defamed person's reputation in the eyes of the community. To succeed in a defamation action, the defamed person must show that there was communication to a third party. Truth of the statements is a defense, as is privilege. If the defamation occurs during a privileged communication—such as during confidential communications between spouses or in a talk with a priest or minister—defamation is not found as long as the statements are made without malice (evil intent). Defamation cases in health care are unusual, but they do occur, especially in the context of medical staff credentialing and granting of privileges, when the defamed party argues that the defamatory remarks were made with malice. Professionals who are called incompetent in front of others generally have a right to sue to defend their reputation. If the person making the remark cannot prove that the comment is true or that some other privilege applies, he or she may be held liable for damages. For that reason, it is generally wise to refrain from making disparaging remarks about other health professionals and colleagues.

Invasion of privacy is an intentional tort with which HIM professionals must be concerned. By the very act of submitting to treatment, patients give up some privacy. However, negligent disregard for patients' privacy can and does result in actions against health care providers and organizations, and it can also result in regulatory penalties such as fines for violations of those regulations, and even criminal penalties. This is discussed later in the chapter. Because HIM professionals and other health professionals work with sensitive information on an almost constant basis, it is easy to become callous to privacy issues. Those who have visited friends or family members in the hospital and overheard staff members talking casually about patients and their conditions in hallways, elevators, and the cafeteria have witnessed what may have been an invasion of privacy or breach of confidentiality. Health care providers who divulge confidential information from a patient's record to an improper recipient without the patient's permission have invaded the patient's privacy and breached their duty of confidentiality. A great deal of this chapter is devoted to identifying what health information is confidential and who is a proper or an improper recipient. HIM professionals must learn these principles well and become expert in applicable state and federal laws so that they not only avoid violating patients' privacy themselves but also can help other health professionals understand how to respect patients' privacy and confidentiality rights.

Fraud is a willful and intentional misrepresentation that could cause harm or loss to a person or the person's property. In addition to fraud associated with improper billing for procedures not performed or deliberately coding incorrectly to gain a higher payment (criminal fraud), fraud can occur in health care facilities when a physician promises a certain surgical result, although he or she knows that the result is not so certain. For example, a physician who promises that there is no chance of a complication resulting from plastic surgery, although such complications can occur, is guilty of misrepresentation.

Intentional infliction of emotional or mental distress can also result in claims against health care facilities. In a 1975 case, a court found that a physician and hospital (through its employees) were guilty of intentional infliction of emotional distress. In this case, the mother of a premature infant (who died shortly after birth) had gone to her physician for a postpartum checkup.[6] She noticed a report in her medical record stating that the child was past 5 months' gestation and therefore could not be disposed of as a surgical specimen. On questioning her physician about what had happened to the body, the physician told his nurse to take the mother to the hospital. At the hospital, the mother was taken by a

---

**See, for example, *Perna v. Pirozzi*, 457 A.2d 431 (N.J. 1983) in which the supreme court of New Jersey held that a patient who consents to surgery by one surgeon but who is actually operated on by another has grounds for an action for battery!

hospital employee to a freezer. The freezer was opened, and the mother was handed a jar containing her baby. The mother was awarded $100,000 damages, upheld on appeal. The cases are not always so dramatic. In 1985, a Georgia court found a physician guilty of intentional infliction of emotional distress for yelling at a patient and her husband.[7]

Products Liability

Products liability cases sometimes involve health care facilities. Products liability is the liability of a manufacturer, seller, or supplier of a product to a buyer or other third party for injuries sustained because of a defect in the product. The injured party may sue the seller, manufacturer, or supplier. If, for example, a hospital improperly processes or stores blood in its own blood bank, it may be liable to any patient who is harmed as a result. If the staff of a research hospital designs a new type of medical equipment that is tested on patients, any harm resulting from product defects can result in product liability claims. Products liability is a complex subject beyond the scope of this chapter. It is included here simply as a reminder that there are many potential sources of liability for today's health care organizations.

Contractual Disputes

Breach of contract is a common claim in litigation that involves health care providers and organizations. Typically, the claims arise when one party to a contract fails to follow the terms agreed to in the contract. Interestingly, courts have been willing to enforce ethical standards prohibiting breach of confidentiality (such as the American Hospital Association's [AHA's] patient right's statement titled *The Patient Care Partnership: Understanding Expectations, Rights and Responsibilities,* and ethical standards of the American Medical Association) as part of a contractual relationship between health care providers and their patients. Thus, improper disclosure of health information can give rise to a breach of contract claim and an invasion of privacy or breach of confidentiality claim. (Invasion of privacy and breach of confidentiality claims are discussed later in this chapter.) In an important case on this subject, *Hammonds v. Aetna Casualty and Surety Co.* (1965), the court found that a physician breached an implied condition of his patient–physician contract when he disclosed health information to a hospital's insurer without the patient's authorization.[8]

Antitrust Claims

Although such claims have decreased in recent years, health care providers and organizations have been targets of antitrust claims. Most of these claims revolve around mergers and acquisitions and alleged anticompetitive behavior in medical staff credentialing activities. For example, if the obstetricians on the medical staff of a local hospital seek to remove an obstetrician's staff privileges so that there is less competition for patients, that hospital may find itself entangled in an antitrust suit. These suits usually do not directly involve the HIM department or service, but sometimes HIM professionals are involved to the extent that they support the medical staff's peer review and credentialing functions.

Crimes and Corporate Compliance

Criminal activity can take place in any health care facility. A nurse practicing in a hospital is probably able to tell of mysterious discrepancies in narcotic counts (counts done on each unit that stores narcotics to ensure that no drugs are missing). Angel-of-death murder scenarios have been sensationalized in books and television, but they have their basis in actual events in which the weak and ill have become prey for criminal or deviant behavior by facility employees. For example, in 2004, Charles Cullen, a registered nurse, pled guilty to the murder of 29 patients he had cared for at various health care facilities. Patient abuse and sexual improprieties are also terrible phenomena that can occur in health care facilities. In addition, falsification of business or patient records (e.g., by billing Medicare for patients not seen or services not performed, or by deliberately assigning incorrect codes to maximize payment) may be grounds for criminal indictment.

DID YOU KNOW?

In 1999, five people were convicted of felonies for their role in a drug diversion scheme where approximately $3 million worth of pharmaceutical drugs were stolen from the SUNY Health Science Center and Crouse Hospitals in New York from 1988 to1995. SUNY Health Science Center pharmacy department employees stole cancer medications from the department, then sold them to other external pharmacies, a physician's group, and a wholesaling company. A pharmacy buyer from Crouse Hospital stole drugs from that organization and sold them to a drug company.

Concerns about improper billing practices have led to the passage of laws and regulations targeting health care providers who submit false claims, engage in fraudulent coding practices, and otherwise fail to comply with statutory and regulatory mandates. The Health Insurance Portability and Accountability Act of 1996 (Public Law 104-191; HIPAA), the Balanced Budget Act of 1997 (Public Law 105-33), and even the Federal False Claims Act (1863, with 1986 amendments) and its subsequent interpretation by the DHHS are examples of laws imposing penalties—up to and including criminal sanctions—against health care providers who engage in fraudulent practices.

The growth in prosecution against health care providers has led to a profound interest (and need) among provider organizations in developing corporate compliance plans with the goal of preventing, detecting, and resolving wrongdoing in health care organizations. Ideally, the compliance program not only discourages unlawful activity but also promotes a culture in which suspected problems can be safely raised internally, preventing the need for "whistleblowers" to go to outside regulatory bodies to raise concerns. These whistleblower-based prosecutions, called *qui tam* prosecutions, have been particularly attractive to employees (disgruntled or otherwise) because the whistleblower is entitled to a share of the government's winnings in these cases. Health care leaders have recognized the sense of solving suspected problems internally and rapidly.

The health care organization's compliance plan should focus on all areas of regulatory compliance, with special emphasis on preventing fraudulent coding and billing practices. The Office of the Inspector General (OIG) of the DHHS has issued model compliance plans for various types of health care organizations (such as clinical laboratories and hospitals), which provide organizations with a logical starting point in developing their own corporate compliance plans. The OIG also issues periodic advisory opinions and fraud statistics to show its prosecutorial priorities, which is useful to health care organizations in planning their own fraud prevention efforts. In addition, the American Health Information Management Association (AHIMA) has published numerous articles on the subject, a model Health Information Management Compliance Program, and a practice brief that is available on AHIMA's Web site. Common to all compliance programs is the need to address and establish internal standards of conduct, education for staff on compliance, regular auditing of coding and billing practices, continual monitoring of practices, and methods of further developing and updating the organization's plan.

Issues germane to the HIM professional take center stage in these compliance plans. Not only must HIM professionals be concerned with accurate coding and billing, they must also focus on other areas of regulatory compliance, such as ensuring the confidentiality and security of health information. HIM professionals must also guard against outside contracts with vendors containing terms that could lead to risks of noncompliance.

Noncompliance with Statutes, Rules, and Regulations

As mentioned earlier, health care organizations that fail to follow government-imposed mandates run the risk of a variety of potential penalties, including monetary or criminal penalties, removal from participation in the Medicare program, and even loss of licensure.

SELF-ASSESSMENT QUIZ

4. Which of the following elements are key to a finding of negligence? (choose best answer below)
   a. Strict liability
   b. Foreseeability
   c. Breach of professional ethics
5. Liability of a manufacturer, seller, or supplier of a product to a buyer for injuries sustained because of a defect in the product is an example of: (choose best answer below)
   a. Negligence
   b. Crime
   c. Products liability
   d. None of the above

With this information as a backdrop, the remainder of this chapter looks at the most common legal obligations and risks that face health care facilities, health care providers, and HIM professionals in particular. Next are the legal obligations and risks that involve HIM professionals most directly.

LEGAL OBLIGATIONS AND RISKS OF HEALTH CARE FACILITIES AND INDIVIDUAL HEALTH CARE PROVIDERS

Duties to Patients, in General

Patients have numerous rights associated with their health care. Some of these rights are discussed in detail in this section. Laws, rules, or regulations establish some rights; others are based on ethical codes and even the federal Constitution. Beyond the specific rights discussed in the following, HIM professionals should be aware of patient rights granted in the AHA's patient rights statement discussed earlier, the Ethics, Rights and Responsibilities chapter of the accreditation manuals issued by The Joint Commission (if applicable to the employer), and specific laws governing access to care, such as the Emergency Medical Treatment and Active Labor Act (EMTALA; 42 USC 1395 dd). The EMTALA imposed new obligations on health care facilities to provide medical screening examinations and stabilizing treatment to patients before transferring them to other facilities. The purpose of the law was to reduce inappropriate transfers (such as those done primarily for financial reasons when the patient has no insurance) that put the patient at risk of harm. The net effect of these various bills or rights, codes of conduct, and laws has been to alert patients to their rights and to provide remedies when their health care providers fail to respect those rights. We are entering the era of empowered health care consumers. This should lead to more interaction between patients and the HIM department as patients seek more information about their care and treatment.

SELF-ASSESSMENT QUIZ

6. Which Act imposed new obligations on health care facilities to provide medical screening examinations to patients before transferring them to other facilities? (choose best answer below)
   a. HIPAA
   b. EMTALA
   c. ARRA
   d. Freedom of Information Act

Duty to Maintain Health Information

One of the most fundamental duties that involve HIM professionals and their health care facility employers is that of maintaining health information about patients. This duty is imposed explicitly by state and federal statutes and regulations as well as accreditation standards. In some states, the hospital licensing statutes specify not only that a medical record must be kept for every patient but also what that record must contain at a minimum. Failure to meet the requirements of these licensing statutes could subject a facility to loss of licensure and closure. The law and regulations setting forth the Conditions of Participation in federal payment programs such as Medicare also require that medical records be kept, and they outline in broad terms what those records must include.[9] Accreditation standards of The Joint Commission also require accredited facilities to maintain medical records, and the HIPAA privacy rule also speaks to what documents must be maintained for patient access and use as part of a designated record set (DRS)—defined in that rule as a group of records maintained by or for a covered entity—as follows:

- The medical records and billing records about individuals maintained by or for a covered health care provider
- The enrollment, payment, claims adjudication, and case or medical management record systems maintained by or for a health plan or
- Used, in whole or in part, by or for the covered entity to make decisions about individuals

Patients must be able to access that information for at least 6 years, and even longer if state or other federal laws require longer retention periods.

The duty to maintain health information is also implied in other laws. For example, vital statistics laws require the reporting of births and deaths. Under federal and state statutes, health care facilities must report to various data banks certain disease conditions and medical events, such as the treatment of gunshot wounds, suspected child abuse, elder abuse, industrial accidents, certain poisonings, abortions, cancer cases, and communicable diseases.

Mandatory reporting requirements vary from state to state. These statutes have in common that reporting is required and the authorization of the patient is generally not needed. In fact, even if the patient expresses the wish not to have information released, the health care organization must comply with the reporting requirement. This tension between the reporting statutes and confidentiality often arises with state requirements for reporting actual or suspected child abuse. Reports made in error admittedly cause much pain and embarrassment for the family involved. Many states, recognizing the natural reluctance of people to make such reports when the abuse is not proved, have exempted the party making the report from liability for erroneous reports as long as the report is made in good faith (in other words, without malice or evil intent).

The reporting statutes attempt to encourage reporting in another important way. For example, failure to report child abuse can result in liability for injuries a child later sustains when discharged home to the suspected or actual abuser.

The problem becomes even stickier when mandatory reporting statutes conflict with other laws, such as state laws that bar disclosure of mental health treatment records and federal laws that bar disclosure of substance abuse treatment. If in the course of therapy a child or an elderly person indicates that he or she has been abused, what must the therapist do? Some court decisions have permitted the protection of these confidentiality laws to be circumvented, but only to the extent necessary to fulfill the requirements of the reporting statute.[10] In addition, some state confidentiality laws permit exceptions in cases of imminent harm, in which the child or abused party is in immediate danger. Other statutes, however, do not provide convenient solutions to this problem. HIM professionals who face such a situation should consult legal counsel, who may seek direction from the court in reconciling all the interests involved.

These examples illustrate why compliance with mandatory reporting statutes is not always as simple as it may seem. HIM professionals must determine their state's requirements and how those requirements may conflict with other confidentiality obligations so that appropriate reporting procedures are in place.

Duty to Retain Health Information and Other Key Documents and to Keep Them Secure

Just as there are requirements to create patient records, there are also requirements to retain that information. Health care facilities take guidance from federal and state record retention laws and regulations and from state statutes of limitations in setting their own record and information retention policies. Facilities must also take into account the uses of and needs for that information, the space available for hard copy storage if the records include paper, and the resources available for microfilming, creating optical disks, or electronic storage. In addition, there are evidentiary considerations in record retention, including most recent amendments to the Federal Rules of Civil Procedure for the preservation of electronically stored information (referred to as "e-discovery rules"). Remember, however, that record retention regulations and rules are only a baseline; in other words, facilities must meet these minimum retention periods but may establish longer retention schedules if desired.

It is not enough simply to keep these records. HIM professionals must ensure that the records are kept in a way that minimizes the chance of their being lost, destroyed, or altered. Plaintiffs have won negligence suits against facilities that failed to safeguard their records from loss or destruction.[11] Security of health information has taken on new and more complex dimensions as more and more health information is stored in various electronic and other media. Medical records security used to be a relatively straightforward matter of controlling access to the areas where paper records were kept and having adequate safeguards against physical threats such as fire, flood, and severe weather. Now, with each new form of data storage and retrieval technology, HIM professionals must be alert to the new security threats that may accompany those technologies.

HIPAA security regulations, which went into effect in 2005, assist in avoiding those security threats. In 1996, Congress passed the act commonly referred to as HIPAA. As part of that act, Congress added a new section to Title XI of the

Social Security Act, titled "Administrative Simplification." The purpose of the Administrative Simplification amendment was to improve the efficiency and effectiveness of the health care system by stimulating the development of standards to facilitate electronic maintenance and transmission of health information. The act directed the secretary of DHHS to adopt standards for electronically maintained health information and standards for electronic signatures and other matters such as unique health identifiers and code sets.

The standards, which went into effect in April 2005, apply to health care providers, health plans, and health care (data) clearinghouses.

Certain administrative procedures, physical safeguards, and technical security services and mechanisms are required under these regulations. Those obligations have been extended not only to the entities covered by HIPAA but also to their business associates, through a new provision within ARRA. See Chapter 8 for an in-depth discussion of security safeguards. The regulations apply to all electronically maintained health information in health care organizations, and it is important for HIM professionals to become familiar with the final standards.

Health information is valuable only if it is accurate, complete, and available for use when needed. Therefore, HIM professionals must design safeguards that not only protect the information from loss or destruction and prevent the corruption of electronically stored data from power losses or surges but also protect the integrity of the information itself. In other words, the information must be protected from inappropriate alteration.

Why would anyone want to alter health information or documentation in a patient's record? In some situations, such as when a health professional is sued for malpractice, he or she may be tempted to alter the record to make the documentation appear more complete than it originally was. Some health professionals have not yet learned the importance of thorough contemporaneous documentation (i.e., documentation made while care is being provided, while the information is fresh in the care provider's mind), and as a result, when the time comes to defend the provider's actions, the record may not reflect the care of the patient in a positive light. HIM professionals must guard against inappropriate alterations to health information by controlling access to records with extra precautions for records that are involved in litigation. If presented with a request to make a change to a patient record involved in litigation, an HIM professional should refer that request to the facility's defense counsel. Rather than "improving" the documentation, a health professional who makes later alterations often ends up harming the case because the plaintiff's attorney may have already gotten a copy of the original, unaltered record from the patient before filing suit. Imagine how it might appear to a jury if the plaintiff's attorney can show that the defendant altered the record when the suit was filed and that the health facility took no steps to protect the record from alteration.[12] For these reasons, it is wise to supervise all access to patient records

that are involved in litigation. By doing so, the integrity of the record can be maintained while appropriate access is permitted.

Falsification of records can lead to other problems as well. In some states, it is a crime if it is done for the purpose of cheating or defrauding and may lead to sanctions against health professionals' licenses, as well as prison sentences.

Error Correction

Errors that are made in documenting information must be corrected as soon as they are detected with use of proper error correction methods. These methods should be outlined in the facility's policy and procedure manual and taught to all people who document patient health information.

Generally, the person who made an error should correct it. If the correction is a major one (e.g., erroneous laboratory results were entered on the record and resulted in a problem in the patient's care), the person making the correction should consult the HIM manager, risk manager, and perhaps even facility legal counsel to ensure that the correction method complies with facility policy and that all appropriate steps that need to be taken are followed. Most corrections are not so dramatic. A nurse begins to chart patient A's information on patient B's record but instantly realizes the error. Or, in the course of making up a new medication administration record, the unit clerk misspells the name of a medication or picks the wrong medication off of a computerized list of drugs and the nurse who double-checks the record quickly catches it. In situations that involve paper-based health information, the person making the error should simply draw a single line through the incorrect entry, enter the correction and initial it, and note the time and date of the correction (Figure 15-1). Under no circumstances should the original entry be erased, scribbled over, or hidden, because an obliteration can raise suspicion in the minds of jurors about the original entry and whether it is an attempt to cover up a major problem.

> **? DID YOU KNOW?**
> The Joint Commission provides a "do not use" list of abbreviations as part of their Information Management standards. Such abbreviations include "IU" (International Unit) because it could be mistaken for "IV" (intravenous) or even the number "10."

Error correction methods are different for electronic health record systems. A system's procedures should clearly specify how errors are to be handled. Errors that are caught immediately at the time they are made can simply be changed, with no need to preserve the original entry. Errors that are caught after the point in time when someone has relied on the erroneous information pose a problem; the system must provide some way to save the original entry but clearly show the new entry and the date and time it was made. Health information systems software varies, and procedures differ with each system. HIM professionals should insist that

FIGURE 15-1 Correcting errors in documentation.

the system they use permits appropriate error correction and addendum procedures so that the integrity of the information is preserved.

Addenda

In some circumstances, simple error correction methods are insufficient. For example, if a substantial portion of a patient's history and physical examination was left out of the original dictated report, it would be impossible to squeeze in the missing information on the original typed report. When new information is being added to a record, an addendum is used. The person making the addendum should create an electronic link or enter a reference to the addendum near the original entry or information (e.g., "1/3/06—See addendum to H&P" —signature) and then file the linked addendum.

Sometimes, after they have reviewed their health information, patients ask that their records be amended. The Privacy Act (discussed later in the chapter) permits such amendments, but it applies only to health care organizations operated by the federal government, such as Department of Defense health care facilities, Veterans Administration health facilities, and Indian Health Service facilities. HIPAA's privacy rule also permits such requests and requires covered entities to consider them. In fact, there are few circumstances under which a facility may deny an amendment request under the HIPAA privacy rule. Requests for amendment may also arise in the context of mental health therapy, when patients have said something during therapy that they later wish they had not said. Facility policy should outline how these requests are to be handled. Ordinarily, requests for amendments should be discussed with the attending physician or the health professional who authored the original entry that is in dispute, if that is the reason for the amendment. If the physician believes that the request is inappropriate, and his or her reasoning falls under one of the permissible reasons under the HIPAA privacy rule for denying an amendment request, he or she should discuss the matter with the patient. Otherwise, the patient's amendment should be handled as an addendum to the record without change to the original entry and identified as an additional document appended to the original patient record at the request of the patient. Section 164.526 of the HIPAA privacy rule outlines an appeal process that must be made available to the patient if the request for amendment is denied and the patient wishes to appeal that denial.

Authentication and Authorship Issues

One aspect of protecting the integrity of health information that has become increasingly controversial is the issue of authentication. In other words, how can facilities identify the author of a particular record or computer entry into a health information system? In a paper record system, this is done through the original signature or through the use of a personal signature stamp (under written agreement with the facility not to delegate the use of the stamp to another person). Authentication not only serves to identify the author of an entry but also indicates that the author has reviewed the entry or report for accuracy and attests to it. In electronic health record systems, authentication of documentation is often achieved through a unique identification code (often called "user ID") and password entered by the person making the note or report. As is true with the use of signature stamps, it is important to ensure that the user's identification code and password are not shared with others; if they are to be reliable indication of authorship, they must be used only by the person to whom they belong.

HIPAA's regulations include a section proposing electronic signature standards. These proposed standards would require that any electronic signature systems for health care information provide a reliable way to identify the signer, ensure the message's integrity, and provide for nonrepudiation (to prevent a signer from later denying having signed the message).

The proposed standards noted that the only current electronic signature system that meets all these requirements is cryptographically based digital signature technology.[†] Any system used would have to guarantee the identity of the signer and prevent changes to the document in question after it is signed. We are still awaiting the final rule on electronic signature standards.

Validity of Health Information as Evidence

One of the reasons it is important to protect the integrity of health information is so that the information or record may be used as evidence in court proceedings as an exception to the hearsay rules, which generally bar out-of-court unsworn statements from being used in court as proof. State laws governing the admissibility of health information as evidence vary.

In some states, health information can be admitted as an exception to the hearsay rule. The **hearsay rule** bars the legal admissibility of **evidence** that is not the personal knowledge of the witness. For example, a defendant physician may want to use the patient record to defend a malpractice claim, but the record contains information beyond the physician's personal knowledge—statements of nurses, descriptions of treatments given by respiratory therapists, recording of laboratory results prepared by medical technologists, and so on. In some states, however, medical records and health information may be admitted either as a business record or as an explicit exception to the hearsay rule in the state's rules of evidence. Business records are presumed to be reliable because they are routinely prepared in the course of business and are created as business is transacted, not specially prepared months later for use in court. In any event, it is up to the judge to decide whether any record is admissible in court proceedings according to the applicable rules of evidence.

When submitting the record for use in court as a business record, the HIM professional must attest that the record was made in the normal course of business. If anything has happened to that record or information that departs from the normal course of business, such as an alteration of original documentation, the information no longer has that presumption of reliability and may no longer be admissible. As discussed earlier, this action can cripple a malpractice defense and destroy the information's value as evidence in other types of proceedings, such as personal injury cases.

What if a record has been microfilmed or put onto other storage media, such as an optical disk or a CD-ROM, and the original destroyed? Can the information still be used as evidence? Rules of evidence require that when originals are still available, they must be produced. This is called the **best evidence rule**. When it becomes necessary to prove the contents of a document, the original must be produced or its absence accounted for. The best evidence rule was adopted

to prevent fraud or mistake as to the contents of a document or record. If the original has been destroyed pursuant to a facility's records retention program and only copies of that information remain, that secondary evidence (e.g., the microfilm or optical disk) is probably admissible if the court is satisfied that the secondary record accurately reflects the original and that destruction of the original was done in good faith (e.g., as part of a facility-sponsored record retention program and not specifically to prevent the information's use in court). The testimony of the HIM professional is important in explaining the retention program and the secondary information or record system. Because of the length of time microfilming has been used, most courts admit microfilm copies without much question, but more recent technologies often must be explained by the HIM professional before the information can be used. This is one of the reasons that careful thought must go into the selection of new technology for information storage and retrieval. Obtaining the opinion of legal counsel about the admissibility of information stored in new ways and forms is a wise step to take before adopting new technology.

Retention of Other Records and Information

Patient records and information are not the only important documents to retain. Medical staff credential files, incident reports, surgical videos that identify patients, peer review data and minutes, radiographs, surgery schedules, and emergency department logs are just a few of the items for which a retention schedule must be established.[13] (See Chapter 7 for a full discussion of record retention.)

> ## ✓ SELF-ASSESSMENT QUIZ
>
> 7. When documents/evidence are needed in court and the originals are available, the originals must be produced. This is an example of: (choose best answer below)
>   a. The best evidence rule
>   b. The substitute doctrine
>   c. A grand jury summons
>   d. A subpoena to testify

Duty to Maintain Confidentiality

Think about a past visit to a physician. What information was shared? If a patient discovered that his or her physician repeated that information to another patient, a neighbor, or the local newspaper, wouldn't that patient be angry? Might that not deter patients from sharing all relevant health and history information with their care providers, thus threatening the quality of care they receive? Today's society considers communications between patients and their health care providers to be confidential. For the sake of discussion, this chapter defines a confidential communication as one that transmits information to a health care provider as part of the relationship between the provider and the patient under circumstances that imply that the information shall remain private. Patients rely on that promise of confidentiality in disclosing intimate details to health care providers.

[†]For a good overview of digital signatures, see Ballam H: HIPAA, security, and electronic signature: a closer look, J Am Health Inform Manage Assoc 70:26-30, 1999.

Health care providers are bound by various laws and ethical standards to maintain the confidentiality of private health information. Physicians, for example, are required by their Hippocratic Oath to maintain confidentiality: "What I may see or hear in the course of the treatment, or even outside of the treatment in regard to the life of men, which on no account one must spread abroad, I will keep to myself."

The AHA's patient rights statement, called *Patient Care Partnership: Understanding Expectations, Rights and Responsibilities,* addresses the health facility's obligation. One of the key elements in that statement addresses the protection of the patient's privacy by the health care organization. AHIMA's own Code of Ethics sets the standard for HIM professionals to "advocate, uphold and defend the individual's right to privacy and the doctrine of confidentiality in the use and disclosure of information." Protecting the confidentiality of protected health information is one of the primary aims of the HIPAA privacy rule (45 CFR Section 164.530). As part of the rule, organizations covered by the rule must provide patients with a notice of privacy practices. This notice is intended to explain to patients how their protected health information is used—both with and without their permission. The HIPAA privacy rule and the HITECH provisions of ARRA specify certain issues that must be addressed in the notice. The actual privacy notice is most often developed by the organization's privacy officer, who often is an HIM professional. In addition, handling requests related to the use and disclosure of health information is most often a function of the HIM department. Also, numerous state laws address the subject, as do Medicare's Conditions of Participation, The Joint Commission standards, and a growing body of court decisions.

To understand fully their obligation to keep patient health information confidential, health care providers need to understand what information is and is not confidential, or, in the language of HIPAA, "protected." Some of the information that may appear in patient records is not "protected" health information.

Determining what information is confidential is not always as straightforward as it might seem. For example, for substance abuse treatment facilities, the very fact of a patient's admission for treatment is confidential, according to federal law, and may not be disclosed without patient authorization except under limited circumstances.[14] Under the HIPAA privacy rule, however, the fact of admission could be shared without completing an authorization, as long as the patient has agreed to inclusion in the facility's directory and as long as applicable state laws are not more restrictive. The HIPAA privacy rule does not preempt (or override) more protective privacy laws and regulations—either federal or state, unless they are in conflict with HIPAA's provisions. So, if HIPAA were to permit the release of directory information, but the applicable state law required patient authorization before release of directory information, that state law would be followed and not be preempted by the HIPAA privacy rule.

HIPAA's provisions protect a broad range of health information. The HIPAA privacy rule defines "protected" health information (PHI) as "individually identifiable health information that is transmitted by electronic media; maintained in any medium described in the definition of *electronic media* at § 162.103 of the rule; or transmitted or maintained in any other form or medium" (45 CFR Sections 160.103).

Thus, the decision as to whether an item is considered protected depends largely on the definition of individually identifiable health information (IIHI). The rule defines IIHI as information that is a subset of health information, including demographic information collected from an individual, and the following:

- is created or received by a health care provider, health plan, employer, or health care clearinghouse and
- relates to the past, present, or future physical or mental health or condition of an individual; the provision of health care to an individual; or the past, present, or future payment for the provision of health care to an individual;
- that identifies the individual or
- with respect to which there is a reasonable basis to believe the information can be used to identify the individual

Originally, HIPAA's privacy rule provisions only apply to "covered entities," as defined by the rule. (Certain aspects of the privacy rule now also apply to the covered entity's "business associates." This was one of the many changes to HIPAA found in Title XIII of ARRA, as noted later in the chapter.) The definition of covered entities includes any entity as follows:

- A health care provider that conducts certain transactions in electronic form
- A health care clearinghouse
- A health plan

So although this covers the majority of health care organizations (because electronic transactions are the most common methods of billing for services), the definition did not cover all organizations that may have access to protected health information, such as personal health record sites on the Internet,‡ companies that provide services related to health information storage and processing, and so on. Covered entities using outside agents or organizations (not part of the facility's own workforce) to handle or process PHI on their behalf must use a special agreement with that agency to ensure that the agency follows rules set by the covered entity for handling PHI. This agreement is called a business associate agreement, and the HIPAA privacy rule and HITECH provisions of ARRA outline what must be addressed in these agreements, at a minimum. ARRA has modified HIPAA in a variety of ways. One of the most important changes is extending certain privacy- and security-related obligations to the business associates of covered entities.

Still, there are many recipients of health information that are neither covered entities nor business associates and are

---

‡On August 25, 2009, the Federal Trade Commission published a "health breach notification" final rule that requires personal health record vendors and certain related parties to notify individuals whose personal health record–related information has been subject to a breach of security. See Federal Trade Commission: Final rule: health breach notification rule (16 C.F.R. Part 318), *Federal Register* 74, August 25, 2009. Available at http://www.ftc.gov/os/2009/08/R911002hbn.pdf.

therefore not governed by the HIPAA privacy rule. This issue has been of great concern to many privacy advocates, who argue that the legal protection should follow the protected health information, regardless of who possesses that information.

Beyond health information, there are other documents in the health care facility that must be kept confidential if they are to serve their purpose adequately. Incident reports in which adverse occurrences are reported and investigated must be kept confidential to the extent permitted by state law so that staff members feel free to report such occurrences. Peer review records, such as committee minutes and credentialing files, must also be kept confidential to encourage candor in monitoring, managing, and improving the quality of clinical care.[15] HIM professionals are often involved in developing facility policies to protect the confidentiality of this information and in teaching staff to follow those policies.

In developing facility policies to protect the confidentiality of health information, HIM professionals must ensure that those policies adhere to federal and state laws and regulations on the subject. Many state HIM associations publish excellent legal guides to cover the basic tenets of individual states' laws. Plan to become familiar with these resources. Additional federal laws and regulations are described next.

Privacy Act of 1974

The Privacy Act was designed to give citizens some control over the information collected about them by the federal government and its agencies. It grants people the following rights:

- To find out what information about them has been collected
- To see and have a copy of that information
- To correct or amend the information
- To exercise limited control of the disclosure of that information to other parties[16]

Health care organizations operated by the federal government (e.g., military hospitals, Veterans Administration health facilities, Indian Health Service facilities) are bound by the act's provisions. The act also applies to record systems that are operated pursuant to a contract with a federal government agency—for example, a disease registry operated under a grant from the DHHS.

Freedom of Information Act

The Freedom of Information Act (FOIA) became law in 1966. It requires that records pertaining to the executive branch of the federal government be available to the public except for matters that fall within nine explicitly exempted areas. Under certain circumstances, medical records may be exempt from the act's requirements. One of the nine exempt categories includes "personnel and medical files and similar files, the disclosure of which would constitute a clearly unwarranted invasion of personal privacy."[16] To meet the test of being an "unwarranted invasion of personal privacy," the following conditions must exist:

- The information must be contained in a personnel, medical, or similar file
- Disclosure of the information must constitute an invasion of personal privacy

- The severity of the invasion must outweigh the public's interest in disclosure

Interpreting this three-part test has been the subject of a number of court cases[18-20]

Regulations on Confidentiality of Alcohol and Drug Abuse Patient Records

These regulations, restricting disclosures of patient health information without patient authorization, apply to facilities that provide alcohol or drug abuse diagnosis, treatment, or referral for treatment—a substance abuse program in the language of the regulations. For a health care facility to be considered such a program, it must offer either an identified unit that provides alcohol or drug abuse diagnosis, treatment, or referral for treatment or medical personnel or other staff whose primary function is the provision of alcohol or drug abuse diagnosis, treatment, or referral for treatment and who are identified as such providers.[20] General hospitals and clinics are not considered to be such programs unless they have either an identified unit for this type of diagnosis or treatment or providers whose primary function is the provision of those types of services.

The regulations apply only to health information obtained by federally assisted programs, but because the definition of this is quite broad (e.g., all Medicare-certified facilities or those that receive funds from any federal department or agency, among other things), it applies to virtually all programs that meet the other requirements of the definition.

The regulations are important for several reasons. They prohibit the disclosure of substance abuse patient records unless permitted by the regulations or authorized by the patient. The regulations require specific content in an authorization to release health information; those issues are discussed later in this chapter.

These regulations are lengthy and detailed. HIM professionals who work in health care facilities that qualify as a "program" under these regulations must become very familiar with the key provisions.

✓ SELF-ASSESSMENT QUIZ

8. What sort of agreement is necessary for covered entities to have with outside agents or persons that handle or process protected health information on their behalf? (choose best answer below)
   a. Business associate agreement
   b. Subcontractor agreement
   c. Adhesion contract
   d. Notice of privacy practices

Internal Uses and External Disclosures of Health Information

When one is sorting through the maze of parties who request health information, it is sometimes useful to categorize the requests as internal uses or external disclosures. Why? Because in a few, but by no means all, circumstances, internal uses may not need patient authorization for access to that information, whereas external disclosures often (but not always) do. Under the HIPAA privacy rule, internal uses for treatment, payment, or health care operations do not require patient authorization, unless other applicable laws or regulations require their use. For example, sharing patient information with employees on the facility's quality improvement staff would be an internal use for health care operations. Those staff members would be entitled to review the records of patients in the course of their duties. Staff physicians, nurses, and therapists caring for the patient would have access to the patient's information as an internal use for treatment. The health care organization's in-house counsel who is coordinating the defense of a malpractice claim would be an example of an internal use for health care operations, whereas a lawyer who represents a patient, a physician, or an employee of the health care organization would be considered an external disclosure and would require patient authorization.

Do not fall into the trap of thinking that just because a person works for the facility, he or she has carte blanche access to all patient information. Although it is true that health care personnel involved in the treatment of a patient should have access to the information they need to know, it does not follow that nurses should know the medical details of patients for whom they are not caring. This can be a serious problem in health care facilities and has taken on special significance with the growing number of patients who test positive for the human immunodeficiency virus (HIV). Is there any reason for a dietary aide who delivers food trays to each nursing unit to know whether a patient on that unit is HIV positive? Certainly, it can be argued that key staff involved in the patient's treatment should know, but often this knowledge goes far beyond the boundaries of those who need to know. The issue goes well beyond HIV status, however. HIM professionals should provide leadership and training to their coworkers on the appropriate and inappropriate uses of health information.

In addition, the HIPAA privacy rule recognizes and incorporates the principle of minimum necessary. (See section 164.514(d) of the privacy rule.) Generally, only the minimum necessary amount of information necessary to fulfill the purpose of the request should be shared with internal users and external requestors. There are only a few situations in which the minimum necessary standard does not apply (e.g., uses or disclosures for treatment purposes, when the patient has specifically authorized the release of more information, and in a few other circumstances).

SELF-ASSESSMENT QUIZ

9. Which of the following uses of protected health information generally do NOT require patient authorization? (choose best answer below)
   a. Uses for treatment purposes
   b. Uses for health care operations
   c. Uses for research
   d. Uses for payment
   e. Uses for 1, 2, and 4
   f. None of the above

General Principles Regarding Access and Disclosure Policies

Health Information Ownership

As a prerequisite for discussing specific access requests, it is important to have a basic understanding of health information ownership. Who owns the record and information? It is generally accepted that the health facility owns the record itself, but the exercise of those ownership rights is subject to the patient's ownership interest in the information within that record. Health information is, after all, a legal record of what was done for the patient and proof that billable services were rendered and that standards of care were (or were not) met. On the other hand, patients have a right to control, to the extent possible given state and federal laws and regulations, the flow of their private health information. This is one of the reasons why every health care facility needs policies and procedures to guide employees in handling health information access and disclosure requests. Those who violate the patient's right to control the flow of his or her health information may be liable to that patient.

Resources on Releasing Patient Information

Various sources are available for setting policies and writing procedures to guide staff in handling health information and in responding to requests for information. As mentioned before, many state HIM associations have published excellent legal manuals. Peers in other local facilities are usually willing to share samples. AHIMA publishes various guidelines and practice standards, updating them and addressing new issues through position statements and practice guidelines. HIPAA's privacy rule required almost all health care organizations to update their practices on release of information. With the passage of ARRA in 2009 and the subsequent issuance of final rules in 2013, more updates were necessary, and the need for changes will continue as new regulations are published. Because laws can change and case law evolves over time, it is important to use the most up-to-date sources available when establishing policies and procedures and to revisit those policies periodically to ensure that they reflect current legal and regulatory standards. Many health care facilities use in-house or outside legal counsel to review such policies.

Authorizations for Disclosure of Patient Information

As mentioned earlier in this chapter, both the HIPAA Privacy Rule and the regulations on Confidentiality of Alcohol and Drug Abuse Patient Records contain standards for what must be present in an authorization form for the authorization to be considered valid. (See Figure 15-2 for the privacy standards.) In addition, many state laws also have requirements for authorization content and timeliness of presentation. The HIM professional must ensure that the forms and processes for handling authorizations meet all applicable standards. Authorizations that do not contain all required elements are considered invalid authorizations, and releasing

(c) *Implementation specifications: Core elements and requirements*

(1) *Core elements.*
A valid authorization under this section must contain at least the following elements:
(i) A description of the information to be used or disclosed that identifies the information in a specific and meaningful fashion.
(ii) The name or other specific identification of the person(s), or class of persons, authorized to make the requested use or disclosure.
(iii) The name or other specific identification of the person(s), or class of persons, to whom the covered entity may make the requested use or disclosure.
(iv) A description of each purpose of the requested use or disclosure. The statement "at the request of the individual" is a sufficient description of the purpose when an individual initiates the authorization and does not, or elects not to, provide a statement of the purpose.
(v) An expiration date or an expiration event that relates to the individual or the purpose of the use or disclosure. The statement "end of the research study," "none," or similar language is sufficient if the authorization is for a use or disclosure of protected health information for research, including for the creation and maintenance of a research database or research repository.
(vi) Signature of the individual and date. If the authorization is signed by a personal representative of the individual, a description of such representative's authority to act for the individual must also be provided.

(2) *Required statements.* In addition to the core elements, the authorization must contain statements adequate to place the individual on notice of all of the following:
(i) The individual's right to revoke the authorization in writing, and either:
(A) The exceptions to the right to revoke and a description of how the individual may revoke the authorization; or
(B) To the extent that the information in paragraph (c)(2)(i)(A) of this section is included in the notice required by §164.520, a reference to the covered entity's notice.
(ii) The ability or inability to condition treatment, payment, enrollment or eligibility for benefits on the authorization, by stating either:
(A) The covered entity may not condition treatment, payment, enrollment or eligibility for benefits on whether the individual signs the authorization when the prohibition on conditioning of authorizations in paragraph (b)(4) of this section applies; or
(B) The consequences to the individual of a refusal to sign the authorization when, in accordance with paragraph (b)(4) of this section, the covered entity can condition treatment, enrollment in the health plan, or eligibility for benefits on failure to obtain such authorization.
(iii) The potential for information disclosed pursuant to the authorization to be subject to redisclosure by the recipient and no longer be protected by this subpart.

(3) *Plain language requirement.* The authorization must be written in plain language.

(4) *Copy to the individual.* If a covered entity seeks an authorization from an individual for a use or disclosure of protected health information, the covered entity must provide the individual with a copy of the signed authorization.

FIGURE 15-2 Standards governing the content of a valid authorization. HIPAA Privacy Rule Section 164.508 (c) (1).

information on the basis of an invalid authorization is a violation of the HIPAA privacy rule and can result in penalties.

Each disclosure from records covered by the federal regulations on confidentiality of alcohol and drug abuse patient records must be accompanied by a notice specified in the regulations. That notice is a prohibition against redisclosure. In other words, recipients of the original disclosure are put on notice that they may not redisclose the information to anyone else or use the information for anything but its intended purpose because the records are protected by federal confidentiality rules in 42 Code of Federal Regulations (CFR) Part 2. The notice states the following:

This information has been disclosed to you from records whose confidentiality is protected by Federal regulations (42 C.F.R. Part 2) which prohibit you from making any further disclosure of it without the specific written consent of the person to whom it pertains, or as otherwise permitted by such regulations. A general authorization for the release of medical or other information is not sufficient for this purpose.

There are some exceptions to the general prohibition against disclosure from alcohol and drug abuse patient records. In a medical emergency, for example, the regulations permit disclosure to medical personnel to treat a condition that "poses an immediate threat to the health of the patient."[21] Records of these disclosures must be maintained, including the following:

- Patient's name or case number
- Date and time of disclosure
- Description of circumstances that require emergency disclosure
- Description of information disclosed
- Identity of the party receiving the information
- Identity of the party disclosing the information

There are also some provisions for interagency disclosures (e.g., to the Food and Drug Administration), research, and Medicare or Medicaid audits.[22]

This list of required elements for authorization is similar, but not completely identical, to the requirements for a valid authorization under the HIPAA privacy rule. This means that HIM practitioners who work in facilities considered covered entities under the HIPAA Privacy Rule, which are also covered by the regulations on the confidentiality of alcohol and drug abuse patient records, must take care to ensure that their authorization forms meet the requirements of both sets of regulations (Figure 15-3).

Who should sign the authorization depends on the patient and his or her status. See Figure 15-4 for some general guidelines.

Disclosure for Direct Patient Care

When patients come to a health care facility or provider for treatment, it is reasonable to assume that they authorize their care providers to have information about their conditions and treatments. The HIPAA privacy rule supports this and allows internal uses of protected health information for treatment purposes without specific patient authorization. What is not reasonable to assume is that patients are granting access to anyone in the facility who may be curious to know that information as well. Internal uses for patient care

---

Requirements for a Valid Authorization

According to the regulations on Confidentiality of Alcohol and Drug Abuse Patient Records, all authorizations must include the following:

- Specific name or general designation of the program or person permitted to make the disclosure
- Name or title of the person or name of the organization to which disclosure is to be made
- Name of the patient
- Purpose of the disclosure
- How much and what kind of information is to be disclosed
- Signature of the patient and, when required for a patient who is a minor, the signature of a person authorized to give consent under §2.14 of the regulations or, when required for a patient who is incompetent or deceased, the signature of a person authorized to sign under §2.15 in lieu of the patient. For minors, state law matters. If state law permits minors to obtain substance abuse treatment without parental or legal guardian consent, then only the minor can authorize the release of that information. If, however, the state does not allow minors to obtain substance abuse treatment without parental or legal guardian consent, both the minor and legal guardian's signatures are required to release this information.
- Date on which the consent (authorization) is signed
- Statement that the consent is subject to revocation at any time, except to the extent that the program or person that is to make the disclosure has already acted in reliance on it. Acting in reliance includes the provision of treatment services in reliance on a valid consent to disclose information to a third-party payer.
- Date, event, or condition on which the consent will expire if not revoked before. This date, event, or condition must ensure that the consent will last no longer than reasonably necessary to serve the purpose for which it is given.

FIGURE 15-3 Requirements for a valid authorization from the Confidentiality of Alcohol and Drug Abuse Regulations.

SITUATION	AUTHORIZING INDIVIDUAL
The patient is:	
An adult of sound mind (age of majority defined in state statutes)	Patient
A minor	Parent or legal guardian
Deceased	Legal representative Executor of estate
Legally judged incompetent	Legally appointed guardian
Emancipated minor 　Married 　Pregnant, or treated for pregnancy 　Treated for: (varies for each state) 　• Venereal disease 　• Birth control 　• Drug or alcohol abuse	Patient
Minor and his parent is also a minor	Parent

FIGURE 15-4 The individual who can sign the form to authorize release of confidential information depends on the patient's situation.

purposes should be on a need-to-know basis. This means that those who really need to know the patient's health information to diagnose or treat that patient should have access.

Sometimes requests for disclosure of health information for patient care purposes come from outside the health facility where the information was originally collected. For example, if the patient chooses to begin seeing a new physician or is treated at another health facility, it may be important for that new health care provider to obtain a copy of the patient's health history, a test result, or the entire record. In fact, certain regulations (such as Medicare's *Conditions of Participation*) anticipate and require the transfer of relevant patient information on direct transfer of a patient from a hospital to a nursing facility. HIPAA's privacy rule permits disclosures of protected health information for treatment purposes without authorization. (However, some state laws continue to require authorization for external disclosures for treatment.) Some HIM professionals cite arguments in favor of obtaining written authorization for any disclosure under this category, which involves releasing information outside the original facility, unless there is an emergency situation in which patient authorization *cannot* be obtained (e.g., the patient is unconscious and the care providers cannot wait for the information until the patient recovers enough to authorize release). In facilities that take that conservative view, however, steps must be taken to ensure that emergency patient care is not delayed by withholding information that is needed, pending the receipt of an authorization.

Disclosure for Performance Management and Patient Safety

Health information can be used to evaluate the quality of care and services provided to patients. The information provides evidence of exactly what was done, when it was done, why it was done, and how things turned out. For that reason, it is a valuable tool in quality management and improvement activities. Using the information in quality management is an impersonal use. In other words, committee members are interested not in who the patient is but in the quality of services provided. Specific patients are referred to by record or identification numbers when individual cases must be mentioned in peer review or quality management minutes and records. Members of the medical and professional staff may have access to patient health information, without patient authorization, in this context. The HIPAA privacy rule classifies this use as part of "health care operations," and uses for health care operations do not require patient authorization. Even so, it is unwise to hand over records to someone just because that person happens to be on a peer review committee. Do not assume that quality management is the purpose for which all requests are made. A simple inquiry as to why the record or information is needed can help to ensure that the request is indeed related to the requester's quality management responsibilities.

One other caveat on this point: it is not unheard of for health professionals to attempt to use health records to gather unflattering evidence of a competitor's professional skill. Although records may be released without patient authorization for bona fide quality management activities, these informal "research" requests may not be sanctioned, official quality management activities. HIM professionals who are approached by a physician or other health professional with a request for records pertaining to other physicians or health professionals should ask the purpose of the request. If the answer does not indicate that the activity is official quality management business, then the requester should be asked to seek the approval of an appropriate committee or department chairperson. This protects the interests of all concerned.

Disclosure for Educational Purposes

Health information is a valuable teaching tool, both for student health professionals who are involved in formal training programs and for staff members who must continue their education. Because some student health professionals may not be employed by the facility or otherwise bound to abide by the facility policies on confidentiality, it is important to ensure that any students with access to patient-identifiable health information agree to follow facility policies on confidentiality. Some facilities write such an agreement into the contract or in a separate agreement between the facility and the educational program or school; others require students to sign individual confidentiality agreements, or to do both. The HIPAA privacy rule permits outside students to be considered as part of the organization's workforce and treated as an employee for the purposes of information access. However, if the organization chooses to classify the students as part of the workforce, they must then be responsible for training those students in the privacy-related policies and procedures relevant to the student's role.

The educational use of the record is, like quality management, an impersonal use. It matters little who the patient is; what matters is what can be learned from the case. Teaching tools, such as case summaries, test results, photographs, surgical videos, and the like, should not identify the patient. Photographs and videos should be made in such a way that the patient cannot be identified, unless authorization to do so is obtained. Valid educational uses of health information are considered health care operations under the HIPAA privacy rule and do not require patient authorization.

Again, care must be exercised in responding to these requests. Facility procedures should provide for some way to verify the validity of a student's request for information access. Sometimes this is done by having the student's preceptor or supervisor sign off on all student record requests. If no such controls are in place, students may be tempted to review health information about friends, relatives, and other people in whom they have no valid interest.

Disclosure for Research

Research, like educational purposes, usually involves an impersonal use of health information. The researchers are not interested in the identity of the patient, just that the patient falls within some predefined research population or control group. Even so, facility policies should define the circumstances under which researchers may have access to health information without patient authorization. Under the HIPAA privacy rule, those circumstances are fairly limited. Ordinarily, authorizations would not be required only if an institutional review board (described in the next paragraph) has waived the requirement, if the request involves a review that is preparatory to research (e.g., the use is simply to help researchers prepare a research proposal and they will not use the information in any other way), or if the research involves decedents' information.

In many facilities, researchers must have their projects approved by an institutional review board (IRB), an advisory board that reviews the proposed research project for its objectives and proposed methods. If the researchers will have access to patient-identifiable data, it may be important to specify expected data security provisions in a written research agreement between the facility and the researcher. For example, the facility may want to require researchers to do all data collection on site in the HIM department and not remove original records or copies of records from the health facility. The HIM professional may expect to review proposed data collection forms to ensure that patient-identifiable data are not being collected. Be aware that the HIPAA privacy rule contains a number of provisions to guide the decision-making process of IRBs in deciding whether to waive the requirement for patient authorization.

Research projects in which the researchers want to contact patients directly pose a special problem because the simple act of verifying whether a patient is part of a specified group may, in many circumstances, be a breach of confidentiality. For those research projects believed to have sufficient merit to warrant cooperation, some facilities agree to act as intermediaries, notifying selected patients of the planned research and giving them the opportunity to determine whether they want to be contacted by the researchers. Only the addresses of patients opting to participate are then provided to the researchers.

Uses for Administrative Purposes

Uses for administrative purposes refers to the many internal activities that support the day-to-day functioning of the health care facility other than direct patient care, billing, and quality management. For example, a department manager or administrator may need access to certain limited patient information if he or she is responsible for responding to a complaint about the services provided to that patient by an employee of that department. Or a security manager may need access to a patient record to review an inventory of patient valuables to determine the validity of a patient's claims of lost property. A health care organization's professional liability insurer may want to review a sample of records to evaluate documentation practices and then use its assessments in determining the organization's insurability, although in this case, because the insurer is not part of the facility's own workforce, a business associate agreement would also be required. The health care organization's attorney, in preparation for expected litigation, may need to review the record of a patient who was involved in a serious incident. These activities generally qualify as health care operations under the HIPAA privacy rule and may use patient information without authorization (and are subject to the minimally necessary provision), but facility policies should define the situations in which patient authorization is required. In addition, all such requests should be funneled through the HIM department to facilitate consistency in handling them.

One of the more potentially problematic administrative uses of health information involves marketing activities. Ordinarily, the use of the patient information for marketing requires authorization, but there are certain exceptions under the HIPAA privacy rule. In some marketing strategies, specific health care services are marketed to patients who are most likely to have a need for those services. For example, brochures that describe a facility's new cardiac catheterization laboratory are mailed to patients who have been treated for cardiac-related problems or who are known to be at risk for such problems. HIPAA and its subsequent regulations handle that by carving those activities out of the definition of marketing. Because of the complexity of the marketing-related regulations, they must be handled carefully, or they run the risk of breaching confidentiality by publicly identifying patients as belonging to certain disease categories.[23] The HIPAA privacy rule has a very complex set of rules surrounding what activities qualify as marketing, the need to provide "opt-outs" so that patients can remove themselves from certain marketing lists, and when authorizations are required. HIM professionals should be involved in defining policies about the use of health information for marketing purposes and educating potential users about the risks. HIM professionals should also be evaluating proposed marketing uses of patient information to guard against abuses.

Disclosure for Payment Purposes

One of the most frequent disclosures of health information involves billing insurers for services provided to patients. Through clinical codes on the bill, and through claims attachments, information about the patient's diagnoses and procedures is relayed to the insurer, who then pays for the services provided. Under the HIPAA privacy rule, disclosures taking place for payment purposes do not require patient authorization, but some state laws may still require authorization. Be aware, however, that ARRA and its subsequent regulations included a new option for patients who wish to shield certain health information from their health insurer. Under Section 13405 of ARRA, covered entities must comply with an individual's request to restrict disclosures to the health insurer, if the requested restriction fits within these circumstances (ARRA Section 13405(a)(1)(2)):

- except as otherwise required by law, if the disclosure is to a health plan for the purpose of carrying out payment or health care operations (and is not for purposes of treatment); and
- the protected health information pertains solely to a health care item of service for which the health care provider involved has been paid out of pocket in full.

This provision will permit patients to avoid sharing health information with their insurer if they choose to pay directly (and fully) for the care out of pocket. Covered entities will need to establish new procedures for segregating, for the purposes of disclosures to health plans for nontreatment uses, the information pertaining to care paid for by the patient versus that paid for by the plan. Although it may sound straightforward on its face, the practical reality is that this restriction could apply to an entire encounter, or just a single test among many, so the process will need to take this granularity into account.

Disclosure for payment purposes is a controversial subject because quite frequently the patient who receives the services is not the same person who authorized disclosure as part of the application for insurance coverage. Therefore, the person whose information is being disclosed may not have given written authorization for disclosure. Many facilities try to handle this situation by making authorization for disclosure of health information part of the general consent to treatment signed by all patients on admission for treatment. HIM professionals should always exercise caution in disclosing information on the basis of a release that was signed before the information was collected. Probably the most practical way to exercise such caution is to make it clear to all patients before treatment that information will be released to their health insurer. If a patient does not want information to go to the health insurer for this treatment episode, he or she can make other arrangements for payment of the bill. Keep in mind that under the ARRA section described earlier, a covered entity could insist on full payment of the bill before honoring such a restriction request.

Disclosure to Attorneys

Written authorization from the patient or the patient's legal representative or a valid subpoena that meets HIPAA's special requirements is required for release of health information to an attorney, unless that attorney represents the health care provider that owns the record. In other words, the hospital's legal counsel does not require patient authorization to obtain access to a specific record, but the attorney for the respiratory therapist employed by the hospital and involved in the case does. If the records sought are from a physician's office, that physician's attorney does not require authorization, but the attorney of a codefendant hospital does require patient authorization.

HIM professionals should take care in reviewing authorizations submitted by attorneys. Some attorneys use blanket authorizations with their clients, general statements that permit just about anyone to give an attorney just about any document related to the client. As with all other authorizations, the content of the authorization should be reviewed to make sure it complies with the health care facility's and applicable laws' requirements as to form and content.

Disclosure to Law Enforcement Personnel and Agencies

Occasionally, law enforcement representatives, including the medical examiner, are interested in gaining access to health information. For example, a police officer who accompanies an unconscious injured patient to the emergency department may need access to the patient's past records to contact family members. Federal Bureau of Investigation and Internal Revenue Service investigators have also been known to request access to health information. The HIPAA privacy rule, in section 164.501, defines law enforcement officials quite broadly: an officer or employee of any agency or authority of the United States, a state, a territory, a political subdivision of a state or territory, or an American Indian tribe, who is empowered by law to investigate or conduct an official inquiry into a potential violation of law or prosecute or otherwise conduct a criminal, civil, or administrative proceeding arising from an alleged violation of law.

Ordinarily, patient authorization is required for disclosures to law enforcement officials, but there are numerous exceptions (e.g., reporting of certain abuse, neglect, or domestic violence situations; compliance with mandatory state reporting statutes for conditions such as gunshot wounds and communicable diseases; limited information for identification and location purposes; and information sought in response to law enforcement inquiries where deidentified (in other words, data that have been stripped of certain patient identifiers specified in the HIPAA privacy rule at 164.514(b)) data could not be used and the official makes those representations in writing). In addition, there are exceptions for certain situations involving the reporting of crimes on the health care facility's premises, crimes in emergency situations, and crimes in which the patient is the victim. All these situations require certain conditions to be met, so the facility needs to have clear policies on release of information to law enforcement to guide staff members when they receive those requests. Many such requests come to staff other than the HIM department, such as the emergency department or nursing units, so it is important for those policies to be well known throughout the organization. Involve the facility's legal counsel if health care facility policies do not address the particular situation that presents itself. In any event, it is wise to verify the credentials of anyone representing him- or herself as a law enforcement officer by checking badge number or ID card or making a phone call to the agency involved, if there is a question as to identity.

In circumstances in which a suspicious death has resulted in the medical examiner or coroner being called in to conduct a postmortem examination, the medical examiner may have access to the patient's health information for use in conducting the autopsy, and no authorization for release of information is required from the next of kin or legal representative.

Disclosure to Family Members When the Patient Is a Minor

Generally, patients control access to their own health information. They may review the information themselves and choose either to share the information with family members or to withhold it. However, there are some exceptions, one of which is when the patient is a minor. Before a child reaches the age of majority, his or her parents or legal guardian generally make(s) authorization decisions on behalf of the child. In some limited circumstances, there are exceptions under various state and federal laws, such as when a minor child seeks treatment without parental involvement or consent (e.g., sexually transmitted disease, alcohol or substance abuse treatment) and when the minor is emancipated. Except in those circumstances, parents or guardians have access to the health information of their child or ward, and they may sign an authorization for disclosure on behalf of their unemancipated minor or ward. In cases of divorce and separation, disclosure decisions are typically made by the parent who has legal custody of the child. Unless one of the parent's parental rights has been terminated by the court, both parents retain the right to access and authorize the release of their child's information. In foster care situations, parental rights are generally terminated, albeit temporarily, and the foster parents assume those rights. The HIPAA privacy rule generally defers to state laws on matters involving parental rights.

Disclosure to Family Members When the Patient Is an Emancipated Minor or an Adult

State laws permit certain minors to make their own health care decisions without parental or guardian involvement. In other words, they are treated as adults, under the law, and have the right to consent to treatment and authorize disclosure of their own health information. Although the conditions vary, they generally involve minors who are married, living away from their parents and family, and responsible for their own support. In those circumstances, that person is considered to be an emancipated minor and can obtain proof of that emancipation. An emancipated minor can consent to treatment without parental involvement and may authorize disclosure of his or her health information. Because many state laws do not specifically state this, caution should be exercised in drafting facility procedures.

Disclosure to Family Members in Cases of Incompetence or Incapacity

A sad comment on the treatment of America's elderly population—especially those who are involved in residential treatment programs such as nursing facilities—is that sometimes health care providers assume that the patient is incompetent to make decisions, so younger family members are consulted about all treatment and disclosure issues. This is a mistake. Patients typically control access to and disclosure of their protected health information. Confidential information should not be shared indiscriminately with family members without the patient's authorization. It should never be assumed that a patient is incapable of making such decisions unless that patient has been legally declared incompetent. The patient should be capable of deciding what health information, if any, is to be shared with family members or others, subject to applicable laws or regulations.

The HIPAA privacy rule does permit health care providers to make certain assumptions about sharing information with family members who are involved in the care of the patient. For example, if a person comes to the pharmacy to pick up prescriptions for a patient, the pharmacy may assume that the patient wished the information about those prescriptions to be shared with that individual. The rule does, however, support the practice of asking the patient directly—when the patient is present—whether he or she wishes his or her information to be shared with others, including family members.

Incapacity is a different issue altogether. Competent patients may otherwise be unable to make access and disclosure decisions for various reasons. They may be unconscious, under anesthesia, comatose, and so on. In cases of temporary incapacity, health care providers should use common sense, good judgment, and some restraint in sharing appropriate health information with family members who are concerned for their relative. It may be appropriate to discuss the basic facts of the patient's condition and what the immediate plan is, but it may not be appropriate to disclose each and every detail. In cases of lengthy or permanent incapacity, a legal guardian for the patient may be appointed through court proceedings. When incapacity is anticipated, a person may grant power of attorney (the legally recognized authority to act and make decisions on behalf of another party) to another person, which authorizes the designee to act on behalf of the person who is now incapacitated. The person with power of attorney or the legally appointed guardian is then responsible for making decisions regarding the disclosure of health information to others. Be mindful, however, of the fact that there are different types of power of attorney. Some grant very broad powers to the holder; others are limited to specific issues, such as consenting to care. Reviewing the documents associated with the power or attorney will make it clear whether that person has the right merely to consent to treatment or to authorize the release of information as well.

Patient Access to Personal Health Information

Although the health care organization or provider owns the physical record of care, state statutes grant patients varying degrees of ownership interest in the health information in their records or data sets. Patients have no constitutional right to that information.[24] However, the HIPAA privacy rule does grant patients fairly broad rights to access their health information held by entities that are covered by the rule. In general, subject to any statutory prohibition or qualification such as those found in the HIPAA privacy rule and as modified by ARRA, patients have a right to review and obtain copies of their health information.

Partly because of the variation in state requirements, health care organizations' practices with respect to granting patients access to their health information differ considerably. Even within states, some health care organizations take a consumer-oriented approach, whereas others try to discourage access requests by imposing additional hurdles for the patient to jump, such as inconvenient hours for accepting and handling such requests. The HIPAA privacy rule has helped to make these practices more uniform and patient friendly, but striking differences are still found. Some hospitals, for example, permit patients to review their health information during their hospitalization (with the attending physician present to answer questions), whereas others require a brief waiting period before such access is granted. The HIPAA privacy rule requires that covered entities act on patients' request for access within 30 days of the request. HIM professionals must ensure that their facility policies comply with state and federal laws governing patient access. Within those limitations, the facility may have some latitude in the handling of patients' requests for information.

Whatever approach is taken, the HIM professional must establish reasonable safeguards for the security and confidentiality of the information. For example, before information is handed over in response to a patient request, there should be some reliable means of identifying the requester as the patient. It may be reasonable to obtain the patient's request in writing by way of a signature on an authorization for release of information form, although this is not required by the privacy rule, and lack of a signed authorization form should not serve as an arbitrary barrier for acting on the patient's request. This form may also be used to document that the review or release occurred. If the original hard copy record is being reviewed, that review should be closely supervised to guard against alterations or destruction of the record. If an electronic health record is being reviewed, similar security provisions are necessary to guard against alterations. Some facilities notify the attending physician or other health care practitioner that his or her patient has requested record access. Facilities may also choose to set certain reasonable hours for such on-site reviews. Again, any facility-imposed restrictions should not conflict with relevant laws.

Interesting questions can arise in the context of patients' requests for access to their health information. For example, what should the HIM professional do if the attending physician thinks that allowing patients to see their health information would be harmful to their recovery? Sometimes this question arises with respect to mental health therapy. Some state laws severely restrict access to mental health records. Some require attending physicians to document in the record that they believe that access to the information would harm their patients. Under the HIPAA privacy rule, if a licensed health care professional has determined, in the exercise of professional judgment, that the access requested is reasonably likely to endanger the life or physical safety of the individual or another person, the facility may then refuse such a request; however, this is a reviewable decision that affords the patient an appeal option.

Other Patient-Directed Disclosures

There are many other situations in which patients authorize other parties to receive their health information. For example, when patients apply for life insurance, disability insurance, or admission to certain schools or programs, they may authorize disclosure of health information. Provided the authorization meets the facility's valid requirements as to form and content, these requests should be promptly honored. Although HIM professionals do not encounter these requests every day, former patients occasionally want to examine their birth records to gain information about their natural parents if they were adopted. Problems may arise because of conflicts between some state laws that grant patients access to their records and adoption laws that may require sealed records to protect the privacy of the birth parents. The sealing of adoption-related records is common. Only a few states permit the adoptee to access these records, and a few provide for the disclosure of health information to the adoptee but strict confidentiality regarding the birth parents' identities. Disclosure of health information about the parents can be important to the adoptee when health conditions that may be genetically based arise later in life. Courts are often sympathetic to these "good cause" requests to open adoption-related records, but this is a decision to be made by a court, not by an individual facility. Keep in mind that not all requests for birth records necessarily require the identity of the parents to be revealed. If the former patient is interested only in time of birth, for example, the facility may be able to honor the request without jeopardizing the privacy rights of the birth parents.

> **? DID YOU KNOW?**
>
> According to AdoptUSKids, more than 250,000 children in the United States enter the foster care system every year (http://www.adoptuskids.org/meet-the-children).

Redisclosure Issues

Once a patient authorizes the disclosure of health information to other parties, such as insurers, control of the information is out of the facility's—and often the patient's—hands. For this reason, health care organizations often include a notice along with the information being disclosed that advises the party receiving the information that redisclosure of the information is prohibited. Through this notice, the third-party recipient is informed of its responsibility not to disclose the information further and to protect it from unauthorized use. Many health care facilities try to discourage redisclosure by stamping a redisclosure prohibition on all information sent out of the facility to alert the recipient that redisclosure issues must be referred to the facility's HIM department. However, except with respect to information covered under the Confidentiality of Alcohol and Drug Abuse Patient Records regulation, the receiving party is not generally bound by that prohibition on redisclosure. In fact, the HIPAA privacy rule anticipates redisclosure in many circumstances, such as in the case of a covered entity that receives another provider's records about a particular patient and then incorporates that information into his or her designated record set. If a valid request was received for release of that information, the second covered entity would be expected to release it.

Another interesting practice with respect to redisclosure involves the insurance industry and the Medical Information Bureau (MIB). The MIB has been described as a kind of medical "credit bureau."[25] Its data bank contains files on millions of people that are shared among hundreds of member insurance companies. The purpose of the MIB is to alert insurers to certain information about applicants for insurance within the past 7 years—information that could be used as the basis for denying insurance. Insurers cooperatively share health information they receive through the claims payment process, pooling it in the MIB for use by all members. How can they do this? The fine print on insurance contract applications generally gives the insurer both the right to use the MIB to access health information (if any

information is on file there) and to redisclose information about any health claims into the MIB. The person signing the insurance application may not have been the patient. Thus, information about any given patient may end up being redisclosed into the MIB without the patient's knowledge or permission.

It is possible for patients to contact the MIB to see whether the bureau contains information about them. After contacting the MIB, patients are required to complete and sign a written request form.

Disclosure to Outsourcing Firms Handling Health Information Functions

External release-of-information vendor services are being used with increasing frequency in HIM departments, and outside contractors have been used over the years to microfilm records, digitally image records for storage, and perform medical transcription, coding, and other functions. Many departments use release-of-information vendors to handle routine release-of-information tasks. Some managers have found that these services can supply a staff person on site in the HIM department to do the job more economically and efficiently than the HIM department personnel can.

Regardless of whether these services make financial sense, their use raises some interesting disclosure issues. The function that these outside contractors perform, by its nature, involves access to confidential health information. HIM professionals who use these services must take steps to oversee the confidentiality, security, and appropriate handling of health information. They must also ensure that the vendor executes a business associate agreement with the covered entity, as required by the HIPAA privacy rule. The vendor (and any subcontractors) should also be contractually bound to handle the confidential information appropriately. In situations in which confidential health information (e.g., dictated reports or hard copy records) must be physically removed from the facility, such as when data are manually delivered to an outside transcription firm or dictation is digitally transmitted over telephone lines to off-site locations, the HIM professional must ensure that adequate security measures are in place to prevent theft, loss, alteration, or destruction of the information. The HIM professional must also ensure that the removal of health information from the facility under this circumstance does not violate state laws. Check state laws to determine what restrictions apply to the removal of health information from the originating facility without patient authorization. Recently, several states have considered bans on sharing patient information with vendors outside the United States.

Disclosure to the News Media

A health care organization has no legal duty to disclose health information to the news media. In past years, hospitals often released basic information about admissions and births to the news media, but many facilities have discontinued this practice. Under the HIPAA privacy rule, no such routine disclosure to the news media of admissions and births should take place without patient authorization. A patient's right of privacy, however, does not bar the publication of information that is of public interest. Courts hold that with regard to a public figure, the celebrity's right to privacy must be weighed against the public's right to know and the freedom of the press. Therefore, if the patient is a public figure, health care organizations usually try, when releasing information to the media, to balance the public's need to know with the patient's need for privacy. For this reason, many health care facilities have adopted policies that permit a spokesperson merely to confirm admission and classify the public figure patient's condition (e.g., critical, poor, fair, stable, good), except under extraordinary circumstances (e.g., treatment of the president or other key public figures, or where the patient requests that absolutely no information be shared or has opted out of the facility's directory). Disclosure of more detailed information should be avoided to minimize the risk of liability to the organization. At the same time, even confirming a patient's admission to a program for alcohol or drug abuse treatment would violate federal law if it were done without the patient's permission. HIPAA's privacy rule offered facilities some assistance in sorting through these issues by establishing rules allowing patients to opt out of directory listings of patients, and this option must be referred to in the facility's notice of privacy practices.

Some segments of the media have been known to use unusual measures to try to obtain health information on celebrity patients. Staff members may even be approached with bribes. Facility policies should address the measures to be used in handling celebrity records. Special security procedures for preserving the confidentiality of these patients' health information may be appropriate. Some facilities use special code names or an alias on printed reports, with the code known only to the HIM director, physician, and chief executive officer, but these procedures may conflict with the laws of some states with regard to identifying the patient. Some facilities remove such records from their regular filing or information systems and store hard copy reports in a locked file in the HIM department with limited access. The HIM professional should work with the organization's legal counsel or risk manager to devise an appropriate strategy for dealing with celebrity records.

Disclosure Pursuant to Legal Process

When health information must be used in court, the request for information comes in the form of a subpoena *duces tecum*, a subpoena (which may also be called a subpoena *ad testificandum)*, a written court order, or simply a verbal order issued in court to the health care organization's attorney. A subpoena is a written order that requires someone to come before the court to testify. A subpoena *duces tecum* is a written order that requires someone to come before the court and to bring certain records or documents named in that order. When health information is needed in court or in pretrial discovery, such as a deposition, those orders are typically directed to the HIM department director.

State laws vary on who is empowered to issue subpoenas; judges, court clerks, and other officials may be authorized—even attorneys. The form and process that the subpoena must follow to be valid is also a matter of state law and is also addressed in the HIPAA privacy rule, but generally a subpoena must contain the following:

- A docket number (an identification number assigned by the court, generally referring to the year the lawsuit was filed and the numerical order in which the cases are filed; for example, the 318th case filed in that jurisdiction for 2001 might have a docket number of 01-318 with some other identifiers appended)
- The names of the parties (plaintiffs and defendants) involved in the case
- The name of the court or agency before which the proceeding is being held
- The details as to when and where the HIM director's appearance is being requested
- The documents that must be brought
- The signature and seal of the official issuing the subpoena

State laws vary with regard to the method through which and the time limits within which subpoenas can be properly served. Some court systems require service by sheriffs or other public officers. Other jurisdictions permit service by mail or messenger. In still other jurisdictions, service must be accomplished in person, by handing the subpoena to the HIM professional. There are also jurisdictions in which the service must be accompanied by a fee to reimburse the person subpoenaed for his or her time and expense. This nominal fee (called a witness fee) is usually set by statute or court rules. HIM professionals must become familiar with the requirements applicable to their state and federal jurisdictions to ensure that they respond properly to the subpoenas received.

There are also some special rules associated with a subpoena of information from organizations covered by the Federal Regulations on Alcohol and Drug Abuse. Any subpoena of this specific information must also be accompanied by a court order before it can be released. For a subpoena *duces tecum* for health information to be valid under the HIPAA privacy rule, it must be accompanied by a court order, or the covered entity must receive satisfactory assurance from the party seeking the information that reasonable efforts have been made to ensure that the individual who is the subject of the protected health information that has been requested has been given notice of the request or that the party seeking the information has made reasonable efforts to secure a qualified protective order that meets the requirements of the HIPAA privacy rule. The HIPAA privacy rule outlines the qualifications for this satisfactory assurance at section 164.512(e)(1)(iii).

Responding to any subpoena that requires the production of health information usually involves the same basic steps, outlined below. These steps, especially when electronic health records are involved, vary somewhat depending on the design of the facility's information system. Most state HIM associations' legal manuals offer good step-by-step procedures for responding to subpoenas, based on the statutes and rules of that jurisdiction. Roach and the Aspen Health Law and Compliance Center recommend that the procedures include the following steps at a minimum:

- Examine the information subject to subpoena to make certain that it is complete, that signatures and initials are legible, and that each page identifies the patient and the patient's identification number. (If the information is not yet complete, try to complete it. However, do not ignore a subpoena because the information is not yet complete.)
- Examine the information to determine whether the case forms the basis for a possible negligence action against the health care organization; if so, notify the appropriate administrators, legal counsel, or risk manager.
- Remove any material that may not properly be obtained in the jurisdiction by subpoena, such as, in some cases, notes referring to psychiatric care, copies of information from other facilities (unless they have been properly incorporated into the patient's information), and correspondence.§
- Number each page of the patient record, and write the total number of pages on the record folder.
- Prepare a list of the record contents to be used as a receipt for the information if it must be left with the court or an attorney. (Most facilities use a standard form for this purpose.)
- Whenever possible, use a photocopy of the record rather than the original in responding (in person) to legal process. (A certificate of authentication can be helpful in convincing the court to accept the photocopy as a true and exact copy of the original.)[26]

The facility's procedures should describe these steps and the steps to follow if a subpoena is defective in some way (e.g., issued by the wrong party, conflicts with state or federal law, asks for records not in the facility's possession, or fails to provide satisfactory assurance where required). Ignoring a subpoena or court order creates trouble, possibly serious trouble. Involve the facility's legal counsel in drafting procedures for dealing with subpoenas and court orders, and do not hesitate to refer unusual problems to your facility's legal counsel. Legal counsel may decide to file a motion to quash the subpoena or order in which the court is asked to set aside the subpoena or order.

As mentioned earlier, court orders can be issued in writing or verbally in court to the facility's attorney. A health care organization should make every effort to comply with a court order as long as the order does not place the facility in the position of violating a statute or regulation. Again, as with the subpoena, if the court order is defective in some way (e.g., would force the facility to violate state or federal law), legal counsel must be involved immediately to work out a solution and to help the facility's leaders avoid being cited for contempt of court.

The fact that health information has been subpoenaed does not mean that it will be admissible as evidence. Here again, state laws vary concerning the admissibility of health information. As explained earlier, admissibility issues have become somewhat murky as new technologies for collecting, storing, and retrieving health information are put into use.

HIM professionals are occasionally called on not only to produce the subpoenaed health information but to testify as well. This process typically involves being sworn in and answering questions that lay the foundation for introduction of the patient's record into evidence. HIM professionals may be asked questions about whether the record or information was prepared in the normal course of daily business or according to established policies and procedures for documentation and record keeping. It is important for them to answer honestly and not speculate on matters that are beyond their knowledge. They should not guess at the "correct" answer to a question. When the answer to a question is not known, the proper response is simply to say, "I don't know" or "I am not qualified to answer that."

Health Information Management Department Security Measures to Prevent Unauthorized Access

Ensuring that all formal releases of information are appropriately handled is only one aspect of protecting the confidentiality and security of health information. Careful, thorough release-of-information policies are ineffective if internal security measures and systems are inadequate to protect health information from loss, theft, destruction, and alteration. One important aspect of protecting health information is preventing unauthorized access. In other words, how can facilities and HIM professionals keep health information out of the hands of unauthorized users?

Who might that "unauthorized user" be? It may be a curious employee or coworker who knows that his or her neighbor was recently admitted and wants to find out what is wrong with the person. It may be a private investigator who is trying to get information about someone on behalf of a client. It may be a computer hacker who breaks into the facility's health information system just for the challenge. It may even be a physician who is reviewing the records of a competitor's patients and trying to collect ammunition for a battle over delineation of privileges or medical staff membership. One of the most important responsibilities of HIM professionals is to keep confidential health information out of the hands of unauthorized users through appropriate policies and procedures, facility and space planning, information systems design and selection, staff education, security management, and other measures.

HIM policies and procedures should specify who has access to what—ideally, as specifically as possible. In an issue of the AHIMA's former confidentiality newsletter, *In Confidence*, information system security expert Dale Miller recommended that information security policies define, by specific job function, information access. "An individual should have full and timely access to the information they need to perform their current tasks, but only for the purposes of fulfilling their responsibilities."[27] This advice is consistent with the approach taken by HIPAA's security regulations, which require access control decisions to be based on need, for

§For a discussion of the issues involved in relying on other health care facilities' tests and records and incorporating them into the patient's record, see King PD: Inclusion of reports from other sources in hospital records, *Top Health Record Manage* 5:81-88, 1984. Many health care facilities are handling these questions by defining, via policy, the "legal medical record" that will be produced in response to a subpoena *duces tecum*. AHIMA has published a number of excellent resources on the subject of the "legal medical record."

example, by the role or function that person fulfills within the organization. When a facility employee asks to review a patient's health information, HIM professionals should not hesitate to inquire about the employee's purpose or need, if that need is not known from the circumstances of the request. Many times, legitimate information needs can be handled by less intrusive means than handing over a complete record. The question itself may discourage or defeat illegitimate or suspicious requests. Likewise, HIM professionals should not hesitate to verify the propriety of a request. Anyone can buy a laboratory coat and walk into a nursing station where health information is readily displayed. A person so attired may even be able to stroll unchallenged through an HIM department if staff are not adequately trained in security measures. Many health care organizations are so large that it is impossible for HIM department employees to know all the employees in other departments. Verification of employee identification is a legitimate security measure, as is checking with the employee's supervisor about the validity of certain requests. Locked access to information technology or server storage areas is a legitimate security measure, as is locked access to record or data storage areas. Sometimes even these basic security measures are not observed. Part of an HIM professional's job is to insist on adequate security measures for both manual and electronic health information systems.

See Chapter 8 for a more in-depth discussion of security issues.

✔ SELF-ASSESSMENT QUIZ

10. If subpoenaed to testify, an HIM professional is likeliest to be asked questions about: (choose best answer below)
    a. His or her opinion about medical negligence
    b. The reputation of the defendant
    c. How the information/record was prepared
    d. All of the above

11. If a fellow health care organization employee asks to view health information he doesn't normally have access to, which actions below would be appropriate? (choose best answer below):
    a. Ask the employee his purpose in seeking the information;
    b. Verify the stated purpose with his supervisor
    c. Go ahead and share the information since he is a fellow employee
    d. Answers a and b only
    e. All of the above

Duty to Provide Care That Meets Professional Standards

In addition to a health care organization's or provider's duty to maintain the confidentiality of a patient's health information, there is a duty to provide care that meets professional standards. Simply put, health care providers must provide a reasonable quality of care to patients—care that meets professional standards. Liability can and does arise when providers fail to meet professionally accepted standards of

quality, such as the practice guidelines and standards issued by various medical specialty societies, professional associations, and other consensus groups and those dictated by statute or regulation.

Before liability can be found, the claimant or plaintiff must meet certain requirements and overcome certain obstacles. First, the complaining party must file the claim within the statute of limitations. For this chapter's purposes, this means that once a plaintiff knows (or reasonably should have known) that he or she has a potential claim against a health care organization or provider, that claim must be filed within a certain period of time (e.g., within 2 years of discovering the malpractice). Otherwise, the claim will not be heard by a court. Statutes of limitations are designed to encourage the timely filing of claims, when evidence is fresh and witnesses are likely to be available. Through prompt filing of claims, the search for the truth is facilitated.

In some states, the plaintiff must also obtain a statement from a neutral health care provider (such as a physician) before filing a malpractice claim, certifying that the claim has some merit. Some states use this approach to discourage the filing of nuisance and groundless claims.

For any negligence or malpractice claim to succeed, the plaintiff must show that all the following elements of negligence or malpractice are present:

- *Duty.* The defendant must have had some duty to the plaintiff to use care. A physician, for example, owes a duty to his or her patients to use care that meets professional standards but owes no professional duty to the letter carrier who delivers the office mail.
- *Breach.* The defendant must be shown to have breached that duty (by action or inaction). In other words, the defendant's conduct must have failed to conform to the applicable standard of care.
- *Proximate cause.* The breach must be the "proximate" cause of the harm that befell the plaintiff.[28]
- *Harm or damages.* The plaintiff must show that he or she was harmed in some way (e.g., physical pain, suffering, emotional distress, monetary losses).

How does a judge or jury decide whether a defendant acted unreasonably—breaching his or her "duty" to the plaintiff? If the claim involves simple (not professional) negligence such as in a personal injury suit, the judge or jury uses the "reasonable man" standard. In other words, the jury is told to evaluate the defendant parties' conduct in light of the jury's own general experience and background. In professional negligence (malpractice) cases, the jury has no experience and training to draw from in evaluating the parties' actions. Therefore, the standard used to judge a professional's actions is the generally accepted standard of care for that profession. For example, orthopedic surgeons' actions are judged against the current standard of care in orthopedics. Pediatricians' actions are judged against pediatric standards of care and so on. These guidelines can be established by expert testimony, professional literature, or published standards. The applicable standard of care is often determined by referring to current standards published by the relevant specialty society and the professional literature. Sometimes referring to accreditation and licensing standards determines it. By pointing to deficiencies in meeting those standards, plaintiffs' attorneys hope to bolster their allegations of negligence.

When a plaintiff brings a civil suit against a defendant, the plaintiff has the burden of proof. In other words, unless the plaintiff can convince the judge or jury by a preponderance of evidence (making it more likely than not) that the claims against the defendant are valid, the defendant will prevail. The preponderance of evidence standard is not a particularly high one—unlike the "beyond a reasonable doubt" standard found in criminal cases. In a case in which the standard of proof is a preponderance of evidence, it may be helpful to think of it as a "51%" requirement. In other words, in weighing whether something is true or not true, if it is just 51% or more likely to be true (vs. 49% or less likely that it is false), then the standard is met.

In a malpractice case against health care providers or organizations, the burden of proof often shifts to the defendant under a concept called *res ipsa loquitur* ("the thing speaks for itself"). An inference of negligence or malpractice is permitted simply because an injury to the plaintiff occurred under the following circumstances:

- The event would not normally have occurred in the absence of negligence.
- The defendant had exclusive control over the instrumentality (e.g., instrument, equipment, procedures) that caused the injury.
- The plaintiff did not contribute to the injury.[29]

For example, if postoperative abdominal adhesions developed in a patient after a surgical sponge was inadvertently left in the abdomen during surgery, the burden of proof would shift to the defendants (probably the surgeon and facility) for the following reasons:

- Surgical sponges are not supposed to be left in the operative site and sewn up inside a patient.
- The sponge, surgical technique, and sponge-counting procedures were within the exclusive control of the defendants.
- The patient did nothing to contribute to the injury.

All three elements must be present to shift the burden of proof in a negligence or malpractice case to the defendant. Otherwise, the plaintiff retains the burden of proving the defendant's negligence by a preponderance of the evidence.

Health information is extremely important in cases that revolve around the health care providers' and organizations' duty to provide care that meets professional standards. In many cases, the documentation of the care provided is the most important evidence available to the trier of fact (the jury, or the judge in cases without a jury). As health care providers soon come to realize, their documentation practices can either help them or hurt them in defending against malpractice claims. Care taken in thorough documentation can make all the difference in the outcome of malpractice litigation.

Incident or occurrence reports can be important pieces of documentation in investigating, pursuing, and defending against claims against health care organizations and providers. These reports, which should not be treated as part of the patient's health information, are factual summaries of unexpected events that have resulted (or could have resulted) in injury or harm to patients, staff, or visitors. They are used by health care organizations' risk managers or attorneys to investigate incidents that have the potential to become claims against the organization or individual provider and to identify areas where improvements are needed. In many facilities, these reports serve as an important data source for the performance measurement or patient safety program by identifying shortcomings and suggesting possible solutions.

State laws vary considerably with respect to protecting the incident report from discovery by plaintiffs and their attorneys. In some states, the reports are protected as part of the attorney–client privilege as long as the incident report is handled as a document prepared in anticipation of possible litigation and not used for other purposes (e.g., performance measurement or patient safety). In other states, the incident report may be protected from discovery as part of the facility's peer review and quality improvement efforts. In still other states, the incident report is not protected, and therefore users must be extremely careful about what is documented in the report. Facility legal counsel should be actively involved in defining incident report preparation and handling procedures so that the maximum protection possible can be obtained for these reports.

Duty to Obtain Informed Consent to Treatment

One important duty to patients that HIM professionals must be aware of is the physician's duty to obtain the patient's informed consent to treatment. Many times, when health professionals refer to obtaining consent, they mean getting a permit signed by a patient. Actually, obtaining consent refers to a communication process between the health professional and the patient. Unless that communication successfully informs the patient about the anticipated treatments and meets certain basic requirements, it cannot be considered a valid informed consent.

For practical purposes, the duty to obtain informed consent splits into the following two parts:

- The duty to obtain a general consent for treatment (a largely administrative process that consists of obtaining the patient's signature on a form, often preprinted on the back of the facility's "face" sheet or emergency department record)
- The attending physician's or surgeon's duty to obtain a separate informed consent before the performance of surgery or other invasive procedures

Because the patient has presented at the facility for treatment and that implies (to a certain extent) his or her consent to at least basic care, obtaining a signature on the general consent to treatment is typically a simple process. Obtaining an informed consent before the performance of surgery or other invasive procedures is often much more complex. How, for example, does the care provider know that the patient is truly making an informed decision?

For a consent obtained by a health care provider to be valid, the health care provider must meet certain requirements. These requirements may be specified in state law and commonly include the following:

- The informed consent should be obtained by the person who will carry out the procedure. In other words, the process of communicating the planned procedure or treatment and its risks, benefits, and alternatives should be handled by the person who will do or supervise the procedure. In the case of surgery, it would be the surgeon. Keep in mind that some states and case law permit the physical act of obtaining a signature on the consent form to be delegated to others, provided the process of informing the patient has already taken place.
- The patient must be capable of giving an informed consent. In other words, the patient must be legally and mentally capable of understanding what is being proposed and making a decision. If the patient has been judged legally incompetent or because of certain emergency circumstances (such as unconsciousness accompanied by a life-threatening injury) cannot give an informed consent, the guardian or next of kin (designated by state law to act in the patient's stead) must receive the information and sign the consent.

    Are minors capable of giving informed consent? In some circumstances and for some treatments, they are. But how young is too young? This criterion varies from state to state. Barring any state law that prohibits this action, minors may indeed be capable of giving informed consent. Yet another aspect of this question is whether the otherwise competent patient can understand what is being said because of language barriers, hearing impairment, literacy problems, or other issues. Care providers must ensure that a patient can understand the risks, benefits, and alternatives to the proposed procedure before they obtain the patient's signature. Many facilities maintain a list of employees who can speak a foreign language and who can use sign language. In locations where there are large populations of patients for whom English is not their native language, it may be important to prepare patient educational materials and consent forms in the most common non-English languages.
- The patient must be free from coercion or undue influence when giving consent. The consent of a patient who agrees to an incidental tubal ligation during gynecologic surgery because her husband threatens not to pay the hospital bill unless she does so is considered invalid.
- The consent should be granted for a specific procedure or treatment. In other words, if the physician asks for permission to do "abdominal surgery," it would be difficult to argue that the patient is giving a truly informed consent. If the diagnosis is uncertain, however, and exploratory surgery is required, the patient may indeed grant valid consent for the physician to do exploratory surgery and to proceed with more extensive surgery if, in the surgeon's opinion, it is warranted (e.g., when frozen-section results indicate cancer). The key issue is whether the patient has been adequately informed of this possibility and agrees to proceed.

- The patient must indeed be adequately informed. State laws provide some guidance on the standard to be used in judging questions as to whether the patient was given enough information. In some states, it is within the caregiver's discretion to decide whether enough information has been given. In other states, a "reasonable man" standard is used. Generally, the standards require that the patient receive information about the nature and purpose of the proposed procedure, the risks and benefits of the proposed treatment, any reasonable alternatives to this procedure, and the risks of refusing the proposed procedure or treatment.[30]
- The patient is given an opportunity to ask and receive answers to questions. This is a fairly common problem faced by health care facility staff when trying to obtain the patient's signature on the consent form after the physician has discussed the procedure with the patient and left. The patient may have been reluctant to pose certain questions to the physician or may not have had time to think through all his or her questions, and the facility staff are faced with a dilemma. Does the fact that the patient still has questions mean that he or she has not been adequately informed? Facility policies should define how far staff should go, if they should be involved at all in answering questions, or whether they should immediately notify the physician so that the patient might speak with the physician directly. Most facilities take an intermediate approach: if the question is not really related to the decision-making process (e.g., the patient wants to know about how long the procedure will take), staff may attempt to answer without questioning the validity of the consent. In cases of doubt, however, the physician should be involved. Otherwise, staff members may find themselves involved in a postprocedure suit alleging a lack of informed consent.

There are a few circumstances in which informed consent is not required. In life-threatening situations in which the patient is incapable of expressing consent, consent is implied by law. In addition, there are situations in which although consent is required, it need not be accompanied by the normal disclosure of risks, benefits, alternatives, and so on. For example, if there is not time for full discussion of all relevant facts because treatment must begin immediately, some care providers have been excused for giving only a brief summary of the facts as long as the patient agrees to the treatment itself. In limited circumstances, some care providers have been excused from providing all relevant facts when the provider believes that full disclosure would be harmful. "Therapeutic privilege" could apply when a patient is clearly beyond his or her ability to cope with the details of needed treatment, but this would have to be clearly documented to withstand court scrutiny. Patients may also waive the right to be informed. For example, if the physician attempts to inform the patient, but the patient says that he or she would rather not know, just go ahead, the physician should clearly document the patient's waiver and all attempts to inform the patient. In addition, some patients may have had similar procedures or treatments before and may already be familiar with the relevant facts. Again, this situation should be documented.

Along with the right to grant consent is the right to refuse any treatment. Public attitudes toward death with dignity and outcries over heroic attempts to keep patients alive at all costs (both financial and human) have led to the enactment of the Patient Self-Determination Act.[31] This legislation requires health care facilities to query patients about whether they have already documented their life support and treatment-related wishes (called advance directives) on admission. These wishes are documented as advance directives to health care providers in the event they become necessary. An advance directive can be either a living will, a written document that allows a competent adult to indicate his or her wishes regarding life-prolonging medical treatment should he or she be unable to consent, or a durable power of attorney for health care, in which a competent adult names in writing another adult to make any medical decisions on his or her behalf in the event he or she becomes incapacitated (although the extent of the decision-making power varies according to state law). The documentation requirements for these advance directives vary by state. The directives, if they exist, are then maintained with the patient's health information.

In some locales, HIM professionals have been faced with patients wanting to put their advance directives on file, although the patient has not been treated at that facility and does not have a health record. Although the facility is not legally obligated to file materials and create records for people who are not yet patients, it does seem prudent to develop a simple filing system (perhaps an alphabetical file separate from the health record) so that those directives can be retained and retrieved if the individual subsequently becomes a patient. This is a service to the community and may speed the location of the advance directives if or when that person is seen in the facility for treatment in the future.

 SELF-ASSESSMENT QUIZ

12. If an existing patient wishes to file advance directives in his health information/records, the health care organization should: (choose best answer below)
   a. Agree to file the information
   b. Only agree to file the information if the patient has paid his bills
   c. Instruct the patient to file the document at his attorney's office instead
   d. Refuse to file the information, since it is the patient's record, not the health care organization's record

Duty to Provide a Safe Environment for Patients and Visitors

A common duty of health care facilities and providers is to provide a safe environment for patients and visitors. If a patient is dropped and injured while being moved from an emergency department stretcher to an x-ray table, the facility (as employer of the people involved) is likely to be held liable for any damages. If a visitor stumbles in the facility's parking lot because the lot lights were not functioning and lawn care equipment was carelessly left in the lot's walkways by the facility's maintenance employees, the facility is liable for damages. If an infant is abducted from the neonatal nursery because the nursery was short staffed and the babies were momentarily left unsupervised, the facility is likely to be held liable for damages.

When health care facilities open themselves up to the public and to patients for "business," they assume a duty to provide a reasonably safe environment. That is not to say that any injury is compensable. For example, if a visitor who is not watching where she is going stumbles over a clearly marked step and crashes through a plate glass window, the facility may not be responsible. Likewise, if a distraught person enters the facility's emergency department with a gun and begins firing, killing patients and employees, the facility might not be liable.

The key issue in determining whether the facility breached its duty to provide a safe environment is whether the facility's actions (or lack of actions) were reasonable under the circumstances. What is reasonable? How much is enough? That determination is often difficult to make in advance. Certainly, at a minimum, the public expects health care facilities to meet the following criteria:
- To comply with life safety and building codes and other recognized standards
- To provide certain training to employees
- To make sure that the equipment and materials used on patients are clean and functioning properly

Duty to Supervise the Actions of Employees and the Professional Staff

Just as health care organizations must take reasonable steps to provide a safe environment for patients and visitors, they must also supervise the actions of employees and the professional staff (including medical staff). As discussed earlier in the chapter, a health care organization can be held liable for damages when its employees fail to perform their duties adequately, under the doctrine of *respondeat superior* ("let the master answer").

This does not just apply to patient care duties. A health care organization can be liable for an employee's failure to perform other duties as well. For example, if an employee of a large physician group practice inappropriately releases confidential information to an unauthorized party, the group practice could be held liable in a breach of confidentiality suit filed by the patient. Employers are responsible for training their staff to exercise their duties properly. Using this example, a health care organization should certainly ensure that staff members understand proper release-of-information practices and follow them. In fact, training in privacy and security-related issues germane to the employee's job is required by HIPAA. Many facilities go even further and insist that employees with access to confidential information sign an agreement to keep that information confidential and to follow facility policies on confidentiality. Numerous examples of such forms can be found in a Web search for HIPAA confidentiality agreements.

Medical Staff Credentialing Process

Under the doctrine of corporate negligence, a health care organization can also be held liable for the acts of its non-employee staff, such as the medical staff. In one of the most important cases on the doctrine of corporate negligence, *Elam v. College Park Hospital* (1982), the court held that a hospital is liable to a patient for the negligent conduct of independent physicians and surgeons who are neither employees nor agents of the hospital.[32] A hospital owes patients a duty to ensure the competence of its medical staff and to evaluate the quality of medical care rendered on its premises. This is one of the main reasons behind medical staff credentialing programs, in which prospective members of the medical staff apply for membership and request that certain privileges to practice medicine at that facility be granted. Likewise, current members of the medical staff periodically (usually every 2 years) renew or request new or changed privileges to render certain types of care and services at the facility.

The purpose of the medical staff credentialing process is to ensure that only qualified physicians and other credentialed health professionals practice within the facility. During the appointment and reappointment process, the applicant's background is reviewed, licenses and certifications are checked, proof of current liability insurance is verified, and practice patterns and quality review data are evaluated to determine whether the applicant should be granted the privileges he or she seeks to gain or renew. If the evaluation is done poorly, medical staff credentialing decisions can result in liability for the health care organization. In *Rule v. Lutheran Hospitals and Homes Society of America* (1987), a hospital was liable for birth injuries that occurred during an infant's breech delivery.[33] The jury found that the hospital had failed to investigate adequately the background and qualifications of the attending physician before granting him delivery privileges. The hospital had, in fact, failed to check with other hospitals in which the physician had practiced. If that check had been made, the hospital would have discovered that the physician's privileges to perform breech deliveries at one of those other hospitals had been substantially curtailed. This probably would have led to similar restrictions on the physician at the defendant hospital and perhaps would have made the physician ineligible for that privilege altogether.

The actual investigative and documentation procedure that is followed in acting on initial appointment and reappointment applications is outlined in the facility's medical staff bylaws and medical staff rules and regulations. Some state statutes address credentialing requirements, and The Joint Commission standards impose certain criteria that should be met. The Health Care Quality Improvement Act of 1986 also imposes some credentialing-related requirements on health care organizations. These requirements are discussed in Chapter 12, "Performance Measurement and Patient Safety."

Payers also have similar systems to verify the credentials of the physicians and other providers that they admit to their panels of "preferred" providers (in the case of preferred provider organizations) or the providers who participate in their health maintenance organization.

There is another body of federal and state laws that can affect the credentialing process. These laws are related to antitrust liability. Antitrust laws were developed to protect and encourage competition. Antitrust liability can arise in this context when the medical or professional staff credentialing process interferes with a physician's or health professional's ability to pursue his or her profession. This interference may be alleged to be a restraint of trade. This claim could arise, for example, when the only hospital for miles around enters into an exclusive employment agreement for certain specialty care consulting services and declares that any inpatients who need this specialty care may use only the employed specialist. The following laws protect against restraint of trade:

- The Sherman Act, which prohibits monopolies created by agreements among competitors[34]
- The Clayton Act, which prohibits certain arrangements that tend to lessen competition, such as certain "tying arrangements" that deny freedom of choice in selecting services and products[35]
- The Federal Trade Commission Act, which prohibits unfair methods of competition that affect commerce

Sometimes physicians try to use these acts to support their claims that their denial of staff privileges has the effect of reducing competition. Probably the best defense to actions that arise out of the denial of staff membership to an individual is for the health care organization to show a valid basis for the denial of privileges (e.g., quality-of-care problems). The defense strategy is different when the complaint involves the denial of privileges to a whole class of plaintiffs, such as podiatrists, but that is beyond the scope of this chapter. Be aware, however, that physicians and other health professionals are increasingly sensitive to antitrust problems and that the avoidance of antitrust liability should be considered when developing credentialing-related policies and procedures.

The credentialing process has its own set of confidential information: the credentials file and the practitioner's quality profile. The credentials file is basically a dossier on each medical or professional staff member. It typically contains at least the following:

- Completed medical staff application for appointment or reappointment
- Copies of the practitioner's license, diplomas, board certifications, controlled substances permit (for prescribing certain drugs), proof of current professional liability insurance, response to the facility's query of the National Practitioner Data Bank (NPDB; established by the Health Care Quality Improvement Act of 1986) and perhaps other organizations (e.g., the Federation of State Medical Boards and American Medical Association Physician Masterfile), and other documents required by the bylaws (e.g., results of any proctoring or observation of the practitioner that is done during the initial "provisional" appointment to the staff)

- Completed references from various sources (e.g., program directors for residencies, department chairpersons at other facilities where the practitioner works)
- Specific listing of the privileges requested by the physician and approved by the medical staff

This background information is supplemented with a quality profile for the practitioner, which is usually kept apart from the credentials file. The profile typically contains statistical information on the volume and type of cases treated in the past by the practitioner at that health care organization. It also contains information on the number and type of cases that have been subjected to quality reviews and the results of those reviews. Department chairpersons and credentials committee members use this information in evaluating the practitioner's competence. This helps them to decide whether to grant the requested privileges. The practitioner may treat only the kinds of cases and perform only the kinds of procedures for which he or she possesses clinical privileges in that facility. For this reason, credentialing and privileging decisions often involve sensitive issues and may be the subject of debate, disagreement, and even litigation (if requested privileges are denied).

Accessibility of Credentials Files and Quality Profiles

Because of their sensitive contents, the credentials file and quality profile are treated as confidential information. As a result, health care organizations need to establish clear policies on who may have access to the files and information, how the files and information are kept secure, and how long the information must be retained. HIM professionals are often involved in developing such policies.

To develop appropriate access policies that govern credentialing-related information, the HIM professional needs to understand who plays a role in the credentialing and privilege delineation process. Although the scenario may vary with individual organizations' medical staff bylaws, the following key players are commonly involved:

Applicant or practitioner. This refers to the person who is applying for either initial appointment or reappointment and is requesting certain clinical privileges. The practitioner has the right to review the contents of his or her own credentials file and quality profile.

Department chairperson. This is the clinical chairperson of the medical or professional staff department to which the applicant or practitioner belongs or wants to belong. The department chairperson must meet with the applicant or practitioner, review the contents of his or her credentials file and quality profile, and make a recommendation to the credentials committee or medical executive committee with respect to the application or request for privileges.

Credentials committee. Members of this medical staff committee are charged with responsibility for reviewing the contents of the credentials file and quality profile and recommending action to the medical executive committee or governing body. Credentials committees are usually made up of a cross-section of the medical and professional staff and provide a sort of check and balance on the appointment and privilege delineation process. For example, if the department chairperson of pediatrics does not want a new pediatrician added to the staff because this would mean more competition for patients, the chairperson might recommend against appointment of an otherwise qualified pediatrician. A cross-sectional credentials committee would probably not have the same biases and therefore could help prevent claims of unfairness.

Medical executive committee. This committee, commonly made up of the officers of the medical staff and clinical department chairperson, is often involved in reviewing the recommendations of the individual department chairperson and credentials committee and then passing that information along to the facility's governing body with its own recommendation. Access policies should define whether executive committee members should have direct access to credential files and quality profiles in their capacity as committee members or whether their review and recommendations should be limited to the information presented by the credentials committee and department chairperson. Because the executive committee often has major responsibilities for supervising the quality of clinical practice in the facility, members often have direct access to related files and information.

Governing body or board of directors. As the group ultimately responsible for ensuring the quality of services provided by the facility and its professional staff, the governing body makes the final decision on requests for appointment or reappointment and clinical privileges. This group often relies heavily on the recommendations made by the medical executive committee, department chairperson, and credentials committee but need not be bound by those recommendations. Facility access policies should define whether board members have direct access to credential files and quality profiles.

Medical staff coordinator. This person is responsible for collecting, organizing, filing, and controlling access to information within the credentials file and, often, the quality profile. By the nature of his or her responsibilities, this person must have access to the files and information. Some facilities choose to separate the handling of the quality profile, delegating that responsibility to the staff who coordinate all quality management and improvement activities. In those cases, the person responsible for the credentials file might not have access to quality profile data.

To the extent that HIM professionals are involved in credentialing-related activities, they have some access to credential and quality profile information. In some facilities, HIM professionals serve as medical staff coordinators. In other facilities, those responsibilities are separate from the HIM function, and HIM staff do not have access to this information.

Legal Risks

As mentioned earlier, the tasks of professional staff appointment, reappointment, and delineation of clinical privileges are fraught with potential problems. Physicians who are dissatisfied with the decisions made by a facility may choose to sue the facility, using a wide variety of legal theories. The elements essential to a successful defense vary with the legal theories involved, but generally, in defending these attacks, it is important to be able to show the following:

- That the facility's bylaws, rules, and regulations related to credentialing and privilege delineation were carefully followed and that those provisions meet relevant state and federal requirements
- That the complaining party was not singled out for special treatment but was treated in the same way as other similarly situated people were treated
- That the adverse decision was clinically justified (e.g., supported by something more than just the hunches of the decision makers) and that the justification for the decision was documented in the credentials file, quality profile, or related papers

The procedures for granting medical and professional staff membership and delineating clinical privileges are closely tied to the facility's performance management and improvement activities. Health care organizations use quality management and improvement monitors and indicators not only to improve the systems that support the provision of patient care but also to gather data about the clinical performance of staff members. In this way, the governing body can fulfill its responsibilities to supervise the actions of both employees and the professional staff.

 SELF-ASSESSMENT QUIZ

13. Which of the following documents/elements would often be found in a medical staff credentials file? (choose best answer below)
    a. Medical staff application
    b. Copies of physician license, controlled substance permit(s), proof of professional liability insurance
    c. References
    d. All of the above
14. True or False? Health information professionals are never permitted to serve as medical staff coordinators, because of certification restrictions imposed by law. (choose best answer below)
    a. True
    b. False

Contract Liability Issues and the Health Information Management Department

Contracts (actual and implied) are another common source of liability for health care facilities and providers—even HIM professionals. Some courts have begun to enforce ethical and statutory obligations regarding the confidentiality of patients' health information as part of the contractual relationship between health care providers and their patients. In the *Hammonds* case cited earlier, the court found that the physician breached an implied condition of his physician–patient contract when he disclosed patient information to an insurer without the patient's authorization.[8] Thus, breach of contract is another theory under which a patient may seek relief for breach of confidentiality.

Contract liability typically arises in response to more traditional scenarios. For example, one party to a contract fails to abide by the terms of the agreement, and the other party sues for damages or specific performance (basically, a court order that requires the losing party to do what it contractually agreed to do). Health care organizations enter into written contracts every day, e.g., the business associate agreements discussed earlier are an example of a contract. Organizations may contract for certain professional services, such as emergency medicine or anesthesia services. They may sign contracts for the purchase or lease of equipment or supplies. Sometimes breach of contract problems arise because a contract has been entered into without careful, advance review by legal counsel or risk manager, and, as a result, the health care organization has agreed to unfavorable terms that may be difficult or impossible to meet.

How can this apply to a manager of an HIM department? Think of the potential contracts with which a typical HIM professional may be involved. There may be a contract with a transcription service. There may be a contract with a consulting company. There may be a contract with a release-of-information service or an imaging service. There may be contracts with local schools and educational programs in which liability issues regarding student-trainees are discussed. There may be managed care contracts in which the facility agrees to share certain health information with the managed care company. There may be a contract for purchase of hardware or software to support the facility's information system—and the list goes on. If the HIM professional signs an agreement without benefit of legal or risk management review, he or she may be agreeing to terms that will later come back to haunt the facility.

The following are some of the typical things attorneys and risk managers look for in contracts:

- *Independent contractor clauses.* In signing a contract for professional services, the facility may want to clarify that the professional is not an employee but an independent contractor who is responsible for his or her own actions.
- *Hold harmless or indemnification clauses.* In these clauses, the health care facility generally wants the other party to accept financial and legal responsibility for its own actions and to agree to indemnify or compensate the health care facility for any claims against the facility that are the result of the other party's actions or inaction.
- *Termination or notification clauses.* Health care facilities typically want the process for terminating the contract to be clearly specified, including responsibility for advance notification of the other party of plans to terminate. The wording of such a clause is extremely important, and the health care facility will want as much latitude and flexibility as can be negotiated.
- *Confidentiality obligations.* Particularly with respect to contractors who will have access to confidential health information, the facility and HIM professional will want to specify the contractor's obligations to safeguard the confidentiality and security of that information. In fact, the HIPAA privacy and security rules require that these issues be addressed in a business associate agreement

between the covered entity and all contractors and sub-contractors who qualify as business associates under the rules. Although certain clauses are required in the rules, the actual language of the agreement is up to the covered entity to develop. The HIM professional may even want to specify the exact procedures that must be followed in handling the information.

In determining the safeguards and clauses that should be included in any contract, the HIM professional should use a variety of resources. Literature searches can locate articles specifically devoted to negotiating certain types of agreements, such as transcription contracts. The health care organization's risk manager and in-house counsel, if they exist, also can be of great assistance. The HIPAA and ARRA privacy rules and security regulations should also be referenced. Because of the expense involved in obtaining legal review of a contract, many facilities establish a policy describing the characteristics of contracts that must be reviewed by counsel versus those that can be entered into with just a departmental review or risk management review; such as requiring all contracts involving protected health information, or contracts involving more than a certain dollar amount, to obtain multiple levels of review.

Legal Resources for Health Information Management Professionals

No one expects HIM professionals to be lawyers. They are, however, expected to understand basic legal concepts, such as those described here. They are also expected to know how to find the information needed to help avoid legal problems for the HIM department, the health care organization, and, to a certain extent, the facility's professional staff. In larger facilities, HIM professionals may have access to a risk manager, in-house counsel, and outside attorneys to assist them in finding answers and developing appropriate policies, procedures, and system safeguards. Smaller facilities probably have fewer internal resources, and HIM professionals may need to work more closely with outside counsel on the most important questions, recognizing that there are often limited budgets for outside legal services.

Regardless of the setting, HIM professionals should use important external resources that are available, such as the following:

- The *Journal of the American Health Information Management Association* and other professional journals and newsletters
- AHIMA's Library, where professional staff are available to assist in literature searches and to loan library materials to members
- AHIMA's online body of knowledge, where articles and other AHIMA publications are available to members, including practice briefs
- The state's HIM association and any legal manuals it may have compiled
- Law firms' client newsletters and client advisories (Some firms with health law departments are glad to put HIM professionals and other health care providers on their free distribution list.)
- State hospital associations or other health care industry groups, which keep members up to date on medicolegal issues
- The loss-control staff of any professional liability carriers that insure the health care organization
- Reference librarians at the public library or at law libraries, who can assist in locating and obtaining copies of legislation and regulations
- The *Federal Register*, a daily government publication that keeps the public apprised of proposed federal rules and regulations so that all interested parties have an opportunity to comment or prepare
- State government Web sites
- The HIPAA and ARRA Web pages of the DHHS's Health IT Web site, where copies of the regulations and the answers to frequently asked questions about privacy can be reviewed
- HIM peers in local health care facilities, who are usually more than glad to share information, either in person or via the AHIMA Communities of Practice online community

With all the information that is available, there is no excuse for ignorance. HIM professionals have important responsibilities in today's health care organizations. Patients, health care organizations, and colleagues rely on HIM professionals to protect their confidential information and to assist them in successfully navigating a maze of standards, rules, regulations, laws, and guidelines related to health information, confidentiality, and patient care issues. In so doing, HIM professionals earn their professional credentials, achieve professional success, and improve the quality of health care.

CHAPTER REVIEW

1. What groups/parties typically rely on HIM professionals to understand health information disclosure rules and related regulations? Choose the best answer.
   a. patients/clients of the health care organization
   b. the health care organization that employs the health information professional
   c. external users of health information from that organization
   d. all of the above

2. Which of the following is the best definition of the right to privacy?
   a. the right to vote
   b. the right to be left alone, to make decisions about one's own body, and to control one's own information
   c. the right to due process
   d. the right to free speech

3. Which of the following are agencies/departments at the federal level that affect health care? Choose the best answer.
   a. DHHS, CMS, and HUD
   b. FDA, IRS, Department of Justice, CMS, DHHS, Department of Labor
   c. Department of Commerce, Medicare, Congress

4. Which of the following is the best definition of "false imprisonment"?
   a. the wrong person goes to jail
   b. using physical force to imprison someone
   c. unlawful restraint of a person's personal liberty, or unlawful restraining or confining of a person
   d. none of the above

5. A spoken communication that tends to damage the defamed person's reputation in the eyes of the community, if communicated to a person other than the person defamed, is an example of:
   a. free speech
   b. libel
   c. slander
   d. all of the above

6. A health care organization's compliance plan should focus on which of the following? Choose the best answer:
   a. employee compliance with regulations
   b. potentially fraudulent practices
   c. both of the above
   d. none of the above

7. Documentation that is made while care is being provided can be described as:
   a. contemporaneous
   b. prospective
   c. retrospective

8. In electronic systems, the authorship of documentation can be traced back to the person making the entry because the author used which of the following?
   a. indelible ink
   b. signature stamp
   c. user ID and password
   d. all of the above

9. A patient who has HIV is admitted to the hospital due to complications resulting from foot surgery. Which person is most likely to be allowed under the HIPAA privacy rule to access this patient's health record information?
   a. housekeeping staff
   b. staff member delivering meals
   c. patient's nurse
   d. the patient's close friend who is also a nurse
   e. the pediatrician for the patient's child

10. What is the best description of an advisory board that reviews proposed research projects for their objectives and methods?
    a. privacy board
    b. board of directors
    d. institutional review board
    e. research committee

11. Which of the following scenarios would be an example of when a minor patient can consent to his or her own treatment without parental involvement?
    a. when the minor is emancipated
    b. when the minor wishes to retain privacy
    d. when the minor is over 14 years of age
    d. never

12. Risk managers or legal counsel commonly look for which of the following elements in contracts in order to minimize risks?
    a. hold harmless or indemnification clauses
    b. name of the law firm drafting the agreement
    c. automatic renewal clauses
    d. all of the above

REFERENCES

1. *Griswold v. Connecticut*, 381 U.S. 479 (1965).
2. 42 U.S.C. 12101-12213.
3. Sec. 51(a), (b) of the Federal Food, Drug and Cosmetic Act, as amended, 21 U.S.C. 360i.
4. *Darling v. Charleston Community Memorial Hospital*, 33 Ill. 2d 326, 211 N.E. 2d 253 (1965), cert. denied, 383 U.S. 946 (1966).
5. *Peete v. Blackwell*, 504 So. 2d 22 (Ala. 1986).
6. *Johnson v. Women's Hospital*, 527 S.W. 2d 133 (Tenn. Ct. App. 1975).
7. *Greer v. Medders*, 336 S.E. 2d 329 (1985).
8. *Hammonds v. Aetna Casualty and Surety Co.*, 237 F. Supp. 96 (N.D. Ohio 1965) and 243 F. Supp. 793 (N.D. Ohio 1965).
9. 42 U.S.C. 1395x(e)(2) (1974); 42 C.F.R. 482.24(c) (1994).
10. *Minnesota v. Andring*, 342 N.W. 2d 128 (Minn. 1984).
11. *Fox v. Cohen*, 84 Ill. App. 3d 744, 406 N.E. 2d 178 (1980).
12. *Pisel v. Stamford Hospital*, 180 Conn. 314, 340, 430 A.2d 1, 15 (1980).
13. Tomes J: *Healthcare records: a practical legal guide*, Westchester, IL, 1990, Healthcare Financial Management Association.
14. 42 C.F.R., Chapter 1, Part 2, Section 2.13, Revised (1983).
15. McCann R: Protecting the confidentiality of peer review information, *JAHIMA* 64:52, 1993.
16. 5 U.S.C. 552a(b) (1977).
17. *Plain Dealer Publishing Co. v. U.S. Dept. of Labor*, 471 F. Supp. 1023 (D.D.C. 1979).
18. *Florida Medical Ass'n, Inc. v. U.S. Dept. of Health, Education and Welfare*, 479 F. Supp. 1291 (M.D. Fla. 1979).
19. *Washington Post Co. v. U.S. Dept. of Health and Human Services*, 690 F. 2d 252 (D.D.C. 1982).
20. 42 C.F.R. Part 2, Subpart B, 2.51.
21. 42 C.F.R. Part 2.51, Subpart B, 2.12.
22. 42 C.F.R. Part 2, Subpart B, 2.51.
23. Dennis JC: Profits and patient information: does database marketing breach confidentiality? *In Confidence* 1:4-6, 1993.
24. *Gotkin v. Miller*, 379 F. Supp. 859 (E.D.N.Y. 1974).
25. Are you "on file" in the Medical Information Bureau? *In Confidence* 1:11-12, 1993.
26. Roach Jr WH: *Aspen Health Law and Compliance Center: medical records and the law*, ed 3, Gaithersburg, MD, 1998, Aspen Publishers.
27. Miller D: Glad you asked: Answers on information security and confidentiality, *In Confidence* 1:2, 1993.

28. *Palsqraf v. Long Island R.R. Co.*, 248 N.Y. 339, 162 N.E. 99, rehearing denied, 249 N.Y. 511, 164 N.E. 564 (1928).
29. Pozgar GD: *Legal aspects of health care administration,* ed 7, Gaithersburg, MD, 1999, Aspen Publishers.
30. Carroll R, editor: *Risk management handbook for health care organizations,* Chicago, 1997, American Hospital Publishing.
31. Public Law 101-508, 4206 (Medicare) and 4751 (Medicaid), 104 Stat. 1388.
32. *Elam v. College Park Hospital,* 183 Cal. Rptr. 156 (Ct. App. 1982).
33. *Rule v. Lutheran Hospitals and Home Society of America,* 835 F. 2d 1250 (8th Cir. 1987).
34. *Patrick v. Burget,* 108 S. Ct. 1658 (1988).
35. *Jefferson Parish Hospital District No. 2 v. Hyde,* 466 U.S. 2, 104 S. Ct. 1551 (1984).

HUMAN RESOURCE MANAGEMENT

Susan Helbig

This is a revision of the chapter originally written by Rebecca J. Harmon and Wesley M. Rohrer III

ⓔ Student Study Guide activities for this chapter are available on the Evolve Learning Resources site for this textbook. Please visit http://evolve.elsevier.com/Abdelhak.

CHAPTER CONTENTS

OBJECTIVES

After reading this chapter, the reader will be able to do the following:

✓ Define key words.

✓ List and explain the human resource management responsibilities of all managers.

✓ Differentiate functions and responsibilities of an organizational human resources management department and those of a health information management department.

✓ Discuss external and internal environmental challenges that face a health information department manager in the 21st century.

✓ Apply the legislative and regulatory agency requirements for managing employees in a health care organization.

✓ Describe the societal, organizational, functional, and personal objectives and activities of human resource management in health care organizations.

✓ Understand the systems model of human resource management as it applies to a health information management department.

✓ Develop methods of recruiting, selection, retaining, and terminating employees who staff a health information services department.

✓ Describe various performance evaluation and compensation management programs used in health care organizations.

✓ Identify and evaluate effective strategies for building a health information management team.

✓ Describe orientation and training needs for health information management departments.

✓ Define and explain career planning programs for health information management personnel.

KEY WORDS

Affirmative action programs
Behaviorally anchored rating scales
Cafeteria benefit plan
Career counseling
Career planning
Compensation management
Counseling and referral
Critical incident method
Employee assistance program
Employee handbook
Employment at will
Equal employment opportunity

Factor comparison
Flex time
Graphic rating scales
Grievance procedure
Halo effect
Human resources audit
Job analysis
Job description
Job evaluation
Job grading
Job performance standards
Job ranking

Job sharing
Key indicators of demand
Layoffs
Management by objectives
Performance appraisal
Point system
Power
Preventive discipline
Progressive discipline
Reasonable accommodation
Recruitment
Recruitment pool

Replacement charts
Selection process
Self-appraisal
Sexual harassment
Staffing table
Transactional leadership
Transformational leadership
Undue hardship
Values clarification

ABBREVIATIONS

ADA	Americans with Disabilities Act	**FMLA**	Family and Medical Leave Act
ADEA	Age Discrimination in Employment Act	**FTE**	Full-Time Equivalent
AFL-CIO	American Federation of Labor-Congress of Industrial Organizations	**HIM**	Health Information Management
		HIPAA	Health Insurance Portability and Accountability Act
AHIMA	American Health Information Management Association	**HIS**	Health Information Services
BARS	Behaviorally Anchored Rating Scales	**HMO**	Health Maintenance Organization
BFOQ	Bonafide Occupational Qualification	**HRM**	Human Resource Management
BLS	Bureau of Labor Statistics	**IRCA**	Immigration Reform and Control Act
CEO	Chief Executive Officer	**ISO**	International Standards Organization
CQI	Continuous Quality Improvement	**LAN**	Local Area Network
EAP	Employee Assistance Program	**MBO**	Management By Objectives
EEO	Equal Employment Opportunity	**NLRA**	National Labor Relations Act
EEOC	Equal Employment Opportunity Commission	**NLRB**	National Labor Relations Board
ERISA	Employee Retirement Income Security Act	**OFCCP**	Office of Federal Contract Compliance Program
FLSA	Fair Labor Standards Act	**OSHA**	Occupational Safety and Health Administration/Act
FMCS	Federal Mediation and Conciliation Service	**PHI**	Personal Health Information

POS	Point of Service	**SQC**	Statistical Quality Control
PPO	Preferred Provider Organization	**TJC**	The Joint Commission
QWL	Quality of Work Life	**TQM**	Total Quality Management
SEIU	Service Employees International Union	**WAN**	Wide Area Network

HUMAN RESOURCE MANAGEMENT

Navigating Through Turbulent Times

Employees (human resources) are a health care organization's most valuable resource. Managing human resources is a necessary and critical skill for any health information management (HIM) professional working in the 21st century whether one is in a management, staff, or line position. No matter in what organization a HIM professional is working, it is important to grasp both the overall organizational human resources management (HRM) department responsibilities and the individual HIM department human resources responsibilities. Sometimes the responsibilities and functions overlap; sometimes they are separate. Both HRM and HIM department management teams, however, need knowledge and skills about how to deal with the human beings who make up the organization.

This chapter introduces HRM as both an organization-wide function administered by a human resources (personnel) department and a departmental function administered by HIM. This shared, collaborative but sometimes separate function is analogous to some of HIM's departmental functions such as privacy, confidentiality, clinical documentation, and release of information. In other words, some HIM functions are completed (or not) by clinicians, administrators, or maintenance workers and some functions are completed by HIM staff.

As we settle into a 21st-century mindset, we would be wise to reflect on the dramatic changes in organization structure, technology, incentive structure, and strategies that have occurred in health care over the past several decades. Many of these changes can be classified as organizational responses to broad environmental influences that have had a pervasive impact across all industries and enterprises, including those in health care, rehabilitation, and long-term care. We have witnessed the emergence of the "informated" organization,[1] the learning organization, the horizontal organization,[2] the virtual organization, and the consumer-driven health care organization. Every manager, worker, and professional has been considerably affected by the explosion of access to information from links to local area networks (LANs) to wide area networks (WANs), data warehousing, and the virtually unlimited resources of the Internet. Benefits as well as excesses of reengineering have been chronicled and experienced by both the victims and survivors of corporate "downsizing" and outsourcing work to offshore sites. A bewildering variety of philosophies,

methods, and buzzwords—continuous quality improvement (CQI), statistical quality control (SQC), total quality management (TQM), quality of work life (QWL), employee participation teams, empowerment, benchmarking, the Toyota manufacturing quality program, lean management, Baldrige awards, International Standards Organization (ISO) 9000, and Six Sigma certification among others—have competed for managerial and scholarly attention during this period of the transformation within the health care industry.

Broad Environmental Forces

Continuing Challenges in the 21st Century

Although the dawn of the new century will be forever marked in time with the events of September 11, 2001, more than a decade later, the rapidity with which change has settled on the United States, and indeed the world, continues to add complexity to societies great and small. Beyond the profound geopolitical, economic, religious, and cultural repercussions that the horrific events of September 11 exerted across the globe, less than a decade later, the world grapples with economic turmoil, emerging potential pandemics—real and forecasted—as well as a continuing shift in demographics that have forever changed business as usual. See Box 16-1 for ways 21st century issues have impacted society and the workplace. With the election of the first African American president of the United States, the face of the American workforce—an important issue for the past 50 years—has changed.

The complexity and risk that all organizations face in this century of terror, economic uncertainty, and turmoil is exemplified by the increasing threat of pandemics (e.g., avian influenza A, H1N1). The public health community is poised to mobilize considerable resources to prevent the onset of a pandemic with global health and economic implications. Not only could such an epidemic have devastating effects on the health of populations (according to the World Health Organization, 30% of the world's population might be affected in the first year of a pandemic, resulting in 2 million deaths)[3] but it also would likely have severe, if temporary, effects on the economic, social, and political infrastructure. The *Harvard Business Review* (May 2006) devoted a lengthy Special Report to alerting the business community to the importance of monitoring and planning for a pandemic.[4] This is a telling indicator of the breadth and severity of the likely impact of such a public health assault on the individual organization and the corporate community. Clearly, because health care organizations will be on the front lines

BOX 16-1 · 21st Century Issues and the Impacts on Society and the Workplace

Issue	Impact (Real or Potential)
Acts of terrorism, war	Immigration, terrorism, security
Global economic downturn	Economic stability, job security, salary freezes, layoffs and downsizing, benefits in jeopardy
Hurricane Katrina (aftermath) and Super Storm Sandy	Preparedness, planning for emergencies, work contingencies, family/personal versus professional responsibility in a crisis
Continuing demographic shift in the United States	The "postracial" environment; growing numbers of Hispanics, new Americans (immigrants); more attention to work–life balance, English as a second language
U.S. population reached 313.9 million in 2012	Ability of existing social programs to support burgeoning population
Health care reform in the United States	The great unknown—how will this affect the business of health care as we know it today?
Pandemic concerns	Planning, prevention, work contingencies for times of acute crisis
The "graying" workforce	Generational staffing, managing work–life balance that spans birth to death, accommodating the older employee, managing a increasingly multigenerational staff

DID YOU KNOW?

In 1978 a class action lawsuit was filed on behalf of present and former female employees of the Los Angeles Department of Water and Power. Allegedly, the Department required female employees to make larger contributions to its pension fund than male employees. The Department's pension plan was based on mortality tables and its own experience proving that female employees lived longer than male employees, therefore they should pay more for their pensions because more monthly payments would be eventually paid out to the female employees. The District Court held that this violated § 703(a)(1) of Title VII of the Civil Rights Act of 1964, which, inter alia, makes it unlawful for an employer to discriminate against any individual because of such individual's sex. The District Court ordered a refund of all excess contributions and the Department's pension plan was amended to eliminate sexual distinctions in the plan's contributions and benefits.

of addressing the consequences of a pandemic along with its public health partners, the organizational effects of such an event would almost certainly be immediate and profound. Although it is impossible to predict the future in detail, it is likely that the new level of heightened awareness, sense of insecurity, and vulnerability throughout the West will have long-lasting consequences in the workplace as well as across society.

The Federal Regulatory Context

Although the pace of regulatory growth affecting HRM slowed somewhat after the explosion of legislative initiatives and regulatory mechanisms of the 1960s and 1970s, subsequent federal legislation continues to have a significant impact on the workplace. Most notable of these federal policies are the Americans with Disabilities Act (ADA) of 1990, the Civil Rights Act of 1991, the Family and Medical Leave Act (FMLA) of 1993, and the Lilly Ledbetter Fair Pay Act of 2009. Although the ongoing elimination of legal and attitudinal barriers to women and minority participation in the workplace has led to formal recognition of diversity programs, in other arenas the philosophical justification for equal employment opportunity (EEO) and especially affirmative action (AA) programs is being challenged. (See the section on Civil Rights and Equal Employment Opportunity Legislation for more information on affirmative action programs.)

The Demographic Imperative

The phenomenon of an aging population is beginning to affect the workplace acutely, in the United States and other highly developed societies worldwide. This demographic trend, coupled with the legislative constraints on employer discretion embodied in the Age Discrimination in Employment Act (ADEA; 1967, as amended), has led to a "graying" of the workforce, at least in some regions of the United States. Also, the cultural and ethnic mix of workplaces in the United States and abroad are feeling the effects of sustained growth and migration. By mid-2007, the Hispanic population in the United States reached 41.3 million, growing almost 4% from the year before, and comprising just over 15% of the total U.S population.[5]

Although demographics continue to shift, other forces, like the steady erosion of union representation within the U.S. workforce (from 25% of the private sector workforce in 1973 to 7.6% in 2008)[6] remain a major theme of labor relations through the end of the 20th century and into the 21st century. Although no major national legislative developments have affected collective bargaining significantly during the past decade, recent political events portend significant changes in the near future. There have been continual skirmishes over management's right to hire replacement workers and the ramifications of team participation in quality management efforts for traditional labor relations. However, the separation in 2005 of roughly 4 million members of three major collective bargaining structures, including the Service Employees International Union (SEIU) and the American Federation of Labor–Congress of Industrial Organizations (AFL-CIO),[7] posits a strong challenge for the future of organized labor. The long-term decline in union membership as a proportion of the workforce and the decline in political power of organized labor at least at the national level begs the question of whether traditional collective bargaining structures and processes will be able to adapt to and survive the environmental and workplace changes discussed.

Forces Transforming Health Care

Beyond these broad influences affecting all organizations are the constellation of forces that have reshaped traditional health care and rehabilitation. The traditional model of health services delivery focuses on acute care (hospital) services and was orchestrated by independent physicians. This model has been radically transformed into an environment of competing managed care networks coordinating an array of linked services and settings across the continuum of care. "Managed care" includes an increasingly diverse set of institutional structures and affiliations, including the established health maintenance organizations (HMOs), physician provider organizations (PPOs), point-of-service (POS) agreements, integrated delivery systems, and other types of health plans and networks. A common element for managed care across these variations of organization design is the commitment to accept the financial and other risks of providing cost-effective services of high quality to enhance the health and well-being of a defined population. This commitment has resulted in priority given to aggressive cost control, organizational consolidation, system integration, market concentration, and image marketing on the basis of perceived differences in quality.

These rather profound changes in health care organization, provider incentives, and relationships among providers, consumers, and purchasers have had a considerable impact on HRM within health care and rehabilitation service organizations. As provider organizations have reduced staff to lower personnel costs, thereby increasing labor productivity in the short term, the potential for work-related stress, conflict, erosion of employee commitment and loyalty, and professional "burnout" has increased accordingly. Concomitantly, the implementation of new technologies, especially information technology, entails greater demands on employees to develop and continuously upgrade their skills and knowledge base to adapt to the plethora of information management tools and resources. Managers especially are faced with the pressures of maintaining their own professional and clinical competence while accommodating the new developments in information technology and information systems and adapting their leadership style and philosophy to the realities of changing employee values and expectations and to innovative structures (i.e., the horizontal, loosely linked, team-based organization) coupled with technological innovations in how health care is delivered and documented.

The inevitability of change, if not of its specific forms or trajectory, is perhaps the only safe prediction about health care organization and delivery in the long term. Consequently, it can be argued that the most critical competencies of the health care manager and professional of the 21st century are the capacity to do the following:

- Exercise flexibility in response to continuous environmental change.
- Communicate effectively with various stakeholders representing multiple and often conflicting priorities.
- Direct the efforts of an increasingly diverse and mobile workforce resistant to traditional forms of control and comfortable with technological change to the workplace.

Challenges for Health Information Management Professionals

Managing health information in the 21st century places special demands on HIM professionals to obtain, train, retain, use, fully develop, and direct the efforts of HIM human resources required to achieve the goals of health care organizations. Several serious studies have concluded that the health care labor force of the future will demand multiskilled workers who have the flexibility of working in interdisciplinary teams in various provider settings within integrated health care systems and networks. Almost 20 years ago, the Pew Commission concluded that "the evolving nature of our health care system will require health professionals with different skills, attitudes and values. . .creating a growing demand for the skills of collaboration, effective communication and teamwork."[8] Health information managers, professionals, and technologists will be required to serve health care delivery systems that emphasize preventive, rehabilitative, and long-term care and will increasingly coordinate services across providers, disciplines, levels, and loci of care. Much of the ability to coordinate the services relies on the implementation of sophisticated use of electronic health record systems and health information exchanges. As community-based and home health services expand, there will be increased demands for integration of clinical and financial data and capture of information relevant to various outcome measures at the individual patient or client level—that is, the health record—and aggregated at the service population or community level. In the presence of considerable uncertainty about exactly how health care will be organized and delivered in the next generation, it can be predicted with confidence that health information managers must be prepared to respond to accelerating changes in technology, public policy, competitive markets, population distribution, employee diversity, technological changes and organizational structures.

Leadership and Human Resources Management

Leadership and *management* are closely related terms that convey different but complementary aspects of the behavior associated with ensuring effective organizational performance. Bennis and Nanus make the distinction in this way: "Managers are people who do things right and leaders are people who do the right things."[9] One implicit difference suggested by this characterization is that managers focus on efficiency and control, whereas leaders focus on the "big picture" (i.e., communicating a vision of the organization and inspiring and influencing people to invest in achieving it). Both perspectives and the associated activities of working managers and leaders at all levels are necessary to sustain effective, high-performance organizations. Although this applies to all complex organizations, it might be argued that in no sector of society is the need for visionary leadership and effective management of organizational resources more important than in health care in the 21st century.

One of the most obvious but surprisingly complex questions is: "What is leadership, actually?" A massive volume of literature in leadership theory and practice has attempted to address this question during the past century, including controlled social science research studies and more descriptive, intuitive narratives from practicing leaders and executive managers. Some researchers have concluded, on the basis of a lack of reliable findings about the nature of leadership in thousands of studies, that its usefulness as a research variable may no longer be warranted. Nonetheless, common wisdom among practicing managers would suggest that leaders do make a difference in influencing the satisfaction, motivation, and achievements of their followers and in effecting organizational outcomes—even if the effects of leadership alone on desired outcomes are difficult to measure reliably. Most working professionals would agree that, even if they are not absolutely certain about what makes leaders effective, they know that we need effective leaders, especially when we face difficult challenges, rapid change, and crises.

DID YOU KNOW?

According to www.mastersinleadership.org, the following are among the "21 Surprising Facts About Leadership Research":[10]

1. In 1974, Ralph Melvin Stogdill, one of the pioneers of leadership research, determined six categories of personal factors associated with leadership: capacity, achievement, responsibility, participation, status, and situation. But, even with this discovery, researchers warned that the information was too narrow, saying that no person becomes a leader simply by possessing a certain list of character traits.
2. Research has determined that effective leaders are those who are able to address two different kinds of needs within their organizations: efficiency needs and human needs. Good leaders are effective at both planning and implementation tasks and at working with the people in their organizations.
3. According to Barnes and Krieger, leadership is more of a reflection of an organization, rather than a person. In other words, in the most successful organizations, leaders' roles overlap, and different people take on leadership roles at different times.
4. *Transformational leadership* is one of the hot terms in leadership research. It is defined as a process by which leaders and followers raise one another to higher levels of morality and motivation.
5. The *Journal of Leadership Studies* recently concluded that the more a company focuses on internal leadership growth, the better its sales, profits, and profit margins.

Overview of Leadership Theory

A thorough review of the themes and models of leadership developed during the past 75 years would go beyond the limits of this chapter. An overview of the key themes and approaches to leadership, however, should be useful in demonstrating the direct relevance of HRM to leadership. One basic difference in the evolving models of management has been the distinction between those that focus on the characteristics of leaders independent of other factors affecting leadership and those that emphasize leadership as a set of relationships. The former is the "trait" approach, which is based on the assumption that leadership could be fully explained by identifying a cluster of personality and character traits that are necessary and sufficient for the leader to be effective. Stogdill's[11] meta-analysis of many such studies found that there was little correlation among the various sets of traits, although some characteristics (e.g., intelligence, initiative, and self-confidence) were frequently identified.

Beyond the lack of agreement about a common and sufficient core of traits was the recognition that different situations seemed to call for different kinds of leadership. For example, the ideal leader for handling a true crisis (i.e., effective decision making under fire) may not necessarily have the best qualities for gaining commitment to a pervasive and long-term process of organization change. This contingency approach to leadership recognizes that other variables in the leadership situation or context are likely to influence the leader's behavior and effectiveness. Among the variables identified in research studies using this model are the nature of the task, the expectations and maturity of followers, and the stability of the environment.[12] One implication of a contingency approach to leadership is recognizing that what it takes to be an effective leader all depends on the situation the leader faces.

Relationships and Leadership Style

The fact that the nature of followers is recognized by the contingency approach as being an important variable suggests the importance of considering the relational nature of leadership. On one level, it is obvious that the concept of leadership entails that some others participate as followers. A credentialed health information manager might be an exceptionally competent and knowledgeable professional, but unless he or she has responsibility for directing the efforts of others, he or she is not a leader. So the aspect of relationship is inherent to a full understanding of leadership. This is also suggested by the leadership style approaches to leadership exemplified by the University of Michigan[13] and Ohio State studies[14] of leadership style or behavior. In both these classic studies, researchers attempted to determine which leadership styles were associated with effective group and organization performance. In these studies, two dimensions of leadership behavior were identified as characterizing different leadership styles: the Ohio State study identified these behavioral aspects as "initiating structure" and "consideration," whereas in the Michigan State studies, the comparable dimensions were called "production orientation" and "employee orientation." The first dimension focused on task behaviors and structuring and organizing work, whereas the second emphasized maintaining supportive relationships, especially between the leader (supervisor) and the followers (subordinates). These same

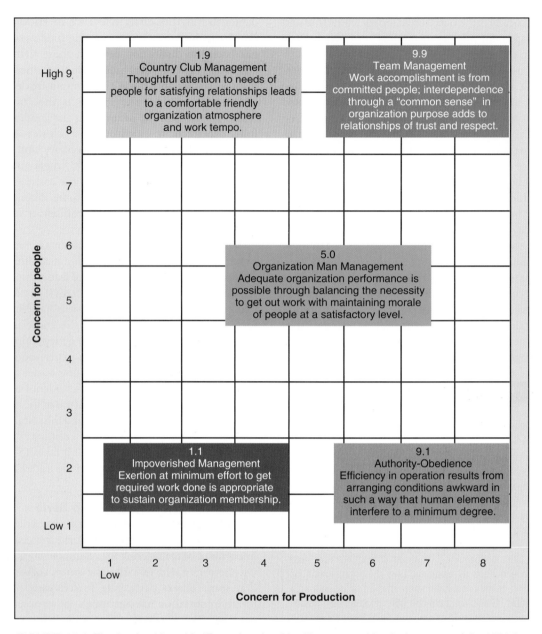

FIGURE 16-1 The leadership grid. (From *Leadership dilemmas-grid solutions*, copyright 1991 by Robert R. Blake and the estate of Jane S. Mouton, Austin, TX. Gulf Publishing Co.)

dimensions are also the basis for the popular Managerial Grid, developed by Blake and McCanse,[15] which describes five contrasting leadership styles (Figure 16-1).

A more sophisticated and dynamic approach to leadership is the situational leadership model developed by Hersey and Blanchard,[16] which builds on the task behavior and relationship behavior vectors. However, this model also incorporates a situational variable, the maturity of followers, to suggest which leadership style might be most appropriate in a given situation. The quadrants on the charts (see Leadership Roles Matrix, Figure 16-2) correspond to four distinctive leadership roles: controller, coach, partner/colleague, and delegator. The effectiveness of these roles, in terms of individual and team satisfaction and productivity, will depend on the degree of team development and maturity of the followers (Figure 16-2).

Although by no means conclusive, the leadership style studies collectively suggest that effective leaders generally are those who exhibit both a high concern for productivity and for people. Fiedler's[17] research linking leadership behavior to similar dimensions suggested that a structuring style was more appropriate when the leadership situation was either very favorable or very unfavorable to the leader, whereas a more people-oriented behavior was more appropriate when the leader faced ambiguous circumstances. What seems clear is that over the long term, the leader must attend to both production and people concerns to continue to be effective.

Human resource management can and should provide support to the operating manager to enhance his or her efforts in both domains. For example, effective employee recruitment and selection and job analysis processes can

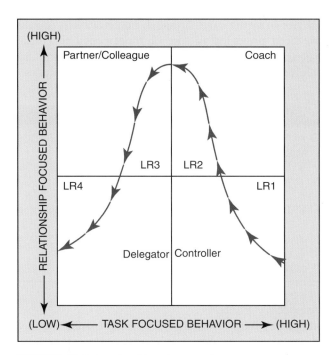

FIGURE 16-2 Leadership roles matrix.

be useful tools in task structuring, whereas diversity management training can enhance the manager's relational skills. Even a significant investment in the HRM function cannot guarantee effective leadership in the specific case, but without effective HRM processes, the manager may be at a distinct disadvantage. It could be argued that the more effective and efficient the HRM technical functions are, the more time and energy the manager should invest in his or her relationship building activities with employees and peers.

Transformational Leadership

Another useful perspective on leadership is provided by Burns in his historical and psychological analysis of leadership.[18] Burns contrasts two aspects or types of leadership: transactional and transformational. Transactional leadership refers to those behaviors associated with the more routine and continuing exchanges of effort and commitment between managers and employees in carrying out the business of the organization and sustaining effective working relationships. The transformational role of the leader refers to the visionary, motivational, and charismatic aspects of leadership. The transformational leader is able to articulate a vision of the organization's future, to convince followers that they have a stake in the achievement of that vision, and to achieve commitment to change (personal and organizational) as not only inevitable but also beneficial both to the organization and to the employee's self-interest. Schein[19] focuses on the role of the leader as a change agent transforming organizational cultures by destroying dysfunctional ones and stimulating cultures supportive of growth and innovation. Hunt and Conger[20] site Tosi's insistence that these aspects of leadership are complementary and necessary: "Supporting most successful charismatic/transforming leaders is their ability to effectively

manage (transact with subordinates) the day-to-day mundane events that clog most leaders' agendas. Without transactional leadership skills, even the most awe-inspiring transformational leader may fail to accomplish his or her intended mission." Rohrer[21] has proposed a third dimension, translational leadership, that allows for the effective communication of the charismatic vision into practice at the operating level, and that this aspect of leadership is an especially important responsibility of the middle manager as the key liaison between executive management and the first-line supervisory and operating staff. From this perspective the HRM director can be viewed as playing a "translational" role in establishing, communicating, and helping to implement HRM policies and procedures that support the strategic direction and goals of the health care organization. Similarly, the HIM director is a "translational" leader in establishing, communicating, and helping to implement HRM policies within his or her span of control and influence.

 SELF-ASSESSMENT QUIZ

1. The HRM director plays which type of leadership role?
  a. Transactional
  b. Translational

Leadership Development

Another aspect of leadership that has direct implications for HRM is that of emerging leadership and leadership development. If leadership is viewed primarily as being most characteristic of executive-level management, then leadership identification and development efforts are narrowly focused. Yet, if leadership is viewed as a capacity that is more widely distributed throughout the organization, the issues of emerging leadership and leadership development become more challenging and complex. Although a useful distinction has been made between management as a set of technical and control activities focused on maintaining day-to-day operations and the status quo in the short term and leadership as entailing a proactive, visionary, strategic, and empowering perspective, it could be argued that both aspects are required to some degree at all managerial levels in the organization. Health care organizations present additional challenges in this respect because of the professional specializations that go with the territory so that each health professional is subject to the claims and influences of both clinical and administrative leaders. Both training and development and performance appraisal functions within HRM should play a critical role in leadership development at the lower and middle management levels, including the early identification of potential leaders as executive managers from lower in the ranks.

The Ethics of Leadership

Although not necessarily recognized as an HRM responsibility, the development of ethically responsible managers and leaders has profound implications for HRM. A justification for serious consideration of the ethical dimension of leadership, specifically in health care, is expressed by Darr.[22] "For the health services manager, a personal ethic is a moral framework for relationships with employees, patients, organization, and community. In these relationships, the manager is not, and cannot be, a morally neutral technocrat. The manager is a moral agent." What follows from Darr's claim is that all managerial behavior—at least all activity that is relational rather than purely technical—must be considered from an ethical or moral perspective. This also entails that ethical decision making is complicated by the fact that the manager must consider his or her decisions in terms of the interests of various constituency groups. Burns'[23] theory of transformational leadership also places the ethical dimension at the core of leadership in that it is rooted in individual, organizational, and societal values. He contends "transforming leaders 'raise' their followers up through levels of morality." He notes that transformational leaders are more concerned about "end values" such as justice and equality, whereas transactional leaders focus more on modal (means) values such as honesty and fairness. Characteristic of both types of leadership is the leader's role in serving a common purpose that transcends individual needs and interests of the leader and the followers.

Normative ethics may be defined as the science or art of determining principles, rules, and guidelines for right conduct (i.e., how one should behave responsibly in the community). For example, the preamble to the American Health Information Management Association (AHIMA) Code of Ethics (2004) states:[24]

> The ethical obligations of the HIM professional include the protection of patient privacy and confidential information; disclosure of information; development, use, and maintenance of health information systems and health records; and the quality of information. Both handwritten and computerized medical records contain many sacred stories—stories that must be protected on behalf of the individual and the aggregate community of persons served in the health care system. Health care consumers are increasingly concerned about the loss of privacy and the inability to control the dissemination of their protected information. Core health information issues include what information should be collected, how the information should be handled, who should have access to the information, and under what conditions the information should be disclosed.

Ethical obligations are central to the HIM professional's responsibility, regardless of the employment site or the method of collection, storage, and security of health information. Sensitive information (genetic, adoption, drug, alcohol, sexual, and behavioral information) requires special attention to prevent misuse. Entrepreneurial roles require expertise in the protection of the information in the world of business and interactions with consumers.

It would be difficult to argue with this statement of ethical accountability, and these standards for HIM professionals could be applied to all health care professionals and managers through the health care system. Yet what specifically are the exemplary values that are to ground and guide ethical

behavior in health care? Although numerous lists of values have been presented as core or fundamental to ethically responsive behavior in health care, the following have achieved a broad consensus as prima facie ethical duties.

✓ **SELF-ASSESSMENT QUIZ**

2. According to the AHIMA Code of Ethics, the HIM professional is obligated to the following:
   a. Protection of patient privacy and confidential information
   b. Disclosure of information
   c. Development, use, and maintenance of health information systems and health records
   d. Quality of information
   e. a and c
   f. All of the above

Respect for Person

This value entails regarding each person (patient, subordinate, boss, peer, neighbor) as an end in himself or herself rather than as a means to some end or as an impersonal stereotype. This value entails granting the other person the maximum freedom that the nature of the relationship allows without impairing the freedom or welfare of others.

Beneficence (Service)

This value represents a commitment to doing good for, or providing service to, the other person, community, or broader society. A disposition toward competent, caring service to specific individuals (e.g., clients) or the broader community seems to be intrinsic in the health care professions. Although the focus of the direct care provider, physician, or therapist is usually on the health and well-being of the individual patient, the HIM manager must also consider the effects of his or her decisions on the organization, the population or community it serves, and the broader society, including the global impact, if any. That the interests of the individual and the community may differ and cause conflict is a challenge faced often by the ethically responsive public health professional.

Nonmaleficence

This value forbids the ethically responsive person from doing harm or injury to the person or welfare of another. In one sense, this represents the other side of the coin of the duty to do good. This is represented by the Hippocratic oath, which indicates that the physician's primary responsibility is to "do no harm." Like beneficence, this value challenges the ethical HIM manager to consider and balance the needs and interests of all his or her key constituencies in making decisions with ethical consequences.

Justice

Often regarded as synonymous with fairness, acting justly in practice is almost always more complex than it appears. A more elaborate definition of justice is ensuring that equals are treated equally, whereas "unequals" may be treated differentially. For example, all patients presenting with diabetes symptoms at the same stage of the disease should be given equivalent (if not strictly identical) treatment by the physician. However, if two patients present in an emergency department at the same time, the one with massive head trauma from an automobile accident should be given priority attention over the patient with a broken toe. The grounds for making these distinctions are addressed in discussion of the concept of distributive justice. For example, if the manager is allocating the end-of-year salary increases, which factors should be given most weight: past performance, recent acquisition of new skills, seniority, or some other consideration?

 SELF-ASSESSMENT QUIZ

3. Which value represents a commitment to doing good for, or providing service to, the other person, community, or broader society?
   a. Beneficence
   b. Respect for Person
   c. Justice
4. Which value forbids the ethically responsive person from doing harm or injury to the person or welfare of another?
   a. Justice
   b. Respect for Person
   c. Nonmaleficence

Other Core Values in Health Care Management

Northouse[25] adds two other values critical to leadership that are certainly worth consideration: honesty and building community. A compelling argument could be made that honesty or truth telling is a bedrock value on which all others are founded. Certainly our entire social fabric and the stability and integrity of our organizational culture depends on the assumption that most people, most of the time, are telling the truth as they see it. Without this ethical foundation, we could not make any reliable assumptions about the link between intentions, speech, and behavior of ourselves or of those with whom we interact. Honesty is not only the best policy ethically; it is the only reasonable basis for group behavior, organizational effectiveness, and managerial decision making in the long run.

If honesty is seen as a necessary precondition for ethical behavior, community building may be viewed as an outcome of ethical leadership. Northouse[26] argues that ethical leadership requires a community-oriented perspective. "Transformational leaders and followers begin to reach out to wider social collectivities and seek to establish higher and broader moral purposes. ... An ethical leader is concerned with the common good—in the broadest sense." Implicit in this statement is that ethical leaders will attempt to align their actions to the extent possible with the good of the community and broader society. For example, the board of directors and executive management team of a hospital should consider the impact of a potential relocation of the facility from the urban core to a growing suburb on both communities affected.

 DID YOU KNOW?

Instrumental values: Identify behavioral attributes such as "ambitious" and "responsible"; often viewed as a means to achieve terminal values.
Terminal or end-state: Identify ideals such as "wisdom" and "a world at peace"; often seen as achievable through implementation of instrumental values.

Ethics of the Ordinary

Students of HIM often assume that the really important ethical issues in health care are those "life, death, and well-being" decisions made primarily by physicians and other hands-on practitioners and that most health care managers and support professionals would have little or no direct involvement in such ethical decisions. Historically, the focus of ethics as applied to health care has been on the problems of biomedical and clinical ethics faced by the practitioner or researcher. Although these issues are of considerable concern to society as a whole and to ensuring ethical practices in medicine and research involving human subjects, this perspective is too narrow because it ignores the ethical implications of managerial practice in health care. Worthley[27] emphasizes the need for greater attention to the "ethics of the ordinary" in health care and for developing ethically responsive health care providers and managers at the level of the "routine and humdrum in which many less visible [ethical] challenges surface on a daily basis." Worthley focuses instead at the "microlevel" of ethical behavior—the innumerable ethical decisions faced in the midst of the daily routine of the health care manager and HIM professional. He argues for the importance of this largely ignored realm of behavior on the basis that "the life of the individual healthcare provider—doctor, nurse, technician, administrator—is largely one of routine and humdrum in which many less visible challenges surface on a daily basis, and in which many ordinary, indirect, and subtle actions must be and are taken." It is within this domain of "the ordinary" that health information professionals will be making most of their ethical decisions, including ones of real consequence to the welfare of the patients, their coworkers, their bosses, and their own families. Even in the midst of their routine work, the HIM professional and the health care manager are moral agents, and this responsibility goes with their professional territory.

Power and Ethical Decision Making

In this context, the concepts of power and values clarification on the decision-making process are fundamental. Power has famously been defined as the ability of person A to influence person B to do something he or she would otherwise not decide to do.[28] Understanding the effects of power, especially differences in the power held or sought by key players in the decision-making situation, is necessary in sorting out the ethical implications of alternative decisions. For example, the ethical health information manager should consider as a criterion in his or her decision making about a coding strategy the implications for the most vulnerable groups affected (i.e., the self-paying, uninsured). Those decision makers who are relatively powerful on the basis of their positions in the organization or their expertise have special responsibility for considering the ethical consequences of their behavior as it affects those with less power and influence, including their staff and clients within and outside the organization.

Values Clarification

Values clarification is also an essential process as a precondition for ethically responsive decision making and leadership. Rokeach[29] has characterized values as "standards that guide ongoing activities" and value systems as "general plans employed to resolve conflicts and to make decisions" (p. 21). He goes on to identify two sets of values, the instrumental, which identifies behavioral attributes such as "ambitious" and "responsible," and terminal or end-state values, such as "wisdom" and "a world at peace," with the former set of values seen as means to achieving the latter. Rokeach's instrumental approach to ethics suggests the practical nature of values and the real advantage, if not absolute necessity, of reflecting on and being clear about our own value commitments and priorities. For example, if we are forced to make a decision that seems to sacrifice "respect for persons" or individual autonomy for societal justice, are we willing to make that trade-off? What, in fact, are our own ethical "nonnegotiables"? We are likely to be more confident, dependable, and balanced decision makers (and perceived to be fair and trustworthy leaders) to the extent that we continue to engage in thoughtful values clarification internally and with our employees.

Servant Leadership

Servant leadership is a paradoxical approach to leadership behavior developed by Robert K. Greenleaf[30] that has a clear ethical foundation and spiritual undertones. Greenleaf argues that the essence of leadership is rooted in effectively serving, nurturing, and empowering one's followers. By taking on the role of servant, the emerging leader would gain the trust, respect, and loyalty of his or her followers. Also by serving to empower his or her followers, the leader should increase the productive capabilities of those to whom he or she is accountable. In this way ethical responsiveness is linked directly to performance improvement. Greenleaf also extends the scope of the leader's servant role to encompass social responsibility, equity, and justice. Ideally, the leader also serves by championing those outside the organization who are marginalized, powerless, and disadvantaged.

? DID YOU KNOW?

Servant leadership: Rooted in effectively serving, nurturing, and empowering those whom you lead.

Greenleaf's primary contribution is to give serious attention to the ethical and good citizenship dimensions of leadership and to provide a foundation for a "business case" for altruistic and ethically responsive leadership. The core concept is certainly not new because it draws on early Christian sources (e.g., "Rather let the greatest among you become as the youngest, and the leader as one who serves" [Luke 22:26]). The servant leader perspective, which was consistent with the countercultural ethos of the 1970s, may seem somewhat anachronistic today. Nonetheless, given the leadership failures and financial crises in the last decades of the 20th and the early 21st centuries, both in corporate boardrooms and in health care (e.g., Allegheny Health, Education and Research Foundation [AHERF], Columbia/Hospital Corporation of America [HCA], and HealthSouth), a reexamination of the servant leader model is timely.

Applications to Human Resources Management

The preceding discussion of ethics highlights the pervasiveness of the ethical aspects of decision making in health care both for the hands-on provider, other support professionals, health care managers, and the HIM professional. It could be argued that, despite its absence in many discussions of HRM, ethics is critical to effective management of people at all levels of the organization. For example, ethical responsibility or maturity should be included as a criterion in managerial recruitment and selection processes if we indeed give priority to the ethical conduct of our managers and intend to inculcate or reinforce a set of core ethical values in our organization's culture. Certainly the training and development function is an appropriate venue for addressing managerial ethics in formal supervisory training. HRM can also play a role in communicating and monitoring policies and procedures with ethical implications (e.g., ensuring due process in the disciplinary function, fair and justifiable allocation of employee compensation, etc.). Perhaps just as important, HRM leaders should serve as advocates for and models of ethical responsiveness in decision making by emphasizing the organization's core values in the implementation of top management's vision, the organizational mission, and strategic direction.

Although role modeling of ethical behavior must flow from the top of the organization, as being an explicit and high priority endorsed and sanctioned by the board of directors and the chief executive officer (CEO), it must be evident in practice at the supervisory level if employees are to regard this commitment seriously. One way to ensure that ethical behavior is given priority by management is to include it as a behavioral dimension within the formal performance appraisal process. This presents a challenge in developing clear criteria and objective measures that allow for valid and reliable assessment of the employee on this dimension. Nonetheless, if management is genuinely committed to fostering ethical sensitivity and behavior in decision making, these goals must be given more than token endorsement. Managers, clinicians, and all staff within the organization must be held accountable for ethical behavior in practice.

Codes of Ethics

Methods to encourage ethical practice in an administrative environment include specific organizational policies and procedures to ensure compliance, formal expressions of core values, and organizational and professional codes of ethics. For example, Mercy Hospital of Pittsburgh, formerly a member hospital of the Catholic Health East system, operated by the Sisters of Mercy, and now a component of the UPMC, makes its value commitments explicit as a set of core values directly related to its mission statement (see http://www.upmc.com/HospitalFacilities/Mercy). These core values (i.e., reverence for each person, community, justice, commitment to the poor, stewardship, courage, and integrity) reflect the values of the Roman Catholic faith and the religious community that sponsors and supports the hospital. However, these values as understood by the organization can also be used as standards to develop criteria and measures for evaluation of organizational and individual performance. Many health care professions have defined their own code of ethics within their sphere of practice. The health information management profession is no different.

The following excerpt from the AHIMA Code of Ethics suggests the tenor and scope of professional codes of ethics and the profound implications for managerial behavior and decision making:

> The mission of the HIM profession is based on core professional values developed since the inception of the Association in 1928. These values and the inherent ethical responsibilities for AHIMA members and credentialed HIM professionals include providing service, protecting medical, social, and financial information, promoting confidentiality; and preserving and securing health information. Values to the healthcare team include promoting the quality and advancement of collaboration.

A code of ethics sets forth values and ethical principles and offers ethical guidelines to which professionals aspire and by which their actions can be judged. Ethical behaviors result from a personal commitment to engage in ethical practice. Professional responsibilities often require an individual to move beyond personal values. For example, an individual might demonstrate behaviors that are based on the values of honesty, providing service to others, or demonstrating loyalty. In addition to these, professional values might require promoting confidentiality, facilitating interdisciplinary collaboration, and refusing to participate in or conceal unethical practices. Professional values could require a more comprehensive set of values than what an individual needs to be an ethical agent in his or her personal life.

The most notable aspects of this section of the AHIMA code is the pervasiveness of the ethical accountability suggested (i.e., that the ethical HIM professional lives an ethical life in every respect and venue as opposed to making occasional ethical pronouncements). Also, this statement explicitly grounds the ethical imperative to the employer, the public, and the individual—the primary constituencies of the health care system (i.e., the patient, resident, and client of services). This standard, then, serves not only as the ultimate criterion of quality, it also serves to ground all ethical decision making in health care.

Organizational Human Resource Management: A Systems Perspective

This treatment of HRM adopts the image or metaphor of the organization as an open system, that is, the organization as a living organism that attempts to achieve and maintain equilibrium with its ever-changing environment.[31] Within this conceptual framework, HRM is viewed as a subsystem linked to and interdependent with other subsystems, such as financial management and health information management, within the internal environment of the organization. Each subsystem and the organization as a whole are subject to continuing influences from the external environment. To survive and thrive, the organization must respond and adapt effectively to these environmental forces. The latter can be distinguished as an unstable array or irregular flow of resources, constraints, threats, and opportunities. To maintain equilibrium with its environment, the organization must ensure an adequate flow of resources to sustain energy for continuing activities and growth. It must adapt to constraints on its access to resources, its decision making, and its actions. The organization must maintain environmental sensing and intelligence functions to answer the questions "what is out there?" and "how is it going to affect us?"

Technology (or throughput) can be defined as the hardware and software (means) by which the organization transforms inputs into outputs (products, services, and benefits to the community). Technology, however, can also be regarded as an environmental factor that affects the organization as a potential resource or constraint. During the last quarter of the 20th century up to the present, the impact of technology on health care and rehabilitation in general and HIM in particular has been dramatic and pervasive. The almost incredible developments in information technology have not only changed the way that we access, process, distribute, store, manage, and exchange data but have also transformed the fundamental structures and processes of organizations in virtually every industry, including health care. The impact of technology, especially information technology, is recognized as a most important factor affecting HRM practice within health information services.

From a systems perspective, then, we can identify inputs, technology, outputs, and environmental influences as system variables that must be addressed in the organization's strategic management and planning processes. The human resources of a health care organization are arguably the most critical strategic variable. Consequently, this systems perspective should be useful in our examination of HRM with applications relevant to the health care environment and especially to the health information manager.

Health Information Management: A Systems Viewpoint

A systems approach to managing human resources is useful in understanding the organization and dynamics of any human collective enterprise including HIM services because

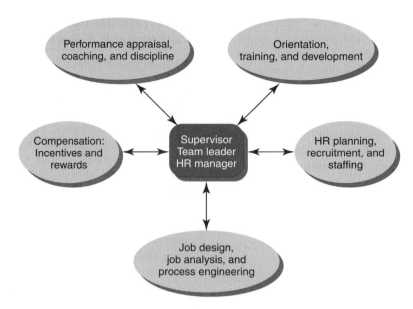

FIGURE 16-3 Activities and objectives of human resource management.

this perspective enables our recognition of the complex interrelationships of individual parts to the whole organization (Figure 16-3). It also encourages viewing the organization as being nested within one or more larger, more comprehensive systems, for example, a HIM department within an acute care hospital within a comprehensive medical center affiliated with a managed care network as part of a regional health care system. When this systems framework is applied, the interdependence of subsystems within the organization and the important boundary relationships with and among relevant sectors of the environment must be considered. For example, applying a systems perspective, the HIM manager must deal not only with the relationships between HIM and financial management (internal) but also with a state-level regulatory agency (external).

As information technology becomes increasingly complex, pervasive, and central to the mission of the health care system, the typical HIM department might be more appropriately conceived as a "service center" for the whole enterprise rather than being limited within the confines of a traditional department. This makes a systems view especially useful in understanding how health information services fit within the organization and might be linked to both internal and external constituencies, including patients, providers, insurers, legal offices, regulatory staff, and other clients.

Systems Perspective Applied to Human Resource Management

Although there are various bases for distinguishing subsystems within any system, the following clusters of human resource functions represent a reasonable and familiar approach:

- Recruitment and employee selection
- Job analysis, job design, and process engineering

- Training and career development
- Performance appraisal and employee development
- Quality management and team building
- Employee and labor relations
- Compensation management
- Employee health and safety
- Regulatory compliance and reporting (e.g., EEO, Occupational Safety and Health Administration [OSHA])

All these subsystems have distinct territories based on historical practice, regulatory scope, and professional or specialist role identification, training, and, in some areas, certification. However, all are interrelated processes, each one addressing some aspect of maintenance and development of the human resources of the system. The health information professional must understand the purpose of these interdependent functions and his or her role in supporting and using these processes. As discussed earlier, these human resource subsystems can be associated with the dynamics of the open systems model: obtaining inputs (employee skills, knowledge, and energy) and transforming these inputs through HRM processes and technologies into outputs (desired results, outcomes, or impact).

Applying a systems view to HIM can assist in defining the key variables that affect production within the department (Figure 16-4). The process of scanning (digitizing), indexing, and performing quality control on clinical documents provides a good example of the interdependence inherent in the systems model. After the patient has been seen and the handwritten documentation completed by the clinician, the paper documents must be collected from the clinics within an appropriate time frame. The documents must be analyzed for readability and for appropriate clinician authentication. They must then be sorted by the appropriate date and/or document type. Next, they will be scanned and indexed appropriately so that the document can be retrieved when needed. A quality control step on a planned and selected number of

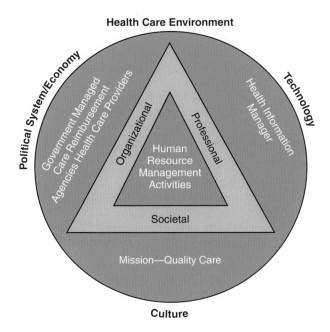

FIGURE 16-4 Systems model diagram.

documents is often inserted into the process. Unless the volume of scanning transactions is very small, one person cannot perform all these functions. Employees with different skills and roles are necessary to perform these various functions in the required sequence at the right times. If the documents are not collected, reviewed, scanned, indexed, and quality control performed as planned, the documents will not be available for continuing care or other authorized purposes. This may result in late digitizing in the electronic health record, decreased productivity, and even, perhaps, less than optimal patient care.

Various human resource activities in both HRM and HIM can also be considered by using the same systems approach. For example:

- Job analysis including the creation or revision of a valid and useful job description, should provide the foundation for setting and communicating performance standards and expectations to the employee. Using the job description as a blueprint, the supervisor can prepare for an effective performance review and appraisal with the employee.
- The performance appraisal process should be completed and documented before sound decisions can be made concerning compensation adjustments and promotions, transfers, or (when circumstances warrant it) disciplinary actions.
- Effective planning for employee orientation and training programs depends on information generated by the recruiting, selection, and performance appraisal processes and, in some organizations, the quality management subsystem.
- Environmental challenges from regulatory and legislative changes, economic conditions, and employee lifestyle and cultural influences continually affect all of the subsystems that constitute HRM in health care.

A systems model facilitates a comprehensive and integrated approach for HRM at the departmental level. To provide highly skilled and high-achieving workers, it is critical for the health information manager to match qualified employees with the positions that best fit their knowledge, skills, and job-related personal characteristics. The manager must take responsibility for maintaining staff competence and motivation through continuing education and staff development activities. In addition, it is important to facilitate career ladders and professional or career growth pathways. These programs should be planned, implemented, and evaluated continually to promote qualified and productive HIM professionals and support staff who will facilitate the delivery of high-quality health care and represent their employers and their profession effectively. By applying a systems perspective, managers, consultants, and students in training to be professionals can better appreciate how these processes and roles are linked and interdependent and the implications for addressing organizational problems and challenges strategically.

Environmental Influences and Human Resources Management

The structure and function of health care organizations and providers are continually changing to adapt to the external environment. The organization is limited in its capacity to control these outside forces, so it must develop appropriate HRM solutions in response to external challenges. These responses are more likely to be successful and persist to the extent that they (1) address the problem, (2) are efficient and cost-effective, and (3) are perceived as compatible with the core beliefs and values of the organization culture. The number of potentially relevant influences on the health care organization in general and the health information manager in particular is great, ever changing, and uncertain because what is "relevant" depends on the individual's and the organization's local context and circumstances. Consequently, we must be selective in which environmental influences to address. The following factors are discussed below in further detail: women's participation in the workforce, technological change, health policy and industry developments, economic forces and trends, demographic change and diversity, health policy and competition in health care, and the legal and regulatory constraints on HRM.

Women's Participation in the Workforce

Over the past four decades, there has been a rapid increase in the participation of women in the workforce. This trend has had profound consequences for the family, including reallocation of responsibilities for child care and other aspects of parental gender roles, as well as for the economy and the workforce. The increasing level of women seeking work outside the home not only has increased the labor pool for the traditionally "female" jobs, including health care and related jobs of housekeepers, food service workers, and clerical staff, but also has led to pressures for expanding employment and career opportunities for women.

As more women with children assumed full-time jobs and careers outside the home, demand for different types of employee benefit programs and more flexible work schedules grew apace. The increasing presence of women in highly professional, managerial, and executive roles has resulted in a raised level of expectations for equal opportunity, equal compensation (for work of comparable value), and the elimination of irrelevant barriers based on gender rather than on ability to perform the job. From an HRM perspective, employment processes, including recruitment, selection, training, promotion, and compensation, should be gender neutral. Although progress has been made in this regard, the existence of a "glass ceiling" for women managers in some organizations across industries, including health care, and the barriers that women still face in some occupations (e.g., public safety) affirms that we have not yet achieved this desirable goal.

According to the Labor Department, during the period between the onset of the recession in 2008 to 2013, the number of women in the workforce increased from 67.4 million to 67.5 million. This contrasts to 69 million men who currently are in the workforce, which is below their high of 70.9 million in June 2007.[33] The primary reason for this contrast is because women tend to hold jobs in health, education, hospitality, and retail while male-dominated sectors suffered more acutely during the recession. Men lost more than six million jobs during the recession while women lost 2.7 million jobs (www.wsj.com, Women Reach a Milestone in Job Market).[34]

These changes in women's participation in the workforce and in the prevailing societal attitudes about women's (and men's) roles contributed to the passage of the FMLA in 1993. This legislation forced many employers to examine and revise policies and procedures about the granting of appropriate leave time and ensuring job security for the employee facing new child care responsibilities or serious illness of a family member.

❓ DID YOU KNOW?

Did you know that a 2012 Catalyst study of 1600 business school graduates (www.catalyst.org)[32] found that men get more significant assignments that lead to advancement than women do? For projects, the average size of men's budgets was twice as big and three times as many staffers as women's.

The increasing number of women in the workforce accompanied by the greater number of single working mothers and of families with both parents working outside the home has affected employee benefits and work schedules. See Box 16-2 for a Benefits Table. Cafeteria benefit plans, in which employees can choose from an array of benefits to fit their needs or lifestyles, were a response to these changes in family roles and expectations. For example, working parents may choose a subsidy for on-site child care, whereas a childless worker may choose additional dental insurance. Family leaves for both mother and father and increased number of

BOX 16-2	Benefits Table
Cafeteria benefit plans	Allows employees to choose from an array of benefits to fit their needs or lifestyle
Job sharing	A staffing option in which a full-time position is shared by two or more persons
Flex time	Allows employees to control their work schedule within parameters established by management
Telecommuting	Allows employees whose jobs make this a reasonable approach to work from a remote location (usually home), thereby eliminating commute and in-office time; can reduce in-office crowding, parking congestion, and traffic; adds an "intangible" benefit for employees

personal days (which might be used to care for sick children) are other examples of how employers have responded to this profound sociocultural trend.

Job sharing and flex time have been offered by employers to accommodate the needs and preferences of working women. Job sharing is a staffing option in which a full-time position is shared by two or more persons. This can provide advantages for both the employer and the employee. The employer gains some staffing flexibility and potential cost efficiency, for example, to ensure reliable coverage for vacations, illness, jury duty, and family emergencies. If additional work hours are required for the short term, two job-sharing employees could be scheduled to perform the job without incurring overtime pay. Advantages for the employee include work schedules that may be arranged to accommodate child care or other lifestyle situations.

Flex time allows employees to control their work schedule within parameters established by management. The employer usually defines an essential core structure of hours of the day and days of the week in which the employee must work to provide needed services and coverage. The employee's preferred schedule can be arranged flexibly around these requirements. Other employers allow flexible scheduling but require employees to submit their schedules in advance, to ensure adequate coverage. The use of flex time often depends on the nature of the work to be performed—that is, the predictability of work flow and how flex scheduling affects overall department operations. If, for example, a project must be completed by a given deadline regardless of the hours expended, the employee or project team may be allowed to schedule work hours at will, provided that the project is completed within the required time period.

✓ SELF-ASSESSMENT QUIZ

5. The cafeteria benefit plan allows employees to choose from:
   a. Any item in the organization's cafeteria.
   b. An array of company benefits to fit their needs or lifestyles.
   c. Flex time or job sharing.

Technological Change

Technology continues to be a significant influence on HRM, especially within HIM. Increasingly, routine and standardized tasks, such as most clerical and filing functions, previously performed by lower-skilled employees are being converted to computer-based processing. Because this evolving information technology facilitates more time-efficient and cost-effective methods of collecting and displaying data for analysis, expanded opportunities and new positions are being created for HIM professionals to manage and use information generated by these decision support tools. Examples of these new positions include:

- Transcriptionists who now act as documentation editors for clinician dictators who use voice recognition programs to "start" their documentation. The transcriptionists finalize the document before it is uploaded to the organization's EHR for clinician authentication.
- Data management specialists who use various databases to collect, analyze, write, and present both quantitative and narrative reports and recommendations to physician and administrative committees on a myriad of topics concerning health data informatics and information: accreditation readiness, revenue cycle report cards, various quality indicators, etc.
- Release of information specialists who work with an EHR and a fully automated release of information computer program that tracks everything from the initial request to the final release (or not) to the authorized requester.
- Information assurance specialists who are responsible for an organization-wide records program of which the medical record is but one subset.

New medical equipment and procedures are changing the way medicine is practiced. Increasingly, clinical practice is becoming evidence or outcome based. These trends have had considerable effects on the type of data and methods of data collection that are required for medical practice and rehabilitation. Health care providers continue to explore ways to free clinicians' time to provide patient care and education rather than spending unnecessary time and effort in extensive documentation and administrative procedures. Event-capturing information systems, such as videotape or handheld data entry devices, can provide more accurate and timely information capture with less effort and can provide a greater benefit to patient care than retrospective, narrative documentation can. Digitized documentation can be transmitted over fiber-optic or wireless networks, which will allow facilities to manage incoming and outgoing data from other organizations as well as internally generated information. Such information management tools and methods have begun to change the job titles, job descriptions, and allocation of responsibilities within health information services units. Human resource managers at both organizational and departmental levels must recognize, understand, and accommodate these changing approaches to information capture, transfer, retrieval, applications, and the impact on managing the workforce.

Economy Forces and Trends

The state of the economy and the values of key economic variables, such as inflation, unemployment, business growth, and interest rates, have a profound if somewhat indirect effect on HRM. These and other relevant economic variables shape the size and fluidity of the labor markets for health care workers, stimulate or inhibit the health care organization's capital expansion and enterprise development, and influence the organization's staffing plans and management's ability to use compensation to recruit and retain skilled employees. Normal economic cycles and periodic perturbations in the local, national, and increasingly, the global economy will continue to affect the management of human resources.

It is critical that HIM managers continually anticipate economic trends in relation to the organization's strategic plans, technological developments, and health policy and regulatory changes. Organizations that monitor economic trends can avoid being blindsided by sudden crises that directly affect their HRM goals and activities. If, for example, the regional economy enters a recession because of the contraction or relocation of a dominant business or industry, the multiplier effects could be experienced as lower patient volumes, reduced revenue streams, changes in case mix, and less favorable credit and lending terms of local vendors. Longer-term or chronic economic downturns could result in the health care organization's contracting its business objectives and reducing employment levels. The health care organization might increase its use of contracted services, including temporary staffing, to lower its personnel costs and avoid long-term commitments. However, this approach also threatens the development of relationships of trust and long-term commitment. In certain areas of health care, including imaging and information technology services, contracts are being extended overseas and services outsourced that were once kept in house. The multitude of cost-saving measures can reduce the stress and anxiety associated with uncertainty and instability of the organization's continued economic presence but can increase anxiety among staff for fear of replacement. The financial system crisis of 2008 to 2009 and the resulting economic recession had severe repercussions for the health care industry as investment portfolios were hard hit and profit margins narrowed or became negative.

As we saw in the 1990s, downsizing of organizations' workforces was a common, if not always well considered, component of a more comprehensive corporate reengineering. These often extensive and hurriedly implemented reductions in force were typically justified on the basis of process rationality, enhanced productivity, and gains in operating and financial performance. In too many cases, however, these draconian measures were an attempt to provide a "quick fix" to "bottom lines," stock market values, and shareholders' impatience. In all too many cases, management discovered in the following business cycle that these drastic cuts in positions led to understaffing, employee burnout, and threatened lower quality of service.

The human costs and dislocation experienced by laid-off workers may be addressed in part by severance pay and outplacement assistance to ease the terminated employee's transition to another job, career retraining, or period of unemployment. To preserve the values of trust, mutual respect, and commitment within the organization—all of which have been severely eroded by "downsizing," outsourcing, and layoffs—executive management must ensure that managers at all levels demonstrate respect for each employee as a valued person and recognize the contributions of all employees, including those exiting the organization. All too often, however, employees are given abrupt notice of their termination and in some cases, especially in key management positions, the employees are treated as pariahs, and escorted from the facilities by security guards. This can only erode the fabric of the corporate culture and sense of trust and common purpose of the surviving employees.

Organizationally, HRM must assume responsibility for ensuring that the appropriate number and type of staff with necessary skills and knowledge are obtained and retained to carry out the mission of the organization effectively and efficiently while sustaining the core values of the organization's culture. This responsibility also pertains to the HIM department's management team to clearly understand and anticipate what type and how many HIM staff are needed to carry out the organization's mission. It is also HIM's responsibility to continuously and proactively educate the HRM department on HIM needs.

Demographic Changes in the Workforce
Multicultural Workforce
A number of demographic changes evident in U.S. society present challenges in HRM. The population continues to become more diversified in most if not all areas of the country because some minority groups have higher birth rates than the majority. Accordingly, we are experiencing a greater representation of minority group persons in the workforce. The U.S. Department of Labor Statistics predicts a continuing influx of Asians, Hispanics, African Americans, and women into the workforce, along with a decline in the proportion of white males. Among current workers scheduled to retire, the majority will be male, and almost half will be white. The Bureau of the Census predicts that by 2050 non-Hispanic whites will represent only 53% of the population, a decline from 72% in 2000.[35] It can be reasonably predicted that in the 21st century, the white male of working age will indeed be in a minority position in the U.S. workforce.[36]

Gender Roles
The continued growing prominence of women in the workforce, not only in numbers but also by attainment of managerial and executive leadership roles, is a cultural phenomenon that has had and will continue to exert a profound impact on power and interpersonal relationships in most organizations, including health care. As the roles of men and women in our society have become less narrowly defined and more fluid and ambiguous, we have experienced considerable tension and potential for conflict in the workplace. An obvious example

in health care is the changing perception of gender roles and power relationships between physicians and nurses. At midcentury, the majority of physicians were men and almost all nurses were women. Subsequently, increasing numbers of women have become physicians and men have become nurses. Furthermore, nurses, regardless of sex, are asserting their claims to professional recognition and autonomy. At the same time, many physicians are feeling frustration from threats to their economic well-being and constraints on their decision-making authority and independence imposed by managed care and other regulatory mechanisms.

DID YOU KNOW?
The *Wall Street Journal* ("Women Reach Milestone in Job Market," Jonathan House[37]) reported that in 2013 about 56.9% of American women are either working or looking for work, versus 69.2% of men. Did you know that despite the fact that more women are obtaining college degrees than men, a wage gap persists? Women earned 76.5 cents for every dollar men earned in 2012.

In HIM historically, women have filled most positions—managerial, technical, and clerical. Almost certainly this gender segregation has suppressed salary levels and career mobility for health information managers and professionals. As our societal distinctions between male and female roles, capabilities, and career expectations continue to blur, we can anticipate more opportunities for women in HIS and greater upward mobility into executive management and less gender restriction within HIM.

Age Distribution
As more and more individuals work beyond the typical retirement age of 65 years and the children born in the latter years of the 20th century begin entering the workforce, the workplace will see a continually lengthened age distribution. Many senior workers of the World War II era have entered retirement, but a significant number are continuing to work beyond the traditional retirement age of 65 years. In health care, it is not uncommon to see physicians either practicing or serving on advisory boards well into their 80s. This cohort models a traditional work ethic and values of loyalty, responsibility, and dedication to coworkers, employers, and patients. This cohort is often referred to as "traditionalists."

Baby boomers, born between 1946 and 1963, are well advanced in their careers. Some have already assumed executive management and professional leadership roles, whereas others have experienced midcareer dislocations as victims of downsizing. This group tends to be goal oriented but more skeptical about and less motivated by allegiance to an organization or industry than their predecessor generation.

The next major age cohort was born and reared after the societal turmoil of the 1960s and is often called "Generation X." They have experienced general economic affluence, the information revolution, and a backlash against the countercultural values of the 1960s. This generation tends to be politically more conservative than their parents' generation, motivated by personal development, self-actualization, and consumption. As employees, this generation responds to workplace autonomy, loose structure and controls, participatory supervision, and non–work-related goals and priorities. In contrast to the World War II generation, the post-1960s employees are less likely to define themselves by their jobs and more likely to engage in multiple careers in the course of their working lives.

Children born in the last two decades of the 20th century, sometimes labeled the "Millennials" or "Generation Y" are now becoming a formidable presence in the workplace. This generation has grown up in an era dominated by information technology, telecommunications, and the entertainment culture. Many have been perceived as being antagonistic to or apathetic about formal authority, bureaucratic routine, and deep or long-term commitment to a job, organization, or cause. A more balanced appraisal may be that members of this generation are accustomed to frequent and dynamic changes in their environment and expect unrestricted and real-time access to unlimited sources of information and communication (e.g., text messaging and "tweeting"), as well as a sense of entitlement to immediate gratification of personal needs and wants. This generation expects to assume positions of authority in the organization rapidly and is likely to be impatient with corporate policies and norms that appear rigid and hierarchical. These attitudes and behaviors that suggest that information is increasingly viewed as a market commodity are reflected in the health care setting as more health information is accessed online and a consumer-driven approach to health care is adopted across society.

Each age group shares some characteristics and values based on the impact of societal, cultural, and economic factors that have affected its generation uniquely, and each suffers to some degree from the stereotypes imposed by other generations. These differences in beliefs, attitudes, and expectations, especially about the relationship among work, career, and personal lives, affect how they approach their jobs, coworkers, and managers. This is not a new phenomenon. The members of the 50- and 60-year-old preretirement generation have a work ethic and value commitments related to careers not necessarily shared by subsequent generations. Intergeneration tensions and conflicts can be anticipated, especially at points of transition, as younger managers assume authority over older employees. The potential for conflict between generations is likely to be exacerbated by the shifts in, and confusion about, the gender roles discussed earlier.

SELF-ASSESSMENT QUIZ

6. The cohort that models a traditional work ethic and values of loyalty, responsibility, and dedication to coworkers, employers, and patients is referred to as:
   a. Traditionalists
   b. Nontraditionalists

Diversity in the Workplace

Diversity issues and diversity management are receiving more and more attention from businesses and the health care sector. Many believe that the term *diversity* translates only to the terms *multicultural* and *multiethnic*. Although each workplace will pinpoint a unique definition, the concept

---

Case Study: Diversity Management in St. Luke's Health System

Institutional Accreditation

A market survey done by St. Luke's Health System (SLHS) revealed that the populations served by the system would be dramatically changing. Over a 5-year span, certain facilities would face a 23% increase in the Hispanic population and a 17% increase in the African American population compared with an 8% increase in the white population. The population over age 65 years would increase by 19%, and those aged 45 to 64 years would increase by 22%.

The first step taken by SLHS was to create a diversity council to provide direction to the senior management on diversity policy issues. The president and CEO sit on the diversity council and appoint new members from within the system. SLHS then created and recruited a system vice president for diversity to spearhead change throughout the organization.

The SLHS diversity council identified six functional areas in which to target diversity efforts: communications, education, patient relations, employee recruitment and retention, medical staff recruitment and retention, and supplier diversity. A diversity council committee was created within each functional area, cochaired by a director-level staff person and a council member. Successes of the diversity council committees include regular publications on diversity topics in both Web-based and paper forms, production of an exceptional new-hire orientation video,

development of a new diversity training curriculum, design of cultural tool kits for nurses' stations, and partnerships with local career-building organizations and health care professional institutions such as "Welfare to Work" or the Women's Employment Network.

Cultural tool kits contain a quick reference for nurses and other health care providers to make patients feel comfortable. The correct contacts for interpreter services within the hospital are listed, as well as contacts for appropriate community or religious organizations. A basic "Do and Don't" list will also be included with room for nurses to add notes about their personal experiences. For example, for new Hispanic prenatal patients, *do* involve the father and other members of the family in the decision-making process involving care of the mother or new baby.[39] Many Native-American populations have a more holistic view of health care and often use herbal remedies that are not considered "medicine" but would still have implications regarding drug interactions that clinicians should take care to note.[40]

Overall success of the diversity initiative within SLHS can already be quantified by the increased number of women in various positions and lower staff turnover throughout the system. These short-term gains speak well of future achievements.

encompasses just as much variation as the term implies: differentiation by sex, gender, race, ethnicity, age, sexual orientation, and cognitive or physical abilities.

Until recently, encouraging diversity in the workplace was more or less a "feel-good" tactic. Many organizational leaders will agree that increasing or supporting diversity is strong ideologically and possibly beneficial economically. Supporting diversity allows workers to feel respected and valued for the qualities each can individually bring the organization. Economically, a more diverse workforce should provide more flexibility and adaptability toward the changing needs of the consumer population. Increasingly, large organizations, including health care systems, have instituted diversity management units and/or programs to encourage diversity in employment within the organization and to recognize internal diversity as a competitive advantage in marketing and community relations.

Since 2000, diversity management has become an HRM paradigm.[38] While many organizations struggle to realize any economic benefits of their transformation, St. Luke's Health System of Kansas City, Missouri, has emerged as a diversity leader in the health care arena.

SELF-ASSESSMENT QUIZ

7. Diversity encompassing which of the following:
   a. Ethnicity
   b. Gender
   c. Race
   d. Age
   e. Sexual orientation
   f. Cognitive or physical abilities
   g. All of the above

Legal, Regulatory, and Accreditation Requirements Affecting Human Resources Management

The primary mission of the health care organization is to address the health needs of a given community or defined population. Because it is a labor-intensive industry, health care is especially dependent on the full and cost-effective use of its human resources in fulfilling this mission. Society's values and priorities are expressed in a formal way through legislation, policies, and regulations. Compliance with these statutory and regulatory requirements, such as the Conditions of Participation for Medicare and Medicaid, is an important example of the organization's need to be responsive to relevant forces and constraints in its environment.

Another societal expectation that health care and other organizations must address is the right of employees to experience a safe and healthy work environment. Safety is not limited to the physical environment alone; private information used for identification and benefit information also requires a number of safeguards. Furthermore, during the last fifty years of the 20th century, public policy has established that all employees have equal opportunity to satisfy their economic and psychological needs by participation in the workforce generally and through jobs and professions

of their choosing without facing barriers of discrimination and exclusion. Most human resource activities either directly support or are affected by compliance with legislation and regulatory mechanisms furthering the societal objectives of equal opportunity and fair employment, employee health and safety, and effective union-management relations.

A complex, evolving array of legal and regulatory requirements mandated as public policy through federal, state, and local legislation has pervasive effects on HRM in health care organizations (Table 16-1). These laws, judicial determinations, regulatory agency actions, and administrative guidelines influence and constrain HRM in all its functions, from recruitment and hiring through employee evaluation, promotion, and compensation to the termination process. These legal and regulatory factors impose a considerable administrative burden on line managers, who depend on support from human resource professionals to avoid preventable exposure to legal and financial risk and to provide efficient and cost-effective systems for resolving human resource problems. It could be argued that HRM has become the most regulated set of functions and activities in the workplace. Some of the most pertinent legislation, regulatory processes, and agencies with greatest impact on HRM in health care and rehabilitation are discussed in the following section.

Institutional Accreditation
The Joint Commission
Many health care organizations submit themselves to voluntary accreditation by agencies such as The Joint Commission, which publishes standards, rationales, and elements of performance to measure the effectiveness of leadership, HRM, and organizational performance in health care organizations. The Hospital Accreditation Standards published by The Joint Commission addresses standards and performance elements that relate specifically to the organization's HRM functions. Some of these have evolved in recent years, moving certain specific topics outside of the HRM area to other subject areas (e.g., leadership, environment of care, performance improvement, and others). As of 2014, The Joint Commission includes several areas of human resource functions.

Hospitals must both identify staff qualifications related to their assigned job responsibilities and verify individual staff qualifications such as experience, education, credentials, health status, and criminal record, etc. Hospitals must also describe how hospital staff function within the health care organization. TJC speaks specifically to assessing and planning for an adequate number and mix of staff for the various functions in the hospital.

Safety is of paramount importance and mandated safety training must include information that is hospital wide as well as specific to individual organizational units.

Education requirements include orientation, training and education of staff so that they understand and can act appropriately regarding the environment of care. Required education also means that staff must participate in various continuing education and training activities that relate to their maintaining job-specific competencies. Data from various

TABLE 16-1 Federal Regulations and Agencies That Affect Human Resources in Health Care

Legislation or Agency	Effective Date	People Affected and Key Points
The Joint Commission	Continuing	Voluntary accreditation Leadership and organizational performance
Occupational Safety and Health Act	1970	Safe and healthy environment for all workers
Fair Labor Standards Act	1938; amended 1963	Sets minimum wage, overtime pay, equal pay, child labor, and record-keeping requirements for employers; 1963 Equal Pay Amendment forbids sex discrimination in pay practices
National Labor Relations Act (Wagner Act)	1935	Gives employees the right to collective actions and outlaws unfair labor practices by management
Labor Management Relations Act (Taft-Hartley Act)	1947	Outlaws unfair labor practices by unions
Labor Management Reporting and Disclosure Act	1959	Forces unions to represent properly their members' interest
Civil Rights Act of 1964 (Title VII)	1964, amended 1972, 1991	Prohibits discrimination on the basis of race, color, religion, sex, or national origin and ensures equal employment opportunity
Health Care Amendments to the National Labor Relations Act	1974	Extends the coverage and protection of the act to employees of nonprofit hospitals and other health care organizations
Vietnam Era Veterans' Readjustment Assistance Act	1974	Affirmative efforts to provide employment for qualified disabled veterans and veterans of the Vietnam era
Age Discrimination in Employment Act	1967	Protects employees from age 40 and beyond
Americans with Disabilities Act	1990	Outlaws discrimination against disabled people and ensures reasonable accommodation for them in the workplace
Family and Medical Leave Act	1993	Grants unpaid leave and provides job security to employees who must take time off for medical reasons for themselves or family members
Lilly Ledbetter Fair Pay Act	2009	Amends the Civil Rights Acts of 1964, extending the 180-day statute of limitations previously applied to the filing of an equal-pay lawsuit; this legislation allows for the resetting of the 180-day limit with the issuance of each subsequent discriminatory paycheck

evaluation activities performed within the hospital are to be used as indicators to assess and improve staff effectiveness.

These standards and performance elements are then used as the basis for the organization's self-assessment and scoring to determine compliance with The Joint Commission's quality standards. See The Joint Commission Web site at www.jointcommission.org for information regarding the most current standards.[41]

Civil Rights and Equal Employment Opportunity Legislation

Civil Rights Act of 1964, Title VII (as Amended)

Title VII of the Civil Rights Act of 1964, which prohibits discrimination in employment on the basis of race, color, religion, sex, or national origin, was the legislative culmination of a growing societal consensus that the vestiges of racial, gender, and other forms of discrimination and segregation had to be eliminated in the workplace as well as in housing and public accommodations. The Equal Employment Opportunity Act of 1972 expanded the scope of Title VII and increased the powers of the Equal Employment Opportunity Commission (EEOC), the federal agency created to monitor and enforce compliance with Title VII. Equal employment opportunity requirements were mandated during the 1960s and 1970s

through federal, state, and local legislation and through Executive Orders of the President of the United States, which, although not requiring Congressional approval, have the force of law. An example of the latter is EO 11246, which prohibits job discrimination on the basis of race, color, religion, sex, or national origin by contractors and their subcontractors doing business with the federal government and requires that they take certain affirmative action in employment. The Office of Federal Contract Compliance Program (OFCCP) has the responsibility of monitoring and ensuring compliance among enterprises covered under the order.

Affirmative action programs are systematic human resource plans that outline goals for hiring, training, promoting, and compensating minority groups and women who are protected by EEO laws. Although critics have argued that affirmative action goes beyond the legislative intent and language of Title VII, affirmative action plans are specifically mandated in EO 11246 for businesses under federal contract to address past discrimination and to achieve a workforce that reflects the diversity of the population. In the 1990s, affirmative action plans and other forms of preferential treatment, especially those that set quotas for hiring or selection, were under increasing assault as representing reverse discrimination. The overturning of affirmative action programs based on racial or ethnic identification for admission to public higher education in California, Texas, and other states reflected unresolved tensions in society about EEO. The conflict can be regarded as one between advocates of providing an even playing field for all citizens (nothing more, nothing less) and those attempting to ensure specific socioeconomic outcomes for one or more preferred groups.

In response to some decisions of the Supreme Court that shifted the burden of proof in alleged discrimination cases to the plaintiff, Congress passed the Civil Rights Act of 1991. This legislation, which represents the current phase in the evolution of the statutory foundation for EEO, requires the employer charged with discrimination to demonstrate that the alleged discriminatory employment practices are job related and justified on the basis of business necessity. Furthermore, the act holds the employer liable for discrimination in "mixed motive" cases in situations in which the employer uses the defense that an employment decision would have been the same (against the interests of the employee) even absent the discriminatory practice. However, the law also prohibits "race norming," in which the employer uses different cutoff scores as employment criteria for the Title VII–protected classes, for example, holding Hispanics to lower cutoff scores than whites on a standardized cognitive test.

In summary, the thrust of the civil rights movement in the workplace as embodied in EEO legislation was to remove artificial, irrelevant, and unfair barriers to full employment opportunity not relevant to performance in the job. It is recognized that employers may and should make distinctions among workers on the basis of effort, skills, productivity, merit, and other job-related criteria in making employment decisions. The law is not intended to discourage employers from rewarding excellence or penalizing employees for unacceptable performance. The law requires, however, that employment actions be related to work-related criteria rather than gender, race, religion, or any other prohibited factors.

> **? DID YOU KNOW?**
>
> In June 2009 the Supreme Court found, in *Ricci vs. DeStefano*, that white firefighters had been subjected to race discrimination when their promotions were overturned based solely on the fact that no black firefighters qualified for promotions based on test scores.[42] These decisions and others add complexity to the decisions and constraints of the manager in today's increasingly complicated workforce, and there are no indications that this trend will abate.

Gender Discrimination and Sexual Harassment

Pregnancy Discrimination Act of 1978
The Pregnancy Discrimination Act of 1978 extended Title VII prohibitions against discrimination on the basis of gender by broadening the definition of this form of discrimination to include pregnancy status, childbirth, and related medical conditions. Essentially, the act prohibits the employer from providing the covered employee less favorable benefits than other employees eligible for short-term sick leave or extended disability benefits.

Sexual Harassment
Sexual harassment is not a new problem in the workplace but has been given greater legal scrutiny and media attention as women's participation in the workforce has grown, especially in professional, managerial, and executive positions. According to the Supreme Court's interpretation, sexual harassment falls under the prohibitions against gender discrimination of Title VII of the Civil Rights Act. The EEOC guidelines (www.eeoc.gov/facts/fs-sex.html) state it is unlawful to harass a person (or an applicant or employee) because of that person's sex. Harassment can include "sexual harassment" or unwelcome sexual advances, requests for sexual favors, and other verbal or physical harassment of a sexual nature. Harassment does not have to be of a sexual nature, however, and can include offensive remarks about a person's sex. For example, it is illegal to harass a woman by making offensive comments about women in general. Both the victim and the harasser can be either a woman or a man, and the victim and the harasser can be the same sex. Although the law doesn't prohibit simple teasing, offhand comments, or isolated incidents that are not very serious, harassment is illegal when it is so frequent or severe that it creates a hostile or offensive work environment or when it results in an adverse employment decision (such as the victim being fired or demoted). The harasser can be the victim's supervisor, a supervisor in another area, a coworker, or someone who is not an employee of the employer, such as a client or customer or vendor.[43]

The groundbreaking legal decision in this area was the Supreme Court's decision in *Meritor Savings v. Vinson* (1986), in which the Court held that the plaintiff did not need to demonstrate a quid pro quo relationship between accepting or rejecting sexual advances and employment decisions (e.g., promotion or termination). Rather, the Court determined that the plaintiff had the burden only of showing that the harassment resulted in an unfavorable or hostile working environment for the victim.

Sexual harassment as one form of gender discrimination can produce a number of negative effects in the workplace, including decreased productivity, increased worker stress and illness, higher turnover and absenteeism, lower morale, interference with team building, additional recruitment and training costs, and potential legal liabilities. Although it is generally viewed as a "women's issue," both men and women can claim protection against sexual harassment under Title VII, and the victim and alleged harasser may be of the same sex.

Given the Court's interpretation of the prohibitions of sexual harassment law extending to "hostile environment" cases, management's potential liability to such complaints is significant. Indeed, the employer may be held liable for sexual harassment on the basis of employee, supervisory, or managerial behavior even when specific complaints were not brought before management. Consequently, from both a risk management and an ethical perspective, it is clearly in management's interest to take assertive action to prevent such behavior and to take quick action to address any complaints that are reported.

To prevent problems with sexual harassment in the workplace, specific policies should be developed and communicated to all employees prohibiting such behavior and explaining the procedures for reporting, reviewing, and resolving complaints. All supervisors and managers should have training in these policies and procedures and in how to respond effectively to both complaints and observed incidents of sexually offensive behavior. Management must ensure that all complaints of sexual harassment are fully and fairly investigated. The employer's legal liability will be influenced by whether management knew or should have known about the harassment and by what actions, if any, were taken to prevent or stop it. As in most other areas of HRM with consequences for employees' rights and welfare, complete documentation of the relevant facts of the situation and management's actions to respond to the complaint is essential.

 SELF-ASSESSMENT QUIZ

8. In order for an organization to defend itself in a sexual harassment suit in a court of law, it is in the employer's best interest to:
   a. Establish a written policy prohibiting harassment.
   b. Communicate the policy and train employees in what constitutes harassment.
   c. Establish an effective complaint procedure and quickly investigate all claims.
   d. Take remedial action to correct past harassment.
   e. Make sure the complainant does not end up in a less desirable position if s/he needs to be transferred.
   f. All of the above.

Protecting the Rights of Persons with Disabilities

The Individuals with Disabilities Education Act (1970), the Rehabilitation Act of 1973, and the Americans with Disabilities Act (1990) form the legislative foundation for equal opportunity for individuals with disabilities in the workplace, in school, for transportation services, and for other public accommodations. The Rehabilitation Act, comprehensive legislation that prohibits discrimination against "the handicapped" and encourages equal access in employment, education, and medical and rehabilitation services for those with disabilities, is limited in its scope to institutions receiving federal funds and federal agencies.

DID YOU KNOW?

Did you know that when addressing a person with disabilities, it is respectful to put the person first? Say, "person with a disability" rather than "disabled person." For specific disabilities, saying "person with Parkinson's" or "person who has Tourette's syndrome" is usually all right. Individuals, of course, have their own preferences. If you are not sure what words to use, ask. Avoid outdated terms like "handicapped," "crippled," or "retarded."

Section 504 prohibits discrimination by any organization or program receiving federal funds against otherwise qualified individuals on the basis of their disability. Because

Medicare Part A and Medicaid are considered to be federal financial assistance, most health care organizations are covered by this act.

The Americans with Disabilities Act extended and expanded the protections of the Rehabilitation Act and has been viewed by advocates of those with disabilities as the culmination of decades of effort and as a crowning achievement of public policy in this area. The National Council on Disability affirms that "the ADA is about enabling people with disabilities to take charge of their lives and join the American mainstream. It seeks to do so by fostering employment opportunities, facilitating access to public transportation and public accommodations, and ensuring the use of our nation's communication systems."[44] Title I of the ADA makes it illegal for organizations with 15 or more employees to discriminate against an otherwise qualified person with disabilities if that person can perform the significant job duties with or without reasonable accommodation. Recruitment, hiring, promotion, compensation, termination, leaves, layoffs, job assignments, and benefits are all covered under this act.

The definition of disability is broad, stating that a disabled person is one who has a physical or mental impairment that substantially limits one or more of his or her major life activities, has a record of substantially limiting impairment, or is regarded as having a substantially limiting impairment. The courts have tended to interpret disability narrowly within the breadth suggested by the legislative language, although several test cases heard by the Supreme Court in April 1999 would significantly widen its coverage to those with correctable conditions, including visual impairment and hypertension.[45] Recent Supreme Court decisions have tended to narrow the scope of application of those covered by the act, however.

Although the ADA could be regarded as the most sweeping civil rights legislation since Title VII of the Civil Rights Act of 1964, the language of the act does not require the employer to commit to affirmative action initiatives for those in the workforce with disabilities. The applicant with a disability must be qualified by meeting all the job requirements with or without accommodation. The act requires that qualified employees with disabilities receive reasonable accommodation in the workplace to perform the essential job functions without causing undue hardship to the employer. If a job description has marginal functions included, the person with a disability cannot be screened out because of inability to perform the nonessential duties if they could reasonably be assigned to someone else (Box 16-3).

Because the ADA gives individuals with disabilities federal civil right protection similar to the rights provided to individuals on the basis of race, color, sex, national origin, age, and religion, organizations need to develop internal policies and procedures when a current employee contracts AIDS or some other chronic illness, begins going blind, or loses motor skills in his or her hands. When these policies and procedures are being developed, they should be communicated to all staff so that they can give input on ways to improve them.

BOX 16-3	Examples of Reasonable Accommodation

- Modifying existing facilities to be readily accessible to and usable by a person with a disability (e.g., widening a cubicle for wheelchair access)
- Restructuring a job to facilitate the employee's disability (e.g., minimizing travel by use of conference calls and online conferencing)
- Modifying work schedules (e.g., providing flex time to accommodate outpatient therapy)
- Acquiring or modifying equipment (e.g., adapted computer keyboards)
- Providing qualified readers or interpreters
- Appropriately modifying examinations, training, or other programs (e.g., online vs. paper-and-pencil responses)
- Reassigning a current employee to a vacant position

What constitutes **undue hardship**? Any action that would require significant difficulty or expense when considered in light of the nature and cost of the accommodation in relation to the size, resources, technology, and structures of the employer's operation is viewed as undue hardship. The courts have tended to place a narrow interpretation on this condition because most accommodations have proved to be easily implemented and neither disruptive nor costly.

The health information manager can comply with the intent of this law by taking the following actions:

- Determine and document the essential functions of each job.
- Review job applications to eliminate questions or statements regarding people with disabilities that would make the employer legally liable.
- Inform and train anyone doing employment interviews about the ADA regulations.
- Review the justification for physical examinations as a requirement for employee selection. If medical or physical examinations are necessary, they can be required only after a conditional job offer is extended and must be required of all applicants in this situation as a condition of employment.
- Increase supervisory awareness about the ADA and issues affecting employees with disabilities; for example, post an appropriate ADA poster in a location and format accessible to applicants, employees, and visitors.

Age Discrimination

The Age Discrimination in Employment Act of 1967 (as amended) protects employees and applicants aged 40 years and older from discrimination on the basis of age. From a public policy perspective, the ADEA can be regarded as a regulatory response to the negative and largely false cultural stereotypes about the aging process generally and about older workers specifically. These stereotypes portray an employee who is transformed into a low-energy, apathetic, cynical, injury-prone, and disengaged hanger-on with nothing of

value left to contribute to his or her organization or profession. It can be argued that in general older employees who choose to maintain or seek employment tend to be highly motivated and responsible and can apply their experience and wisdom in serving as experienced mentors to their younger colleagues.

Several exceptions are recognized in the act to the prohibitions against age discrimination. The employer may be able to demonstrate that age is a bona fide occupational qualification (BFOQ), an otherwise prohibited factor construed to be reasonably necessary to the operation of the enterprise. Also, the ADEA makes allowances for forced retirement at age 65 years for "bona fide executives" or those in "high policy-making positions."

With the graying of the U.S. population, congressional discussion about increasing the age for Social Security benefit eligibility, and the decline in the value of retirement portfolios due to the financial crisis of 2008–2009, a higher proportion of older employees can be anticipated in the workforce. This might lead to more intergenerational conflict over jobs and economic security and to increased litigation under the ADEA.

Immigration Control and Employment

The Immigration Reform and Control Act (IRCA) of 1986 was primarily designed in response to growing public concern in certain regions of the United States about the influx of illegal aliens, including those from Mexico, Central America, and the Far East. Concerns were raised about the impact of these illegal immigrants on employment opportunities for U.S. citizens and legal aliens and on the social service network. The IRCA prohibits employers from hiring or retaining unauthorized and undocumented workers after the effective date of the legislation. However, the act also prohibits discrimination in employment against noncitizens who can document their legal right to work in the United States. The impact of this legislation has been somewhat localized, affecting California, Texas, other southwestern states, and Florida more than other areas. However, political debate periodically arises about the impact of illegal and undocumented aliens in the context of homeland security and economic concerns, making this a major public policy issue with direct implications for human resource management.

Employee Health and Workplace Safety
Occupational Safety and Health Act

Growing concern about worker health and safety in the workplace, especially in manufacturing and the extractive industries, with strong backing by organized labor led to congressional passage of the Occupational Safety and Health Act in 1970. In passing OSHA, Congress intended that "certain [occupational and health] standards would define the conduct expected from employers covered by the OSHA, and that adherence to these standards would bring about a safe and healthy workplace."[46]

OSHA covers all workers except those who are self-employed or protected under other federal agencies and those who work on family-owned and -operated farms. It has jurisdiction over every chemical substance, piece of equipment, and work environment that poses even a potential threat to worker health and safety. The extremely detailed OSHA standards are administered by the Occupational Safety and Health Administration, the regulatory agency that issues work and safety standards and schedules inspections to ensure employer compliance.

Health care organizations are also subject to OSHA's regulatory oversight. They are required to communicate to their employees information on the known risks associated with any hazardous materials encountered on the job and to label all hazardous materials. A written orientation and training program must be developed and used to educate all employees. Examples of hazards that may affect HIM are electronic equipment operation and exposure to hazardous materials, such as alkaline batteries. Efforts to guarantee protection from exposure to communicable disease may also be required by OSHA for employees who have patient contact. Record keeping requirements are extensive because such documentation constitutes the only effective method of tracking, identifying, and correcting safety and health hazards. Detailed reports must be filed for all occupation-related injuries, illnesses, and deaths.

In its early years of implementation, OSHA was much criticized by the employer community as an example of heavy-handed overregulation. Although business associations and smaller business enterprises might be especially likely to complain about the administrative burden imposed, the general consensus among both management and organized labor is that OSHA has increased the overall awareness of safety and occupational health issues in the workplace.

> ✓ **SELF-ASSESSMENT QUIZ**
>
> **9.** What federal law governs workplace safety?
>   **a.** Americans with Disabilities Act
>   **b.** National Labor Relations Act
>   **c.** Occupational Safety and Health Act
>   **d.** Title VII of the Civil Rights Act

Security and Privacy of Information

The Health Insurance Portability and Accountability Act of 1996 (HIPAA) has affected employees in the health care sector in two distinct ways. First, HIPAA has mandated the ways in which patients' medical information should be stored and transmitted electronically to ensure that it remains private and is only used for appropriate means. Second, and perhaps more relevant to the HRM functions in an organization, the HIPAA Security Rule applies to many employer groups. The Security Rule has implications related to the provision of group health, dental, and vision plans but also applies to flexible spending accounts and employee assistance programs. Whereas the HIPAA Privacy Rule covers protected health

information (PHI) in any format, the Security Rule applies specifically to information that is stored or transmitted electronically. PHI created or received by a covered entity (e.g., health plans, other similar organizations) that documents a member's physical or mental health, treatment, or payment for treatment is explicitly protected under this rule, and beyond basic health information, this rule covers information pertaining to enrollment, the processing of claims, any dispute resolution, and payments (premiums, member fees, etc.). Finally, covered entities are required to protect electronic health information against "reasonably anticipated threats or hazards and against reasonably anticipated uses or disclosures by unauthorized persons or by authorized employees in an unauthorized manner."[47]

HIPAA also affects the employees of the health care entity as protected under this law. The HRM functions of benefits enrollment and management, employee assistance programs (EAP), and even OSHA compliance will require that employee PHI is handled in an appropriate way. The same caution that employees of the health care entity use to protect their patients and consumers must be used by internal HRM staff when dealing with the employee's PHI. See Chapter 15 for further discussions about HIPAA.

Employee Compensation

The Fair Labor Standards Act (FLSA) of 1938 was passed at the end of the Depression era to address a number of employer abuses involving the compensation of employees in various industries. This act (sometimes referred to as the Wage and Hour Law) establishes minimum wage, overtime pay, child labor restrictions, and record-keeping requirements for employers. For every "covered" job, overtime compensation must be paid at one-and-a-half times the employee's regular rate of pay for every hour over 40 worked in a week or over 80 hours for some health care organizations that use a 14-day pay period—that is, the 8/80 plan. Several categories of employees—executive, administrative, and professional—are exempt from the overtime provisions of the act.

> ❓ **DID YOU KNOW?**
>
> Did you know that the Fair Labor Standards Act of 1938 addresses minimum wage, overtime pay, and child labor provisions, but does not address gender wage?

The Equal Pay Act of 1963 amended the Fair Labor Standards Act to eliminate gender-based discrimination in pay practices. It requires employers to pay men and women equal wages when the jobs they perform are equal in skill, effort, and responsibility and are performed under equivalent working conditions. Exceptions are allowed for valid merit or seniority award systems and when individual productivity determines compensation, such as in sales commissions or piece rate work. Some advocates of gender equity have promoted the comparable worth doctrine, which calls for equivalence of wages for jobs that, although not identical in content, require comparable skills, knowledge, training, and responsibility. However, the federal courts have not been sympathetic to this expansion of the equal pay logic.

Congressional passage of the Family and Medical Leave Act of 1993 reflects the increasing role of women, especially working mothers, in the workforce and the implications for child care arrangements. The FMLA grants up to 12 weeks of unpaid leave annually and affords job security to employees of either sex to address family health care needs and childbirth. Specifically, the FMLA authorizes either parent who is eligible under the act to take leave associated with the birth or adoption of a child. The act also covers leave for care for a spouse, child, or parent, as well as for the employee's own extended illness. The FMLA is administered by the U.S. Department of Labor, which enforces compliance with the FMLA for all private, state, and some federal employees.

On return from FMLA leave, employees must be restored to their original jobs or equivalent positions with equivalent pay, benefits, and other terms and conditions of employment. Advance notice of leave of at least 30 days is required from the employee for "foreseeable" circumstances. An employer may require medical certification to support all medical leave requests, including second or third opinions and a fitness-for-duty report to return to work.

The Employee Retirement Income Security Act (ERISA) of 1974 is a comprehensive and exceedingly complex federal law governing the administration of employee pension and welfare benefit plans. ERISA evolved in response to increasingly widespread and cynical corporate abuses of employees' pension rights and funds. Although the original version of ERISA passed in 1974 was derided as "lawyer's dream" legislation and as being so complex that employers would not be able to comply even with good intention, the law has furthered the goal of reducing the more notorious examples of pension fund abuse. Among the major objectives of this legislation are to ensure that (1) retirement funds are adequately safeguarded, (2) future benefit obligations are ensured through prudent financing, and (3) benefits are provided to all employees, not just the highly placed and highly paid.

ERISA establishes the fiduciary responsibilities of pension plan administrators and specifies conditions of employee participation, eligibility, vesting, funding, and reporting. The law stipulates management's obligation to communicate clearly to all employees about their pension and welfare benefit rights and options.

Labor-Management Relations and Collective Bargaining Legislation

The National Labor Relations Act (NLRA), also known as the Wagner Act, has served as the foundation for U.S. labor law and collective bargaining since it became law in 1935. The major legislative intent was to establish as national policy the need to "eliminate the causes of certain substantial obstructions to the free flow of commerce and to mitigate and eliminate those obstructions...by encouraging the practice and procedure of collective bargaining and by protecting the exercise by workers of full freedom of association, self-organization, and designation of representation of their own choosing, for the purpose of negotiating the terms and conditions of employment or other mutual aid or protection."[48]

Several factors led to the passage of this legislation at the end of the Great Depression, including growing public concern about the disruptive effects of labor-management conflict and violence and the recognition that workers had legitimate rights to organize to better represent their interests. In striking contrast to the English common law principle, which considered unions to be a criminal conspiracy against property rights of owners, the NLRA established a formal justification for and mechanisms to implement collective bargaining. The latter was established as an effective and preferred means of formalizing labor-management relations and resolving conflict between these two forces in the workplace.

Specifically, the NLRA gives employees the right to collective action free of employer interference or repercussion. It gives employees the right to form labor unions and bargain with management about wages, hours, and other terms and conditions of employment with the goal of achieving written agreement. When ratified by both sides, the written agreement or contract becomes the basis for managerial actions, employee behavior, and mutual expectations for the life of the agreement.

The NLRA originally prohibited the unfair labor practices directed toward management listed in Box 16-4.

To monitor and enforce the NLRA, the act established the National Labor Relations Board (NLRB). The role of the NLRB is to determine an appropriate bargaining unit for elections and negotiation, to conduct secret ballot elections that determine whether a union will be recognized, and to investigate and adjudicate any unfair labor practices claimed by the employer or the union.

✓ SELF-ASSESSMENT QUIZ

10. The Equal Pay Act of 1963 requires that
- **a.** Men and women are paid equally for similar work in all like organizations.
- **b.** Men and women receive the same pay if they do the same job in the same organization.
- **c.** Individuals receive similar pay for jobs within a similar grade of the organization.
- **d.** Individuals of a protected class are paid equally for similar work in all like organizations.

BOX 16-4   Unfair Labor Practices

- To interfere, restrain, or coerce employees from engaging in or refraining from collective action covered in the law
- To dominate or interfere with the formation or administration of any labor organization by contributing money or other support to it
- To discriminate against anyone in hiring, retention, or any other condition of employment because of his or her union activity or noninvolvement
- To discharge, discipline, or otherwise discriminate against employees who have exercised their rights under this act
- To refuse to bargain in good faith with employee representatives

The Labor Management Relations Act (1947), commonly referred to as the Taft-Hartley Act, is a set of amendments to the NLRA passed in response to public concerns about renewed labor conflict threatening the post–World War II economic prosperity and perceptions in the business community that "big labor" had gained unfair advantage under the NLRA. The Taft-Hartley Act addressed these concerns by specifying unfair labor practices committed by unions (Box 16-5).

BOX 16-5 Illegal Union Conduct

- To restrain or coerce employees or employers in the exercise of their legal rights under the National Labor Relations Act
- To force an employer to discriminate against an employee because of the employee's membership or nonmembership in the union
- To refuse to bargain with an employer in good faith
- To engage in certain kinds of picketing and strikes, such as recognition picketing to force the employer to recognize or bargain with an alternative union than the one already certified
- To engage in "featherbedding," in which management agrees to pay for work not actually performed
- To demand excessive or discriminatory initiation fees
- To engage in secondary boycotts and "hot cargo" agreements

The Labor Management Reporting and Disclosure Act was passed in 1959 as additional amendments to the NLRA in response to reported corruption and abuse of power of some influential union leaders. Its major provisions include the following:

- An employee bill of rights
- Financial reporting requirements
- Fair election practices for union offices
- Other measures to curtail and correct abuses of power of union leaders

The Health Care Amendments of 1974 represent the most recent revisions of the NLRA and those of special interest to health care organizations. In passing this legislation, Congress attempted to balance its desire to bring most health care workers under the protection of the NLRA with the need to protect health care from the potential conflict and instability associated with some aspects of collective bargaining. In fact, it is estimated that the 1974 amendments covered about 1.5 million health care workers who had not been afforded NLRA protection by extending the act to all voluntary, nonprofit, nongovernmental health care institutions.

The health care amendments include several constraints on collective bargaining unique to health care in recognition of congressional concern and that of the broader public about preserving stability and reducing conflict within health care organizations and ensuring continuity of service delivery. The most notable of these amendments is the 10-day strike notice, which requires the union to provide written notice to the employer and the Federal Mediation and Conciliation Service (FMCS) 10 days in advance of a strike, picketing, or other collective action disrupting work. The 1974 amendments also contain an extended notice period for resolving disputes before contract expiration. Another mechanism is provided to facilitate contract dispute resolution through establishing a board of inquiry when negotiations reach an impasse and a strike or other disruptive action is threatened. The board of inquiry is selected by the director of the FMCS to investigate the facts in dispute, allow a cooling-off period, and make a written report of findings of fact and recommendations to resolve the dispute. Although the recommendations are nonbinding, they can be instrumental in highlighting and narrowing differences between the two parties and pointing toward resolution. Finally, this legislation recognizes the historical roots of health care in religious tradition by exempting individuals with faith-based, conscientious objection from showing allegiance to labor or other secular organizations by permitting a waiver of paying union dues.

Built on these foundation blocks of labor legislation are innumerable judicial decisions and administrative law rulings and guidelines that collectively have shaped the process and boundaries of collective bargaining both across industries and within health care. One example is the Supreme Court's decision in 1991 to uphold the NLRB regulations issued in 1988 that reversed the board's former logic concerning the appropriate composition of bargaining units in health care organizations. This court decision resolved a long-standing conflict between the federal courts and the NLRB over the impact of bargaining unit determination on health care delivery and resulted in establishing clear rules that specified eight narrowly defined bargaining units (e.g., RNs, other professionals, office clericals, etc.), rather than the broader bargaining units preferred by management as being more difficult to organize and to win union representation. Although dealing with an apparently narrow and technical issue, this judicial decision has had significant effects on the direction of collective bargaining in health care with implications for human resource managers.

✓ SELF-ASSESSMENT QUIZ

11. Which of the following is prohibited under the Taft-Hartley Act?
    a. Interfering with employees' rights to form unions
    b. Discriminating against an employee who has filed charges under the act
    c. Refusing to bargain with the union
    d. Coercing employees

Managing Human Resources Within the Unionized Environment

The primary objective of labor unions is to become a counterbalancing power to management by presenting a unified and assertive voice calling for improved wages, benefits, job security, or working conditions for the employees represented. Unions justify their claims on workers' support and loyalty by promising to achieve economic and well-being objectives (Box 16-6).

Management almost always vigorously opposes any new attempt at union organization affecting its enterprise or facility. At one level, it could be argued that no individual or group holding power would choose rationally to dilute

---

| BOX 16-6 | Examples of Union Benefits |

- Protect jobs within the bargaining unit
- Negotiate the best possible total compensation package for the life of the contract, that is, wages and benefits
- Preserve against the erosion of economic benefits in the future
- Defend workers' rights, including the right to engage in political activity
- Ensure a safe and healthy working environment for all workers

---

| BOX 16-7 | Guidelines for Managers and Supervisors During a Union Organizing Campaign |

Management has both the right and the obligation to:

- Tell employees that the organization does not believe that union representation is in their best interest and therefore encourage them to vote "no" on the ballot.
- Answer employees' questions honestly about organizational policy, strategy, and goals in relation to the union's campaign issues.
- Explain the costs of unionization to the employees personally—for example, the necessity of paying union dues and fees.
- Assure employees that with or without the union, management is committed to providing high-quality health care and a desirable working environment and culture for all employees.
- Explain that if the employees choose to recognize the union, any improvements in wages, benefits, and working conditions will thereafter be subject to negotiation and not guaranteed, as the union might suggest.
- Administer appropriate disciplinary action against any employee who threatens or coerces other employees, whether for or against the union.
- Enforce the organization's policy against solicitation and distribution of union literature in compliance with prevailing National Labor Relations Board rules.

Management should not risk unfair labor practice charges or the erosion of mutual trust and respect of the majority of the employees by engaging in any of the following:

- Surveillance of employees or other kinds of espionage to determine the level of union sentiment or to "finger" employees as union activists
- Interrogating individual employees about their union sympathies or union activity
- Threatening, coercing, or intimidating any employees because of their union support or activities
- Making any specific promises contingent on the outcome of the election
- Offering unilateral improvements in wages, benefits, or working conditions during the election campaign

Data from Werther WB Jr, Davis K: *Human resources and personnel management,* ed 3, New York, 1989, McGraw-Hill, pp. 500-519.

---

or give up that power except by force or subterfuge. Consequently, executive management collectively (and probably most managers individually) operates so as to preserve and, if possible, expand its sources of power and degree of control. Consequently, management's response to a unionization drive is predictably assertive opposition.

However determined management is to defeat a union effort, its capacity to mount an aggressive campaign is constrained by the NLRA and the union's right to file unfair labor practice charges with the NLRB. Furthermore, management (more so than union leadership) must consider the long-term effects of its actions on employee satisfaction, morale, and productivity; workforce stability; and quality of service. Accordingly, the employer's wisest campaign strategy is to provide complete, objective information in presenting management's arguments against unionization within the organization. Management has the right under the law to counteract the union's claims but should do so with facts rather than appeals to emotion or unsubstantiated claims. Probably the most important factor is the attitude management demonstrates toward all its employees, those favoring the union and those opposed. Management is best served if it maintains a genuine attitude of respect, trust, and commitment to the welfare of all its employees. If the employer cannot make these value claims authentically, it probably deserves the constraints and costs associated with dealing with a union at the bargaining table. It could be argued that weak, ineffective, and unresponsive management is a good predictor of successful unionization.

Management may and should provide facts that place its past efforts for the employees in a favorable light and, conversely, that show the adverse effects of unionization in general or the union seeking representation in particular. For example, management can communicate information about union dues; history of picketing, strikes, and election "win rates"; salaries of union officers; and any other relevant facts about the union and its likely behavior and effects on the organization (Box 16-7). However, the ultimate outcome will be influenced by local circumstances and cannot, of course, be guaranteed.

The Changing Work Environment and Employee Expectations

In today's environment of geographical, career, and social mobility, it is rare for an employee to hold the same job in one organization for longer than several years. The erosion of organizational loyalty and identification was aggravated by aggressive downsizing efforts associated with the corporate reengineering movement of the early 1990s. Furthermore, we have witnessed increasing "externalization" of the workforce in the form of part-time and casual employees, off-site work, and contracting for temporary workers and outsourcing the work itself to another organization. These actions have further eroded the expectations of the traditional employment relationship.[49]

College graduates are cautioned to maintain a high level of current and transferable skills, to "travel light" without making or expecting long-term commitments, and to anticipate a career of continuing transitions from one project to another with an ever-changing set of team members and rotating leaders. Organizational identities blur as mergers, buyouts, and restructuring leave the outsider (and perhaps even the employees and other stakeholders most affected) confused and frustrated. As traditional organizational structures seem to "morph" rapidly into new, less-familiar ones, defining accountability, maintaining controls, and sustaining vision over the long term (i.e., beyond the end of the quarter) seem increasingly elusive goals. In health care, it is especially important that managers, health care professionals, technologists, and support staff all stay focused on the mission of providing high-quality health care and related services continuously while doing so cost effectively.

Internal Environment of the Health Care Organization

Organizational Culture

Every organization has its own unique culture that maintains and symbolically represents the meaning and value of organizational roles and functions and managerial and employee activities. Organizational culture is shaped primarily by the organization's leadership, historical factors, core technology, mission, and key environmental forces. Schein[50] has argued the leader's key function is to transform organizational culture by eliminating destructive, obsolete, and dysfunctional aspects of culture that no longer fit its mission and environment and creating new cultural forms and symbols that better match the threats and opportunities it faces (Box 16-8).

The challenge for management in the 21st century is to create a culture of receptivity to change because this will be necessary for survival given the likelihood of accelerated developments in science, technology, and the global economy. At the same time, leadership must preserve the cultural linkages to its past heroes and achievements and to a clear sense of mission, ties that provide and maintain a sense of greater purpose and commitment among the members of the culture. Preparing the organization for inevitable change, while remembering and appreciating the traditions and legacy of the past, is essential for effective management of organizational culture.

Another challenge is based on the existence of multiple subcultures in all complex organizations. The existence of subcultures with associated differences in values, beliefs, norms, language, style preferences, and so forth creates potential misunderstanding, tension, and conflict. For example, accountants in the financial management division are likely to have different values, priorities, jargon, and dress codes than software design engineers. Managers above the unit level, especially human resource managers, must be able to recognize, understand, and respond to this source of potential conflict. Organization leadership must try to channel the potential energy and creativity associated with cultural diversity in productive efforts to further the broader goals of the organization. As a leader, the HIM director's responsibility is to be aware of the organization's culture within HIM and to be able to articulate, model, teach, and communicate the organization's vision, mission, values, and behaviors to HIM staff and customers.

Information Systems

Information systems continue to improve in power, efficiency, accessibility, and ease of use. For efficient management of human resource functions, appropriate use of information systems and technology is necessary. Because managing people requires an increasingly large base of relevant information, an adequate information system should be developed to facilitate decision making and to accomplish more work of higher quality with less effort. In most health care organizations, electronic processing has replaced much of the manual paperwork formerly used for most HRM functions. Increased use of electronic, online processing of information should result in better services to employees (as internal clients), more powerful planning tools for the manager, and more cost-effective and accessible information processing for all users in the organization.

HIM managers and supervisors have an important, continuing responsibility to maintain complete and accurate information concerning their human resources for whom they are responsible. The amount of information that must be maintained for each employee has grown exponentially along with the dramatic growth in regulatory oversight and demands for compliance affecting HRM. For example, the FLSA requires that accurate records be maintained on all employees to include the employee's identifying information, hourly rate of pay, total hours worked, total earnings, and other data relevant to administering the compensation system.

In addition to compensation system data, other types of information relevant to HRM are required for each employee. For example,

- Hire dates and anniversary dates of promotions are needed for performance appraisal and ERISA administration.
- The employee's pay rate and range, job grade classification, current job title, and position number must be recorded.
- Copies of performance appraisals, job descriptions, disciplinary actions, commendations, and other performance-related documents must be maintained consistent with

---

BOX 16-8 Major Components of an Organization's Culture

- Foundation assumptions about the person and his or her world
- Basic ideology about the organization's role within society and the economy
- Core values and beliefs that define membership in or affiliation with the organization
- Visible symbols that reflect organization membership and allegiance
- Norms, customs, rituals, and taboos that reflect core values and beliefs

management policy and (if applicable) terms of the prevailing written agreement.

- Documentation of participation in orientation, training, or management development programs is important in maintaining a workforce skills inventory and in making decisions about promotions, transfers, and job sharing.

These records are essential to provide a justification of and legal defense for various staffing decisions and actions affecting individual employee's compensation and terms and conditions of employment.

Role of Human Resources Management System in Health Care Organization

Human resource activities in the HIM department mirror the activities found in enterprises in other industries (Figure 16-5). A common set of HRM functions, processes, and activities are required to obtain, maintain, and sustain a competent, motivated HIM workforce that through individual and team efforts accomplishes tasks to achieve the goals associated with satisfying the needs of the internal and external consumers of health information services.

HRM systems are also used to assist an organization in fulfilling its specific mission, strategic goals, and business plans. Human resource planning, recruitment and selection, job analysis, training and development, performance appraisal and productivity measurement, quality management, compensation management, employee assistance and counseling, discipline, and occupational health and safety are essential human resource processes maintained to further the organization's objectives while addressing broader public policy goals.

The Employee as Client of the Human Resources Management System

Human resource functions can also be seen from the perspective of the individual employee with unique needs, goals, concerns, and priorities. The employee typically attempts to satisfy various needs through participation at work. In Abraham Maslow's model of human motivation, the individual responds to a hierarchy of needs ranging from lower-order physiological and safety needs to higher-order ego and spiritual (peak experience) needs.[51] At least to the degree that the employee's individualized needs and objectives are congruent with the goals of the organization, which must be given priority, HRM systems can be expected to address the individual's needs also. Indeed, not only is it ethically well founded for management to consider the employee's welfare in its decision making, it is essential in the long term for attracting, retaining, and motivating knowledgeable and skilled workers in today's dynamic health care market.

If the organization routinely fails to satisfy the individual's needs, employee satisfaction is eroded, performance and productivity decline, and turnover rates increase. These adverse trends are likely to result in increased costs to the organization both in the direct costs of recruitment, selection, and training and in indirect costs of lost productivity and, ultimately, lower quality patient care. High turnover rates and low employee morale may result in lower levels of customer satisfaction, adverse public relations, loss of market share, and decline in financial viability.

The personal goals and objectives of employees may be addressed through the following human resource activities:

- Supervisory coaching
- Training and development programs
- Career ladders and job rotations
- Performance appraisal and feedback
- Team development and empowerment
- Compensation management
- Employee discipline (linked to a progressive improvement plan)
- Employee assistance services (matched to individual needs)

Clearly, the importance of competent and responsive first-line supervision is paramount because the supervisor often serves as either the facilitator of the employee's growth and well-being in the workplace or as an obstacle to the individual's development.

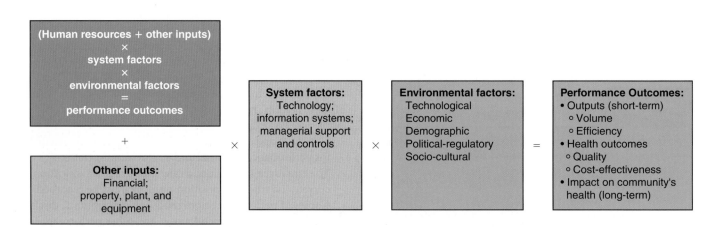

FIGURE 16-5 Application of the systems model to productivity.

Employee Assistance Programs

Employees experiencing personal problems may obtain support and referral services through an employee assistance program (EAP) in most health care organizations. EAPs have emerged as specialized in-house service centers, staffed by professionals such as social workers, counselors, and health educators. Increasingly, the health care organization provides the employee seeking assistance referral to an external provider under contract to ensure professionally competent and confidential services. The purpose of these programs is to help employees who have personal, family, or community-based problems that interfere with and detract from job satisfaction and performance. Some common employee problems that might lead to EAP services are alcohol and substance abuse, gambling, financial problems, intrafamily conflicts, difficulty coping with stress, and chronic physical and mental health conditions.

Employees may seek these confidential services on their own initiative or be referred by a supervisor. Whichever route is pursued, maintaining strict confidentiality is a key element in achieving effective EAP services. The primary goal of the EAP approach is to help employees help themselves. In addition to the personal rewards and problem solving facilitated by this assistance, these programs can be justified as cost-effective investments for the organization to the extent that they lower the costs of excessive absenteeism, lost productivity, interpersonal conflict, and turnover. An EAP referral may result in retention of an employee who would otherwise leave the organization, perhaps with diminished capacity, or it might eliminate or lower barriers to optimal performance of the employee.

SELF-ASSESSMENT QUIZ

12. Employee assistance programs (EAPs) typically deal with which of the following?
   a. Alcohol and/or alcohol abuse
   b. Compulsive gambling
   c. Eating disorders
   d. All of the above

Strategic HIM Workforce Planning

Human Resource Planning and Forecasting

One of the most important roles the HIM director and management team can assume is that associated with strategic human resource planning, also called workforce planning. HIM departmental HR planning must, of course, be consistent with organization-wide HR planning for both short-term and long-term needs. A useful strategic HR planning tool for the HIM manager is one adapted from an approach recommended by the state of Minnesota's Human Resource Reengineering Project Strategic Staffing Team.[52]

Future staffing requirements (the demand) are determined by strategic and operational planning efforts (issue identification). Simultaneously, the model takes current staff data and forecasts what the future staff (the supply) will be. These two pieces of information (the supply and the demand) are compared to determine what the gap or surplus will be. The results are measured for efficiency and effectiveness.

The purpose of strategic planning is to identify and develop a skilled workforce to meet the changing needs of the health care organization in general and individual departments, including HIM. Strategic human resource planning ought to be a proactive rather than a reactive HRM process in which HIM managers with the collaborative assistance of HRM specialists continually forecast and coordinate the supply of qualified HIM human resources with predicted demand based on work-flow cycles in HIM and in any external and internal changes affecting HIM services. This strategic approach to planning anticipates and prepares for future staffing needs on the basis of key indicators of demand, which are measures of program operations (i.e., volume, activity, or output) that can be reliably linked to staffing levels. Ultimately, a HIM strategic HR planning process includes all managed movements into, around, and out of the HIM department including,

- Recruitment
- Hiring
- Promotion
- Transfer
- Redeployment
- Attrition, as well as
- Other HRM activities such as employee development and classification.

Planning improves use of resources by providing a systematic and reliable method of matching personnel requirements with organizational and departmental goals and priorities. As HIM services become more distributed with organization-wide as well as department-level accountability, astute and reliable planning becomes an essential role for the HIM professional. Issues that drive the need for HIM strategic planning include:

- Changes in HIM requirements
- Shortage of qualified HIM professionals to fill HIM positions
- A functional skill shortage in current staff
- Obsolete employee skills
- Changes in reimbursement systems
- Expansion/downsizing of the health care organization's services
- Mergers, centralization of organization services, including HIM
- Changes in the organization's local health care environment
- Increased internal and external customer expectations for responsiveness
- Need for development of career paths and systems that will attract/retain qualified and diverse HIM applicants

Strategic staffing requires a collaborative effort among the HIM management team, HR professionals, IT experts, and other key stakeholders to identify critical HR issues in strategic and operational plans. One obvious HIM issue in 2015 is the now imminent implementation of ICD-10-CM, which requires HIM coders to learn a different coding system, the

IT department to technically support the implementation of the new required software, clinicians to learn and apply more precise documentation in their paper and/or electronic health records, and the HRM department to support the overall effort. The HIM director and project and/or line managers are leading the development and implementation of staffing plans while HRM staff is providing consultation for needed staffing activities.

Human resource planning can provide useful tools to the HIM professional for developing and justifying staffing supply and demand projections. These include trend (demand) analysis, replacement charts, flow (Markov) analysis, and staffing (census) tables. These and other techniques support strategic HRM and encourage contingency thinking in which the decision maker can pose and respond to a number of "what if" questions related to future HR supply and demand. For example, as electronic patient records increasingly replace written notes, the need for manual record filing positions will decline, and proactive human resource actions can be taken in anticipation of new staffing requirements. If a feasible and current human resource plan is prepared and periodically reviewed and updated, recruitment, transfer, retraining, promotion, and lay-off actions can be implemented more efficiently and with greater sensitivity to the employees affected. Continuous human resource planning ensures that external environmental challenges and opportunities can be addressed by effective use of available human resources and support systems. Strategic human resources planning must also include analysis of the physical space and all materials, equipment, and technology relative to the planned HR changes, whether increasing, downsizing, or otherwise changing where the work takes place.

Staffing management always requires timely and thorough planning to support short-term operations and long-term strategies. Thoughtful human resource planning to maintain the desired level of service is essential in a competitive environment, especially when facing significant resource constraints, for example, after a drastic "downsizing" or an especially tight labor market for critical skills. As expense budgets tighten to meet anticipated shortfalls in revenue, departments are likely to be required to do as much or more work with a smaller staff. This not only reduces the available "hands and minds" but also places greater demands on line managers, supervisors, and human resource specialists (Box 16-9).

Effective staffing is dependent on useful and reliable forecasting. Forecasting or prediction ranges in sophistication from a manager's intuitive "guesstimates" to the scenarios generated by computer simulations of complex systems using multivariable algorithms. The most appropriate forecasting method depends on the nature of the problem. In real-world situations, the forecasting method used and the priority given to it are often driven by time and resource constraints. It is incumbent on the HIM manager, however, to create enough time in his or her busy work schedule to think about forecasting on a regular basis. The most common

BOX 16-9   Human Resource Planning Process

- Forecasting (predicting or estimating) key staffing variables
- Volume of activity or output for the period projected
- Application of productivity measures or targets
- Level of staffing required for that volume— that is, demand estimate
- Staff available to satisfy demand for labor— that is, supply estimate
- Reconciliation of supply and demand estimates (a process of validating the net shortfall or excess of available staff)
- Developing or revising external recruitment plan
- Projection of training needs and schedules
- Identifying or reviewing promotion, transfer, and retirement opportunities
- Continuous evaluation of planning activities

approach is to extrapolate from past trends and current values of key variables into the short-term future. In other words, we base our forecasts on the assumption that the future will most likely resemble the past.

Staffing projections and plans are needed to ensure that a supply of educated workers is available to meet the demand for information services at the time and place required. Cross-training technical staff through a regular rotation of job duties and assignments accomplishes several objectives. It not only ensures a pool of potential substitutes for employees on leave or for position vacancies but also alleviates the boredom, frustration, and declining motivation that have been associated with turnover in positions with highly structured and routine activities.

A human resource strategic plan for staffing the coding function, for example, should be based ultimately on the projected volume of patients and the associated workload for coding staff. In 2015, however, training in ICD-10-CM also needs to be included in the staffing plan for both current coders and any newly hired coders. This training would also encompass whatever new software the coders will be using. This can be translated into demand estimates for coding staff based on employee or unit productivity standards. And, because of ICD-10-CM, productivity estimates for the initial implementation may not be as accurate as in the past. A comparable supply estimate can be determined by adjusting the current census for projected flows into and out of these jobs and by considering the size of the recruitment pool for these positions from traditional sources, such as local colleges and technical institutes. After the demand and supply estimates are verified and reconciled, specific recruitment, training, and internal promotion and transfer plans and schedules can be developed or revised (Figure 16-6). An unexpected gap in projected supply of trained coders or analysts could result in more aggressive campus recruitment or increased in-service and external training activities. Another response might be increased reliance on temporary staffing agencies to address peak workload needs for transcriptionists (for example) on a short-term or as-needed basis. Such solutions can lower the overall costs of staffing in the long term while addressing fluctuations in

Supply Estimate	Reconciliation Process
• Current census • +/− Inflows/outflows = **Net Available Supply** **Demand Estimate** • Key demand indicator/productivity/labor-hour = • Demand for labor hours/2080 hours = • Demand for FTE labor • +/− % Adjustments = **Net Projected Demand**	• Are supply and demand estimates realistic? • If not, reanalyze; if so, compare estimates • If supply = demand, focus on retention • If supply > demand, consider staff reduction • If supply < demand, consider recruitment, retraining, and pay

FIGURE 16-6 Reconciliation of supply and demand estimates.

the workload—both those that are cyclic and those that are less predictable. With the development of such plans, staffing levels can be managed cost effectively by minimizing lost productivity and any compromising of essential services.

In summary, an HIM strategic staffing process model includes these stages:

- Continuously identifying and defining critical and strategic HIM operational issues within the strategic planning process of the organization.
- Recognizing and documenting the internal and external environments, resources, and other factors that impact current HIM staffing.
- Quantifying measurable HIM activities; i.e., volume, activity, timeliness, or other output that can be reliably linked to staffing levels.
- Reviewing current HIM employee skills, knowledge, and abilities essential to operational issues.
- Determining skills and knowledge bases that differentiate HIM employees from each other.

From the information collected, the HIM management team will be able to predict staffing levels and competencies needed to address HIM future critical issues. The next stage is to assess differences—the gap, or surplus—between current staffing levels and the predicted future staffing levels.

✔ **SELF-ASSESSMENT QUIZ**

13. Why is it critical to understand HIM workforce planning (strategic human resource planning) for anyone working in the HIM field?
  a. Organizations must adjust to a rapidly changing environment.
  b. Technology innovations will continue to transform HIM processes.
  c. HIM professionals must commit to lifelong learning and willingly seek new challenges in order to stay competitive.
  d. All of the above.

Tools for Human Resource Planning

Some of the methods and tools useful in developing a human resource or staffing plan are described next.

Replacement Charts

Replacement charts present a visual representation of employees available to fill projected vacant positions. Typically, these charts are reserved for key managerial or highly professional positions. The replacement chart identifies individual incumbents, the most likely (or all potential) replacements, and summary measures of performance and promotion potential. The information in the chart should include that obtained from supervisory performance appraisals, assessment centers, training and career development activities, skill inventories, performance audits, and other sources relevant to the employee's career mobility. For example, the replacement chart in Figure 16-7 shows that if there is a vacancy at the manager level (M. Jones leaves), J. White is more likely to be promoted than B. Benson. If J. White moves to manager, then B. Benson succeeds White as assistant manager, and presumably both F. Brown and S. Green would be considered for an upcoming vacancy.

Staffing Table

A staffing table also provides a graphic representation of job titles and anticipated position vacancies (Figure 16-8). Because of increased computerization of health records processing, management predicts that additional data entry clerks must be hired in February, May, and October. A total of six full-time equivalent (FTE) clerks will be needed in the current budget year.

Human Resources Audit

A human resources audit is conducted to assess which openings can be filled with internal candidates already employed within the organization. An audit results in the integration of relevant information about the skills, knowledge, abilities, and leadership potential of all employees in the workforce into one document. This report should be useful in developing and coordinating effective recruitment, selection, orientation, training, and career-planning activities.

	Possible HIS Position Vacancies	Name of Employee	Attributes
Date Compiled: _____			
Manager, Health Information Services		M. Jones	A, 1
C. Smith, Incumbent		B. Benson	B, 2
		J. White	B, 1
Assistant Manager, HIS		J. White	A, 1
M. Jones, Incumbent		B. Benson	B, 2
Supervisor, Clinical Data		F. Brown	A, 1
J. White, Incumbent		J. Jones	B, 2
Supervisor, Medical Language Division		S. Green	A, 1
B. Benson, Incumbent		C. Black	B, 1

Key to Attributes:
A = Ready for Promotion
B = Needs More Experience Before Promoting
C = Not Suitable for Promotion at Present
1 = Performance Appraisal Rating Excellent
2 = Performance Appraisal Rating Acceptable
3 = Performance Appraisal Rating Unacceptable

FIGURE 16-7 Replacement chart.

Job Title	J 1	F 2	M 3	A 4	M 5	J 6	J 7	A 8	S 9	O 10	N 11	D* 12	Total FTE's
HI Analysts			2						1		1		4
Data Entry Specialists		3			1					2			6
Optical Imaging Specialists								1					1
Release of Information Coordinators					1				1				2
Director of HIS													
												Total	13

*Months of the year.

FIGURE 16-8 Staffing table. Anticipated openings for this budget year by month of the year.

Skill Inventories

These profiles of employee skills, knowledge, and capabilities can be developed for both nonmanagerial and supervisory-management employees. Demographic information, such as job title, job experience, and length of service with the organization, is typically provided. The most essential data presented in the inventory characterize the employee's performance history, current assessment of the employee's performance, and managerial judgments about the employee's potential for promotion. This tool should provide a coherent and comprehensive summary profile of the employee's credentials, including specific skills, areas of expertise, capabilities, and potential for professional growth.

SELF-ASSESSMENT QUIZ

14. Which of the following is not one of the most common types of flexible work schedules?
    a. Flexible work hours
    b. Condensed-compressed workweeks
    c. Core workweeks
    d. Telecommuting

Job Analysis and Design

Job analysis is a key human resource function that is often undervalued and misunderstood by many managers and employees. Although job analysis is generally viewed as a technical function performed by HRM specialists, it cannot be implemented effectively without the active involvement of supervisors and the employees whose jobs are subject to analysis. Because first-line supervisors and the employees themselves are in the best position to understand what is required to perform the job, how it can be performed most efficiently, and what outcomes are expected from doing the job effectively, these individuals must be recognized as primary sources of information. Consequently, every supervisor and line manager must understand the purpose, processes, and outcomes associated with job analysis and his or her responsibilities in ensuring that it is done effectively for all jobs within that area of accountability. Ultimately, job analysis should result in the design of jobs and work processes that maximize the cost-effective use of human resources to support the mission and goals of the organization while addressing the individual employee's needs, concerns, and goals.

Specific outcomes of job analysis include but are not limited to the following:

- Job requirements necessary for performing the job
- Essential functions of the job for ADA compliance
- Job specifications or qualifications (required of the employee)
- Selection criteria (based on the job specifications)
- Formal job description
- Performance standards (established or reviewed)
- Productivity measures (established or reviewed)
- Training needs and priorities
- Data to inform job evaluation or "pricing"

This representative list of outcomes of job analysis suggests the importance of this function to the organization.

Indeed, it can be argued that job analysis, if done well, serves as the foundation and "glue" for the HRM system as a whole. Consequently, managers must be held accountable for fulfilling their responsibilities to support this process. The supervisor or manager should also directly benefit from this process by having current and accurate job descriptions as tools useful in managing individual and team performance and coaching. It should be noted, however, that the focus for job analysis is not on the performance of the employee holding the job but on the job itself as a component of the total structuring and coordination of effort within the whole organization.

The following tools are some of those more commonly used to conduct formal job analysis:

- Job analysis forms (Figure 16-9)
- Questionnaires
- Interviews (individual and group)
- Checklists (supervisor or employee)
- Employee logs or diaries
- Work process, activity, and output records
- Direct observation (by supervisor or consultant)
- Video recording or taping (infrequent, special circumstances)

Any one or a combination of these methods may be used, but some form of survey or checklist is typically used as the basic data collection instrument. When teamwork is inherent in the work process, observation of the team process or group interviewing is appropriate. Direct observation of a complex work process may be useful but is also time-intensive, costly, and subject to perceptual bias of the observer. Self-reported activity or incident logs can be effective in analyzing managerial and professional positions characterized by a high degree of flexibility, exercise of discretion, and complex behavior. However, this method can be disruptive and also prone to bias and subjective reporting.

FIGURE 16-9 Sample job analysis form.

Position Title:	Health Information Secretary
Department:	Health Information Services
Supervisor:	Manager, Health Information Services
Current Supervisor's Name:	Kathy Castlerock

General Job Objectives:
- Acts as department receptionist and first telephone contact.
- Processes daily work schedules.
- Demonstrates effective relationships with coworkers, patients, public, physicians, administration, and outside agencies.

Essential Job Duties:
(List all tasks required to perform the routine functions required for the position.)
Example:
- Greets visitors to the department.
- Routes incoming phone calls and takes messages when intended party is unavailable.

Meets Standards of Performance By: (Example)
(For Greeting Visitors) Receiving no complaints in the performance period concerning discourteous service.

Exceeds Standards of Performance By: (Example)
(For Greeting Visitors) Receiving compliments by visitors, coworkers, or physicians on helpfulness and courteous service.

Job analysis should be an established human resource activity scheduled so that all jobs in the organization are subject to review and analysis on a predictable cycle. With the rapid changes in technology, regulation, and other environmental factors, it can be argued that the job analysis cycle should be no longer than 3 to 5 years, although organizational and industry factors will determine the appropriate frequency of formal job analyses. Certainly the job description should be reviewed at least once a year, preferably as part of the performance appraisal process, by both the employee and the supervisor.

In addition to the organization-wide rationale for conducting regular job analysis, individual managers might want to perform job analysis to do the following:

- Evaluate the effects of external challenges, such as a change in Medicare reimbursement regulations, on a specific job (e.g., billing clerk).
- Identify and eliminate irrelevant or potentially discriminatory job requirements and specifications.
- Identify job elements and working conditions that can be addressed to enhance the quality of work life.
- Develop an effective staffing plan to respond to changes in departmental mission, technology, or workload.
- Ensure better match of applicants with projected job vacancies and new positions.
- Develop a unit-wide training and career development plan and schedule for in-services.
- Rotate an employee to another position in the unit in which he or she will learn new skills and use already developed skills more fully.
- Determine whether the salary difference between two employees with different jobs but similar responsibilities and performance records is fair and reasonable.
- Initiate a unit-wide study to establish realistic productivity standards.
- Develop untapped potential in a specific position.

For example, a review of the position of insurance clerk at a neighborhood health clinic reveals that basic knowledge of the current edition of the coding manual is required. The clinic often faces a backlog in coding outpatient service records. By identifying this untapped resource, the clinic director can obtain training for the insurance clerk to prepare the clerk to help with backlog coding. This job redesign not only enhances the facility's capacity to provide more efficient service but also may improve the job satisfaction and career opportunities of the employee.

SELF-ASSESSMENT QUIZ

15. A job analysis inquiry precedes writing a job description.
   a. True
   b. False

Job Descriptions

A job description is the most tangible output of the job analysis process. The job description is a written document of the essential requirements, responsibilities, reporting relationships, qualifications, working conditions, and other significant aspects of the job. Within the organization, all job descriptions should normally follow the same format for ease of comparison and analysis. Form and content of job descriptions among health care organizations vary, however. Some job descriptions also include job performance standards that are used as the primary criteria for performance evaluation. For the job description to be a useful supervisory tool, the performance factors applied in practice must be consistent with the job description, even if these standards are not included in the text of the job description.

The job description can be a relatively brief summary or outline of the job requirements or a more comprehensive and detailed narrative. All job descriptions should contain, at a minimum, a set of key elements to serve the many purposes discussed earlier (Table 16-2).

TABLE 16-2 Structure and Key Elements of the Job Description	
Element Required	Purpose
Date	Date it was created and most recently revised
Author/responsible manager	Establishes accountability and source to refer any questions
Organization level/unit (department, division, office, etc.)	Places the job within the organizational structure
Job grade or classification	Ranks the job's level and importance for compensation purposes
Supervisory relationships	Identifies immediate supervisor and employees supervised (if any)
Job status	Exempt or nonexempt from overtime and other Fair Labor Standards Act requirements
Job summary	Concise description of the basic purpose and functions of the job
Essential functions, duties, and activities	Major tasks and responsibilities of this position; estimated time and effort distribution; "essential functions" must be identified for Americans with Disabilities Act compliance
Job specifications	Qualifications in terms of education, experience, skills, knowledge, certification, etc., needed to perform the essential job responsibilities
Working conditions	Physical and psychological demands of the work environment; any unusually challenging aspects should be addressed, such as handling hazardous materials or need to maintain strict confidentiality

SELF-ASSESSMENT QUIZ

16. A job description is a written portrait of a job that identifies, defines, and describes a position in terms of its duties, responsibilities, working conditions, and specifications, including minimum qualifications.
   a. True
   b. False

Employee Handbooks

The **employee handbook** provides a written reference manual of organizational policies and procedures covering employee rights, benefits, obligations, norms and standards of conduct, and other expectations of and constraints on employee behavior. With increasing challenges to the employment-at-will doctrine, the content and language of employee handbooks have come under considerable scrutiny by employers, unions, their respective legal counsel, and individual employees. For example, in some state courts, employee terminations have been challenged on the basis that language in the employee handbook implied a contractual obligation to offer continuing employment to the employee unless specific grounds for due cause of termination were proved. Subsequently, most employers have screened and revised such language to reduce the likelihood of a successful legal challenge on the basis of the handbook.

The following guidelines pertain to their appropriate content and use. Employee handbooks should be:
- Presented to communicate precisely and clearly the relevant policies and procedures established by management
- Reviewed periodically by legal counsel to minimize legal risk
- Updated continually to reflect changes in policy and procedures
- Distributed to all employees at orientation and following any significant policy revisions
- Covered as an essential component of supervisory training

All employees, at the time of orientation or distribution of revisions to the handbook, should be required to sign a statement to be maintained in the employee's file indicating that they have received a handbook and reviewed its contents within a predetermined time period. Management must assume the burden of ensuring that employees have access to the handbook and understand its scope and purpose. Also, employees must be informed that it is their responsibility to inquire of their managers or supervisors if they need clarification about any material in the handbook.

Job analysis should yield accurate and useful job descriptions that describe the essential functions of the job, how these are to be performed, and what qualifications the employee must present to perform the position effectively. Management policies and procedures governing employee conduct and working conditions should be clearly communicated through employee handbooks, personnel manuals, and supervisory coaching. These human resource processes and tools should provide the foundation for recruiting and selecting qualified individuals to fill the target positions consistent with human resource staffing plans and current needs.

 SELF-ASSESSMENT QUIZ

17. The *primary* reason that employee handbooks should be carefully reviewed is that they:
   a. Provide new employees with an impression of the organization.
   b. May be the primary method of employee communication.
   c. May be viewed by the company's competitors.
   d. May create an enforceable contract.

Recruitment

Recruitment is the process and set of activities performed to identify and maintain a **recruitment pool** of potential applicants presumably qualified and willing to perform one or more target positions in the organization. The recruitment function includes setting specific targets and schedules for filling vacant positions, selecting appropriate media for communicating the staffing needs, notifying external recruitment sources, announcing position vacancies, and identifying a group of potentially eligible applicants.

Key Activities in the Recruitment Process

The following key activities involved in employee recruitment must be performed whether recruitment is provided under contract with external agencies or is conducted in-house:
- Identify a position vacancy or need.
- Review and (if needed) revise the job description.
- Develop a recruitment plan, including appropriate internal and external communications about the position.
- Create and maintain a recruitment pool of eligible applicants.

The job opening has been identified either in the human resource plan or by request of a manager facing an immediate or foreseeable future need. The recruiter becomes familiar with the job requirements by reviewing the current job description, job specifications, and related information developed during the job analysis process. This review enables the recruiter to achieve a better match between the job requirements and the applicant's qualifications. The recruiter (staff or contractor) should discuss this job with the immediate supervisor or other responsible managers to ensure that they have a common understanding of the organization's expectations for filling this position. If necessary, the job description should be revised to reflect any changes in requirements or other aspects of the job before the position is advertised.

Once a common understanding of the essential requirements and expectations of the job has been achieved, recruiting specialists must consider and select appropriate recruitment sources and media for communicating the position opening. Cost-benefit considerations should be applied on the basis of systematic and continuous evaluation of the recruitment effort. A pool of potentially qualified applicants should be identified among those who respond to the position announcements and those referred by employees or external agents.

SELF-ASSESSMENT QUIZ

18. Recruiting is the process of choosing the most qualified candidate from a pool of applicants to fill a position.
   a. True
   b. False

Sources of Applicants

Newspaper and trade journal advertisements, walk-in and online inquiries, or employee referrals are commonly used in filling entry-level positions. Health care organizations may also use professional recruiters, such as executive search agencies, for managerial and highly skilled professional positions. If a professional recruiter is used, the employer must be sensitive to any intentional or unintentional biases of the recruiting agency, such as referring only applicants younger than 40 years, which might unnecessarily limit the applicant pool and expose the employer to legal risk. Executive search and other professional recruiting agencies typically charge fees for their services to the hiring organization, and the employer must understand its obligations and include such expenses in any cost-benefit analysis of its recruitment program.

Recruitment channels that are both available to most health care organizations and relatively cost-effective include walk-ins, self-initiated applications (write-in and online), and employee referrals. The latter process might be especially useful and even encouraged by management if it proves to be a reliable source of appropriate applicants. Not only are current employees likely to be effective recruiters for desirable positions, management can also signal its respect for the employees by welcoming such referrals.

Another recruitment tactic often used by today's health care organizations is to include job opportunities within the organization's Web site. Often a potential applicant is asked to "register" on the Web site before access is granted to the list of employment opportunities. Frequently, an applicant can apply on the Web site and may be able to attach his or her resume.

Targeted advertising is the most common channel of recruitment and can be cost-effective. Local daily newspapers, professional journals, and trade periodicals are the most likely places to advertise. Many organizations post or publish new positions on bulletin boards and in in-house newsletters, often in advance of externally focused efforts to encourage internal applicants. Increasingly, organizations announce position openings online. Increasingly, employers and job seekers rely on online recruitment and application processes to accomplish the initial screening.

Local and regional educational institutions, including community colleges, are usually excellent sources of recruitment for HIM positions at all levels. Medical assistant, medical transcriptionist or secretary, physician office management, nursing administration, HIM, information sciences, and business administration programs are likely sources of potential employees, depending on the nature of the position and level of training and certification required. Often, graduates from entry-level health profession and technologist programs have been required to complete supervised clinical placements in health care, rehabilitation, or health administrative settings. These applicants should have an easier transition to the health care environment and a shorter learning curve than others who lack this experience.

Constraints on Effective Recruitment

Constraints arise from the organization's strategic plans and objectives, current financial position, compensation policies, environmental conditions, job requirements, departmental or unit budgets, and federal and state regulation and legislation, including EEO requirements.

Management's human resource policies in support of long-term strategic plans and short-term operational objectives can constrain line managers and the recruitment staff by limiting the recruitment pool or by increasing the cost of maintaining an adequate pool of qualified applicants. For example, a promotion-from-within policy that mandates that qualified employees in place be given preferential consideration for promotion before external applicants are considered will probably be justified on the basis of effective employee relations and lower recruitment and training costs. However, this policy might also make the filling of any one position more difficult. A hire-from-within policy also might work against some organizational and public policy objectives, such as achieving a more diverse workforce, while supporting other values and policy objectives, such as extending the working life of older employees before retirement. Awarding preference to military veterans for civil service positions—for example, municipal, state, or federal agencies—is another constraint affecting the discretion of the recruiting staff or manager.

Certainly, compensation policies may constrain recruiting and influence the performance levels and productivity within the organization. For example, if the pay range for coders is significantly below the prevailing market rate or that of a key competitor, the recruiting effort for these jobs could be adversely affected. However, if the pay rate cannot be improved at least in the short term because of organizational constraints, the job might be made more attractive to applicants in other ways, such as flex-time scheduling, on-site child care, or subsidized parking.

Employee Selection

After an adequate pool of applicants has been recruited, the selection process begins. As a practical matter, the line between recruitment and selection processes is a fuzzy one. The **selection process** involves a sequence of activities that should result in the hiring of a well-qualified employee to fill the target position. The number of available and qualified applicants for the position is an important consideration. For example, if there is a surplus of trained medical transcriptionists in the region given the number of competing health care providers and total number of position vacancies, the hiring health information services unit is likely to identify and hire a qualified candidate without great difficulty. However, if the local or regional labor market is tight, the hiring unit may need to take very aggressive measures to fill open positions, for example, by making recruitment trips to colleges and job fairs outside the region to identify and recruit health information managers and technical staff. In the latter situation, recruiting methods should be reviewed to determine which recruitment sources, communication channels, and strategies for widening the recruitment pool are most effective. Consideration must be given to increased use of online recruitment methods, especially for positions related to information services.

Each health care organization must implement a set of activities essential to effective employee selection within regulatory and budgetary constraints. The process is sufficiently flexible that each organization can develop a recruitment and selection plan appropriate for its own needs and constraints. For example, some employers take aggressive steps to increase staff diversity by targeting recruitment and selection efforts to attract minority group applicants to fill key positions, such as by sending mailings to leaders of African American and Hispanic churches or other social organizations.

Components of the Employee Selection Process
Initial Contact

The screening process actually begins during the first interaction, usually face-to-face or by telephone, between the employer (as represented by an HRM departmental receptionist or interviewer) and applicant in which the applicant and employer's representative each form initial impressions of the other in terms of a potential match. These initial perceptions may be quite robust, especially in influencing the applicant's decision to continue pursuing the open position. As mentioned earlier, it is indicative of the dramatic changes brought about by the "information revolution" and the development of the Internet that the applicant's initial encounter with the organization is increasingly likely to be through its Web presentation or by e-mail.

Application Review

Research has shown that the standard application form may be the single most valid and reliable selection tool commonly used, especially if used in conjunction with personal contact reference checks.[53] If the application form has been developed to meet the hiring needs of the organization, it is essential to the completion of the initial screening phase of the selection process. The application could be developed to produce weighted scores based on selection criteria identified during job analysis. A rating cutoff score could be established to screen out applicants who do not meet the basic criteria of eligibility for the position. Structuring the selection process as a set of increasingly rigorous screens should increase the

efficiency of the process and validity of the final selection decisions. It is important for HIM professionals to know when it is the HRM department's responsibility to contact an initial review of an applicant's documentation and at what point the applicant's documentation is sent to the HIM department.

Although some organizations consider career resumes to be a substitute for the application form, this approach is not advisable. Because all applicants should be evaluated fairly and objectively against the same set of criteria, it is essential that the same information is collected and considered for each applicant. Failing to do so could subject the employer to legal liability under Title VII or other EEO legislation and lead to an inconsistent and unreliable selection process; that is, poor decisions might be made about both well-qualified and less-qualified applicants.

Furthermore, there is some evidence that applicants distort, exaggerate, or otherwise misrepresent their academic attainments, work experience, or other credentials in the prepared resumes. Some notorious cases have been documented of individuals creating separate and fraudulent identities through their resumes and paper record. Of course, applicants can also embellish or present false information on the application. Consequently, the use of reference checks should be considered an essential component of the selection process. In the case of verifying credentials of HIM professionals, the validity of the certification or registration should be confirmed with AHIMA.

Reference Checks

References are checked to accomplish two objectives: (1) to obtain new information about the applicant's performance history and likely future performance and (2) to verify information already obtained from other sources, including information disclosed by the applicant during an interview. For various reasons, including concerns of employers about exposure to legal liability, it is difficult although not impossible to obtain useful and accurate information about performance history and personal characteristics of an applicant from previous supervisors or coworkers. Many organizations have adopted a policy that requires the supervisor or other manager asked to provide a reference by another employer to refer that request to an HRM specialist. Typically, HRM staff limits its response to verifying dates of employment with that organization, the last position held, and (perhaps) whether the person left the job voluntarily or was terminated. The organization is often reluctant or unwilling to provide relevant and useful performance-related information and subject itself or its managers to the risk of legal liability if that information could be regarded as prejudicial or defamatory to the applicant. Consequently, it is more likely that the HRM staff specialist or manager will at best be willing to verify the accuracy of the work history reported by the applicant.

If the person conducting the reference check is able to reach the previous supervisor directly, he or she might obtain more candid feedback about performance strengths and deficiencies, disciplinary or interpersonal problems, and the circumstances of the applicant's separation from the previous position. However, it is increasingly unlikely that such important information can be obtained. It is notable that employers are also subject to legal liability for failing to obtain information relevant to job performance or behavioral problems of an applicant who is hired during or subsequent to the selection process. These competing legal principles place the hiring official between the proverbial "rock and a hard place" and certainly impede the organization's ability to base its selection decisions on what is usually considered the most effective predictor of future performance, that is, past performance in similar situations.

Testing

All selection tools normally used to make assessments about the applicant can be considered "tests" of some aspect of the applicant's abilities, knowledge, or personal characteristics. In effect, the entire selection process can be seen as an elaborate process of prediction of future performance: which applicants are likely to perform the job successfully and which ones are not likely to do so? The various selection tools in this respect serve as tests or predictors of some aspect of future job performance. From this perspective, even the application form and personal interview should be regarded as tests.

However, in common usage, "tests" refer to evaluative devices—written, oral, and electronic—that measure some skill, knowledge capability, interest, or psychological trait. In the HIM environment, such tests would include but not be limited to instruments or methods measuring knowledge of coding and medical terminology, quantitative analysis ability, keyboarding and transcription skills, and understanding of effective supervisory or management principles.

Employers are subject to demonstrating the validity of all selection tests in the event of a Title VII charge of discrimination in the selection process. The acid test legally is whether the challenged test can be demonstrated to be job related, the principle established in the Supreme Court's decision in the landmark EEO case of *Griggs v. Duke Power* (1971). In this case, the Supreme Court held that a test not demonstrated to be job related could be considered illegal under Title VII if it had adverse (discriminatory) effects on members of a protected class—in this case, African Americans—even if the test was not intended to do so. Management has the burden of proving that all selection tests used are valid and reliable indicators of some aspect of future job performance and that all applicants for the position are administered the test(s) under the same testing conditions. In the language of the Supreme Court, "Congress has forbidden giving [testing or measuring procedures] controlling force unless they are demonstrably a reasonable measure of job performance."[54] For example, requiring applicants to achieve some target score in a mathematics proficiency test would probably not be considered appropriate if the position does not require numerical calculations or use of statistical methods.

Although once commonly used as screening tools, aptitude, intelligence, personality type, and other psychometric measures are not considered performance tests and, except in special situations, would be difficult to justify as being job related. Aptitude tests and interest inventories presumably predict the probability of a person's being successful in some activity independent of his or her training or experience. Psychometric tests provide measures of a range of psychological, personality, and cognitive characteristics and predispositions, some of which might be linked to job-related behavior. Such tests should be administered and results interpreted only by testing experts and only if the test(s) has been validated in terms of measuring specific job or performance requirements. In no case should a line manager apply a test "locally" to an applicant or employee without review and approval by the appropriate human resources professional.

Selection Interview

The personal interview is regarded within management circles as the most important of all selection tools or predictors, and many managers have great confidence in their ability to use this technique effectively. Unfortunately, the interview is considered by many HRM professionals and scholars to be often unreliable and prone to bias and errors of judgment.

The justification for using the personal interview is that it gives the supervisor or other interviewer the opportunity to get a "good look" at the applicant, to determine whether the applicant will "fit in" with others in the unit, and to confirm whether the applicant can really get the job done. The problem with the personal interview is its susceptibility to various distortions and bias. In a personal interview the applicant's physical appearance and ability to communicate orally can dominate the interviewer's impressions. This can result in a halo effect bias in which the observer's perception of one characteristic of an individual dominates other perceptions. This perception can result in either a positive (halo) impression or negative (horns) impression. For example, the HIM applicant appears to be physically attractive and well dressed, which leads the interviewer to judge that the applicant is intelligent, well-educated, and will make an excellent HIM leader, which may or may not be reality. The interviewer, of course, should have already read and digested the applicant's resume, cover letter, and application form before the interview. The interview, then, becomes a subsequent impression, which can mitigate a halo or horns effect.

Some research has shown that dominant impressions are formed within the first several minutes of the interview. If the interview process is regarded as a data collection tool as well as a test, it will be inefficient and invalid to the degree that data that are available after the formation of the initial impression are discounted or ignored. Consequently, the validity and reliability of the interview as a test of future job performance could be severely compromised by halo effect bias.

Many managers believe that they are good interviewers, that they know how to make accurate and reliable judgments of the person's fit with the organization, intelligence, integrity, dependability, leadership potential, and other strengths and weaknesses on the basis of one relatively brief interaction. The manager may indeed be able to assess fit with the organization's culture, the applicant's ability to "think on his or her feet," and other characteristics relevant to the job on the basis of the interviewer's wisdom and years of experience. However, without training in interviewing, effective listening, and other human relations skills, as well as knowledge of the implications of Title VII, the ADA, and other legal constraints on the selection interview, the manager may misperceive and inflate his or her abilities in this role. It is essential that HIM managers and specialists gain specific knowledge, skills, and practice to become effective interviewers. An organization's HRM department may offer classes in these areas.

Despite these real concerns about the personal interview as a selection tool, virtually no organization would make a decision to hire for a position vacancy without the interview. Clearly, the interview process can be a useful tool for obtaining job- and performance-related data and for verifying and clarifying information given on the application. To avoid grounds for charges of discriminatory treatment under Title VII, the interview should be structured so that all those interviewed are asked the same array of questions under similar interview conditions to permit fair comparisons of all applicants. In summary, then, training the interviewer, structuring the interview to address important selection factors, and standardizing the process to ensure fair treatment for all applicants can enhance the reliability and validity of the interview process.

We should also recognize the value of the interview as an opportunity for the applicant to assess his or her fit within the job and the organizational culture. Furthermore, the employer has an opportunity not only to evaluate the applicant but also to market the position to a well-qualified applicant. If this two-way communication process is implemented effectively, it can assist both parties in their decision making about the potential employment match.

Typically, individuals conduct a series of interviews with different perspectives on the selection process. An HRM specialist usually conducts an initial screening interview to determine the applicant's eligibility on the basis of essential selection factors. If the applicant meets these criteria, subsequent interviews are scheduled with the immediate supervisor, the unit or division manager, and other managers with a relevant perspective on this position. In some organizations, peers or employees to be supervised by the applicant (if selected) are included in the interview process. For example, in selection of a quality improvement director or tumor registrar, a higher-level administrator or physician may want to participate in the interview process. When there are multiple interviews, the person who retains final hiring authority must be clearly designated. It is essential that the immediate supervisor be given a significant role in the selection process even if not given final or decision-making authority. Certainly, the supervisor has the greatest stake in achieving a good employment match and is usually the person in the best position to predict the applicant's fit within the job and the unit.

Applicants who are deemed eligible for further consideration based on the initial screening process should be scheduled for one or more intensive interviews. The interviewer should review the job description and job specifications with the applicant during the interview and provide a copy to the applicant

for consideration. Additionally, in health care organizations, any required credentials for the position must be verified and background checks performed. The applicant should be encouraged to ask any questions about the job requirements, working conditions, compensation level, work schedule, and other concerns and should be given an orientation tour of the work environment, including introduction to key managers and employees in the unit. Professional, courteous, and informed interviewing can only benefit the employer regardless of the outcome of an individual selection decision.

Medical Examination

The medical examination is provided to evaluate or certify that the applicant is sufficiently healthy and physically fit to carry out the duties and activities of the target position. This step is critical in health care organizations, especially when the employee is likely to have frequent contact with patients. Management and the general public have acknowledged concern about the potentially destructive effects of substance abuse in the workplace.

It should be noted that the ADA has directly affected the use of this selection tool, which had previously been routinely required in many organizations. Under ADA guidelines, the organization may impose a medical examination only after a bona fide job offer has been extended and only if required of all applicants extended job offers for the position.

Probationary Employment

Although not usually considered part of the selection process itself, the period of probationary or provisional employment covering the first phase of the selected applicant's employment in the target position is an important component of selection and retention. This period, typically lasting 3 months for nonprofessional and technical positions and 6 months or longer for professional and managerial positions, gives the applicant an opportunity to become oriented to the job and organization under lower performance expectations than when the employee achieves regular employment status. For the employer, the probationary period provides an opportunity to set expectations and closely monitor the new employee's performance and conduct with his or her supervisor and coworkers. Furthermore, it allows either the employer or the employee to terminate the relationship voluntarily during the probationary period in the case of an unsuccessful match without adverse effects on either party.

SELF-ASSESSMENT QUIZ

19. Which of the following are tools that can be used in the selection process? Check all that apply.
   a. Letters of recommendation
   b. Application forms
   c. Interviews
   d. Reference checks
   e. Background checks
   f. All of the above

Employee Retention

Retention of staff, although not considered to be a separate and distinct function within HRM, is in fact one of management's most important responsibilities. To survive as a system the organization must maintain a reasonable degree of stability in its structures, processes, and staffing. Consequently, the organization must give priority to retention of its productive assets, especially its most productive and valued employees, because employee turnover is so costly to the organization. The costs associated with placing a new employee in a target position ready to perform the job are considerable. These include the costs of reviewing and updating job descriptions, developing recruitment plans, media advertisements, recruiter's travel expenses, employee relocation, separation compensation, interviewing, reference checks, test administration and analysis, and employee orientation and supervisory training. Implicit costs are also incurred, such as decreased productivity associated with position vacancies and the learning curve for employees in training. Various estimates have been made of the total costs of employee turnover. Cascio[55] reported a study of this issue within the pharmaceutical firm Merck & Company that showed turnover costs ranging from 1.5 to 2.5 times the annual salary paid for the affected job. By applying his turnover cost model to hypothetic hospital cost data, Cascio[55] estimated an average turnover cost of almost $8000 per employee.

Supervisory Coaching

All of the HRM functions and activities discussed in this chapter can be considered to have direct or indirect effects on employee retention. Although supervisory coaching is inherent in the supervisor's role and not an HRM staff function, it could be argued that this process has the greatest long-term impact on employee satisfaction, morale, level of performance, and, ultimately, retention.

Providing regular feedback on performance to employees is perhaps the most critical aspect of the supervisor's coaching role in encouraging, developing, and retaining employees. Employees typically want to have constructive and useful feedback about aspects of their performance that require improvement and would benefit from additional guidance, practice, or formal training. Without clear and candid feedback, employees quite naturally assume that their performance is at least satisfactory and that it satisfies the supervisor's expectations.

Orientation

Human resource management involves more than identifying, evaluating, and hiring qualified individuals for positions within the organization. Unless the employer ensures that the new employee has an appropriate and supportive transition into the job and the broader organization, the efforts and cost associated with recruitment and selection may be wasted. When the employee reports for the first day of work, processes must be in place to facilitate the new employee's transition. The process of becoming a productive employee effectively socialized into the culture of the organization is critical to the organization and to the employee. This process includes both orientation to the environment (e.g., locating the restrooms, obtaining an identification card, meeting coworkers) and orientation to the job itself in terms of performance expectations and standards, work process, and cultural norms. Various methods are used in the orientation process, including formal group presentations, self-guided instructional media including online modules, supervisory "walk-throughs," review of orientation manuals and employee handbooks, and the shadowing of veteran employees and supervisors. New employee orientation is usually a collaborative effort between the HRM department and the individual department in which the new employee will work.

Formal orientation programs may be provided for all new employees within a health care organization through scheduled group or individual sessions conducted by the human resources department. This formal orientation should complement but never substitutes for the job-specific departmental orientation and personal interactions among the new employee, the supervisor, and the peer group.

Orientation programs are key for new employee satisfaction in an organization. The central objectives of orientation are to reduce a new employee's anxieties about acceptance into the work group and to ensure that the employee is sufficiently familiar with the job requirements and expectations so that she or he may begin to make a positive contribution in the position without undue delay. An effective program should address all aspects of the work environment including the social, technological, cultural, and political dimensions relevant to performance in the position so that the employee can effectively adapt to her or his new role.

One of the major benefits to the employer of a formal, integrated orientation program is to provide accurate, relevant, and consistent information to all new employees in contrast to their obtaining information and misinformation piecemeal from new coworkers and acquaintances. An effectively designed HIM orientation program utilizes HRM staff, HIM supervisors, and well-respected coworkers to provide a comprehensive and participatory learning experience.

Performance Appraisal Systems

Performance appraisal is one of the most critical and problematic of all the human resource subsystems. Most employees and many supervisors approach the performance appraisal process with suspicion, cynicism, frustration, and anxiety. Typically, neither employees nor supervisors expect any positive or lasting outcomes, at least for most employees. It is not uncommon for supervisors to regard the process as something to get out of the way so that more productive and less unpleasant work might be accomplished. All too frequently, performance appraisal has been done carelessly, unreliably, and even destructively in terms of the employee's motivation, productivity, and relationship with the supervisor. Indeed, sometimes performance appraisal as a systematic method for observing, evaluating, documenting, and giving feedback to employees about their performance is not done at all. Effective performance appraisal is not something that happens once a year. It is an ongoing process in which the supervisor has conversations with the employee about how well he or she is doing his or her job.

Given the importance of performance appraisal and its potential benefits to both the employee and the organization, its negative characterization is especially unfortunate. When the process is understood by supervisors and employees (both the evaluators and the evaluated), assuming the process has been well designed and is effectively managed, performance appraisal should further the goals of individual employees, managers, and other stakeholders of the organization. For the health care organization, among the outcomes of effective appraisal is enhancing and ensuring the quality of health care provided to the community.

Performance appraisal entails three interrelated processes: measurement, judgment, and communication. Although each of these processes must be done competently to achieve the objectives of appraisal, it can be argued that the last is the most critical because it has the most pervasive impact on the supervisory relationship. The measurement dimension is addressed by the determination of the assessment method, for instance, quantitative rating of performance factors, and the design of the appraisal instrument(s). Graphic rating scales, one of the most common rating techniques in practice, calls for the rater to assess performance according to numerical scales often anchored by brief descriptors of performance. This measurement aspect of appraisal is a technical specialization performed by HIM staff or under contract. The judgment aspect is a special (and especially challenging) case of the supervisory coaching function. The effectively trained supervisor, who understands the supervisory role, has gained the respect of his or her team, and typically exercises good sense in day-to-day decision making, is likely to demonstrate good judgment in the performance appraisal process.

? DID YOU KNOW?

Did you know that a problem with performance appraisal is that personal biases and many other factors affect how a manager views someone at a particular point in time? If the manager is upset with someone, he or she may think of him or her as a lower performer. If the manager is pleased with someone, he or she may think more highly of his or her performance.

Communication is a fundamental supervisory-management process and organizational dynamic. Effective multidirectional and reciprocal communication is a requirement for any open system to sustain itself and maintain internal coordination. Communication as a critical aspect of performance appraisal entails the presentation of clear performance expectations, attempts to validate the employee's understanding and "buy in" to enhancing performance, and the supervisor's feedback on performance, such as encouragement, identifying deficiencies, and praising notable effort and meritorious performance. Unless the supervisor provides the employee with ongoing, specific, action-oriented, candid, but supportive, feedback, investment in other aspects of the process is likely to be wasted, and the primary objective—shaping employee behavior in achieving individual, unit, and organizational goals—will be frustrated.

Structured and comprehensive evaluation of employee performance should provide valuable information to management to support various organizational systems. Compensation decisions, such as merit-based increases and promotions, are often linked to performance appraisal results. Appraisal results can identify skill, knowledge, and other development needs to plan for individual, team, and unit-wide training. Alternatively, the appraisal process might be used to justify a disciplinary response to a "problem" employee or referral to an EAP for counseling and referral. Managers can monitor output from performance appraisal reviews to identify patterns or trends that reflect strengths and deficiencies in recruitment, selection, or training programs.

A performance appraisal system should produce an accurate and comprehensive profile of the employee's job performance. One approach calls for a 360-degree evaluation[56] that identifies, observes, and assesses the totality of the employee's responsibilities and contributions. For this to be done effectively, job performance factors, standards, weights, and criteria must be established, defined, communicated, and accepted by both managers and employees. The performance appraisal system then uses this information as the foundation for the evaluation process.

Ideally, performance factors, standards, and criteria should be developed through a rigorous consensus process that includes input from those employees with relevant perspectives on the job(s) subject to job analysis. Typically this would include job incumbents, supervisors, peers in jobs linked to those being analyzed, and, when feasible, clients. The 360-degree approach to performance evaluation is built on the assumption that diverse perspectives that "wrap around" the entire job can be obtained. For example, one performance factor for an HIM release of information specialist might be "quality of customer services." The related performance standard might be "providing courteous, accurate patient services that are responsive to the patient's expressed need for health information within resource and time constraints" and the criterion, to establish one or more specific conditions that define success, such as some measure of efficient design or productivity target.

Although some performance factors and standards might be common to many jobs within an organization, such as quality of patient care, no two units or supervisors are likely to apply precisely the same criteria for evaluation in practice.

For performance appraisal to be valid for any one position or unit, the factors, standards, and criteria must be established with the target jobs in mind. Poor fit between the performance appraisal process and the reality of the jobs subject to this process works against valid, reliable, and useful appraisal outcomes.

Methods of Performance Appraisal
Employee Ranking

Although no longer commonly used as the primary appraisal method, employee ranking has been used in the military for leadership assessment and promotional review and in higher education for faculty recruitment and appointment processes. Two types of ranking have been used most often: simple ranking and forced distribution. In simple ranking, all employees (or candidates) are ranked from 1 to *n* on one or more summary or global measures of performance, such as overall contribution to the department's goals. The supervisor should consider and rank all employees under his or her authority, often in descending order from "best" to "least" contributor. This approach has the benefit of simplicity and efficiency, assuming that the number of employees supervised is not so large that it makes meaningful distinctions infeasible. The major disadvantages are that one global performance factor is usually too broad to be a useful measure for employee feedback and performance improvement and that a ranked list of employees does not allow for effective feedback.

DID YOU KNOW?

Did you know in 2013 the *Wall Street Journal* (http://blogs.wst.com/digits/2013/11/12, *Why Microsoft dumped 'stack ranking', Shira Ovida*) announced Microsoft is moving away from ranking on a "bell curve" type of system?[57]

Forced distribution ranking requires the supervisor to place the employees into a set of ordered groups—for example, top 10%, above average 20%, middle 40%, below average 20%, and bottom 10%—on the basis of a global measure. In effect, this forces the employees into a more or less normal distribution along this performance factor. Because it does not require the supervisor to rank within these categories, it eases the ranking burden and may make the ranking more useful as a feedback measure of "where the employee stands." However, it shares the other deficiencies of simple ranking.

If used as the sole or primary method of employee evaluation, ranking is too limited and subjective to be a useful measure of performance in most situations. However, ranking could be applied as a supplement to another method that is considered generally more valid and reliable.

Graphic Rating Scales

Various approaches and tools (instruments) have been used to rate employee performance. A set of graphic rating scales is probably the earliest and most common method in practice (Figure 16-10). A graphic rating scale is a linear, continuous

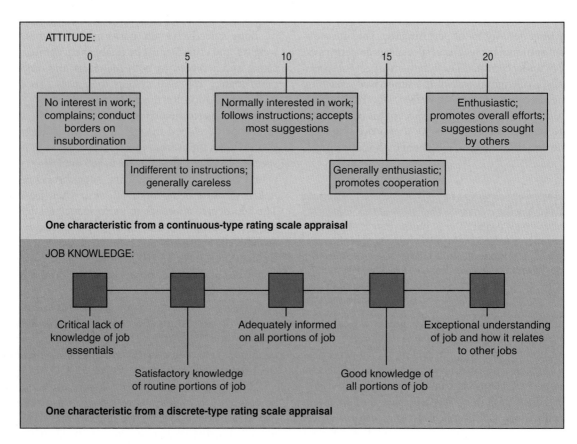

FIGURE 16-10 Sample performance evaluation system rating scale.

scale representing performance for a predetermined performance factor, dimension, component, or personal characteristic. Typically, the scale displays a discrete but arbitrary range of numerical increments, with 4-, 5-, and 7-point scales the most common. Often the scales are labeled by using verbal "anchors," such as "fails to meet standards," "meets standards," and "far exceeds standards," to enhance the reliability of the rating. Some scales are anchored only at the end points, and raters are asked to check the appropriate location on the continuum corresponding to their intuitive rating. To be useful and valid measures of job performance, the scales must be clearly understood, designed to be reliable indicators of performance, and based on the critical behaviors and skills that determine job performance.

Critical Incident Method

The critical incident method of employee performance evaluation requires the supervisor to document exceptional job-related behavior—that is, notably effective or ineffective performance that is actually observed or reported. Such statements, identified as critical incidents, collectively represent the range of behavior typical for that employee. Documented positive critical incidents may be used as the basis for merit pay decisions and negative ones used as the basis for performance correction plans or disciplinary action. Although this method is a potentially powerful source of job-specific feedback, it is prone to various biases and subjectivity in observation and reporting. Nonetheless, documenting exceptional incidents of performance is on balance likely to be worth the supervisor's effort.

Behaviorally Anchored Rating Scales

Behaviorally anchored rating scales (BARS) were developed in part to address concerns about the reliability of traditional graphical rating scales. The BARS method anchors the numerical scales with brief narrative descriptions of a range of behavior from highest to lowest level of performance on that dimension. These narrative descriptions may be drawn from critical incidents documented in real-world supervisory situations. For example, on a scale of "interpersonal effectiveness with clients" as an aspect of the performance of physical therapists, a brief scenario representing especially cordial, responsive, and client-centered behavior could be used to anchor the highest level of performance on this dimension. Other realistic scenarios would be developed and matched to the range of discrete points on the scale. This method offers several advantages over the traditional rating scales in addition to the objective of improving the reliability of the rating itself. When the numerical ratings are anchored in "slices of life" familiar to both supervisor and employee, the employee should have a clear and concrete understanding of how the supervisor views his or her performance. Although this method does not guarantee that the supervisor will rate the employee fairly or "objectively" or that the employee will agree with the supervisor's rating, both parties should have a common ground for discussion on the basis of specific job behavior. It should be noted, however, that research has not demonstrated that the BARS method results in more reliable ratings statistically (Figure 16-11).

FIGURE 16-11 Behaviorally anchored rating performance appraisal system.

Behavioral Anchors	Rating	Score
Manager consistently models the highest standards of ethical behavior as demonstrated in her/his leadership in organizational, professional, and community roles.	Outstanding	4
Manager holds her/himself and her/his staff to high standards of ethical performance by addressing this dimension explicitly in the performance appraisal review with her/his employees.	Excellent	3
Manager periodically acknowledges the core values of the health system and the HIM profession in staff/team meetings and other modes of communication, e-mails, bulletin board postings, etc.	Good	2
Manager's behavior complies overall with organizational policies and AHIMA Code of Ethics.	Satisfactory	1
Manager has one or more documented incidents of violations of organizational conduct and/or professional ethical standards.	Unacceptable	1

Goal Setting and Performance Improvement Plans (PIP)

During the 1970s and 1980s, management by objectives (MBO) dominated corporate thinking as the model paradigm or system to integrate business planning, productivity management and control, employee performance evaluation, and supervisory coaching. MBO, developed as an integrated planning process by George Odiorne and popularized by the management guru Peter Drucker, became so pervasive and its advocates so committed that it might be regarded as a total philosophy of management. Although MBO has largely been replaced by waves of alternative approaches, such as strategic management, total quality management, and process reengineering, one of its core principles, the systematic setting and periodic review of performance goals, has survived the passing of management paradigms and fads.

In fact, there would be considerable consensus among scholars and managers that goal setting should be an essential part of any performance appraisal process. When any evaluation method reveals a significant performance or skill deficiency, behavioral problem, or other obstacle to peak performance, the supervisor has a responsibility to address this concern. One effective approach is to set specific, actionable goals within a coherent performance plan, known as a performance improvement plan (PIP). The goals should be clearly understood by both supervisor and employee, as concrete and quantifiable as possible, and their attainment measurable or at least observable. A specific target date for completion of the goal or a sequence of projected progress points must be established for the goal to be effective. Although some flexibility should be built into the performance plan to recognize the effects of factors beyond the employee's control, agreement about projected dates of key milestones is critical. A goal without a time frame for implementation is at best an expression of good intention but not a genuine performance goal statement. The employee should be encouraged to participate actively in the goal-setting process, but at the very least, the employee must "buy into" whatever goals are established for him or her.

Self-appraisal can be a useful complement to traditional rating schemes and goal setting. The employee should be encouraged to reflect on his or her performance for the period, identify strengths and weaknesses, and identify accomplishments and obstacles to progress before the formal performance appraisal review. The employee and supervisor, using the same evaluation tool, can then compare one another's perceptions of the same performance history. Although this process does not guarantee agreement about ratings or the value added by the employee's contribution, it certainly encourages the exploration of common ground, a more objective approach to analysis of performance problems and mutual goal setting.

An example of a performance improvement plan is shown in Figure 16-12.

For professional development and growth, the following goals will be established to improve personal productivity and enhance contributions to department objectives and the hospital mission.

Within each goal, selected objectives are outlined to serve as benchmarks and measure toward that goal.

Area of Accountablilty—Clinical Data Coordination

I.   Reduce unbilled accounts due to coding to 0 days with minimum oversight.
  A.   Report status every Monday to department head using the Health Information Services weekly statistics form.
  B.   Outline reasons for variance from the standard.
  C.   Perform timely follow-up to assure that all records are released for billing within the time parameters established.

II.   Improve productivity in coding and abstracting. Industry standards for coding hospital inpatients are 8 minutes per record and Outpatient Services, 2.5 minutes per record.
  A.   Document obstacles that prohibit this level of performance at this hospital.
  B.   Increase coding expertise through continuing education from a variety of resources.
  C.   Code all patient types to enhance skills.

III.   Use Continuous Quality Improvement (CQI) principles to improve work efficiency in your responsibility area.
  A.   Organize work area to exhibit neatness and efficiency.
  B.   Prioritize daily work to optimize adherence to department CQI standards. Report when not attainable for reasons beyond your control.

FIGURE 16-12 Sample performance development goal plan.

Checklists

Standardized checklists may be used to select statements or words that most clearly describe an employee's performance (Figure 16-13). They may also be associated with weights when scored so that the more critical job duties have greater impact than less important ones. A forced-choice method requires the supervisor to choose the one statement in each pair of statements that is more descriptive of some relevant aspect of the employee's performance being evaluated. Examples of paired statements follow:

1a. The employee is a quick learner.
1b. The employee is often late in completing assigned work.
2a. The employee is a diligent worker.
2b. The employee takes longer than the typical employee to learn new procedures.

Forced-choice methods often use a standardized instrument so that the process is not likely to include job-specific performance factors and criteria. Another disadvantage is

FIGURE 16-13 Representation of a sample weighted performance checklist.

Employee Name _____		Department _____
Position _____		Date _____
Supervisor _____		

Weights	Performance Appraisal Criteria	Check
6.5	Employee is accountable to essential job duties.	
4.0	Employee keeps work area well organized.	
3.9	Employee works cooperatively with others as a team.	
4.3	Employee considers consequences before taking action.	
0.2	Employee adheres to dress code.	
etc.		
Total 100		
	Total of All Weights Checked	

that the supervisor may find this method unfamiliar and difficult to complete by choosing between statements that appear to be unrelated or abstract. Furthermore, it is not obvious that the output of this process lends itself to useful feedback to the employee.

Each of the methods just presented and variations of them have relative strengths and deficiencies as performance evaluation tools. HIM managers have the responsibility of ensuring that a reliable, useful, and credible process is tested, implemented, and monitored for effectiveness. It is critical that all HIM employees are educated about the process and that supervisors are trained to understand their role in the process and how to conduct performance appraisal effectively.

Rater Biases That Affect Appraisal

A major problem associated with the measurement aspect of performance appraisal is the potential for rater bias. The following are common biases that can invalidate any evaluation method if not recognized and addressed:
- Halo effect—when one performance factor or personal characteristic dominates the evaluator's perceptions and judgments. This is one of the most common and difficult to remedy sources of bias.
- Central tendency error—when the evaluator rates all employees similarly as "average" on most performance factors. This predisposition to "play it safe" distorts the process by failing to make valid distinctions among employees in level of performance and among factors of performance for the same employee that are demonstrated in practice.
- Leniency or strictness bias—the tendency to be consistently too lenient or too strict in evaluation relative to the actual level of performance.
- Recency effect—the phenomenon in which the most recent incidents or trends in employee's performance have disproportionate influence on the overall perceptions of and judgments about the employee's

performance. Ideally, the entire range of employee behaviors across all job duties and activities for a specified time period should be reviewed and assessed on the basis of reliable documentation.
- Stereotyping—this is the habit of grounding evaluative judgments on stereotypes on the basis of racial, ethnic, gender, age, disability, or other personal or cultural characteristics. Bias based on these deep-seated stereotypes and attitudes independent of an individual's competence and level of performance has proved to be resistant to change.
- Personal prejudice or favoritism—the supervisor's personal likes and dislikes of employees independent of their performance and conduct should not affect performance evaluation. Assessments should be based as firmly as possible on applying clearly communicated performance factors and criteria to observed and documented performance.

SELF-ASSESSMENT QUIZ

20. When an employee is considered to have a lingering effect that leads her manager to see her as being a good performer long after a specific positive action or high level of achievement is attained, this is called:
   a. Individual focus.
   b. The halo effect.
   c. Recency effect.
   d. Stereotyping.

Implementation of the Performance Appraisal System

Effective implementation of the employee performance appraisal system is one of the most critical and challenging of management's responsibilities because it is so central to the organization's strategic planning and control functions. The system must be demonstrated to be useful and valid both to justify the resources committed to it on a cost-benefit basis and to withstand any legal challenges. An effective system should make a measurable difference in terms of improved performance, whereas an ineffective system can actually result in deterioration of performance, job satisfaction, and supervisory and employee motivation. The risks of ineffective performance appraisal are great indeed. The key element in the process resides in the fabric of the supervisory relationship itself. If the supervisor applies effective coaching and interpersonal skills, understands team process, and has earned respect among the employees as a fair, competent, and ethical leader, this will provide a solid foundation for the performance appraisal system. Without this foundation of consistently effective supervision, even a technically sound method backed by strong top management endorsement is likely to fail.

 SELF-ASSESSMENT QUIZ

21. The identification, measurement, and management of human performance in organizations is known as:
   a. Employee coaching
   b. Performance appraisal
   c. Employee development
   d. Performance improvement

Adverse Outcomes of Employee Performance

Although the goals of the HRM system are focused on the effective use and full development of all the individuals participating in the organization, it is a fact of our organizational experience that too often these objectives are not fulfilled for some employees. Employees fail to live up to supervisory expectations, and perhaps their own as well. Individuals with an excellent work history suddenly demonstrate declining performance or erratic behavior. After a generally positive but somewhat critical supervisory evaluation, employees become less enthusiastic about the job, distance themselves from coworkers, and begin to miss work frequently without clear justification. On failing to obtain an expected promotion, a manager "retreats" into the technical aspects of work and becomes increasingly absorbed in Internet stock investment or Facebook searches. A single parent has an interruption of child care coverage and begins to leave before the shift ends, spends excessive time on the phone, and periodically displays fits of temper with coworkers. Such signs of performance failure, career frustration, or personal and family problems interfering with on-the-job performance can point to adverse consequences to follow for the employee and for the organization. Instead of promotions, career mobility, compensation increases, and job satisfaction, many employees experience the anger, frustration, and erosion of self-confidence and credibility among their peers associated with career plateaus or performance decline.

Adverse organizational responses to real or perceived deterioration of performance and problematic behavior—for example, inappropriate sexual references or abusive conduct—can lead to invoking of the employee discipline process, referral to an EAP, demotions, or job transfers. In the extreme case, the employee may be terminated for cause

BOX 16-10   Examples of Employee Behavior That Might Justify For-Cause Termination

- Prolonged absence from work without notification
- Chronic history of irregular attendance and failing to report
- Threatening behavior directed toward patients, coworkers, or managers
- Reporting for work under the influence of drugs or alcohol
- Being caught in the act of theft, embezzlement, or fraud against the employer or clients
- Extremely offensive or chronic acts of sexual harassment
- Significant use of the organization's resources for private business or gain without prior approval

on the basis of performance deficiencies, unacceptable conduct, or failing to provide net benefit to the organization. Because of a disruptive personality, poor work ethic, refusal to accommodate to the organizational culture, or some other factor, management has determined that the employee's behavior incurs higher costs to the organization than the benefits gained.

Most organizations have termination-for-cause events that require immediate dismissal. These situations are usually clearly defined and, although unpleasant, not usually as troublesome for the manager as subtler and more chronic problems (Box 16-10).

Wrongful Discharge

The employer almost always justifies an employee termination on the basis of "just cause," that is, the employee's outrageous, dangerous, negligent, or insubordinate behavior or chronically deficient performance. Despite the legal tradition of "at-will" employment discussed next, employees increasingly (and in some state courts, successfully) have challenged presumed just-cause terminations. Because this legal doctrine is evolving and differs among states, this remains an ambiguous and therefore risky area for HRM professionals and the employer.

An attempt to negotiate a resolution with the problem employee is recommended if an employee is likely to take court action to pursue a wrongful discharge. A negotiated severance payment, outplacement assistance, and transfer to another, more suitable position in the organization are some alternatives to termination that may be mutually acceptable and beneficial. Whatever the facts of a specific situation, the health information manager must be aware of the legal constraints and consequences imposed on employers to protect employees from wrongful discharge.

At-Will Employment

Historically, employers and employees have operated under the English common law doctrine of employment at will. Under this doctrine, either party with or without cause could terminate an employment contract without a specified length of term. Recently, this doctrine has been eroded in the courts in some states as a reflection of the expanding scope of employee rights initiated by the EEO revolution.[54]

Such claims of unjust termination are generally based on one of these legal foundations:

Tort law. The termination is based on the premise that the employee has economic injury or damages from the action of the employer. This application of civil law principles does not entail breach of contract.

Implied contract. Courts in many states have recognized claims based on statements made in employee manuals and handbooks or oral statements made by managers. The managers' statements or the handbooks are interpreted with the implication that an employee would be retained for a certain length of time or indefinitely as long as he or she meets standards of satisfactory performance.

Implied covenant of good faith and fair dealing. This approach challenges the termination on the basis that the employee was discharged for reasons other than just cause, violating an implicit covenant. The good faith and fair dealing principle would most likely be recognized on the basis of an employee's seniority, record of satisfactory performance, and positive representations of the employee's performance by supervisory management. Relatively few states recognize such an implied covenant in the employment context.

Public policy exception. This covers a situation in which a termination for any cause conflicts with the intent of another public policy. For example, an employee demonstrating irregular performance is discharged for filing a Workers' Compensation claim or for threatening to report abuse of hospital patients to state authorities.

It must be emphasized that differences in legal precedent and interpretation among state courts make this area uncertain and difficult. In general, management is in the best position by treating terminations as a last resort, being prepared to prove just cause, and by applying this remedy equitably to all employees under similar circumstances.

For additional safeguards for management contemplating disciplinary action, please refer to Figure 16-14.

Prior to taking disciplinary action, a manager may complete this checklist. If one or more "no's" are checked, it is a good idea to discuss the action with the Director of Human Resources or someone from Administration to assure the disciplinary action planned is appropriate under the circumstances.

		Yes	No
1.	Has the work rule or the policy that was violated been published or otherwise clearly communicated to this employee?	☐	☐
2.	Did this employee ever receive a written copy of this rule or policy?	☐	☐
3.	Is the rule posted on bulletin boards or similar areas?	☐	☐
4.	Is the infraction reasonably related to the orderly, efficient, and safe operation of the unit, department, or organization?	☐	☐
5.	If others have similar infractions, did they receive the same disciplinary action as is being contemplated for this employee?	☐	☐
6.	Are there factual records available on all employees covering violation of the rule or policy in question?	☐	☐
7.	Does this employee have the worst record of all employees on violation of this rule or policy?	☐	☐
8.	Have there been any previous warnings for violation of this rule or policy given to this employee?	☐	☐
9.	Does the documentation surrounding the infractions include dates, times, places, witnesses, and pertinent facts on all past violations?	☐	☐
10.	Is there a factual written record showing the steps taken by the manager to correct the improper conduct of all employees?	☐	☐
11.	Is the degree of discipline to be imposed related to the seriousness of the offense, the degree of fault, and any mitigating factors?	☐	☐
12.	Has this employee had an opportunity to tell his or her side of the story?	☐	☐

FIGURE 16-14 Disciplinary checklist.

Layoffs

Involuntary separation occurs whenever the employer terminates the employment relationship for whatever reason, sometimes as a result of low patient volume, restructuring, or adverse economic conditions. As previously discussed, layoffs should be avoided when possible if the same result can be achieved by reduction of the employee's hours, early retirement, or job sharing. Involuntary separation usually provides the employees affected with no direct benefits other than eligibility for unemployment compensation administered by a state agency. If layoffs affecting a significant number of employees can be anticipated, it is sound management policy and ethically responsive to notify the affected employees as early as possible to give them the opportunity to plan for the economic dislocation involved.

Retirement

Retirement is another type of separation, which may be voluntary or involuntary. The number of involuntary retirements is likely to decrease in large part because of amendments to the ADEA, which eliminated forced retirement at an arbitrary age for most employees, with the exception of some highly paid executives. The adverse effects of the recent financial crisis on pension investments and personal savings are likely to result in delayed retirements and reentry of retired workers into the workforce. It will be the responsibility of HRM staff to track retirement patterns and identify key individuals facing retirement so that recruitment and replacement plans and targets may be developed. It would also be wise for the HIM management team to track individual HIM employee retirement plans. In some environments, including health care, some older professionals may choose to negotiate contacts on a part-time or per-project consulting basis. This could provide advantages to the employer by reducing employee benefit costs while retaining access to the considerable knowledge, skills, and experience that the senior employee has to offer the organization. At the same time, this arrangement could ease the older employee's transition into his or her later career.

Employee Counseling and Discipline

Employee counseling and referral and progressive discipline are problem-solving processes to halt the decline in a troubled employee's performance and to prevent excessive employee turnover through termination or supervisor-initiated transfers. Whatever managers can do to prevent unnecessary terminations is likely to provide net benefit to the organization. Employees do not resign voluntarily, except under exceptional circumstances, if they enjoy a satisfying work environment, a challenging job, communication with their supervisors, and personal opportunities for growth.

All organizations have policies, procedures, and standards for employee conduct that serve as guidelines to expected employee behavior. These policies and procedures are usually documented in organizational and departmental policy manuals and in employee handbooks. These personnel policies should include a description of a progressive disciplinary process and the grievance procedure. The disciplinary process should be invoked when neither performance appraisal nor assertive supervisory coaching has been an effective remedy for problem behavior. The grievance process, on the other hand, provides a communication and problem-solving mechanism for employees to express a complaint that management has violated one of its own policies (or the union contract) with adverse consequences for the employee. The proactive health information manager communicates these policies and procedures to current staff and to new employees in orientation, staff in-services, and periodic performance reviews. Critical incidents of problem behavior and violations of management policies must be documented for follow-up actions, such as initiating the disciplinary process. When employees fail to follow these policies and rules of acceptable conduct, it is the manager's responsibility to assist the employee in taking corrective action and achieving an effective level of performance.

 SELF-ASSESSMENT QUIZ

22. Which of the following is not a step that might be used in disciplining a difficult employee?
   a. Ignoring the undesirable behavior
   b. Examining the facts of the situation
   c. Confronting the employee to discuss the situation
   d. Looking at the situation from both sides

Counseling and Referral

Employee counseling is provided to assist the employee in addressing personal and other problems that might originate outside the workplace but affect job performance and behavior in the workplace. Referral is the process of linking the employee with an array of resources to address the problem(s) identified. Informal counseling and referral on a limited basis has traditionally been regarded as a supervisory role. However, within the past three decades, most large organizations, including those in health care, have recognized the need to provide counseling and referral services on a more professional and consistent basis by establishing employee assistance programs (EAPs). EAP services may be provided in-house through a centralized staff of trained counselors who provide counseling and referral to address an array of problems and issues, including financial concerns, family and community conflicts, depression, eating disorders, alcohol and substance abuse, and other behavioral problems. Alternatively, EAP services may be provided under contract with one or more external agencies. This arrangement might reduce the total costs of providing these services and should mitigate concerns about maintaining strict confidentiality for employees who seek these services.

In either approach, the supervisor has a key role in providing a link between the troubled employee and appropriate resources to address the employee's problems. One of the most critical aspects of this role is that the supervisor recognizes employee verbal and nonverbal behavior that indicates more serious problems and responds to any employee's suggestions that he or she requires assistance and resources in handling problems interfering with work performance and overall well-being. The other obligation is to ensure that the supervisor and all others involved in any referral to the EAP maintain complete confidentiality to preserve the integrity and credibility of the program.

Employee Discipline

Although it may be uncomfortable, maintaining employee discipline is a prerequisite for organizational effectiveness and even viability in a competitive, uncertain environment. Every system must maintain internal order to survive and grow. An employee disciplinary process must be invoked in cases in which that basic order is threatened or disrupted by challenges to authority, insubordination, dangerous or abusive behavior to coworkers or clients, chronic violation of management policies, criminal activity, or other behavior that brings discredit or legal liability to the organization.

Progressive Discipline

There is a consensus among practitioners that a progressive discipline process is most effective, one in which there is a planned sequence of managerial responses of increasing severity to correct continuing violations of policy regarding acceptable employee conduct and performance standards. Its purpose is to give the employee subject to the disciplinary process several opportunities to correct the offensive behavior before the final irrevocable step of termination is invoked. It is in the best interests of both management and the employee to have the problem(s) resolved satisfactorily at one of the earlier stages in the process. When the infraction is of a less disruptive nature, such as chronic tardiness or absenteeism, employees may be motivated to take corrective action without additional incentives, having realized the risks entailed by continuing the challenged behavior. In other situations, progressive discipline may not be appropriate, for example, in response to outrageous behavior endangering the lives of others.

The progressive disciplinary process usually includes at least the following stages after the supervisor has identified a chronic or emerging behavior problem:
Oral warning (with a note to the employee's file)
Written warning and reprimand
Suspension with final warning
Termination

It should be noted that depending on the severity of the infraction, the employee's history of conduct, and his or her response to the disciplinary warning, steps in the process may be adjusted or omitted. However, management should ensure consistency of disciplinary response in like situations to avoid charges of favoritism or discriminatory treatment.

For example, a HIM release of information (ROI) specialist discovers she has sent health information requested by one patient to another patient in error. Instead of telling her supervisor about this breach, she prepares the information again and sends it to the right patient. While doing this, she tells one of her coworkers what happened but warns the coworker not to tell their supervisor. The coworker decides to let the supervisor know, as is part of the organization's HIPAA policy. The supervisor confronts the ROI specialist, talks with her about her failure to follow policy and procedure. She gives the specialist an oral warning and documents the incident in the specialist's file. Nine months later, the same ROI specialist makes a similar mistake, does not report it to her supervisor, but again tells a coworker. The coworker reports this to the supervisor. Before scheduling a meeting with the ROI specialist, the supervisor confers with an HR specialist and prepares a written warning and reprimand for the ROI specialist. The supervisor then schedules a meeting with the specialist. Before the meeting occurs, the specialist resigns, having found a new position in another organization.

Oral Warning
Progressive discipline is initiated by an oral warning from the supervisor to the employee about the offending behavior. The warning should include a candid description of the problem, what measures are required to correct it, and the deadlines or target dates to accomplish the behavior change. A summary of this conversation should be documented in the manager's records but not placed in the employee's permanent personnel file.

Written Warning and Reprimand
If the behavior is not corrected within the expected time frame, the next step is a written warning and reprimand. The written warning must clearly indicate the following information:
- Nature of the problem behavior
- Reference to the specific policy, guidelines, or standards violated
- Record of the date of the verbal warning

- Documentation of any critical incidents of the employee's behavior subsequent to the initial warning
- Restatement of the corrective action required
- Explanation of the consequences of failure to correct the sanctioned behavior

A separate statement reprimanding the employee for engaging in the offending behavior might be provided as well. The purpose of this stage is to put the employee clearly on notice that pursuing the unacceptable behavior or failing to take the corrective action specified will result in clear and certain disciplinary consequences, including termination if circumstances warrant it.

Suspension or Final Written Warning
Suspension from work without pay may be an appropriate "last resort" disciplinary action before termination. This step might be especially appropriate in situations involving the threat of violence or especially disruptive behavior because it provides a "cooling off" period for all parties involved. Suspension (usually for a 3- to 5-day period) also gives management an opportunity to do a thorough investigation of the facts of the situation when the employee's presence might interfere with that process. This should facilitate management's making a more informed decision about whether to proceed to termination or alternative disciplinary actions. It should be noted that suspension per se should not be invoked as a punishment of the employee. In fact, the employee facing further disciplinary action would probably be feeling considerable stress and might welcome a temporary separation from the workplace.

#5 Termination or Discharge
Termination should be reserved as a last resort when other good faith efforts have failed. It is only partly in jest that this step is referred to as the workplace "death penalty" because of the adverse personal, economic, and career consequences. Although in some extreme cases, it might be appropriate to skip other stages in the disciplinary process and proceed to termination, this should be done only with caution and strong justification because it appears to conflict with the "progressive" aspect of the process. Termination in one sense represents a system failure, a waste of organizational resources, even when the employee is given full and fair opportunity to correct the problem. Furthermore, termination decisions are subject to employee grievances and the risk of legal action. Consequently, this disciplinary action should never be taken without the most serious deliberation and after all other options have been explored.

Progressive discipline works well with violations of policy and rules of acceptable conduct but may not be appropriate or effective in problems involving skill deficiency or quality of work performance. In fact, invoking the disciplinary process may produce a negative reaction that would complicate efforts to help the employee develop a performance improvement plan. In-service education or focused counseling is likely to be more effective in these situations. It should be recognized that in some "gray-area" situations, the determination of whether to treat a performance problem as a disciplinary issue may be difficult. In these cases, the supervisor should seek advice from his or her manager and/or the designated HRM professional to make a fully informed decision. It should be emphasized that the objective of the disciplinary process is not punishment but correction and compliance.

Preventive discipline is another approach consistent with the purposes of the disciplinary process already discussed. A preventive approach encourages understanding of the rationale for and compliance with policies, standards, and rules so that significant violations of policy are avoided. These efforts might be most effectively incorporated within continuing team development activities, such as quality team leadership training. However, it is reasonable for the employer to expect self-discipline and that all employees will make reasonable efforts to comply with organizational policies, rules of conduct, and expected standards of performance.

Grievance Process

 DID YOU KNOW?

Did you know that a grievance procedure is a formal means of internal dispute resolution by which an employee may have his or her grievances addressed?

Management must ensure that employees have full access to an effective mechanism for expressing their concerns and the opportunity to obtain satisfaction when they believe that management has violated organization policy in taking some adverse action against them. The grievance process is provided to facilitate communication and problem solving when management or the supervisor is in conflict with the employee. A grievance is a formal charge that management has violated a specific management policy or provision of the written agreement (labor contract) that results in denial of some benefit to the employee or an infringement of some alleged right or privilege of employment. Not infrequently, a grievance is filed in response to a disciplinary action taken against the employee, especially in a unionized environment.

Employee grievance or complaint procedures are established because no matter how clearly defined or well communicated an organization's policies and procedures might be, they are always subject to misunderstanding, being applied inappropriately, overlooked, or, less frequently, intentionally disregarded. Questions of interpretation and application of policies or contract language often arise that require a systematic investigation and structure for problem resolution and redress.

Critical to an effective process for handling complaints and disagreements that arise over policies and rules governing the workplace is that prompt and fair action be taken on the basis of informed and balanced judgment. The employee must perceive that a fair hearing will be given and that the final judgment will be equitable and impartial. Ideally, employees who believe that they have been unfairly treated should be able to discuss their concerns with their supervisors. However, the employee's grievance is often directed against the behavior of the immediate supervisor. In these circumstances, it may be difficult to resolve the problem at this level in one-to-one negotiation. When this occurs, a progressive grievance process ensures that the employee will have a fair hearing, that the issue will be thoroughly and fairly investigated, and that a good faith effort will be made to resolve the grievance reasonably and efficiently at the lowest level possible.

The progressive grievance process gives an employee the opportunity to present his or her case to increasingly higher levels of management, recognizing that the problem may not be resolved at the supervisory level. The grievance is presented first to the immediate supervisor for resolution. Failing that, the case may proceed through a sequence of higher levels of authority in the hierarchy for subsequent review and decision. In the nonunion environment, the final decision is typically made at the top executive level, by (for example) the vice president for HRM/labor relations or ultimately the CEO.

In a unionized environment, the grievance process is negotiated as part of the labor contract and usually parallels the process for nonunion employees. The presentation of a grievance by an employee or a group of employees is a protected activity under the NLRA. This entails that the employer cannot fire, penalize, or otherwise discriminate against an employee because the employee has filed a grievance. If the employer takes such an action, the employee has the right to file a complaint with the NLRB.

The primary difference between the nonunion and the unionized environment is that the grievance procedure achieved through collective bargaining almost always includes external arbitration as the final stage. This entails vesting authority for ultimate disposition of the grievance in an impartial third party from outside the organization. The arbitrator, who is typically knowledgeable about the industry and experienced in the role, makes a judgment (award) that is "final and binding" on both sides. Because final arbitration places the decision beyond the control of either party and the costs are split equally between management and the union, there is some incentive to settle the grievance at a lower level in the process. Indeed, the logic of the process at least from management's perspective calls for resolution of the issues at the lowest possible level to avoid unnecessary costs and emotional escalation of the dispute.

Developing an Effective Grievance Policy

When communicating a grievance procedure through a policy statement, management must ensure that the following topics are clearly addressed:

- Stating the purpose and goals of the process.
- Identifying which complaints may be handled through the grievance process and which may not—for example, terminations for active drug abuse.
- Describing each stage of the process and the respective time frames for review and decision.
- Specifying who is to participate in the presentation of and response to the grievance.
- Describing the mediation and final arbitration process, if applicable.

- Communicating critical time limits for grievance handling to encourage prompt action, investigation, and resolution.
- Clarifying the responsibilities of management at each level for documentation, notification, and subsequent action.

A representative (and condensed) model of an effective grievance process for nonunionized employees that is appropriate for most health care organizations is provided next.

Sample Health Information Management Complaint Procedure
Goal of the Complaint Procedure

This procedure intends to create an avenue for problem resolution so that questions or conflicts can be investigated and resolved quickly, thoroughly, and within the appropriate organizational structure.

Valid Complaints

- Questions about or concerns with policies and procedures
- Disagreement with performance appraisal
- Concerns about the physical work environment
- Questions about or concerns with compensation and benefits management

Invalid Complaints

Appeal of termination for cause as specified in the organization's policies and procedures manual is an invalid complaint.

Procedure

- Employee orally presents complaint to immediate supervisor. *Note:* The employee may present complaint personally or may organize a group to present the complaint.
- The supervisor hears complaint and makes every effort to resolve the problem at this step. The supervisor documents the complaint, whether resolved or not, signs it, and then asks the employee or the employee group representative to sign so that the complaint is documented and clearly defined. *Note: If the employee or employee groups refuses to sign, then the supervisor documents this non action as well.*
- If the outlined plan or the resolution proposed by the supervisor is unsatisfactory to the employee or group, the supervisor sends a copy of the report to the HIM departmental director and requests a review of the complaint and outlined plan.
- The departmental director conducts a review and responds to the employee or employee group representative within 3 working days (or in whatever time is stated in the policy) with a plan for problem resolution.
- If, after this step, the employee or group still believes that the problem is not resolved, the next step is to present the issue to the HRM director or personnel action committee for consideration. This committee convenes in special session within 10 working days. The decision of this interdisciplinary committee is binding, and no other appeals will be heard. *Note*: This process would, of course, be modified depending on the organization-wide HRM policies governing nonunion complaint procedures.

SELF-ASSESSMENT QUIZ

23. The first step in a grievance procedure is arbitration in hopes that a reasonable agreement satisfying all parties can be met.
a. True
b. False

Compensation Management

Compensation management involves understanding the organization's wage and salary administration, payroll systems, employee benefits, knowledge of applicable federal and state legislation and regulation, and effective communication strategies. It can be argued that the most critical aspect of compensation management is to effectively communicate the goals, procedures, and constraints associated with the organization's compensation policies and to maintain the credibility of the system as being managed fairly and with integrity. Employees at the least expect to see some stable relationship between their training and experience, level of effort, productivity, and quality of performance (as their contribution) and their total compensation (as their return). Unfortunately, various constraints on the organization often make it difficult, if not impossible, for management to achieve, sustain, and demonstrate this relationship convincingly. The HIM director and management team are key in understanding the organization's compensation program and communicating compensation policies to department employees.

Compensation Management and Other Human Resource Management Functions

Compensation management is interdependent with all the other HRM functions, but especially with recruitment, performance appraisal, and retention of valuable employees. If the health care organization is not able to offer competitive salaries and benefit packages to the qualified applicants for health information services, nursing, physical therapy, occupational therapy, dietetics and food service, business office, and other positions, its recruitment efforts are considerably constrained. This affects not only recruitment but also the capacity of the organization to retain its high-performing employees. Inability to maintain competitive compensation almost inevitably has adverse effects on the quality of care provided. If employees have no faith in the fairness of the merit pay or pay-for-performance (P4P) program and believe instead that favoritism dominates annual pay decisions, this perception can stimulate or reinforce cynicism, frustration, and declining motivation and performance. When the department manager is committed to rewarding superior performers, to acknowledging performance improvement in underachievers, and to correcting historical salary inequities but is given no significant increase in the department's personnel budget, what are the likely effects on the manager's morale and credibility with the staff?

By fairly rewarding meritorious performance, productivity gains, extraordinary effort, notable commitment to customer (patient) service, and other desired outcomes, the organization is more likely to attain employee behaviors over the long term that are consistent with the organization's goals and strategic plans. Human resources planning, recruiting, selection, placement, career planning and development, and performance appraisal also contribute to furthering the organization's mission. However, compensation management programs are somewhat unique in the immediacy of their effects, positive and negative, on individual employees' perceptions of their value to the organization, motivation to perform, and sense of economic security and well-being.

Objectives of Compensation Management

The following objectives are anticipated as a consequence of effective compensation management:

- Attracting well-qualified applicants for positions when needed
- Retaining and motivating employees who are making positive contributions to the organization's mission
- Ensuring high-quality health care services are continually provided
- Rewarding desirable work behaviors and attitudes
- Controlling costs by managing human and financial resources effectively
- Complying with laws and regulations governing wage and salary administration and employee benefits
- Communicating the goals and policies supporting compensation management programs to sustain employees' understanding and acceptance
- Achieving a system that is perceived by the employees to be fairly and prudently managed

Job Evaluation

Job evaluation, a technical function at the foundation of the compensation management system, provides a formal procedure to determine the relative worth of each position in the organization. In other words, job evaluation results in the fair "pricing" of all jobs in the organization. To be effective, the job evaluation process must be based on a current and useful job description. In fact, job evaluation can be regarded as a process parallel to job analysis that translates a hierarchy of jobs into a pay structure for the organization. Because job evaluation requires special expertise and training, it is usually performed by human resource staff or contracted out to a consultant specializing in compensation systems.

It is critical, however, that the HIM director understands the organization's hierarchy of jobs and how the positions in the HIM department compare with similar positions in other departments. Understanding the process used by the organization to determine the worth of a job to the organization is important for the HIM director. The director has a responsibility to ensure that the pay and benefits established for health information services positions is equitable with that for comparable positions in the organization and competitive in the relevant labor market. If health information services managers and staff are paid significantly less than staff in similar positions within or external to their organization, the health information manager faces a major constraint in attracting and retaining well-qualified and highly motivated employees. This results in higher costs for recruitment, orientation, and training and the lost productivity because of excessive turnover and supervisory stress and burnout.

Job ranking, job grading or classification, factor comparison, and the point system are alternative methods used to evaluate jobs. Figure 16-15 compares these methods along two matrices: whether they consider the job as a whole or divide the job into factors for comparison and whether jobs are compared against one another or against some relevant standard.

Job Ranking

The simplest method, but also the least precise, is the ranking method. In this approach, whole jobs are ranked by comparing them with other positions within the organization on the basis of one or more key characteristics. A file clerk in the health information services department may be ranked near the bottom, whereas the diagnosis-related group coordinator is closer to the top. This ranking is based on the relative levels of responsibility of these positions and their impact on revenue generation. The ranking method is best used in organizations with a small number of positions.

Job Grading

Job grading is more sophisticated than ranking but not necessarily any more precise. This process classifies each job by assigning it to the narrative description of a grade that it most closely resembles. A common example of this method is the traditional civil service classification as used in the federal bureaucracy. This method is not precise because the jobs are compared and categorized on the basis of broad

	COMPARES EACH JOB AS A WHOLE	COMPARES EACH JOB ONE ELEMENT AT A TIME
Measures job against job	Ranking methods	Factor comparison methods
Measures job against predetermined scale	Classification or grade methods	Point methods

FIGURE 16-15 Job evaluation systems chart.

descriptions and judgments about overall similarity. This intuitive assignment process is likely to be least reliable when classifying new jobs that are unlike any of those already classified. The health information manager in an organization using this system must be knowledgeable about the distinctions between job grades to ensure that the jobs within the department are fairly classified and valued.

Factor Comparison

The factor comparison method requires identification of essential factors or elements common to all jobs and comparison of jobs on the basis of rating those elements, not the job as a whole. Factors typically applied in this method are as follows:

- Level of responsibility, including supervision
- Essential skills and knowledge
- Mental effort (demands)
- Physical effort
- Working conditions, including hazardous situations and confidentiality

When these factors have been determined, a set of key or benchmark jobs are identified on the basis that they reflect the array of jobs in the organization. Generally, the pay level of these jobs should reflect market wages for similar positions. The key jobs are then ranked by applying a rating scale to each of the common factors. By using a current average salary or prevailing market rate for each job, weighting the common elements, and distributing this wage rate among the job factors, a pay level or range is established for each job. Finally, all other jobs are evaluated and priced using the key jobs as benchmarks.

Point System

A point system evaluates jobs by analyzing key elements of the job and assigning point values to these factors on the basis of predetermined descriptive standards or criteria. The latter define each factor and specify the levels or degrees within the factor. For example, if education were one of the evaluation factors, degrees within this factor would be assigned to the level of education required for this position from doctoral degree or postdoctoral training (most points) to high school diploma or equivalent (least).

Points are then assigned to each degree within the factor for each job. Job grades or levels are established by specifying a range of evaluation scores for each grade. Pay ranges are then associated with each job grade by establishing arbitrary but reasonable bands (e.g., ± 15%) around some average or target wage, which might be based on a prevailing market rate for such jobs. Actual jobs in the unit are then matched to the pay grades and priced. By applying the linear regression technique, a statistical relationship between the point scores and target prices (wages) can be established. Current pay levels for all jobs or those being given priority attention can be plotted against their point scores to identify any "outliers," those significantly above or below the established pay range for that grade. This analysis could support managerial action to address any jobs whose pay levels seem inappropriate.

To manage effectively under the constraints associated with this method, the health information manager needs to be familiar with the logic of the pricing procedure, the factors and degrees identified, and the relationship between points assigned and pay ranges for the job grades. The appropriate compensation specialist within the HRM department should be a useful resource to the line manager who needs more information about the point system or other method of pricing jobs in the organization.

Many variations of these methods are tailored to meet the strategic goals, financial health, and environmental and market challenges faced by the organization. The Hay plan has been a popular proprietary method commonly used in health care organizations. This job evaluation method is a variation of the point and factor approach that uses a committee process for evaluating critical job factors to determine each job's relative worth.

Importance of Job Evaluation

Regardless of the specific method used, all job evaluation approaches seek to determine a position's relative worth to maintain pay equity within an organization and competitive compensation for target jobs within the relevant labor markets. No matter which method of job evaluation is in place, the responsible manager should review all wage rates for employees under the manager's authority and advocate adjustments for any pay levels that do not appear reasonable and fair compared with the job requirements. For example, health record analysts review the patient record after discharge and identify missing documents or data. The supervisor of the health record analysts might determine that workers doing comparable jobs in the outpatient surgery center were ranked two job grades above the health record analysts. Investigation reveals that the inpatient health record analyst position had been ranked lower because the current job description fails to reflect the medical terminology skills, data entry experience, and frequency of interaction between this position and the medical staff. After the job descriptions have been revised to better reflect the actual skills, knowledge, and responsibilities of this position, the job is reevaluated. The newly determined "price" might result in a pay adjustment for the health record analysts to correct this inequity.

Wage and Salary Surveys

Some organizations use data from wage and salary surveys to determine the market value of a given position. These surveys are often conducted by industry or professional associations, such as state hospital associations. In using this information in managing compensation, management determines how it wants to be positioned competitively relative to its labor markets. For example, if the director of health information services has had difficulty retaining coding analysts, she may argue on the basis of regional wage and salary data that her organization needs to bring the average salary for these positions above the regional mean salary.

The organization typically uses such data when overhauling its compensation program through a comprehensive job evaluation program. Management must be cautious in using survey data to ensure that the jobs included in the survey data are comparable to the target positions within the organization. A position of "data analyst" can represent quite different responsibilities, tasks, and skill requirements from one organization to another. Also, if the study was based on small samples of jobs or otherwise not representative of the relevant labor market, the survey pay ranges might provide misleading and unreliable benchmarks. It is also important to understand what other types of monetary compensation are being used by organizations; for example, productivity bonuses for coding analysts and/or medical transcriptionists, which may or may not be captured in a survey.

Another concern is that survey data should not necessarily be imposed as standards, overriding the organization's unique circumstances and compensation experience. For example, if the average salary data for clinical coders reflects a shortfall in supply of qualified applicants statewide, then this standard may be inappropriate (too high or too low) given their relative worth in the organization. When any unit within the workforce has been unionized, the negotiated wages in the contract covering that bargaining unit could have an escalator effect on comparable positions outside the bargaining unit. Negotiated wages that exceed their value relative to other nonunionized positions in the organization could cause an imbalance in the organization's wage and salary program that eventually should be identified and addressed through job evaluation.

Training and Development

Training and development is a critical function for maintaining the health care organization as a productive system in a competitive environment. The importance of training and development has grown with the explosion of information technology, telecommunications, and health-related technologies during the past several decades. The focus of training and development has traditionally been on individual skill building and growth of knowledge to facilitate upward mobility along some career track or pay scale. With the growth of quality management programs, employee empowerment, and innovative, "looser" forms of organizational design, such as the horizontal organization, the emphasis today is more on team development. In his model of the learning organization, Senge[56] defines the learning organization as one that "is continually expanding its capacity to create its future," and this requires commitment to five disciplines including team learning. Senge claims "team learning is vital because teams, not individuals, are the fundamental learning unit in modern organizations." HIM managers must look for opportunities to assure HIM staff are up-to-date with the changing knowledge and skills needed for a high-performing HIM department.

Rationale for In-Service Training and Development

Credible and cost-effective training programs must be linked to the mission and strategic goals of the organization, leadership priorities, environmental challenges, and needs for training and development identified at the operating level. Clearly, employee development is not only desirable but also a necessary investment for the long-term survival and growth of the organization. However, as aggressive competition and changes in federal health care policy constrain traditional revenue streams for many health care providers, management increasingly focuses on areas to control costs. Unfortunately, some organizations look first to cut back or eliminate educational and training programs on the basis that they are an expendable employee benefit. This view is shortsighted and likely to prove unwise in the long term. The failure to make sound investments in full development and use of its human resources threatens the organization's ability to retain well-qualified employees, respond effectively to environmental change and market pressures, and fully utilize technological developments.

Historically, hospitals have emphasized skill building and maintenance by keeping staff current with the latest clinical, technological, and regulatory developments affecting the health care professions through regular in-service, targeted, on-site training. Although training and development programs can entail a significant operating expense, failure to provide continuing investment in training can result in an even higher cost in the long term. For example, if the coding staff has not kept up to date with ICD-10-CM diagnosis-related group coding and reimbursement changes, a hospital could have huge revenue losses as a result of inappropriate code assignment or denied claims because of incorrect coding. Failure to keep abreast of changing regulatory and accreditation requirements may place an organization in danger of unfavorable accreditation decisions or sanctions. At the same time, management must practice systematic assessment to determine its most important training needs and match these needs with appropriate training and development opportunities, in-service and externally based. Furthermore, each training and development program and activity should be subject to cost-benefit consideration to maximize the net benefit of the total investment in this area.

Designing a Training Program
Needs Assessment

A needs assessment provides the foundation for a well-designed training program and should precede curricular development and scheduling. Programs already in place should be evaluated periodically to ensure that they continue to be relevant to identified training needs. Teaching and instructional methods should be reviewed to ensure that content is effectively presented and learning reinforced consistent with established principles and practices for the adult learner. Special attention should be given to incorporating new online technologies into the training programs to ensure an active learning experience for the employees. As discussed earlier, the importance of team building and team learning to new organization designs, relationships among coworkers, and work processes is likely to require the development of new training models and materials appropriate for team approaches (Box 16-11).

BOX 16-11

Potential Training Needs for the Health Information Services Organization

- Monitor professional journals and other relevant information sources to identify changing requirements in the collection, analysis, dissemination, and regulation of health information.
- Survey employees to assess their need for new skills or knowledge.
- Identify skill, knowledge, and interpersonal strengths and deficiencies within the performance appraisal and disciplinary processes.
- Access and analyze training need indicators from other sources including quality assessments, management and peer feedback, grievance reports, claims denial reports, productivity monitoring systems, and accreditation reviews.
- Observe and review employee participation in quality management activities and other team-based processes, presentations, and project reports.

Staff Development

After the formal orientation of the new or promoted employee as the employer's initial training investment, HIM managers must be responsive to any training need that is identified for the employee to remain competent, knowledgeable, and responsive to changes in clinical practice, technology, and regulatory and accrediting requirements. During the initial departmental or unit orientation, the manager should review the job description in detail and emphasize the expectations of performance for every significant job responsibility. The employee cannot be expected to perform at or above standards if those expectations and standards are not clearly communicated and reinforced. Many employees become frustrated, dissatisfied, and demotivated because they were reprimanded by a supervisor for performance deficiencies and failed expectations that were never adequately communicated. The supervisor must never assume that employees can "read the manager's mind" or intuitively understand the organizational priorities. Job responsibilities, work procedures, productivity standards, performance criteria, and management's goals and priorities must be communicated clearly, explicitly, and often. The supervisor has the responsibility to take the guesswork out of performance.

Training and development programs may be provided by in-house staff, by external consultants, by funding employees' participation in external educational programs, or by a combination of these approaches. Instructional methods and designs include but are not limited to the following:

- Traditional lecture and discussion
- Group role playing and problem solving
- In-service demonstrations by supervisors and experienced clinicians
- Professional mentoring and partnering
- Programmed instruction
- Online interactive learning (LAN or Internet based)
- Participation in part-time external degree or certificate programs
- Accredited continuing education, such as workshops and conferences

Career Planning

Career planning enables employees to be promoted from one job in a career path or ladder to another within an organization. It also provides an incentive for motivating and retaining effective performers and identifying potential managers and leaders for appropriate training and placement. It should support and encourage a learning culture in which all employees have the opportunity for challenging work, responsibilities, and social interaction that sustain job satisfaction, motivation to achieve, commitment to quality service, and desire for career-long learning and skill development. Effective career planning activities benefit the organization by ensuring a continuous supply of qualified workers to accomplish the objectives of the organization.

The health information manager can assist in career planning within the organization and within the profession. Executives from the organization can be asked to give presentations on developments in health information technology and systems and career and leadership opportunities within and outside the organization. Career counseling may be offered formally by the human resources staff, through an EAP, or less formally by the mentoring of veteran professionals and managers. Mentoring is an often underappreciated and rarely formalized professional development process that has considerable value-added for both the seasoned mentor and the new employee or manager.

An organization in-service resource center with current materials relevant to professional advancement and educational programs should be provided to supplement the employee's access to the wealth of resources and linkages available through the Internet. Another means of promoting career planning is to post job descriptions within the department so that job requirements and specifications for position openings are communicated and accessible to all employees. Trainee or transitional positions can be created for people who want to advance but lack the job experience to apply for a desirable, higher-level position.

Training and development programs are especially helpful in preventing obsolescence and career plateaus. Obsolescence threatens when employees no longer have the skills required to perform successfully in an ever-changing workplace, for example, medical transcriptionists who have not kept current with medical terminology or financial analysts who have not mastered the latest generation of electronic financial analysis software.

Career plateaus represent stages in an employee's career when a decline in performance or failure to achieve a newly imposed, higher standard of performance or level of commitment might place the employee at risk for demotion, termination, or career stagnation. The employee may be labeled fairly or not as a burnout, an individual who has peaked and will no longer be considered for promotional, professional development, or other career-building opportunities. Key signs of career plateaus are reluctance or refusal to adapt to new technology and insistence that "this is the way we've always done it here." These employees may lose interest in volunteering for professional growth activities and may require assertive supervision, including mandatory training in conjunction with realistic goal setting and career planning.

Employees at this stage who have a proven record of good performance and continuing value to the organization should be identified and given consideration for developmental opportunities as an investment in career prolongation. The costs of career rejuvenation are likely to be far less than the "hidden" costs of losing the potential benefits of work experience, expertise, professional relationships, and mentoring associated with the older employee at a plateau stage. However, supervisory management should candidly but humanely discuss future prospects within or outside the organization with employees who are not perceived by their managers to have much potential for career renewal and performance improvement. EAP counseling or outplacement services might be appropriate resources in these situations.

Employee Health, Safety, and Well-Being

The work environment consists of the physical, psychological, sociocultural, and political factors associated with a community of diverse individuals participating together more or less voluntarily to perform work to achieve their own personal and career objectives, consistent with furthering the mission and goals of the organization. These individuals are motivated by physiological, social, and psychological needs as well as by their economic objectives. Today's workforce expects the employer to provide a working environment that addresses this array of needs, one that is at least comfortable, safe, hygienic, and accessible.

The influence of social and psychological factors in the workplace on employees' job satisfaction, sense of well-being, and motivation has been a recurring focus of research and managerial concern.

Hertzberg demonstrated that some groups of professional employees regarded working conditions, including the physical and psychological factors of the work environment, as factors that, if not perceived to be adequate or sufficient, would act as "dissatisfiers" and erode employee motivation and performance. In contrast, the presence of a positive working environment would serve as a foundation necessary for management to address factors associated with job performance itself, that is, the "satisfiers,"[58] that could enhance employee motivation. This accords with our common work experience: when the work environment is perceived to be comfortable, pleasant, and safe, we are more likely to be satisfied with our job and organization and less likely to have our working conditions interfere with our performance and productivity.

Legal Requirements and Recommendations

Some of the laws and regulations previously discussed in this chapter affect the design, safety, and accessibility of the workplace. OSHA (1970) requires that employers furnish a workplace that is free from health and safety hazards that are likely to cause injury, harm, or death. The ADA expands the scope of organizations covered by such accessibility requirements to include most types of service establishments, including hospitals; rehabilitation facilities; physician's, dental, and other health providers' offices; pharmacies; insurance offices; banks; and virtually all others that provide "public accommodation."

The employer is required under ADA to make reasonable accommodations in the workplace to the individual's ADA-relevant disability, including physical disability, mental health, and other medical conditions. Adjustments to the workplace to accommodate the employee's disability are usually simple and inexpensive to implement without being disruptive to the normal work processes. Of course, if more elaborate facilities' renovation is required—for example, making restrooms ADA accessible for wheelchair users—the initial investment will benefit all future applicants, employees, clients, and visitors with disabilities using these facilities.

"Green Building" Design in Health Care

A relatively recent development related to employee health and satisfaction is the use of "green building" design and construction for health care facilities. "Green" or "high-performance" architectural design and construction approaches and standards have been applied for decades in commercial facilities but have only recently been implemented in health care. The argument for green buildings in industry has been based largely on cost efficiencies and environmental protection concerns. However, there is some evidence that green facilities also are associated with employee and customer or patient satisfaction, improved health, and enhanced performance and productivity. An architect's perspective on these relationships follows: "The most compelling argument for improving building efficiency and performance may be found in the relationship between occupant comfort and worker productivity [given]...that worker salaries comprise the major cost of operating a commercial building."[59]

Limited evidence is available beyond industry testimonials to support the link between green buildings and employee satisfaction and outcomes in health care. However, the Center for Health Design, a research and advocacy organization whose mission is to "transform health care settings...into healing environments that contribute to health outcomes through the creative use of evidence-based design,"[60] has funded research and advocacy efforts to encourage best practice in facilities design that will enhance employee satisfaction and performance and health care outcomes. This is an area that seems promising for health care system managers as they face the challenge of controlling costs, retaining productive and well-motivated employees, and increasing patient satisfaction and other desired performance measures.

FUTURE ISSUES

The opportunity to lead and manage human resources within a health information management context is an exciting and challenging endeavor. This chapter has provided an overview of the dynamic and complex field of HRM at both organizational and HIM departmental levels. The continuous rate of accelerating change of technological development in both information services and clinical knowledge in health care delivery, uncertainties about the implementation of new national health care policies, challenges to the national and local economies, continuing pressures for accountability on all health care providers to maintain quality improvement in health care delivery and doing so cost effectively—all these forces and others not foreseeable will only increase the complexity of managing human resources effectively, especially because priorities often differ among various key constituencies.

An effective health information leader and manager must proactively engage in lifelong learning to further develop technical HRM knowledge, leadership skills, and personal mindsets to become successful in managing an organization's most valuable asset: human resources.

CHAPTER REVIEW

1. What are four distinctive leadership roles?

2. Differentiate between transactional and transformational leadership.

3. The identification, measurement, and management of human performance in organizations is known as:
   a. employee coaching
   b. performance appraisal
   c. employee development
   d. performance improvement

4. What concepts or practices presented in the Human Resources chapter do you envision using in your current or future jobs?

5. When an employer makes sure that its coders are receiving pay similar to that received by coders in similar positions in other organizations, it is making sure that there is _____ in pay levels.

a. internal equity
b. egalitarianism
c. external equity
d. fairness

6. An employee's compensation can have three components: salary, incentive pay, and benefits.
   a. true
   b. false

7. The goal of _____ is to grow, enrich, create, and nurture more capable workers.
   a. career development
   b. training

8. The goal of _____ is improvement in performance.
   a. career development
   b. training

REFERENCES

1. Zuboff S: *In the age of the smart machine: the future of work and power,* New York, 1988, Basic Books.
2. Ostroff F: *The horizontal organization,* Oxford, 1999, Oxford University Press.
3. Staples J: Grist: A new type of threat, hbr.org/web/2009. Last accessed January 2014.
4. Ibid.
5. U.S. Census Bureau, News Release, *U.S. Department of Commerce, U.S. Hispanic population surpasses 45 million now 15 percent of total,* May 1, 2008: http://www.census.gov/newsroom/releases/archives/population/cb08-67.html. Last accessed January 2014.
6. U.S. Department of Labor: *Union members in 2004,* (USDL 05-112. 27), January 2005: http://www.bls.gov/news.release/History/union2_01272005.txt. Accessed January 2014.
7. Matthews RG, Maher K: Labor's PR problem: as more workers find unions weak and irrelevant, leaders seek to restore positive image, *Wall Street Journal,* August 15, 2005, p. B1.
8. Health Professions Education for the Future Schools in Service to the Nation: *Report of the Pew Health Professions Commission,* San Francisco, February 1993, p. 7.
9. Bennis WG, Nanus B: *Leaders: The strategies for taking charge,* New York, 1985, Harper & Row.
10. www.mastersinleadership.org. 21 Surprising facts about leadership research. Last accessed January 2014.
11. Stogdill RM: *Handbook of leadership: a survey of theory and research,* New York, 1974, Free Press.
12. Fiedler FE: *A theory of leadership effectiveness,* New York, 1967, McGraw-Hill.
13. Cartwright D, Zander A: *Group dynamics research and theory,* Evanston, IL, 1960, Row, Peterson.
14. Health Professions Education for the Future Schools in Service to the Nation, Report of the Pew Health Professions Commission, San Francisco, February 1993, p. 7.
15. Blake R, McCanse A: *Leadership dilemmas—grid solutions,* Houston, TX, 1991, Gulf Publishing.
16. Hersey P, Blanchard K: *Management of organization behavior: utilizing human resources,* ed 6, Englewood Cliffs, NJ, 1993, Prentice Hall.
17. Op. Cit. A Theory of Leadership Effectiveness.
18. Burns JM: *Leadership,* New York, 1978, Harper & Row.
19. Schein E: *Organizational culture and leadership,* San Francisco, 1985, Jossey-Bass.
20. Hunt JG, Conger TA: From where we sit: an assessment of transformational and charismatic leadership research, *Leadership Q* 10:335–343, 1988.
21. Rohrer W: The three T's of leadership: leadership theory revisited, *Top Health Record Pract:* 914–925, 1989.
22. Darr K: *Ethics in health services management,* ed 4, Baltimore, MD, 2005, Health Professions Press.
23. Op. Cit. Leadership.
24. American Health Information Management Association: Code of ethics, *American Health Information Management Association,* Chicago, 2004, Revised and approved by AHIMA House of Delegates on July 1, 2004.
25. Northouse PG: *Leadership: theory and practice,* ed 3, Thousand Oaks, CA, 2004, Sage.
26. Ibid.
27. Worthley JA: *The ethics of the ordinary in healthcare: concepts and cases,* Chicago, 1997, Health Administration Press.

28. Robbins SP: *Essentials of organizational behavior,* ed 8, Upper Saddle River, NJ, 2005, Pearson/Prentice Hall.

29. Rokeach M: *The nature of human values,* New York, 1973, Free Press.

30. Greenleaf RK: *Servant leadership: a journey into the nature of legitimate power and greatness,* New York, 1977, Paulist Press.

31. Morgan G: *Images of organization,* Thousand Oaks, CA, 1998, Sage.

32. Silva C, Carter N, and Beninger A: "Good intentions, imperfect execution? Women get fewer of the hot jobs to advance", *Catalyst* www.catalyst.org 2012.

33. U.S. Department of Labor, Bureau of Labor Statistics: *Women in the labor force: a datebook (Report No. 985),* Washington, DC, 2005, U.S. Department of Labor, Last accessed January 2014.

34. House, J: "Women reach a Milestone in job market", www.wsj.com updated 20 November 2013.

35. U.S. Census Bureau: *Men's and women's earnings by state: 2008 American community survey,* September 2008: http://www.census.gov/prod/2009pubs/acsbr08-3.pdf. Last accessed January 2014.

36. Day JC: Population projections of the United States by age, sex, race, and Hispanic origin: 1995 to 2050, *U.S. Bureau of the Census (Current Population Reports, P25-1130),* Washington, DC, 1996, U.S. Government Printing Office.

37. Op. Cit. "Women reach milestone in job market."

38. Gilbert JA, Stead BA, Ivancevich JM: Diversity management: a new organizational paradigm, *J Bus Ethics* 21:61–76, 1999.

39. Sanchez TR, Plawecki JA, Plawecki HM: The delivery of culturally sensitive health care to Native Americans, *J Holist Nurs* 14:295–307, 1996.

40. Ling, Sally: "Baby plan targets dads", South Florida Sun-Sentinel. (Accessed 05.11.04.)

41. The Joint Commission: One Renaissance Blvd, Oakbrook Terrace, IL 60181. www.jointcommission.org.

42. Liptak, Adam: "Supreme Court Finds Bias Against White Firefighters", The New York Times www.nytimes.com 6/30/2009.

43. U.S. Equal Employment Opportunity Commission www.eeoc.gov/facts/fs-sex.html. Last accessed October 2014.

44. Young J: *Equality of opportunity: the making of the Americans with Disabilities Act,* Washington, DC, 1997, National Council on Disability. Last accessed January 2014.

45. Kaufman L: Adjusting the legal bar for disability, *New York Times,* April 18, 1999. Last accessed October 2014.

46. Kahn S, Brown B, Zepke B et al.: Legal guide to human resources, Boston, 1996, Warren, Gorham & Lamont.

47. Gordon PL: *HR's role in HIPAA security compliance,* 2005: http://library.findlaw.com/2005/May/19/174544.html. Last accessed January 2014.

48. Leslie D: *Labor law in a nutshell,* St. Paul, MN, 1986, West.

49. Pfeffer J: *New directions for organization theory: problems and prospects,* New York, 1997, Oxford University Press.

50. Schein E: *Organizational culture and leadership,* San Francisco, 1985, Jossey-Bass.

51. Maslow A: A theory of human motivation, *Psychol Rev* 50:370–396, 1943.

52. Human Resource Reengineering Project Strategic Staffing Team, January 1999: http://www.beta.mmb.state.mn.us/doc/wfp/stratstf.pdf. Accessed November 16 2013.

53. Cascio W: *Applied psychology in personnel management,* Reston, VA, 1982, Reston.

54. Douglas J, Feld D, Asquith N: *Employment testing manual,* Boston, 1989, Warren, Gorham & Lamont 1989.

55. Cascio W: *Costing human resources: the financial impact of behavior in organizations,* Boston, 1991, PWS-KENT.

56. Senge P: *The fifth discipline,* New York, 1990, Doubleday/Currency.

57. "Why Microsoft Dumped Stack Ranking". Wall street journal. http:blogs.com/digits/2013/11/12. Last accessed January 2013.

58. Pugh D, Hickson D: Frederick Hertzberg in *Writers on organization,* Thousand Oaks, CA, 1997, Sage Publishing, p 105.

59. Lehrer D: Building a case for building performance, *AIA SF Newsletter,* August 2001: http://techstrategy.com/lineonline/aug01. Last accessed January 2014.

60. Center for Health Design: *Fact sheet, 2006.* http://www.healthdesign.org/aboutus/press/factsheets/. Last accessed January 2014.

CHAPTER 17

OPERATIONAL MANAGEMENT

Carol Venable • Anita Hazelwood

This chapter contains revised information from a previous edition authored by Peter M. Ginter and W. Jack Duncan.

ⓔ Student Study Guide activities for this chapter are available on the Evolve Learning Resources site for this textbook. Please visit http://evolve.elsevier.com/Abdelhak.

CHAPTER CONTENTS

OBJECTIVES

After reading this chapter, the reader will be able to do the following:

✓ Define key words in operational management.

✓ Describe various methods of organizing work.

✓ Define productivity, productivity standards, and a productive unit of work.

✓ Describe the various methods of measuring output to establish productivity standards.

✓ Apply the work simplification process to improve a system.

✓ Explain the concepts applied to the systems model.

✓ Utilize the systems analysis and design process to analyze and improve a system.

✓ Differentiate between the formal and informal organization.

✓ Introduce the concept of strategic management and how it concerns the achievement of a fit between the organization and its environment.

✓ Examine the characteristics of projects and project management.

✓ Utilize the project management process to achieve an organizational goal.

✓ Define reengineering.

✓ Outline the considerations that must be examined in designing work space for health information services.

✓ Apply the employee's individual needs to the design of the work space.

✓ Describe the components of a workstation.

KEY WORDS

Accent lighting
Adaptive strategies
Ambient lighting
American plan of office design
Benchmarking
Carpal tunnel syndrome
Critical path
Decision grid
Decision matrix
Decision table
Decision tree
Directional strategies
Ergonomics
External environmental analysis
Flow process chart
Flowchart

Functional strategies
Gantt chart
Informal or unwritten organization
Internal environmental analysis
Linkage strategies
Market entry strategy
Methods improvement
Mission
Movement diagram
Office landscaping
Open office design plan
Operation flowchart
Operational strategies
Organization chart
PERT network
Policies

Population
Procedures
Process
Productive unit of work
Productivity
Productivity standards
Project management
Proximity chart
Random selection
Reengineering
Relative humidity
Sample
Staff hour
Stopwatch study
Strategic control
Strategic implementation

System
Systems analysis and design
Systems flowchart
Task lighting
Task-ambient lighting
Trip frequency chart
Values
Vision
Work breakdown structures
Work distribution chart
Work sampling
Work simplification
Workstation

ABBREVIATIONS

ADA Americans with Disabilities Act
BLS Bureau of Labor Statistics
CMS Centers for Medicare and Medicaid Services
CTD Cumulative Trauma Disorder
CTS Carpal Tunnel Syndrome
DRG Diagnosis-Related Group
EPA Environmental Protection Agency

HIM Health Information Management
HVAC Heating, Ventilation, and Air-Conditioning
TJC The Joint Commission
NIOSH National Institute for Occupational Safety and Health
OSHA Occupational Safety and Health Act
RSI Repetitive Stress (or Strain) Injury

INTRODUCTION

Health information is not limited to one department or even to one organization. It is developed, disseminated, and used throughout organizations and communities. The effective use of health information depends on the systems that can create, analyze, disseminate, and use it. To be effective, the systems must effectively use the resources of people, processes, and equipment.

An important skill for the health information manager is the ability to analyze the processes that create and handle health information to be sure that they are functioning in the most efficient and effective manner. These processes could involve paper, computer systems, or both. There are numerous software programs available to assist with the various operational functions.

This chapter describes the tools that can help to analyze and improve the methods used in health information systems. The discussion begins at the micro level of individual jobs and procedures and moves through a midlevel look at systems analysis and design and organizational concepts to a larger macro or organization-wide level with the concepts of project management, reengineering, and design.

INDIVIDUAL WORK PROCESSES (MICRO LEVEL)

Organizing Work

The method of organizing, or allocating, the work among the employees depends somewhat on the type of organization and the nature of the work to be accomplished. Work division can be accomplished using any of the following methods:

Function—Similar tasks are performed by one unit within a department or an organization.

Project—A work unit performs all steps for a particular project (an example is a task force).

Product—In a manufacturing company, one unit performs all the work to produce a single product.

Territory—Sales forces are divided in this manner, with each representative responsible for a certain geographical area. Another example may be the organization of the hospital nursing service by patient care units.

Customer—This concept can be applied in a health information management (HIM) department when teams are organized to work on patient records of particular physicians.

Process—Similar work processes or procedures are grouped together and performed by a particular unit or group of employees.

Work processing can be further subdivided to the individual employee level. This subdivision can be classified into serial, parallel, and unit assembly (Figure 17-1).

Serial Work Division

The serial work division is one of consecutive handling of tasks. A series of small tasks is grouped together. Each task in the series is performed by a specialist in that type of work. The work passes from one employee to another until all tasks have been performed and the work is complete. An example of the serial arrangement is an assembly line in a factory, in which each step in the process is performed by a different person.

Parallel Work Division

Parallel work division demonstrates a concurrent method of handling work. One person performs a series of tasks. The tasks may be, but are not necessarily, related. Several employees may be performing the series of tasks at the same time. An example of this method in an HIM department is one in which four persons are employed to assemble and analyze patient records. Each employee assembles and analyzes records.

Unit Assembly Work Division

In unit assembly work division, each employee specializes in a particular task, as in serial work division, but the sequence of tasks on each unit is not identical. For example, in Figure 17-1, Poly Ester specializes in tasks 1 and 2. She may perform these tasks before anyone else works on a particular item, after tasks 3 and 4 are done, after tasks 5 and 6 are complete, or even after all steps—3, 4, 5, and 6—are done. A great deal of coordination is necessary in the unit assembly method because the amounts of time needed to perform individual tasks differ. The advantages and disadvantages of the three methods of organizing work are delineated in Table 17-1.

Work Distribution Chart

The **work distribution chart** is a useful tool that provides data to analyze the processes performed by a work group and the individual employee within the work group. Examination of the data assists in identifying problems but not solutions. The work distribution chart is a matrix that

Serial Work Division			
Employee	Raquel Simpson	Justin Walker	Cindy Dunnings
Processes	Tasks 1 & 2 on all records	Tasks 3 & 4 on all records	Tasks 5 & 6 on all records
Sequence	Before tasks 3, 4, 5, & 6	After tasks 1 & 2 and before tasks 5 & 6	After tasks 1, 2, 3, & 4

Parallel Work Division			
Employee	Raquel Simpson	Justin Walker	Cindy Dunnings
Processes	Tasks 1, 2, 3, & 4 on 1/3 of the records	Tasks 1, 2, 3, & 4 on 1/3 of the records	Tasks 1, 2, 3, & 4 on 1/3 of the records
Sequence	First to work on this group of records	First to work on this group of records	First to work on this group of records

Unit Assembly Work Division			
Employee	Raquel Simpson	Justin Walker	Cindy Dunnings
Processes	Tasks 1 & 2 on all records	Tasks 3 & 4 on all records	Tasks 5 & 6 on all records
Sequence	First to work on record, or after tasks 3 & 4, or after tasks 5 & 6, or after tasks 3, 4, 5, & 6.	First to work on record, or after tasks 1 & 2, or after tasks 5 & 6, or after tasks 1, 2, 5, & 6.	First to work on record, or after tasks 1 & 2, or after tasks 3 & 4, or after tasks 1, 2, 3, & 4.

FIGURE 17-1 Methods of organizing work.

TABLE 17-1   Advantages and Disadvantages of Work Division Methods

Serial	Parallel	Unit Assembly
Advantages		
Employees are skilled in their own tasks.	Because employees know all functions, absences and volume fluctuations are managed.	Saves time; employees can work on the item without waiting for others to finish their tasks.
Causes of delays are easily identified.	Work is more interesting to the staff because they see it through to completion.	Employees are skilled at their own tasks, and the method encompasses a wider variety of functions.
If one step in the process requires a specialized skill or use of specialized equipment, fewer skilled staff or pieces of equipment are needed.		
Disadvantages		
Employee absences can cause backlogs.	If one or more of the steps require specialized skills or equipment, more skilled staff or pieces of equipment are needed, making the process more expensive.	Work can become boring because employees' work has limited variety and scope.
Slow employees can delay the final product.	Recruiting and training of staff to complete multiple functions may be difficult.	Difficult to use unless work can be easily divided into tasks that do not depend on the results of other tasks.
Work can become boring because employees' work has limited variety and scope.		Coordination of work flow and scheduling of completion of individual items would be difficult.
The work items are handled numerous times because each step is performed by different employees. This may increase the total processing time for all steps.		

displays the tasks being performed in a work group, the employees who perform them, and the amount of time spent on each task by each employee and the work unit as a whole.

Preparation of the work distribution chart requires the following steps:

Each employee prepares a task list (Figure 17-2). The employee should be instructed that the task list should reflect what the employee actually does, not what he or she should be doing. To gain cooperation from the employees, the supervisor should explain the purpose of gathering these data. The purpose is not punitive but to analyze how time is spent in the work group to improve the jobs. Over a 1-week period, each employee lists the tasks he or she performs and the amount of time spent on each. The task statements should be brief and specific and include no more than 15 statements. The duties should be listed in order of importance. Every minute need not be accounted for. Hours should be entered to the nearest 15 minutes, and breaks and other nonproductive time should be included in a miscellaneous category.

Supervisor prepares a list of the major activities of the work group (Figure 17-3). This is a list of general categories into which all activities of the employees can be classified. As a rule, no more than 10 activities should be listed. They should be listed in order of importance with the most

important listed first. When the activity list is completed, each task shown on the individual employee's task lists should be classified under one of the major activities. It may be necessary to add a miscellaneous category to accommodate all the tasks that may not fall under one of the major activities of the section.

Supervisor combines the employee task list and the activity list into the work distribution chart (Figure 17-4). The work distribution chart is complete when the following entries are made:

- The major activities are listed in the left-hand column.
- The employees are listed across the top of the chart; the columns should be assigned in the order of responsibility starting with the department head or supervisor at the left.
- The tasks performed by each employee, and the amount of time required for the performance of each task are listed in the column under the employee's name.
- The total time spent on each major activity by all employees is recorded in the right-hand column.

Analysis of the work distribution chart can answer the following questions:

- ***What tasks are employees performing? Are these tasks important to achieving organizational goals?*** Question the total time of the group on a particular activity and then that of individual employees. Are the activities that

FIGURE 17-2 Task list.

Name of employee: Janet Doe
Job title: Incomplete Medical Records Clerk
Department/area: Incomplete Medical Records Area
Date compiled: 02/01/XX-02/05/XX

Task number	Activities	Hours per week	Posted to activity #
1.	Designating records for physicians to complete	10	
2.	Checking physicians' completed records after completion	6	
3.	Updating the deficiency analysis tracking system	4	
4.	Preparing the delinquent records list	4	
5.	Compiling delinquent statistics for the medical staff	2	
6.	Notifying physicians of delinquencies	5	
7.	Faxing copies of discharge summaries and operative reports to designated physicians	3	
8.	Miscellaneous (lunch breaks, other assigned tasks)	6	

FIGURE 17-3 Activity list.

Department: Health Information Management
Area: Incomplete Medical Records Area
Number of employees: 4

Task number	Activities	Hours per week
1.	Designating records for physicians to complete	21
2.	Analyzing completed records and updating computer system/folder	24
3.	Preparing delinquent list	7
4.	Distributing completed discharge summaries and operative reports	21
5.	Filing/storing discharge summaries and operative reports in medical records	13
6.	Supervising employees	20
7.	Auditing incomplete medical records	7
8.	Analyzing records from the OB-GYN unit	9
9.	Answering the telephone	12
10.	Miscellaneous incomplete area activities and nonproductive time	26
	Total Hours	160

TASKS	SUPERVISOR	HR	JANET DOE	HR	CLERK 3	HR	CLERK 4	HR	TOTAL HOURS
Supervise	Supervisory duties	20							20
Access computerized delinquent list; makes copies to distribute			Accesses computerized delinquent list; makes copies to distribute	10	Accesses computerized delinquent list; makes copies to distribute	5	Accesses computerized delinquent list; makes copies to distribute	6	21
Analysis of completed records			Checks each completed record; puts on shelf for filing; makes changes in computer	10	Checks each completed record; puts on shelf for filing; makes changes in computer	8	Checks each completed record; puts on shelf for filing; makes changes in computer	6	24
Access computerized delinquent list to printing; verifies completion of records			Prints delinquent list; checks for accuracy; makes copies	6	Distributes new delinquent lists to administrative staff	1			7
Copy and distribute reports	Receives transcribed reports; makes copies and distributes to originating physician	4	Receives transcribed reports; makes copies and distributes to originating physician; notifies physicians of deficiencies	8			Receives transcribed reports; makes copies and distributes to originating physician	9	21
Filing					Files transcribed reports	10	Files transcribed reports	3	13
Audit of files	Audit of records for quality	4			Physical audit of files	3			7
Log records received					Analyzes records from OB-GYN	6	Analyzes records from OB-GYN	3	9
Answer phone	Manages complaints from physicians	4					Receives physicians' requests to gather records for completion	8	12
Miscellaneous	Orders supplies; attends/conducts meetings; breaks	8	Assists supervisor; breaks	6	Gathers records for medical staff committee; breaks	7	Messenger duties; breaks	5	26
Total		40		40		40		40	160

FIGURE 17-4 Work distribution chart.

take the most time really the most important ones? Is a lot of time spent redoing work that had errors? Handling complaints?

- *How are tasks distributed among employees of the work group?* Does each employee do a little bit of one task?

Does any one employee do the bulk of one task, while the others are not using their time effectively?

- *Are employees' qualifications being used?* Are highly skilled, highly paid employees using those qualifications? For example, are medical transcriptionists filing the reports that they type? On the other hand, are employees doing tasks that they are not qualified to do—for example, does a person with only knowledge of medical terminology assign codes to Medicare patients' diagnoses and procedures?

- **How are individual jobs constructed?** Are employees performing too many unrelated tasks, or are they doing one thing all day long? Performing too many unrelated tasks wastes effort and is costly. Changing from one task to another decreases productivity because of the time spent setting up and ending each task. The monotony of performing one or a few tasks for most of the work time causes boredom and, possibly, dissatisfaction with the job.

Analysis of the work distribution chart may also aid the manager in choosing one of the types of work division (serial, parallel, or unit assembly). By including the number of units produced in the work distribution chart, managers can use the chart to establish productivity standards in an organization.

Productivity

Productivity is the process of converting an organization's resources (labor, capital, materials, and technology) into products and services that meet the organization's goals. Productivity is also defined as the number of items produced per staff hour that meet established levels of quality.[1] A productive organization is one that produces quality products or services with the least expenditure of resources.

Productivity is often expressed as a ratio:

$$\frac{\text{Output (services or products)}}{\text{Input (resources consumed)}}$$

Or

$$\frac{\text{Quantity and quality}}{\text{Staff hours}}$$

Some related definitions are important to the understanding of productivity. A staff hour is defined as 60 minutes of time during which an employee is working on a task or a particular function and being paid for that work. A productive unit of work is an item produced that meets established levels of quality. The quality (or accuracy) level is an important aspect of this definition. When a product does not meet the quality level, it often has to be redone. Therefore, if products that do not meet the quality level were counted as output, the number of products would be inflated because of counting the rework and the original work as outputs. Quantity, in the preceding ratio, generally refers to the number of work units that are produced by an employee who is trained and who is working at a normal pace. Examples of outputs in an HIM department are coded patient data, completed response to a request for information, and a transcribed report.

Productivity Standards

Productivity (also known as performance or work) standards are the tools that are used to specify the expected performance and to measure actual performance. Productivity standards have many uses in managing an HIM department. They can assist in determining the number of personnel and supplies and the amount of equipment that are necessary to accomplish the projected workload; in scheduling completion and distribution of tasks; in evaluating proposed changes in processes or systems to see whether a savings in personnel time would occur; in setting goals for a work group or individual employee; and in evaluating the performance of a work group or individual employee. Productivity standards can also be used to determine the actual cost of producing a given product or service.

Setting Productivity Standards
Getting Started

When a productivity program is designed, the work requirements and resources of the department must be clearly understood and the following should be addressed:

- All departmental activities should be identified and defined.
- An area of productivity focus should be selected.
- For the specific functions that are studied, quantity and quality must be defined.
- Current and past performance should be reviewed.
- Staff members should be involved in the establishment of the expectations of the program.
- Reporting mechanisms should be developed, and then performance should be monitored.
- As a final step, the improvements identified should be implemented.

Measuring Input

To set productivity standards, certain determinations must be made. First, the methods of quantifying inputs must be determined. This is usually in terms of employee time expressed in paid staff hours worked. Second, the unit of work for measuring output must be established. For given processes, this can take various forms. For example, for the coding function, should the number of codes be counted or the number of records? Should the output be classified by level of difficulty (e.g., outpatient vs. inpatient, Medicare vs. non-Medicare)?

Measuring Output

Actual Performance. Various methods are used to measure output, ranging from using past performance data to using time studies and work sampling. Using data from actual performance is the most common method of measuring output, as well as the easiest, quickest, and least expensive. Data can be collected by the organization's own staff; therefore, specialists are not needed. Methods used to collect this information include employee-reported logs in the form of time ladders or diaries, as shown in Figure 17-5. Equipment can also be used to count items of work; for example, dictation equipment can record the number of minutes transcribed or characters entered.

Work Sampling. Work sampling is another method of collecting actual performance data. This method is based on the statistical laws of probability. The research concepts

Employee's name: Mary Knowles   Date: July 1, 20xx
Employee's job: Medical Record analyst

Time	Task	Time	Task
8:00	Receive records from floor	3:20	
8:05	Place discharged records (40) in alphabetical order	3:25	
8:10		3:30	Input deficiencies into computer system
8:15	Assign service assignment on each record	3:35	
8:20		3:40	
8:25		3:45	
8:30	Place each record in order	3:50	
		3:55	
10:30	Analyze records for deficiencies	4:00	Place records in doctors' incomplete chart area
10:35		4:05	
10:40		4:10	
		4:15	
11:00	Coffee break	4:20	Clean up work area
11:05		4:25	
11:10		4:30	Head for home
11:15	Continue record analysis		
12:30	Lunch break		
1:30	Continue record analysis		
3:00	Coffee break		
3:05			
3:10			
3:15	Search for reports and append to records		

FIGURE 17-5 Time ladder.

of **population**, **random selection**, and **sample** must be comprehended to understand the work sampling method.

Population. All items or members of the group to be studied.

Sample. The group of items chosen to represent the whole population. The size of the sample is important because it must be large enough to represent all members of the group but small enough to be manageable and cost effective.

Random selection. The method of choosing the sample that gives each item in the population an equal chance of being chosen.

In work sampling, the supervisor observes employees at times randomly selected, as opposed to continuous, all-day observations, and records the task the employee is doing at the time of the observation. The observations are tallied to determine the percentage of all work time (the population) spent on each task. Combining these percentages with the number of items produced determines the productivity standards for these tasks. Advantages of the sampling method as opposed to the use of continuous observations are as follows:

- Detailed information can be gathered that might otherwise be difficult to obtain by using continuous observations.
- Data can be obtained in less time and with less expense by using the sampling method.
- Personnel who are being studied complain less often than individuals being observed continuously.
- Data can be easily obtained without any interruption of the normal work routine by using the sampling method.
- The sampling method is likely to produce more accurate results than continuous observations.

Using actual performance data has several problems. These productivity standards are based on existing procedures, processes, employee performance, and qualifications, all of which might not be the most effective for this **process**. Therefore, expected results would be based on poor performance and ineffective processes.

Benchmarking. **Benchmarking**, another method of setting standards, is the comparison of one organization's performance with that of another organization that is known to be excellent in that area. Benchmarking is beneficial because it is more than comparing productivity. It involves discovering how the benchmark organization achieves its goals and then incorporating these methods into the other organization. The aim of benchmarking is the improvement of the organization's processes.

Stopwatch or *time-and-motion.* **Stopwatch** or time-and-motion studies are the most expensive techniques for setting productivity standards. Stopwatch studies require a skilled analyst to observe the employee performing the task and to record stop and start times for each portion of the task. The selection of the employee to be observed is an important element of this technique. The employee should be one who performs the task at an average speed, not the fastest or the slowest. This method is a poor public relations tool. Having to watch every move an individual makes can be unsettling and puts the individual on edge.

Whichever method is used to collect data and set productivity standards, the concept of quality cannot be overlooked. Techniques for ensuring the expected quality level of the output must be built into the methods for measuring the quantity.

Efficiency is as important in setting work standards as it is elsewhere in the organization. If it becomes too expensive to set standards and measure work, the goal of productivity monitoring is defeated.

Productivity standards must be understandable, realistic, reliable, and attainable under normal working conditions. Clear communication between employers and employees is important for the program to be a success. An effective productivity management program is based on accurate, reliable standards that have earned credibility with the employee.

Increasing Productivity

Productivity can be increased through the following methods:

- Increasing output while holding input constant
- Decreasing input (resources) while maintaining the same level of output
- Increasing output while decreasing resources
- Increasing resources and output but with a proportionately greater increase in output
- Decreasing output and resources with a proportionately greater decrease in resources

Research findings on productivity improvement show the following:[2]

- Productivity goes up when it is measured.
- Productivity improves as it becomes a primary goal of management.
- Productivity increases as managers and staff are held accountable for its measurement and evaluation.
- Productivity increases as its benefits are shared with the employees responsible for the increase.
- Productivity increases as employees are rewarded for extra output.
- Productivity increases as the resources allocated are in direct proportion to the productivity improvement potential.

Implementing a Productivity Program

For the program to be useful, an organization needs a focused approach to improving productivity. A productivity improvement program needs well-defined goals. To be effective, as many employees as possible should be involved in the development of the program. Organizational goals should be integrated with employee goals. All employees should be part of the program and should be accountable for productivity improvement in their own work areas. Employees should share in the benefits of improved productivity and should be rewarded and reinforced for their contributions. Implementing a productivity improvement program is a six-step process.

1. Identify an area in the organization for improvement.
2. Establish a unit of measurement (productivity ratio) and measure current performance in that area.

Productivity Improvement Area:	Coding
Productivity Ratio	Number of records coded per man hour
Current Level of Productivity	6 correctly coded patient records per man hour
Productivity Objective	10 correctly coded patient records per man hour
Improvement Strategy	Weekly educational programs on coding. Each coder will attend a coding seminar each year.
Time Frame	Six months
Checkpoints	Monthly
Evaluation and Feedback	Measure productivity; if level meets goal, praise and congratulate. Establish incentive pay program.

FIGURE 17-6 Productivity improvement program for coding.

3. Develop a measurable productivity objective.
4. Identify a strategy for meeting the objective.
5. Establish time frames and identify checkpoints.
6. Analyze results and provide feedback.

An example of a productivity improvement program in an HIM department is shown in Figure 17-6.

Monitoring and Improving Performance
The department head or supervisor should develop a mechanism for analyzing the productivity of each employee and a means for summarizing overall section or departmental productivity. Depending on the specific management needs, reporting may be done on a daily, weekly, or monthly basis.

After overall productivity is established, management should review the areas that are in need of improvement. This improvement may be in the form of additional staff or training, improvement of work methods or individual work performance, or a change in the structure of the section or department. Time management and motivational techniques for employees may also prove to be beneficial in many cases.

Motivation
Managers in the workplace today often forget how important a role motivation plays with their employees. To be effective, managers need to understand what motivates employees in the context of the job they perform in the department or facility. Greater productivity and increased employee morale is a natural result of properly motivated employees. In general, motivation for better job performance depends on job satisfaction, individual recognition, personal achievement, and professional growth.

According to Kovach,[3] managers should ask themselves the following 10 questions when attempting to provide a more positive motivational climate for employees:
Do you personally thank staff for a job well done?
Is feedback timely and specific?
Do you make time to meet with and listen to staff on a regular basis?
Is your workplace open, trusting, and fun?
Do you encourage and reward initiative and new ideas?
Do you share information about your organization with staff on a regular basis?

Do you involve staff in decisions, especially those that will affect them?
Do you provide staff with a sense of ownership of their jobs and the unit as a whole?
Do you give associates the chance to succeed?
Do you reward staff on the basis of their performance?[3]

Aside from motivational theories and information published by notable authors such as Douglas McGregor, Frederick Herzberg, and Abraham Maslow, managers must understand that they are dealing with human beings and that basically, motivation involves getting people to do something simply because they want to do it. The manager's reward is productive employees.

SELF-ASSESSMENT QUIZ

1. Productivity standards are also known as _____ standards.
2. When setting productivity standards, what determinations should be made?
3. _____ is a method of collecting performance data based on the statistical laws of probability.
4. (Quantity + Quality)/staff hours is an expression of _____.

DID YOU KNOW?

- Productivity standards are tools that are used to specify expected performance and to measure actual performance.
- To set productivity standards, the methods of quantifying inputs must be determined and the unit of work for measuring output must be established.
- Measuring output or actual performance can be accomplished by:
  - Using data from actual performance
  - Work sampling
  - Random sample
  - Benchmarking
  - Stopwatch or time-and-motion studies
- Productivity standards must be understandable, realistic, reliable, and attainable.

Work Simplification or Methods Improvement

An organizational goal is to provide the best service or make the best product with the least expenditure of resources while maintaining a healthy and contented workforce. The effectiveness of the individual employee depends on the effectiveness of the processes used. Work simplification, sometimes called methods improvement, is an organized approach to determine how to accomplish a task with less effort in less time or at a lower cost while maintaining or improving the quality of the outcome. It uses commonsense concepts to eliminate waste of time, energy, material, equipment, and space when performing work processes. Sometimes work simplification is misunderstood to mean work speed up. When work simplification tools are correctly used, the rate of production is enhanced by performing only the essential steps in the best way possible at a standard pace.

The fundamental objectives of work simplification are as follows:

- Simplify
- Eliminate
- Combine
- Improve

The simplest means of performing the work is usually the easiest and most practical.

Questioning is fundamental to improving work processes. The first question that must be asked is, "Does this process assist in achieving the organization's goals?" When the answer is no, the process should be eliminated. Remember to question the statement, "That's the way it has always been done." The questions of who, what, when, where, and how must be answered.

The philosophy of work simplification is that there is always a better way to perform every task. The statement that the process has always been done this way is a red flag that the process could use change and that the employee does not understand why the procedures are done in this way. The goal of a work simplification program is to increase efficiency through the elimination of unnecessary work and through the optimal structure of necessary work.

The individual who performs the tasks must be given significant attention when individual jobs are dissected. Employees need to be involved in the process because they are the experts in their own work processes. If they are involved in change, they are more likely to accept it. However, care must be taken so that the content of the job does not become oversimplified and boring.

The steps in the work simplification method are similar to those in the scientific method:

Identify a problem area or select a work process or function to improve.
Gather data on the problem.
Organize, analyze, and challenge the data gathered on the problem.
Formulate alternative solutions or improvements.
Select or develop the improved method.
Implement the improved method and evaluate the effectiveness of the improvement through follow-up.

Identifying a Problem Area or Selecting a Work Process or Function to Improve

Identification of a problem is not an easy task. A competent manager must be able to differentiate between a symptom and its cause or problem. What appears to be the problem may only be a symptom. This step is essential because if the symptom's cause is not correctly identified, the problem will not be solved, and the symptom may be only temporarily eliminated.

In health care, distinguishing between symptoms and diagnoses (problems) is a familiar process. The patient comes to the emergency department with the symptom of abdominal pain. On testing and evaluation, the patient is diagnosed with acute appendicitis. When the cause of the abdominal pain is identified, treatment can be initiated to remedy the symptom.

By use of the same approach of symptom versus diagnosis, common work symptoms can be examined to find the diagnosis or problem. For example, the symptom of poor productivity may be traced to the problem of inefficient work flow. High employee turnover may be a symptom of low morale caused by poor workload distribution.

The following list indicates potential problems that should be investigated:
- Duplication of work processes
- Overlapping of responsibilities
- Frequent backtracking
- Inconsistencies
- Frequent delays and interruptions
- Poor workload distribution (congestion and clutter)
- Inaccuracies and errors
- Lack of controls
- Lack of instructions or procedures
- Low employee morale
- High absenteeism or turnover
- Complaints from customers and employees
- Apparent waste of materials, effort, personnel, time, and space
- Obvious fatigue
- Poor safety record
- Excessive time required to carry out an activity in comparison with results achieved
- Chronic backlog
- Regular overtime

Managers need to be sensitive to cues from their employees and their surroundings. When managers are not responsive to these cues, a potential problem may develop into a crisis situation. After a sign has been recognized as a potential problem, the manager must proceed to investigate and move to resolution of the problem. Nothing is more discouraging to employees than to raise a concern and have no response from management. After a while, employees complain among themselves and fail to make management aware of problem areas.

Another approach to selecting an area of work to be simplified is to review areas with high labor requirements and a large number of diverse work activities and those in which excessive time is needed to perform the work, the costs are high, or the end product is inadequate.

Gathering Data About the Problem

Data collection methods vary with the type of problem and the work performed. Data-gathering methods include the collection of blank forms used in the process, completed forms, office or work layout, organizational charts, job descriptions, work logs, manuals/standards/procedures, interviews with employees, and observation. Additional facts may be obtained from supervisory staff.

The key to gathering data is to ask the right questions to find out how the work is being performed. The following are key questions to ask:

- Why is this process performed? How does it move the organization toward achievement of its goals?
- Who does the work? Why this particular individual? What are the individual's qualifications for performing these processes?
- What work is currently being done and why is it being done?
- When (in what sequence) is the work being performed and why in this manner?
- Where is the work being performed and why there?
- How is the work being done? Why is it being done this way? Is there a better way to achieve the same result?
- At what rate does the work flow to the employee? Is the rate consistent?

A flow process chart can be used to analyze procedures and to determine opportunities for improvement through eliminating, combining, or resequencing any part of the process.

Flow Process Chart

A **flow process chart** is a tool used to collect information on the steps of a work process and to analyze and improve the process. It is especially helpful in analyzing manual operations. The flow process chart is used to show the steps or actions involved with respect to a single person (job), a single material, or a single form.

There are several basic steps in constructing a flow process chart:

- Accurately describe the job or activity that is being studied, for example, "Processing a request for copies of medical records." Flow process charts may be constructed for current or proposed jobs.
- Select the employee, material, or form to be followed.
- Determine the beginning and ending points of the process to be studied.
- List each step in the procedure or job. A separate line should be used for each step, no matter how insignificant it may seem.
- Select the symbol that best describes the activity. The symbols used to represent each step in the process are shown in Figure 17-7. The symbols that represent each step are connected with a line to facilitate analysis.
- Indicate distance traveled if the transportation symbol is selected. The amount of time should be indicated when there is a delay in the process or whenever indicating the time would be of some use in analyzing the process.
- Each of the operations should be counted and entered in the summary box. The distance traveled and the minutes delayed should also be entered.

Each step in the process should be subjected to the following questions:

- Is that particular step necessary or of value?
- Can the step be eliminated?
- Can the step be streamlined or combined with another step?
- Is the step properly sequenced within the process?

This analysis of the flow process chart can identify problems such as duplication of effort, too much travel time from one workstation to another, and delays in transferring work.

Figure 17-8 shows a completed flow process chart for a current and a proposed release-of-information function.

Flowcharts

Additional types of **flowcharts** are used to verify and obtain information about how a procedure is being performed. Flowcharts are essentially road maps that show the logical steps and the sequence involved in a procedure. Flowcharts are used to

SYMBOL	PROCESS	END RESULT	EXAMPLE
○	Operation Make-ready	Get-ready to do	Sorting
○	Operation Do	Produces or accomplishes	Coding, data entry
➡	Transportation	Moves	Walking
▽	Storage	Keeps	Object placed in permanent storage
■	Inspection	Verifies	Proofreading
▷	Delay	Interfaces	Object is in temporary storage or waiting

FIGURE 17-7 Flow process chart symbols.

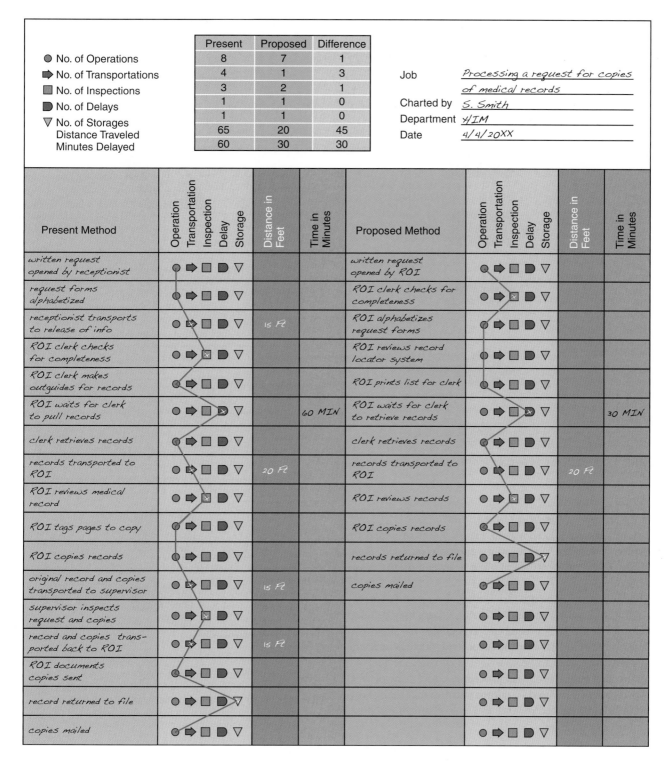

FIGURE 17-8 Flow process chart for release of information (ROI).

depict all levels of operations from whole systems that involve many departments and people, as in a systems flowchart, to the work of one person or procedure, as in an operations or procedure flowchart. The systems flowchart depicts the flow of data through all or part of the system, the various operations that take place within the system, and the files that are used to produce various reports or documents. Figure 17-9 shows an example of a systems flowchart for the master patient index.

Operation or Procedure Flowchart

The operation flowchart is a graphical representation of the logical sequence of activities in a procedure. In addition, it points out the decision points encountered in carrying out that function. The operation flowchart should specify how a function is performed, not the methods used. This type of flowchart is a superb communication tool between employees and management (Figure 17-10).

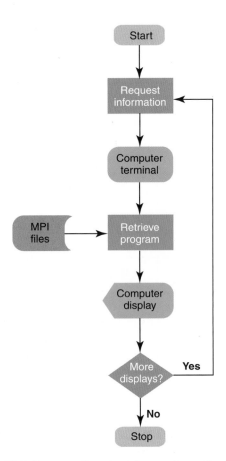

FIGURE 17-9 Systems flowchart for master patient index.

Flowchart Symbols and Guidelines

The standard symbols shown in Figure 17-11 are used to construct flowcharts. When unique symbols are used, their meaning should be identified in a key or legend on the flowchart (Box 17-1).

The flowchart can be used for both planning and controlling activities. As a planning tool, the flowchart may be used to help develop a new procedure. The chart will show the linkage points among the various aspects of the task and will show areas that need to be changed. It can also be used to compare current and proposed procedures. As a control tool, the flowchart can be used to compare the actual work flow with the original procedure and also as a means of constant evaluation of processes.

Movement Diagrams

The **movement diagram**, sometimes called a layout flowchart, represents graphically the physical environment in which the processes are performed. The purpose of a movement diagram is to depict the flow of work activities through the desks and equipment. A movement diagram can show movement of paper or an employee. This type of chart can be beneficial in identifying the problem of backtracking or bottlenecks in procedures. With a graphical display of the physical layout, a more efficient route for accomplishment of the task can be achieved.

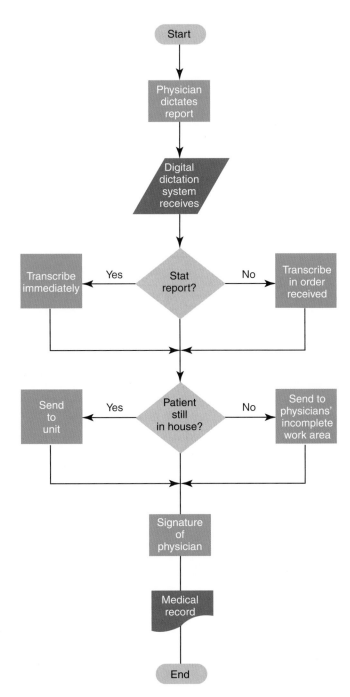

FIGURE 17-10 Operation flowchart for transcription.

Movement diagrams or layout flowcharts are especially useful in the analysis of manual systems (Figure 17-12).

Organizing and Analyzing Data Gathered on the Problem

The third step of the process entails organizing and analyzing the facts or data obtained from step 2. As with all steps in work simplification, the employees who perform the work need to be included in this process.

Data can be organized in many ways. One is by chronological sequence of the work under study. Another is by

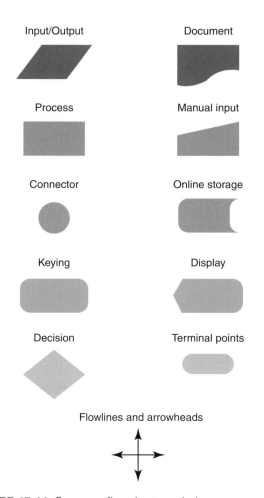

Input/Output

Document

Process

Manual input

Connector

Online storage

Keying

Display

Decision

Terminal points

Flowlines and arrowheads

FIGURE 17-11 Common flowchart symbols.

BOX 17-1   Guidelines for Constructing a Flowchart

- Title the chart with the name of the procedure or system, the name of the department and organization, and the date.
- Describe each step of the process, using concise, brief phrases (e.g., file record, transcribe discharge summary). If possible, write the step description inside the symbol for the step.
- Write decision steps in a question form that can be answered with a yes or no (e.g., Is record complete?). Decision steps are usually followed by two steps: one leading from the yes response and one leading from the no response.
- Draw the flowchart from top to bottom and from the left-hand side to the right-hand side of the page. Use on-page connectors to show flow without drawing lines over the diagram. Use off-page connectors to show the links to subsequent pages. Note the start and end of an activity.

problems or source of problems, such as the department or function in which they originate.

Formulating Alternative Solutions and Improvements

By use of the fundamental belief of methods improvement that there is always a better way along with the information

gathered, questioned, organized, and analyzed from the prior steps, several alternatives should come to mind. Employees who are close to the situation might not see the value of making changes, but their input must be acquired. Journal articles and conferences with colleagues within and outside the organization may stimulate some new and different thinking.

Selecting the Improved Method

To identify the best alternative for rectifying the problem, several decision-making tools are available.

Decision Grid or Matrix

The decision grid or matrix (Figure 17-13) is the most basic of the decision support tools. The alternatives are compared with one another by various criteria. The alternatives are listed down the left side. The elements or criteria are listed across the top. Examples of criteria frequently considered in selecting alternatives are cost, feasibility, desirability, acceptance, effect on productivity, and effect on quality.

This grid may be used to arrive at a decision concerning any type of problem after the alternatives are defined and the criteria selected. Another option is to weigh the criteria. The element of cost may be weighted three times that of any other element. This would mean that cost is the first priority in this decision-making process. The grid's primary advantage is that all relevant information can be displayed and viewed at the same time. This is useful when a committee or group is attempting to arrive at a consensus.

Decision Table

A decision table is an analytical tool that provides a means of communication of the logical sequence of a particular operation. This type of decision support tool can be used in situations in which the logic and sequential flow of data cannot be clearly shown on a flowchart. The decision table was originally designed to explain the logic found in computerizing a manual process.

A basic decision table is divided into four segments:

Conditions segment. These are usually questions that form the conditions that may exist in a system. Condition statements or questions are assigned row numbers and entered in the left-hand column. A heavy line separates the condition statements or questions from the action statements.

Condition-entry segment. This is the set of rules (or scenarios) that provides yes or no answers to the questions in the conditions segment. The rules should be numbered. The rule numbers are then assigned horizontally across the top of the form. The condition entries are entered opposite the applicable condition questions.

Action segment. This lists the action to be taken for fulfilling each condition. Action statements are assigned row numbers and are entered below the condition statements below the heavy line.

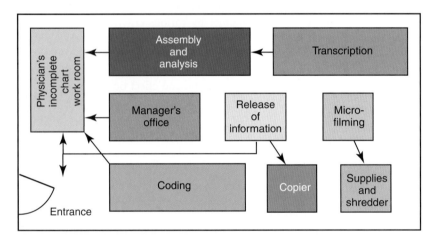

FIGURE 17-12 Movement diagram or layout flowchart. *Top,* an inefficiently arranged section of a health information management department. The release-of-information employees are not located near the photocopier, and the manager and coding staff are far removed from physician access. *Bottom,* improved physical layout, making movement and work flow more efficient.

Alternative	Cost	Feasibility	Desirability & Acceptance	Decision
1 Hire new coding supervisor	$58,200 for this new position	Requires recruitment; few qualified applicants; usually new grad	Coding staff will resist new graduate	3rd priority
2 Promote lead coder to coding supervisor	Current Salary: $42,400; Raise: $8,000; Total Salary: $50,400; Savings: $7,800	Places heavy burden on workload	Coding staff may resist	2nd priority
3 Promote operations supervisor to assist. director supervising both operations and coding	Current Salary: $40,000; Raise: $10,000; Total Salary: $50,000; Savings: $8,200	Excellent; supervisor has previous coding experience	Poses minor acceptance problem with coders; very desirable to operations supervisor	1st priority

FIGURE 17-13 Decision matrix or grid showing the elements considered by the director of the health information management department in the hiring decision for a coding supervisor.

Action-entry segment. This section uses an "X" to indicate the suitable action concluded from the answers entered in the condition-entry segment.

A decision table may be simple and characterize only a few conditions. It can, however, be complex and contain dozens of conditions and actions. Examples of the usage of decision tables in the HIM department may involve a complex process within the department or may assist in employee decisions. For example, in Figure 17-14, employees who are employed less than 1 year will receive no raises, whereas individuals who have been employed for 1 to 3 years will receive 3% raises.

FIGURE 17-14 Decision table used to determine employee raises.

Employee Raises	Rule 1	Rule 2	Rule 3	Rule 4
Employed less than 1 year	Y	N	N	N
Employed 1–3 years	—	Y	N	N
Employed 3–5 years	—	—	Y	N
Employed 5 or more years	—	—	—	Y
No Raise	X			
3% Raise		X		
5% Raise			X	
7% Raise				X

Conditions / Actions (left); Condition Entry / Action Entry (right)

Decision Tree

Decisions are often linked to other decisions. In effect, sometimes one decision necessitates future decisions. A **decision tree** is used to chart alternative courses of action for solving a problem. It also depicts some of the probable consequences or risks resulting from each course of action. Decision trees are a valuable tool for evaluating decisions that are linked together over time with assorted potential outcomes. As an example, the transcription supervisor has an unanticipated heavy load of dictation. He or she has insufficient staff to handle the workload. The obvious alternatives in this situation include (1) hiring more transcriptionists, (2) paying overtime to current transcriptionists, (3) contracting work out to a transcription service, and (4) hiring temporary help (Figure 17-15).

When this decision tool is used, the decision centers on the objective of making the wisest expenditure of money. This decision tool is effective when probabilities can be determined for the various outcomes. In this example, it would be helpful for the transcription supervisor to determine the probability of an increased demand for transcription services or the probability of continuation of the heavy load of dictation. After evaluating additional services rendered and considering previous year figures, the supervisor may estimate that there is a 70% probability that the workload will increase next year and a 30% probability that the workload will decrease. Monetary values have to come into play in evaluating the risks compared with the alternatives.

FIGURE 17-15 Decision tree.

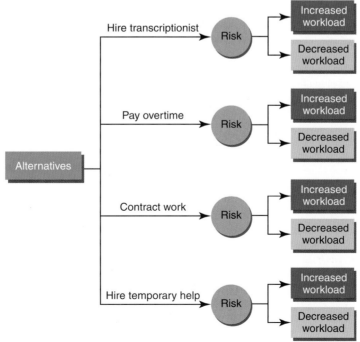

Implementing the Improved Method and Evaluating the Effectiveness of the Improvement

Provided that the employees have participated in the entire process, this step should be easy and simple to apply. The improved method should result in a more simplified, better, faster, more convenient, and less costly method of performing the task. The purpose of the work simplification and the reasons for its importance should be made clear to every employee it affects.

To ensure success with the improved process, the new procedures should be documented and reviewed with all employees involved. People, by nature, tend to resist change. However, if employees realize that this change is part of their own efforts, resistance should be minimal. Sometimes it is helpful to demonstrate work simplification examples from other departments. If the employees can see results in reducing waste and accomplishing the work effectively, they will work together to meet the challenge that work simplification offers (Box 17-2).

BOX 17-2 Guidelines for Work Simplification

- Encourage employee participation in planning for work simplification. Promote employee knowledge of work simplification objectives, process, and results. In-service training may be necessary.
- The series of work activities needs to be simple and productive. Each adopted activity must be justified for its necessity. All unnecessary or duplicative activities should be eliminated. The activities that contribute directly to the goal should be maximized.
- Whenever reasonable, combine work activities. Duplication of effort is frequently found in evaluating a procedure. In various activities, certain data are copied over and over. If feasible, these writing activities should be combined into a single method or operation.
- As much as possible, reduce the distances traveled. Sometimes the movements of people and paper are costly and may be wasteful. Closely examine such movements and attempt to reduce them to the shortest distance possible. However, when movement is essential, it is typically a more efficient process to move the paper than to move the person. Some specific guidelines are as follows:
  Equipment, materials, and supplies often used should be located within an individual's normal grasp area.
  The quickest way to move small objects is usually by sliding rather than carrying.
  Hand motions should begin simultaneously and be completed at the same time, motions should be as simple as possible, and individuals should work to achieve rhythm.
  Continuous curved motions are more desirable than straight-line motions requiring sudden changes in direction.
  Strive to arrange activities to provide a smooth work flow. When more than one clerical step is included in the process or activity, a pattern of steady, constant flow of work is ordinarily desirable. The employee may feel overwhelmed by workloads that are too heavy. On the other hand, the employee may become frustrated and bored if workloads that are too light occur frequently. Hesitations and delays in the flow of work should be minimized.

SELF-ASSESSMENT QUIZ

5. A step on a flow process chart that states "arranges sheets in alphabetical order" would be characterized as a(n)_____.
6. What are some common tools used in the data gathering stage of work simplification?
7. A step on a flow process chart that states "record brought to physicians' incomplete area" would be characterized as a(n)_____.

DID YOU KNOW?

- Work simplification is an organized approach to determine how to accomplish a task with less effort in less time or at a lower cost while maintaining or improving the quality of the outcome.
- Six steps are involved in work simplification:
  - Identify the problem.
  - Gather the data using
    - flow process chart
    - flowcharts
    - movement diagram
  - Organize, analyze, and challenge the data.
  - Formulate improvements or alternatives.
  - Develop the improved method.
  - Implement the improved method and evaluate effectiveness.

SYSTEMS AND ORGANIZATIONAL LEVEL (MIDLEVEL)

Systems Analysis and Design

Systems analysis and design is a method used to evaluate and study all types of systems. This process is usually used at an organizational level involving several departments and functions. The main benefit of using this process is that it is a defined and accepted method for gathering and "analyzing a great quantity of data in a logical, documented format" (p. 118).[4] Like work simplification, it follows the scientific method of problem solving, using tools of description, investigation, research, creativity, and judgment. The analysis portion involves examining the way things are currently done and defining the users' requirements for the system. The design segment determines the best way to meet the users' specified requirements for the system.

The systems analysis and design process can be used for various types of systems, ranging from paper-and-pencil to paperless computer-based systems. The process can be lengthy and time-consuming, and it requires dedication of staff and financial resources. It is usually used when an existing system no longer meets the organization's needs or when new needs are identified.

The health information manager can be involved in this process in a variety of ways, including being a user of a system, defining its requirements with a systems analyst, or even assuming the systems analyst role.

The use of the systems analysis and design method does not guarantee success. The choice of solutions (designs) is still a human one and fraught with possibilities of human bias and error.

Systems Model Concept

The process of systems analysis and design is based on the systems model concept. A system is an assemblage of things that form a connected whole, a complex but ordered whole, a plan or scheme, or a method. A system refers to various elements that are interrelated according to a plan for achieving a well-defined goal. In an organization, the elements are employees or human resources, equipment and supplies, and raw material. These elements are linked together by processes or procedures to achieve the organization's goals or desired outcomes (Figure 17-16).

Hierarchical Structure

The systems model concept also recognizes the hierarchical structure of systems. Large systems are composed of subsystems, which in turn are composed of subsystems. For example, the human body is a system composed of subsystems of the digestive, respiratory, and cardiovascular systems. The digestive system is composed of the stomach system, the small intestine system, the large intestine system, and so on.

Unity of Purpose and Boundary Concepts

Embedded in the systems model concept are the principles of unity of purpose and boundary or integrity of the system. These concepts are important for effective application of the systems analysis and design process. A system has unity of purpose when the system and its subsystems all focus on achieving a single purpose. The boundary concept refers to separating the system from other systems. It identifies what is included and what is excluded in the system being studied. The boundaries define the scope of the study and the possible limits of the system. For example, the process under study may involve several departments, but the study may be limited to the part of the process that occurs only within one department. Determination of the system's boundaries is often an administrative or management decision.

Input-Output Cycle

Systems are composed of input, processing, output, feedback, and control.

Input

The flow of work through a system begins with some type of input. Examples of input include labor, energy, money, and attitudes. In a health information system, the types of input are commonly data, information, or materials. Examples of materials include the mail, demographic data on the health care facility's patients, and telephone calls received by the receptionist. Incorporated in this input are employees' skills and knowledge and the equipment and supplies needed to perform the task.

Processing

The processing element transforms the input into a desired output. Sometimes this phase is called the transformation process. The following are traditional processing activities:

- Classifying
- Storing
- Sorting
- Filing
- Calculating
- Retrieving data and information

Processing refers to the procedures and methods involved in the system. Procedures are an established series of work steps used to accomplish a goal and commonly include the efforts of several people. Procedures handle recurring transactions consistently and uniformly. In viewing procedures microscopically, we see that they consist of a progression of methods. Procedures consist of related methods that are essential to complete various work processes. Methods apply to the tasks of an individual employee and may represent a manual, mechanical, or automated way of performing a procedure. An example of a method is alphabetizing the names of the physicians on the medical staff by their last names.

Output

The ultimate goal of a system is output. Output is a result of transforming input into a desired form. For example, the transcriptionist transforms the physician's dictation into a typed report. Other output examples are release-of-information correspondence, coded diagnoses and procedures, and productivity reports. Output is usually in paper or computer screen format and is needed as the input for another process or system.

Feedback

Feedback is crucial for the success of the entire system. It compares the output with expected standards of performance.

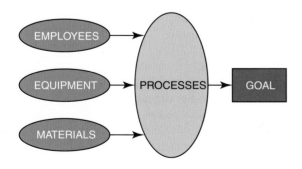

FIGURE 17-16 Diagram of a system.

In other words, feedback contrasts what was produced with what should have been produced. An example of feedback would be the physician's evaluation of the typed report or the quality improvement plan. If the feedback shows that the quality standards were not met, a modification is sent back to the input phase for improvement of the system.

Feedback can also occur concurrently with the input–processing–output cycle. The input and processing are evaluated and improved before the preparation of the output.

Controls and Constraints

Systems do not operate in a vacuum; they are controlled and constrained by internal and external factors. These factors dictate what can and cannot be done in every phase of the system. An internal dimension of controlling encompasses the organizational policies, procedures, and standards that affect the system. An example of an internal control for a health information process is the policies and procedures that govern the release of health information. This policy stipulates the type of information that may or may not be released without the patient's written authorization. Additional internal controls may be those required for profit as a profit margin or for quality of service and those required by the customer.

The external controls include the local, state, and federal rules and regulations and social, economic, and ethical values. External controls that affect the HIM department are the federal regulations on the confidentiality of drug and alcohol patient records, the information management standards of The Joint Commission, and the diagnosis-related group (MS-DRG) weights published in the Federal Register.

Goals of Systems Analysis and Design Process

The goal of the systems analysis and design process is to produce a well-designed system that can be described as follows:

Effective. The system accomplishes its purpose and achieves its established goals.

Efficient. The system accomplishes its purpose while remaining cost-effective.

Dependable. The system meets established time frames.

Flexible. The system can accommodate unusual circumstances.

Adaptable. The system can absorb changes, if necessary.

Systematic and logical.

Functional. The system serves its intended purpose.

Simple.

Resourceful. The system is useful within the organization.

Accepted. The system is accepted by those who work with it.

Components of Systems Analysis and Design

The major components of systems design are as follows:
- Determination of the need and objectives of the system
- Systems analysis
- Design of the system
- Evaluation of the proposed system
- Implementation of the system

Determining the Need for the System

Before the analysis process is begun, the users must determine the need for the system. The needs, which are often determined by management, are in the form of objectives. They should provide answers to the following questions:
- What information is needed?
- Who needs the information?
- When do they need it?
- In what format do they need it?

Systems Analysis

The analysis of the system has three components: accumulation of facts, organization of facts, and evaluation of facts.

Accumulating the Facts

Gathering of data is made possible by envisioning the course that a piece of paper follows in a process and then tracking each step in that particular process. The tracking can begin at any point and work backward or forward from there. Sources that may be used in the accumulation or gathering of facts include the following:
- Organization charts
- Procedure manuals
- Job descriptions
- Flowcharts
- Financial data

Investigation methods include group discussions and interviews with managers and operations employees and questionnaires to all affected personnel and users of the system. Before the investigation is begun, the existing manuals and charts should be reviewed. The interview should focus on obtaining facts pertinent to the system analysis. At this point in the process, solutions should not be suggested. Strategic questions should be devised to verify facts from previous sources.

Organizing the Facts

The facts obtained in the previous step must be organized or classified in some way. Conventional ways to organize facts are in the following categories:
- Interrelated objectives
- Organizational structure
- Input and output
- Processing modes
- Major complaints or problems disclosed

Organizing facts by organizational structure can be advantageous because it shows not only who has authority to make decisions but also the flow of data among organizational units. Organizing facts by major complaints or problems is also beneficial because only valid problems and significant complaints should be included. The organization of facts is helpful in proceeding with their evaluation. The means of organization should also show meaningful relationships.

Evaluating the Facts

As much as possible, the facts should be ranked, rated, measured, weighed, and evaluated. The assignment of quantitative values to facts should be accomplished in as many areas as possible. In reality, some evaluation may be subjective and based on opinion. Information tends to include some non-quantifiable components. Again, try to adhere to the facts, not to feelings or beliefs. At this point in the process, possible solutions to the problems may be examined.

Designing the System

After the facts have been gathered, organized, evaluated, and analyzed, a design of a new system or a proposed revision to an existing system is explored. People must be committed to this process. The design of a system should be a team effort that includes management, operations personnel, and users of the system. Often, numerous systems could fit the requirements. However, they can differ in many aspects, especially cost.

The following factors should be considered when designing the new system:
- Effects on employees (retraining, layoffs, transfers, schedules)
- Profits and costs (salaries, space, materials, and supplies)
- Customer service

System design should not be performed in a rush. Various possibilities must be considered with their strengths and weaknesses. The term *trade-off* is routinely used in this part of the process. In other words, sometimes one need must be sacrificed for another.

Evaluating the Proposed System

In this step of systems design, the proposed system should be evaluated to determine whether it is satisfactory. A review of the overall arrangement and a specific check of the design's critical areas are crucial. The proposed system must meet the needs of the employees and managers as well as the organizational needs.

Implementing the System

The last step in systems design is the implementation phase. This phase may be time-consuming. To implement a new system smoothly, it is imperative that the employees have a stake in the new system. Again, the employees and management should have been actively involved in the entire system design process. The new system may be implemented on a trial basis by a few employees. Employee acceptance should be taken into consideration. Some retraining may need to take place at this time. Modifications to the new system may occur during this trial period. If the new system involves a large operation, parallel operations may be conducted. This procedure allows the old system to continue to function while the new system "bugs" have been worked through and removed or modified. After the trial period, the old system can be phased out.

Organizational Structure

Organizational structure can be either formal or informal.

Formal Organizational Infrastructure

The formal organizational infrastructure is designed to plan work, assign responsibility, supervise work, and measure results. The formal relationships between various people and the organizational structure are identified on an organization chart. This chart clearly identifies hierarchical relationships, the lines of authority, responsibilities, and span of control. In an organization chart, the primary functions of the organization and the subfunctions within each primary function are identified. It should also aid in the identification of any areas of overlap in responsibility. The major disadvantage of the formal organization chart is its inability to show the informal interaction between employees as they carry out their everyday activities.

Informal Organization

The informal or unwritten organization refers to the many interpersonal relationships that occur in an organization that do not appear on the formal organization chart. A typical informal organization is composed of two or more persons who develop mutually satisfying interactions pertaining to personal or job-related matters. An informal organization develops over time.

Positive Aspects of Informal Organization

The most positive aspect of an informal organization is its blend with the formal organization to produce an operable system for the accomplishment of the work. If management can motivate the informal leaders to accept a new procedure, these leaders may be able to convince others to accept it. The informal organization provides the necessary social values and stability to work groups.

A well-known benefit of informal organization is that it provides an additional channel of communication. It is capable of efficiently sending and receiving communications. This informal channel is called the "grapevine." The grapevine can be described as the informal oral communication network that aids employees in learning more about what is happening in the organization and how it might affect them. Often it is more effective than the formal line of communication in distributing information, obtaining feedback, solving problems, and revising procedures.

Negative Aspects of Informal Organization

Informal organizations can also be a hindrance to management. In some organizations, the disadvantages far outweigh the benefits. A common example of abuse of the informal organization is one in which the employees find opportunities to work together even when no such work assignments have been made.

When an informal group loses confidence in a manager, they may combine forces to make life miserable for the manager. On occasion, informal groups may develop cross-purposes with the goals and objectives of the formal organization.

Potentially negative impacts or conflicts resulting from informal organization must be weighed against its constructive and practical function in nurturing creativity and innovation. A relatively conflict-free organization tends to be rigid, static, and inflexible.

Acceptance and Balance

Managers must accept three additional facts about the formal and informal organizations:

1. Informal organization is inevitable. Management creates the formal organization and can alter it as it so desires. The informal organization is not created by management. As long as organizations are composed of people, informal organizations will exist.

2. Small groups are the central component of the informal organization. Group membership in the informal organization strongly influences the overall behavior and performance of its members. Many sociologists agree that the group, not the individual, is the basic component of the human organization.[5]

3. Informal organization always coexists within the formal structure. This is a fact of organizational life. The formal and informal organizations must be balanced to achieve optimal performance and attain organizational objectives. Management trying to suppress the informal organization creates a destructive situation that results in reduced effectiveness. On the other hand, if the formal organization is too weak to accomplish its objectives, the informal organization can grow in strength, resulting in abuse of power, insubordination, and disloyalty.

The ideal situation is one in which the formal organization is strong enough to achieve its objectives and at the same time permit a well-developed informal organization to maintain group cohesiveness and teamwork. The informal relationships that exist in an organization deserve attention from employees and managers concerned with the organization's effectiveness.

✓ SELF-ASSESSMENT QUIZ

8. A system is composed of several elements. What are these?
9. What are the three components of systems analysis?
10. The formal relationship between various people and the organizational structure can be identified on the _____.

❓ DID YOU KNOW?

- Systems analysis and design is a method used to evaluate and study all types of systems.
- Systems are composed of input, processing, output, feedback, and control.
- The major components of systems design are the following:
  - Determining the needs and objectives of the system
  - Systems analysis
  - Design of the system
  - Evaluation of the proposed system
  - Implementation of the system

ORGANIZATION-WIDE LEVEL

Change Management

Simply put, change management can be defined as the task of managing change. One meaning of managing change refers to "the making of changes in a planned and managed or systematic fashion."[6] This is a proactive approach in which an organization plans to implement new systems or processes to grow and thrive. Managing change may also refer to a reactive response "to changes over which the organization exercises little or no control."[6] This may include implementing new systems or policies in response to new Joint Commission standards or Centers for Medicare and Medicaid Services (CMS) directives. There are various methods for managing change, including strategic management, project management, and reengineering.

STRATEGIC MANAGEMENT

One useful model of the strategic management process is illustrated in Figure 17-17.

Strategic management involves four primary stages. These stages are situational analysis, strategy formulation, strategic implementation, and strategic control.

Situational Analysis

Analyzing and understanding the situation is accomplished by three separate processes: (1) external environmental analysis, (2) internal environmental analysis, and (3) the development of the organization's directional strategies or its mission, vision, and values. The interaction and results of these processes form the basis for the development of strategy.

Issues in the external environment directly and simultaneously affect all three situational analysis processes. Issues in the external environment affect the process of environmental analysis, provide the context for internal analysis, and influence the mission, vision, and values. For example, a regulatory change may well independently affect the analysis of the external environment, the determination of factors to be considered strengths or weaknesses of the organization, and the way managers view the mission, vision, and values.

External Environmental Analysis

To operate in today's changing environment, health care managers need a method for obtaining and assessing external information that will affect the organization. This process is referred to as external environmental analysis. As information is accumulated and classified, managers must determine the environmental issues that are significant to the organization. In addition, they must monitor these issues, collect additional information, evaluate their impact, and incorporate them in a strategy.

FIGURE 17-17 Overview of strategic management process.

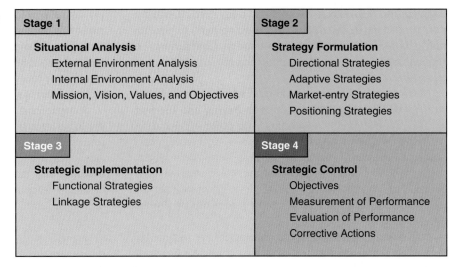

An overview of the strategic management process with four stages:

Stage 1

Situational Analysis
- External Environment Analysis
- Internal Environment Analysis
- Mission, Vision, Values, and Objectives

Stage 2

Strategy Formulation
- Directional Strategies
- Adaptive Strategies
- Market-entry Strategies
- Positioning Strategies

Stage 3

Strategic Implementation
- Functional Strategies
- Linkage Strategies

Stage 4

Strategic Control
- Objectives
- Measurement of Performance
- Evaluation of Performance
- Corrective Actions

External environmental analysis is the process by which an organization crosses the boundary between itself and the external environment to identify and understand changes (issues) that are taking place outside the organization. These changes represent both opportunities and threats. Health care managers need to understand the nature of these opportunities and threats before they affect the organization. These external opportunities and threats represent the fundamental issues that will spell success or failure for the organization. Opportunities and threats should influence the strategy adopted by the organization, that is, what the organization should do.

Internal Environmental Analysis

The organization itself has an internal environment that represents the resources, competencies, and capabilities of the organization (what the organization can do). An understanding of these factors requires an extensive, in-depth analysis of the internal functions, operations, structure, resources, and skills.[7]

An internal environmental analysis should reveal the strengths and weaknesses of the organization. An understanding of the strengths and weaknesses provides a foundation for strategy formulation and is essential if a strategy is to be developed that optimizes strengths and deemphasizes and overcomes weaknesses.

Mission, Vision, and Values

The mission, vision, and values of an organization greatly affect the strategy it ultimately adopts. The organization's mission represents the consensus and articulation of the organization's understanding of the external opportunities and threats and the internal strengths and weaknesses.[8] It is a general statement of what distinguishes the organization from all others of its type and answers the questions "Who are we?" and "What do we do?" Vision, on the other hand, is the view of the future that management believes is optimal

for the organization (ideally, it is based on an understanding of the external opportunities and threats and internal strengths and weaknesses) and is communicated throughout the organization. Vision profiles the future and constitutes what the organization wants to do.

The values of an organization are the fundamental beliefs or "truths" that the organization holds dear. Values are the best indicator of the philosophy of the organization and specify what is important (honesty, integrity, customers, and so on) in the organization. Values are sometimes referred to as guiding principles. These become the directional strategies of the organization and the basis for setting organizational objectives.

Mission, vision, and values are considered part of the situational analysis because they rely on and influence external environmental analysis and internal environmental analysis. Taken together, these directional strategies express an understanding of the situation, what the organization is now, and what it wants to be. They are also a part of strategy formulation because they provide a definition of the broadest direction for the organization.

Strategy Formulation

Situational analysis involves gathering, classifying, and understanding information. Strategy formulation involves making decisions using that information.[9] These decisions result in a strategy for the organization.[9] As noted earlier, the first set of decisions concerns the mission, vision, and values and provides the general direction for the organization. Next, more specific strategic decisions must be made. These decisions include determination of the adaptive strategies, market entry strategies, and the positioning strategies.

The adaptive strategies are more specific than the directional strategies and indicate the method for carrying out the directional strategies. The adaptive strategies specify how the organization will expand (diversification, vertical integration, market development, product development, or penetration), contract (divestiture, liquidation, harvesting, or retrenchment), or stabilize (enhancement or status quo) operations.

Market entry strategies indicate whether the adaptive strategy will be accomplished through buying into the market (i.e., acquisitions), cooperating with other organizations in the market (i.e., mergers and alliances), or internal development. Positioning strategies delineate how the organization's products and services will be positioned vis-à-vis competitors' products and services in a given market and might include strategies such as cost leadership or product differentiation.

Decisions concerning these strategies are sequential. Directional strategies are developed first, then adaptive strategies are formulated. Next, market entry strategies are selected. Finally, positioning strategies are formulated. These strategic decisions explicitly answer the following questions: What business(es) are we in? What business(es) should we be in? How are we going to compete? At this point, the broad organizational strategies have been selected.

Strategic Implementation

After the directional, adaptive, market entry, and positioning strategies have been formulated, operational strategies that support these organizational strategies are developed and the process of strategic implementation is initiated. Operational strategies are made up of strategies developed within the functional areas of the organization and strategies that link the functional areas and develop the capabilities of the organization. Functional strategies and supporting programs and budgets must be developed for the key areas in the organization, such as marketing, information systems, finance, and human resources. These functional areas are directly and independently affected by the strategy formulation process, yet functional strategies must be integrated to move the organization toward realizing its mission. In addition to the functional strategies, organizations often develop linkage strategies that enhance the general capabilities and link organizational processes. These operational strategies include initiatives such as changing the organization's culture, reorganization, upgrade of facilities and equipment, and social and ethical strategies. These strategies generally affect the entire organization and cut across all functional areas.

Strategic Control

The final stage of strategic management is strategic control. Strategic control is similar to the general management control process discussed later in this chapter. Strategic control is a process that includes (1) establishment of standards (objectives), (2) measurement of performance, (3) evaluation of organizational performance against the standards, and

(4) taking corrective action, if necessary. However, strategic control is much broader and, in turn, affects the operational strategies, the organization's general strategy, and situational analysis processes. As managers monitor these various organizational processes, they learn what is effective and take corrective action as necessary.

Sometimes it is difficult for managers to plan or envision the long-term future of an organization in a dynamic environment. Managers often need to react to unanticipated developments and new competitive pressures. Strategy becomes an intuitive, entrepreneurial, political, culture-based, or learning process. In these cases, previous experience is of limited value. Managers must create and discover an unfolding future, using their ability to learn together in groups and to interact politically in a spontaneous, self-organizing manner. When there are provocative atmospheres conducive to complex learning, organizations may change and develop new strategic directions. In such atmospheres, the destination and the route may turn out to be unexpected and unintended. As a result, strategy emerges spontaneously from the chaos of challenge and contradiction through a process of real-time learning and politics.[10] At the center of this process is the manager, who must carefully craft the decisions that will contribute much to the success or failure of the organization. Therefore, we must understand the manager if we are to understand management.

SELF-ASSESSMENT QUIZ

11. In situational analysis, analyzing and understanding the situation is accomplished by three separate processes. What are these processes?
12. An internal environmental analysis should reveal the _____ and _____ of the organization.
13. State the differences between adaptive strategies, market entry strategies, and positioning strategies.

DID YOU KNOW?

- The four primary stages of strategic management are:
  1. Situational analysis
  2. Strategy formulation
  3. Strategic implementation
  4. Strategic control
- The organization's *mission* is a general statement of what distinguishes the organization from all others of its type and answers the questions "Who are we?" and "What do we do?"
- An organization's *vision* profiles the future and constitutes what the organization wants to do.
- The *values* of an organization are the fundamental beliefs or "truths" that the organization holds dear. Values are sometimes referred to as guiding principles.

Project Management

Project management as defined by some experts is management plus planning.[11] It uses the basic management principles of planning, organizing, directing, and controlling (with an emphasis on planning) to bring a project to a successful conclusion. Because projects are unique and demand that people do things differently from before, the team is following an unknown path and must plan ahead.

Project management techniques are used by many professions, including engineering, construction, and military and government agencies. Today's health care managers also find project management techniques helpful in confronting the conflicting responsibilities of completing continuous and routine work while exploring and implementing new health care delivery models and technologies with less resources, greater time constraints, and continuous communication links across organizational units.

Characteristics of a Project

To understand the concepts of project management, the characteristics of a project must be defined.

Unique

This process has never been done before. It is a one-time event or one-of-a-kind activity. It will never be repeated in precisely the same way again. There is no practice or rehearsal. Experience can be gained from previous projects. However, this particular combination of time, place, people, and project is unique.

Product or Result

The outcome of the project is a single, definable product, such as a bridge that is built, a rocket that is launched, or a hospital that is constructed. Projects are goal oriented and work through the process to achieve that goal. The product is different for each project.

Finite

The project is usually on a fixed time scale with start and finish dates. It can be viewed as a temporary activity. The project is undertaken to accomplish a goal within a set period of time. After the goal is achieved, the project ceases to exist.

Complex, Numerous, and Sequenced Activities

Projects involve a variety of complex and sequenced activities used to achieve the goal or objective.

Team

Projects are completed by a team of people from diverse professions and organizational units. Projects may be task interdependent and may use advanced technology. However, projects are human endeavors and cannot be performed by technology alone.

Cross-Functional

Often projects cross several functional areas in an organization, involving multiple skills and talents of many people. The actual work may be performed by many functional areas. Because of this, the project does not neatly fit into the organizational structure.

Limited Resources

Projects usually have a set limit of resources and budget. The end result is specified in terms of cost, schedule, and performance requirements.

Change

Projects have the characteristic of being somewhat unfamiliar. Projects may comprise innovative technology and possess pivotal elements of uncertainty and risk. However, the essence of project management is to create change. When the project is completed, the world (i.e., organization, department) is a little different.

Characteristics of Project Management

The following are some characteristics of project management:[12]

- A single person, the project manager, administers the project and operates independently of the normal organization chart or the chain of command. The project manager has the authority to plan, direct, organize, and control the entire project from start to finish.
- Decision making, accountability, results, and rewards are shared among the members of the project team.
- Although the project activities are temporary, the functional areas performing the work are usually a permanent part of the organization. After the completion of the project, the individual workers are returned to their original assignments or reassigned to a new project.
- The project focuses on delivering an end product or end result at a certain time, with certain resource allotments, and to the satisfaction of performance or technical requirements.
- Project management can set into motion other support functions, including personnel evaluation, accounting, and information systems.

Project Planning

Planning is essentially thinking ahead. In project management, planning involves two phases: defining the project and planning the project.

Defining the Project

Defining the project is often called project overview. Four areas are detailed in the definition phase.

1. The *problem statement* answers the following questions:
   - What is the problem?
   - What is the opportunity?
   - What is to be done?
   - Who is responsible for the project?
   - When must it be completed?

2. The *goal statement* is the final outcome of the project. It serves as a point of focus and reference that keeps all activities on track. A goal statement tells precisely what the outcome will be and when it will be done. It needs to be action oriented, short, simple, and straightforward. An example of a project goal is to implement a computer-based patient record by 2014.

3. To achieve the stated goal, several steps have to take place. These steps represent milestones in the project and are considered *objectives*. They define major components that must be accomplished to achieve the overall goal. Objectives are more precise and measurable than the goal statement. A project objective for the goal of implementation of a computer-based patient record is an online connection between the hospital computer system and the medical staff offices within 6 months.

4. *Resources* include people (human resources), materials, space, and money that are needed to achieve the goal.

Plan

A project is initiated with the preparation of a written plan. The purpose of the plan is to direct and guide the project manager and the project team members through the project. Basically, planning is thinking ahead, communicating the plan, and using the plan as a yardstick to measure the progress toward achievement of the goal. The five areas detailed in the planning phase are as follows:

Project activities. Every objective of the project should encompass separate activities. These activities define the work to be accomplished to attain the objective. The method of work breakdown structures is often used in projects. It divides the project into major objectives, partitions each objective into activities, further divides the activities into subactivities, and creates work packages that must be done to complete the project.

Time and cost. The time and cost for completion of each activity are estimated. Variations in time may be due to the skill level of the people performing the activity, material availability, technology or machine variations, and unexpected events, such as illness and employee turnover. Estimates of time may contain the most optimistic completion time, the most pessimistic completion time, and the most likely completion time. Cost estimates are typically categorized into labor, materials, other direct (e.g., telephone, postage) costs, and indirect costs or overhead.

Activity sequence. After the activities have been identified, along with their time and cost estimates, they need to be sequenced. Some activities are dependent on others; that is, one activity cannot be started until another is completed. They must be done sequentially. Other activities may be done simultaneously.

Critical activities. Management tools such as the Gantt chart and PERT network can be used to determine the sequence and the amount of time needed to complete the project. The sequence of activities that makes up the longest path to complete the project is called the critical path. When activities are completed on schedule, the whole project will be completed on time. However, sometimes activities take longer than anticipated or materials cannot be obtained, and then the project completion time is extended.

Project proposal. The purpose of a project proposal is to provide a complete description of the project activities, time lines, and resource requirements. It is a statement of the general approach being taken and the results expected. It is a decision-making tool, a key to management control, a training aid for new project team members, and a reporting document. The project proposal portrays the transition from project management planning to project management implementation.

Project Implementation

After the project has been approved, the work begins. The implementation process contains three phases: organize, control, and termination.

Organize

Organizing includes the assembly of the required resources (materials, personnel, and money) to accomplish the work defined in the plan. Organizing also includes the development of the structure needed to administer the plan. The following three areas are detailed in the organization phase:

1. *Project manager.* The most important element of project management is the project manager. This person has the responsibility to integrate work efforts and plays a major role in planning and executing a project. The project manager is accountable for the project and dedicated to achieving its goals. The criteria for selection of a project manager vary according to organizations. The usual characteristics include the following:
   - Background and experience
   - Leadership
   - Strategic expertise
   - Technical expertise
   - Interpersonal skills
   - Managerial capability

   Selecting the most qualified project manager can be the key to the project's success or failure.

2. *Project team.* Project management entails bringing individuals and groups together to form a single, cohesive team working toward a common goal. Project work is teamwork accomplished by a group of people. After the project manager is selected, he or she can assist in the selection of the project team members. The size and composition of the project team depend on the resources allocated to the project. The following characteristics are desirable in a member of a project team:
   - Commitment to the project goal
   - Communication skills
   - Flexibility
   - Technical competence
   - Task orientation

- Ability to be a team player
- Experience with project management tools
- Dependability, history of meeting deadlines

3. *Work activities.* Now that the planning and organizing have been done, work on the project gets started. The project manager assigns responsibilities for completing activities to members of the project team. As discussed previously, activities can be subdivided into subactivities and work packages. A work package as one continuous activity is assigned to a project team member who has the authority, expertise, and access to the appropriate resources necessary to complete the assignment. A work package has beginning and ending tasks with a definitive description of each task. The project manager schedules the start dates of each work package. Because many activities are interrelated, work packages must be clearly documented so that their completion can be tracked.

Control

Controlling is the monitoring and maintenance of the structure of the project. Part of control is the reporting at specified points throughout the project. The reports should indicate potential problems. The following two areas are detailed in the control phase:

Effective project leadership. The project manager and the project team must work together to reach the project goal. Group cohesiveness, open communication, team development, and empowerment of members are top priorities for the project manager (Box 17-3).

Control tools. Controls focus on performance levels, cost, and time schedules. Controls also track progress, detect variance from the plan, and allow the project manager to take corrective action.

The project manager reports the status of every activity in the project at least monthly. This report summarizes the

BOX 17-3 Guidelines for Effective Project Leadership

- Do not overdirect.
- Recognize individual differences.
- Allow individual team members the freedom to guide their own work.
- Become a resource person instead of a controller.
- Become a facilitator instead of a boss.
- Become a buffer between team members and outside problems.
- Insist on feedback.
- Do not over-observe.
- Appreciate each project team member for his or her unique characteristics and contributions.
- Develop conflict resolution strategies.
- Improve communication techniques.
- Maintain group cohesion.
- Facilitate effective meetings.

progress for that month and for the length of the entire project. The project manager should also report the variances from the plan. These variances may be related to budget, labor, time, or materials. Positive variance examples are being ahead of schedule or under budget. Negative variances may include an extended time schedule or a greater budgetary item than anticipated. Negative cost variances, such as unexpected equipment failure or increased cost of supplies, may not be under the project manager's control.

When each milestone of the project is completed, the project manager should review the project. Despite all the extensive planning, things will not automatically happen according to the plan. To get back on schedule, the project manager may have to reallocate resources, consider alternatives, and reevaluate activities. This is where good project managers prove their worth by getting the project back on schedule.

Termination

There are three types of project termination.

Termination by extinction. The project work as scheduled is either successfully or unsuccessfully done and the decision to terminate is agreed on.

Termination by inclusion. The successful project is institutionalized or transformed into the organization as a unit.

Termination by integration. A common way of closing successful projects occurs when equipment, material, and personnel are distributed back into the organization.

Termination Process

The four phases in the termination process are as follows:

Approval. Obtain the client's or administration's approval of the project. The termination or closing down of the project depends on their satisfaction and the quality of service the project provided.

Logistics. Assign a termination manager and team to assist in the termination phase, conduct a termination meeting, prepare personnel reports, and terminate work orders and contracts.

Document. Document the entire project. Document the completion and performance of all team members and the performance of vendors, consultants, and contractors.

Final report and audit. The final project report is a history of the project. Items included in the final project report are the overall success and performance of the project, techniques used, strengths and weaknesses, organization, and recommendations from the project manager and project team. An audit of the project should be conducted after implementation. The essential questions that need to be asked in evaluating the success of the project are the following:

- Was the goal achieved?
- Was the work done on time? Within budget? Within specifications?
- Was the client or administration satisfied with the results?

Project Tools

Project tools may be used in the planning or controlling phase of project management. The two most common tools are the PERT network and the Gantt chart.

PERT Network

PERT is the acronym for Program Evaluation Review Technique. It is a scheduling device that was originally developed early in the Space Age as a tool for missile development programs. It is a system of diagramming the steps or component parts of a large, complex project that is usually nonrepetitive in nature. The various components of a PERT network and the estimated completion time for each component must be identified. All events in the network and all subsequent activities that are performed flow from and are aimed toward the completion of a specific goal. The basic components of a network (goal, events, and activities) are discussed further as follows:

Goal: The acknowledgment and statement of the goal is the most basic concept of the PERT network, and all major events and activities flow toward this goal. The network is essentially a diagram representing the overall plan for achieving the final goal. An example of a goal statement in the construction of a PERT network is the following: *Conversion of the computer system in the HIM department is fully operational.*

Events: Events in the network are discrete control points in time and reflect either the starting or ending points for one activity or a group of activities. Events are usually represented on the network by circles, rectangles, or ovals and usually contain the descriptive wording of an element. For ease of reference, events are usually numbered, but letters can also be used if there is a limited number of events. Examples of the wording of an event are as follows: *Computerized coding system selected* and *Renovation of department begun.*

Activities: In the network, activities must be performed to move from one event to the next and finally to the actual goal. Activities generally require time, money, and resources for completion and usually represent the work or action required to move from one event to another. Activities may also involve staff members. Remember that activities connect events in the network and along with events constitute the diagram reflecting the starting point through the accomplishment of the actual goal. Activities in a PERT network are generally depicted by a solid line (or a solid line with an arrow on one end) between the events to which they are related. Because activities reflect work being done, examples of the wording of activities would be as follows: *Developing job procedures* and *Training file clerks.*

Included in the preparation of a PERT network is the determination of a critical path. The critical path is the longest route and estimated completion time in the PERT network for a given project. This route would consist of the events and activities that must be completed, the order in which they must be completed, and the time

frame in which they must be completed for the project to be accomplished (Figure 17-18). The critical path therefore controls the time required to complete the project.

In Figure 17-18, the circled letters represent events, and the solid line with the arrow at one end represents an activity or a group of activities that leads to the next major event. The goal is represented by the letter N in this network. The critical path is the A-B-D-G-J-M-N path, and the time needed to complete this project is 66 days.

The following steps are suggested for constructing a PERT network:

- The final goal should be stated in detail and then worked forward from the beginning to the end.
- All possible events should be listed, followed by a description of all activities for each of the events in the network.
- All events should be analyzed and should be placed in the proper sequence. At this point, relationships between events, logical flow of events, and dependencies should be considered.
- Remember that the length of the line representing an activity or a group of activities does not represent time. There may be burst events (events that stem from one event) or merge events (events that merge together into another event). For example, in Figure 17-18 events C and E would be burst events, and events J and I would be merge events.
- The flow of events and activities is always forward because there can be no backward loops or backtracking in a PERT diagram.

Advantages of a PERT Network and the Critical Path

A PERT diagram is a valuable tool for the systems analyst because it can be used to plan an individual, detailed project or to plan an entire department's workload. The advantages of such a diagram are as follows:

- The analyst is forced to determine and define all the individual events that must take place from the start of the project through its completion.
- The analyst is also required to predict time estimates for the completion of each activity in the network.

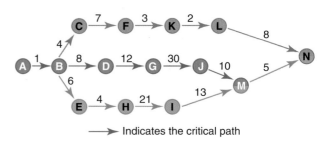

FIGURE 17-18 PERT (Program Evaluation Review Technique) network.

- After the diagram is drawn, the analyst can determine the critical path or the longest time needed to complete the project.
- Because estimated times are listed on the diagram for completion of each event, the analyst can determine whether the project is moving along according to schedule. If more time is needed than indicated on the diagram, then that extra time taken must be made up during some other event for the project to remain on schedule. (See the following example of setting up a PERT schedule.)

As shown in Figure 17-18, some activities may occur at the same time. Other activities must wait for an activity to be completed before they can begin.

Gantt Chart

Named after the famous management consultant Henry Gantt, a Gantt chart is a common project scheduling tool. Gantt charts are appropriate for complex projects with multiple steps. The chart consists of a horizontal scale divided into time units (days, weeks, months) and a vertical scale depicting project work elements (tasks, activities, work packages). The length of the horizontal bar corresponds to the expected length of time to complete the activity. As time progresses, the bar is filled in with symbols related to projected completion, actual progress, and actual completion (Figure 17-19). When the chart is used as a visual control tool, shading or color coding could be used.

The Gantt chart can also be used for personnel planning, resource allocation, and budgeting, and it is often used to track the progress of computer-based projects. It provides an excellent view of project status and it is a useful tool for monitoring progress. As with the PERT network, the Gantt chart plays an important role in the planning and controlling of projects.

Example of Setting Up a PERT Schedule

The director of a health information management (HIM) department in XYZ Hospital is responsible for supervising the enlargement and renovation of the reimbursement section of the HIM department. The director must determine the length of time needed to complete the project. The following events must be accomplished to complete the project:

START (A): A meeting is called to discuss thoroughly the plans for the departmental renovation.

STEP (B): During the meeting, a committee is established to oversee the renovation of the reimbursement section.

STEP (C): One duty of the committee is the recruitment of additional employees for this section. Recruitment ads must be written and approved before advertising in professional journals, newspapers, and so forth.

STEP (D): A second duty of committee members is to finalize the departmental layout for this section.

STEP (E): Finally, the committee must make decisions regarding the additional equipment needs of the reimbursement section.

STEP (F): Prospective applicants for the reimbursement section are interviewed by committee members and the director of the HIM department.

STEP (G): After the approval of the layout, construction on the new renovation begins.

STEP (H): Additional office equipment and furniture must be ordered for the renovated section.

STEP (I): When all equipment is received, it must be thoroughly checked and installation must be scheduled.

STEP (J): This step involves the completion of all construction on the new section.

STEP (K): After the applicant interviewing phase, a decision is made to hire four new employees.

STEP (L): Orientation and training sessions are scheduled for the four newly hired employees.

STEP (M): All equipment is installed in the renovated section of the department.

FINISH (N): The reimbursement section of the HIM department begins operation.

Information Technology Applications

According to Wayne Niemi, "Project management software is designed to improve communications between the project manager and project team members, transfer information about project deadlines, and track the status of multiple projects. One of the many benefits of these programs is that they allow users to manage more projects and accounts with fewer staff members. With a more organized approach to project management, job tasks are simplified with improved communication."[13] Some programs allow the manager to break out each participant's tasks, goals, and deadlines so that they have their own project program. Software programs also give managers the ability to help keep track of action items from several projects at once.

There are various types of software packages available that will assist with project management. Charting software provides tools for drawing flowcharts, organizational charts, and other types of diagrams. Specifically, these tools can help a supervisor see whether the steps of a project have problems or miscommunications, define the boundaries of a process, and develop a common base of knowledge. They will often bring to light redundancies, delays, dead ends, and indirect paths that can go unnoticed or ignored. Time lines, PERT and Gantt charts, and cause–effect diagrams can also be used in this process.

SELF-ASSESSMENT QUIZ

14. In project management, planning involves what two phases?
15. What are the three phases of the implementation process?
16. What are the three types of project termination?
17. What are the two most common tools used in the planning or controlling phase of project management?
18. What are the basic components of a PERT network?
19. Name a common project scheduling tool.

Begin date: March 1, 20XX
Meeting date: December 15, 20XX

Activity	Individual assigned	March	April	May	June	July	August	September	October	November	December
Initial appointments	Susan	▪									
Prepare Gantt chart	Bill	—									
Agenda is prepared	Susan		▪								
Committee meeting	Susan		▪								
Committee on site selection appointed	David		—	—							
Committee on meals/entertainment appointed	Vanessa		—	—							
Program committee is appointed	Nick		—	—							
Speakers arranged	Nick					—	—	—			
Facilities arranged	David				▪	—	—	—			
Luncheon arrangements	Vanessa							—			
Arrangements for entertainment	Vanessa					—	—	—			
Print forms and address to mail	Bill								—		
Mail program/reservation forms	Nick/Bill								—		
Confirm speakers	Nick								▪	▪	
Reservations for meals reported	Vanessa									—	
Reservations for hotels reported	David								▪	—	
Registration materials prepared	Bill					—	—	—			
Registration is accepted	David/Susan								—	—	▪
Morning session held	Nick										—
Evaluation of speakers	Nick										—
Luncheon	Vanessa										▪
Afternoon sessions are held	Nick										▪
Coffee breaks are held	Vanessa										—
Conference report is filed	Susan										▪

FIGURE 17-19 Gantt chart.

? DID YOU KNOW?

1. The characteristics of a project are:
   - Unique
   - Product or result
   - Finite
   - Complex, numerous, and sequenced activities
   - Team
   - Cross-functional
   - Limited resources
   - Change
2. The problem statement answers the following questions:
   - What is the problem?
   - What is the opportunity?
   - What is to be done?
   - Who is responsible for the project?
   - When must it be completed?
3. The *goal statement* is the final outcome of the project.
4. *Project resources* include people, materials, space, and money that are needed to achieve the goal.
5. The most important element of project management is the *project manager.*
6. Controlling is the monitoring and maintenance of the structure of the project.
7. *Effective project leadership* and *control tools* are the two areas that are detailed in the control phase of project management.
8. *PERT* is the acronym for Program Evaluation Review Technique.

Reengineering

Reengineering (also known as business process reengineering) has been used in the business world and is now finding its way into health care. Business process reengineering is a theory in which the way business is done is radically reevaluated to achieve dramatic performance improvement. It encourages streamlining functions to reduce time, cost, and effort while enhancing the quality of service. In health care, this means meeting the challenges of becoming efficient and productive while providing quality care. This concept is new and different in health care, possibly because the terms *radical* and *health care* usually do not go hand in hand.

Reengineering means challenging every aspect of the way of doing business to improve performance substantially. Reengineering the process means "starting with a blank sheet of paper," starting all over, starting from scratch, and challenging the status quo with the goal of vast improvements.[14] It explores new ways of doing the work and questions why processes are done at all. Each process performed should contribute to achieving the organization's goals. The processes that do contribute are called value-added activities.

After a process is determined to be necessary, each step of the process is questioned. Does the step add value? Can it be simplified? Would resequencing the steps smooth the work flow? When practical, can the steps be automated?

Objectives

The main objectives of reengineering are as follows:
- Reduce cost
- Increase revenue
- Improve quality
- Reduce risk

Reengineering is a complete rethinking and transformation of key processes. With use of the reengineering approach, a key hospital process of admitting an inpatient could be transformed or virtually eliminated, perhaps by using an interactive computer process from the patient's home.

Reengineering emphasizes streamlining of cross-functional processes to achieve organizational objectives. Patient-focused care is an example of a cross-functional process in a health care environment. The nursing units are transformed into self-contained mini hospitals in which the delivery of care is closer to the patient. The unit might contain a mini laboratory, a mini radiology department, and a mini pharmacy. A health care team is selected according to the patient's diagnosis, procedure, or severity of illness. That health care team delivers all the care to the patient. The actual number of health care workers the patient has contact with is fewer than in the traditional health care delivery models. Business process reengineering entails the assimilation of several interrelated changes, including policies and procedures, organization and staff, facilities, and technology.

Use of Policies and Procedures in the Reengineering Process

Policies and procedures are important at all times as controlling tools, but they are especially useful during departmental reengineering.

Policies

Policies are the guides that managers use to make decisions. Policies translate the mission statement and corporate objectives into practical and easily understood terms. Policies within an organization should be clearly written and consistently applied so that as similar situations arise, they are handled in a like manner. Thus, policy making is usually the responsibility of upper management, although individual department heads may develop policies specific to their department. When this is the case, these department-specific policies must not conflict with the policies of the organization as a whole. In time, implied policies may be developed. Implied policies are those that, although not officially approved, are generally accepted by management. A problem may arise when management tries to enforce the official policy after the implied policy has become the norm.

Although policies must be consistent, they should be flexible enough to accommodate a dynamic workplace and should permit, even require, interpretation, as appropriate. Organizations generally have policy manuals so that employees are aware of all policies. Personnel policies are often included in the employee handbook. An example of a policy might be: "All discharge summaries will be directly entered into the computer and electronically signed by the attending physician no later than 24 hours post discharge."

Upper management should be certain that all policies conform to applicable state and federal laws and to the requirements of various accrediting and certifying agencies or organizations.

Procedures

Procedures are the guides and plans for action. Although policies outline a general course of action, procedures are the step-by-step instructions for accomplishing a specific task or job. A well-written procedure explains what is supposed to be done, who is to do it, and exactly how it is to be done. Procedures ensure uniformity of practice, make training of personnel easier, and can be used as a controlling tool to ensure that the job is being done as planned. Written procedures can establish benchmarks to compare with past or future operating practices.

When procedures are written or evaluated (or existing ones are redesigned), several steps may be followed (Box 17-4).

Procedures are generally written in narrative, step-by-step outline, or playscript style. In narrative style, the procedure is written in story or paragraph format and includes all of the parts of the procedure. It is usually the hardest style to write because there must be transition statements between all of the parts of the process.

The step-by-step procedure is written in outline format and takes the employee through each individual task in the procedure. It is generally the easiest style for the employee to follow.

The playscript format is often used when several employees are involved in a particular task. In this method, a number is assigned to each step in the procedure and action verbs are used to describe the key steps in the task. It also identifies which employee or "actor" completes each step. (See Example of a Statement Written in Playscript Style.)

Example of a Statement Written in Playscript Style

Actor	Step Sequence	Action Word	Action Sentence
Receptionist	1	Greets	Greets visitors as they enter the health information department

After all procedures are written, they should be organized into a procedure manual. Effective communication and writing skills should be used in creating this manual. Clarity and brevity are essential elements of the procedure manual, as is the use of action verbs to convey the steps in the procedure. The purpose of the manual and the intended audience are factors in deciding on the writing style used, the level of detail, and the kinds of examples used.

How the procedure manual is to be arranged and disseminated must also be considered. The procedure manual should be accessible, easy to read, and arranged so that information is easily found. It should be updated frequently. It is often distributed in a binder for ease in updating.

Relationship to Quality Improvement

Because reengineering advocates radical change that might be too risky for health care organizations, the more cautious and acceptable approach of quality improvement is often used in conjunction with reengineering. Sometimes total quality management is used in conjunction with reengineering to restructure a process to create the most efficient operation model for delivering an outcome. Total quality management starts with minor successes and builds.

Applications to Health Information Management

HIM professionals need to become involved in the organization-wide reengineering process. They need to look at processes and procedures in a whole new light. Looking forward to the computer-based patient record, HIM professionals need to view how it will radically change the delivery of patient care and management of information. For its full potential to be realized, HIM professionals have to be willing to let go of old ways and change things dramatically.[15] The same forms that are used in paper records cannot simply be computerized and expected to meet the information needs of the future. Given the HIM role in the health care field and the dramatic changes in health care delivery systems, HIM professionals need an understanding of and commitment to the reengineering process.[16]

BOX 17-4 ▸ Steps in Writing Procedures

- List each step in the procedure.
- Determine a logical sequence for the steps.
- Eliminate unnecessary steps.
- Determine whether some steps are too difficult for employees' skills.
- Review potential bottlenecks or obstacles to completion.
- Determine the impact of this procedure on other procedures.
- Test the procedure for several weeks.
- Ask for employee input.
- Evaluate the effectiveness of the procedure.
- Make changes as necessary.
- Implement the new procedure.

SELF-ASSESSMENT QUIZ

20. Define the use of policies and procedures in the reengineering process.
21. When writing procedures in this format, a number is assigned to each step in the procedure, and action verbs are used to describe the key steps in the task. It also identifies which employee or "actor" completes each step of the procedure. What is the name of this format?
22. What is the definition of reengineering or business process reengineering?

DID YOU KNOW?

- The main objectives of reengineering are:
  - Reduce cost
  - Increase revenue
  - Improve quality
  - Reduce risk
- *Clarity* and *brevity* are essential elements of a procedure manual.
- Procedures are generally written in either *narrative*, *step-by-step outline*, or *playscript style*.
- *Quality improvement* is often used in conjunction with reengineering.

DESIGN AND MANAGEMENT OF SPACE IN HEALTH INFORMATION SERVICES

This section focuses on the arrangement of the physical components of furniture, equipment, and environment with the goal of providing maximum effectiveness and coordinating these physical components into a comfortable work area, thus contributing to maximum efficiency of the department and organization.

Work-Space Design

When the work space is designed, the following aspects should be considered.

Work Flow

Considering the purpose of the organization, the primary objective in work-space design is efficient and effective work flow. Is the work moving to the next person with a minimum of backtracking and bottlenecks? Work flow is a greater concern in an environment where paper is used than in a totally computerized system. As discussed earlier in the chapter, several tools are available to use in analyzing and improving work flow, including flowcharts.

Traffic Patterns

Along with work flow, the traffic patterns of employees and visitors to the area are important considerations. To determine these patterns, the location of entrances to the area, the employees who work together, and the employees who frequently receive visitors or leave the area need to be identified. A **trip frequency chart** shows which employees frequently interact with one another (Figure 17-20). The various employees and locations are listed along the horizontal and vertical axes. The number indicates how many times one employee visits the work space of another employee. Low numbers indicate which employees do not

FIGURE 17-20 Trip frequency chart.

FROM \ TO	Director	Secretary	Health Information Analyst	Release of Information Specialist	Clinical Coder	Optical Image Specialist
Director		14	5	3	7	8
Secretary	30		4	9	2	10
Health Information Analyst	8	3		4	12	20
Release of Information Specialist	16	9	5		5	14
Clinical Coder	12	4	10	6		9
Optical Image Specialist	25	19	9	11	7	

interact frequently and, therefore, do not need to be close to one another, whereas high numbers indicate a need for closeness.

Work groups or teams are commonly found in today's workplace. Space design must facilitate the work of these teams, not prohibit it. Supervisors or team leaders also need to be located in proximity to their staff to provide more effective supervision and to facilitate communication.

The work space allotted to a particular departmental function or work group should conform to the number of employees performing that function. Equipment, references, and other materials needed to perform the job can then be located in one central area so that they are easily accessible to all employees performing similar tasks.

Functions Performed in the Work Space

When the work space is designed, an obvious consideration is the type of function performed in the space. Some specific functions beyond those of the data entry-clerical type must be considered. The reception area has a public relations aspect. Because visitors see this area first, it should be neat, well organized, and functional. It should be located so that visitors do not interrupt the work flow. Serving as a buffer zone between the outside and the place of work, the reception area provides privacy for the staff. This area should be monitored constantly to assist and screen visitors, letting only those people enter who have legitimate business.

Another special-purpose area is a conference room. This area is needed for meetings that are too large to take place in a private office, that might disturb others in the office, or that need special equipment (e.g., an overhead projector). This area can also be used for training.

In the overall design of a department, it is often desirable to place certain areas next to each other and other areas far away from each other. A restaurant designer would not place the patron waiting area near the garbage dump. This would be undesirable. A proximity chart shows the need to place some areas close to or far from each other (Figure 17-21). It can also show why the proximity is important.

FIGURE 17-21 Proximity chart.

Scales			
Importance of proximity		Reason for proximity	
Code Importance		Code Reason	
A Absolutely necessary		1 Flow of materials	
E Especially important		2 Share equipment	
I Important		3 Share personnel	
U Unimportant		4 Supervision	
X Undesirable		5 Noise; distraction	
		6	
		7	
		8	

Need for Confidentiality of Work Performed

If the work being performed is of a confidential nature, access to the work area may need to be controlled. If the confidential information is audible—for example, physicians dictating reports for the patient record or employee conferences—then the space design must provide for this speech privacy. If the work is performed on a computer, the use of screens or panels around work areas may be advisable to prevent others from reading information displayed on the computer screen. The location of a fax machine also involves security concerns. In a health care organization, confidential information is often transmitted by way of fax machine. Fax machines should be located in areas that are secure from access by unauthorized employees.

Shift Workers—Sharing Work Space

Sometimes it is necessary to divide a particular job function into shifts. This is true if space is restricted or if equipment to perform the job is costly and limited in supply. Shift work may mean that employees must share their work space. Under these circumstances, each employee should have some private space in the work area that is his or her own for displaying photographs and for storage of personal items. Employees sharing work space need to respect one another's privacy. Adjustability of chairs and other work equipment is important so that the needs of all may be met.

Flexibility for Future Needs

Work-space design should be as flexible as possible to accommodate the future needs of the organization. These needs might include downsizing, expansion, or further computerization. The use of partitions instead of solid-walled offices is recommended for organizations that anticipate change, either in size or in the work functions being performed. Workstations in which components may be added or subtracted as necessary (i.e., modular furniture) increase the capability of organizations to implement change without loss of efficiency.

Expanding technology demands increase the need for power capabilities of the work space. Regular electrical power and "clean" power for computers and telecommunications systems are located beneath access floors so that necessary power is available at any given location. This system allows for flush-to-floor outlets and flexible placement of furniture and equipment.

Employees' Personal Needs

The work environment is composed of people gathered together to perform work that will accomplish the objectives of an organization. These people have physical, safety, social, and psychological needs that must be met as well as the need to collect a paycheck. Today's workforce wants a comfortable, safe, and user-friendly environment.

Physical Size and Structure

Because employees vary in physical characteristics such as height, weight, and length of torso and extremities, workstation components should be as flexible and adjustable as possible. More information on the workstation and its components is presented later in the chapter.

Age

Older people may require special considerations in the workplace regarding lighting, sound, and temperature.

Medical Conditions

In addition to the special considerations of age, workplace requirements for physical handicaps or other medical conditions of the worker must be addressed. The Vocational Rehabilitation Act of 1972 requires that federal buildings and buildings that were built with more than $2500 in federal funds be accessible to handicapped people. These requirements include wide aisle space for wheelchairs, 28-inch height for desks, 32-inch-wide doors, ramp entrances to buildings, and appropriate (time-delayed) entry doors.

The Americans with Disabilities Act (ADA), which became effective in 1992, provides that if a facility is a "public accommodation," it must take "barrier removal" steps. Public accommodations include many types of service establishments, such as professional offices of health care providers, pharmacies, insurance offices, banks, and hospitals. Barriers that affect work space access can be modified in the following ways:

- Installing ramps where steps are located
- Repositioning shelves
- Installing flashing alarm lights
- Widening doors
- Installing offset hinges to widen doorways
- Installing accessible door hardware
- Removing high-pile, low-density carpeting[17]

Adjustments to the work space to accommodate special equipment or handicaps without causing the employer undue hardships are required by the ADA.

Safety Needs

A safe work environment is important to management and to workers. It reduces the number of work-related accidents, which are costly to the organization in terms of lost work time and workers' compensation claims.

Management is responsible for providing a safe work environment for employees. These responsibilities include the following:

- Maintaining a favorable climate for safety
- Ensuring that the equipment and furniture are in the best working condition
- Being a good example
- Teaching principles of safety (see Basic Safety Principles)
- Stressing an orderly work environment
- Stopping unsafe acts

The Occupational Safety and Health Act (OSHA) requires that employers furnish a workplace that is free from hazards that are likely to cause serious harm or death. OSHA has safety requirements for equipment, noise level standards, and lighting requirements for computer users.

Basic Safety Principles

- Cords for telephones or electrical equipment should be out of sight, if possible. Furniture often contains cable channels to accommodate the multitude of cords required in today's workplace. Cords should never be draped across aisles or walkways. Whenever unplugging an electrical appliance, always pull on the plug, not the cord. Yanking on the cord breaks insulation or loosens terminals.
- File and desk drawers should not be left open for people to trip over or walk into. They should not be used as a step stool because they will not hold a person's weight.
- Office tools such as scissors, staples, razor blades, and pencils should be used only for their intended purpose. Pencils are not to be used as hole punchers. Letter openers are not to be used for prying open stuck drawers.
- Paper cuts are an annoying type of injury that can be avoided by proper handling: using rubber finger guards, picking up individual sheets of paper at the corner instead of the side, and encouraging the use of hand lotion for dry skin, which is more susceptible to paper cuts.
- Drawer files can tip over if more than one drawer at a time is opened or if heavy objects are placed in top drawers or far in the front of a drawer.
- Stepladders should be fully open and locked before use. Move the ladder to the desired location instead of reaching from the ladder. Do not use boxes, chairs on rollers, or tables in place of ladders.
- Open-shelf files should be bolted to a wall or to the back of another file. Trying to remove records from files that are too tightly packed can cause the files to sway or topple if they are not bolted to some other support.

Social Needs

The atmosphere in the office affects employees' happiness and feelings of well-being. A positive environment can motivate employees to improve productivity and decrease use of sick days.

Employees, especially those engaged in similar activities, like to work in proximity to one another, where they can easily ask questions or otherwise confer on the work at hand. Workstations in clusters are effective in encouraging the team approach concept.

Personal Space

Personal space is the private area that surrounds an employee and is felt to belong to him or her. Personal space requirements vary among cultures, with those from Middle Eastern countries, for example, typically requiring less personal space than Americans do.

Territoriality is another concept that should be considered in office-space planning. Territoriality refers to the physical area that is under the control of the employee or is specifically for his or her use. It may be the employee's workstation or a private office.

Employees take pride in their physical surroundings. The workstation becomes a reflection of employees' personalities. They like the freedom to decorate or personalize it to suit themselves.

Reflection of Status in the Organization (Is the Corner Office Dead?)

The status of an employee within an organization, especially the managerial staff, used to be reflected by whether the employee had a private office, the size of that office, and whether the office had windows. The large corner office in a building or suite was seen as the most desirable space in terms of status within the organization.

Private offices are not as common or as widely used as they were in past years. The trend is toward a more open type of office landscaping. The private office still denotes prestige, however, and most managers prefer to have some degree of privacy in their work setting. The work may be of a personal or confidential nature that requires a location in which business matters cannot be overheard by other employees. The work may also require a high degree of concentration. Such a case would require locating the workstation in an area free from distractions and interruptions.

The disadvantages of private offices are interference with heat and air-conditioning systems, a decrease in supervisory effectiveness, and increased construction costs.

Managers can enjoy almost as much privacy with an open plan as with a private office by using high divider panels to surround the office furnishings. Panels with doors are available in a wide variety of fabrics and materials, including glass.

Evaluation of individual needs is necessary to decide whether a private office is needed. Combining the conventional office plan with private offices with the open plan maintains the status and privacy needs of the executive. Such a combination is referred to as the American plan of office design.

Design of the Workstation

Ergonomics

Ergonomics is the science concerned with the relationship of people to their working environment and more particularly to the study of how to design a work environment that promotes comfortable, safe, and injury-free work. The science of ergonomics includes the analysis of psychological and physiological influences.

Background

Repetitive strain (or stress) injuries (RSIs), also called cumulative trauma disorder (CTD), are the fastest growing workplace injuries in the United States today. The most common RSIs are carpal tunnel syndrome (CTS) and tendinitis. CTS often occurs in workers who spend long hours using computers or workers who perform repetitive tasks. According to the Bureau of Labor Statistics (BLS), the median of days missed from work was highest for carpal tunnel syndrome.

Employers are becoming increasingly interested in workplace design as the absenteeism rate related to CTD increases and workers' compensation claims soar.

OSHA is committed to achieving safer workplaces and is in the process of developing industry- and task-specific guidelines that assist employers and employees in recognizing and controlling potential ergonomic hazards. A guideline is a voluntary tool and is designed to be flexible so that employers can adopt innovative programs to suit their workplaces. OSHA is developing these guidelines for a select number of industries taking into account injury and illness incidence rates.

The National Institute for Occupational Safety and Health (NIOSH) sets standards in office design, construction, and use of equipment, especially in the use of computers. The results of a NIOSH study showed that computer users have various types of health complaints. Among them are optical problems (thought to be brought on by stress), painful or stiff muscles and joints, and loss of strength in arms, hands, wrists, and fingers. After the study, NIOSH stressed ergonomic solutions to these problems. In other words, they recommended that managers provide employees with furniture and equipment that can be adjusted to the physical traits of each worker to eliminate strain. NIOSH sets standards for lighting as well.

Successful Ergonomics Programs

Organizations that have implemented ergonomic programs report decreases in work-related injuries and subsequent health care costs and increases in productivity and worker morale. A successful ergonomics program requires a strong commitment from management. Education and training are important parts of any such program. Workers and supervisors should have an understanding of the potential risks of injuries, symptoms to be aware of, and prevention and treatment. Managers should attend training sessions with the employees. Sharing the responsibility for a comfortable and productive work area increases the success of the ergonomics program.

Identifying ergonomic risk factors (situations in which extra demands are placed on the employee) is essential for preventing ergonomics-related injuries and illnesses.

There are several ways to identify risk factors:

- Use employee interviews or questionnaires. Employees are asked to identify what they consider risk factors present in their jobs. Anonymous written questionnaires may elicit more honest responses than one-on-one interviews.
- Use an ergonomics checklist to survey the workplace. Many commercial checklists are available for purchase. The types of questions asked include:
  1. Does the work area allow a full range of motion?
  2. Is the height of the work surface adjustable to accommodate varying heights of employees?
  3. Is the employee able to vary posture?
  4. Are objects within easy reach?
  5. Is the chair adjustable to assist in maintaining good posture?
  6. Does the chair have an adjustable backrest?
  7. Is there sufficient leg and knee room?
  8. Is the lighting sufficient for comfort?
  9. Are employees trained in handling and lifting heavy objects?
  10. Are materials and forms moved over minimal distances?
- Examine the absenteeism rate.
- Review employee grievance logs.
- Look for signs of stress among workers.

Components of the Workstation

The workstation is a collection of desks or work surfaces, equipment, storage facilities, and chairs shaped by technology, the tasks to be performed, and various human needs.

Desk or Work Surface

The office desk serves as a work space, storage space, filing area, and place where office and communications equipment rests. Efficiently organized, the desk can enhance productivity. Made-to-order drawer arrangements facilitate storage and make supplies accessible.

The height of the work surface should be adjustable, if possible, to accommodate the height of the user and the task to be performed. Work surface height should be about 28 inches for tasks other than keyboarding. Keyboard or typing tasks require a lower work surface than other tasks. Keyboards should be at least 2 to 3 inches lower than the regular work surface so that the users' arms do not have to be raised to type. Keyboards may be attached under the desk in a pull-out arrangement, or a special lower work surface may be built into the workstation to accommodate the keyboard.

There should be adequate knee clearance to accommodate a full range of movement, and feet should lie flat on the floor or on a footrest so that the knees are parallel at a 90- to 110-degree angle.

The size of the desk often depends on employees' organizational levels and the tasks assigned. The work surface should be at least 30 inches wide. When possible, the desktop should not be crowded with equipment. Managers who do many types of desk work may require a larger work area.

Guidelines for Work Surface of Desktop Arrangements

The positioning of key workstation components is extremely important in an organization concerned with efficiency and ergonomics. Employees should be able to reach all work surfaces and equipment with a minimum of movement. Frequent stretching to reach key workstation components causes fatigue and other musculoskeletal problems related to the arms, neck, and back. Short, frequent breaks and rest pauses assist in reducing these problems. Employees should incorporate exercises, stretches, and movement into these short breaks or rest pauses. Software programs are available to remind workers to take a break. Some flash instructions on the screen for simple neck, shoulder, wrist, and arm exercises. For example, medical transcriptionists commonly sit at word processing stations for many hours without changing position or routine. Breaks do not always have to be rest breaks. Interspersing different functions into the transcriptionist's day can also alleviate the strain and muscle fatigue that come from sitting for long hours in the same position. Transcriptionists should break their routine occasionally by doing other tasks to relieve the boredom and fatigue. Changing the routine may not work well if an incentive or other type of productivity program is in place.

The positioning of the components on the work surface depends on the frequency, sequence, and duration of the task. The more frequent and longer-duration tasks are done in the primary zone; the materials that are used to support the more frequent tasks are stored in the secondary zone.

Writing, keying, and reading use the primary zone or front area of the work space. This is the area of the work surface that is within bent arm's reach. Computers may be located in the primary space in the workstation for full-time computer operators and in the secondary space for managers and others who operate computers only part of the time.

Supporting materials and equipment only occasionally used or waiting to be used are placed in the secondary area or the area of extended arm's reach.

Space that does not fall into the primary or secondary zone categories should be used for storage.

The Chair

The office chair is probably the single most important component of the workstation because of its ergonomic impact. Ergonomic chairs have positive effects on posture and circulation and minimize stress placed on the back. Chairs should be adjustable to support the body. Chairs should have the following adjustments:

- Seat pan tilts forward and backward
- Pneumatic height adjustment
- Independent back adjustment
- Individualized lumbar support in both height and firmness

Chairs should be adjusted so that the forearms are parallel to the floor with both feet flat on the floor or on a footrest with thighs parallel to the floor. When the chair is too high, the feet lack the proper support and the chair places pressure on the blood vessels in the thighs, leading to pain and poor circulation. A seat that is too low increases back fatigue.

Backrests support and distribute the upper body weight. The back support should follow the natural curve of the back. A towel or lumbar pad can be used if the chair does not provide adequate support.

Computer and Peripherals

As with the chair, flexibility and adjustability are prime factors in monitor selection and placement. Monitors should swivel and tilt and, if possible, be adjustable in height. The top of the monitor screen should be just slightly below eye level when the employee is sitting. Employees who wear bifocals or trifocals may need to have the monitor at a lower position. The center of the screen should be about 20 degrees below eye level. Maintaining a distance of 18 to 28 inches between the eyes and the monitor allows easy focusing and reduces eyestrain and fatigue. The employee should refocus the eyes periodically by looking away from the monitor. Blinking, yawning, and moving the eyes up and down and right and left also help. Source documents should be positioned to be at the same height as the screen to reduce neck and eye movements, thus reducing neck discomfort and eyestrain. Hanging document holders may be provided with the monitors or purchased separately. Finally, filter screens reduce glare and relieve eyestrain.

Printers should be located so that the user does not have to get up from the chair to retrieve printed pages.

The design of the keyboard should allow the hand to be in a neutral position while keying. A neutral position is similar to a handshake position. Traditional keyboard design forces the palm downward and the wrist outward, called an ulnar deviation. New designs for keyboards attempt to alleviate these problems. Newer detachable keyboards can be positioned for ergonomically correct keyboarding. Wrist rests or supports help to keep the wrists in a straight position while allowing freedom of movement.

Ergonomic software that monitors how much the computer is used and prompts the employee to take a rest break at appropriate intervals and even suggests simple exercises is available.

Partitions

Partitions surrounding the workstation are usually less than ceiling height and designed to house shelves or closed-in storage space, bulletin boards, and other components that may be useful to the employee. Such panels or partitions provide privacy and diminish distractions from the surroundings.

Shelving, Filing, and Storage Space

The efficiently designed workstation contains filing and storage space located conveniently for the seated worker. Shelves may be located above the workstation within easy reach of the worker, and drawers for supplies can be attached to the work surface for easy accessibility.

Telephone

The telephone and any accessory equipment should be positioned so that they are convenient to the user but do not interfere with the primary work space. Telephone cords should be long enough to permit the employee to reach the phone from any position in the workstation. Cordless telephones and headsets are useful for various applications.

Shared or Multifunction Workstations

Workstation furniture or components must accommodate a number of functional tasks. Many workstations used by general or technical employees are shared, either on the same shift or between shifts. This means that it is even more important to purchase furniture with as many adjustable features as possible.

BOX 17-5 **Guidelines for Allocating Office Space**

- Generally, each clerical employee should be allocated at least 60 square feet for his or her work area (this includes the desk, aisle space, and storage space). The amount of space allocated depends on the job assignment, total space available, need for privacy, and number of pieces of equipment used. When space permits, 75 to 85 square feet per clerical worker is allocated.
- Space standards for aisles:
  - Main aisles: 4 to 5 feet wide
  - Secondary aisles: 3 to 4 feet wide
  - Aisle space between desks: not less than 36 inches
- Spacing of filing cabinets depends on the frequency of use and the type of cabinet.
- Equipment used should be placed near the user.
- A supervisor should be placed at the back of the group of workers whom he or she supervises.
- The file area should be placed in a location that is inaccessible to unauthorized personnel.
- Do not have employees working too near a heat source, in an air-conditioning draft, or facing a window.
- Provide sufficient floor electrical outlets for office machines.
- Paper or forms should move to the employee rather than having the employee move to the paper.
- Movable files are the most space-efficient type of filing units.

Space Standards and Guidelines for the Office

One of the first steps that should be done is to secure a drawing or blueprint of the available area. Blueprints are generally drawn to scale; for example, one quarter inch on the blueprint is equal to 1 actual foot of space. Many variables must be considered when allocating space in an office, but there are some guidelines to assist the supervisor in making decisions (Box 17-5).

Environmental Considerations

Ergonomics encompasses many aspects of the workplace, including lighting, sound, air temperature, air quality, and color. Workers who participated in the Steelcase Study II on office comfort stated that, if they could change physical conditions in their offices, they would most often make improvements in the heat and air-conditioning, regulate temperature, reduce noise, obtain more space and privacy, and acquire more comfortable chairs.

Given a choice between getting a raise with no improvements in the office environment and getting a smaller increase with improvements, more than half the employees in the Steelcase Study selected the larger raise. A substantial number, however, stated that they would select a smaller raise if they could control heat and air-conditioning (30%) and general office comfort (27%), had a chair with back support (26%), had a private office with a door (21%), and had a quieter place in which to work (20%). It is interesting to note that heat and air-conditioning ranked highest as the item employees most wanted to control; it ranked eleventh as the item that executives believed that their company would consider a motivator or reward for high employee performance. Employers greatly underestimated the need of employees to control their own environment.

Air Quality

Heating, ventilating, and air-conditioning (HVAC) systems are an integral part of office design. Heating and air-conditioning systems are easier to operate in the **open office design plan** of most modern offices than in the traditional or closed plan.

Good air quality improves productivity. Air pollution (stale, dusty air), on the other hand, produces undesirable effects, such as headache and fatigue. Air circulation is important in the work environment. Fifteen cubic meters of fresh (outside) air per hour per person is desirable in a nonsmoking environment. Air-conditioning not only cools the air but also removes undesirable pollutants such as smoke, asbestos, soot, dust, and chemicals. Clean air is important for equipment operation as well as for its effects on employees. Mechanical air filters are helpful, as are frequent cleaning, sweeping, and vacuuming.

OSHA has set indoor air quality standards and can take action against employers who fail to comply. The Environmental Protection Agency (EPA) lists indoor air pollution as one of its top five environmental issues, causing a wide range of problems such as bronchitis, asthma, emphysema, cancer, and heart disease. The EPA states that a common problem in businesses is that the HVAC system operates only on weekdays and not when the building is unoccupied. It suggests starting the system several hours before workers arrive and continuing it for several hours after they leave for maximum effectiveness. The EPA also promotes restricted areas for smokers. The agency recommends regular inspections of the building and the HVAC system. Data on symptoms suffered by building occupants and likely contamination sources should be collected and analyzed periodically.

Temperature

Temperature means the hotness or coolness of the air. A comfortable office temperature is about 70°F or lower, with older employees requiring a slightly warmer environment. Thermostats are often set at 65°F during the heating season to conserve energy. Human bodies in large numbers generate heat, especially when they are performing physical tasks such as walking and typing. A computer also generates heat equal to that generated by one person.

Humidity

The percentage of moisture in the air is called **relative humidity**. The most comfortable standard for office workers is 30% to 60% with a temperature ranging between 65°F and 70°F. Automated equipment requires a relative humidity range between 20% and 80%. Too much humidity causes short circuiting in equipment, and too little humidity produces static electricity.

Lighting

Proper lighting is more important today than ever before with so many people using computers. Lighting affects not only productivity but also employee health.

In planning a good lighting system, the following factors should be considered:

- Flexibility and adjustability
- Ease of installation
- Low energy use
- Low initial cost
- Efficiency of the system
- Safety
- Effect on employees (comfort level)
- Integration of sunlight into lighting systems

Amount and Type of Light

The amount and type of light should be evenly diffused over the work area. Moving from areas of greater light intensity to areas of lesser intensity causes eyestrain, fatigue, and headache because of pupil expansion and contraction.

The amount and type of light used depend on the color scheme of the office decor, the type of work being performed, and the age of the worker. Less light is needed in areas that are decorated with light colors because light colors reflect light, whereas darker colors absorb light.

High levels of illuminance are needed for many tasks that involve paper documents, whereas lower levels are needed in computer-user environments, reception areas, storerooms, and stairways. In areas where work is both paper-based and done on computers, appropriate lighting is difficult to achieve because of the different lighting needs.

Also, older workers require more light to perform the same tasks as younger workers. After age 50 years, light requirements may be 50% higher and after age 60 years 100% higher than for younger workers.

Light Source Design

Light sources are designed as direct lighting, indirect or reflective lighting, or combinations of the two. Direct lighting reflects directly on the work surface. Semidirect lighting reflects some light off the ceiling, but most shines directly on the work surface. Indirect lighting reflects all light off the ceiling. Lights may be suspended from the ceiling, recessed in the ceiling and enclosed, placed in troughs near the top of the wall, suspended from partitions, or attached directly to modular furniture.

Task Lighting

The number one priority for lighting is to achieve the best task visibility possible. A second priority should be to create the most comfortable visual environment possible. Task lighting, also referred to as accent lighting, often involves building the light fixtures into the furniture or workstations to illuminate specific work areas. Task lighting is especially important in an open office design.

Sometimes variable-intensity task lighting is used in work areas. Variable-intensity lighting achieves adjustability by using a plastic cylinder with a network of dark lines enclosing a fluorescent lamp. By turning the cylinder, employees can adjust the illumination to suit themselves or the tasks.

Ambient Lighting

Indirect lighting fixtures provide ambient lighting. Light is directed upward so that it is reflected off the ceiling onto the work area. It provides light for a large area, but the light is insufficient to work by. Ambient lighting is often combined with task lighting to provide a lighting system that is flexible, lower in energy cost, and easier to install than direct overhead lighting. Task-ambient lighting can be used with reduced overhead lighting, or it can supply light by means of fixtures that emit light both upward and downward. It is an attractive and economical means of providing adequate light for an open office design.

? DID YOU KNOW?

1. The primary objective in work-space design is efficient and effective *work flow*.
2. When the work space is designed, an obvious consideration is the *type of function* performed in the space.
3. The work environment is composed of people gathered together to perform work, and these individuals have *physical*, *safety*, *social*, and *psychological* needs that must be met along with the work they perform.
4. Barriers that affect work space access can be modified in the following ways:
   - Installing ramps where steps are located
   - Repositioning shelves
   - Installing flashing alarm lights
   - Widening doors
   - Installing offset hinges to widen doorways
   - Installing accessible door hardware
   - Removing high-pile, low-density carpeting
5. *Territoriality* is another concept that should be considered in office space planning and refers to the physical area that is under the control of the employee or is specifically for his or her use.
6. *Ergonomics* is the science concerned with the relationship of people to their working environment and more particularly to the study of how to design a work environment that promotes comfortable, safe, and injury-free work.
7. The *workstation* is a collection of desks or work surfaces, equipment, storage facilities, and chairs shaped by technology, the tasks to be performed, and various human needs.
8. The *office chair* is probably the single most important component of the workstation because of its ergonomic impact.
9. The *Environmental Protection Agency (EPA)* lists indoor air pollution as one of its top five environmental issues, causing a wide range of problems such as bronchitis, asthma, emphysema, cancer, and heart disease.

Lighting and Computers

The lighting at computer workstations should be lower than for areas in which concentrated work on paper documents is performed. Glare on the monitor from lights and windows can be avoided by using antiglare filters with proper placement and by having the capability of adjusting the computer screen. Computers should be placed at right angles to outside windows. The user should not directly face the window when working at the computer. Window coverings such as louvered blinds can be used to adjust the amount and glare of sunlight.

Sound and Acoustics

Sound control is important for a healthy and productive work environment. Without a sound control program, employees experience physiological and psychological problems such as increased blood pressure, accelerated heart rate, increased muscle tension, mental stress, and irritability.

Sound is measured in decibels. One decibel equals the smallest degree of difference or change in loudness that is detectable by the human ear. Maximum sound levels for various types of office environments are as follows:

- General offices—60 dB
- Private offices—40 dB
- Data centers (with computers, printers, copiers, telephones, and other equipment)—70 dB

The sound control system has two main goals: speech privacy and controlling noise generated inside and outside the work area.

Levels of Speech Privacy

Various levels of speech privacy can be attained through the use of construction materials, acoustic decorations, and sound-masking devices. Levels of speech privacy are as follows:

- Absolute: Nothing can be heard, not even mumbling. It is the most difficult and expensive level to achieve.
- Confidential: Cannot understand what is said but mumbling can be heard.
- Normal: Sound of incoming conversation is loud enough to distract people from their work; a fair amount of conversation could be heard if one concentrated on listening; recommended where the confidential level is not needed.
- None: Most common level; incoming speech is distracting and easy to understand.

Guidelines for Controlling Sound

Controlling sound can be done by confining the source of the noise within a separate room, muffling the sound source with acoustic materials, or submerging it in the background hum

---

BOX 17-6 Guidelines for Controlling Sound

- Use barriers to block sound.
- Locate desks so that employees do not face traffic.
- Use sound-absorbent materials.
- Position overhead lights so that sound reflection is minimized.
- Angle windows outward if possible.
- Use acoustic covers on printers and other equipment to reduce noise levels.
- Use felt or rubber cushions under equipment.
- Carpet the work area where equipment is being used.

---

of a white noise system. Some additional guidelines for controlling sound should be considered in work-space design (Box 17-6).

Pleasant background noise such as music is often used in the workplace. Music has a calming effect, reduces fatigue, and lessens monotony. Music appropriate for the office environment and the type of work being performed should be selected.

An effective sound control system results in increased efficiency, decreased errors, a higher level of concentration, increased physical comfort, and elimination of distractions.

Color

Using color appropriately not only adds to the attractiveness of the office but also contributes to the efficiency and productivity of the workers. Certain colors cause employees to have positive feelings, whereas other colors have the opposite effect.

One popular approach to selecting colors is the monochromatic approach, which uses various shades of one color for floors, walls, and draperies with one bright accent color for furniture, pictures, or lamps. Color choices vary depending on the task of the employees and the function of the area.

Light colors are appropriate in offices where close paperwork is done. White is a neutral color and is nonthreatening as long as it is not too bright a shade of white. Earth tones evoke a feeling of safety in the environment. Blue is a good color for a break area because it is relaxing and reduces blood pressure, pulse, and respiration. Violet is the most restful color but should not be used as a solid color for walls. It is a good accessory color that helps people to relax. The color red is rarely used in offices because it has such a strong stimulating effect that it can cause headaches and increased blood pressure.

An ergonomically designed health information department contributes to the overall efficiency of the organization. Considering all the factors mentioned here in the design of the department will accomplish this goal.

CHAPTER REVIEW

1. What type of chart is used to indicate which employees frequently interact with one another?

2. What are some of the considerations needed in the workplace for older employees?

3. The _____ Act, which became effective in 1992, provides that if a facility is a "public accommodation," it must take "barrier removal" steps.

4. What is the name of the specific act that requires employers to furnish a workplace that is free from hazards that are likely to cause serious harm or death?

5. The _____ sets standards in office design, construction, and use of equipment, especially in the use of computers.

6. What is the proper temperature for a "comfortable office"?

REFERENCES

1. Amatayakul MK, Schraffenberger LA: *Productivity: a handbook for health record departments,* Chicago, 1988, American Medical Record Association.

2. John Sheridan Associates: *Management for productivity.* Presented at the Southeastern Medical Record Conference, Miami, May 13, 1981.

3. Kovach K: *Employee motivation: Addressing a crucial factor in your organization's performance,* Ann Arbor, MI, 1999, University of Michigan Press.

4. Waters K, Murphy GF: Systems analysis and computer applications. In *Health information management and systems analysis,* Rockville, MD, 1983, Aspen Systems p. 118.

5. Longest Jr. B: *Management practices for the health professional,* ed 3, Reston, VA, 1984, Reston Publishing, p. 122.

6. Nickols F: *Change management 101: A primer,* 2008: http://www.nickols.us/change.htm (Accessed 20 August 2010).

7. Duncan WJ, Ginter PM, Swayne LE: Competitive advantage and internal organizational assessment, *Acad Manage Exec* 12:6–16, 1998.

8. Duncan WJ, Ginter PM, Kreidel WK: A sense of direction in public organizations: an analysis of mission statements in state health departments, *Admin Soc* 26:11–27, 1994.

9. Duncan WJ, Ginter PM, Reeves T, et al: Consensus building about the future in a local public health organization: from strategic thinking to strategy formulation, *J Public Health Manage Pract* 4:13–25, 1998.

10. Senge PM: *The fifth discipline,* New York, 1990, Currency Doubleday.

11. Reiss G: *Project management demystified,* ed 3, New York, 2007, Taylor & Francis.

12. Cleland D, Kin W: *Systems analysis and project management,* New York, 1983, McGraw-Hill.

13. Niemi W: Personal Information Managers organize business appointments and enhance communications, Foodservice Equipment & Supplies Specialist, *Newton* Vol. 50, (Iss. 3):10, Mar 25, 1997.

14. Hammer M, Champy J: *Re-engineering the corporation: a manifest for business revolution,* New York, 1993, Harper Business.

15. Brandt M: Re-engineering—starting with a clean slate, *J Am Health Inform Manage Assoc* 65:61–63, 1994.

16. Fox L: Organizational change: re-engineering the work flow, *J Am Health Inform Manage Assoc* 65:35–36, 1994.

17. *American jurisprudence,* ed 2, New York, 1992, Lawyers Cooperative Publishing.

CHAPTER 18

REVENUE CYCLE AND FINANCIAL MANAGEMENT

Bryon D. Pickard

ⓔ Student Study Guide activities for this chapter are available on the Evolve Learning Resources site for this textbook. Please visit http://evolve.elsevier.com/Abdelhak.

CHAPTER CONTENTS

OBJECTIVES

After reading this chapter, the reader will be able to do the following:
- ✓ Define key words.
- ✓ Use fiscal terms with understanding.
- ✓ Describe the various stages of the revenue cycle.
- ✓ List different reimbursement methodologies.
- ✓ Explain the differences between financial and managerial accounting.
- ✓ Calculate key financial ratios.
- ✓ Understand the difference between cash and revenue.
- ✓ Explain the role of the health information professional in the budgeting process.

- ✓ Recognize that organizational planning drives financial management activities.
- ✓ Prepare a business plan and a budget.
- ✓ Explain the purpose of each budget type.
- ✓ Use capital evaluation methods.
- ✓ Describe various cost allocation methods.
- ✓ Assist in charge master updates.
- ✓ Review and analyze variance reports.
- ✓ Define general principles of accounting.
- ✓ Review and apply ratios to financial reports.
- ✓ Understand the potential financial implication of noncompliance with Medicare fraud and abuse regulations.

KEY WORDS

Accounting rate of return	Controlling	Managerial accountant	Profit
Accounts receivable	Current ratio	Managerial finance officer	Prospective payment system
Accounts receivable turnover ratio	Days of revenue in patient accounts	Master budget	Ratio analysis
Accrual basis accounting	receivable ratio	Master charge list	Revenue
Action steps	Depreciation	Matching concept	Rolling budget method
Activity ratio	Disclosure	Medicare	Simultaneous-equations method
Assets	Discounting	Mission	Stable monetary unit
Balance sheet	Double-distribution method	Net	Statement of cash flow
Budgets	Entity	Net operating revenue	Statement of revenues and
Business plan	Equity	Net present value	expenses
Capital expenditure	Fee schedule	Objectives	Statistics budget
Capital expenditure committee	Financial accountant	Operating budget	Step-down method
Capitalization ratios	Financial accounting	Operating margin ratio	Third-party payer
Capitation	Financial analysis	Opportunity costs	Time value of money
Cash basis accounting	Flexible budget	Participating provider	Turnover ratio
Certificate of need	Fund balance	Payback method	Variance report
Charge description master	Goals	Per case	Whole service
Charge master	Liabilities	Per diem	Zero-based budget
Chart of accounts	Liquidity ratios	Performance ratio	
Compounding effect	Long-term debt/total assets ratio	Productive time	

ABBREVIATIONS

ACA	Affordable Care Act	**COB**	Coordination of Benefits
ACO	Accountable Care Organization	**DRG**	Diagnosis-Related Group
AHA	American Hospital Association	**DSS**	Data Security Standard
AICPA	American Institute of Certified Public Accountants	**EDI**	Electronic Data Interchange
ANSI	American National Standards Institute	**EFT**	Electronic Funds Transfer
ARRA	American Recovery and Reinvestment Act	**EOB**	Explanation of Benefits
CCI	Correct Coding Initiative	**ERA**	Electronic Remittance Advice
CDM	Charge Description Master	**FASB**	Financial Accounting Standards Board
CFO	Chief Financial Officer	**GAAP**	Generally Accepted Accounting Principles
CLIA	Clinical Laboratory Improvement Amendment	**GASB**	Government Accounting Standards Board
CMS	Centers for Medicare and Medicaid Services	**HCPCS**	Healthcare Common Procedure Coding System

HIM	Health Information Management	**PCI**	Payment Card Industry
HIPAA	Health Insurance Portability and Accountability Act	**PHI**	Personal Health Information
HITECH	Health Information Technology for Economic and Clinical Health Act	**PPACA**	Patient Protection and Affordable Care Act
		PPO	Preferred Provider Organization
HMO	Health Maintenance Organization	**PPS**	Prospective Payment System
IRS	Internal Revenue Service	**PQRS**	Physician Quality Reporting System
MIPPA	Medicare Improvements for Patients and Providers Act	**RAC**	Recovery Audit Contractor
NCQA	National Committee for Quality Assurance	**RBRVS**	Resource-Based Relative Value Scale
NPI	National Provider Identifier	**RVU**	Relative Value Unit
PCAOB	Public Company Accounting Oversight Board	**UB-04**	Uniform Billing Code of 2004

An explanation of why health information management (HIM) is of widespread interest is that the field itself is so broad. Health information professionals have long been considered experts and industry leaders when it comes to understanding health care information regulations, statutes, data standards, and clinical vocabularies and terminologies. The role of information management and documentation principles is essential to the successful application of technology and ensuring an effective health information infrastructure. It is the assurance of reliable standards, data integrity, and ethical principles and guidelines that makes health care information of use for organizations and individuals. Health information is utilized in clinical decision making, improving quality and safety, consumer empowerment, research, and fulfilling administrative and policy needs. In the same manner, financial management and accounting principles exist to ensure the quality, integrity, and reliability of financial data and information. Generally accepted accounting principles (GAAP) provide a common set of rules and procedures recognized as the accepted standard for financial management and reporting.

In this chapter, we examine a number of concepts, tools, and decision-making approaches to understand and effectively use health care financial information as a strategic resource. Now more than ever is a time to recognize and make use of these concepts in light of the economic climate we live in and the many challenges facing health care organizations. We also highlight a broad number of roles and responsibilities health information managers may find themselves engaged in pertaining to the management and stewardship of an organization's financial resources. Financial management principles apply not only to finance department staff and accountants but to an organization's entire management team. The precise scope and nature of the role of HIM professionals in regard to financial management responsibilities will vary from one organization to another; however, a common theme prevails. First, the information found in health care records is at the core of patient care, clinical decision making, and ultimately delivering quality outcomes. At the same time, the economic aspects of providing health care and being able to communicate financial and monetary matters effectively, covering every facet of health care delivery, are essential. Health information managers have always contributed to the organization's fiscal viability through productive and proficient data collection and information processing for patient care, reimbursement, research, and by management of the resources under their control. In today's data-driven health care environment, it becomes increasingly clear that clinical and financial health information go hand in hand, and being able to analyze, interpret, communicate, and use this strategic resource offers even greater opportunities for health information professionals to flourish.

HISTORICAL PERSPECTIVE

Financial management in health care has become increasingly complex over the past 25 years. Concurrently, the roles held by the HIM professional and health information services have become pivotal positions in the fiscal success of any health care organization. The dependence on the health record's content to define accurately and completely the services provided and conditions treated for reimbursement purposes have contributed to this escalation in status. Skilled HIM professionals have the expertise to analyze the health record and interpret for pertinent data and information to maximize reimbursement without compromising the integrity of data quality.

During this dynamically changing period, the financial aspects of health care organizations have become much more important. Health care managers not only must know how to adjust their operations to respond to the dynamics of a shifting economy and constantly changing regulatory requirements but must also understand the many concepts and principles of financial management. To use a sports analogy, a football quarterback must understand the entire playbook to throw the football to the exact yard line on the field where the wide receiver is expected to run.

Payment for Health Care Services

Perspectives on the significance of financial management in health care show no signs of a slowdown, especially as reimbursement for health care continues to receive increased focus. One only needs to look back at the substantial change that has occurred over the years. Back in the 1930s, the customary method of paying for health care was direct, out-of-pocket remuneration. Some payments were monetary, others were in goods. When hospitals started being used more often than physician offices or house calls, both hospitals and industry explored ways to insure for the cost of health care. This exploration resulted in the establishment of insuring agents that served as the forerunner for what became Blue

Cross and led into multiple private insurance companies, both nonprofit and for profit. These companies provided a new service to the public: coverage for health care expense.

As more people paid health care insurance premiums, they began exercising their "right" to make use of services paid for by their premiums. Health care premiums are the dollars individuals and organizations pay to insurers in return for health care insurance coverage. The increasing use of health care services contributed to rising premiums and greater than anticipated demands on health care providers and organizations. The demand was but one factor leading to building more hospitals and more people seeking training in health care as physicians. Insurance provided an avenue that not only insured the individual but also assured the hospital that it could receive payment for the care provided. Such assurances were atypical before the 1930s. Those insured had no incentive to limit or judiciously seek health care services. Access to full or nearly full payments for services did not encourage hospitals to limit the realm of services provided or control duplication of services within the same community.

By the mid-1960s, social reform required the establishment of a government-subsidized health care program. This program became known as Medicare. The Medicare program further encouraged hospitals to provide services without regard to cost because most costs were reimbursed under the Medicare reimbursement program. Over the past 50 years, the government's perspective has become one that embodies the philosophy that all citizens have a right to health care. This trend began with the passage of Titles 18 and 19 to the Social Security Act in 1965.

As health care expenditures continued to increase (Figure 18-1), the federal government found it necessary to impose controls on its insurance costs. It was not until the 1980s that the reimbursement formula was modified to restrict reimbursement and control the government's expenditures for health care. In 1982, the Health Care Finance Administration

(since restructured to become the Centers for Medicare and Medicaid Services [CMS]) implemented the Tax Equity and Fiscal Responsibility Act. The law mandated a prospective payment system (PPS) for most hospital inpatient services. The PPS became effective in 1983. This program attempted to balance the payments made for the same services rendered by different providers and pay the providers on the basis of the diagnosis at a fixed rate. Diagnosis-related groups (DRGs) were established in the United States and case mix groups in Canada.

Reimbursement modifications occurred in the private insurance industry as well. Some contracts established between insurance companies and hospitals paid the hospital a specific rate for care provided to its subscribers (covered insureds). Different reimbursement methods now exist, including prenegotiated amounts, reimbursement based on a discount off billed charges, per diem payments, reimbursement based on audited costs, DRGs, ambulatory care groups, resource utilization groups, and payment for services at full billed or discounted charges. Reimbursement at billed or full charges seldom occurs anymore. Some insurance organizations provide payments directly to the insureds or subscribers, who then must pay the health care provider.

The sequence of events that has occurred over the past 50 years has created the third-party payer concept. A third-party payer (the insurance company) pays for services provided by health care organizations or practitioners to the "insured." In addition, the "payer" often receives premium payments from the insured's employer. Health insurance has become entwined with employee benefits rather than insurance purchased by the individual, as is the case for automobile or homeowner insurance. The employers have gained considerable purchasing power in regard to health insurance and, at the same time, have a significant interest in the cost of health care services. The federal government and state governments also cover or insure nonemployees in significant programs such as Medicare and Medicaid.

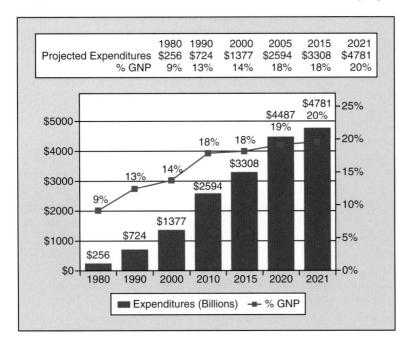

FIGURE 18-1 Growth of national health expenditures. (From the *National Health Expenditure Amounts by Type of Expenditure and Source of Funds: Selected Calendar Years 1980–2021:* http://www.cms.gov/Research-Statistics-Data-and-Systems/Statistics-Trends-and-Reports/National HealthExpendData/Downloads/Proj2011PDF.pdf.)[1]

Reimbursement modifications have extended beyond hospital providers to home health agencies (converted from **whole service cost** based to discipline cost based), skilled nursing facilities (resource utilization groups), outpatient departments (ambulatory patient classifications), ambulatory surgery centers, rehabilitation facilities (case mix function-related groups), and pharmacies (prescription drug tiered formularies).

The philosophical change in reimbursement to control costs affected physicians and other independent practitioners as well. The resource-based relative value scale (RBRVS) was implemented in 1992. The intent of the RBRVS was to ensure equity in payment for like services. The scale assigns a certain number of units (or partial units) to each procedure of service. In effect, payments were based on current procedural terminology (CPT)–4 codes, regardless of the practitioner's specialty.

Example of Work-Based Relative Value Unit (RVU)

Description of Service	CPT Code	Associated Work RVU
Chest x-ray	CPT 71010	RVU 0.18
Evaluation and management, new patient, comprehensive office/ outpatient visit— approximately 30 minutes	CPT 99203	RVU 1.42
Arthroscopically aided anterior cruciate ligament repair/augmentation or reconstruction	CPT 29888	RVU 14.30

*Source for work RVU: CMS National Physician Fee Schedule Relative Value File 2013.[2]

Other attempts at controlling costs included reducing the options available to a person to obtain health care services. In the 1980s, the growth of managed care programs (e.g., health maintenance organizations [HMOs], preferred provider organizations [PPOs], and prepaid group practice plans) was significant. Growth continued through the 1990s. Some communities had as much as 60% of their insured population enrolled in a managed care program. The programs require the insured person to comply with specified rules of access, obtain approval for routine care, seek services from a preselected directory of providers, and fulfill other utilization requirements. Substantial financial disincentives are imposed on those who choose to receive services outside the predefined network of providers or without obtaining the necessary approvals.

In truth, health care costs increased uncontrollably when health care was paid for "in full." Controls using a variety of methods, fee structures, prospective rates, access mandates, and so on have slowed the rate of increase in expenditures to some degree. Provider dropout through hospital closure and state-mandated authorization processes such as **certificate**

of need programs to set up new services or purchase expensive equipment has reduced some duplication of services. However, even with the advancements and efforts that have been made in an attempt to control and maintain health care expenditures, most experts agree that the U.S. health care system is still considered to be one of the most costly and inefficient (Box 18-1).[3] Even with more recent health care reforms, it is projected that health care expenditures will continue to outpace the rest of the economy and by 2021 will reach nearly 20% of gross national product (see Figure 18-1).

In 2010, there were more than 50 million individuals with no health insurance coverage, representing 16.3% of the U.S. population.[4] One of the principle drivers for the increased numbers of uninsured is the high cost to employers offering health care benefits to employees. In 2010 much of health care insurance continued to be employment based, and businesses found it necessary to share the burden through increased cost to employees. The growth of personal out-of-pocket expenses continued to accelerate through higher employee premiums as well as the expansion of high deductible and consumer driven health plans with greater copayments, coinsurance, and spending caps. Simply put, employers have limited financial resources and seemingly endless competing needs for these same resources. In many cases, employers discontinued offering health benefits completely. This is particularly seen in small businesses or companies that are able to use greater numbers of part-time workers—employees who may not qualify for health care benefits.

✓ SELF-ASSESSMENT QUIZ

1. What are the periodic payments patients and employer organizations make to insurance companies for health care coverage?
2. List and describe three other types of personal out-of-pocket costs a patient might owe when receiving health care services.

The high cost of health care and how to make health care more affordable while expanding insurance coverage to all citizens escalated to the top of most business agendas and political policy debates. In 2009, the federal government passed economic stimulus legislation known as the American Recovery and Reinvestment Act (ARRA), a big piece of which

BOX 18-1 Factors Driving Health Care Costs[3]

- Fee-for-service payment model
- Fragmented care delivery
- Administrative complexity
- Demographics and inflation
- Chronic disease and lifestyle
- Medical technology advances
- Legal, regulatory, and tax environment
- Market forces and demand
- Fraud and abuse
- Workforce supply and scope of practice

Source: Bipartisan Policy Center; What Is Driving U.S. Health Care Spending 2012.

invests in health information technology. Formally known as the Health Information Technology for Economic and Clinical Health (HITECH) Act, the law advances the creation of a nationwide health information network to assist in lowering health care costs and strengthening the economy. There is widespread consensus that information technology and the ability to deliver health information where and when needed is a centerpiece to answering the question of controlling health care costs. HITECH laid the foundation for further regulatory and payment reform provisions of the Patient Protection and Affordable Care Act (PPACA), enacted in 2010. Together, these two pieces of legislation put forward a framework to significantly expand health care insurance coverage and coordination of care. Ultimately, the desired outcome of the legislation will be to achieve accountable care with high-quality outcomes at the best possible cost. As new accountable care rules for government-sponsored pilot programs and demonstration projects continue to evolve, and market-based transformation accelerates, controlling costs and accepting greater levels of risk will continue. The ability to track performance and accurately report financial data will be of utmost importance for organizations of all types. New payment and quality incentives will impact every player in the health care industry, including patients, providers, payers, employers, system vendors, and other entities. It is essential for health care managers to provide services efficiently and effectively, at a cost lower than or equal to the payment that will be received. The health information manager's role now includes many different skill sets and disciplines and much more than effective and efficient management practices.

? DID YOU KNOW?

Accountable Care is an emerging concept and a key provision in the PPACA for achieving health reform. An Accountable Care Organization (ACO) is created by hospitals and physician groups entering into contractual agreements to provide health care to specified populations. Delivering care through clinical integration and greater collaboration among providers and payers is expected to lead to improved quality and lower costs. Better coordination of care with a heightened focus on primary care and patient engagement are essential elements to reducing costly hospitalizations. ACOs are held accountable for patient outcomes and are incentivized to keep people healthy rather than being paid for the volume of services provided. CMS has established multiple programs and ACO models for treating Medicare beneficiaries, each with alternative payment arrangements and varying levels of risk.[5]

- **Advance Payment ACO Model**—Includes up-front and installment payments for smaller eligible providers to invest in coordination of care infrastructure.
- **Medicare Shared Savings Program ACO**—Rewards coordination and cooperation to encourage lower costs and improved measures of quality.
- **Pioneer ACO Model**—Carries higher levels of shared savings and risk for health care organizations and provider groups experienced in coordinating care.

✓ SELF-ASSESSMENT QUIZ

3. Research the CMS Web site and distinguish between each type of ACO.
4. Differentiate between fee-for-service and bundled payments.

MANAGING THE REVENUE CYCLE

Because of the high cost of health care and corresponding financial pressures faced by most health care provider organizations and individual practitioners alike, significant emphasis is placed on generating revenue and maximizing potential sources of revenues. In accounting terms, an organization's revenues can be classified as either operating revenue or nonoperating revenue. When we speak of accounting terms, we are referring to GAAP mentioned earlier. For the purposes of our discussion of managing the revenue cycle, we focus on operating revenues, which include those revenue sources generated from the actual delivery of clinical patient care activities and services; that is, charges for the services that are provided. Nonoperating revenues can also be important in contributing to the bottom line of health care providers and may include such items as gifts and donations, income from endowment funds, research grants, interest from investments, and other miscellaneous income.

Health information professionals have learned as part of their biomedical education that human beings are complex organisms comprising multiple interrelated systems; without the nourishment of constant blood flow, the human body would stop working. Much in the same manner as red blood cells and white blood cells make up the lifeblood contributing to the growth and overall health of the human body, organizations cannot survive without sufficient streams of revenue. Applying a similar analogy to financial management and specifically to the revenue cycle, without a constant flow of revenues and subsequent cash flow, health care organizations would cease to exist. For most health care organizations or providers, revenues result from performing the services and equate to the charges for services provided. Cash results from the collection of payments for services provided. You can think of revenue as what is earned and cash as what has been collected. A health care organization's revenue stream and subsequent cash flow enable its ability to acquire and retain sufficient operational and capital resources for providing ongoing patient care services.

It is well documented that the revenue cycle and the management of an organization's revenue streams can be a rather complicated process, particularly when striving to keep up with complex and constantly changing regulatory requirements, technology enhancements, and specific detailed reimbursement contracts. The scope and breadth of interrelated functions making up the revenue cycle comprise many essential HIM competencies, making HIM professionals well positioned to step in at almost any point in the revenue cycle. In many cases, HIM professionals may oversee the entire revenue cycle process for an organization.

✓ SELF-ASSESSMENT QUIZ

5. Distinguish between operating and nonoperating sources of revenue.
6. Give at least three example sources of nonoperating revenue.

Front-End Activities

Most traditional forms of health care are not cash and carry that is paid for at the time of service but rather a complex network or group of operations and systems interwoven with multiple participants and administrative processes. Movements toward retail health care solutions, consumer-driven health plans, and point of service collection initiatives enabled by technology enhancements are beginning to change this dynamic for some consumer segments. In either case, when revenues are generated, any outstanding accounts receivables (dollar amount owed) that result are often an organization's largest asset following its physical plant and facilities. The actual makeup of the revenue cycle can vary greatly from organization to organization and often is best described by breaking down into component front-end and back-end activities. The revenue cycle consists of all previsit and postcare activities and systems associated with a patient or consumer entering the health care system, the receipt of services, and eventually the provider being paid for the service (Figure 18-2).

Contracting

Because the major source of revenue for most health care organizations comes not from patients or the consumer but from third-party insurance companies, it is important for providers to understand and negotiate the best reimbursement contract terms up front. Of course, the effectiveness in negotiating payer contracts is often dictated by the power of the major health care players in the local market. Individual physicians in private practice may find it more difficult bargaining with a payer dominating the market. On the other hand, if the payer needs a certain hospital, medical specialty, or provider group in their network, the tables may be turned as far as negotiating. In addition to actual negotiated payment rates, it is important that specified reimbursement rules and such items as technical coding and billing requirements be identified beforehand and agreed to by both parties. Payer contracts are legally binding documents describing the obligations for both providers and payers in providing health care services to patients (e.g., insurance plan members or beneficiaries in the case of government payers). Contract language will typically include essentials for submission and payment of claims, including reimbursement specifics for modifiers, CMS's Healthcare Common Procedure Coding System (HCPCS), medical necessity determination, services to be carved out (e.g., behavioral health, vision, or dental), and any contract exclusions. Language provisions will also be included describing provider requirements for granting payer access to confidential patient records and other personal health information (PHI). There are numerous opportunities for health information professionals to lend their expertise as part of the contracting process. Traditional contracted methods of reimbursement might include the following:

- Percent of billed charges
- RBRVS or percent of Medicare
- Per diem arrangement
- DRG or case rate
- Per unit
- Predefined fee schedule
- Capitation

More contemporary methods include pay-for-performance, bundled payments and evidence-based care

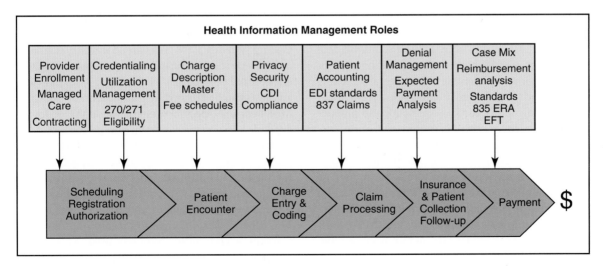

FIGURE 18-2 The revenue cycle process. The revenue cycle begins with the patient entering the health care system for treatment and services, includes the flow of patient financial and health information through the system, and culminates with reimbursement for services provided.

rates designed to provide reimbursement directed at improving quality of care rather than based solely on volume, or the amount of services and treatments provided. Economic, demographic, and regulatory forces will drive the change to more value-based methods of reimbursement. Both government and nongovernment payers may make available incentive payments for achieving agreed-on outcomes and levels of reporting for specified quality measures and measures groups, e-prescribing activities, and other evidence-based metrics. Federal legislation called the Medicare Improvements for Patients and Providers Act of 2008 (MIPPA) authorizes incentive payments to physicians and other eligible professionals who make use of new e-prescribing technology. Beginning in 2012, the program also applies an escalating payment adjustment to eligible professionals who have yet to adopt e-prescribing or do not fulfill reporting requirements.[6]

After a provider has come to terms with a payer and is under an approved contractual agreement, the provider is considered a participating provider and agrees to provide services to covered plan members or Medicare beneficiaries and must abide by established payment rates. A nonparticipating (noncontracted) provider is considered out-of-network by the payer, which most frequently results in a reduced payment or nonpayment. Most payers offer out-of-network benefits, enabling the patient to receive care from a nonparticipating provider at a higher rate of coinsurance, which must be collected directly from the patient. In the case of Medicare, if an individual provider is considered nonparticipating, government regulations specify a limit on how much the patient can be charged.

Licensure and Provider Enrollment

Apart from actual payer contracts, government and nongovernmental commercial payers alike require providers rendering health services to patients to be fully licensed and fulfill rigid credentialing requirements. The credentialing process enables both payers and providers to document a certain standard of quality of care. Provider enrollment documentation must be completed before a payer grants billing privileges to individual providers. The National Committee for Quality Assurance (NCQA) establishes accreditation standards that payers and providers use to oversee the credentialing process. The credentialing process essentially provides a screening mechanism for verifying provider education, credentials, licenses, board certifications, clinical experience and practice history, and malpractice coverage and professional claims history. In the case of clinical laboratories, the Clinical Laboratory Improvement Amendment (CLIA) of 1988 mandates completion of a certification process before obtaining billing privileges. Payers also require that a specific tax identification number be included as part of their enrollment information. The Internal Revenue Service (IRS) requires health care business organizations and individual provider or group entities conducting business to file an application for obtaining a federal tax identification number. Depending on the terms of payer contracts, delays in completing and submitting provider enrollment licensing and credentialing information

to a payer can delay or possibly prevent reimbursement all together. The Health Insurance Portability and Accountability Act (HIPAA) requires health care providers to obtain and use a unique 10-digit National Provider Identifier (NPI) for health care transactions. HIM professionals already engaged in handling medical staff credentialing responsibilities will note that many of the same licensing and credentialing source documents already used in the medical staff office are needed for this integral front-end revenue cycle function.

Charge Master—Fee Schedule

Because health care services rendered generate revenues, it is imperative that services be priced (charged for) effectively and that the price be consistent with the cost to provide the service and at a level above contracted rates for each given service. This requires regular analysis of contracted reimbursement rates and expenses associated with services or product costing. HIM professionals have access to all data associated with various clinical treatment and procedures to resolve health conditions because they have access to the health record. The HIM professional can be key to collecting and classifying tests and procedures performed for the various conditions treated. Likewise, HIM professionals can assess the various expenses (costs) associated with a service. Charges must be assigned so that costs are covered for the various supplies and services used. Each health care organization has a master charge list, sometimes called the charge master, charge description master (CDM), or fee schedule. This list reflects the charge for each item that may be used in the treatment of a patient and the charge for most services—that is, respiratory therapy treatments, physical therapy services, laboratory tests, and so on. The charge description master is most always automated and linked with the billing system. In some organizations, it is also linked with the clinical data system maintained by HIM services and can be used to perform fiscal-clinical analyses (Table 18-1). In many organizations, information system logic may be established to generate both technical and professional charges automatically.

Associated with each service is a charge and either a CPT-4 code or an HCPCS code from the CMS Common Procedural Coding System. CPT-4 codes are an industry standard, updated annually by the American Medical Association. HCPCS codes are updated periodically by the CMS. Also, individual charge amounts can be affected by the addition of clinical modifiers. Modifiers are specific numeric or alpha codes that when appended to a given line-item charge can affect the level of reimbursement. The HIM professional's knowledge of classification systems can be beneficial in ensuring that the master list is accurate and up-to-date at all times. Organizations may also maintain an expanded list of zero-charge house codes to gauge or report certain activities and services that are performed. This expanded list may assist in measuring activity and service volumes or account for resources used. An example of these nonbillable codes might comprise specific CPT Category II codes used for measuring quality indicator usage as part of the physician quality reporting system (PQRS) sponsored by the Centers for Medicare and Medicaid Services (CMS).

TABLE 18-1 Example from Pine Behavioral Health Charge Master

CHARGE MASTER—PINE BEHAVIORAL HEALTH (PROVIDERS ARE ALL EMPLOYEES OF PINE BEHAVIORAL HEALTH)						
UB Code	CPT Code	Description	Provider	Facility Charge	Provider Charge	Comments
915	90791	Diagnostic psychological assessment	MD/clinical psychologist	20.75	198.25	Split bill for Medicare
915	90853	Group Tx	CSW	15.75	45.00	Split bill for Medicare
915	90853	Group Tx	MD/clinical psychologist	15.75	55.00	Split bill for Medicare
915	90853	Group Tx	Other clinician	50.00		
510	90862	Medication management	MD	15.75	72.25	Split bill for Medicare

CSW, Clinical social worker; *MD,* medical doctor; *Tx,* therapy.

Registration and Admitting—Access Management

The health care delivery system requires that numerous front-end activities take place before a patient ever receives treatment or health care services. For a patient to be effectively scheduled and registered for admission to a hospital or other health care facility, or for the patient to be seen by an individual medical provider, numerous previsit verification processes are used to capture necessary information for billing purposes. In addition to appropriately handling all the clinical aspects of a patient registration leading up to the actual encounter, the registration function requires the collection of complete and accurate demographic, financial, and insurance information. The actual process of obtaining this information can be cumbersome and may include accessing a multitude of varying sources and systems to effectively gather. Not only must providers verify whether a patient is covered under a given health plan, they must also determine what specific benefits are available. This task becomes even more complex when considering the increasing variations of copayments and deductibles and other complexities coinciding with the growth of consumer-driven health plans. Providers are strongly encouraged to make use of the HIPAA standard code sets for eligibility inquiry (ASC X12 270) transactions and eligibility response (ASC X12 271) transactions to electronically verify patient eligibility and benefits with payers. The American National Standards Institute (ANSI) Accredited Standards Committee (ASC) X12 plays an instrumental role in electronic information exchange standards impacting the revenue cycle. Failure to register a patient accurately and obtain all necessary demographic, financial, and insurance information on the front end can lead to missed insurance authorizations, costly claim errors, claim denials, and subsequent reimbursement delays later on in the revenue cycle.

Health care payer policies set administrative standards that necessitate that some treatments and services require a referral (formal request) from a physician before the patient can be seen by another specialist provider. Other policies mandate that hospital or physician services be precertified (preapproved) by the payer before the patient receives services. This is particularly true for hospital admissions and surgical procedures, and enables the payer to monitor and control potential costs (expenditures) before services are performed.

Utilization Management—Case Management

Because health care is expensive, payers and providers alike expend significant resources and efforts toward determining the medical necessity and appropriateness of patient care. A patient's insurance and coverage requirements can change quickly, making it essential that services be constantly evaluated and authorized in advance. A payer may deny services or refuse to reimburse providers if a patient's care or course of treatment does not meet certain clinical protocols and established benchmarks. Services that are not authorized result in lost patient revenues. Using the documentation found in the patient's health record, utilization management staff can evaluate the appropriateness and necessity of medical services on the basis of established guidelines and clinical criteria. Utilization staff members perform upfront prospective reviews and concurrent and retrospective reviews to evaluate the medical necessity of procedures, admissions, treatment plans, length of stays, and discharge plans.

Patient Encounter

Whether it is an admission to the hospital, skilled nursing facility, a surgical procedure, clinical lab test, x-ray examination, physician office visit, home health visit, or any other mode of patient treatment, it is the actual service and corresponding documentation that provide the ability to generate revenue. Not only is documentation of the patient encounter necessary for continuity of care purposes, it also serves as a source document for billing purposes. Source documents may be in the form of electronic health records and automated information systems or traditional paper health records and encounter forms. The adage that "if it is not documented it is not done" holds true. Billable services must be appropriately documented, and failure to do so can result in nonpayment and lost revenue.

Coding-Charge Capture

In many health care organizations, there can be one distinct information system with billing and financial functions tied seamlessly to the electronic health record. Alternatively, there may be several order entry and ancillary clinical systems interfacing with the core billing system. Many of these information systems may include system logic established to automatically generate both technical facility charges and professional charges. In some organizations, charges may be manually entered from encounter forms decentralized in provider offices or input centrally in data control. In yet other cases, complex manual coding or computer-assisted coding may be required before a charge being released to the billing information system and for a claim or patient bill to be generated. In these cases, a reasonably complete clinical health record must be accessible to coding staff to meet the goal of timely and accurate coding and submission of data for billing. Physicians and other clinicians support this activity by timely, accurate, and complete documentation. Coding staff may also confer with physicians and other practitioners to obtain information to clarify a code assignment.

As we mentioned earlier, cash flow is the lifeblood of any organization. The HIM manager holds an important key to expediting the time lapse between the recording of revenue and the receipt of cash. This key is in the coding and classification function. The health information manager must implement systems and appropriate procedures to monitor work flow to ensure the timeliness and quality of coding, and avoid causes for any delays (Box 18-2). In fact, clinical documentation improvement (CDI) programs have become the standard for accurately recording and communicating clinical indicators that may impact diagnosis coding, DRG assignment, patient severity of illness, and risk of mortality. A strong multidisciplinary CDI program with an effective query process built into the clinical workflow and improved documentation can have a positive impact on coding, billing, and reimbursement.[7]

Because codes are required for proper billing and complete accurate codes are required for optimum reimbursement, the health information manager must ensure that the coding and CDI staff members are up-to-date in their work and in the application of coding rules and principles. This holds true whether manually assigning codes from paper or electronic record documentation or functioning to validate and edit codes generated from computer-assisted coding tools. As detailed in an earlier chapter, the importance of training and preparation for the transition to ICD-10 and potential impact on billing, payment policies, and subsequent reimbursement cannot be underestimated.

Back-End Activities

Keeping in mind that the revenue cycle is composed of an interwoven system with multiple participants and systems, the actual distinction between front-end and back-end revenue cycle activities will vary depending on such reasons as organizational structures, staffing patterns, historical performance, or information systems within the organization.

Patient Accounting

The patient accounting department, patient financial services, or business office typically has primary responsibility for the back-end billing, collection, and cash processing associated with patient accounts. Many patient accounting departments also have responsibility for the front-end registration or patient access function. With the advent of DRGs, a cooperative relationship has evolved between the HIM department and patient accounting. The need to keep each other informed of accounts receivable status requires that each area's manager and staff work closely and respect the other's constraints. Each area has expertise that should be shared with the other. The HIM department has a good working relationship with medical staff members. Patient accounting has extensive experience working with patients and insurance companies to collect balances due on the accounts. Sharing techniques with each other on how best to get results from people benefits both departments. Each department receives newsletters, regulatory notices, and other information that can be shared with the other to allow both departments to be more knowledgeable.

Each area works with medical terminology. The staff members in patient accounting are often trained from within. HIM professionals can teach medical terminology to the patient accounting staff and educate them in medicolegal aspects, such as patient confidentiality and proper release rules concerning personal health information (PHI).

Patient accounting is expected to manage billing and collection of revenue earned by the organization, otherwise known as managing the accounts receivable. The HIM department can also support increased reimbursement by ensuring that the organization's CDM (master listing of services) is kept up-to-date with current CPT-4 codes.

Claims Processing

Generating clean and accurate claims has become complex with the number of payers and the variety of administrative and technical reimbursement rules associated with obtaining payment for health care services. In the same manner, accurate submission of administrative claims to report performance measures can be essential in determining incentive payments and avoiding undesired payment adjustments. Health care providers use secure in-house billing systems and external clearinghouse vendors to define specific claim billing formats and edit checks unique to particular clinical services and individual payers. Example claim edits might include the following:

- Correct patient or subscriber information
- Valid subscriber number formats
- Correct coding initiative (CCI) edits
- Local coverage determination (LCD) edits
- Confirmation of accident date when diagnosis code indicates an accident

> **BOX 18-2** **Causes for Delays in Coding and Billing**
>
> - Untimely receipt of health records after care or service
> - Incomplete health records
> - Lost records or misplaced records
> - Inadequate coding staff or scheduling
> - Untimely transcription or key reports

- Confirmation that age- or sex-related procedure codes match
- Valid authorization number present

Claims for health care services are most often billed to insurance companies with a standardized health insurance claim form and are submitted electronically or by the traditional paper format. As a rule, hospital technical charges are submitted with a UB-04 (Uniform Billing Code of 2004) claim format for institutional health care providers, whereas physician professional charges are submitted to payers using the CMS 1500 claim format. See examples of UB-04 and CMS 1500 claim forms in Figure 18-3.[8] In the current electronic data interchange (EDI) environment driven by HIPAA, the recommended standard transaction set to define electronic claim formats and data content is the American National Standards Institute (ANSI) Accredited Standards Committee ASC X12 837 health care claim. An understanding of paper claim field definitions and corresponding ASC X12 837 loop and segments, contained in electronic claims, are invaluable skills to possess. Providers are required to use a new ASC X12 5010 version of the UB-04 health claim form and CMS 1500 health claim form beginning in 2012. The new ASC X12 5010 version is a precursor and requirement for the use of expanded ICD-10 code sets to be implemented in 2014.

Patients covered by multiple insurance plans may necessitate the submission of both primary and secondary health care claims. Primary insurance coverage provides reimbursement to providers regardless of other insurance coverage. Secondary coverage reimburses providers after considering benefits paid by the primary insurance plan. Specific coordination of benefit (COB) rules determine which payer is responsible for paying full benefits and which becomes the secondary payer for a given claim.

Collection Follow-up and Claim Denial Management

Submission of clean health care claims and collecting the proper reimbursement of what is owed are common and essential goals among all health care providers. With that stated, defining what constitutes a clean claim and being paid accurately and on time can be elusive goals for providers and payers alike. A novice might come to expect that accurate and timely payment would follow the submission of clean claims. Although advances have indeed been made in standardizing electronic systems and work flows to verify eligibility, provide coding edit checks, adjudicate third-party claims, and remit payments, health care reimbursement is still fraught with potential pitfalls. There are a number of reasons payers may delay or deny a claim, resulting in the provider having to file an appeal or resubmit the claim to receive payment. Common denial reasons might include lack of coverage, bundled services, coordination of benefits, missing referral or authorization, or additional information needed to process a claim. Patient accounting collection staff must frequently coordinate with the HIM department to obtain requested clinical documentation to support a claim. In addition to delayed reimbursement,

the added cost of reworking denied claims makes it essential that denial trends be scrutinized for root cause and corrective action. Denial reasons can also evolve from internal information systems, from payer systems, or within the systems of an external clearinghouse. HIM professionals can be exceptionally helpful in formulating appeal letters to address medical necessity and coding related denials.

The collection of self-pay balances after insurance pays or for those patients without insurance coverage can be a resource intensive and elaborate task. For accounts not paid on a timely basis, providers may have to file liens, handle probate matters, and assist with the collection of delinquent accounts. This may include giving depositions to stipulate that charges are reasonable and customary and that charges coincide with documented clinical services. In the case of delinquent patient accounts, sometimes the remaining accounts receivable balance will be referred (outsourced) for professional collection. When a patient balance is referred to collection and written off as a bad debt, it is no longer an active accounts receivable. An unpaid patient balance may also be written off as a charity allowance should the patient be eligible for a health care organization's financial assistance program. Determination of financial eligibility is based upon income levels and family size using Federal Poverty Guidelines published annually by the Department of Health and Human Services.[9]

Payment Processing

The patient accounting office is also responsible for handling daily deposits, bank reconciliations, and cashiering duties, as well as accurately recording insurance and patient payments. Because of the volume of transactions, providers may use a bank lockbox service to receive individual insurance and patient payments. Insurance payments are accompanied by a remittance advice (RA) or explanation of benefits (EOB), defining the amount adjudicated (paid) by the payer. The remittance advice may vary from payer to payer, although it will typically include the following:

- Charges billed amount
- Amount allowed by insurance
- Payment amount
- Patient liability (balance)
- Amount disallowed by insurance

The HIPAA ASC X12 835 electronic remittance advice (ERA) standardizes claim payment formats enabling health care payment transactions to be electronically transmitted and posted to provider billing systems. Actual payments are deposited either by hardcopy check or wired through electronic funds transfer (EFT) directly to the provider's banking institution. Updated standards and operating rules adopted by Health and Human Services make the use of ERA and EFT a mandated requirement for all HIPAA covered entities in 2014. The patient accounting office may also be responsible for issuing insurance and patient refunds for accounts with overpayment credit balances, providing cashier services, and maintaining patient valuables.

FIGURE 18-3 UB-04 claim form and CMS 1500 claim form. (From the National Uniform Billing Committee: UB-04 claim form: http://www.nubc.org; the National Uniform Claim Committee: CMS 1500 form: http://www.nucc.org.)

HEALTH INSURANCE CLAIM FORM

APPROVED BY NATIONAL UNIFORM CLAIM COMMITTEE (NUCC) 02/12

CARRIER

| | PICA | | | | | | | PICA | |

1. MEDICARE	MEDICAID	TRICARE	CHAMPVA	GROUP HEALTH PLAN	FECA BLK LUNG	OTHER	1a. INSURED'S I.D. NUMBER	(For Program in Item 1)
(Medicare#)	(Medicaid#)	(ID#DoD#)	(Member ID#)	(ID#)	(ID#)	(ID#)		

2. PATIENT'S NAME (Last Name, First Name, Middle Initial)

3. PATIENT'S BIRTH DATE MM | DD | YY SEX M F

4. INSURED'S NAME (Last Name, First Name, Middle Initial)

5. PATIENT'S ADDRESS (No., Street)

6. PATIENT RELATIONSHIP TO INSURED Self Spouse Child Other

7. INSURED'S ADDRESS (No., Street)

CITY   STATE

8. RESERVED FOR NUCC USE

CITY   STATE

ZIP CODE   TELEPHONE (Include Area Code) ( )

ZIP CODE   TELEPHONE (Include Area Code) ( )

9. OTHER INSURED'S NAME (Last Name, First Name, Middle Initial)

10. IS PATIENT'S CONDITION RELATED TO:

11. INSURED'S POLICY GROUP OR FECA NUMBER

a. OTHER INSURED'S POLICY OR GROUP NUMBER

a. EMPLOYMENT? (Current or Previous) YES NO

a. INSURED'S DATE OF BIRTH MM | DD | YY SEX M F

b. RESERVED FOR NUCC USE

b. AUTO ACCIDENT? PLACE (State) YES NO

b. OTHER CLAIM ID (Designated by NUCC)

c. RESERVED FOR NUCC USE

c. OTHER ACCIDENT? YES NO

c. INSURANCE PLAN NAME OR PROGRAM NAME

d. INSURANCE PLAN NAME OR PROGRAM NAME

10d. CLAIM CODES (Designated by NUCC)

d. IS THERE ANOTHER HEALTH BENEFIT PLAN? YES NO If yes, complete items 9, 9a, and 9d.

READ BACK OF FORM BEFORE COMPLETING & SIGNING THIS FORM.

12. PATIENT'S OR AUTHORIZED PERSON'S SIGNATURE I authorize the release of any medical or other information necessary to process this claim. I also request payment of government benefits either to myself or to the party who accepts assignment below.

SIGNED _____ DATE _____

13. INSURED'S OR AUTHORIZED PERSON'S SIGNATURE I authorize payment of medical benefits to the undersigned physician or supplier for services described below.

SIGNED _____

PATIENT AND INSURED INFORMATION

14. DATE OF CURRENT ILLNESS, INJURY, or PREGNANCY(LMP) MM | DD | YY QUAL.

15. OTHER DATE QUAL. MM | DD | YY

16. DATES PATIENT UNABLE TO WORK IN CURRENT OCCUPATION FROM MM | DD | YY TO MM | DD | YY

17. NAME OF REFERRING PROVIDER OR OTHER SOURCE

17a.

17b. NPI

18. HOSPITALIZATION DATES RELATED TO CURRENT SERVICES FROM MM | DD | YY TO MM | DD | YY

19. ADDITIONAL CLAIM INFORMATION (Designated by NUCC)

20. OUTSIDE LAB? YES NO $ CHARGES

21. DIAGNOSIS OR NATURE OF ILLNESS OR INJURY Relate A-L to service line below (24E) ICD Ind.

A. |_____ B. |_____ C. |_____ D. |_____

E. |_____ F. |_____ G. |_____ H. |_____

I. |_____ J. |_____ K. |_____ L. |_____

22. RESUBMISSION CODE   ORIGINAL REF. NO.

23. PRIOR AUTHORIZATION NUMBER

24. A. DATE(S) OF SERVICE						B. PLACE OF SERVICE	C. EMG	D. PROCEDURES, SERVICES, OR SUPPLIES (Explain Unusual Circumstances)		E. DIAGNOSIS POINTER	F. $ CHARGES	G. DAYS OR UNITS	H. EPSDT Family Plan	I. ID. QUAL.	J. RENDERING PROVIDER ID. #
From			To					CPT/HCPCS	MODIFIER						
MM	DD	YY	MM	DD	YY										
1														NPI	
2														NPI	
3														NPI	
4														NPI	
5														NPI	
6														NPI	

PHYSICIAN OR SUPPLIER INFORMATION

25. FEDERAL TAX I.D. NUMBER SSN EIN

26. PATIENT'S ACCOUNT NO.

27. ACCEPT ASSIGNMENT? (For govt. claims, see back) YES NO

28. TOTAL CHARGE $

29. AMOUNT PAID $

30. Rsvd for NUCC Use $

31. SIGNATURE OF PHYSICIAN OR SUPPLIER INCLUDING DEGREES OR CREDENTIALS (I certify that the statements on the reverse apply to this bill and are made a part thereof.)

SIGNED _____ DATE _____

32. SERVICE FACILITY LOCATION INFORMATION

a. NPI b.

33. BILLING PROVIDER INFO & PH # ( )

a. NPI b.

PLEASE PRINT OR TYPE   APPROVED OMB-0938-1197 FORM 1500 (02-12)

FIGURE 18-3, cont'd

? DID YOU KNOW?

Electronic payments and the proliferation of credit and debit card usage represent a growing percentage of all health care payments. The value of payment cards and electronic processing has a profound effect on overall cash flow, convenience, handling costs, productivity, and how health care operations are managed. The Payment Card Industry (PCI) Data Security Standard (DSS) provides a framework and set of tools for handling sensitive cardholder information. In the same fashion as HIPAA, internal policies and procedures as well as contractual agreements with third-party processors must contain clear and strong language regarding how cardholder data are transmitted and stored, and overall obligation for PCI compliance. PCI DSS offers guidance for preventing, detecting, and responding to potential security incidents.[10] A robust PCI DSS compliance program can minimize the consequences of a breach, which might include:
- Payment card issuer fines
- Government fines
- Lawsuits
- Insurance claims
- Loss of credit card processing privileges
- Damage to reputation

✓ SELF-ASSESSMENT QUIZ

7. Name the standards development organization that defines HIPAA electronic transaction standards.
8. List three standard HIPAA transactions and describe the purpose of each.

Reimbursement Analysis

Achieving success in managing the revenue cycle to a great extent involves understanding and effectively utilizing data to make decisions. Decision support systems provide comprehensive reporting tools to help health care managers track and report on all aspects of reimbursement and financial performance. These are the systems that unite both clinical and financial information, which is useful to measure, for example, revenue cycle performance, case mix, budgeting, cost accounting, clinical protocols and pathways, and outcomes. Many of these performance measurements can occur annually, monthly, weekly, or daily (Table 18-2) and may be trended over time to compare with historical performance and available benchmark information.

It is essential that accounts be reviewed to ensure that correct payment was made according to the terms of each individual payer contract. Configuring information systems to coincide with the language found in each individual reimbursement contract can be difficult for payers and providers alike, making it necessary to monitor payment trends closely. As mentioned earlier in the chapter, insurers pay for services in one of several ways, including the following:
- Percent of billed charges
- RBRVS or percent of Medicare
- Per diem arrangement
- DRG or case rate
- Per unit

TABLE 18-2 Common Revenue Cycle Performance Measures

Measure	Description	Example
A/R days	Average time to receive payment	Accounts receivable/average daily revenue
A/R aging	Distribution of accounts receivable by aging days	1–30 days, 31–60 days, 61–90 days, >90 days
Collection rate	Effectiveness of collecting	Cash collections/revenue
Payer mix	Distribution of revenue by payers	Commercial, Medicare, Medicaid, private-pay
Denial rate	Number or dollars of denied claims	Denied charges/total revenue
Bad debt rate	Write-offs due to bad debt	Bad debt write-offs/total revenue
Charity rate	Write-offs due to charity	Charity write-offs/total revenue

A/R, Accounts receivable.

- Predefined fee schedule
- Capitation

Routinely analyzing paid claims to determine how much was paid by the insurer for a service, test, procedure, and so on and comparing the payments with the charge master are important also. If the insurer pays full charges, no variances are noted, but for other arrangements, the payments may be less than or more than the amount charged by the health care provider. Frequently, charges must be compared with health record documentation to ensure accuracy.

DRGs are an example of a **per case** or fixed payment system. Care provided for a given condition classified into a DRG may cost more than the approved payment for the given DRG. If payment rates are less than the amount charged, a revenue deduction or adjustment occurs. If adjustments are significant, expenses may not be fully covered. If expenses are not covered, management must consider alternatives to providing the care, such as modifying the supplies and services included in the treatment of a condition. Coding professionals who recognize the effectiveness of different tests in treating a condition can identify the more effective tests for utilization management professionals and physicians to consider in establishing treatment guidelines for other physicians to follow. It is important to consider possible outlier payments in addition to the contracted DRG payment. A day outlier can occur when a patient's length of stay extends beyond what is considered normal (standard) for a particular DRG.

If payment rates are higher than the amount charged by the health care provider, the provider should assess its charges. Typically, health insurance companies set their rates on the basis of community averages. If the amount paid by the insurance company is higher than the provider's charges, then the provider's charges are lower than the community average. Insurers also pay based on a practice of paying the lower of the insurance company's fee schedule or the provider's charges. Whenever charges are paid, the same analysis of the provider's charges should occur. This type of periodic review of payments and charges helps the provider maximize reimbursement for the organization.

In some areas of the country where managed care is a dominant method of insurance, another payment arrangement known as capitation may apply. Capitation payments are used in health maintenance organizations (HMOs). Insured members enroll with an HMO. For each month an insured remains with the HMO, the HMO's providers are paid a fixed amount (capitated payment), usually at the beginning of the month. The providers (physicians, therapists, and sometimes facilities such as hospitals and ambulatory surgery centers) are required to provide any care needed by the insured during this period, regardless of whether the capitation amount is sufficient to cover the cost to do so.

Case Mix Analysis

When the DRG system for payment was introduced, hospitals began looking not only at the number of services provided (e.g., the number of days of care) but also at the "case mix" or types of care classified by estimated resource use.

A case mix value is assigned to each DRG. The values may vary by payer. Medicare values are published each year in the Federal Register. For example, if a DRG has a case mix value or weight of 1.4 and the hospital's payment for 1.0 value of service is $4000, then the hospital will receive $5600 as payment for the entire hospital stay. The system allows some flexibility for unusual cases that are "outliers," which consume more than the normal amount of resources.

Aggregating the case mix data for a group of patients allows the hospital to compute a case mix average or "index."

Example of Case Mix

Number of DRG	Total Value of Case Mix Value	Cases in Period	Service
DRG XX1	1.2	45	54.00
DRG XX2	0.95	15	14.25
DRG XX3	1.4	60	84.00
DRG XX4	2.1	10	14.25
Case mix index	1.3	130	173.25

Case mix index for the period = total value of service/total number of cases. Total value of service = case mix value × number of cases in the period.

Analyzing the case mix for all inpatients for a given period of time is useful for tracking trends. Is the overall case mix increasing (or decreasing)? Is the hospital treating sicker patients? Are patients consuming more resources? Does the case mix vary by payer? Does the case mix vary by type of service? When you compare case mix with other data (length of stay, age groups of patients, charges for services, actual reimbursement for services), what do you find?

FINANCIAL ASPECTS OF FRAUD AND ABUSE COMPLIANCE

As a result of improprieties among the ranks of some publicly traded companies, the Sarbanes-Oxley Act of 2002 was created to provide greater and much needed financial accountability. Now an organization's management must attest annually to the effectiveness of internal controls and undergo an external audit, attesting to the effectiveness of internal controls. This legislation is of particular interest to nonprofit organizations as well because they evaluate their own internal controls and financial reporting. The Public Company Accounting Oversight Board (PCAOB) was created as a result of Sarbanes-Oxley to oversee the audit of public companies and guard the public interest.

Because of the overall magnitude of the cost of health care and the ever-increasing dollars being spent, there is a tremendous interest in detecting and preventing fraud and abuse. The federal government, through the Centers for Medicare and Medicaid Services (CMS), is focusing on eliminating fraud and abuse in its health care program. With annual health care expenditures topping $2.9 trillion in 2013, national health care fraud estimates place annual financial losses in the tens of billions of dollars.[11] Major efforts have been put in place to recover these potential losses from health care providers. To identify and recover many of these improper or inadvertent payments, CMS has instituted a Recovery Audit Contractor (RAC) program. The Tax Relief and Health Care Act of 2006 (TRHCA) charges official RAC contractors with detecting and recouping improper payments, which may be attributed to noncompliance with complex Medicare coverage, coding, billing, and payment rules. Providers must have effective operational processes in place to swiftly respond to any RAC notices of overpayment, due to the time constraints for requesting a redetermination or reconsideration and to prevent automatic recoupment of payments. The Affordable Care Act (ACA) expands RAC efforts to coordinate with State Medicaid agencies as well. With health record coding, CDI programs, medical necessity, and release of information such integral components of the RAC initiative, this has resulted in new RAC coordinator roles for many HIM professionals.

As identified in a number of publicly traded companies in other industries, some of the financial losses identified in health care have been due to dishonest providers and outright calculated efforts to defraud. The federal government has won judgments against health care providers and settled cases with others without any admission of guilt. For some health care providers, it was a better decision to settle a potential case for an agreed-on dollar amount—that is, pay a fine—than to engage in detailed and prolonged scrutiny. Justice department involvement in whistleblower lawsuits under the False Claims Act has resulted in criminal fines and civil damages in many cases totaling in the tens and hundreds of millions, and even billions, of dollars. The Office of the Inspector General publishes an annual work plan that details its focus for Medicare fraud and abuse. The work plan

---

BOX 18-3   Definitions and Examples of Fraud and Abuse

Medicare fraud is defined as "making false statements or representations of material facts to obtain some benefit or payment for which no entitlement would otherwise exist." Fraud is committed knowingly.[12]

Medicare abuse is defined as "any practice that is not consistent with the goals of providing patients with services that are medically necessary, meet professionally recognized standards, and are fairly priced."[12] It is not required that the acts were committed knowingly.

Examples of fraud:

Claim submitted for services not rendered

Bill submitted for more costly procedures than those actually rendered

Examples of abuse:

Misuse of codes on a claim

Providing services that are not medically necessary

Billing Medicare on a higher fee schedule than used for non-Medicare patients

---

gives health care providers an indication of general and specific areas that are targets for review (Box 18-3).[12]

Providers have set up compliance programs within their organizations to implement necessary programs that meet the complex Medicare requirements. The American Health Information Management Association (AHIMA) has information and resources designed to help organizations set up and administer compliance programs. Health information managers often manage or actively participate in their organization's compliance program.

Medicare laws and regulations are promulgated by the federal government. The federal government contracts with fiscal intermediary organizations that help process and adjudicate bills for services. These organizations are referred to as Medicare Administrative Contractors (MACs) and oversee administrative rules and guidelines related to claims processing. Health care providers must become familiar with and use the laws, rules, regulations, and guidelines from both federal and local levels in designing and maintaining their workflow processes and information systems.

Health care providers that participate in the Medicare program are expected to have systems for coding diagnoses and procedures and for submitting claims that meet Medicare requirements. The documentation in the clinical record must accurately describe the service provided and justify the need for the service. The diagnoses, and any services or procedures, must be coded correctly according to national guidelines. The bill for services must be submitted with sufficient information in the correct format. As stated, interpretation of these complex and changing rules can be a complicated process, and reconciling the appropriate action to take may not always be clear for every practice-related decision that is faced.

One of the ways for HIM professionals, or any professional for that matter, to stay focused in carrying out day-to-day responsibilities without sacrificing ethical principles is to rely on their core values. Professionals have an ethical obligation to do what is right and, by their nature, recognize a standard code of ethics. HIM professionals have an obligation to follow a specific code of ethics as put forth by AHIMA. One key ethical principle included in the code of ethics clearly articulates the HIM professional's responsibility to "refuse to participate in or conceal unethical practices or procedures."[13] These ethical principles hold true regardless of whether handling clinical or financial health information. The American Institute of Certified Public Accountants (AICPA) adheres to a similar code of professional conduct for certified public accountants.

Unfortunately, not everyone involved in health care adheres to a professional code of ethics, and the potential for fraud is a growing concern. The Office of the National Coordinator for Health Information Technology (ONC) recognizes that the transition to electronic health records and a national health information network will go a long way toward minimizing health care fraud. At the same time, there is an awareness of new challenges this may bring as well. Health information technology is being looked upon to accelerate efforts to hardwire necessary internal controls and combat health care fraud.

 SELF-ASSESSMENT QUIZ

9. Distinguish between "fraud" and "abuse."
10. What government program is intended to identify payment errors so CMS can implement actions to prevent in the future?

SETTING PRIORITIES FOR FINANCIAL DECISIONS

Up until this point in our discussion, we have concentrated on effectively and appropriately managing an organization's revenue cycle. We have examined how the revenue cycle bridges the gap between clinical practice and the attainment of necessary economic resources. Managing the revenue cycle is just one component of overseeing an organization's financial resources, and it does not happen in a vacuum. Health care leaders are also responsible for planning future activities and must learn to use and interpret many types of financial accounting information.

Management Accounting

Managerial accounting provides economic information and an internal framework to enable health care leaders to make effective decisions concerning the activities and overall performance within an organization. Information in the form of internal accounting reports, budgets, business plans, cost analysis, and other reports measuring an organization's performance make up management accounting. In establishing priorities, planning and controlling are essential management functions. Health care organizations and individuals engage in planning to provide a framework for their actions. The strategic and operational plans set the targets for performance. Budgets are plans for the financial resources associated with these performance plans. Most organizations have a mission, goals, and objectives that departmental managers use as an umbrella for developing and linking departmental objectives and budgets to organizational goals.

Mission

The mission is a statement of the organization's purpose in broad terms. It defines the geographic environment and population that the organization serves—for example, "The mission of Citywide Surgi-Centers, Inc. is to provide convenient, state-of-the-art, surgical services for all residents of the City of Citywide and its surrounding neighborhoods."

Goals

To implement the mission, organizational leaders define goals to support the mission. A goal is a statement of what the organization wants to do. One of Citywide's goals may be "to increase the number of nontraditional surgeries performed at the center by supporting research into safe surgery techniques." The goals established by senior leaders or administration serve as a foundation, offering the direction management needs to determine the organization's intent.

Objectives

Once the intent is known, management can formulate objectives. Objectives are more specific statements that define the expectations or outcomes given the goal direction. One of Citywide's objectives may be "to begin performing laser eye surgery as a new service next year." Objectives provide clear guidelines for management and supervisors to define the action steps to achieve the objective. The action steps define the dates when certain activities are to be completed, how much labor or funding will be required, how resources will be used, and the expected outcomes or results. During action step formulation, budgets are developed.

THE BUDGET AND BUSINESS PLAN

Budgets

Budgets are detailed numeric documents that translate the goals, objectives, and action steps into forecasts of volume and monetary resources needed. The managerial accounting process includes the activities of planning and preparing budgets consistent with the strategic plan. Just as we have an accounting component responsible for recording transactions as they occur (financial accounting), there are other people who work with administration and management to assign the anticipated fiscal resources of the organization. These individuals may work in the budget or controller's office. Their primary responsibilities include helping management to prepare budgets, conducting cost-finding studies to set rates, and determining productivity. The reports they produce include the budget, the budget variance reports, cost reports, and third-party reimbursement reports. The types of

budgets that result from the planning process include the statistics budget, the operating budgets, and the master budget.

Statistics Budget

The first of several budgets developed from the planning process is the statistics budget. Future volumes are often predicted by assessing data from historical trends. The HIM department is the primary source of historical data, such as discharges by clinical service, payer type, DRG, and physician; operative procedures by type and surgeon; length of stay by DRG, diagnosis, clinical service, and physician; number and type of ambulatory visits; number and type of home health visits; number and type of ambulatory surgery cases; number and type of emergency department visits; and many other volume indicators. Unless significant changes have occurred in the regulatory and external and internal environments, relying on historical data to predict the future is appropriate. History should not be the only source of volume predictions, however.

Key medical and other clinical staff members should be interviewed for their prediction of future demands for services. The medical staff is a valuable source of information and may be aware of plans for service changes and expansions of competing organizations. The staff members also have access to literature that describes technological advances in patient care. Such advances could drastically reduce volumes experienced in the past. In the 1990s, it was not uncommon for patients who had coronary artery bypass surgery to be hospitalized for 6 or more days. Today, cardiac stents can be implanted to open a blocked artery as an outpatient procedure.

The statistical analysts in the HIM department can also predict declining volumes by comparing data from month to month and identifying trends in utilization of the enterprise by different physicians or by geographic location. Sometimes physician utilization declines as a physician ages and cuts back his or her practice, or when a physician brings patients to a health care facility that is more convenient to his or her practice.

When new services are contemplated, the staff involved in providing the service should be involved in predicting the utilization of the services or the volumes anticipated. Staff optimism should be tempered by management querying staff and the anticipated users of the service. Sometimes health care leaders use marketing research firms to predict volumes on the basis of the demographics of the community. If a health care organization is anticipating opening a long-term care or skilled nursing facility, an analysis of the age demographics of the local area should be done to ascertain the number of elderly people residing in the community today and the number expected to be residing in the community in the next 5 to 10 years. Furthermore, an assessment of the competition would be completed.

If a departmental activity is directly tied to the volume of activity of the organization, then statistical projections can form the base for a departmental budget. For example, if the organization projects a 15% increase in the volume of home health encounters because of a new service market, what HIM activities are related to this statistic? How will the HIM budget reflect these data in budget planning?

Operating Budgets

Once patient, physician, and procedure volumes are determined, managers can begin building their **operating budgets**. These budgets predict the labor, supply, and other expenses required to support the work volume predicted.

Example of Budgeting for a New Service

If Citywide implements an outpatient service with a projected annual volume of 4500 laser eye surgeries, what does Citywide's HIM department need to do to support this new service? The supervisor may predict the following:

- An average of 15 surgical procedures will occur per working day.
- The department will be responsible for gathering pre-service information by telephone or other means.
- A coder will need to be trained to code laser and alternative nonlaser types of eye surgery services.
- Four additional desktop computers will need to be purchased to access the organization's electronic health record (EHR) and other information systems.
- A scanner will be necessary to scan hardcopy records into the EHR.
- If some of the eye surgeries involve implants, the HIM department may need to set up and maintain a registry component in the organization's patient information system.

The supervisor must now assign costs to each of these items and budget them in the correct categories as they apply: labor, supplies, training and education, hardware, and software.

When budgeting for supplies and services it is helpful to segregate expenses into at least two categories: (1) fixed expenses (those that are not related to the volume of business) and (2) variable expenses (those that fluctuate as a result of changes in volume).[14] If managers must adjust their budgets because of a reduction or an increase in volume, it will be easier to identify the supplies and services that are volume dependent.

The departments that provide direct patient care prepare both the expense portion and the revenue portion of their operating budgets. To determine their revenue budget, the patient care departments assign estimated charges and estimated payment to the services they will be delivering on the basis of the statistics budget.

Master Budget

After all departments develop their operating budgets, the same categories of expenses (e.g., labor, supplies, training, and education) and revenues (patient care, nonpatient care [e.g., cafeteria, gift shop]) are rolled up and consolidated into one **master budget** with each of the operating account's combined balances.

When the organization has aggregated this information, organizational leaders determine whether the budget will go forward as constructed or whether it needs rework in certain areas.

Additional information on budgeting for capital expenditures is covered later in this chapter.

Who Participates in Budget Development?

Many people participate in the budgeting process. Organizations find it advantageous to include supervisory and frontline staff members in the development of budgets because they are closer to the consumption of resources. This is known as the participatory approach to budgeting. However, management is ultimately responsible for the budget and its compliance with organizational objectives, goals, and mission. Because the budget is a prediction of expenses, revenues, services, and volumes to come some time in the future, it cannot be exact but should be used as a guide to measuring and improving management's predictive capability.

Budget Periods and Types

The budget period may differ from organization to organization. Budgets may be prepared for 1 year or several years. Typically, budgets are prepared for 12 months, running parallel to an organization's fiscal year. Some organizations use a **rolling budget method**. This method requires management to prepare a budget for a period of time and add another month to the end of that period when a month is consumed. For example, a budget may be prepared for 6 months (January through June), and when the first of the 6 months (January) ends, the manager would prepare the budget for the new sixth month (July).

Flexible Budget

Another type of budget is the **flexible budget**. This budget is predicated on volume. All supplies, labor, and other variable expenses are budgeted in proportion to the anticipated volume. If the volume anticipated is not reached, labor and other expenses are expected to decrease accordingly, and vice versa if the volume exceeds expectations.

Zero-Based Budget

Because many facilities are experiencing reduced reimbursement for their services, modified approaches to budgeting are being considered. One such approach is the **zero-based budget**. In the zero-based budgeting approach, management must complete a program assessment and define consequences if specific programs are terminated or reduced. Cleverley et al.[14] defined the seven steps of zero-based budgeting:

1. Define the outputs or services provided by the program or department (statistical reports, coding, quality assurance study preparations, responses to requests for information, transcription, filing, and so on).
2. Determine the costs of these services or outputs.
3. Identify options for reducing the costs through changes in outputs or services (modify current procedure, eliminate an activity).
4. Identify options for producing the services and outputs more efficiently (use of a contracted service, voice recognition, optical imaging, and so on).
5. Determine the cost savings associated with options identified in steps 3 and 4.

Budgeting for Staff

Because staffing expenses usually consume a major portion of any health care organization's budget, careful attention is given to preparing the supporting detail for this component of the budget. A detailed staffing plan is useful for comparison during the year with staffing utilization and other reports. Calculating staffing needs is accomplished by carefully analyzing productivity data and merging with activity levels. Many HIM departments have a number of functions that have associated productivity data that can be gathered and used in budgeting.

Example Analysis of Merging Productivity Data and Volume Data

A department has an annual volume of 9500 requests for information per year. A staff person can usually complete about 15 request responses per day. Each staff person uses an average of 11 holidays, 8 sick days, and 12 days of vacation per year. How many full-time equivalents (FTEs) should be included in the budget?

15 requests per day × 5 days × 52 weeks = 3900
9500 requests/3900 = 2.4 FTEs (without productivity adjustment)
Nonproductive time = 11 holidays
8 sick days
12 vacation days
31 days off
× 8 hours a day
248 hours/year
Productive time 2080 hours per year − 248 nonproductive time = 1832 hours
Productivity rate 1832/2080 = 0.88 or 88%
FTEs needed 2.4 FTEs/88% = 2.7 FTEs
Also see Table 18-3.

Using the Budget As a Control

The activity of **controlling** is one of several management duties. In this chapter, it refers to the activities that management typically pursues when what was planned does not occur financially. The chapter on human resources management (see Chapter 16) identifies the budget as a feedback tool. Once established, the budget is a "non–self-correcting feedback control" that managers can use to make decisions.

Variance Reports

One tool that most organizations have is a **variance report**. This document reflects the budget that was prepared and approved and shows the actual results on at least a monthly basis. Given financial pressures and the need to control the use of resources, variance analysis is an important item to have in a managers' toolbox.

Variances may occur for a variety of reasons. Reviewing the reports and identifying areas where the variance is significant (material) in either a positive or negative fashion is appropriate. Significance or materiality of any discrepancies can be determined by a dollar amount and/or a percentage. Commonly, variances are due to volume and rate differences from what was planned. It is helpful to be able to determine how much of the variance is due to volume and how much is due to rate or cost. Some variances are due to a combination of factors, and may even be due to incorrect account or center classification of specific transactions. Various approaches are used to identify variances—some more basic, others more complex.

If the real cause of the variance is understood on a timely basis, then the management action taken, if any, is more likely to be informed and appropriate (Tables 18-4, 18-5, and 18-6).

PREPARING A BUSINESS PLAN

As mentioned earlier, the organizational planning process links departmental objectives and budgets to the overarching goals. In some cases, organizations may require their managers to prepare business plans in addition to compiling a

---

TABLE 18-3 Example of Salary Budget for Departmental Staffing (Partial Worksheet with Estimated Totals)

LEALAND CLINIC
SALARY BUDGET WORKSHEET FOR HEALTH INFORMATION DEPARTMENT

Classification of Position	Staff Name	FTE	Hourly Pay Rate	Current Year Base Salary	Increase Planned Next Year	Date of Increase	Amount of Increase	Total Next Year
Manager	Hansen	1.0	42.00	87,360	7%	3/1	6,115	92,460
Supervisor	Holden	1.0	25.00	52,000	7%	5/1	3,640	54,426
Data Specialist	Hillier	0.8	25.00	52,000	7%	1/1	3,640	44,512
Tech I	Hardy	1.0	20.00	41,600	7%	7/1	2,912	43,056
Totals		32.5		954,000			66,800	1,006,000

Example of calculations: 87,360 × 0.07 = 6115/12 = 510 × 10 months = 5100+87,360 = 92,460.
FTE, Full time.

TABLE 18-4 Basic Variance Analysis—Sunshine Hospital

Service	Actual	Budget	Variance
Inpatient revenue	190,000	180,000	10,000

SUNSHINE HOSPITAL VOLUME AND RATE DATA

Inpatients	Actual	Budget	Variance
Patient days	950	900	50
Average rate per day	200	200	0

This reflects a positive variance because of an increase in volume.

TABLE 18-5 Variance Analysis with an Adjustment for Volume—Melrose Outpatient Clinic

INITIAL REPORT

Outpatients	Actual	Budget	Variance
Visits	16,500	13,500	3,000
Salaries (variable item)	460,000	360,000	(100,000)
Supplies (variable item)	75,000	55,000	(20,000)

ADJUSTED REPORT

	Budget	Actual	Adjustment	Adjusted Budget
Salaries	360,000	460,000	79,200	439,200
Supplies	55,000	75,000	12,100	67,100
Total	415,000	535,000	91,300	506,300

Outpatient is over budget; however, there is an increase in service, and there should be a corresponding increase in revenue unless this is a capitated or managed care contract environment. If the report is adjusted for volume, it presents a different picture.
3000 visits/13,500 visits = 22% higher volume than budget plan
Melrose Outpatient Clinic budget with a 22% increase in the variable cost items
When the adjusted report is compared with the actual expenses, the salary variance is $20,800 instead of $100,000, and the supply variance is $7900 instead of $20,000. The clinic is exceeding anticipated expenses given the 22% increase in volume; however, the variance is significantly less when adjusted for volume. The unexplained variance is now $20,888 + $7900 = $28,700 instead of $100,000 + $20,000 = $120,000.

TABLE 18-6 Product Line Variance Report Using DRGs As a Product Line

	ACTUAL			BUDGET		
DRG	Net Revenue	Cost	Profit	Net Revenue	Cost	Profit
XX1	75,500	63,400	12,100	81,200	61,000	20,200
XX2	61,400	44,500	16,900	59,300	38,800	20,500
XX3	82,800	84,700	(1900)	63,600	61,200	2,400
Totals	219,700	192,600	27,100	204,100	161,100	43,100

DRG, Diagnosis-related group.

BOX 18-4 Common Data Sources for the Health Information Management Department

- Monthly discharge, operations, and visit statistics by payer type (e.g., Medicare, public aid, commercial, managed care)
- Monthly discharge, operations, and visit statistics by service type (e.g., medical, surgical, obstetric)
- Length of stay by clinical service and payer type
- Incomplete medical records, per week or month, per physician, per clinical service, and so on
- Requests for records from insurers, patients, other health care providers
- Average pages per records, number of pages generated by automated sources, number of pages handwritten
- Lines, minutes, or words of diction per month, per physician, per report type
- Records requested and pulled
- Discharges by diagnosis-related group
- Cases by physician (encounters, discharges, operations)
- Records and loose sheets filed
- Research studies (e.g., organized, searches)
- Quality improvement studies (e.g., organized, supported)
- Records, encounters scanned, and quality reviewed

budget. A **business plan** is a formal written document that evolves from the input of others, listing objectives that support the organizational goals. The plan includes the following:

- Specific action steps
- Quantifying resource requirements and cash flow benefits
- Prediction of expected outcomes
- Programmatic outline that may span a fiscal year or a longer time frame

All budgets and business plans rely on data. Collected data must be in a format that conveys information to the manager. There are many sources for data useful in the development of budgets and business plans (Box 18-4).

Identifying Trends

For the business plan data gathering to be completed, the statistics gathered should be compared with those of prior periods to identify trends that imply a need to change operations or staffing. For example, in the health information department if the statistics showed that the number of minutes of dictation was increasing by 10% per month, it could be anticipated that additional transcriptionists would be required or external assistance would be needed to transcribe the dictation.

Staffing Information

Staffing information is a necessary component of business planning and budgeting. Staffing information maintained by the HIM manager should include the following:

- Current organizational chart by function and by name
- Productivity standards
- Skills assessment inventory for each staff member
- Training obtained or needed
- Average time off by categories of staff (nonproductive time)
- Salary or hourly wage for each position or staff member

- Hire dates or planned raise dates and amounts
- Accrued vacation and sick leave (if accrual is allowed)
- Staffing utilization reports

Maintaining these data allows management to know which staff members are prepared to assume new duties, what training must be planned or budgeted for to allow other staff members to take over activities, what amounts of staff resources were actually used during a period, how much vacation time and sick time are accrued for this department, and the true productive time of staff members. Productive time is the time a worker is present and working. A full-time position is typically 2080 hours annually (40 hours per week × 52 weeks). Yet a full-time position does not equate to 2080 productive hours. Some hours are not worked because of vacation, holidays, sick time, and so on and thus would be considered nonproductive time. Productive hours are further reduced by training and meeting hours. Monitoring time off and nonproductive time allows management to estimate more closely the productive hours available to meet workload demands.

Program and Automation Assessments

Two assessments may be completed before proceeding with a business plan and budget: automation assessment and program assessment. These assessments are similar to doing an internal environment assessment of the HIM department. When the assessments are completed, the health information manager knows whether the tools are available to achieve the outcomes necessary. If administration has determined that no additional staff can be added this year, then a manager's dependence on automation may increase. Automation may be less expensive to add than staff and increase productivity as well. The assessment of programs requires the staff to consider seriously the adequacy of each service it offers and decide whether the services meet the users' or customers' needs and how critical the service is to the organization.

The Four Ms

All managers have the responsibility to manage the four M's:
- Manpower
- Machinery
- Materials
- Money

When preparing the business plan and, ultimately, the budget, all proposed expenditures must balance the M's; that is, an increase in one should attempt to offset the cost of another. If we request an upgraded computer to help us do our work, we should be able to do the work faster or with fewer persons. This is a trade-off between machinery and personnel. Sometimes, however, machinery is needed to offset the need for more personnel to meet volume increases.

Developing the Business Plan and Budget

Now that we have gathered and assessed the data, we have identified the needs we want to address. The first step is to figure out whether the needs we identified are consistent with the organization's mission and goals.

If your proposal is consistent with the organization's mission and goals, then you must decide what you want to do and how you want to do it. Several questions can be answered during the process (Figure 18-4).

Example of Departmental Objectives for Budget Planning

Develop an implementation, training, and evaluation plan for a clinician electronic signature program for transcribed reports and other electronic components of the electronic health record (new objective).

Meet or exceed the state-regulated time frame for response to release-of-information requests (ongoing).

Continue to receive, prepare, image, index, and do a quality review of all outpatient documentation within 24 hours of receipt, 7 days a week (ongoing).

As each objective is developed and linked to organizational goals, the action steps must be prepared in detail to ensure that the objective is attained. Costs to do each step of the planned objective must be determined and associated with the timing of the steps. Some expenses may be evenly distributed throughout the year. Other expenses may be "one time" expenses planned for a particular month. Some objectives will be new objectives, and others will be ongoing objectives.

COST ALLOCATIONS

Another important tool in management accounting is cost analysis and being able to measure the impact on various subunits within an organization. To determine the approximate costs to provide services, an organization must develop and maintain a cost allocation system. The cost management system allocates direct and indirect costs. Costs are classified by department or responsibility center. Non–revenue-generating departments are considered indirect cost departments, whereas revenue-generating departments are considered direct cost departments. Cost allocation allocates the costs of indirect, non–revenue-generating departments to direct, revenue-generating departments.

Why Does Allocation Occur?

Some payers reimburse on the basis of the full costs of direct departments and permit the allocation of indirect departments to the direct departments only to the extent that the indirect departments contribute to the direct departments' provision of care or generation of revenue. Many indirect departments support the provision of care through the assistance provided to the direct departments. For example, telecommunications is an indirect department. If no one answers the organization's phone during an emergency, services are not provided. The HIM department supports the efforts of the nursing service, the therapy departments, and the ancillaries by serving as the central controller of all records and reports. The HIM department is considered a nonpatient revenue-generating department. The total costs

The organization's goals include increasing cash flow. Your proposal is to establish a courier service to deliver incomplete records to physicians' offices to decrease the number of incomplete records.

Objective

To decrease the number of incomplete records by 25%.

When do you plan to do it?

By second quarter of next year.

What will be achieved?

- Reduction in accounts receivable days by 2 or $140,000 by delivering records to physicians' offices. This will reduce the time for the physician because he/she does not have to come to the HIM department to do his/her records.
- Reduction in physician complaints or increase in compliments.
- Avoidance of purchase of additional file shelving units to store incomplete records.

What is needed to achieve the objective?

Resources: Capital: Small Car*: $10,000

Operating Expenses:
    Labor: 0.5 FTE $17,200
    Auto Costs: 4,000

Collaboration Required: Security, Personnel, and Purchasing Departments

*Car to be used by courier. Courier must be licensed driver.

How does the hospital benefit from this objective?

Cash flow impact: The reduction in incomplete records will result in 2 fewer days in accounts receivable or the equivalent of $140,000. Invested annually at 10%, the $140,000 will yield at least $14,000 in interest income.

FIGURE 18-4 Questions to ask when preparing a business plan.

of the department are therefore considered indirect and must be allocated to patient revenue-generating departments such as nursing, therapy, and laboratory.

The HIM department does have revenue-generating opportunities. Some departments charge for copies of health records provided to insurance companies and lawyers. Other departments provide transcription services for their physicians and charge accordingly. These services are revenue generating; however, they are not directly related to the primary mission of the organization—patient care.

Allocation Methods

Step-Down Method

The step-down method is a common technique that is supported by Medicare in its cost-reporting requirements. In this method, the indirect department that receives the least amount of service from other indirect departments and provides the most service to other departments has its costs allocated first.

The chaplain service is an indirect department that may offer less service to other departments than the HIM department offers to direct departments. Both provide services to nursing, but seldom does the chaplain provide services to the therapy departments or the laboratory. So the HIM department costs would be allocated before those of the chaplain service.

The allocation is made on the basis of the ratio of services provided to each department or some other basis, such as square footage, employees, or worked hours.

Example of Step-Down Cost Allocation

Housekeeping serves more indirect departments than laundry/linen or health information services. Housekeeping's services are used 20% of the time by laundry/linen, 5% of the time by health information services, 5% by radiology, and 70% by nursing. Laundry/linen's services are used 3% by health information services, 5% by radiology, and 92% by nursing. This results in allocation of the costs of the indirect departments to the direct departments of nursing and radiology.

The step-down approach is most common in health care institutions. The steps in the allocation table's appearance show how the approach was named.

Double-Distribution Method

The double-distribution method is similar to the step-down method. This method assumes that the allocation of costs cannot be linear and that some indirect departments need to be allocated to less commonly dispersed departments before the costs of these departments are fully allocated. In the example discussed earlier, housekeeping was fully allocated to the remaining departments of laundry/linen, health information services, radiology, and nursing. Then laundry/linen's costs were fully allocated. In the double-distribution method, we would now have the opportunity to distribute some of laundry/linen's costs back to housekeeping. In the step-down method, that option is not available.

Simultaneous-Equations Method

The simultaneous-equations method (also known as the algebraic or multiple apportionment method) permits multiple allocations to occur through sophisticated mathematical software and the use of simultaneous mathematical equations. This method may require 10 to 12 distributions of costs.

Why Is Cost Allocation Methodology Important for the HIM Professional?

Some forward-thinking organizations provide comprehensive budgeting reports to their department managers. The managers see not only the direct costs incurred by the department—that is, the supplies they order and pay for, the labor they paid for, and so on—but also the allocations of costs from other departments. The HIM department may find it unusual to see costs for the laundry department allocated to the HIM department. If the HIM department uses no laundry services, then the allocation should be removed

and reallocated to the departments that use this service. The health information manager must fully investigate the services of laundry before removing the allocation because the laundry department may assist housekeeping in removing stains that may appear on the carpet in the HIM department.

Furthermore, the HIM department should assess whether costs are being properly allocated to its user departments. This may require HIM department management to monitor the user demand for several months, perhaps by counting the number of records, reports, or statistics requested and then determining what percentage of all requests should be allocated to each user department. For example, the HIM director may decide that the simplest method for allocating the HIM department costs is by record requests (Figure 18-5).

Given this information, the HIM professional can now approach the cost accountant and review current allocations to the new data and then may make adjustments as indicated on the basis of the factual data provided.

Some organizations allocate costs in a less scientific manner for simplicity. Some methods include allocating costs of other departments to user departments based on the total square feet occupied by all user departments. In our example, if the HIM department represented 5% of the total square feet served by housekeeping, then 5% of housekeeping's costs would be allocated to the HIM department. Clearly, one could argue that the HIM department area requires less

FIGURE 18-5 Example of record request.

RECORDS REQUESTED FOR FIRST NINE MONTHS OF YEAR		
Requestor	Number Requested	Percent of All
Administration	5	.004
Fiscal Services	210	.16
Quality Management	400	.30
Risk Management	17	.01
Nursing Service	323	.24
Respiratory Therapy	105	.08
Physical Therapy	90	.07
Anesthesiology	47	.04
Surgery	143	.11
Medicine	180	.13
Social Work	12	.01
Total	1340	1.01 (due to rounding)

Example of Cost Allocation Method

	Department Total Costs	Housekeeping	Laundry/Linen	HIS	Total
Housekeeping	$ 30,000	$30,000			
Laundry/linen	$ 15,000	$6,000 (.20)	$32,000*		
Health information services	$100,000	$1,500 (.05)	$630 (.03)	$102,130	
Radiology	$135,000	$1,500 (.05)	$1,050 (.05)	$10,213 (.10)	$147,760
Nursing	$270,000	$21,000 (.70)	$19,320 (.92)	$91,917 (.90)	$402,240
Total	$550,000	$30,000	$21,000	$102,130	$550,000

*The laundry/linen department costs were $15,000, and the allocated housekeeping costs were an additional $6,000. HIS, Health information systems.

cleaning than perhaps the operating room, but the allocation method is simple to apply and keep up to date.

? DID YOU KNOW?

Calculating key financial ratios and preparing management and financial reports is most commonly accomplished using Microsoft Excel spreadsheet software. Using Excel spreadsheets to access, view, and edit large amounts of data for producing financial reports, graphs, and analyses of all types is a valuable tool for HIM managers. Integrating raw data from legacy clinical, billing, finance, and budget systems and organizing into meaningful information allows for more effective decisions. Pivot Tables within Excel offer an additional dynamic reporting tool enabling users to rearrange data to examine different perspectives and quickly spot patterns and trends. The knowledge and skill demands to be considered an effective user of Excel vary widely dependent upon reporting needs and job roles. Recognition as an expert may range from understanding basic formulas and filters, to more advanced VLOOKUP, IF function and macros, or even advanced certifications.

FINANCIAL ACCOUNTING

The role of managerial accounting was explained previously in our discussion of how budgets, business plans, and cost allocations are linked to organizational goals and provide financial information to internal decision makers. Financial accounting, in contrast, refers to recording and reporting the financial transactions of the organization for both internal management and users outside of the organization. External users might include loan officers, creditors, investors, and payers. For the purposes of financial accounting, organizations must adhere to generally accepted accounting principles promulgated by the Financial Accounting Standards Board (FASB). FASB is a rule-making body of the American Institute of Certified Public Accountants (AICPA), which establishes general accounting principles for all types of financial accounting transactions and reporting. A separate Government Accounting Standards Board (GASB) provides financial accounting and reporting standards for state and local governments.

Fundamental Accounting Principles and Concepts

It is these basic underlying concepts and principles that help ensure the quality of financial accounting information made available to users. Generally accepted accounting principles and assumptions provide a common framework for both recording individual accounting transactions and communicating financial information. An understanding of these important concepts will provide a foundation for understanding how financial accounting information develops and is communicated. Some of the more important accounting principles and concepts follow.

Entity

General accounting principles define an entity as the business unit or activity for which accounting records are maintained. Separate financial statements must be prepared for each individual business entity. Just as a physician in private practice should not combine funds with his or her own personal household finances, an individual hospital as part of a large publicly traded health care corporation should not combine accounts with the parent corporation. Each entity must keep its own unique set of books and prepare separate and distinct financial statements.

Going Concern

According to GAAP, an assumption is made that an entity will continue for the foreseeable future. The going concern concept assumes that the owners of a business entity will continue operating indefinitely to fulfill the business plans of the organization.

Stable Monetary Unit

Accounting entities use a stable monetary unit of measure to record and report financial transactions. In the United States, this stable monetary unit is represented by the U.S. dollar. It is understood that inflation could affect the reporting of financial information; however, for the purposes of accounting standards, it is assumed that this would not be significant enough to cause alarm.

Matching Concept

The importance of recognizing revenues and expenses in the same accounting period is represented by the matching concept. Earlier in the chapter during our discussion of the revenue cycle, we mentioned that revenue is accounted for when the actual charge is posted to a patient account. The matching concept recognizes that any associated expenses such as labor, supplies, and travel would be recorded in the same accounting period and matched with the revenue for that accounting period.

Objectivity

Because of inflation and market dynamics, there can be considerable differences between the current value of an asset and its original cost. For this reason, accounting principles recognize the historical cost of an asset as the most objective measure for financial reporting. As an example, a physician office building currently valued at $1.5 million that was purchased 5 years ago for $500,000 would be recorded on the balance sheet at $500,000. Even though the market value of the office building is $1.5 million, the objectivity concept states that historical cost is a more objective measure than current value.

Disclosure

An entity's financial statements provide a mechanism to communicate the economic activities of an organization. In the event supplemental data are available to better clarify or offer additional information for decision makers, this should be disclosed on pertinent financial statements. Disclosure of additional information through the use of footnotes on an organization's financial statements is a commonly accepted accounting practice.

Financial Management Duties

When the HIM professional interacts with the financial accounting staff of the organization, it might be to request a payment to a publisher for a departmental reference book. The payment is recorded as an expense to the HIM department and classified by the type of expense, for example, books and subscriptions. Besides recording the expense, financial accounting professionals must reduce the cash balance to allow for the payment to be issued to the publisher. The people employed in the financial accounting section of fiscal services capture the data necessary to build the foundation for reports used in understanding the financial management of the organization. Just as there are numerous diverse job roles within the HIM profession, the duties of the financial accountant, managerial accountant, and managerial finance officer cover different aspects of financial management (Table 18-7).

Cash and Accrual Systems

The financial transaction processing associated with financial accounting can be accomplished in one of two manners: cash basis accounting or accrual basis accounting. In a cash basis environment, each transaction is recorded when cash is exchanged, as with one's personal finances. Revenues are

TABLE 18-7   Financial Management Duties

Financial Accounting	Managerial Accounting	Managerial Finance
Record financial transactions (e.g., payments, orders, expenses, revenues, accruals)	Prepare reports such as budgets, cost reports, productivity, and volume schedule; set rates or charges; monitor variances	Financing and funding activities; planning for future expenditures; investment decisions and planning
When: Past and current activities	When: Current and future activities	When: Future activities
Titles: Staff accountant, accountant, bookkeeper	Titles: Cost accountant, budget coordinator	Titles: Chief financial officer, treasurer

recognized when money is received for services provided, and expenses are recognized when money is paid out for the resources used to provide those services. The cash basis accounting method may have worked for health care providers in years past, but it does not work today because services rendered today are seldom paid for today. Instead, health care providers often must wait 30 or more days to receive payment from a third party, typically an insurance company.

Accrual basis accounting uses the matching concept, enabling revenues to be matched with the actual expenses incurred to produce the revenue. The accrual method records the revenues expected as "revenues," although the "cash" has not yet been received. The revenues are matched as closely with the expenses as possible. For example, if an operation occurred today, the expenses associated with performing the operation are operating room staff, anesthesia, medications, disposable medical-surgical supplies, and so on. The charges associated with each of these items are recorded as revenue, and the actual cost or expense of these items is recorded as expenses of the operation.

Profit represents the amount of money (cash) actually received from the payer (patient or insurance company) less the actual cost to do the service, assuming that the cost is less than the cash received.

Each financial transaction must be recorded during the financial accounting process. Transactions are assigned to designated accounts. Several health care associations, such as the American Hospital Association (AHA), have developed a standard chart of accounts, although there may be slight variations from one health care organization to another. Typically, the largest expense items are in the lower number account categories, whereas the expense categories that have limited expenses appear in the higher number account groups. Labor expenses may be classified in the 100 series, and dues expenses may be classified in the 900 series. A chart similar to the standard chart of accounts for expenses exists for revenues.

Financial accounting using the accrual basis requires the accountant to comply with the double-entry method of transaction recording. This means that when revenues and expenses are matched and recorded, another set (double) of entries must occur simultaneously. These entries typically record an amount equivalent to the revenue in a category called accounts receivable; the expense amounts reduce categories of assets, such as medical-surgical supply inventory and pharmaceutical inventory, or increase liability categories, such as wages payable. The statement of revenues and expenses and balance sheet results from the double-entry activities.

Fiscal Periods

Organizations can choose a calendar year as a fiscal year—that is, it begins January 1 and ends December 31. Or a fiscal year may not coincide with a calendar year. It may be July 1 through June 30. Fiscal periods are selected by organizations because they more consistently conform to activity cycles of the organization. A teaching institution may choose the fiscal period of July 1 through June 30 because students finish one level of training in June and are ready to start the next level in July. Budgets often correspond to fiscal periods. Specific IRS rules require that a health care organization's fiscal year must coincide with the tax year for tax accounting reporting purposes.

✓ SELF-ASSESSMENT QUIZ

11. True or False? Budget preparation, cost allocation, and productivity analysis are key principles for effective financial accounting.
12. How is the "matching concept" used in accrual basis accounting?

USING FINANCIAL REPORTS TO PROVIDE MANAGEMENT INFORMATION

The balance sheet displays the organization's assets, liabilities, and fund balance or equity at a fixed point in time—for example, December 31 of a given year (Figure 18-6). The balance sheet may be computed at any time. It is a snapshot at that time and may vary considerably during a time period. The balance sheet lists assets and liabilities and the difference between them. This financial report is best represented by the following basic accounting equation:

$$\text{Assets} - \text{Liabilities} = \text{Fund Balance (Equity)}$$

Assets are cash or cashlike items or other resources that can be converted to cash. Assets may be considered as short-term (those easily converted to cash) or long-term (items more difficult to convert to cash quickly or items needed to operate the business). Liabilities are the debts or obligations the organization owes. They may include

FIGURE 18-6 Balance sheet.

RKK Memorial Hospital Balance Sheets for Year Ending December 31 (thousands of dollars)		
	Year 2	Year 1
Cash and securities	7,250	5,850
Accounts receivable (estimated net)	22,760	20,850
Inventories	4,780	3,440
Total current assets	34,790	30,140
Gross plant and equipment	152,420	145,780
Accumulated depreciation	26,930	21,550
Net plant and equipment	179,350	167,330
Total assets	214,140	197,470
Accounts payable	5,680	5,250
Accrued expenses	5,790	5,420
Notes payable	945	2,870
Current portion of long-term debt	2,670	2,200
Total current liabilities	15,085	15,740
Long-term debt	29,420	30,800
Capital lease obligations	1,720	2,140
Total long-term liabilities	31,140	32,940
Fund balance	167,915	148,790
Total liabilities and funds	214,140	197,470

wages accruing between paydays and mortgage payments owed to the bank. The fund balance category is the residual category that collects the profits and losses that result from the differences between revenues and expenses.

The statement of revenues and expenses reports the expected or earned income and the associated expenses for an accounting period (Figure 18-7). This financial report may also be referred to as the income statement and is best described by the basic equation:

$$\text{Revenue} - \text{Expense} = \text{Net Income}$$

The statement of cash flow is an important financial report that provides additional detailed information about the source and use of funds (Figure 18-8). This report documents the change in cash balance for a given accounting period and is useful in evaluating an organization's ability to pay its bills. The statement of cash flow looks at sources and uses of cash based on the organization's operating, investing, and financing activities.

USING RATIOS TO EVALUATE FINANCIAL DATA

The statement of revenues and expenses, the balance sheet, the statement of cash flow, and other reports allow management to compare the success of providing services cost effectively. Financial analysis or ratio analysis is the management process of formulating judgments and decisions from the relation between the numbers represented on two reports: the balance sheet and the statement of revenues and expenses.

A ratio expresses the relation between two numbers, such as one asset category, cash, to all assets. Professional associations, such as the Healthcare Financial Management Association, the Medical Group Management Association, and the AHA, and health care systems collect data from their member organizations and members and publish average or benchmark ratios. Sometimes the data are reported by region, facility size, and facility type. The publication of average ratios permits organizations to compare their individual ratios with the average to determine how well they compare with others. Benchmarking performance against peer data provides a good yardstick for measuring performance.

When conducting ratio analysis, it is important to be consistent in defining the ratio components. When HIM professionals calculate the average length of stay of adult patients, they must be careful not to include infant discharges or infant days. This means that the definition for adult length of stay demands that the composition of the denominator and numerator be consistently determined. In addition, one should not assume that published average ratios are developed in the same way by all who submitted data to the collecting organization.

FIGURE 18-7 Statement of revenues and expenses.

RKK Memorial Hospital—Income Statements for Year Ending December 31 (Revenues and Expenses) (thousands of dollars)		
	Year 1	Year 2
Net patient services revenue	110,500	98,500
Other operating revenue	7,300	8,800
Total operating revenue	117,800	107,300
Operating expenses		
Nursing services	54,300	50,200
Dietary services	5,200	4,640
General services	12,680	11,450
Administrative services	11,290	10,360
Employee health and welfare	9,560	9,240
Provision for uncollectibles	4,220	3,980
Provision for malpractice	1,450	1,220
Depreciation	4,200	4,050
Interest expense	1,890	2,300
Total operating expense	104,790	97,480
Income from operations	13,010	9,860
Contributions and grants	3,290	890
Investment income	540	345
Nonoperating gain or loss	3,830	1,235
Excess of revenues over expenses	16,840	11,095

RKK Memorial Hospital Statement of Cash Flow for Year 2 (thousands of dollars)	
Cash flow from operations	
Total operating revenue	117,800
Total cash operating expenses	(100,590)
Change in acounts receivable	(1,910)
Change in inventories	(1,340)
Change in accounts payable	(430)
Change in accruals	370
Net cash flow from operations	13,900
Cash flow for investing activities	
Investment in plant and equipment	(6,640)
Cash flow from financing activities	
Repayment of long-term debt	(1,380)
Repayment of notes payable	(1,925)
Capital lease principal repayment	(420)
Change in current portion of long-term debt	470
Net cash flow from financing	3,255
Nonoperating cash flow	
Contributions and grants	3,290
Investment income	540
Nonoperating cash flow	3,830
Net increase (decrease) in cash	7,835
Beginning cash and securities	5,430
Ending cash and securities	14,285

FIGURE 18-8 Statement of cash flow.

There are four commonly recognized ratio categories:
- Liquidity
- Turnover
- Performance
- Capitalization

Liquidity and capitalization ratios focus on balance sheet numbers (assets, liabilities, and equity/fund balance accounts). They measure the ability of the health care organization to meet its short- and long-term financial obligations. Performance ratios use data from the statement of revenues and expenses. Ratios in this category evaluate the effectiveness of resource use to deliver services and products. Turnover or activity ratios use data from the balance sheet and the statement of revenues and expenses. These ratios measure the organization's ability to generate net operating revenue in relation to its various assets.

Liquidity Ratio

One of the most common liquidity ratios is the current ratio. This ratio compares current assets with current liabilities. Both categories appear on the balance sheet. What the current ratio tells a manager is whether there are sufficient cash and cashlike assets to cover the immediate liabilities (bills) that will come due in the short term (1 year).

Example of Liquidity Ratio

The Citywide Surgi-Center has cash, marketable securities, and accounts receivable of $300,000. Citywide has payroll liabilities, payables due to their suppliers, and the mortgage on the surgery equipment and building due this year in the amount of $150,000.

Current assets = $300,000
Current liabilities = $150,000
Current ratio = 2:1 or 2.0

The ratio says that Citywide can meet its current obligations twice. It has twice as much cash and other liquid assets as it needs to meet its bills.

Turnover Ratio or Activity Ratio

One ratio that is affected by the activities of the health information services department is the days of revenue in patient accounts receivable ratio.

This turnover ratio, or activity ratio, divides patient accounts receivable by the average daily patient revenues. Patient revenues are found on the statement of revenues and expenses, and patient accounts receivable are found on the balance sheet because accounts receivable are considered an asset to an organization. Accounts receivable are eventually paid and converted to cash. Patient revenues can be expressed as either net or gross. Gross patient revenues, sometimes referred to as patient services revenues, refer to the value of services provided at full billed charges. Net patient revenues, sometimes referred to as net patient services revenues, refer to the amount the health care provider expects to receive as payment for the services. Therefore, net revenue is gross revenue less any contractual discounts or adjustments agreed to between the insurance company and the provider or the difference between full charges and fixed fees established by the government (e.g., DRG) or insurer. The 1990 American Institute of Certified Public Accountants' audit and accounting guide, *Audits of Providers of Health Care Services*, requires that reports prepared for public use reflect net patient revenues, not gross patient revenues.

When using net patient revenues in the accounts receivable turnover ratio (AR days ratio), one must be certain to use net accounts receivable. For consistency, if gross patient revenues are used, then the divisor must be gross accounts receivable. Most reports are now expressed in terms of net patient revenues and receivables.

Net days of revenue in patient accounts receivable
= Net patient accounts receivable/Average daily net patient service revenue

Average net daily patient service revenue
= Net patient service revenue for the period/Days in the period

The days of revenue in the patient accounts receivable ratio provide a measure of the average time that receivables are outstanding or the period for which a health care organization extends credit to its debtors. High values for this ratio imply longer collection periods and may signal a need for the health care organization to seek cash or financial resources from other sources to pay its ongoing day-to-day expenses until the receivables are collected.

Example of the Average Number of Days of Revenue in Accounts Receivable

Compare Citywide Surgi-Center's days of revenue in patient accounts receivable (also known as AR days) with the hypothetical average published by U.S. Surgi-Centers:

Citywide Surgi-Center's AR Days

	May	June	July	August	Sept	U.S. Surgi-Center Average
AR Days	37.6	37.9	38.4	39.1	39.7	45.8

Conclusion: Citywide is collecting their receivables effectively, yet the collection period is increasing. Management should assess the causes for this trend.

Performance Ratio

The **performance ratio** evaluates the use of resources to achieve a goal. A common performance ratio is the **operating margin ratio**. This ratio displays the relation between the net revenues received and the expenses required to supply the revenues. **Net operating revenue** is the amount of revenue expected to be received or total charges less the deductions expected by third-party payers resulting in revenues **net** of deductions or net operating revenue. If Citywide had net operating revenue this month of $100,000 and expenses of $96,000, the revenues in excess of expenses would be $4,000 ($100,000 − $96,000). Citywide's operating margin ratio would be 0.04 or 4%.

Capitalization Ratio

There are several **capitalization ratios**. One that may be experienced by anyone who works in an organization that has an anticipated building project is the **long-term debt/total assets ratio**. This ratio compares the amount of long-term debt the organization has (bills that will come due in a period more than 1 year from now [e.g., mortgages]) with the amount of assets (things the organization can convert to cash [e.g., furniture, land, inventories, marketable securities]) it has to pay those debts. The banks will consider the organization's ability to pay back the estimated additional debt it will incur.

CAPITAL EXPENSE AND INVESTMENT DECISIONS

You may ask who has the overall responsibility for capital decisions. This responsibility is another component of the fiscal services area. The overall capital planning function is part of the managerial finance role. Some institutions assign this duty to a chief financial officer (CFO); others, a treasurer. The role of the **managerial finance officer** is one of planning for the future. We have discussed the role of the financial accountant. It is one of recording what has happened today or in the past, such as paying staff for work performed. We have also discussed the role of the managerial accountant during the budget review. This person helps record what is happening currently or previously (variance analyses) against what was anticipated and what is still anticipated to happen (the budget).

The managerial finance officer, CFO, or treasurer works with financial organizations (e.g., banks or investors) to obtain funding and financing for an organization's plans. If an organization wants to build a new building, financing support is required. This person may also make investment decisions to maximize the income on idle money the organization may have at any given time. The thrust is to ensure that the organization is effective in delivering the services suggested by the mission statement while doing so efficiently so that funds are not being spent on inappropriate items. The following reports result from these activities:

- Balance sheet
- Statement of changes in financial position
- Investment reports
- Financing reports

Capital Expenditures

Some facilities establish a capital expenditure committee to evaluate all capital requests so that cash resources are used to purchase the high-cost items that will yield the most benefit to the organization. When the final list is approved, proposed acquisition dates are assigned. The proposed acquisition date does not guarantee that a manager will be able to purchase the item on that date. The CFO or controller must assess the condition of the cash budget to determine whether sufficient cash will be available to meet not only the upcoming expenses to support the upcoming service levels but also the one-time expense associated with the piece of capital.

Because capital requests are typically considered by a committee, it is important for department managers to know how to prepare a well-developed and justified request for the equipment needed for their departments. To do so requires an analysis of the opportunity cost of funds.

The capital expenditure committee considers all requests received. A capital investment should be evaluated in terms of the following:

- From the perspective of its contribution to the mission and from a financial perspective relative to the cost of the capital acquisition
- Revenues it may generate for the organization
- Period of time the acquisition will contribute to the organization (economic life)
- Cost to the organization to borrow the funds or loss of interest on the funds
- Regulatory hurdles, such as requirements to obtain approval from planning or rate-setting agencies, and any reimbursement opportunities through Medicare or taxation

Any organization has limited funds to invest in new capital. Each decision to use funds for one acquisition means that another must be foregone. Financial managers describe this process as weighing opportunity costs. Opportunity costs are benefits that would be received from the next best alternative use of the investment funds. Some providers use as a measure of opportunity cost the interest rate received on invested funds. Cleverley et al.[14] define opportunity costs as "values foregone by using a resource in a particular way instead of in its next best alternative way."

The health information manager is obligated to contribute to conserving the facility's cash and adjusting the department's operations to meet the actual levels of service.

Capital Request Evaluation Process

In most organizations, there is a formalized process for obtaining approval of a capital expenditure. The process is usually initiated by a department manager preparing a written request on a capital expenditure approval form (Figure 18-9).

Some request forms are elaborate, requiring the manager to calculate various financial analyses. Others are more verbiage oriented, requiring the manager to define the need, alternatives considered, volume of business related to the item being requested, analysis of various vendors or suppliers

considered or bids obtained to determine the item's cost, and an economic feasibility study.

Each facility defines its capitalization value. For the sake of this example, Citywide Surgi-Center, Inc. recognizes any expenditure in excess of $5000 for equipment or furniture as a capital expenditure. Capital items usually have a high initial cost and a "life" of more than 1 year.

Time Value of Money

No discussion of capital expenditures would be complete without including the concept of the time value of money. This concept includes several premises. The first is that a person who invests money should be entitled to a return or interest. The return is based on at least two conditions: the length of time the money is invested and the degree of risk associated with the investment. If the investment carries great risk, the rate of return should be higher and vice versa.

The time value of money says to the layperson that it is more beneficial to receive a dollar today than to receive it 1 year from now. The reason is that a dollar received today can be invested and gain interest for 1 year longer than a dollar received 1 year from now. That is, a dollar received today and placed in a savings account at 5% interest accrues a minimum of $0.05 in interest. At the end of the year, the savings account closes at $1.05. If the dollar is not received until the end of the year, there would be $1.00, not $1.05.

Compounding

The value of the investment is determined by the length of time the investment is in place because of the compounding effect. In the example previously discussed, we started with $1, but at the end of the year we had $1.05, simply by selecting a safe bank in which to deposit this dollar. If that dollar was left in the bank for 3 years at the 5% interest rate, we do not end up with $1.15, but rather $1.16. An extra $0.01 is earned because of the compounding effect. By the fourth year, $0.22 is gained. Although the gain may not seem significant in this example, consider the effect if $10,000 is invested. Compounding can mean significant gains for the investor.

Discounting

The concept of discounting is the opposite of compounding. The question we ask ourselves when we are considering discounting is, how much must one invest today at a compound interest rate of x to receive a given amount at the end of N years? What we know is how much we want to have at the end of the period—say, our retirement age. What we do not know is the present value of the money we need to invest today at today's interest rate to accumulate the sum we want by retirement age. For example, if you were to retire next year and today's interest rate is 5% and you want $105,000 next year, what is the present value you would need to invest today? ($100,000)

When the capital expenditure committee evaluates capital requests, they are evaluating the opportunities available to the organization. Should the organization leave its funds in the

CITYWIDE SURGI-CENTER
CAPITAL EQUIPMENT REQUEST FORM

BUDGET YEAR:	DATE:				
BUDGET DESCRIPTION:	REQUESTED BY:				
DEPARTMENT NAME:	Replacement	Yes ☐	No ☐
ACCOUNT / CENTER:			
CER AMOUNT:	New Item	Yes ☐	No ☐
DESCRIPTION OF NEED:			
	Revenue Stream	Yes ☐	No ☐

CAPITAL EQUIPMENT DESCRIPTION AND JUSTIFICATION
List all other associated costs such as additional staffing, maintenance agreements, supplies, etc.

EFFECT ON OPERATIONS
List quality benefits, operational efficiencies, productivity improvements, other rationale

COMPLETE THIS SECTION FOR ALL EQUIPMENT REQUESTS

Quantity	Vendor	Model Number

SIGNATURE APPROVALS

Director: _____ Date: _____

Administrator: _____ Date: _____

FINANCE SCREENING AND PURCHASE AUTHORIZATION

PROJECT CATEGORY	Budget Amount	CER Amount	
Professional Fees			Date: _____
Staff Salaries			☐ Approved
Fringe Benefits			☐ Approved with Modification
Supplies			☐ Disapproved
Computer Support Services			
Training			Comments:
Installation			
Maintenance			
Depreciation			
Trade In (Amount)			
TOTAL PROJECT COST	$ -	$ -	

REVIEW AND APPROVAL

DIRECTOR OF PURCHASING	Date	CHIEF FINANCIAL OFFICER	Date
CHIEF OPERATING OFFICER	Date	FINANCE - RELEASE OF FUNDS	Date

A

FIGURE 18-9 A. Capital expenditure approval form. B. Capital Equipment Request form shall be submitted for any capital expenditure greater than $5000 and must receive Finance authorization prior to purchase.

CAPITAL EQUIPMENT REQUEST (CER) INSTRUCTIONS	
Budget year	Planned date of purchase
Budget description	Complete name and specifications of item to be purchased
Date	Date CER form is prepared
Requested by	Manager's name who initiates request
Department name	Department submitting CER form
Account/center	Ledger to be charged for items purchased
CER amount	Total amount should reflect Quantity × Price, less Discount
Description of need	Explanation of why item is needed; consequences if not approved
Replacement	Note if replaces existing item
New item	Note if does not replace existing item
Revenue stream	Note if generates new revenue (include pro forma)
Description and justification	Document business case why item is needed and any ancillary costs associated with purchase
Effect on operations	Describe anticipated benefits
Quantity	Include number of items requested
Vendor	Include complete name, business address, and contact
Model number	Verify exact model number of item to be purchased
Signature approvals	Signature denotes support for project (does not approve purchase)

B

FIGURE 18-9, cont'd

bank at a certain interest rate, or should it invest in a new program that predicts it may yield yet another level of revenue and do so for several years? Decisions such as these are confronted by managers every day. The managers must weigh the risk associated with the new program against the considerably lower risk of leaving the money in the bank. Unfortunately, it is not this simple because each year many capital requests are submitted and must be compared with one another.

Helping the capital expenditure committee is the fiscal management staff. Financial managers assess or weigh the value of an investment in equipment or other capital request against the interest that would be received on the funds if left in the bank by using one or more of the following capital evaluation methods:

- Accounting rate of return
- Payback method
- Net present value

Net Present Value

In its simplest format, a new piece of equipment or new program will have cash outflows and cash inflows. For example, St. Elsewhere Medical Center has two capital requests. One is

from the HIM department for a new dictation system. The other is from the business office for a new charge auditing program.

We know that capital requests will require some cash outflows. The dictation system vendor will expect to be paid a certain sum at the time of installation. The charge auditing program will require additional staff and training costs before it is fully productive. Both proposals will have cash inflows. The HIM manager predicts that she will be able to eliminate the contract typing service expense and do all work in-house, thus eliminating payments to the outside contract service. The business office manager says he will find items that have been used in the patient care process and not been charged. When they are found, his staff can add these charges to the bill and obtain third-party reimbursement for them.

Both proposals have an expected life of 5 years. That is, the equipment will operate optimally for 5 years before the technology is outdated. Each will be depreciated over 5 years as well. Straight-line **depreciation** is calculated by dividing the capital cost by the years of life (in this example, the life is 5 years). The resulting amount is considered the annual depreciation expense.

The charge auditing program includes a training program for the departments that provide services. It is proposed that the program will use a continuous quality improvement approach to identify where charges are lost and assist these areas in reducing errors. Over a period of 5 years, all departments will have improved their charge-entering procedures to ensure that no charges are overlooked or lost.

The proposals will subtract cash outflows from cash inflows to result in a new cash inflow or outflow at the end of each year for the full 5 years. Depreciation expense is considered an outflow. The proposed annual nets for each project must be evaluated against the rate of interest the moneys would have earned if left in the bank. Because the net amounts are the remaining amounts received at the end of each year, we must use a discounting factor to determine the present value of each net amount or **net present value**.

To find this factor, use a table that can be found in most finance textbooks. Table 18-8 represents a portion of such a table.

TABLE 18-8 Internalizing the Copy Service Proposal

Year	New Cash Flows	Present Value 13%	Value of Cash Flows Today
1	1,000	0.88496	885.00
2	3,000	0.78318	2,349.54
3	7,000	0.69305	4,851.35
4	12,000	0.61332	7,359.84
5	15,000	0.54276	8,141.40
Total	38,000		23,587.13

is $23,587.13. In other terms, if we had $23,587.13 today and invested it at 13% interest, at the end of 5 years, it would yield $30,000. If we need $25,000 in capital to start this program, the investment ($25,000) would not be recovered in the 5 years and may be turned down. If we need only $19,000, perhaps to buy a personal computer and a big copy machine to support the logging effort, then the project may be approved because the investment is less than the net present value of the cash flows ($23,587).

Accounting Rate of Return

This evaluation method uses averages. The annual net inflows or outflows are averaged over the project's life for each project. The asset value or investment value is averaged over the life of the project as well. The asset value is depreciated on a straight-line basis for the life of the program.

Example Comparing Competing Projects-Net Present Value

	HIM	Patient Accounts
The project	Dictation system	Auditing program
Net cash flows	$25,000/year	$15,000/year
Project life	5 years	5 years
Initial capital	$75,000	$60,000
Annual depreciation	$15,000	$12,000
Return required	10%	10%
Net present value (NPV)	$94,775	$56,865
NPV-initial capital	$19,775	($3,135)

Decision: The health record project meets the criteria to have a 10% return and exceed the initial capital outlay.

Example of Net Present Value Evaluation-Copy Service

You want to bring the copy service in-house. Because you know the volumes intimately, you can accurately forecast the service's growth. Your current contracted copy service pays your organization a retrieval fee, but your staff does all the logging, pulls all the records, and answers all the calls about the records requested. On the basis of the volumes you have experienced in the past and anticipate in the future, you can estimate the revenues from the copies and the related expenses. The revenues less the expenses are the net cash flows.
1. Prepare your pro forma (expected revenues and expenses) to provide this service internally.
2. Meet with your CFO and ask what interest rate he expects on investments or what return he expects from new programs. Review the table in a finance book labeled "Present Value of One Dollar Due at the End of *N* Years" and the interest column that corresponds to the CFO's expectations. He expects 13%.

From the copy service example, one can see that even though the program is projected to generate $38,000 in net cash flows, the real value of those flows in today's dollars

Example of Accounting Rate of Return—Copy Service

If we use our same copy service example's facts, we can use the following **accounting rate of return** formula:
Average net income $38,000/5
Initial investment = $19,000
$38,000/5 years/$19,000 = 40%
Accounting rate of return: 40%
Before proceeding further, we need to revisit the CFO and determine whether an accounting rate of return of 40% is acceptable.

Example Comparing Competing Projects— Accounting Rate of Return

	HIM	Patient Accounts
Net cash flows	$25,000/year	$15,000/year
Depreciation	−15,000/year	−12,000/year
Average net income	$10,000/year	$3,000/year
Average investment	$75,000/year	$60,000/year
Accounting rate of return	13%	5%

Decision: The HIM project has a higher accounting rate of return.

Payback Method

The **payback method** is probably the simplest of all methods. The payback period determines the number of years it will take for the cash inflows from each project to pay back the initial investment (cash outflow).

Example of Payback Method—Copy Service

Year	Net Cash Flows	Initial Investment	Remaining
0		$19,000	
1	$ 1,000	−1,000	$18,000
2	$ 3,000	−3,000	15,000
3	$ 7,000	−7,000	$48,000
4	$12,000	−12,000	
5	$15,000		
Total	$38,000		

We can see that by year 4, our initial investment will be paid back. To calculate the portion of year 4 that it consumes, we divide the remaining amount ($8,000) by the net cash flow ($12,000). Therefore, this investment will be paid back in 3.67 years.

Example of Payback Method—Comparing Competing Projects

The HIM project's initial investment is $75,000. Annual cash flows of $25,000 will result in a payback period of 3 years ($75,000/$25,000).

The patient accounts project's initial investment is $60,000. Annual cash flows of $15,000 will result in a payback period of 4 years ($60,000/$15,000).

Arguments Pro and Con for Evaluation Methods

Each of the evaluation methods has advantages and disadvantages. No one method is more effective than the others, and occasionally financial managers use more than one method to weigh the opportunities. The payback method is the simplest to use. No special tables are required, but it ignores the basic concept of money management—the time value of money.

The accounting rate of return is simple to use. No special tables are required, but it ignores the time value of money and does not take into consideration when inflows are received. The same average could result if the heavier inflows are received later in the project's life or earlier. If the time value of money was considered, a money manager would want to receive the larger inflows earlier rather than later.

The net present value approach requires calculations of the discounted amounts or the use of special discounting tables. It assumes, however, that net inflows are reinvested at the same rate as the cost of capital or the interest rate the investment would have received had the money been left in the bank. It also requires the evaluators to assume a rate of return.

✓ SELF-ASSESSMENT QUIZ

13. The difference in the value of an investment today compared to the future refers to what financial concept?
14. List and describe three methods an organization might use to maintain tight controls over capital and equipment planning.

OTHER PHASES OF FINANCIAL MANAGEMENT

Implementing

The implementation process is probably the most rewarding activity of management because it confirms whether your ideas were correct, your plans were accurate, and your achievements are worth reaching. It requires support from your entire staff and from administration and organizational leaders.

Because of the high cost of health care and the continuing impact on the overall economy, reimbursement pressures are certain to increase. Even in an economy operating under ideal conditions and in an environment of health care regulation and reform, the need to monitor closely all activities to ensure that services are delivered as cost effectively as possible is management's greatest challenge.

Seeking Alternatives

No manager can identify all alternatives to doing a task. Just as the composition of the business plan requires the involvement of all staff, during times of high growth and increasing volumes, all staff members need to be involved to find new and better methods to achieve the same outcome. This holds true for periods of economic downturns and lower volumes as well. Management should meet with staff (in teams if the staff size is large or as a whole if the staff size is small) at regular intervals to brainstorm alternatives to performing tasks. Ideally, this process should occur before the budgeting process so that management can fully investigate the options that surface and prepare any justification materials at budget time. This participative management approach is becoming more common in health care with the increased awareness of continuous quality improvement processes and need to hardwire excellence.

ROLE OF THE HIM PROFESSIONAL IN FINANCIAL MANAGEMENT

The need for HIM professionals to be more adept in fiscal activities is apparent. The ability to understand, use, and communicate both financial and clinical information continues to take on a new level of importance in health care organizations. This chapter cannot review all aspects of financial management. To be truly successful, HIM professionals of tomorrow must be able to communicate as easily with the CFO as they are able to deal with the medical staff. If the HIM professional is to gain this level of expertise, additional training must be sought beyond the contents of this chapter.

CHAPTER REVIEW

1. When evaluating health plan options, the upfront costs patients and employers make to payers for health care insurance coverage are:
   a. copayments
   b. coinsurance and deductibles
   c. premiums
   d. all of the above

2. Health care providers increasingly look to nonoperating revenues as a significant source of revenue, examples of which might include:
   a. durable medical equipment
   b. investment interest
   c. prescription drugs
   d. all of the above

3. A primary role of the federal government's Recovery Audit Contractor (RAC) program is to:
   a. identify false hospital cost reports
   b. identify payment errors due to noncompliance with billing and payment rules
   c. detect deliberate upcoding of cases or billed services not actually performed
   d. all of the above

4. Which of the following are key principles for effective financial accounting practices?
   a. budget preparation
   b. productivity analysis
   c. cash and accrual systems
   d. all of the above

5. The managerial accounting process of forecasting volume and monetary resources needed by the organization is best accomplished through:
   a. financial ratio analysis
   b. budget preparation
   c. matching concept
   d. capital expenditure planning

6. Timely and accurate coding in the HIM department has an impact on what key revenue cycle performance metric?
   a. accounts receivable aging
   b. days in accounts receivable
   c. claim denial rate
   d. all of the above

7. Capitation, DRGs, per diems, and predefined fee schedules are all examples of:
   a. reimbursement methods
   b. accounting rate of return
   c. profit
   d. chart of accounts

8. When a small physician practice organization reports AR days of 30.5 days:
   a. the average payment turnaround is 30.5 days
   b. average daily charges are $82,000 and total accounts receivables are $2.5 million.
   c. outstanding accounts receivables are $2.5 million and average daily revenue is $82,000
   d. all of the above

9. To prepare for a new CDI program, an HIM manager must include 4 new FTE coders in the department labor budget. At an average salary of $25 per hour, non productive hours of 15%, and anticipated 50% productivity reduction due to ICD-10, what is the projected annual salary expense?
   a. $104,000
   b. $176,800
   c. $208,000
   d. $353,600

10. A health care organization's statement of revenue and expenses will show:
    a. estimated accounts receivable
    b. actual accounts receivable
    c. accrued expenses
    d. net income

REFERENCES

1. Centers for Medicare & Medicaid Services: *National health expenditures by type of expenditure and source of funds: Calendar Years 1965-2021*:2011: http://www.cms.gov/Research-Statistics-Data-and-Systems/Statistics-Trends-and-Reports/NationalHealthExpendData/Downloads/Proj2011PDF.pdf.
2. Centers for Medicare & Medicaid Services: *National Physician Fee Schedule Relative Value File 2013*: http://www.cms.hhs.gov/physicianfeesched/.
3. Bipartisan Policy Center: *What is Driving U.S. Health Care Spending?*: 2012. http://bipartisanpolicy.org/sites/default/files/BPC%20Health%20Care%20Cost%20Drivers%20Brief%20Sept%202012.pdf.
4. U.S. Census Bureau: *Income, poverty and health insurance coverage in the United States: 2011*: http://www.census.gov. 2012: http://www.census.gov/prod/2012pubs/p60-243.pdf.
5. Centers for Medicare & Medicaid Services: *Accountable Care Organizations*, 2012: http://www.cms.gov/aco/.
6. Centers for Medicare & Medicaid Services: *Physician Quality Reporting System*: http://www.cms.hhs.gov/pqrs. 2013: http://www.cms.gov/ERxIncentive/.
7. American Health Information Management Association: *Clinical Documentation Improvement Toolkit*, 2010: http://library.ahima.org/xpedio/groups/public/documents/ahima/bok1_047236.pdf.
8. National Uniform Billing Committee: UB-04 claim form: http://www.nubc.org; National Uniform Claim Committee: CMS 1500 claim form: http://www.nucc.org.
9. Department of Health and Human Services. *2013 Federal Poverty Guidelines*: http://aspe.hhs.gov/poverty/13poverty.cfm.

10. Payment Card Industry Security Standards Council: 2013 *For Merchants*: https://www.pcisecuritystandards.org/merchants/index.php.

11. National Health Care Anti-Fraud Association: *The Challenge of Health Care Fraud*: http://www.nhcaa.org. 2013: http://www.nhcaa.org/resources/health-care-anti-fraud-resources/the-challenge-of-health-care-fraud.aspx.

12. Department of Health and Human Services: *Medicare Learning Network: Medicare Fraud & Abuse: Prevention, Detection and Reporting*, 2012: http://www.cms.gov/Outreach-and-Education/Medicare-Learning-Network-MLN/MLNProducts/downloads/Fraud_and_Abuse.pdf.

13. American Health Information Management Association: Code of ethics, Chicago, 2011, American Health Information Management Association Revised and approved by AHIMA House of Delegates on October 2, 2011.

14. Cleverly WO, William O, Cameron AE: *Essentials of health care finance*, ed 5, Sudbury, MA, 2003, Jones and Bartlett Publisher p. 236.

ADDITIONAL RESOURCES

American Health Information Association: *Foundation of Research and Education: A study of health care fraud and abuse: implications for professionals managing health information*, 2010: http://www.ahima.org.

American Health Information Association: *Foundation of Research and Education: report on the use of health information technology to enhance and expand health care anti-fraud activities*, 2005: http://www.ahima.org.

American Health Information Management Association: Fraud and abuse compliance programs (journal articles and seminars). Chicago, 1998, 1999, 2000, 2011, AHIMA.

Berger S: *Fundamentals of healthcare financial management: a practical guide to fiscal issues and activities, Healthcare Financial Management Association*, New York, 1999, McGraw-Hill.

Department of Health and Human Services. *Office of Inspector General: Fiscal Year 2013 Work Plan*: http://oig.hhs.gov/publications/docs/workplan/2013/WorkPlanFY2013.pdf.

Development of automated coding software: development and use to enhance anti-fraud activities, 2005: http://www.ahima.org.

Kovner AR, Jonas S, editors: *Health care delivery in the United States*, ed 6, New York, 1999, Springer.

Newmann BR, Suver JD, Zelman WN: *Financial management—concepts and applications for health care providers*, ed 2, Baltimore, 1988, National Health Publishing.

Nowicki M: *The financial management of hospitals and healthcare organizations*, Chicago, 1999, Health Administration Press and Washington, DC AUPHA Press.

Robinson-Crowley C: *Understanding patient financial services*, Gaithersburg, MD, 1997, Aspen Publishers.

Ward WJ Jr: *Health care budgeting and financial management for nonfinancial managers*, Westport, CT, 1994, Auburn House.

GLOSSARY

Abbreviation list An official list of approved abbreviations maintained by health care organizations, to avoid misunderstandings from either poor handwriting or the fact that many abbreviations have more than one meaning.

Abstracting (1) A process by which a set of predetermined data is obtained from the patient record and related sources; (2) the process of selecting specific data items from medical records for clinical and administrative decision making. Abstracting has a wide range of uses, from billing and case-mix analysis to selection of cases for quality review. Also known as statistical analysis.

Accent lighting (See Task lighting.)

Accountable Care Organizations ACOs are groups of providers that collaborate with the goal of giving high quality, coordinated care to Medicare patients. The providers involved in ACOs may include physicians, hospitals, home health agencies, and other health care delivery organizations.

Accounting rate of return An evaluation method that uses averages. The annual net inflows or outflows are averaged over the project's life for each project, and the asset value or investment value is averaged over the life of the project as well. The asset value is depreciated on a straight-line basis for the life of the program.

Accounts receivable The revenue (dollar amount) owed to an organization.

Accounts receivable turnover ratio A ratio that provides a measure of the average time that receivables are outstanding or the period for which a health care organization extends credit to its debtors.

Accreditation A voluntary process by which a private nongovernmental organization or agency performs an external review and grants recognition to a program of study or institution that meets certain predetermined standards.

Accredited record technician A credential offered in the early 1950s after completion of a 9- to 12-month technical program and successful completion of a certification examination. This was eventually replaced by the RHIT (Registered Health Information Technician) credential.

Accrual basis accounting Financial transaction processing method that uses the "matching concept," enabling revenues to be matched with the actual expenses incurred to produce the revenue. The accrual method records the revenues expected as "revenues," although the "cash" has not yet been received. The revenues are matched as closely with the expenses as possible.

Action steps Define the dates when certain activities are to be completed, how much labor or funding will be required, how resources will be used, and the expected outcomes or results.

Active case ascertainment surveillance systems Identify cases in all hospitals, clinics, or other medical facilities through systematic review of patient records, surgery records, disease indexes, pathology reports, vital records, and hospital logs (obstetrical, newborn nursery, neonatal intensive care unit, postmortem) or by interviewing health professionals who may be knowledgeable about diagnosed cases.

Active record Based on the date of the patient's last treatment or activity associated with their health record. Active records are stored in a location commonly referred to as the active files.

Activity ratios Ratios that use data from the balance sheet and the statement of revenues and expenses to measure an organization's ability to generate net operating revenue in relation to its various assets. Also referred to as turnover ratios.

Acute care The treatment of common illnesses and injuries, such as nausea, vomiting, and abrasions.

Adaptive strategies More specific than directional strategies; indicate the method for carrying out the directional strategies.

Advance directive (1) A documented life support or treatment-related wish of a patient that is given to health care providers to follow in the event they become necessary; (2) a legal written document that specifies patient preferences regarding future health care or specifies another person to make medical decisions in the event the patient has an incurable or irreversible condition and is unable to communicate his or her wishes. The patient must be competent at the time the document is prepared and signed.

Adverse events Negative side effects or complications a patient may experience associated with health care.

Advocacy The support or promotion of something.

Affinity diagrams Affinity diagrams often are used to organize and prioritize information into clusters or categories.

Affirmative action programs Written, systematic human resource planning tools that outline goals for hiring, training, promoting, and compensating minority groups and women who are protected by EEO (Equal Employment Opportunity) laws. Affirmative action plans are specifically mandated in EO 11246 for businesses under federal contract to address past discrimination and to achieve a workforce that reflects the diversity of the population.

Aggregate data Data that have been collected or combined from many different sources.

Alphabetical identification Identifying the record by patient name.

Alternative dispute resolution Rather than settling a dispute in court, a neutral party or panel hears both sides of a dispute and renders a decision, or settling claims by negotiating a direct payment to the parties bringing the claim in exchange for the claimants' dropping the claim. Also referred to as arbitration or mediation.

Alternative hypothesis In a test of statistical significance, an alternative hypothesis states that there is a difference or relationship and that the observations are the result of the effect plus chance variation.

Alternative medicine Those practices that are used in lieu of conventional or what might be thought of as "Western Medicine."

Ambient lighting Light is directed upward so that it is reflected off the ceiling onto the work area. It provides light for a large area, but the light is insufficient to work by.

Ambulatory care A comprehensive term for all types of health care provided in an outpatient setting; the patient travels to and from the facility on the same day and is not hospitalized, institutionalized, or admitted as an inpatient.

Ambulatory payment classification system System of assigning groupings and weights to ambulatory care services. The groupings and weights are used by third-party payers such as Medicare to determine payment for services.

American plan of office design (1) Evaluation of individual needs is necessary to decide whether a private office is needed. Combining the conventional office plan with private offices with the open plan maintains the status and privacy needs of the executive. (2) The combination of the conventional office plan with private offices and the open plan which allows the executive needed privacy.

Analytic study (1) In an analytic study, a disease or health condition is examined to determine possible causes. Intensive research related to the disease is necessary to determine characteristics that may cause the specific disease. (2) A type of epidemiologic research study design that includes case-control or retrospective, cohort or prospective, and historical-prospective. It examines diseases and health conditions to determine characteristics that may cause the disease or condition.

Ancillary services Departments that provide diagnostic and therapeutic services at the request of a physician to both inpatients and outpatients; the departments include radiology (medical imaging), clinical laboratory, physical therapy, occupational therapy, respiratory therapy, cardiographics, pharmacy, and so on. Ancillary services differ from other areas of the hospital because the hospital is able to charge patients or third parties directly and, therefore, generate revenue for the hospital. They are under the direction of physicians.

Anesthesia death rate A rate that indicates the number of deaths that are due to the administration of anesthetics for a specified period of time.

Antitrust Laws that prohibit anticompetitive behavior such as price discrimination, restraint of trade, and monopolies.

Applets Programs that are allowed by JAVA to run on top of HTML pages and are more efficient than CGI scripts. Applets, which run on the client side, are available through the user's Web browser. After the user clicks on the submit button, the JAVA applet is downloaded to the user's machine temporarily.

Application gateway A type of firewall solution that allows only certain applications to run from outside the network. This is applicable if an organization wants to prohibit outside entities from transferring files to its network.

Application software Sets of instructions used to accomplish various types of business processes. For example, software written to process laboratory orders.

Applied research Uses accumulated theories, knowledge, methods, and techniques to solve the practical problems identified in a clinical setting.

Arbitration The settling of a dispute outside of court through a neutral party or panel. (See also Alternative dispute resolution.)

ARDEN Syntax language for medical logic modules (MLMs) that allows encoding of medical knowledge (e.g., laboratory values, medication orders).

Ascension number A unique identifier.

Ascertainment Identification.

Assault A deliberate threat, coupled with the apparent ability, to do physical harm to another person without that person's consent. No contact is required.

Assets Cash or cashlike items or other resources that can be converted to cash. Assets may be considered as short-term assets (those easily converted to cash) or long-term assets (items more difficult to convert to cash quickly or items needed to operate the business).

Assisted living facility A type of long-term care facility that typically offers housing and board with a broad range of personal and supportive care services.

Attending physician The senior physician primarily responsible for the care and treatment of the patient, particularly during an acute care hospital admission.

Attribute A data element that describes the entity. It is generally represented as a column in a table (e.g., city).

Authentication (1) The process of identifying the source of health record entries by attaching a handwritten signature, the author's initials, or an electronic signature. (2) The process of verifying or confirming the identity of a user who is requesting access to the information.

Authorization In the context of patients authorizing disclosure of their protected health information, the term refers to the written permission that meets the requirements of the applicable law that is required to be able to disclose the information.

Autopsy rate A rate computed so that health care facilities can determine the proportion of deaths in which an autopsy was performed. This enables a facility to examine why a higher or lower autopsy rate may be seen from one month to another.

Average daily inpatient census The average number of inpatients in a facility for a given period of time.

Average length of stay The average length of stay of inpatients discharged during a specified period.

Backward mapping Mapping from ICD-10-CM and PCS codes back to ICD-9-CM codes is referred to as backward mapping. Backward mapping is used to map a newer code set to an older code set.

Bailiff Courtroom personnel who are present to assist in keeping order, administering oaths, guarding and assisting the jury, and performing other duties at the direction of the judge.

Balance sheet A financial report that displays an organization's assets, liabilities, and fund balance or equity at a fixed point in time.

Baldrige National Quality Award Established by Congress in 1987 to recognize organizations for their achievements in quality and business performance and to raise awareness about the importance of quality and performance excellence as a competitive edge.

Bandwidth A measure of how much information can be transmitted simultaneously through a communication channel. Bandwidth is measured in bits per second (bps).

Bar chart (See Bar graph.)

Bar code A machine-readable representation of information in a visual format.

Bar code reader Equipment that reads bar codes.

Bar graph A type of graph used to illustrate nominal, ordinal, discrete, and continuous data. The discrete categories are shown on the horizontal, or x, axis and the frequency is shown on the vertical, or y, axis. The purpose of the bar graph is to show the frequency for each interval or category.

Basic interoperability One computer system can send data to another, but that does not necessarily mean that the receiving system can interpret those data.

Basic research Focuses on theoretical concepts and fundamental principles.

Battery Nonconsensual, intentional touching of another person in a socially impermissible manner.

Bed size (bed count) The total number of inpatient beds with which the facility is equipped and staffed for patient admissions.

Bed turnover rate The number of times an inpatient hospital bed, on the average, changes occupants during a given period of time.

Bedside documentation systems Software and hardware located at the patient's bedside that encourages recording of information about patient care at or near the time of its delivery.

Behavioral health Services that include psychiatric, psychological, and social work services to the patient (often referred to as *client*) and characterized as including mental health, alcohol, drug abuse, foster care, case management, and developmentally disabled services.

Behaviorally anchored rating scales (BARS) A method used in employee evaluation that anchors the numerical scales with brief narrative descriptions of a range of behavior from highest to lowest level of performance on that dimension. These narrative descriptions may be drawn from critical incidents documented in real-world supervisory situations.

Benchmarking Comparing an organization's performance against organizations that have been identified as excellent. Benchmarking is a commonly used tool for gathering data and identifying ways to improve processes and initiate change at all operational levels.

Beneficiaries People who are enrolled in Medicare or Medicaid programs.

Benefit period Time frame in which the insurance benefits are covered; varies from insurance policy to policy.

Benefits realization A system evaluation method that determines if the system has delivered all the benefits that were anticipated.

Best evidence rule Rules of evidence require that when originals are still available, they must be produced. When it becomes necessary to prove the contents of a document, the original must be produced or its absence accounted for.

Bias Preference for a particular point of view, a flaw in the system or design caused by methods used in the selection of subjects, nonresponse of subjects, and interviewing techniques are a few examples of bias.

Big data The term used to distinguish data sets that are very large. Refers to data sets that are too big for typical database software tools to capture, store, manage, and analyze, the speed at which the data is acquired and use, and to the variety of different types of data that are available to collect and analyze.

Biomedical device A device (such as automated electrocardiogram systems and patient monitoring systems) that converts data from one form to another and transmits the data to a database.

Biometric A unique, measurable characteristic or trait of a human being that can be used for automatic recognition or identity verification.

Bioterrorism Terrorism using germ warfare, an intentional human release of naturally occurring or human-modified toxin or biological agent.

Brainstorming A structured but flexible process designed to maximize the number of ideas generated. Brainstorming requires a leader who serves primarily as a facilitator and recorder and a team of 6 to 10 persons brought together to generate ideas about a relevant issue. The issue is defined, a time limit for discussion is set, and ideas are recorded for all team members to discuss.

Breach of contract Occurs when one party to a contract fails to follow the terms agreed to in the contract.

Break glass Refers to a quick means for a person who does not have access privileges to certain information to gain access when necessary.

Break-even analysis A cost-benefit analysis (CBA) technique in which costs to operate the current system are compared with those to operate the proposed system. The point at which old system costs equal new system costs is the break-even point. After the break-even point, the proposed system should begin to generate a positive monetary return compared with the old system.

Budgets Detailed numerical documents that translate the goals, objectives, and action steps into forecasts of volume and monetary resources needed.

Burden of proof When a plaintiff brings a civil suit against a defendant, unless the plaintiff can convince the judge or jury by a preponderance of evidence (making it more likely than not) that the claims against the defendant are valid, the defendant will prevail.

Business associate agreement A special agreement required by HIPAA that covered entities must use when using outside agents or organizations (not part of the facility's own workforce) to handle or process protected health information on their behalf. This agreement ensures that the agency follows rules set by the covered entity for handling protected health information.

Business data In a health care organization, this includes ALL aspects of the business, clinical as well as financial.

Business intelligence The general term used for the identification, extraction, and analysis of data.

Business plan A formal written document that evolves from the input of others, listing objectives that support the organizational goals. The plan includes the following: specific action steps, quantifying resource requirements and cash flow benefits, prediction of expected outcomes, and a programmatic outline that may span a fiscal year or a longer time frame.

Business rules (1) As applied to an information systems environment, the rules that determine the user interface and database services that may be required. The business rules reside on the application server; (2) as applied to an organization, business rules describe the operations, definition, and constraints that apply to an organization in achieving its goals.

Cafeteria benefit plan A common type of benefit plan that allows employees to choose from an array of benefits to fit their needs or lifestyles.

Capital expenditure committee A committee that evaluates all capital requests so that cash resources are used to purchase the high-cost items that will yield the most benefit to the organization.

Capital expenditure Items that usually have a high initial cost and a "life" of more than 1 year. Each facility defines its own capitalization value.

Capitalization ratios Ratios that focus on balance sheet numbers (assets, liabilities, and equity/fund balance accounts) to measure the ability of the health care organization to meet its short- and long-term financial obligations.

Capitation (1) A form of reimbursement in which a prepaid, fixed amount is paid to the provider for each person (per capita) served, regardless of how much or how often the patient receives health care services; (2) a type of fixed-payment arrangement used in health maintenance organizations (HMOs). For each month an insured member remains with the HMO, the HMO's providers are paid a fixed amount, usually at the beginning of the month. The providers are required to provide any care needed by the insured during this period, regardless of whether the capitation amount is sufficient to cover the cost to do so.

Career counseling A service that may be offered to employees formally by the human resources staff, through an employee assistance program, or less formally by the mentoring of veteran professionals and managers.

Career planning Enables employees to be promoted within an organization from one job in a career path or ladder to another. Career planning also provides an incentive for motivating and retaining effective performers and identifying potential managers and leaders for appropriate training and placement.

Carpal tunnel syndrome   Swelling of the tendons through the carpal tunnel (located in the front part of the wrist), which puts pressure on the median nerve, causing pain and weakness. The most common repetitive strain (or stress) injury that occurs in workers who spend long hours using computers or workers who perform repetitive tasks.

Cascading style sheets (CSS)   A tool used to optimize the use and appearance of a Web page by allowing users to easily apply personalized formatting to Web documents. With CSS-styled pages, the user can transform Web content into a format that addresses the requirements for accessibility.

Case   A person with a given disease or condition that is under study.

Case-control study   A type of analytic study design where the researcher collects data on the cases (those who have the disease that is under study) and controls (those who are similar to the cases but do not have the disease that is under study) by looking back in time. The intent of the researcher is to establish some association between the disease and the exposure characteristic. Also referred to as a retrospective study.

Case eligibility   All of the organization's patients diagnosed (clinically or histologically) and/or treated for active diseases on or after the reference date or beginning of the registry are eligible for inclusion in the registry.

Case finding   The method by which all of the eligible cases to be included in the registry are identified, accessioned into the registry, and abstracted.

Case law   In deciding on cases when no statutes apply, judges refer to similar cases that have been decided in the past and by applying the same principles, courts generally arrive at the same ruling in the current case as in similar previous cases.

Case management   An aspect of health care that refers to all activities, including assessment, treatment planning, referral, and follow-up, that ensures the provision of comprehensive and continuous services and the coordination of payment and reimbursement of care.

Case studies   Provide a richly detailed portrait of an individual, program, event, department, time period, culture, or community.

Cash basis accounting   Financial transaction processing method whereby each transaction is recorded when cash is exchanged. Revenues are recognized when money is received for services provided, and expenses are recognized when money is paid out for the resources used to provide those services.

Catchment area   A defined geographic area that is served by a health care program, project, or facility such as a hospital or mental health center. Services provided are usually directed at population groups and range from immunizations, diagnostic testing, and screening to nutrition counseling and family planning.

Cause-and-effect diagram   A diagram used for solving complicated problems by helping people consider many factors and the cause-and-effect relationships between those factors. Also referred to as fishbone diagrams.

Censored   The subject in a research study is alive at the time of analysis or was alive when last seen.

Census statistics   Ratios, percentages, and averages related to the length of stay, occupancy, bed turnover, and total number of patients present at a specified time within the institution.

Centralized filing   The filing method where there is a single location for all records created throughout the facility. This centralized file location is staffed by specialized personnel who provide records that have been requested by authorized users.

Certificate of need   A regulatory process that requires certain health care providers to obtain state approval before offering certain new or expanded services.

Certification   Refers to the process by which government and nongovernment organizations evaluate educational programs, health care facilities, and individuals as having met predetermined standards.

Certified coding associate (CCA)   An entry-level coding credential implemented by AHIMA in 2002. The recommended amount of experience for this credential is 6 months or completion of an AHIMA-approved coding certificate program or other formal training program.

Certified coding specialist (CCS)   An advanced coding credential implemented by AHIMA in 1992. To receive this credential, individuals must pass the CCS examination, which focuses on inpatient coding systems. The recommended amount of experience for this credential is 3 or more years.

Certified coding specialist—physician-based   An advanced coding credential implemented by AHIMA in 1997. To receive this credential, individuals must pass the CCS-P examination, which focuses on ambulatory care coding. The recommended amount of experience for this credential is 3 or more years.

Certified health data analyst (CHDA)   In 2009, AHIMA implemented the Certified Health Data Analyst credential to offer individuals who possess these skills an avenue for recognition of expertise in health data analysis and mastery of this domain of practice. Eligibility requirements for this credential includes a baccalaureate or advanced degree and 5 years of experience or an RHIA and a minimum of 1 year health care data experience.

Certified in Healthcare Privacy and Security (CHPS)   A credential offered by AHIMA that validates an individual's expertise in designing, implementing, and administering comprehensive privacy and security protection programs in all types of health care organizations.

Charge description master   (See Charge master)

Charge master (charge description master)   A list used by a health care organization that reflects the charge for each item that may be used in the treatment of a patient and the charge for most services (e.g., respiratory therapy treatments, physical therapy services, laboratory tests, and so on). The list is most always automated and linked with the billing system. (See also Master charge list.)

Charitable immunity   A doctrine that had, until the early to mid-1960s, protected nonprofit hospitals from liability for harm to patients. Courts now permit harmed patients to sue hospitals for their wrongful acts.

Chart of accounts   Used by several health care organizations to assign transactions to designated accounts in the financial accounting process. The largest expense items are in the lower number account categories, whereas the expense categories that have limited expenses appear in the higher number account groups.

Chart order   The reference that defines the facility's standard sequence of pages to be followed in each record.

Checksheet   A form specially designed so that the results can be readily interpreted from the form itself. This form of data collection is ideal for capturing data concurrently (during actual delivery of patient care or services) because the employee can interpret the results and take corrective actions immediately.

Checksum   A special character that is added to the bar code that tells the bar code reader that the bar code is correct. The checksum character is read by the bar code scanner, but it is not passed along as part of the data.

Claim Request for payment by the insured or the provider for services covered.

Claims management Claims management refers to the administrative and legal procedures initiated following an adverse event. These procedures may include an internal audit of the charges billed, examination of the health record for completeness, sequestration of financial and health records, interrogatories, settlement negotiations, preparation for trial, tracking of the status of claims, analysis of aggregate claims and losses, and the objective use of resulting information to improve individual and organization performance.

Classification A scheme for grouping similar things in a logical way, based on common characteristics.

Classification system A scheme for grouping similar things in a logical way, based on common characteristics. Classification systems vary in their level of detail; some offer very general groupings, whereas others allow more detailed groupings and subgroupings, enabling the user to capture a greater degree of specificity, or granularity, of data. (See also Classification.)

Clerk of the court The administrative manager of the court who handles the paperwork associated with lawsuits. Complaints are filed with the clerk, as are other pleadings and documents.

Client A person who receives professional services; a patient in the behavioral health setting, adult day care, or home health care may be referred to as a client.

Clinical case definition A list of signs and symptoms that establish a clinical diagnosis.

Clinical data repository Collects, organizes, and analyzes all institutional business and clinical data that have been summarized and aggregated for that purpose. Clinical data repositories are designed to deliver the individual patient's information to the care team through the clinical workstation.

Clinical decision support systems (CDSSs) Systems that provide diagnostic investigation tools and clinical guideline advice to patient care providers. Basic clinical decision support provides computerized advice regarding drug doses, routes, and frequencies, and more sophisticated CDSSs can perform drug allergy checks, drug laboratory value checks, and drug–drug interaction checks and can provide reminders about corollary orders (e.g., prompting the user to order glucose checks after ordering insulin).

Clinical document ontologies A formalized naming and coding of document types

Clinical interface terminology A systematic collection of health care–related phrases that supports clinician entry of patient-related information into computer programs.

Clinical practice guidelines Specific procedures or protocols for medical professionals to follow for patients with a particular diagnosis or medical condition based on research.

Clinical privileges The permission granted by the appropriate authority (governing board) to practitioners to provide well-defined patient care services in the granting institution, based on licensure, education, training, experience, competence, health status, and judgment.

Clinical reference terminology Terminology that offers a consistent language for capturing, sharing, and aggregating health data across specialties and sites of care.

Clinical terminology Terminology used to represent the information in a medical record, whether that record is in paper form or electronic form.

Clinical Terms Version 3 formerly known as Read Codes Version 3, which was created on behalf of the UK Department of Health and is Crown copyrighted.

Clinical trial A study consisting of two or more groups that have different exposures and that are followed forward to determine their outcomes. A certain medication or treatment is given to a group and the outcomes are compared with those of a control or comparison group (subjects who do not have the intervention). Also referred to as a community trial.

Closed-ended questions Questions that provide a list of responses to choose from, similar to the multiple-choice type questions, dichotomous or yes/no questions, or questions based on level or measurement or ranking. Also referred to as structured format questions.

Code A unique identifier assigned to a specific term, description, or concept.

Code of ethics Guides the practice of people who choose a given profession and sets forth the values and principles defined by the profession as acceptable behavior within a practice setting.

Code set A list of codes and the terms or descriptions with which they are associated.

Coding The assignment of unique identifiers to the terms within a particular clinical terminology. In the field of health information management, coding commonly refers to the selection of alphanumeric codes to represent diseases, procedures, and supplies used in the delivery of health care. Also referred to as encoding.

Coding system A system primarily designed to support the administrative, financial, and regulatory functions associated with care. Coding systems serve as the primary communication tool between those providing services (e.g., physicians and hospitals) and those paying for services (e.g., insurance companies).

Coefficient of variation Used when two samples or groups have very different means. The coefficient of variation compares their standard deviations expressed as percentages of the mean.

Cohort study A study that begins in a community or an industrial setting or within a hospital. Subjects are separated into two groups on the basis of their exposures or health characteristic and then are followed forward to determine whether the disease develops. (See also Prospective study.)

Coinsurance When the insured is partially responsible or liable for the debt (cost of their health care); usually expressed as a percentage of the cost (e.g., insured pays 20% and plan pays 80%).

Collaboration The combined labor of users and information systems staff in the pursuit of electronic health records.

Color coding Used to designate certain letters or digits to help prevent misfiles, aid in rapid storage and retrieval, provide an easy way to distribute workload, and make sorting of folders easier. Color coding methods can also be applied to the use of outguides. Two common methods of color coding outguides are assigning colors for specific request reasons or assigning colors to a specific retrieval time period. Using unique colors for different request reasons alerts the staff to immediately check another location, such as the release of information area or the physicians' incomplete area.

Commission on Accreditation of Health Informatics and Information Management (CAHIIM) The accrediting body established by AHIMA in 2004 that accredits undergraduate HIM programs that were previously accredited by CAAHEP (Council on Accreditation of Allied Health Educational Programs). The CAHIIM also offers an approval process for master's degree programs in HIM which will convert to an accreditation process in the future.

Common law The large body of principles that have evolved from prior court decisions. (See also Case law.)

Common Procedural Terminology (CPT) Used for reporting diagnostic and therapeutic procedures and other services performed by physicians.

Communities of Practice (CoP) An online communication tool offered by AHIMA for connecting association members. The CoP provides up-to-date news and links to resources, helps keep members informed on the latest trends in HIM, helps members solve problems, network, and career build.

Community trial A study consisting of two or more groups that have different exposures and that are followed forward to determine their outcomes. A certain medication or treatment is given to a group and their outcomes are compared with those of a control or comparison group (subjects who do not have the intervention). (See also Clinical trial.)

Community-acquired infection Infection that occurs in the community or less than 72 hours after admission as a hospital inpatient.

Comorbidity A condition that is in addition to a primary condition and affects course or treatment of a condition or length of stay.

Compensation management Entails understanding of wage and salary administration, payroll systems, employee benefits, knowledge of applicable federal and state legislation and regulation, and effective communication strategies. Compensation management should communicate effectively the goals, procedures, and constraints associated with the organization's compensation policies and maintain the credibility of the system as being managed fairly and with integrity.

Complaint A written statement by the plaintiff that states his or her claims and commences the action in a lawsuit.

Complementary and alternative medicine Therapies (usually not included in Western medicine) that may or may not have been proven to be effective, including herbal remedies, massage therapy, natural food diets, acupuncture, and biofeedback. Complementary medicine includes those practices that could be used along with conventional therapies. Alternative medicine includes those practices that would be used in lieu of conventional medicine.

Compounding effect The result of applying an interest rate to the number of compounding periods in a year and the length of the term (i.e., number of years). The more frequent the interval of compounding the greater the effect—$100 invested at 8% after 5 years is $148.98.

Computer-based patient record A term proposed by the Institute of Medicine (IOM) committee in 1991 to describe a patient record system that could be could be part of hospital information systems, medical information systems, or a type of clinical information system. This term has most recently been replaced by the terms *electronic medical record* or *electronic health record.*

Computer-based Patient Record Institute The Institute of Medicine convened a committee of industry experts who reported in 1991 that health care professionals and organizations should be encouraged to adopt computer-based patient records as a standard for all records related to patient care. One recommendation of the study was that the "public and private sectors join in establishing a Computer-based Patient Record Institute to promote and facilitate development, implementation, and dissemination of the CPR."[9] The institute was formed and functioned throughout the 1990s in support of computerizing patient records.

Concept permanence Once a concept has been created within a terminology, its meaning cannot change, and it cannot be deleted. The preferred name of the concept can change, or the concept may be deemed inactive, but its meaning must remain fixed as long as the terminology is in use.

Concurrent review A review process that assesses the need for continued inpatient stay and the provision of care and services while the care is in process.

Conditions for Coverage Regulations that health care organizations must meet in order to begin and continue participating in the Medicare and Medicaid programs. These minimum health and safety standards are the foundation for improving quality and protecting the health and safety of beneficiaries. CMS also ensures that the standards of accrediting organizations recognized by CMS (through a process called "deeming") meet or exceed the Medicare standards set forth in the Conditions for Coverage.

Conditions of Participation (COP) Regulations governing providers of services to Medicare beneficiaries are detailed in the Conditions of Participation. These regulations require that providers develop, implement, and maintain an effective organization-wide, data-driven quality assessment and performance improvement program. The regulation specifics vary according to the provider setting.

Confidence interval An estimated range of values with a high known probability of covering the true population value.

Confidential communication Communication that transmits information to a health care provider as part of the relationship between the provider and the patient under circumstances that imply that the information shall remain private.

Confidentiality An ethical and a legal concept endorsed by health professionals to meet the expectation of patients that their information, when provided to an authorized user, will not be redisclosed or misused.

Confounding variables Variables that affect the dependent and independent variables.

Consent Written permission from the patient allowing care or treatment.

Consultation At the request of one provider, another provider reviews the patient's record, examines the patient, and makes recommendations regarding care and treatment. A medical consultant is a specialist with expertise in a particular medical field.

Contemporaneous documentation Documentation made while care is being provided, while the information is fresh in the care provider's mind.

Context representation Formal, explicit information about how concepts are to be used. Context representation is essential to avoid the misinterpretation of health data.

Contingency table A table that displays the joint frequencies of two qualitative variables used to compute a Chi square statistic.

Continuing record review Hospital medical records should be reviewed on a continuing basis at the point of care and based on organization-defined indicators that address the presence, timeliness, readability (whether handwritten or printed), quality, consistency, clarity, accuracy, completeness, and authentication of data and information contained within the record.

Continuity assessment record evaluation An item set designed to standardize assessment of patients' medical, functional, cognitive, and social support status across acute and post-acute settings.

Continuous data Data on quantitative variables that can assume an infinite number of possible values.

Continuum of care The full range of health care services provided, moving from the least acute and least intensive to the most acute and most intensive or vice versa.

Contract   A formal and binding agreement (actual or implied).

Contracted amount   The amount of reimbursement that is negotiated between the provider and the third-party payer.

Control   A person who is similar to the case, but does not have the disease or condition that is under study.

Control chart   A data display tool used to monitor performance that can determine whether a process is statistically in control. Control charts have three important lines: the central line is the mean or median, and the upper and lower lines are termed control limits. Data points outside the control limits (or unusual data patterns) indicate a special cause that should be found and eliminated.

Controlled clinical reference terminology   A coded vocabulary of medical concepts and expressions used in health care.

Controlled vocabulary   Terms within the vocabulary are carefully selected for their inclusion; terms outside that boundary are not included. Two rules are generally followed: (1) if the same term is commonly used to mean different concepts in different contexts, then its name is explicitly qualified to resolve the ambiguity; (2) if multiple terms are used to mean the same thing, one of the terms is identified as the preferred term, and the others are listed as synonyms.

Controlling   The activities that management typically pursues when what was planned does not occur financially.

Copayment   A type of cost-sharing in which the insured (subscriber) pays out of pocket a fixed amount for health care service.

Core measure   A set of standardized metrics developed and used by The Joint Commission to assess the quality of health care organizations.

Corporate negligence   Under this theory, courts can hold health care organizations liable for their own independent acts of negligence. Organizations are responsible for monitoring the activities of the people who function within their facilities, whether those people are employees or independent contractors, such as physicians, and for complying with appropriate industry standards, such as accreditation (The Joint Commission) standards, licensing regulations, and Conditions of Participation issued by Medicare.

Correlation analysis   Determines the strength, direction, and statistical significance of a relationship between one or more performance variables.

Correlation coefficient   A statistic that shows the strength of a relationship between two variables.

Cost-benefit analysis (CBA)   A system evaluation method that attempts to measure benefits compared with system costs. Cost-benefit analysis is used to determine whether the information system decreases or increases benefits and whether it decreases or increases cost for the organization.

Cost-effectiveness analysis   A system evaluation technique that is used to evaluate certain beneficial consequences in nonmonetary terms. In cost-effectiveness analysis, desirable benefits are not valued in monetary terms but are measured in some other unit.

Council on Accreditation   This body is now the Commission on Accreditation for Health Informatics and Information Management Education. Its mission is to establish and enforce standards for educational preparation of health informatics and information management professionals by recognizing educational programs that meet their standards.

Council on Certification   The certifying body of AHIMA that is responsible for developing and maintaining certification and recertification processes.

Counseling and referral   Problem-solving processes used to halt the decline in a troubled employee's performance and to prevent excessive employee turnover through termination or supervisor-initiated transfers. Employee counseling is provided to assist the employee in addressing personal and other problems that might originate outside the workplace but that affect job performance and behavior in the workplace. Referral is the process of linking the employee with an array of resources to address the specific problem(s) identified.

Court order   A written or verbal order issued by the court.

Court reporter   The individual who is responsible for creating a verbatim transcript of court proceedings.

Covered entity   Any entity that is a health plan, a health care clearinghouse, or a health care provider that conducts certain transactions in electronic form and must comply with the Privacy Rule of the HIPAA.

Credential   Denotes that individuals have met specific standards and demonstrated a level of competence in their field of practice. Individuals who obtain credentials are required to maintain their credentials over time by meeting continuing education requirements as defined by the agency or organization that supports the credential.

Credentialing   (1) Any process by which practitioners are evaluated with the intent to affect control over their professional practice. More specifically within health care organizations, credentialing refers to the policies and procedures used to determine the membership category and clinical privileges to be granted to each member of the professional staff. (2) The process of granting (or renewing) certain privileges to practice medicine to prospective or existing members of the medical staff at a facility. During the appointment and reappointment process, the applicant's background is reviewed, licenses and certifications are checked, proof of current liability insurance is verified, and practice patterns and quality review data are evaluated to determine whether the applicant should be granted the privileges he or she seeks to gain or renew.

Credentials verification organization   Makes the contacts necessary to verify an applicant's education, training, experience, and professional licenses and certifications through primary source agencies.

Critical access hospital (CAH)   A critical access hospital is certified by the state as being necessary to the residents in the community or no hospital or other CAH is within 35 miles of the CAH. The CAH provides acute inpatient care, has no more than 25 beds, and has an annual average length of stay of 96 hours.

Critical incident method   A method of employee performance evaluation that requires the supervisor to document exceptional job-related behavior, either extremely effective or ineffective performance, actually observed or reported. These statements, or critical incidents, collectively represent the range of behavior typical for that employee. Documented positive critical incidents may be used as the basis for merit pay decisions and negative ones used as the basis for performance correction plans or disciplinary action.

Critical path   The sequence of activities on a PERT network that takes the greatest amount of time to complete.

Cross-sectional study   A type of descriptive study that examines the distribution of disease or health characteristics in the population at one point in time. This type of study is used to generate hypotheses and is also referred to as a prevalence study.

Current ratio   This ratio compares current assets with current liabilities to determine whether there are sufficient cash and cashlike assets to cover the immediate liabilities (bills) that will come due in the short term (1 year). The current ratio is one of the most common liquidity ratios.

Data (1) A collection of elements on a given subject; the raw facts and figures expressed in text, numbers, symbols, and images; facts, ideas, or concepts that can be captured, communicated, and processed either manually or electronically. (2) Raw facts, characters, or symbols.

Data analysis The process of evaluating data using analytical and logical reasoning to examine each component of the data.

Data analytics Refers to the field of data analysis and often involves studying past historical data to research potential trends for decision-making.

Data compression A mathematical technique that applies formulas to a file to produce a smaller file. Files are compressed by eliminating strings of redundant characters and replacing them with more compact symbols.

Data dictionary Serves as the central repository for all information about the database and functions as a catalog for identifying the nature of all the data in a system. The data dictionary provides the central resource for ensuring that standard definitions for data elements and data structures are used throughout the system.

Data element It is best described as a single question that demands a singular defined response. The data dictionary describes the nature of the data element sufficiently so that any user of the system will understand what the question and the response means, what it does not mean, and the limits of what it can express.

Data flow diagram (DFD) A diagram used to track the flow of data through an entire system. Data flow diagrams identify the data flow within a system, providing a data map of what data go from an area, what data are received by an area, and what data are either temporarily or permanently stored in an area. In addition to tracking data flow, a DFD identifies transformations on data (processes) and data repositories (data stores).

Data interface standards Agreed on means of transmitting data and connecting data communications equipment. A formal standard is typically the product of a standards development organization and is recognized by the American National Standards Institute.

Data mapping The process of identifying and describing the link between two distinct data models or databases. It is used to identify terms that have the same meaning in two different databases. It may be used in a classification system to identify specific terms that fit within a particular classification. It could be used to consolidate multiple databases into a single database identifying redundant data for consolidation or elimination. It could be used to identify data relationships as part of data lineage analysis.

Data mart A subset of data extracted from the larger database. It is a smaller application with a focus on a particular subject or department.

Data mining The process of searching large volumes of data for patterns using tools such as clustering, classification, and association rule mining. The science of extracting useful information from large data sets or databases. An example is a retail company that can mine its data to identify which products are frequently purchased together. These products might then be placed in proximity to encourage other customers to do the same.

Data repository Brings together information from all or a few of the applications and databases for an organization. Useful when an organization has a number of different databases or systems from a variety of vendors that contain related pieces of information about an individual or a company function. The software can quickly organize the information that is needed and provide access to enable better decision-making.

Data security The technical, physical, and procedural methods by which access to confidential information is controlled and managed.

Data set A group of data items or data elements and their definitions. Data sets frequently also have defined values for each data element. A data set that has defined values for each element is useful for systematic data collection and measurement.

Data sheet A form designed to collect data in a simple tabular or column format. Specific bits of data (e.g., numbers, words, or marks) are entered in spaces on the sheet. As a result, additional processing is typically required after the data are collected to construct the performance measure.

Data standards Documented agreements on representations, formats, and definitions of common data.

Data warehouses Receive clinical data from a transactions system such as a pharmacy system or a radiology system and combine them with other organizational data from administrative and financial systems. Also referred to as information warehouses.

Database A collection of stored data, typically organized into fields, records, and files.

Database management system (DBMS) An integrated set of programs that manages access to the database.

Database model A collection of logical constructs used to represent the data structure and the relationships between the data. The four major database models are relational, hierarchical, network, and object oriented.

Data-driven rules Rules that are applied to data to trigger an outcome, for example, create an alert in an electronic health record.

Days of revenue in patient accounts receivable ratio Measure of the average time that receivables are outstanding or the period that a health care organization extends credit to its debtors.

Decentralized filing A filing method where parts of the record are filed in different locations in the facility. Outpatient and emergency departments (EDs) may file their active records in their own departments. In clinic facilities, decentralized records may be created when specialty departments maintain their own records.

Decision grid Used to compare various alternatives in a decision with criteria that are the basis for making the decision. Also known as a matrix chart.

Decision matrix (See Decision grid.)

Decision support systems Information systems designed to support planning functions of an organization by drawing from multiple databases to analyze the day-to-day business activities of the organization. Decision support systems range from simple analysis of cost per patient for specific departments or clinics to high-level strategic analysis, marketing, and policy development.

Decision table Analytical tool that provides a means of communication of the logical sequence of an operation.

Decision tree Used to chart alternative courses of action for solving a problem and subsequent consequences from each course of action.

Deductible The cost that must be incurred by the patient beneficiary before the insurer assumes liability for the remaining charges.

Deemed status Refers to facilities that are accredited by The Joint Commission and AOA and are in compliance with the Medicare Conditions of Participation (COP) for hospitals.

Defamation Oral (slander) or written (libel) communication to a person (other than the person defamed) that tends to damage the defamed person's reputation in the eyes of the community.

Defendant The party or parties in a lawsuit from whom relief or compensation is sought from the plaintiff.

Deidentified Refers to data that have been stripped of certain patient identifiers.

Demographics Personal data elements, sufficient to identify the patient, collected from the patient or patient representative and not related to health status or services provided.

Dependent variable A variable whose value is dependent on one or more other variables but which cannot itself affect the other variables.

Deposition A sworn verbal testimony.

Depreciation Systematic allocation of the cost of a capital asset over a predetermined time frame in a rational manner. Calculated by dividing the capital cost by the years of life.

Descriptive study A type of research design. In epidemiologic research it is used to describe the frequency and distribution of diseases in populations. Descriptive studies are usually the first study design chosen when little is known about the disease or health characteristics.

Desiderata Desirable characteristics.

Designated Record Set (DRS) A term used in HIPAA to include the records that contain protected health information maintained by or for a covered entity. For a health care facility these records include medical records and billing records about an individual. For a health plan these records include the enrollment, payment, claims adjudication, and case or medical management records.

Diagnosis related group (DRG) A classification scheme to group cases into groups expected to use similar amounts of hospital resources. Developed for Medicare and used since 1983 as part of a prospective payment system for services.

Differentiation A term used for variation from normal tissue. (See also Grading.)

Direct method of age adjustment An age adjustment method that uses a standard population and applies the age-specific rates available for each population. One then determines the expected number of deaths in the standard population. To use the direct method of age adjustment, age-specific rates must be available for both populations, and the number of deaths per age category should be at least five.

Direct pay, self-pay, out-of-pocket Payment by the patient to the health care provider.

Directional strategies Basis for setting organizational objectives.

Disaster recovery An organization's plan detailing how it will restart operations after a natural or human-caused disaster. As part of the plan critical information stored by the organization must be identified and a plan put in place to restore the records, data hardware, and software needed for business operations. In health care the clinical and business records are critical resources.

Discharge days The duration of hospitalization for an inpatient (see Length of stay).

Discharge planning A utilization management (UM) function designed to assist patients in transitioning from one level of care to another. Often UM staff conduct an initial discharge assessment but will refer patients in need of intensive discharge planning to case management services.

Disclosure An entity's financial statements provide a mechanism to communicate the economic activities of an organization. In the event supplemental data are available to better clarify or offer additional information for decision makers, this should be disclosed on pertinent financial statements.

Discounted payback period A cost-benefits analysis method in which an organization determines how much a system costs in future dollars. The basic concept underlying this approach is that today's dollars are worth more than future dollars. Future dollars that are anticipated to be made by installing an information system are discounted in calculations used to determine the discounted payback period.

Discounting The opposite of compounding. Discounting is used to determine how much one must invest today at a compound interest rate of x to receive a given amount at the end of N years.

Discovery A process whereby each party in a lawsuit seeks to discover important information about the case through a pretrial investigation. Discovery includes obtaining pertinent testimony (through depositions and through interrogatories) and documents that may be under the control of the opposing party. The purpose of the discovery phase is to encourage early out-of-court resolution of cases by acquainting all parties with all pertinent facts.

Discrete data Data on quantitative variables that can only take on a limited number of values, typically only whole numbers. Examples of discrete data include the number of medications a person is taking, the number of children in a family, or the number of records that are coded.

Dispersion The extent to which scores within a set vary from each other.

Document A document contains information. A document may be something physical like one or more printed pages or a virtual document in electronic format.

Document naming nomenclature This nomenclature contains five axes: subject matter domain, role, setting, service, and document type. A standard title is created by combining a term from each axis into a composite title. Not all axes are required to create a valid document title; some may be left blank as long as the correct order is maintained.

Documentation Documentation in the health record refers to clinical information in various formats communicated among health care providers. It also serves as the official business record and supports compliance, reimbursement, and other functions.

Domain The domain represents the type of value that is allowable for a specific element.

Double blind Subject and observer blind as to which study group he or she is in or is observing.

Double-distribution method An allocation method that assumes that the allocation of costs cannot be linear and that some indirect departments need to be allocated to less commonly dispersed departments before the costs of these departments are fully allocated.

Downtime The length of time when the computer system is not available to the user community.

Diagnostic related groups (DRGs) Used to categorize patients on the basis of principal and secondary diagnoses, principal and secondary procedures, age, sex, complications, discharge status, and comorbidities.[81] DRGs were designed as a way to group services and estimate costs to support prospective payment under Medicare.

DSM-5 (DSM-IV) includes definitions and diagnostic criteria for mental disorders, with code numbers for each diagnosis.

Due process The right to a full hearing.

Durable medical equipment Equipment such as wheelchairs, oxygen equipment, walkers, and other devices prescribed by the physician.

Durable power of attorney for health care An advance directive in which a competent adult names in writing another adult to make any medical decisions on his or her behalf in the event he or she becomes incapacitated (although the extent of the decision-making power varies according to state law).

E-health   See Electronic-health.

EHR systems   EHR systems will include the ability to collect longitudinal data for and about a person in an electronic format; immediate electronic access to person- and population-level information by authorized users; provision of knowledge and decision-support tools that enhance the safety, quality, and efficiency of health care; and support of efficient processes for health care delivery.

Electronic data interchange (EDI)   The electronic (computer-to-computer) exchange of data.

Electronic health records (EHR)   Patient records that are maintained electronically in a manner that is accessible to caregivers, the patient, and others who need access to specific information or to aggregate information to prevent illness and improve future treatment. (See also Patient record.)

Electronic measures   Some of the NQF endorsed performance measures have been converted to electronic measures (known as e-measures). The data for calculating e-measures are extracted automatically from EHRs without the need for manual review of records.

Electronic medical records (EMR)   Electronic patient records that are developed by individual health care providers/organizations. EMRs are composed of whole files as opposed to individual data elements. The data from the EMR are the source of data for the electronic health record (EHR). (See also Patient record.)

Electronic-health (e-health)   The use of emerging information and communication technology, especially the Internet, to improve or enable health and health care. The field of e-health includes a range of functions and capabilities such as specialized search engines focused on various kinds of health care, provider and payer Web sites, support groups, Web-based physician consultations, self-care or monitoring systems, telemedicine, disease management, and so forth.

Electronic-health information management   The use of emerging information and communications technology to manage health information systems.

Emancipated minors   Minors who can make their own health care decisions without parental or guardian involvement. They are treated as adults, under the law, and have the right to consent to treatment and authorize disclosures of their own health information. Although the conditions vary, emancipated minors generally involve minors who are married, living away from their parents and family, and responsible for their own support.

Emergency department (ED)   Facility that provides emergency services. Functional areas of an emergency department include a trauma area, a casting room, examination rooms, and observation beds. A patient in the ED can be managed in one of the following ways: treated and discharged to home, treated and admitted for observation, treated and admitted to an inpatient unit, assessed and sent to surgery, stabilized and transferred to another facility, or, in the event of death, transferred to the morgue.

Emergency response   A public health activity undertaken in an urgent or emergency situation, usually because of an identified or suspected imminent health threat to the population, but sometimes because the public and/or government authorities perceive an imminent threat that demands immediate action. The primary purpose of the activity is to document the existence and magnitude of a public health problem in the community and to implement appropriate measures to address the problem.

Employee assistance programs (EAPs)   Programs offered by most health care organizations, which provide support and referral services for employees experiencing significant personal, family, or community-based problems that interfere with job satisfaction and performance.

Employee handbook   A written reference manual of organizational policies and procedures covering employee rights, benefits, obligations, norms and standards of conduct, and other expectations of and constraints on employee behavior.

Employment at will   English common law doctrine under which an employment contract without a specified length of term could be terminated by either party with or without cause.

Encoding   The assignment of unique identifiers to the terms within a particular clinical terminology. (See also Coding.)

Encounter   The professional contact between a patient and a provider during which services are delivered.

Encryption   Protects transmitted information by changing readable text into a set of different characters and numbers on the basis of a mathematical algorithm. Computers on either end of the transmissions must have keys to encrypt the information being sent and then decrypt the text at the receiving end into the original text.

Entity/Entities   An entity (or subject) represents a higher level than the data element. It refers to a subject of information that may be a thing, a concept, or a process. The entity may contain many data elements that act as attributes, or descriptors of the entity, and are used to identify the nature of an instance of the entity.

Entity-relationship diagram   A diagram used principally to illustrate the logical design of information system databases by describing diagrammatically the relationship between entities and by identifying entity attributes. Entity-relationship diagrams are composed of three categories of items: entities, relationships, and attributes.

Epidemiologic case definition   A definition set as a reportable condition by the Centers for Disease Control and Prevention. These are of diseases that must be reported to a public health agency.

Epidemiology   The study of disease and the determinants of disease in populations. Also, the study of clinical and health care trends or patterns and the ability to recognize trends or patterns within large amounts of data.

Episodes of care   Care for a specific condition during a period of relative continuous care.

Equal employment opportunity   Requirements that were mandated during the 1960s and 1970s through federal, state, and local legislation that prohibit employers from discriminating on the basis of race, color, religion, national origin, sex, age, and disability status.

Equity   The profits and losses that result from the differences between revenues and expenses. Also referred to as fund balance.

Ergonomics   Study of the relationship of people to their working environment, including the construction and adjustability of equipment and furniture, arrangement of workstations, and design of work processes.

Ethernet   A standard defined by the Institute of Electrical and Electronics Engineers (IEEE) as having a data transmission speed across the LAN of either 10 million bits per second (Mbps) or 100 Mbps. The topology is designed with messages that are handled by all computers in the LAN until they reach their final destination. Ethernet is the most widely used LAN network topology in use today.

Etiology   The study of the causes of disease.

Event engine   A tool that tracks unexpected data and notifies the providers by e-mail and beepers that something unusual has occurred.

Evidence   Refers to information legally presented at trial, which is offered to prove or disprove an issue under contention. If that information is allowed to be used at trial, it can be "admitted into evidence." Both the federal government and individual states have rules of evidence, which are interpreted and applied by the judge in deciding what information may fairly be admitted into evidence.

Evidence-based medicine   Using guidelines developed through research in making clinical decisions.

Ex officio   A member of the governing board or committee who does not have voting privileges.

Experimental epidemiology   Epidemiologic research through two types of studies: clinical trial and community trial.

Expert system   A program that symbolically encodes concepts derived from experts in a field and uses that knowledge to provide the kind of problem analysis and advice that the expert might provide.

Exposure characteristics   Characteristics or risk factors that may cause (or increase the risk for development of) the specific disease.

External benchmarking   Sometimes called performance benchmarking, is used to close the gap between an organization's performance and that of other organizations. External benchmarking may involve examination of processes in industries outside of health care. For example, an HCO might examine the ticket sales and itinerary planning process in the airline industry to improve its patient registration and scheduling processes.

External environmental analysis   Process by which an organization crosses the boundary between itself and the external environment in order to identify and understand changes that are taking place outside the organization.

External users   Health care data users from outside an organization.

Extranet   Allows users outside the network to gain access to the network through a password. Also known as a VPN.

Factor comparison   A method for evaluating jobs that requires identification of essential factors or elements common to all jobs and comparison of jobs on the basis of rating those elements, not the job as a whole. Factors typically applied in this method are level of responsibility, including supervision; essential skills and knowledge; mental effort (demands); physical effort; and working conditions, including hazardous situations and confidentiality.

Failure mode and effects analysis (FMEA)   A risk analysis technique now being used in health care organizations to analyze existing systems and to evaluate new processes before implementation. FMEA is a technique that promotes systematic thinking about the safety of a patient care process.

False imprisonment   The unlawful restraint of a person's personal liberty or the unlawful restraining or confining of a person. Physical force is not required; all that is required is a reasonable fear that force will be used to detain or intimidate the person into following orders.

Federal medication terminologies   A list of terms that will be freely available in its aim to improve the exchange and public availability of medication information and support health information technology interoperability. It is hoped that this effort will provide access to a common language for communicating medication information, processes for maintaining terminologies, and an infrastructure for sharing that information

Federal Register   A Monday-through-Friday publication of the National Archives and Records Administration that reports regulations and legal notices issued by federal agencies, presidential proclamations and executive orders, and other documents as directed by law or public interest.

Fee for service   A reimbursement method in which the cost is based on the provider's charge for each service.

Fee schedule   List that reflects the charge for each item that may be used in the treatment of a patient and the charge for most services; that is, respiratory therapy treatments, physical therapy services, laboratory tests, and so on. The fee schedule is most always automated and linked with the billing system. Also called the master charge list, charge master, or charge description master.

Fellowship of American Health Information Management Association (FAHIMA)   A credential offered by AHIMA that is designed to recognize AHIMA members who have made significant and sustained contributions to the profession over time. Eligibility for fellowship requires that an individual have a minimum of 10 years of full-time professional experience in health information management or a related field, 10 years of continuous AHIMA membership, evidence of sustained and substantial professional achievement, and a minimum of a master's degree. An individual must complete an application that is reviewed for approval by the AHIMA Fellowship Committee.

Fetal death rate   Computed to examine differences in the rates of early, intermediate, and late fetal deaths.

Field   A term that refers to the place in a computer system in which a data element might reside. It is best described as the container for the data. The field container may accommodate the data element in terms of data size or data type, or it may impose limits on how the data element can be defined because of the limits of the system.

File guide   Used to aid in the filing process. These guides list the letter of the alphabet and any vowel subdivisions within the main letter category, such as Da, De, Di, Do, Du, all within the main letter category of D.

Financial accountant   Responsible for recording past and current financial transactions (payments, orders, expenses, revenues, accruals, etc.).

Financial accounting   Recording and reporting the financial transactions of the organization for both internal management and users outside of the organization.

Financial analysis   The management process of formulating judgments and decisions from the relationship between the numbers represented on two reports: the balance sheet and the statement of revenues and expenses. Also known as ratio analysis.

Firewall   A system used to prevent access to a private network from the outside or to limit access to the outside from within the network. All data that enter or leave the organization's network must pass through the firewall, which acts as a filter, providing a single point of entry to a network.

Fiscal intermediary   An organization that has contracted to manage the processing of claims and payments.

Fishbone diagram   A diagram used for solving complicated problems by helping people consider many factors and the cause-and-effect relationships among those factors. (See also Cause-and-effect diagram.)

Flex time   Flex time allows employees to control their work schedules within parameters established by management. The employer usually defines a core structure of hours of the day and days of the week in which the employee must work to provide needed services and coverage. The employee's preferred schedule can be arranged flexibly around these core hours and days of the week.

Flexible budget A type of budget that is predicated on volume. All supplies, labor, and other variable expenses are budgeted in proportion to the anticipated volume. If the volume anticipated is not reached, labor and other expenses are expected to decrease accordingly and vice versa if the volume exceeds expectations.

Flow chart A graphical representation of a specific sequencing of steps in a process. A flow chart can be an outline or schematic drawing of the actual process that needs improving or a picture of the ideal process once improvement actions are taken. A flow chart consists of a series of connected symbols that represent actual or expected process steps.

Flow process chart Chart used to list each step in a work process; identifies the distance traveled and the time consumed by each delay. It is useful to collect information about a manual process, analyze it, and improve it.

Focus groups Interviews that include a small group of people (usually experts in the field or people whose opinion on the topic is being sought) that are brought together to answer and discuss specific questions. Participants can discuss issues, hear one another's viewpoints, and comment on those views. Focus groups enable a researcher to learn more about the topic because a group of experts is brainstorming.

Focused review A review conducted to determine the cause of less-than-desired performance.

Follow-up The processes used by cancer registries to determine the cancer patient's status. The primary purposes of follow-up are to ensure continued medical surveillance to determine outcomes of the treatment and to monitor the health status of the population under investigation. Follow-up information provides the documentation of residual disease or its spread, recurrences, or additional malignancies. Subsequent treatments should be included in the patient hospital database.

Force field analysis Analysis used to identify the variables that help and variables that hinder reaching the desired outcome or solution to a problem. In addition to identifying the causal order, force field analysis estimates the relative effect of each process variable (such as the number of available trained workers) on an outcome variable (such as increasing the number of outpatient visits).

Formal definitions Definitions that follow a formal structure and that are represented in a form that can be manipulated by a computer, as opposed to narrative text definitions intended for human readers.

Forward mapping Mapping from ICD-9-CM codes to ICD-10-CM and PCS codes. Forward mapping maps from an older code set to a newer code set.

Foundation of Research and Education (FORE) A separately incorporated affiliate organization (to AHIMA) that actively promotes education and research in the health information management (HIM) field. The Foundation offers grants-in-aid to support research activities and professional self-development opportunities, scholarships, professional recognition awards, and more.

Frames Vertical and/or horizontal lines that structure the form on the screen. Frames divide the form into logical sections and to direct data entry length and location.

Fraud A willful and intentional misrepresentation that could cause harm or loss to a person or the person's property.

Frequency distribution The number of times that each category of a qualitative variable or value of a quantitative variable is observed within a sample.

Frequency polygon A method used to present a frequency distribution with continuous data. It is constructed by joining the midpoints of the tops of the bars of a histogram with a straight line. The total area under the polygon is equal to the sum of the areas of the bars in the histogram and therefore equal to total sample size multiplied by interval width.

Functional interoperability (syntactic interoperability) Specifies the syntax or format of the transmitted message so that it can be parsed and stored by the receiving system.

Functional model A description of the environment and what happens in that environment that is used to begin the process of developing a specific information system. (See also Use case.)

Functional strategies Developed in functional areas of the organization to support programs and budgets in key areas of the organization.

Fund balance The profits and losses that result from the differences between revenues and expenses. (See also Equity.)

Gantt chart Scheduling and progress chart that emphasizes work time relations necessary to meet a defined goal; a common project scheduling tool.

Gatekeeper The primary care physician who participates in a comprehensive managed care plan and is responsible for coordinating all care provided to the managed care enrollee (patient). The focus of care is on prevention through regular physical examinations and other primary care services. If a patient needs to see a specialist, the gatekeeper must make the referral and thereby controls access to all other care.

General equivalency mappings (GEMs) The GEMs are a comprehensive translation dictionary that can be used to convert, accurately and effectively, any ICD-9-CM–based application or data to ICD-10-CM/PCS, including data for tracking quality, recording morbidity/mortality, and calculating reimbursement. The GEMs can be used to convert large applications with a high degree of complexity and still preserve the essential logic of the application.

General system life cycle A life cycle that can apply to all systems and includes a birth or development period, a period of growth and maturity, and a period of decline or deterioration.

Generalizability The ability to extrapolate or make inferences about a population on the basis of results of a study of a sample of the population.

Goals Statements of what the organization wants to do.

Governing body A group of individuals who have the ultimate legal authority and responsibility for the operation of the health care organization, including the quality and cost of care. Also called the board of trustees, board of governors, or board of directors.

Grading Variation from normal tissue. Also known as differentiation. Used in the description of tumors.

Granularity A term used to describe the level (degree) of detail in the data.

Graphic rating scales When employee performance is evaluated, graphic rating scales require the rater to assess performance by use of numerical scales often anchored by brief descriptors of performance. This is one of the most common rating techniques in practice.

Grievance procedure Provides a communication and problem-solving mechanism for employees to express a complaint that management has violated one of its own policies (or the union contract) with adverse consequences for the employee.

Gross death rate A crude measure that shows the number of hospitalizations that end in death out of all patients who were discharged or who died during the same period of time.

Group decision support software (GDSS)   Usually a network of workstations or portable personal computers that are all located in a conference or meeting room and used to facilitate the joint application design process. GDSS can be used to administer a survey or questionnaire electronically to a group of people at the same time and to facilitate brainstorming or a nominal group technique. GDSS allows anonymity of response, minimizes bias, and speeds up the deliberative process.

Hospital-acquired conditions (HACs)   Conditions that could have reasonably been prevented by following appropriate patient care guidelines.

Halo effect   Bias in which an observer's perception of one characteristic of an individual dominates other perceptions to result in an undifferentiated overall impression, positive or negative.

Hardware   The physical equipment (both electronic and mechanical) that makes up computers and computer systems. It includes electric, electronic, mechanical, and other equipment.

HCPCS   The coding system used to report physician services and other health care services and medical supplies, orthotic and prosthetic devices, and durable medical equipment.

Health   Defined by the World Health Organization as a state of complete physical, mental, and social well-being and not merely the absence of disease or infirmity.

Health care information   Information about wellness strategies, diseases, and conditions associated with treatment options. Information about how to use the health care system.

Health care operations   Under HIPAA's privacy rule, health care operations is a term used to describe activities such as conducting quality improvement activities, contacting patients with information about treatment alternatives, providing educational information, evaluating practitioner and provider performance, accreditation, licensing, and credentialing. These activities may need to use or reference protected health information, but when the use is related directly to the operation of the health care entity and is handled appropriately, no specific authorization is required on the part of the individual(s) whose information is being used.

Health care services   The processes that contribute to the health and well-being of the person. Services may be provided in a variety of health care settings, such as the hospital, ambulatory, or home setting and include nursing, medical, surgical, or other health-related services.

Health informatics   The intersection of information science, medicine, and health care. It deals with the resources, devices, and methods required to optimize the acquisition, storage, retrieval, and use of information in health and biomedicine. Health informatics tools include not only computers, but also clinical guidelines, formal medical terminologies, and information and communication systems.

Health information exchange (HIE)   The Office of the National Coordinator for Health Information Technology (ONC) laid out strategic action to achieve a vision of consumer-centric and information-rich health care. To achieve this vision, the ONC supported numerous efforts to implement EHRs and regional health information organizations, now identified as health information exchanges.

Health information technology   Health information technology is broadly defined as the use of information and communication technology in health care. Health information technology allows the transfer and linkage of data well beyond the walls of a health care facility. This technology is supporting the conversion of patient records to EHRs and EHR systems

Health Insurance Portability and Accountability Act of 1996 (HIPAA)   Legislation enacted in 1996 related to health insurance that also contained provisions for administrative simplification in the handling of health information. A primary focus was the adoption of standards that are required for electronic capture and transmission of billing and health insurance information. The legislation also recognized the need for privacy and security standards for health information. HIPAA regulations also invigorated the government's efforts to reduce health care fraud and ensure that health care organizations are complying with reimbursement regulations and coding guidelines associated with the submission of claims for services rendered to federally funded patients.

Health care data users   Range from individual patients, health care providers, and organizations to epidemiologists, researchers, health care payers, grants funding organizations, politicians, and public agencies.

Healthcare Effectiveness Data and Information Set (HEDIS)   A comparative performance measurement project that evaluates a health plan's clinical and administrative systems. These data are made available to purchasers and consumers to assist them in making choices about health care providers.

Healthcare Integrity and Protection Data Bank   A database of practitioner-specific information available only to managed care organizations. This information source contains the same practitioner-specific data that is in the National Practitioner Data Bank and civil judgments, criminal convictions, and actions taken by licensing agencies.

Health insurance exchange   Electronic marketplaces through which individuals can shop for health insurance. These exchanges provide information about different plans that can be directly compared.

Healthy People 2010   A report generated by the U.S. Department of Health and Human Services (DHHS) that identifies national objectives for disease prevention and health promotion.

Hearsay rule   Bars the legal admissibility of evidence that is not the personal knowledge of the witness.

Hierarchical   A term used to describe a database model that supports a treelike structure that consists of parent (or root) and child segments. A parent can have more than one child segment, but each child segment can have only one parent. A user queries the database, and the search seeks the answer from parent to child. The answer to the query is found by matching the conditions by searching downward through the tree.

Hierarchy chart   A type of decomposition diagram that breaks down problems into smaller and smaller detail by identifying all the tasks in a process and grouping them into various hierarchical levels.

Hierarchical relationships   Define specific concepts as children of more general concepts.

HIM Profession Core Model   Reflects potential roles, settings, and impact of the profession in the next decade.[32] The model consists of five functional components with a sixth under review that relate to a HIM professional's direct interaction with patient health information (Box 2-4). In addition, the model identifies four areas of practice identified as extenders that "support, advance, extend and contribute" to the functional components.[32]

Histogram   A graphic representation of frequency distributions. Histograms are useful for identifying whether the variation that exists in the frequency distribution is normal or skewed.

Historical-prospective study   An epidemiologic research study design that uses past records to collect information regarding the exposure characteristic or risk factor under study. Then, over the next 10, 15, or 20 years, medical records, death certificates, and so on are monitored to determine the number of cases of a particular disease that have developed.

Home health care   The provision of medical and nonmedical care in the home or place of residence to promote, maintain, or restore health or to minimize the effect of disease or disability. Home health care services mainly provide care for rehabilitation therapies and after acute care.

Horizontal integration   A merging of health care organizations offering services at the same point on the continuum of care (e.g., a multihospital system).

Hospice   A multidisciplinary health care program that is responsible for the palliative and supportive care of terminally ill patients and their families, with consideration for their physical, spiritual, social, and economic needs.

Hospital   Defined by the American Hospital Association (AHA) as a health care facility that has an organized medical and professional staff, inpatient beds available 24 hours a day, and the primary function of providing inpatient medical, nursing, and other health-related services for surgical and nonsurgical conditions and usually providing some outpatient services, especially emergency care.

Hospital ambulatory care   "Hospital-directed" health care that is provided to patients who are not admitted as inpatients and for which the hospital is responsible, regardless of the location of the health care. Services include satellite clinics, observation units, outpatient departments, ancillary services, and other specialty clinics.

Hospital cancer data system   The purpose of the hospital cancer data system is to collect and maintain information on every patient with cancer from the initial date of diagnosis or treatment until death. The information collected furnishes the health care team with outcome data that enable them to see the results of their diagnostic and therapeutic efforts and provide them with the tools to improve patient care.

Hospital formulary   Provides information on drugs that are approved and maintained by the health care organization and contains information on drugs including, but not limited to, names, dosages and strengths, packaging, characteristics, and clinical usage.

Hospital inpatient   A patient who generally stays overnight and is provided room, board, and nursing service in a unit or area of the hospital.

Hospital patient   Person who is receiving or using health care services for which the hospital is liable or held accountable. Hospital patients include inpatients, observation patients, ambulatory care patients, emergency patients, and newborn inpatients.

Human resource audit   An audit conducted to assess which openings can be filled with internal candidates already employed within the organization.

Hypothesis   An educated guess about the outcome of a study. A hypothesis is a claim or statement that poses an assertion to be supported and may predict a relationship between two or more variables.

Inactive record   Defined based on the health care activity of the patient. For example, if a patient has not received treatment or had other activity associated with the record for more than 5 years, then the record could be declared inactive. The organization decides the period of time associated with the definition of active record. Inactive records do not need to be as readily available as active records, but do need to be accessible when they are needed.

Incidence   The number of new cases of disease.

Incidence rate   The number of newly reported cases of a disease in a specified time period divided by the population at that time. The quotient is then multiplied by a constant such as 1000 or 100,000. Incident rates are determined to examine the frequency of specific types of disease.

Incident report   A paper-based or electronic report completed by health care professionals when a variance occurs from the usual process of patient care or when a mishap or injury occurs involving a patient, staff member, or visitor. Incident reports are meant to be nonjudgmental, factual accounts of the event and its consequences, if any, and are prepared to assist the organizations in identifying and correcting problem-prone areas and in preparation for legal defense. Also referred to as occurrence reports.

Independent variable   The variable that causes change in the other variables.

Indicator   An indirect measure that describes events or patterns of events suggestive of a problematic process or behavior.

Indigent   Someone who is without the means for subsistence— poor or impoverished.

Indirect pay   Involves payment by a third party to the provider on behalf of the patient. Indirect payers may be the government, insurance companies, managed-care programs, or self-insured companies.

Infant death rate   A rate that is computed to examine deaths of the neonate and infant at different stages. An infant death is death of an infant at any time from the moment of birth through the first year of life.

Inference   A generalization.

Informal or unwritten organization   Composed of two or more persons who develop mutually satisfying interactions pertaining to personal and/or job-related matters. These relationships are not depicted on an organization chart.

Information   Data that have been organized and processed into meaningful form, either manually or by computer, to make them valuable to the user. Information adds to a representation and tells the recipient something that was not known before.

Information governance   The creation of an accountability structure and culture at the enterprise level that minimizes costs, manages risks, and maximizes value of information assets.

Information system development life cycle   See System Development Life Cycle.

Information system life cycle   A life cycle that is similar to the general system life cycle. The information system life cycle consists of the following phases: design, implementation, operation and maintenance, and obsolescence.

Information warehouses   Receive clinical data from a transactions system such as a pharmacy system or a radiology system and combine them with other organizational data from administrative and financial systems. (See also Data warehouses.)

Informed consent   A communication process between the health professional and the patient. The patient must be informed about the anticipated treatment and its risks and alternatives.

Infrastructure (technical)   Technical infrastructure refers to the technology architecture required to maintain systems. Technology infrastructure includes the hardware, software, network, and communication resources required as underpinning to an electronic health record system.

Inpatient   A patient who is receiving health care services and is provided room, board, and continuous nursing service in a unit or area of the hospital.

Inpatient bed occupancy rate   The proportion of inpatient beds that are occupied (the percentage of occupancy).

Institutional review board (IRB)   A research and human rights advisory board that is part of most health care facilities and universities and that meets at least quarterly. The aim of an IRB is to protect human subjects or patients from research risks and invasion of privacy, by reviewing all research studies that involve subjects or patients, including experiments, interviews, and questionnaires, and any study that collects data from a patient's medical record.

Insurance   A purchased contract (policy) in which the purchaser (insured) is protected from loss by the insurer's agreeing to reimburse for such loss.

Integrated delivery system (IDS)   A network of health care organizations that provide or arrange to provide a continuum of services to a population; the network assumes the clinical and fiscal responsibility for the outcomes and health status of the population.

Intensity of service/severity of illness   Criteria that measure a need for health care services that can be provided only in an inpatient facility or define a degree of acute physical impairment that requires inpatient medical intervention.

Intentional tort   Includes assault and battery, false imprisonment, defamation of character, invasion of privacy, fraud or misrepresentation, and intentional infliction of emotional distress.

Interface engine   A type of middleware (software and hardware that serve as a bridge between applications) that allows two applications to exchange information without having to build a customized interface for each application.

Internal benchmarking   Internal benchmarking compares performance between functional areas or departments *within* an organization. The goal is to decrease or eliminate process errors or to improve process efficiency.

Internal environmental analysis   Reveals the strengths and weaknesses of the organization.

Internal users   Individual health care data users that are affiliated with the organization.

Internet   A telecommunications international computer network that serves as the gateway to a multitude of users.

Interobserver reliability   Reproducibility or reliability between more than one research assistant or observer.

Interoperability   The ability of different information systems to communicate. The ability of software programs to exchange data using a common set of business procedures and to read and write the same file formats and use the same protocols.

Interrogatory   A form of testimony. Interrogatories are sworn written answers to questions.

Interval data   Interval data convey more precise quantitative information than do ordinal data because it is assumed that equal differences between numbers correspond to equal differences in the trait or characteristic being measured. Examples of interval data include scores on college examinations and scores on nationally administered tests such as the SAT (Scholastic Aptitude Test).

Intranet   Like an Internet that runs exclusively within a network. An intranet is accessible only by users who can be authenticated as being within a specific network.

Intraobserver reliability   Reliability within one research assistant or observer.

Invasion of privacy   In health care, invasion of privacy is a negligent disregard for patients' privacy. For example, health care providers who divulge confidential information from a patient's record to an improper recipient without the patient's authorization have invaded the patient's privacy and breached their duty of confidentiality.

Inpatient prospective payment system (IPPS)   A system that brings the number of MS-DRGs to 745 and replaces the previous schedule of 538 DRGs. This system adjusts the DRG weights based on the severity of the patient's condition and correlates more closely with resource consumption.

JAVA   A programming language introduced in late 1995 by Sun Microsystems. JAVA is thought to be less complicated than the C programming language. The main objective of a JAVA program is to allow applications to be built as stand-alone applications that can be transferred across the Web and run independently on a client computer. JAVA is an object-oriented language that is compiled into a universal, non-machine-dependent format.

Job analysis   Systematic collection, evaluation, and organization of job performance; understanding of what is required to perform the job, how it can be performed most efficiently, and what outcomes are expected from doing the job properly.

Job description   A narrative presentation of the key responsibilities, activities, and working conditions associated with a designated job.

Job evaluation   A formal procedure used in compensation management to determine the relative worth of each position in the organization. The process is usually performed by human resource staff or contracted out to a consultant specializing in compensation systems.

Job grading   A job evaluation method that classifies each job by assigning it to the narrative description of a grade that it most closely resembles.

Job performance standards   Included in some job descriptions and used as the primary criteria for performance evaluation.

Job ranking   A job evaluation method that ranks whole jobs by comparing them with other positions within the organization on the basis of one or more key characteristics. This ranking is based on the relative levels of responsibility of these positions and their impact on revenue generation. The ranking method is best used in organizations with a small number of positions.

Job sharing   A staffing option in which a full-time position is shared by two or more persons. This option is offered by some employers to accommodate the needs and preferences of working parents.

Joint application design   A data-gathering technique by which a group of people spend a concentrated time together in determining system requirements. The group is usually composed of end users, managers, analysts, and others who may have an impact on or be affected by the system under study. This method is also referred to as joint requirements planning (JRP).

Joint Commission on Accreditation of Healthcare Organizations   (See The Joint Commission.)

Jurisdiction   The power of a court (federal, state, etc.) to hear a dispute.

Key indicators of demand   Measures of program operations (i.e., volume, activity, or output) that can be reliably linked to staffing levels.

Knowledge   Derived from information once information is organized, analyzed, and synthesized by the user.

Knowledge base   A collection of stored facts, heuristics, and models that can be used for problem solving.

Layoffs   Involuntary separation that occurs whenever the employer terminates the employment relationship for whatever reason, sometimes as a result of low patient volume, restructuring, or adverse economic conditions.

Lean thinking   A performance improvement model that is based on the principles of eliminating waste and retaining only value-added activities, concentrating on improving value-added activities, responding to the voice of the customer, and optimizing processes across the organization.

Leapfrog Group   A collaboration of large employers that came together in 1998 to determine how purchasers could influence the quality and affordability of health care. The Leapfrog Group identified four hospital quality and safety practices that are the focus of its health care provider performance comparisons and hospital recognition and reward. The quality practices are computer physician order entry, evidence-based hospital referral, and intensive care unit (ICU) staffing by physicians experienced in critical care medicine.

Legal health record   The data and information within the patient record used to substantiate the care given for reimbursement and quality proposes. It is also a legal document that confirms whether treatment was delivered in a manner appropriate for the given health problem. The record is used to show proof in a court of law of what transpired during the course of a patient's illness and treatment. As a legal document, the patient record is defined as a record that is generated at or for a health care organization as its business record and is the record that would be released upon request.

Legal medical record   (see Legal health record)

Legal record analysis   A review of the clinical records that focuses on the presence or absence or items that are required in clinical records based on state and federal regulations.

Length of stay   The number of calendar days from admission to discharge for an inpatient. Also referred to as the duration of inpatient hospitalization or discharge days.

Level of significance   The criterion or standard a researcher chooses when performing a test of significance—usually 0.05 or 0.01.

Liabilities   The debts or obligations an organization owes. Liabilities may include wages accruing between paydays, mortgage payments due to the bank, and so forth.

Libel   Written defamation of character.

Licensed independent practitioner   Defined by The Joint Commission as "any individual permitted by law and by the organization to provide care, treatment, and services without direction or supervision."

Licensure   The legal approval for a facility to operate or for a person to practice within his or her profession. An individual must meet eligibility requirements defined by the state before the individual is granted a license to practice. Licensure occurs at the state level and is overseen by a state licensing board or agency.

Life care centers   Centers that provide living accommodations and meals for a monthly fee. They offer a variety of services, including housekeeping, recreation, health care, laundry, and exercise programs. Also referred to as retirement communities.

Life-table analysis   Examines survival times of individual subjects and is most appropriate for prospective studies or experimental studies when the researcher has a loss of subjects as a result of follow-up or the study ends before recurrence or death has occurred in some subjects.

Line graph   A graph that provides a simple, yet highly graphic, visual method of monitoring trends over time.

Linkage strategies   Initiatives such as changing the organization's culture, reorganization, upgrade of facilities and equipment, and social and ethical strategies.

Liquidity ratios   Ratios that focus on balance sheet numbers (assets, liabilities, and equity/fund balance accounts) to measure the ability of the health care organization to meet its short- and long-term financial obligations.

Literature review   A review of past research studies on the same subject. A literature review is the second step of a sound research study design (after the hypothesis or question is established).

Living will   A written document that allows a competent adult to indicate his or her wishes regarding life-prolonging medical treatment should he or she be unable to consent.

Location code   Codes that enable systems to identify the source from which data originate. A facility may have 15 different locations or location codes. These code numbers do not have meaning, but make the data easier to handle. The users do not have to enter the codes and are unaware that a unique identifier is being used.

Logical data model   The logical data model represents the structure of the relationship of data elements and entities within an information system. The logical model is crucial to the proper functioning of any system within an enterprise. The logical model allows for elegance in system design so that the system is adaptable to the changing information needs of the enterprise.

Logical system design   Describes the functionality of the system and presents the vision of system performance and its features.

LOINC   The Logical Observation Identifiers, Names, and Codes used for representing laboratory data for ordering and naming specific test results

Longitudinal patient record   The longitudinal patient record is a comprehensive patient record compiled and accessible over the individual's life span from birth to death. It is a valuable resource for clinical decision-making that provides easy access to medical history, contains costs by reducing repeated diagnostic testing and treatments, and promotes patient safety through medical alerts and information on allergies, drug reactions, and drug-drug or drug-food interactions.

Longitudinal record   A comprehensive record that provides the complete history of a patient, from birth to death. This record provides easy access to medical history, reduces repeated diagnostic testing and treatments, and promotes patient safety through medical alerts and information on allergies, drug reactions, and drug interactions.

Long-term care   Health care that is provided over a long period of time (30 or more days) to patients who have chronic diseases or disabilities.

Long-term debt/total assets ratio   A capitalization ratio that compares the amount of long-term debt the organization has with the amount of assets it has to pay those debts.

Loss reduction   A risk management strategy, loss reduction focuses on a single incident or claim and requires immediate response to any adverse occurrence.

Lossless   When data compression reproduces the original file exactly with no information loss.

Lossy   When data compression causes some information to be lost in the translation.

Mainframe   Machines that are used for major applications, to maintain large databases, and for high-volume work.

Major birth defects   Birth defects that affect survival, require substantial medical care, or result in marked physiological or psychological impairment.

Malpractice   Professional negligence.

Malware   Malicious software (can be any unauthorized software that is found in an information system).

Managed care   A generic term for a health care reimbursement system that is designed to minimize utilization of services and contain costs while ensuring the quality of care. The term *managed care* encompasses a continuum of practice arrangements, including health maintenance organizations (HMOs), preferred provide organizations (PPOs), and other alternative delivery systems.

Management by objectives (MBO)   A management planning process popular during the 1970s and 1980s, used to integrate business planning, productivity management and control, employee performance evaluation, and supervisory coaching. MBO has largely been replaced by alternative approaches, such as strategic management, total quality management, and re-engineering. One of its core principles, however, the systematic setting and periodic review of performance goals, is still used today.

Managerial accountant   Helps record what is happening currently or previously (variance analyses) against what was anticipated and what is still anticipated to happen (the budget).

Managerial finance officer   Plans for the future by working with financial organizations (banks, investors, and so on) to obtain funding and financing for an organization's plans. Also referred to as the chief financial officer (CFO) or treasurer.

Mapping   Enables users to use data for multiple purposes without having to capture the data in multiple formats. Mapping is also valuable for retaining the value of historical data when migrating to newer database formats and terminology versions.

Market entry strategy   Indicates whether the adaptive strategy will be accomplished by buying into the market, cooperating with another organization in the market, or internal development.

Master budget   A consolidation of all department operating budgets with each of the operating account's combined balances.

Master charge list   A list used by a health care organization that reflects the charge for each item that may be used in the treatment of a patient and the charge for most services (i.e., respiratory therapy treatments, physical therapy services, laboratory tests, and so on). The list is almost always automated and linked with the billing system. Also known as the charge master, charge description master (CDM), or fee schedule.

Master patient index (MPI)   Index that identifies all patients who have been treated by the facility and lists the number associated with the name. The index can be maintained manually or as part of a computerized system.

Matching concept   Revenue is accounted for when the actual charge is posted to a patient account. The matching concept recognizes that any associated expenses such as labor, supplies, and travel would be recorded in the same accounting period and matched with the revenue for that accounting period.

Maternal death rate   The rate is calculated by dividing the number of maternal deaths by the number of obstetric discharges. A maternal death results from causes associated with pregnancy or its management but not from accidental or incidental causes unrelated to the pregnancy.

Mean   A measure of central tendency that summarizes an entire set of data by means of a single representative value. The mean or average is calculated by adding up the values of all the observations and dividing the total by the number of observations.

Meaningful Use   An incentive program established by CMS using the ARRA. The program provides funds to encourage eligible providers and eligible hospitals to adopt and use certified electronic health record systems.

Median   The middle value within a data set. When the values are arranged from lowest to highest, the number of values above the median is equal to the number of values below the median. For an odd number of observations, the median is the middle number in the ordered set of numbers; for an even number of observations, it is the mean of the middle two numbers.

Medicaid   A joint program between the state and the federal governments to provide health care to welfare recipients in the different states.

Medical informatics   The study of medical computing. (See also Health informatics.)

Medically indigent   People whose incomes are above what would normally qualify for Medicaid but whose medical expenses are high enough to bring their adjusted income to the poverty level.

Medicare   A government-subsidized health care program that provides health insurance for elderly people and certain other groups.

Messaging standard   A consensus-based specification standard for exchange of data among electronic systems.

Metadata   The term *metadata* is defined as "data about data." It defines the structure that will be used to define all of the characteristics about data so that different individuals looking at characteristics of a data element would arrive at the same conclusion as to what the data means and how it is to be used.

Metathesaurus   The core database of the UMLS consisting of a collection of concepts and terms from the various controlled vocabularies and their relationships. It is organized by concepts that are linked to corresponding concepts in various source vocabularies. It comprises more than 1 million biomedical concepts and 5 million concept names.

Methodology   The way a research study is designed so that the hypothesis can be properly tested. Includes a step-by-step process of what is done in the research study and why this process is necessary to test the hypothesis properly.

Methods improvement   (See Work simplification.)

Microcomputers   Based on small microprocessing chips found in individual PCs. Microcomputers are used for desktop applications such as word processing and spreadsheets and, with the increase in computing power available on the PC, can serve as the hardware for a database management system.

Middleware   Software and hardware that serve as a bridge between applications.

Minicomputers   Often used in departmental systems such as laboratory or radiology systems. Minicomputers were popular in the 1980s and early 1990s because they were less expensive than mainframes and had some of the processing power of a mainframe and allowed devices and files to be shared.

Minimum necessary   A principle of the HIPAA privacy rule whereby only the minimum necessary amount of information necessary to fulfill the purpose of the request should be shared with internal users and external requestors. There are only a few situations in which the minimum necessary standard does not apply (e.g., uses or disclosures for treatment purposes or where the patient has specifically authorized the release of more information and in a few other circumstances).

Mission   A broad-term statement of the organization's purpose. The mission statement defines the geographic environment and population that the organization serves.

Mode   The value that occurs most frequently in a given set of values. The mode is the only measure of central tendency that can be used with nominal data.

Morbidity   The extent of illness, injury, or disability in a given population.

Morbidity rates   Complication rates, such as community-acquired, hospital-acquired or nosocomial, and postoperative infection rates. Morbidity rates can also include comorbidity rates and the prevalence and incidence rates of disease.

Morphology   Cell structure and form.

Mortality   The death rate in a given population.

Mortality rates   Death rates, including gross death rate, net death rate, cause-specific death rates, and neonatal and infant death rates. Death rates that are computed because they demonstrate an outcome that may be related to the quality of the health care provided.

Motion to quash   A motion filed by legal counsel in which the court is asked to set aside the subpoena or order.

Movement diagram (layout flow chart)   Graphically represents the movement of paper or people in the physical environment where the processes are performed.

Multimedia   Information content and information processing using multiple formats (e.g., text, graphics, video, audio).

Multiple consistent views   Required to support the different views of the vocabulary depending on the utility.

National Committee for Quality Assurance (NCQA)   A private, not-for-profit organization established in 1991. NCQA accredits a variety of organizations from health maintenance organizations to preferred provider organizations to managed behavioral health care organizations, and each accreditation program has distinct performance management requirements. More than 100 million Americans are covered by an NCQA-accredited health plan.

National Practitioner Data Bank (NPDP)   A database of practitioner-specific information that is used by hospital medical staffs considering applications for membership (either initial appointment or reappointment) or requests for clinical privileges to identify any available adverse quality of care information about the applicant.

National Quality Forum (NQF)   Created in 1999 to develop and implement a national strategy for health care quality measurement and reporting. The NQF, a not-for-profit membership group, includes representatives from a diverse group of national, state, regional, and local organizations, including purchasers, consumers, health systems, health care practitioners, health plans, accrediting bodies, regulatory agencies, medical suppliers, and information technology companies. The mission of the NQF is to improve American health care through endorsement of consensus-based national standards for measurement and public reporting of health care performance data that provide meaningful information about whether care is safe, timely, beneficial, patient-centered, equitable, and efficient.

Nationwide Health Information Exchange

Natural language processing   The processing of data in natural language form. Natural language processing for cardiology, for example, would need to include all the terms and expressions used by cardiologists in their models of thinking. (See also Text processing.)

NDCs   A system that was originally established as part of an out-of-hospital drug reimbursement program under Medicare but has since expanded in scope. The NCD system is currently mandated by HIPAA as the standard medical data code set for reporting drugs and biologics for retail pharmacy transactions. The NDC is owned by the FDA and distributed by the Department of Health and Human Services (DHHS) and is sometimes referred to as the FDA-NDCs.

NDF-RT   The National Drug File—Reference Terminology (NDF-RT) is produced by the U.S. Department of Veterans Affairs, Veterans Health Administration (VHA) and is an extension of the VHA National Drug File (NDF). The NDF-RT is used for modeling drug characteristics including ingredients, chemical structure, dose form, physiologic effect, mechanism of action, pharmacokinetics, and related diseases. It combines the NDF hierarchical drug classification with a multicategory reference model. The metathesaurus representation of NDF-RT includes only concepts above the "packaged product" level. Some attributes of concepts at this level have been attached to the parent product level concept. NDF-RT is updated monthly.

Negligence   Conduct that society considers unreasonably dangerous. Failure to provide a reasonable level of care.

Neonatal death rate   A rate computed to examine deaths of the neonate and infant at different stages. A neonatal death is the death of an infant within the first 27 days, 23 hours, 59 minutes of life.

Net   Income from revenue reduced by all relevant deductions.

Net death rate   A rate that differs from the gross death rate in that it does not include deaths that occurred less than 48 hours after admission to the health care facility. The net death rate is useful because it provides a more realistic account of patient deaths related to patient care provided by a specific health care facility.

Net operating revenue   The amount of revenue expected to be received or total charges less the deductions expected by third-party payers resulting in revenues net of deductions or net operating revenue.

Net present value   Discounted or present value of all cash inflows and outflows of a project as a given discount rate.

Network   A term used to describe a database model. A network model is similar to the hierarchical model except that a child can have more than one parent. In a network database, the parent is referred to as an owner and a child is referred to as a member. In other words, it supports the many-to-many relationship.

Never events   Hospital-acquired conditions considered by CMS to be (1) preventable; (2) high cost or high volume (or both); and (3) resulting in additional costs.

Nursing Interventions Classifications (NIC)   A comprehensive, research-based, standardized classification system used to classify the interventions that nurses perform.

Niche vendors   In health care a company that focuses on one particular market and may focus on particular software products.

Nursing Outcomes Classifications (NOC)   A comprehensive, research-based, standardized classification system used to classify outcome evaluations based on the interventions that nurses perform.

Nomenclature   A system of names that have been assigned according to pre-established rules.

Nominal data   Data collected on variables where qualitative rather than quantitative differences exist between individuals. Nominal data are also called categorical, qualitative, or named data.

Nominal group technique (NGT)   An idea-generating technique, similar to brainstorming, that uses silent generation of ideas and a sequential reporting approach to ensure participation by all group members.

Nonrepudiation   In an electronic system, the electronic signature must ensure the signed document was not modified after the signature was affixed. Additionally, the electronic signature must ensure that only the signer could have created a signature.

Nonsemantic concept identifier   An identifier that does not carry any meaning in itself and does not indicate the hierarchical position of the term it represents.

Nosocomial (infection)   An infection that develops more than 72 hours after hospitalization.

"Not elsewhere classified" (NEC)   Term used to collect concepts that are not covered elsewhere in a terminology.

Null hypothesis   In a test of significance, a null hypothesis states that there is no difference or relationship in the population and the observations are the result of chance.

Numerical identification   An alternative method of identification using a number to identify the patient record.

Nursing care   Nursing care is based on a process that involves assessment, diagnosis, outcomes and planning, implementation, and evaluation of patient care, and the documentation in the health record must reflect this process.

Nursing classification schemes   Classification schemes used to classify the interventions that nurses perform and outcome evaluations based on those interventions. Two nursing classification systems include the Nursing Interventions Classification (NIC) and the Nursing Outcomes Classification (NOC). NIC and NOC are useful for clinical documentation, communication of care across settings, integration of data across systems and settings, effectiveness research, productivity measurement, competency evaluation, reimbursement, and curriculum design.

Nursing facility   A comprehensive term for a long-term care facility that provides nursing care and related services for residents who require medical, nursing, or rehabilitative care.

Object   In programming, an object is an individual unit of runtime data storage that is used as the basic building block of programs. In object-oriented programming a program works with a dynamic set of interacting objects. These objects include a very specific kind of typing that allows for data members to associate with the object and for methods that access the data members in predefined ways. An example of an object would be "my car," which is an instance of a type (class) called "car," which is a subclass of "motor vehicles."

Objectives   Specific statements that define the expectations or outcomes given the goal direction. Objectives provide clear guidelines for management and supervisors to define the action steps to achieve the objective. Objectives are usually measurable.

Object-oriented   A type of database model that embraces the concept of an object. An object-oriented database is a collection of objects. Objects support encapsulation and inheritance. Encapsulation is the technique by which an object such as a patient is defined with certain characteristics. The user does not need to know how the characteristics are stored, just that the object "patient" exists and has certain attributes.

Observation unit   The observation unit of the hospital is a unit, department, or beds for the observation patient who needs assessment, evaluation, or monitoring because of a significant degree of instability or disability that does not require admission to the hospital as an inpatient.

Occurrence report   Factual summaries of unexpected events that have resulted (or could have resulted) in injury or harm to patients, staff, or visitors. Occurrence reports are used by health care organizations' risk managers or attorneys to investigate incidents that have the potential to become claims against the organization or individual provider and to identify areas where improvements are needed. (See also Incident report.)

Odds ratio   An estimate of the relative risk a person has if he or she is exposed to a certain characteristic.

Office landscape   The overall design of the office areas or spaces; the most common type is the open type.

Office of the National Coordinator for Health Information Technology   In 2004 President Bush created the new position of National Health Information Technology Coordinator. This office and role within Health and Human Services (HHS) is charged with providing national leadership in support of government and private efforts to develop the standards and infrastructure to more effectively use information technology to achieve quality health care and to reduce health care costs. The Coordinator reports to the Secretary of HHS.

Omaha System   A research-based, comprehensive, and standardized taxonomy designed to enhance practice, documentation, and information management. It consists of three relational, reliable, and valid components: (1) the Problem Classification Scheme (client assessment), (2) the Intervention Scheme (service delivery), and (3) the Problem Rating Scale for Outcomes (client change/evaluation).

Ongoing record review   The review of a health care facility's clinical records on an ongoing basis, beginning at the point of care and based on organization-defined indicators that address the presence, timeliness, readability (whether handwritten or printed), quality, consistency clarity, accuracy, completeness, and authentication of data and information contained within the record.

Ontology   A formal representation of a set of concepts within a domain and the relationships within those concepts.

Open office design plan   Design for an office arrangement that features open space free of permanent walls. Workstations that are created with the use of partitions and furniture. The open plan focuses on work groups, traffic patterns, and work flow.

Open-ended questions   Questions that do not provide a list of responses to choose from, similar to an essay type question, enabling the recipient to write out his or her thoughts in free form. Also referred to as unstructured format questions.

Operating budget   A budget that predicts the labor, supply, and other expenses required to support the work volume predicted.

Operating margin ratio   A common performance ratio that displays the relation between the net revenues received and the expenses required to supply the revenues.

Operating system   Directs the internal functions of the computer and serves as the bridge to application programs. Operating systems act as system managers that direct the execution of programs, allocate time to multiple users, and operate the input/output (I/O) devices and the network communication lines.

Operation flow chart   A graphic representation of the logical sequence of activities in a procedure. It shows the decision points encountered in carrying out that function.

Operational strategies   Made up of strategies developed within the functional areas of the organization and strategies that link the functional areas and develop the capabilities of the organization.

Opportunity costs   The benefits that would be received from the next best alternative use of the investment funds.

Optical character reader   A device used for optical character recognition.

Optical character recognition   A data entry technique that uses a scanner to read typewritten or specifically formatted data such as bar codes into a computer at high rates of speed.

Order entry   The online entry of orders for drugs, laboratory tests, and procedures, usually performed by nurses or unit clerks.

Ordinal data   Data expressing rankings from lowest to highest according to some criterion.

Organization chart Illustrates the hierarchical relationships between various individuals, lines of authority, accountability, and responsibility; identifies the organization's primary functions and the subfunctions within each primary function.

Osteopathic medicine Based on the theory that all body systems are interconnected and therefore the focus of health care is directed at the whole person. Because two thirds of the body is composed of muscle and bone, osteopathic medicine places a great deal of emphasis on the musculoskeletal system.

Outcard A manual record-tracking system used to determine when a patient record has been purged, or thinned, from the active files and either moved to an alternative storage site or converted to another medium, such as digitally scanned. Outcards are usually cardboard to allow the patient name and record number to be written directly on them. Outcards stay in the file permanently to tell the new location of the paper record or the new medium to which it has been transferred.

Outcome The term *outcome* refers to an indicator of the results of a process. Although that process may be of almost any type, typically it is related to the content and delivery of health care.

Outcome measures Performance measures that examine the end results or product of the patient's encounter with the system.

Outguide A plastic folder used in place of a record when the record has been removed from the files. It can be thought of as a placeholder. Outguides usually contain two separate see-through pockets, one to hold the requisition slip and one to hold any loose papers to be filed in the record that accumulate while the record is out of file.

Out-of-pocket A payment method in which the patient pays directly to the health care provider. (See also Self-pay.)

Outpatient A patient who is receiving health care services at a hospital without being hospitalized, institutionalized, or admitted as an inpatient.

Outsourcing The use of contract services.

***P* value** In a test of significance, the probability that the observed value of the test statistic could occur in the event that the null hypothesis is true. The *P* value can range from 0 to 1. The smaller the *P* value or closer it is to 0, the less likely the null hypothesis is true and the smaller the probability that the observed difference or relationship could be due to chance or sampling error alone.

Packet filter A type of firewall that examines data entering or leaving and accepts or rejects the data on the basis of system-defined criteria.

Palliative care Health care services that relieve or alleviate patient symptoms and discomforts, such as pain and nausea; it is not curative.

Pareto chart A chart that is similar in form to bar charts and histograms. However, unlike bar charts and histograms, occurrences plotted on a Pareto chart are ordered from the largest or most frequently occurring category (and presumably most important) to the smallest or least frequently occurring category. Pareto charts often are used in conjunction with brainstorming as a visual aid to demonstrate where attention to specific problems should be focused.

Participant observation A type of qualitative research in which the researcher is immersed into the subject's environment to learn what the subject experiences firsthand. The researcher pays special attention to the physical, social, and human environment and formal and informal interactions and unplanned activities. The researcher can choose to be disguised or undisguised and is basically there to describe a problem to outsiders on the basis of the understanding of the insider's perspective.

Participating physicians A term that refers to physicians who participate in a preferred provider organization (PPO).

Participating provider Once a provider has come to terms with a payer and is under an approved contractual agreement, the provider is considered a participating provider and agrees to provide services to covered plan members, or Medicare beneficiaries, and must abide by established payment rates.

Passive case A term used to describe reporting systems that rely on reports submitted to the registry by hospitals, clinics, or other facilities, supplemented with data from vital statistics. In some states, staff submits reports voluntarily, but, in general, reporting requirements are established by state legislation.

Password aging The process whereby users must change their password at a specific frequency (e.g., 30 days, 90 days). This process enables the passwords to remain unique and identifies users who do not log in for a period of time.

Patient An individual, including one who is deceased, who is receiving or using or has received health care services.

Patient advocacy The promoting of health care quality and patient safety improvements. Patient advocacy is concerned with ensuring overall patient satisfaction with the process and outcomes of care episodes.

Patient assessment The process of obtaining appropriate and necessary information about each individual seeking entry into a health care setting or service.

Patient-centered care Care that puts the patient in charge and gives him/her as much control as desired. It gives patients choices that allow them to express their cultural traditions, personal preferences and values, family situations, and lifestyles.

Patient-centered medical home A model of primary care that is patient-centered, comprehensive, team-based, coordinated, accessible, and focused on quality and safety.

Patient health record The primary legal record (either paper or electronic) documenting the health care services provided to a person in any aspect of the health care system. The patient health record includes routine clinical or office records, records of care in any health-related setting, preventive care, lifestyle evaluation, research protocols, and various clinical databases. The principal repository for information concerning a patient's health care, uniquely representing patients and serving as a dynamic resource for the health care industry. (Synonymous with clinical record, medical record, health record, resident record, client record. In electronic format, synonymous with electronic health record, electronic medical record.)

Patient portal A secure online Web site that gives patients convenient 24-hour access to personal health information from anywhere with an Internet connection. The portal is hosted by a health care provider (or through a health care entity's contract with a vendor that includes a business associate agreement). The portal typically contains information provided by the health care provider specific to the patient (lab results, visit summaries), options for secure communications with the provider (secure e-mail, appointment requests) and options for the patient to add notes to the portal. The portal belongs to the provider.

Patient record The patient record is a primary source of health data and information for the health care industry. The record can be paper-based, electronic, or a combination of both referred to as a hybrid record. It is the legal documentation of care provided to an individual by the medical or health care professionals who practice in the setting. The data, information, or record may have the term "clinical" preceding it to denote that the data, information, or record relates specifically to the care and treatment of a patient.

Patient record system   The set of components that comprise the system and mechanisms by which patient records, the data in the records, and the data about the records are created, used, stored, and retrieved. The patient record contains administrative, legal, and clinical information about an individual. The individual and aggregate use of this information is essential to the delivery of health care. The patient record system also includes information about the system (e.g., policies and procedures, information on who may use the system, practice standards for clinical documentation). The system may use a paper-based patient record or a hybrid combination of paper and electronic patient record or use a fully electronic patient record. (Synonymous with medical record system, health record system, resident record system, electronic health record system.)

Patient safety improvement   The actions undertaken by individuals and organizations to protect health care recipients from being harmed by the effects of health care services.

Patient safety indicators   Indicators that screen for problems that patients experience as a result of exposure to the health care system and that are likely amenable to prevention by changes at the system or provider level.

Pay for Performance (P4P)   A payment system initiated by some health plans that financially rewards providers who achieve specific quality or patient safety goals. The fundamental principles of Pay for Performance are (1) common performance measures for providers (usually represent a balance of patient satisfaction, prevention, and chronic care management) and (2) significant health plan financial payments based on that performance, with each plan independently deciding the source, amount, and payment method for its incentive program.

Payback method   The payback period determines the number of years it will take for the cash inflows from each project to pay back the initial investment.

Payback period   The time in which a project saves enough money to pay for itself. To determine the payback period, a comparison between total old system (project) costs and total new system (project) costs (including investment) is made. The difference between new and old costs is calculated on a year-by-year (cumulative) basis. When the difference between old costs and new costs reaches zero, the payback period has been reached.

Payer   The party who is financially responsible for the reimbursement of the health care costs.

Pearson correlation coefficient   A statistic used to assess the direction and degree of relationship between two continuous variables. The direction of the relationship between two continuous variables can be either positive or negative.

Peer review   Review of patients' records is a way the medical staff evaluates performance of physicians and LIPs. This is often called peer review because the individual whose practice is being reviewed is evaluated by individuals who have similar training, work in similar environments, and have similar proficiency in a clinical practice area or specialty.

Peer-reviewed journal   A journal with articles that have been extensively reviewed by peers within the specific research area. Peers have provided comments and feedback to the authors to incorporate into their revision of the article before publication.

Per case   A fixed payment system.

Per diem   Established payment for a day's worth of services.

Percentage   A number based on a whole divided into 100 parts.

Percentage of occupancy   (See Inpatient bed occupancy rate.)

Performance appraisal   A systematic method for observing, evaluating, documenting, and giving feedback to employees about their performance.

Performance assessment   An assessment that involves a formal periodic review of performance measurement results. Sometimes called evaluation, appraisal, or rating.

Performance measure   A generic term used to describe a particular value or characteristic designated to measure input, output, outcome, efficiency, or effectiveness.

Performance ratios   Ratios that evaluate the use of resources to achieve a goal based on data from the statement of revenues and expenses.

Performance target   A "stretch goal" that represents a future performance expectation that the health care organization will work toward achieving.

Period prevalence rate   Refers to evaluating a health condition over a period of time, such as 1 year.

Personal health record (PHR)   An electronic or paper record of health information compiled and maintained by the patient. The PHR is not a part of the health record that is compiled by a health care provider's legal health record.

PERT network   The acronym for Program Evaluation Review Technique; a diagram that illustrates the dependency relation of several projects leading to a larger nonroutine goal (e.g., building project); a tool used to plan and coordinate the smaller projects and accomplish the larger goal; used to give likely completion times.

Phishing   A type of security threat that uses e-mail messages that appear to come from a legitimate business or organization. These e-mail messages request personal information, such as an account number, and contain a link to a Web site to submit the information.

Physical system design   Specifies all the characteristics that are necessary so that the logical design can be implemented, including details about the design of hardware, software, databases, communications, and procedures and controls.

Physician advisory   Physicians who participate in the utilization management process by reviewing hospitalized patients whose conditions do not meet criteria for remaining in the hospital. This provides a type of peer review.

Picture archiving and communication system (PACS)   A system that provides rapid access to digitized film images for radiology applications and that can help eliminate the cost of film processing and storage.

Pie chart   Used to represent the relative frequency of categories or intervals within a sample. A pie chart is constructed by drawing a circle, 360 degrees, and dividing that circle into sections that correspond to the relative frequency in each category.

Pilot testing   Testing a survey with a small sample of the potential recipients. Recipients go through the survey as if they are going to answer the questions and provide feedback on any changes or additions to the survey. Once the feedback is received by the research team, the survey should be changed where applicable to meet the feedback received.

Plaintiff   The party that initiates a lawsuit.

Plan-Do-Check-Act (PDCA)   A widely used model of performance improvement developed in the 1920s by Walter Shewhart.

Pleading   When the defendant files an answer to the complaint from the plaintiff. In this answer, the defendant denies or otherwise responds to the plaintiff's claims.

Point of care system   A system by which data are captured at the place where the care is provided. For example, a bedside terminal system that is located where the patient is receiving care, such as the bedside.

Point of service   A type of managed care plan that combines characteristics of both the HMO and the PPO. Members of a POS plan do not make a choice about which system to use until the point at which the service is being used.

Point prevalence rate   Refers to evaluating a health condition at a specific point in time. Therefore, each study participant is assessed only once at one point in time, although the actual point prevalence study may take months or years to conduct.

Point system   A job evaluation method that analyzes key elements of the job and assigns point values to these factors of the basis of predetermined descriptive standards or criteria.

Pointer   In computer science a pointer is a data type with a value that refers directly to (points to) another value stored elsewhere in the computer.

Point-to-point   Refers to the method of connection between two endpoints, usually host computers. The term point-to-point telecommunications is used to refer to wireless data communications for Internet or voice over IP via radio frequencies.

Policies   The guidelines that managers use to make decisions. Policies translate the mission statement and corporate objectives into practical and easily understood terms.

Polyhierarchy   An arrangement that is necessary to support different users and uses of the same terminology.

Population   All items or members of the group to be studied.

Population-based cancer registry   A registry that collects data for a defined geographic area. There are three types of population-based registries: incidence only, cancer control, and research.

Postoperative death rate   A cause-specific death rate that expresses the number of deaths that may have resulted from surgical complications. The number of patients who die within 10 days of surgery is divided by the number of patients who underwent surgery for the period.

Postoperative infection rate   A rate used by the health care facility to determine which infections occur after surgery and are probably due to the surgical procedure.

Potentially compensable event (PCE)   An adverse occurrence, usually involving a patient, that could result in a financial obligation for the health care organization.

Power   The ability of one person A to influence another person B to do something he or she would otherwise not decide to do.

Power of attorney   The legally recognized authority to act and make decisions on behalf of another party.

Practice Act   The state law that defines the rights and scope of practice of each profession and the requirements to attain a license.

Practitioner   An individual who is licensed or certified to deliver care to patients.

Precedent   The rulings of similar previous cases. By referring to similar cases that have been decided in the past and applying the same principles, courts generally arrive at the same ruling in the current case as in similar previous cases.

Preempt or preemption   Override.

Pre-existing condition   A disease, injury, or condition identified as having occurred before a specific date.

Preferred provider organization (PPO)   A network of physicians and/or health care organizations that enter into an agreement with payers or employers to provide health care services on a discounted fee schedule in turn for increased patient volume. Patients are encouraged to use these providers by having a lower

deductible, copayment, and coinsurance for services given by these providers.

Premium   Payment required to maintain policy coverage; usually paid periodically.

Preponderance of evidence   "More likely than not" when weighing whether something is true or not true when the evidence supports the case by 51%.

President's Information Technology Advisory Committee (PITAC)   The President's Information Technology Advisory Committee was authorized by congress under the High-Performance Computing Act of 1991 (P. L. 102-194) and the Next Generation Internet Act of 1998 (P. L. 105-305) as a Federal Advisory Committee. The Committee provides the president, congress, and the federal agencies involved in networking and information technology research and development with expert, independent advice on maintaining America's preeminence in advanced information technologies.

Prevalence   The number of existing cases of disease

Prevalence rate   The number of existing cases of a disease in a specified time period divided by the population at that time. The quotient is then multiplied by a constant, such as 1000 or 100,000. Prevalence rates are determined to examine the frequency of specific types of disease.

Prevalence study   A type of descriptive study that examines the distribution of disease or health characteristics in a population at one point in time. This study is used to generate hypotheses. (See also Cross-sectional study.)

Preventive discipline   A disciplinary approach that encourages understanding of the rationale for and compliance with policies, standards, and rules so that significant violations of policy are avoided.

Primary care   The care provided at the point of first contact (encounter) with the health care provider in an ambulatory care setting; the care is continuous and comprehensive. Primary care encompasses preventive care (comprehensive care) and acute care.

Primary data   The information contained in the actual patient record.

Primary key   In database design, a primary key is a value that can be used to identify a unique row in a table. Attributes are associated with the primary key. In a relational model of data, a primary key is a key chosen as the main method of uniquely identifying a tuple in a relation. A tuple represents some object and its associated data. A key is a constraint that requires that critical information about the object not be duplicated.

Primary patient record   The record that is used by health care practitioners while providing patient care services to review patient data or document their own observations, actions, or instructions.

Privacy   The right of individuals to control disclosure of their personal information.

Privilege delineation   The process of determining the specific procedures and services a physician or other professional is permitted to perform under the jurisdiction of the health care organization. The applicant formally requests specific privileges, and any award of privileges must be supported with documentation of training, education, and other evidence of qualification or competence.

Privileged communication   Statements made to attorneys, priests, physicians, spouses, or others in a legally recognized position of trust. The confidentiality of these statements is generally protected by law from being revealed, even in court.

Proactive risk assessments Patient safety improvement projects that are proactive. These projects are initiated prospectively for the purpose of avoiding an undesirable event.

Procedures The guides and plans for action. The step-by-step instructions for accomplishing a specific task or job.

Process Similar work processes or procedures are grouped together and performed by a particular unit or group of employees.

Process measures Process measures focus on what is done during the delivery of health care services. Some process measures evaluate the quality of the health care professional's decisions as they direct a patient's course of treatment.

Productive time The time during which a worker is present and working.

Productive unit of work An item produced that meets established levels of quality.

Productivity Process for converting the resources of an organization (labor, capital, materials, and technology) into products and/or services that meet the organization's goals.

Productivity standards Tools used to specify the expected performance and to measure actual performance. Also known as work standards.

Profession A profession is an occupation that requires extensive training and the study and mastery of specialized knowledge and skill and usually has a professional association, ethical code, and process of certification or licensing.

Profit The amount of money (cash) actually received from the payer (patient or insurance company) less the actual cost to do the service, assuming that the cost is less than the cash received.

Progressive discipline A process used in response to employee misconduct, in which there is a planned sequence of managerial responses of increasing severity to correct continuing violations of policy. Progressive discipline gives the employee subject to the disciplinary process several opportunities to correct the offensive behavior before the final irrevocable step of termination is invoked.

Project A unit of work to acquire or build and implement a computer system (software, hardware, and all infrastructure) with a definitive start date, targeted stop date, steps, milestones, and outcome.

Project life cycle Refers to the development phases that a project can go through. The project life cycle is tailored to suit individual project needs.

Project management Group of people with expertise in a variety of functions led by a project manager who work to accomplish a single goal.

Project management life cycle Refers to a project management cycle and consists of five sequential stages (initiate, plan, execute, control, and close).

Promulgated Formally made public, most frequently used in relationship to the act of formally, publicly declaring new statutory or administrative law when it receives final approval.

Proportion A proportion is similar to a rate. A proportion, which is a part considered in relation to the whole, is normally expressed as a fraction (20/1000, 2/100, 1/100,000, 10/1,000,000, and so on).

Proprietary Private, for profit, or investor-owned (hospitals).

Proprietary system A system that uses only equipment designed and manufactured by a certain vendor.

Prospective payment A method of reimbursement based on payment rates that are established in advance and reflect an average of what a service should cost.

Prospective payment system (PPS) A reimbursement program in which the amount of payment is determined in advance of services rendered. Rates are established annually by the Centers for Medicare and Medicaid Services.

Prospective review process Review of health care utilization is intended to reduce over- and under-use of services by examining the appropriateness of care. The prospective review process is initiated before a patient actually receives health services. If the patient's health plan requires prior approval of high-cost services (such as nuclear imaging studies or elective surgeries), the provider or facility contacts the utilization management company or health plan to obtain approval on behalf of the patient.

Prospective study A type of study that determines whether the characteristic or suspected risk factor truly preceded the disease or health condition. The prospective study design is the best method for determining the magnitude of risk in the population with the characteristic or suspected risk factor. Also referred to as a cohort or incident study.

Protected health information Under the HIPAA privacy rule, patient health information that could be used to identify an individual and should be kept confidential.

Protocols Computer-based communication protocols are specifications or algorithms for how data are to be exchanged. Protocols may also be used to describe the expected or recommended course of treatment for a particular health condition.

Prototype A draft that is developed to provide a preliminary model or early version.

Provider Any entity that provides health care services to patients, including health care organizations (hospitals, clinics) and health care professionals.

Proximate cause That which, in a sequence unbroken by intervening causes, produced injury, and with which the injury would not have occurred; in other words, the primary or substantial cause of an injury. Whether an action or omission is the proximate cause of an injury is sometimes a difficult question involved in negligence/malpractice litigation.

Proximity chart Matrix that provides information useful in workspace design; shows the desirability of having work areas close to or far apart from one another.

Proxy server A form of firewall that intercepts all messages entering and leaving the network so that the network address is hidden.

Public health Focuses on the threats to the overall health of a community based on population-based health data analysis, as opposed to medical health care, which focuses on the treatment of the individual.

Public health informatics The systematic application of information from public health practice and research, using computer science and technology. The majority of the work in public health informatics in the United States occurs at the local and state level, in the state, county, or parish departments of public health.

Public key One of the most popular forms of encryption. A public key is a key that the user gives to anyone he or she wants to receive the message. Web servers often have a public key available to the requester of a Web document.

Qualitative analysis (1) Part of a quality assessment and improvement study of patient records. Qualitative analysis involves reviewing the record for consistency, completeness, and accuracy of facts including diagnoses found on admission forms, physical examination, operative and pathology reports, care plans, and discharge summary. (2) A review of the patient record that assesses how well a standard is being met. Typically requires training and judgment on the part of the assessor, and is frequently used to assess documentation standards.

Qualitative research   A type of descriptive study design that is used when little is known about a specific topic. Qualitative research provides richer information than can be obtained from quantitative-based studies alone. Qualitative research is most appropriate to use when one is examining attitudes, feelings, perceptions, or relationships.

Quality improvement   Initiatives or efforts to improve the quality of health care and customer satisfaction.

Quality improvement organizations   Organizations contracted by CMS (Centers for Medicare and Medicaid Services) at the state level to direct and oversee nationwide health care performance measurement and improvement initiatives.

Quantitative analysis   (1) Part of a quality assessment and improvement study of patient records. Quantitative analysis involves checking patient records for correctness, presence, and authentication of all authorizations and consents, documented diagnoses, procedures, discharge summaries, histories and physicals, consultation reports, diagnostic tests, physician or practitioner orders, and operative, procedure, therapy, pathology, preoperative, operative, postoperative, and other reports. (2) A review of the patient record to assess whether an item of required documentation is present or absent. This analysis may also apply time requirements to the expectation of required documentation.

Quick response code   A two-dimensional bar code consisting of black modules (square dots) arranged in a square grid on a white background. The QR code can be read faster and contain more information than a traditional bar code. Many mobile devices have an application that can read a QR code directly from the device.

Qui tam   Whistleblower-based prosecutions.

Random sample   A sample in which every member of the population has the same chance of being included in the sample and the selection of one member has no effect on selection of another member.

Random selection   The method of choosing the sample that gives each item in the population an equal chance of being chosen.

Range   The difference between the highest and lowest values of a set of numbers; a way to measure dispersion.

Rapid cycle improvement (RCI)   A performance improvement model that uses an accelerated method (usually less than 4 to 6 weeks per improvement cycle) to collect and analyze data and to make informed changes on the basis of that analysis. This is then followed by another improvement cycle to evaluate the success of the change. RCI relies on small process changes and immediate, careful measurement of the effect of these changes.

Rate   The number of individuals with a specific characteristic divided by the total number of individuals, or alternatively the number of times an event did occur compared with the number of times it could have occurred.

Ratio   A ratio is similar to a rate. A ratio is expressed as 20:1000, 2:100, 1:100,000, 10:1,000,000, and so on. The number of physicians relative to patients or teachers relative to students is normally expressed as a ratio. For example, if a physician group practice has 10 physicians and 1000 patients, the ratio is 10:1000, which reduces to 1:100.

Ratio analysis   The management process of formulating judgments and decisions from the relationship between the numbers represented on two reports: the balance sheet and the statement of revenues and expenses. (See also Financial analysis.)

Ratio data   Ratio data share the property of equal differences with interval data. What is unique about ratio data is that the value of 0 represents the total absence of the trait or characteristic being measured. Examples of ratio data include height and weight of patients and length of stay at a hospital.

Reasonable accommodation   Adjustments made to the workplace to accommodate an employee's disability that allow the employee to perform the essential job functions without causing undue hardship to the employer.

"Reasonable man" standard   If a claim involves simple (not professional) negligence such as in a personal injury suit, the jury uses the "reasonable man" standard to evaluate the defendant parties' conduct in light of the jury's own general experience and background.

Recognized redundancy   Terms with the same meaning are treated as synonyms and are represented by the same identifying code.

Record   A row within the data dictionary table. It contains the data elements within fields that will provide sufficient data to identify a unique instance of the entity.

Recruitment pool   A maintained list of potential applicants who are presumably qualified and willing to perform one or more target positions in the organization.

Re-engineering   Fundamental rethinking and radical redesign of business processes to achieve dramatic improvements in performance, such as cost, quality, service, and speed; management theory in which the way business is done is radically re-evaluated to achieve dramatic performance improvement.

Reference date   The date the registry began accessioning cases.

Regional health information organizations (RHIOs)   Organizations that are working together to develop means of sharing health information for patient care and other uses, typically within a geographic area. Various models exist, including models where the information stays with its originator and is accessed as authorized and models that centralize data and control access as authorized. RHIOs are part of the development of a national health information infrastructure.

Registered health information administrator (RHIA)   A credential offered by AHIMA to individuals who pass a certification examination and successfully meet the academic requirements of a CAHIIM-accredited health information management program at the baccalaureate degree level or have a certificate of completion from a CAHIIM-accredited health information management program plus a baccalaureate degree from a regionally accredited college or university. The RHIA functions in the managerial areas of health services and information systems and the uses of health-related data for planning, delivering, and evaluating health care.

Registered health information technician (RHIT) A credential offered by AHIMA to individuals who pass a certification examination and successfully meet the academic requirements of a CAHIIM-accredited health information management program at the associate degree level. The RHIT typically functions in the technical areas of health data collection, analysis, and monitoring, and often specializes in coding diagnoses and procedures for reimbursement and research purposes.

Registered record librarian (RRL)   A credential first offered to individuals in 1933 when the American Association of Medical Record Librarians (now known as AHIMA) formed a Board of Registration to set standards for its members.

Registration   (1) For the purpose of professional recognition, entails entering on an official list an individual who has been certified as eligible by set qualifications of an organization or agency. (2) The process of gathering information from an individual to assist in providing care. This information consists of administrative data and pertinent clinical data. The data are entered into a computer system that is used to track registration for services, outpatient, emergency, admission to inpatient care, transfers within the care system, and discharge from care.

Registry   A method of systematic and ongoing data collection that is population-based (includes all cases of TBI in a defined population, e.g., a state), includes personal identifying and contact information for each case, and may be used for follow-up of TBI cases over time and/or linking TBI cases to services.

Regression analysis   Analysis used to learn to what extent one or more explanatory variables can predict an outcome variable.

Regulation   Dictates of government agencies charged with enforcing and implementing legislation in a particular area; these dictates are designed to carry out the intent of the law.

Rehabilitation   The processes of treatment and education that lead the disabled person to the achievement of maximum independence and function and a personal sense of well-being.

Reimbursement formula   The agreement between the third-party payers and the providers concerning what will be paid for and how much will be paid to the provider.

Relational model   The most popular database model. Designed around the concept that all data are stored in tables with relationships between the tables. A relationship is created by sharing a common data element; for example, if two tables have a patient identifier, patient identifier relates those tables. Developed by E. F. Codd in 1970.

Relative humidity   The percentage of moisture in the air.

Relative risk   An estimate of risk found by using the odds ratio in an epidemiologic study.

Reliability   Refers to consistency between users of a given instrument or method.

Reliable   A term used to describe a measure that is stable, showing consistent results over time and among different users of the measure. A reliable measure has low levels of random error.

Regenstrief LOINC Mapping Assistant (RELMA)   The tool that is used to view and search the LOINC database. The purpose of the database is to facilitate the exchange of results for clinical care, outcomes management, and research.

Replacement charts   Charts used in human resource planning that present a visual representation of who is available to fill projected vacant positions. Replacement charts usually identify individual incumbents, the most likely (or all potential) replacements, and summary measures of performance and promotion potential.

Request for information (RFI)   Solicits general information from vendors about their products. The RFI may state in general terms what the facility is looking for in system functionality. Vendors then respond with information about their product lines and their experience in the marketplace and provide copies of their annual reports.

Request for proposal   A document that details all required system functionality, including functional, technical, training, and implementation requirements. The document is distributed to a selected number of vendors, who are invited to respond to the proposal.

Requisition   An acknowledgment that someone has taken a record and intends to return it.

Res ipsa loquitur   "The thing speaks for itself" doctrine applied to cases where the defendant had exclusive control of the thing that caused the harm and where the harm ordinarily could not have occurred without negligent conduct.

Research   A systematic investigation, including research development, testing and evaluation, designed to develop or contribute to generalizable knowledge.

Research question   Asks a question to be answered and identifies the goal of the research.

Resident   A patient who resides in a long-term care facility.

Respite care   A type of short-term care that allows caregivers time off while continuing the care of the patient. Respite care is often provided to caregivers of terminally ill patients or severely disabled children or adults.

Respondeat superior   "Let the master answer." Under this doctrine, health care organizations must take reasonable steps to supervise the actions of their employees and professional staff (including medical staff). Organizations can be held liable for damages when their employees fail to perform their duties adequately.

Response rate   The rate of individuals who respond (in a survey).

Restraint of trade   Contracts or agreements that tend to or are designed to eliminate or stifle competition, create a monopoly, artificially maintain prices, or otherwise hamper or obstruct the course of trade and commerce. When the medical or professional staff credentialing process interferes with a physician's or health professional's ability to pursue his or her profession.

Results reporting   Applications designed to retrieve diagnostic test and treatment results from feeder systems such as laboratory, radiology, and other departmental settings such as transcription and present them directly on inquiry to the care provider. Results reporting usually includes a graphical user interface (GUI) for viewing laboratory results, ECG results, and other reports using graphics displays such as flow sheets.

Retention period   The amount of time a health care organization keeps patient records. The retention period varies depending on federal and state regulations and organization needs.

Retrospective payment system   A payment method in which the charges for the health care services are determined after the health care was provided. The actual amount paid may be based on fee for service or on the usual, customary, and reasonable charges.

Retrospective review   A review that occurs after care has been rendered. A retrospective review can provide valuable information about patterns of undesirable practices that can be used to improve future performance.

Retrospective study   One type of analytic study design. The researcher collects data on the cases (those who have the disease that is under study) and controls (those who are similar to the cases but do not have the disease that is under study) by looking back in time (See also Case control study).

Return on investment (ROI)   The money earned from investment at a certain interest rate.

Revenue   Money earned from the services provided (in a health care organization).

Right of privacy   A constitutionally recognized right to be left alone, to make decisions about one's own body, and to control one's own information. Right of privacy is an important constitutional right for the health care industry.

Risk   Any event or situation that could potentially result in injury to an individual or financial loss to the health care organization.

Risk factors   Factors that may increase the risk for development of a disease. Also referred to as exposure characteristics.

Risk management Encompasses all policies, procedures, and practices directed at reducing risk and subsequent liability for injuries that occur in the organization's immediate environment. The policies and procedures that constitute a risk management program are developed in collaboration with the health care organization's legal counsel because judicial interpretation of statutory law in the court system is a continually evolving process. In general, risk management activities are intended to minimize the potential for injury occurrence, ensure prompt and appropriate response to injured parties, and anticipate and plan for ensuing liability when injuries occur. Activities are directed at preventing or reducing financial loss, allocating funds for compensable events, and diminishing negative public image resulting from injury claims.

Rolling budget method A budgeting method that requires management to prepare a budget for a period of time and add to the end of that period another month when a month is consumed.

Root cause analysis A systematic investigation process that occurs after a complication or adverse event that resulted in a patient injury caused by medical management rather than by the underlying disease or condition of the patient.

Run chart A chart used to provide a visual method of monitoring trends over time. A run chart can illustrate performance trends and standards of evaluation over a long time period.

RXCUI A RxNorm concept unique identifier. If there are two drug names that share the same concept, RxNorm assigns the preferred name and a concept unique identifier. The RXCUI always designates the same concept, no matter the source, the form of the name, or in what table it is found.

RxNorm A standardized nomenclature for clinical drugs and drug delivery devices produced by the NLM.

Sample The group of items chosen to represent the whole population. The size of the sample is important because it must be large enough to represent all members of the group but small enough to be manageable and cost effective.

Sample size In a study, the number of subjects included in the sample.

Sampling error The principle that the characteristics of a sample are not identical to the characteristics of the population from which the sample is drawn.

Satellite clinic An ambulatory care facility that is not located on the campus of the main hospital. Satellite clinics are established in areas that are convenient to the patients, such as places of employment, or in areas that are closer to a specific patient population.

Satisfactory assurance For a subpoena *duces tecum* for health information to be valid under the HIPAA privacy rule, reasonable efforts must be made by the party seeking information to ensure that the individual who is the subject of the protected health information has been given notice of the request or that the party seeking the information has made reasonable efforts to secure a qualified protective order that meets the requirements of the HIPAA privacy rule.

Scanner Usually referred to as a bar code scanner, scanners are available in two types: contact and noncontact. A contact scanner is sometimes referred to as a light pen or wand and must come in contact with the bar code to read its contents. Noncontact scanners can be hand-held or fixed.

Scenario A "story," narrative description, or simulation that represents an actual situation. Also referred to as a use case.

Script-based systems An alternative form of structured text, script-based systems combine key words and scripts. Scanning for key words invokes a particular script. The script itself then serves as a building block for the remainder of the text-processing event and may act as a template that specifies necessary components and the properties required.

Secondary care Care by a specialist, usually through referral from the primary care physician.

Secondary data The information that is generated from the patient record.

Secondary patient data The patient record is a valuable source of data for research such as comparative effectiveness research, program evaluation, education, and public health studies. Data from the record that are stored in government and private databases are often termed *secondary patient data* and are used in the aggregate for these purposes.

Secondary patient record A subset that is derived from the primary record and contains selected data elements.

Security of health information HIPAA and good business practices require that health care organizations implement administrative, technical, and physical safeguards to protect the confidentiality, integrity, and appropriate availability of health information maintained in either paper or electronic format. HIPAA's focus is on protected health information in electronic format.

Selection process Involves a sequence of activities that should result in the hiring of a well-qualified employee to fill the target position.

Self-appraisal A method of employee performance evaluation that requires an employee to reflect on his or her performance for the period, identify strengths and weaknesses, and identify accomplishments and obstacles to progress before the formal performance appraisal review.

Self-pay A payment method in which the patient pays the health care provider directly. Also referred to as out-of-pocket pay or direct pay.

Semantic content The meaning of the message.

Semantic interoperability The most sophisticated level of interoperability, incorporating the semantic content of the message. At this level, data received from another system can be displayed, interpreted, and manipulated as if it were generated locally.

Sensitivity A measure of validity, sensitivity is the percentage of all true cases correctly identified.

Sentinel event A term used to describe serious patient incidents that should have a root cause analysis (a systematic investigation as to what, how, and why something happened). Examples of sentinel events include abduction of a baby from the newborn nursery and amputation of the wrong body part.

Serial numbering A system of number assignment in which a patient receives a number for each encounter at the facility. The patient could have multiple numbers, all of which require entry onto the manual index card or maintenance in the computerized database. Each encounter at the facility requires the use of a new file folder in a paper-based system. Each new folder is filed in a different location, requiring the searching of multiple locations to retrieve one patient's entire record.

Serial-unit numbering A numbering method developed to combine the ease of number assignment from serial numbering and the unit record concept from unit numbering. Numbers are assigned serially, but as each new encounter takes place, all the former records in a paper-based system are brought forward to the most recently assigned record number and filed together as a unit in the same folder. Typically, the previously used folder

(s) remain in place and a note is placed on/in the folder noting the newly assigned number.

Servlet   A program that executes itself on the Web server and handles multiple requests simultaneously. Servlets reside on the server side and function by having the user's request run directly on the Web server to generate dynamic HTML pages. This technology is generally used to provide interactive Web sites that interface to databases or other data sources.

Sexual harassment   A form of gender discrimination that can produce a number of negative effects in the workplace including decreased productivity, increased worker stress and illness, higher turnover and absenteeism, lower morale, interference with team building, additional recruitment and training costs, and potential legal liabilities.

Simulation   A technique to replace or amplify real-life experiences with guided experiences that evoke or replicate substantial aspects of the real world in a fully interactive manner. This technique is helpful in preparing people for error-prone, high-risk, or unusual situations. By simulating possible adverse events, people learn to recognize problems and understand the effects of their responses in a safe environment. Simulation forces people to review processes on a very detailed level, which can help to improve patient safety.

Simultaneous equations method   An allocation method that permits multiple allocations to occur through sophisticated mathematic software and the use of simultaneous mathematic equations. This method, also known as the algebraic or multiple apportionment method, may require 10 to 12 different distributions of costs.

Single blind   Subject blind as to which study group he or she is in.

Six Sigma   A performance improvement approach that aims to eliminate defects. Under this approach, results that fail to meet performance standards are called "defects," typically reported as defects per million opportunities. Six Sigma is the performance level attained when a process yields only 3.4 defects per million opportunities. The goal is to achieve an almost perfect level of quality by eliminating these defects.

Skilled nursing facility   A facility providing long-term care is considered to be a nonacute care facility or skilled nursing facility. The type of care a patient can receive is highly variable and ranges from personal care and social, recreational, and dietary services to skilled nursing or rehabilitation care.

Slander   Oral defamation of character that tends to damage the defamed person's reputation in the eyes of the community.

Sliding scale fee   The cost of health care is based on the patient's ability to pay.

Software   The set of instructions required to operate computers and their applications. Software includes programs that are sets of instructions that direct actual computer operating functions, called the operating system, and sets of instructions used to accomplish various types of business processes, known as application software.

Solo practices   Physicians who are self-employed and legally the sole owners of their practices.

Specialist lexicon   A database of lexicographic information for use in natural language processing. The lexicon includes more than 200,000 items and identifies their spelling, form, and structure, as well as how they are put together to create meaning. The lexicon is used in natural language processing applications.

Specific aims   Briefly describes a project's goals or objectives.

Specificity   A measure of validity, specificity is the percentage of all true noncases correctly identified.

Stable monetary unit   Accounting entities use a stable monetary unit of measure to record and report financial transactions. In the United States this stable monetary unit is represented by the U.S. dollar.

Staff hour   Sixty minutes of time during which an employee is working on a task or a particular function and being paid for that work.

Staffing table   A tool used in human resource planning that provides a graphic representation of job titles and anticipated position vacancies.

Stage   In reference to cancer, the stage is the extent of the spread of the disease.

Stakeholder   In relationship to a computer project, any individual who has a stake or real interest in the project and its implementation, regardless of department, position, or functional role in the company.

Standard deviation   The square root of variance. Represented by the symbol σ.

Standard of care   The generally accepted standards of care (for each profession), determined by referring to current standards published by the relevant specialty society and the professional literature. Sometimes determined by referring to accreditation and licensing standards.

Standardized mortality ratio (SMR)   An indirect method of age adjustment.

Standardized terminology   Uniform terms, concepts, and definitions used to create clinical documentation for symptoms, diagnoses, procedures, test findings, health status, problem lists, and plans in the EHR.

Stare decisis   "Let the decision stand." A legal principle that courts should decide similar cases similarly. In other words, cases that have similar facts and questions should ordinarily be decided the same way.

Statement of cash flow   This report documents the change in cash balance for a given accounting period and is useful in evaluating an organization's ability to pay its bills. The statement of cash flow looks at sources and uses of cash based on the organization's operating, investing, and financing activities.

Statement of revenues and expenses   A financial report of the expected or earned income and the associated expenses for an accounting period. This financial report may also be referred to as the income statement and can be described by the following equation: Revenue − Expense = Net income.

Statistical analysis   A process performed to select specific data items from medical records for clinical and administrative decision-making. Uses of statistical analysis range from billing and case-mix analysis to selection of cases for quality review. (See also Abstracting.)

Statistics budget   Budget based on historical data regarding the volume and type of health care services provided, data about the community, and future projection of need for health care services. All available data are used to estimate types and volumes of health care services needed for the projected budget period.

Statute   A law enacted by Congress or state legislatures.

Statute of limitations   A law that requires a claim to be filed within a certain period of time; otherwise the claim will not be heard by a court. Statutes of limitations are designed to encourage the timely filing of claims, when evidence is fresh and witnesses are likely to be available. In most states the statute of limitations begins at the time of the event or (in a health care case) at the age of majority if the patient was treated as a minor.

Step-down method   A common allocation method in which the indirect department that receives the least amount of service from other indirect departments and provides the most service to other departments has its costs allocated first.

Stopwatch study   A technique for setting productivity standards. Stopwatch studies require a skilled analyst to observe the employee performing the task and to record stop and start times for each portion of the task.

Store and forward   Data are initially gathered and then sent at another time.

Strategic control   Final stage of strategic management process that includes (1) establishment of standards (objectives), (2) measurement of performance, (3) evaluation of organizational performance against the standards, and (4) taking corrective action, if necessary.

Strategic human resource planning   A proactive human resource management activity in which managers must continually forecast and coordinate the supply of qualified human resources the predicted demand on the basis of workflow cycles in health information services. This strategic approach to planning anticipates and prepares for future staffing needs.

Strategic implementation   The third step in the strategic management process; based on the operational strategies that have been developed.

Stratified random sample   A random sample that's obtained by dividing a population into groups (strata) and taking random samples from each stratum. Stratified random sampling is done to ensure that the sample is representative of the population.

Structure measures   Indirectly assess care by looking at certain provider characteristics and the physical and organizational resources available to support the delivery of care. Structure measures look at the capability or potential for providing quality care. By their nature, structure measures are static because the organization or individual is evaluated at a unique point in time.

Structured data   A type of data entry that allows users to draw from standard phrases or pick lists and pull-down menus to help guide the entry and ensure that complete information is included.

Subject blind   In a clinical or community trial, the subject has no knowledge as to which group he or she is in.

Subpoena   A written court order that requires someone to come before the court to testify.

Subpoena *duces tecum*   A written court order that requires someone to come before the court and to bring certain records or documents named in that order.

Surveillance   The collection, collation, analysis, and dissemination of data.

Survey design   A type of descriptive study in which the research focuses on collecting data with a survey instrument such as a questionnaire or interview guide.

Swing beds   Designated hospital beds that have the flexibility of serving as acute care or post acute care long-term beds.

Symbiology   The way the lines and spaces in a bar code are arranged.

Syndromic surveillance system   A public health surveillance system that can detect patterns of disease in a population and that is designed to recognize outbreaks on the basis of the symptoms and signs of infection.

System   Series of elements that are interrelated according to a plan for achieving a well-defined goal.

System analysis and design   The activities related to specifying the details of a new system. Typically, this includes making decisions about the logical and physical design of the system.

System development life cycle   The process used to identify, investigate, design, select, and implement information systems. The system development life cycle consists of five principal phases: initiation phase, analysis phase, design phase, implementation phase, and evaluation phase.

System testing   Often called user acceptance testing. For electronic health record applications, information systems staff set up a "test database" that consists of the full system features and functions complete with dummy patients supplied by users. This test database is isolated from the "production" database and made available to selected users who add fake data and then test the system's features and functionality. Performance is measured against test plan criteria established earlier.

Systematic sampling   A sampling method in which the researcher must first decide what fraction or proportion of the population is to be sampled. If a researcher decided to sample one tenth of the population, the researcher would first randomly choose a starting point on a list of the population and then select every tenth record beginning with the designated starting point.

Systems flow chart   Depicts the flow of data through all or part of the system, the various operations that take place within the system, and the files that are used to produce various reports or documents.

Table   The physical representation of the data dictionary entity. Like the field, it is the container that has the data elements that will describe many instances of the entity in the manner established by the logical data model.

Tags   Used to define or describe the text that is contained in them.

Task lighting   Light fixtures that are built into the furniture or workstations to illuminate specific work areas; especially important in an open office design. Also referred to as accent lighting.

Task-ambient lighting   Combination of general light with light directed to the work surface.

Tax Equity and Fiscal Responsibility Act (TEFRA)   A law enacted in 1983 that brought prospective pricing to health care and enhanced the value of the patient record because it became the key document for supporting and determining reimbursements to hospitals.

Template   A pattern used in computer-based patient records to capture data in a structured manner; it may contain both text and data objects.

Terminal   Connected to information systems and used to enter and retrieve information.

Terminal digit filing   A filing method based on a patient identification number that is divided into three parts. Most facilities use a minimum of six digits (filling any unused digits on the left for numbers lower than 100,000 with zeros), and other facilities use the terminal digit method with numbers as large as a nine-digit number.

Terminology   The usage and study of terms. The labeling or designating of concepts particular to one or more subject fields through the research and analysis of terms in context, for the purpose of documenting and promoting correct usage.

Tertiary care   The care provided at facilities with advanced technologies and specialized intensive care units, such as teaching institutions and university medical centers.

Test statistic   Measures the size of the difference or relationship observed in the sample.

Tests of significance   Used to determine whether observed differences between groups or relationships between variables in the sample being studied are likely to be due to chance and sampling error or reflect true differences or relationships in the population of interest.

Text processing The computerized processing of natural language.

The Joint Commission A private entity whose primary function is to develop and assess standards of performance by health care organizations. The organization's goal is to improve the quality of health care. Recent initiatives include data collection and dissemination regarding sentinel events and treatment for certain types of health problems. This organization changed its name from the Joint Commission for the Accreditation of Healthcare Organizations (JCAHO) to The Joint Commission (TJC) in 2007.

The National Committee for Quality Assurance (NCQA) A private, not-for-profit organization established in 1990. NCQA accredits a variety of organizations from health maintenance organizations to accountable care organizations to managed behavioral health care organizations, and each accreditation program has distinct performance management requirements.

Thesaurus A work that lists words grouped together according to similar meaning.

Thick client A device that requires a substantial amount of memory and disk space to perform functions that the application may require. Thick clients are devices that might include a desktop PC or a workstation.

Thin client A device that has minimal or no disk space; it loads its software and data from a server and then uploads any data it produces back to the server. Thin clients are devices that vary from a laptop computer to a hand-held network instrument.

Third-party payer Private insurance companies, managed care organizations (MCOs), and fiscal intermediaries (FIs) that process claims for Medicare and Medicaid.

Three-tier A type of client-server architecture that has three components: user interface, application server, and database server. The user interface is the software that runs on the user or client machine, and it can be customized to the needs of the client. The application server processes the data. The logic behind the database queries is hidden from the user.

Threshold The minimum acceptable quality on the basis of the organization's historical performance.

Time value of money A basic concept of money management that says that it is more beneficial to receive a dollar today than to receive it 1 year from now. A dollar received today can be invested and gain interest for 1 year longer than a dollar received 1 year from now.

Token ring When transmissions travel from one computer to another until they reach their final destination, allowing a single computer to be added to or disconnected from the network without affecting the rest of the computers on the local area network.

Topography Site or location of a neoplasm.

Tort In private law, tort refers to an action where one party alleges that another party's wrongful conduct has caused him or her harm. The party bringing the action to court seeks compensation for that harm.

Training manual Materials that teach concepts that serve as background to hands-on exercises that teach system functionality and outcomes.

Transactional leadership Those behaviors associated with the more routine and continuous exchanges of effort and commitment between managers and employees in carrying out the business of the organization and sustaining effective working relationships.

Transformational leadership The visionary, motivational, and charismatic aspects of leadership. The transformational leader is able to articulate a vision of the organization's future, to convince followers that they have a stake in the achievement of that vision, and to achieve commitment to change (personal and organizational) as not only inevitable but also beneficial both to the organization and to the employee's self-interest.

Trauma center An emergency care center that is specially staffed and equipped to handle trauma patients; most trauma centers are equipped with an air transport system.

Triage The process of sorting out patients in the emergency department to determine the urgency and priority for care and to determine the appropriate source of care. Triage promotes efficiency and effectiveness in the management of the diverse patient group arriving in the emergency department.

TRICARE (formerly CHAMPUS) A health insurance program provided by the Department of Defense for active and retired military personnel and their dependents.

Trip frequency chart Matrix that represents the number of times employees interact with one another in a specified period of time; used in designing a work space.

Triple blind Subject, observer, and statistician blind as to the study group they are in.

Turnover ratios Ratios that use data from the balance sheet and the statement of revenues and expenses to measure an organization's ability to generate net operating revenue in relation to its various assets. Also referred to as activity ratios.

Two-factor authentication Authentication protocol that requires two forms of authentication to access the system (token plus a password). Also referred to as strong authentication.

Two-tier A type of client-server architecture that was developed in the early 1990s in which most of the processing occurs on the server. It reduces network traffic by providing a query response rather than total file transfer. The user interface is located on the user's desktop, and the database management application and data tables are stored on a database server.

Universal Medical Device Nomenclature System (UMDNS) A proprietary, standardized, and controlled international nomenclature and coding system for medical devices that has been adopted by more than 90 countries and more than 5,000 institutions.

UMLS Developed by the U.S. National Library of Medicine to bring together diverse coding schemes with multiple terminologies, UMLS connects scores of vocabularies, classifications, and other sources by concept, allowing users to map data from one terminology to another.

Undue hardship Any action that would require significant difficulty or expense when considered in light of the nature and cost of the accommodation in relation to the size, resources, technology, and structures of the employer's operation.

Unique identifier A number that is assigned to link patients to their records. This number is used on all record forms and views to collect all patient data in the correct record or to be accessed by computer database query.

Unit numbering system A system developed to prevent assigning a new number for each patient encounter and to avoid searching multiple locations for record folders. In the unit numbering system, each patient receives an identification number at the first encounter and retains that number throughout all contacts with the facility.

Use case A scenario, "story," or description that represents an actual situation.

User   A user in computing context is one who uses a computer system. Users typically have an account (a user account), a username, and a password.

User manual   A complete textual documentation of the system that includes all system features and functionality, complete rationale behind use of particular features, complete picture of system usage within organization or user environment, solutions to potential problems with usage, sources of help for users, and so forth.

Usual, customary, and reasonable charges   The physician's usual charge for the service, the amount that physicians in the area usually charge for the same service, and whether the amount charged is reasonable for the service provided.

Utilization management (UM)   Activities that are intended to ensure that facilities and resources (both human and nonhuman) are used appropriately to meet the health care needs of patients. Both underutilization (unmet patient needs) and overutilization (provision of care or services not medically necessary) are undesirable outcomes.

Utilization review   The process of evaluating the efficiency and appropriateness of health care services according to predetermined criteria.

Validity   Assesses relevance, completeness, accuracy, and correctness. Validity measures how well a data collection instrument, laboratory test, medical record abstract, or other data source measures what it should measure.

Value/coding   The value or coding for a data element represents a more specified way that values may be returned to the data element question. In general, it represents a tighter leash on the domain of the element by specifying more specifically what the answer to the data element question can be.

Values   The fundamental beliefs or truths that the organization adheres to.

Values clarification   The idea that reflecting on and understanding our own value commitments and priorities is an essential process as a precondition for ethically responsive decision-making and leadership.

Variance   Measures the deviations of the values from the mean. Variance is computed by squaring each deviation from the mean, summing the deviations, and then dividing their sum by one less than n, the sample size.

Variance report   A document that reflects the budget that was prepared and approved and shows the actual results on at least a monthly basis.

Vertical integration   Network of health care organizations that provide or arrange to provide a continuum of services to a population; the network assumes the clinical and fiscal responsibility for the outcomes and health status of the population.

View   In a computer system a view is a particular way of looking at the data in a database. The view organizes the data visible on the computer screen in a way that meets the needs of a user. Different users may need different views of data from the same database. Different views do not affect the physical organization of the database.

Virtual machine   A virtual machine is a software container with an operating system and application inside. A single computer can run many virtual machines within its hardware.

Vision   View of the future that management believes is optimum for the organization and is communicated throughout the organization.

Vital statistics   Data collected for vital events in our lives, such as births and adoptions, marriages and divorces, and deaths, including fetal deaths.

Vocabulary   A set of terms and their corresponding definitions. Used to represent concepts and to communicate these concepts.

Voice recognition   The computer capability to understand human speech. Voice recognition allows practitioners to talk directly to devices and record findings.

Weighted mean   An overall mean (average) for a total sample when separate means are reported for different subdivisions of the sample.

Whistleblower   An individual who goes outside regulatory bodies in an organization to raise a problem rather than reporting a suspected unlawful activity internally.

Whole service   When facilities or individuals are paid for all services rendered at the rate the facility or individual charges with no discount applied.

Wi-Fi   A type of network that enables computers and other handheld devices to communicate with the Internet and other network servers without being physically connected to the network. Also referred to as wireless.

Wireless   A type of network (popular in health care) that enables computers and other hand-held devices to communicate with the Internet and other network servers without being physically connected to the network. (See also Wi-Fi.)

Work breakdown structures   Divides the project into major objectives, partitions each objective into activities, further divides the activities into sub-activities, and creates work packages that must be done to complete the project.

Work distribution chart   A useful tool that provides data to analyze the processes performed by a work group and the individual employee within the work group. Examination of the data assists in identifying problems but not solutions. The work distribution chart is a matrix that displays the tasks being performed in a work group, the employees who perform them, and the amount of time spent on each task by each employee and the work unit as a whole.

Work sampling   Method of measuring work that collects data about the work being performed on randomly selected times of observations.

Work simplification   Organized approach to determine how to accomplish a task with less effort, in less time, or at a lower cost while maintaining or improving the quality of the outcome.

Workforce   The authorized employees of an organization as used in the HIPAA Privacy Rule.

Workstation   A PC or other device that is connected to an information system. A workstation is used to connect directly with the database in the system and to access and receive information from the system directly. A workstation is well suited for applications that require more memory and disk storage than a desktop PC, and usually functions as part of a hospital network. Also, a collection of desks or work surfaces, equipment, storage facilities, and chairs shaped by technology, the tasks to be performed, and various human needs.

Zero-based budget   A type of budgeting approach that requires management to complete a program assessment and define consequences if specific programs are terminated or reduced.

INDEX

Note: Page numbers followed by *f* indicate figures, *t* indicate tables and *b* indicate boxes.

Information resources management committee, 127
Information system(s)
  implementation phase of, 338
  integrating, 531–532
  life cycle of, 367
  testing of, 341–343
Information system analysis, process modeling, 334
Information technology
  applications, 663–665, 665b
  description of, 588
  in health care, 45
Informed consent, 567
Injury
  deaths by mechanism, 520f
  and violence, 518–522, 519f
Inpatient, 4b
Inpatient prospective payment system (IPPS), 284
Inpatient Rehabilitation Facility Patient Assessment Instrument, 137
Input, of data, 169
Input-output cycle, 653–654
Input-output devices, 297
Institute of Electrical and Electronics Engineers (IEEE) 1073, 200t
Institute of Medicine (IOM), 36
  description of, 6–7, 45
  electronic health record systems, 184
  health information technology infrastructure support by, 64
Institute of Medicine Committee, 528
Institutional review board (IRB), 415, 418, 419, 559
Instrumental values, 585b
Insurance, 32b
  definition of, 31–32
  history of, 44
  terminologies associated with, 32b
Integrated delivery systems, 28
Integrated medical record, 113
Intensity of service/severity of illness, 471–472
Intentional infliction of emotional or mental distress, 546–547
Intentional torts, 545–547
Interdisciplinary patient care plan, 104
  in hospice care, 140
Interface engine, 302, 302f
Interface terminologies, 260–262, 261f, 262b
Intermountain health care system, 489
Internal benchmarking, 458–459
Internal environmental analysis, 657
Internal medicine, 22t
Internal users, 485, 486t
International Classification for Nursing Practice (ICNP), 277, 278f
International Classification of Clinical Services (ICCS), 509
International Classification of Diseases (ICD), 279–281
  derivations of, 281–285
International Classification of Diseases, Ninth Revision (ICD-9), 200t
  description of, 257, 279
  general equivalence mappings, 262, 262b
International Classification of Diseases, Ninth Revision with Clinical Modifications (ICD-9-CM)
  code structure of, 280b
  definition of, 280
  discontinuing, 278
  ICD-10-CM versus, 280b, 281t
  ICD-10-PCS versus, 282b
International Classification of Diseases, Tenth Revision, Procedural Coding System (ICD-10-PCS), 262, 280–281, 282b
International Classification of Diseases, Tenth Revision (ICD-10), 280
  description of, 257

International Classification of Diseases, Tenth Revision (ICD-10) (Continued)
  general equivalence mappings, 262, 262b
International Classification of Diseases, Tenth Revision with Clinical Modifications (ICD-10-CM), 262
  ICD-9-CM versus, 280b, 281t
International Classification of Diseases for Oncology, Third Edition (ICD-O-3), 491
International Classification of Diseases for Oncology (ICD-O), 282–283, 283b
International Health Terminology Standards Development Organization (IHTSDO), 68, 71, 265–268
International Organization for Standardization (ISO), 68b
Internet, 310–313
  fundamentals of, 310–311
  history of, 310
  security for, 319
Internet browsers, 310
Internet Engineering Task Force (IETF), 310
Internet tools, 311–312
Interobserver reliability, 421–422
Interoperability, 249–250
Interrogatories, 544
Interval data, 394
Interval estimation, 408–409, 409b
Interventional radiology, 22t
Interviewer bias, 424
Intranet, 313
Intraobserver reliability, 421–422
Intraorganizational outcomes teams, 506
Invalid complaints, 627
Invasion of privacy, 546
Investment decisions, 705–710

J
JAVA, 312–313
Job analysis, 609–610, 609f
Job applicants
  interview with, 614–615
  selection of, 612–613
  sources of, 612
Job descriptions, 610–611, 610t
Job evaluation, 628–630, 628f
  importance of, 629
Job grading, 628–629
Job performance standards, 610
Job ranking, 628
Job sharing, 590, 590b
Joint Commission on Accreditation of Healthcare Organizations, 5, 6b, 43–44
Joint Commission on Accreditation of Hospitals, 6b, 43–44
Jurisdiction, 543
Justice, 584–585

K
Kaiser Permanente, 33
Kaplan-Meier estimation of survival, 436f
Kaplan-Meier product limit method, 435, 435b, 435t
Kappa statistic (κ), 422
Keyboard, 671
Knowledge, 41, 94, 210, 333–334
Knowledge hierarchy, 93–94, 93f

L
Labor and delivery record, 108
Labor-management relations, 600–601
Labor Management Relations Act, 601
Labor Management Reporting and Disclosure Act, 601

ABBREVIATIONS

AAFP—American Academy of Family Physicians
AAMRL—American Association Medical Record Librarians
AAP—American Academy of Pediatrics
ACA—Affordable Care Act
ACEN—Accreditation Commission for Education in Nursing
ACF—Administration for Children and Families
ACG—Adjusted Clinical Group
ACIP—Advisory Committee on Immunization Practices
ACO—Accountable Care Organization
ACP—American College of Physicians
ACS—American Cancer Society
ACS—American College of Surgeons
ACSCOT—American College of Surgeons Committee on Trauma
ADA—Americans with Disabilities Act
ADEA—Age Discrimination in Employment Act
ADE—Adverse Drug Event
ADL—Activities of Daily Living
ADT—Admission, Discharge, and Transfer
AFL-CIO—American Federation of Labor–Congress of Industrial Organizations
AHA—American Hospital Association
AHCPR—Agency for Health Care Policy and Research
AHDI—Association for Healthcare Documentation Integrity
AHIC—American Health Information Community
AHIMA—American Health Information Management Association
AHIP—America's Health Insurance Plan
AHRQ—Agency for Healthcare Research and Quality
AICPA—American Institute of Certified Public Accountants
AIDS—Acquired Immunodeficiency Syndrome
AIS—Abbreviated Injury Scale
AJCC—American Joint Committee on Cancer
ALOS—Average Length of Stay
AMA—American Medical Association
AMRA—American Medical Record Association
ANA—American Nurses Association
ANOVA—Analysis of variance
ANSI—American National Standards Institute
AoA—Administration on Aging
AOA—American Osteopathic Association
APACHE—Acute Physiology, Age, and Chronic Health Evaluation
APC—Ambulatory Payment Classification
AP-DRG—All Patient Diagnosis-Related Groups
APR—DRG—All Patient Refined Diagnosis-Related Groups
AQA—Ambulatory Quality Alliance
ARLNA—Association of Record Librarians of North America
ARRA—The American Recovery and Reinvestment Act of 2009
ART—Accredited Record Technician
ASP—Application Service Provider
ASTM—American Society for Testing and Materials
ASCP—American Society of Clinical Pathologists
ATM—Asynchronous Transfer Mode
BARS—Behaviorally Anchored Rating Scales
BCBS—Blue Cross and Blue Shield
BFOQ—Bona Fide Occupational Qualification
BI—Business Intelligence

BICS—Brigham Integrated Computing System
BLS—Bureau of Labor Statistics
BMI—Body Mass Index
CAAHEP—Commission on the Accreditation of Allied Health Education Programs
CAD—Coronary Artery Disease
CAH—Critical Access Hospital
CAHIIM—Commission on Accreditation of Health Informatics and Information Management
CAI—Community-Acquired Infection
CAM—Complementary and Alternative Medicine
CAP—College of American Pathologists
CARE—Continuity Assessment Record and Evaluation
CARF—Commission on Accreditation of Rehabilitation Facilities
CASE—Computer-Aided Systems Engineering
CBA—Cost-Benefit Analysis
CCA—Certified Coding Associate
CCBH—Connecting Communities for Better Health
CCHIIM—Commission on Certification for Health Informatics and Information Management
CCHIT—Commission on the Certification for Health Information Technology
CCI—Correct Coding Initiative
CCOW—Clinical Context Object Workstation
CCS—Certified Coding Specialist
CCS—Clinical Classification Software
CCS-P—Certified Coding Specialist—Physician-based
CDC—Centers for Disease Control and Prevention
CDI—Clinical Documentation Improvement
CDM—Charge Description Master
CDR—Clinical Data Repository
CDS—Clinical Decision Support
CDSS—Clinical Decision Support System
CDS—Clinical Documentation Specialists
CEO—Chief Executive Officer
CfC—Conditions for Coverage
CFO—Chief Financial Officer
CFR—Code of Federal Regulations
CGI—Common Gateway Interface
CHAMPUS—Civilian Health and Medical Program for the Uniformed Services
CHAP—Community Health Accreditation Program
CHCA—Child Health Corporation of America
CHC—Community Health Center
CHCF—California Health Care Foundation
CHDA—Certified Health Data Analyst
CHI—Consolidated Health Informatics
CHP—Certified in Healthcare Privacy
CHPS—Certified in Healthcare Privacy and Security
CHS—Certified in Healthcare Security
CHT—Center for Health Transformation
CINAHL—Cumulative Index of Nursing and Allied Health Literature
CIO—Chief Information Officer
CIS—Commercial Information System
CITL—Center for Information Technology Leadership
CLIA—Clinical Laboratory Improvement Amendment
CMS—Centers for Medicare and Medicaid Services
CNA—Certified Nursing Assistant
COA—Council on Accreditation
COB—Coordination of Benefits
COBOL—Common Business-Oriented Language
COBRA—Consolidated Omnibus Reconciliation Act
CoC—Commission on Cancer

COC—Council on Certification
COCA—Commission on Osteopathic College Accreditation
CODEC—Coder/Decoder
COO—Chief Operating Officer
COP—(Medicare) Conditions of Participation
CoP—Communities of Practice
CPOE—Computerized Physician Order Entry
CPOE—Computerized Provider Order Entry
CPRI—Computer-based Patient Record Institute
CPR—Computer-based Patient Record
CPRS—Computerized Patient Record System
CPT—Current Procedural Terminology
CQI—Continuous Quality Improvement
CRNA—Certified Registered Nurse Anesthetist
CT—Computed Tomography
CTD—Cumulative Trauma Disorder
CTR—Certified Tumor Registrar
CTS—Carpal Tunnel Syndrome
CV—Coefficient of Variation
DCE—Distributed Computing Environment
DCG—Diagnosis Cost Group
DEEDS—Data Elements for Emergency Department Systems
DFB—Between-groups Degrees of Freedom
DFD—Data Flow Diagram
DFW—Within-Groups Degrees of Freedom
DHHS—Department of Health and Human Services
DICOM—Digital Imaging and Communications in Medicine
DIKW PYRAMID—Data, Information, Knowledge, Wisdom Pyramid
DMAIC—Definition, Measurement, Analysis, Improvement, and Control
DME—Durable Medical Equipment
DMZ—Demilitarized Zone
DOD—Department of Defense
DO—Doctor of Osteopathy
DOQ-IT—Doctors' Office Quality Information Technology
DOS—Denial of Service
DRG—Diagnosis-Related Groups
DRS—Designated Record Set
DSM—Diagnostic and Statistical Manual of Mental Disorders
DSS—Decision Support Systems
DSS—Data Security Standard
DSTU—Draft Standard for Trial Use
DTD—Document Type Definition
EAP—Employee Assistance Program
EBM—Evidence-based Medicine
ECG—Electrocardiogram
ED—Emergency Department
EDI—Electronic Data Interchange
EDM—Electronic document management
EEOC—Equal Employment Opportunity Commission
EEO—Equal Employment Opportunity
EFT—Electronic Funds Transfer
e-Health—Electronic health
e-HIM—Electronic Health Information Management
EH—Eligible Hospital (Non VA and DOD Hospitals)
EHR—certified Electronic Health Record technology. (sometimes abbreviated EMR or cEHRT)
EHR—Electronic Health Record
EIS—Executive Information Systems

Continued

EMR—*Electronic Medical Record*
EMS—*Emergency Medical System*
EMTALA—*Emergency Medical Treatment and Active Labor Act*
EOB—*Explanation of Benefits*
EO—*Executive Order*
EP—*Eligible Professional (Primary Care Clinics, Dentists, Chiropractor etc)*
EPA—*Environmental Protection Agency*
ERA—*Electronic Remittance Advice*
ERD—*Entity-relationship Diagram*
ERISA—*Employee Retirement Income Security Act*
ERP—*Enterprise Resource Planning*
ERX—*Electronic Prescribing*
ESC—*Evidence of Standards Compliance*
ESRD—*End-Stage Renal Disease*
FAHIMA—*Fellow of the American Health Information Management Association*
FASB—*Financial Standards Accounting Board*
FDA—*Food and Drug Administration*
FDDI—*Fiber-distributed Data Interface*
FI—*Fiscal Intermediary*
FIGO—*International Federation of Gynecology and Obstetrics*
FLEX—*Federation Licensing Exam*
FLSA—*Fair Labor Standards Act*
FMCS—*Federal Mediation and Conciliation Service*
FMEA—*Failure Mode and Effects Analysis*
FMLA—*Family and Medical Leave Act*
FN—*False Negatives*
FOIA—*Freedom of Information Act*
FORDS—*Facility Oncology Registration Data Standards*
FORE—*Foundation of Research and Education (Now AHIMA Foundation)*
FP—*False Positives*
FTE—*Full-time Equivalent*
GAAP—*Generally Accepted Accounting Principles*
GAO—*General Accounting Office*
GASB—*Government Accounting Standards Board*
GDP—*Gross Domestic Product*
GDSS—*Group Decision Support Software*
GPO—*Government Printing Office*
GUI—*Graphical User Interface*
H&P—*History and Physical*
HCFA—*Health Care Financing Administration (now CMS)*
HCO—*Health Care Organization*
HCPCS—*Healthcare Common Procedure Coding System*
HCUP—*Healthcare Cost and Utilization Project*
HEDIS—*Healthcare Effectiveness Data and Information Set*
HFAP—*Healthcare Facilities Accreditation Program*
HGML—*Hyper Graphics Markup Language*
HHS—*Department of Health and Human Services*
HIE—*Health Information Exchange*
HI—*Health Informatics*
HIM—*Health Information Management*
HIMSS—*Health Information Management Systems Society*
HIO—*Health Information Organization*
HIPAA—*Health Insurance Portability and Accountability Act*
HIS—*Health Information Services*
HISB—*Health Care Informatics Standards Board*

HISPC—*Health Information Security and Privacy Collaboration*
HISPP—*Healthcare Informatics Standards Planning Panel*
HISSB—*Health Information and Surveillance Systems Board*
HIT—*Health Information Technology*
HITECH—*Health Information Technology for Economic and Clinical Health Act*
HITPA—*Health Information Technology Promotion Act*
HITSP—*Health Information Technology Standards Panel*
HIV—*Human Immunodeficiency Virus*
HL7—*Health Level 7*
HMO—*Health Maintenance Organization*
HOI—*Health Outcomes Institute*
HRM—*Human Resource Management*
HRSA—*Health Resources and Services Administration*
HTML—*Hypertext Markup Language*
HTTP—*Hypertext Transfer Protocol*
HUGH—*Human Gene Nomenclature*
HVAC—*Heating, Ventilation, and Air Conditioning*
I/S—*Information Systems*
ICCS—*International Classification of Clinical Services*
ICD-10-CM—*International Classification of Diseases, Tenth Revision, Clinical Modification*
ICD-10—*International Classification of Diseases, Tenth Revision*
ICD-10-PCS—*International Classification of Diseases, Tenth Revision, Procedural Coding System*
ICD-9-CM—*International Classification of Diseases, Ninth Revision, Clinical Modification*
ICD-9—*International Classification of Diseases, Ninth Revision*
ICD—*International Classification of Diseases*
ICD O-3—*International Classification of Diseases for Oncology, Third Edition*
ICD-O—*International Classification of Diseases for Oncology*
ICU—*Intensive Care Unit*
IDDM—*Insulin-Dependent Diabetes Mellitus*
IDS—*Integrated Delivery System*
IEC—*International Electrotechnical Commission*
IEEE 1073—*Institute of Electrical and Electronics Engineers 1073*
IEEE—*Institute of Electrical and Electronics Engineers*
IETF—*Internet Engineering Task Force*
IG—*Information Governance*
IHS—*Indian Health Service*
IIHI—*Individually Identifiable Health Information*
IOM—*Institute of Medicine*
IPA—*Independent Practice Association*
IRB—*Institutional Review Board*
IRCA—*Immigration Reform and Control Act*
IR—*Incidence Rate*
IRF-PAI—*Inpatient Rehabilitation Facility Patient Assessment Instrument*
IRS—*Internal Revenue Service*
IS/SI—*Intensity of Service/Severity of Illness*
ISO—*International Organization for Standardization/ International Standards Organization*
IT—*Information Technology*
IWG—*Informatics Working Group*
JAD—*Joint Application Development*
JRP—*Joint Requirements Planning*

JVM—*Java Virtual Machine*
K—*Kappa statistic*
LAN—*Local Area Network*
LHR—*Legal Health Record*
LIP—*Licensed Independent Practitioner*
LOINC—*Logical Observation Identifiers Names and Codes*
LPN—*Licensed Practical Nurse*
LTC—*Long-Term Care*
MACDP—*Metropolitan Atlanta Congenital Defects Program*
MBO—*Management by Objectives*
MCAT—*Medical College Admission Test*
MCO—*Managed Care Organization*
MD—*Medical Doctor*
MDS—*Minimum Data Set*
MESH—*Medical Subject Headings*
MFD—Multifunction device
MHCA—*Mental Health Council of America*
MIB—*Medical Information Bureau*
MIS—*Management Information Systems*
MMA—*Medicare Modernization Act*
MPI—*Master Patient Index*
MSB—*Mean Square between Groups*
MSW—*Mean Square within Groups*
MU—Meaningful Use
MUMPS—*Massachusetts General Hospital Utility Multi-programming System*
NAACCR—*North American Association of Central Cancer Registries*
NACHRI—*National Association of Children's Hospitals and Related Institutions*
NAHDO—*National Association of Health Data Organizations*
NAHIT—*National Alliance for Health Information Technology*
NANDA—*North American Nursing Diagnosis Association*
NBME—National Board of Medical Examiners
NBS—NEDSS Base System
NCCAM—*National Center for Complimentary and Alternative Medicine*
NCDB—*National Cancer Data Base*
NCHS—*National Center for Health Statistics*
NCI—*National Cancer Institute*
NCPCP—*National Council on Prescription Drug Programs*
NCQA—*National Committee For Quality Assurance*
NCRA—*National Cancer Registrars Association*
NCR—*No Carbon Required*
NCVHS—*National Committee on Vital and Health Statistics*
NDC—*National Drug Codes*
NDF-RT—*National Drug File Reference Terminology*
NEC—*Not Elsewhere Classified*
NEDSS—*National Electronic Disease Surveillance System*
NEHC—*National eHealth Collaborative*
NHII—*National Health Information Infrastructure*
NHIN—*National Health Information Network*
NIC—*Nursing Interventions Classification*
NICU—*Neonatal Intensive Care Unit*
NIDDM—*Non–Insulin-Dependent Diabetes Mellitus*
NIH—*National Institutes of Health*
NI—*Nosocomial Infection*